Provided as an

educational

service by

◆

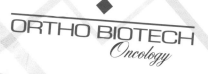
ORTHO BIOTECH
Oncology

Angela Gritton

D1189695

Third Edition

Applied Pharmacokinetics
Principles of Therapeutic Drug Monitoring

Edited by

William E. Evans, Pharm.D.
First Tennessee Professor of
Clinical Pharmacy and Pediatrics
University of Tennessee,
Memphis, TN
 and
Chair, Pharmaceutical Division
St. Jude Children's Research Hospital

Jerome J. Schentag, Pharm.D.
Professor of Pharmaceutics and Pharmacy
State University of New York at Buffalo
Buffalo, NY
 and
Director, Clinical Pharmacokinetics Laboratory
Millard Fillmore Hospital

William J. Jusko, Ph.D.
Professor of Pharmaceutics
School of Pharmacy
State University of New York at Buffalo
Buffalo, NY

Assistant Editor

Mary V. Relling, Pharm.D.
Assistant Member
Pharmaceutical Division
St. Jude Children's Research Hospital
 and
Assistant Professor of Clinical Pharmacy
University of Tennessee
Memphis, TN

Applied Therapeutics, Inc.
Vancouver, WA

Printing and Binding: Edwards Brothers, Ann Arbor, MI
Cover Design: Steven B. Naught

Other Publications by Applied Therapeutics, Inc.:

Applied Therapeutics: The Clinical Use of Drugs, 5th edition
Edited by Mary Anne Koda–Kimble and Lloyd Y. Young
ISBN 0–915486–14–8

Basic Clinical Pharmacokinetics, 2nd edition
by Michael E. Winter
ISBN 0–915486–08–3

Bedside Clinical Pharmacokinetics, revised edition
by Carl C. Peck, Dale P. Conner, and M. Gail Murphy
ISBN 0–915486–10–5

Clinical Clerkship Manual
Edited by Larry Boh
ISBN 0–915486–17–2

Drug Interactions & Updates
by Philip D. Hansten and John R. Horn
ISBN 0–8121–1381–0   ISSN 0271–8707

Handbook of Applied Therapeutics, 2nd edition
by Mary Anne Koda–Kimble, Lloyd Y. Young,
Wayne A. Kradjan, and B. Joseph Guglielmo, Jr.
ISBN 0–915486–16–4

Applied Therapeutics, Inc.
P.O. Box 5077
Vancouver, WA 98668–5077
Phone: (206) 253–7123
FAX: (206) 253–8475

Library of Congress Card Catalog # 91–074098
ISBN 0–915486–15–6

First Printing June 1992
Second Printing October 1992
Third Printing November 1994
Fourth Printing June 1995

Dedication

Dedicated to our colleagues and students, who inspired this book, and to our families, Leslie and Kelli Evans; Rita Sloan and Annie Schentag; and Laura, Suzanne, Marjorie and Katherine Jusko, who are a continuing source of support and inspiration.

Acknowledgments

With any undertaking as large and comprehensive as a textbook, many individuals must make substantial contributions if a successful product is to emerge in a timely manner. Many of these individuals are formally recognized in the list of contributors and reviewers, and we wish to thank them again for their promptness, thoroughness, and attention to detail. In addition, we wish to thank a number of other individuals who have been instrumental in bringing the third edition to fruition. First, our secretaries and the secretaries of our contributors are to be commended for typing and retyping the manuscripts as they evolved over the last year. We also thank our colleagues, post–doctoral fellows and students, especially Lea Anne Johnson, for reading near–final drafts of chapters to ensure clarity and comprehensiveness. Likewise, numerous readers and reviewers have provided helpful comments and insights related to the first two editions of the book. We are also indebted to Drs. Mary Anne Koda–Kimble and Lloyd Y. Young, who made considerable editorial contributions to the style and content of the book.

Contributing Authors

Gail D. Anderson, Ph.D.

Assistant Professor
Departments of Pharmacy Practice and Pharmaceutics
College of Pharmacy
University of Washington
Seattle, WA 98195

Charles H. Ballow, Pharm.D.

Director, Therapeutic Drug Monitoring
The Clinical Pharmacokinetics Laboratory
School of Pharmacy
State University of New York at Buffalo, and
Millard Fillmore Hospital
Buffalo, NY 14209

Robert Alan Blouin, Pharm.D.

Professor
Pharmacology and Experimental Therapeutics
College of Pharmacy
University of Kentucky
Lexington, KY 40536-0082

Michael B. Bottorff, Pharm.D.

Associate Professor and Chairman
Clinical Pharmacy
College of Pharmacy
University of Cincinnati
Cincinnati, OH 45267-0004

Kim L. R. Brouwer, Pharm.D., Ph.D.

Assistant Professor
Division of Pharmaceutics
School of Pharmacy
University of North Carolina at Chapel Hill
Chapel Hill, NC 27599-7360

Stanley W. Carson, Pharm.D.

Associate Professor of Pharmacy, and
Research Associate Professor of Psychiatry
Division of Pharmacy Practice
School of Pharmacy
University of North Carolina at Chapel Hill
Chapel Hill, NC 27599-7360

Mary H. H. Chandler, Pharm.D.

Assistant Professor, Division of Pharmacy Practice and Science, and
Director, Clinical Pharmacokinetics Service
College of Pharmacy
University of Kentucky
Lexington, KY 40536-0084

Robert J. Cipolle, Pharm.D.

Associate Professor, and
Associate Dean for Academic Affairs
College of Pharmacy
Pharmacy Practice
University of Minnesota
Minneapolis, MN 55455-0343

James D. Coyle, Pharm.D.

Assistant Professor
Division of Pharmacy Practice
College of Pharmacy
The Ohio State University
Columbus, OH 43210

William R. Crom, Pharm.D.

Associate Member
Pharmaceutical Division
St. Jude Children's Research Hospital
Memphis, TN 38105

David Z. D'Argenio, Ph.D.

Associate Professor
Department of Biomedical Engineering
University of Southern California
Los Angeles, CA 90033

C. Lindsay DeVane, Pharm.D.

Professor
Department of Pharmacy Practice, and
Department of Psychiatry
University of Florida
Gainesville, FL 32610-0486

Sydney H. Dromgoole, Ph.D.

Manager, Clinical Evaluation
Technical Development
Herbert Laboratories
Irvine, CA 92713

Michael N. Dudley, Pharm.D.

Associate Professor, and
Director, Antiinfective Pharmacology Research Unit
Roger Williams Medical Center, and
University of Rhode Island College of Pharmacy
Providence, RI 02908

George Earl Dukes, Pharm.D.

Associate Professor of Pharmacy
Pharmacy Practice
School of Pharmacy
University of North Carolina at Chapel Hill
Chapel Hill, NC 27599-7360

William Edward Evans, Pharm.D.

First Tennessee Professor of Clinical Pharmacy and Pediatrics
University of Tennessee
 and
Chair, Pharmaceutical Division
St. Jude Children's Research Hospital
Memphis, TN 38105

David J. Edwards, Pharm.D.

Associate Professor
Department of Pharmacy Practice
College of Pharmacy
Wayne State University
Detroit, MI 48202

Daniel E. Furst, M.D.

Director of Clinical Research Programs
Virginia Mason Research Center
Seattle, WA 98101

Douglas R. Geraets, Pharm.D.

Assistant Professor of Clinical/Hospital Pharmacy
College of Pharmacy
University of Iowa
Iowa City, IA 52242

Malcolm R. Hill, Pharm.D.

Assistant Professor of Pediatrics and Pharmacy
Clinical Pharmacology Division
Department of Pediatrics
National Jewish Center of Immunology and Respiratory Medicine, and
University of Colorado Health Sciences Center
Denver, CO 80206

C. Rick Jarecke, Pharm.D.

Clinical Pharmacist
Hastings Regional Center
Hastings, NE 68902-0579

Kenneth E. Johnson, Pharm.D.

Adjoint Assistant Professor
Division of Pharmacy Practice
School of Pharmacy
University of Colorado
Denver, CO 80262

William J. Jusko, Ph.D.

Professor of Pharmaceutics
School of Pharmacy
State University of New York at Buffalo
Buffalo, NY 14260

David J. Kazierad, Pharm.D.

Director, Cardiovascular Research
The Clinical Pharmacokinetics Laboratory
School of Pharmacy
State University of New York at Buffalo
Buffalo, NY 14209

Richard L. Lalonde, Pharm.D.

Director, Pharmacokinetics and Clinical Pharmacology
Phoenix International Life Sciences, Inc.
Montreal, Quebec
Canada H4R 9Z7

Gerhard Levy, Pharm.D.

Distinguished Professor of Pharmaceutics
Department of Pharmaceutics
School of Pharmacy
State University of New York at Buffalo
Buffalo, NY 14260

Rene H. Levy, Ph.D.

Professor and Chairman
Department of Pharmaceutics, and
Professor
Department of Neurological Surgery
University of Washington
Seattle, WA 98195

John Joseph Lima, Pharm.D.

Associate Professor of Pharmacy and Medicine
Pharmacy Practice
College of Pharmacy
Ohio State University
Columbus, OH 43210-1291

Elizabeth A. Ludwig, Pharm.D.

Clinical Assistant Professor of Pharmacy
State University of New York at Buffalo
  and
Assistant Director, Clinical Services
Department of Pharmacy
Buffalo General Hospital
Buffalo, NY 14203

Janis J. MacKichan, Pharm.D.

Associate Professor of Pharmacy
Pharmacy Practice
College of Pharmacy
The Ohio State University
Columbus, OH 43210

Gary R. Matzke, Pharm.D.

Professor, Department of Pharmacy and Therapeutics
School of Pharmacy, and
Center for Clinical Pharmacology
School of Medicine
University of Pittsburgh
Pittsburgh, PA 15261

Michael Mayersohn, Ph.D.

Professor
Department of Pharmaceutical Sciences
University of Arizona
Tucson, AZ 85721

Stephen P. Millikin, Pharm.D.

Associate Director
Pharmaceutical Product Development
Clinical Research Unit, and
Clinical Assistant Professor of Pharmacy
University of North Carolina at Chapel Hill
Durham, NC 27713

Rebecca L. Milsap, Pharm.D.

Clinical Pharmacist
Infusion Therapy
Department of Pharmacy
Nutritional Metabolic Support Associates
Amherst, NY 14228

Gene D. Morse, Pharm.D.

Associate Professor of Pharmacy, and
Research Associate Professor of Medicine
Center for Clinical Pharmacy Research
School of Pharmacy
State University of New York at Buffalo
Buffalo, NY 14260

Milap C. Nahata, Pharm.D.

Professor of Pharmacy and Pediatrics
Colleges of Pharmacy and Medicine
The Ohio State University, and
Wexner Institute for Pediatric Research
Children's Hospital
Columbus, OH 43210

David E. Nix, Pharm.D.

Assistant Director
The Clinical Pharmacokinetics Laboratory
Millard Fillmore Hospital
Buffalo, NY 14209

Joseph A. Paladino, Pharm.D.

Director, Clinical Pharmacokinetics Laboratory
Millard Fillmore Suburban Hospital
  and
Clinical Assistant Professor of Pharmacy
State University of New York at Buffalo
Buffalo, NY 14221

Carl C. Peck, M.D.

Director, Center for Drug Evaluation and Research
Department of Health and Human Services
Food and Drug Administration
Rockville, MD 20857

John A. Pieper, Pharm.D.

Associate Dean and Head
Division of Pharmacy Practice
School of Pharmacy
University of Colorado
Denver, CO 80262

R. Stephen Porter, Pharm.D.

Director, Cardiovascular Pharmacology
Division of Cardiology
Department of Medicine
Hahnemann University Hospital
Philadelphia, PA 19102-1192

J. Robert Powell, Pharm.D.

Director of Clinical Pharmacology
Glaxo Inc.
Durham, NC 27709

Mary Violet Relling, Pharm.D.

Assistant Member, Pharmaceutical Division
St. Jude Children's Research Hospital
  and
Assistant Professor of Clinical Pharmacy
College of Pharmacy
University of Tennessee
Memphis, TN 38105

Richard H. Reuning, Ph.D.

Professor and Chair
Division of Pharmacy Practice
College of Pharmacy
The Ohio State University
Columbus, OH 43210

Mario L. Rocci, Jr., Ph.D.

Director
Pharmaceutical and Chemical Research Division
Oneida Research Services, Inc.
Whitesboro, NY 13492

John H. Rodman, Pharm.D.

Vice Chair and Associate Member
Pharmaceutical Division
St. Jude Children's Research Hospital
Memphis, TN 38105

Keith A. Rodvold, Pharm.D.

Associate Professor
Departments of Pharmacy Practice and Infectious Diseases
Colleges of Pharmacy and Medicine
University of Illinois at Chicago
Chicago, IL 60612

Daniel R. Salomon, M.D.

Clinical Associate Professor
Georgetown University Medical Center
  and
Guest Researcher
Laboratory of Immunology
National Institutes of Health
National Institute of Allergy and Infectious Diseases
Bethesda, MD 20892

William Theron Sawyer, M.S.

Associate Professor
Division of Pharmacy Practice
School of Pharmacy
University of North Carolina at Chapel Hill
Chapel Hill, NC 27599-7360

Jerome John Schentag, Pharm.D.

Professor of Pharmaceutics and Pharmacy
Division of Clinical Pharmacy Research
School of Pharmacy
State University of New York at Buffalo
Buffalo, NY 14209

Karen D. Schlanz, Pharm.D.

Fellow in Cardiology
Division of Clinical and Hospital Pharmacy
College of Pharmacy
University of Cincinnati
Cincinnati, OH 45267-0004

Richard L. Slaughter, M.S.

Professor and Chair
Pharmacy Practice
College of Pharmacy and Allied Health Professions
Wayne State University
Detroit, MI 48202

Stanley James Szefler, M.D.

Director of Clinical Pharmacology
Department of Pediatrics
National Jewish Center for Immunology and Respiratory Medicine
Denver, CO 80206

Thomas Nelson Tozer, Pharm.D., Ph.D.

Professor of Pharmacy
Department of Pharmacy
University of California, San Francisco
San Francisco, CA 94143-0446

Clarence T. Ueda, Pharm.D., Ph.D.

Professor and Dean
Department of Pharmaceutical Sciences
College of Pharmacy
University of Nebraska Medical Center
Omaha, NE 68198-6000

Peter Harris Vlasses, Pharm.D.

Associate Director
Technology Advancement Center
University Hospital Consortium
Oak Brook, IL 60521

Michael E. Winter, Pharm.D.

Professor of Clinical Pharmacy, and
Director, Clinical Pharmacokinetics Consulting Service
Division of Clinical Pharmacy
School of Pharmacy
University of California
San Francisco, CA 94143-0622

Alan J. Wilensky, M.D., Ph.D., F.R.C.P. (C.)

Associate Director, and
Associate Professor
Regional Epilepsy Center
Department of Neurosurgery and Medicine (Neurology)
University of Washington
Harborview Medical Center
Seattle, WA 98104

Gary C. Yee, Pharm.D.

Associate Professor of Pharmacy Practice
College of Pharmacy
University of Florida
Gainesville, FL 32610

Barbara Jeanne Zarowitz, Pharm.D.

Clinical Manager, and
Adjunct Associate Professor of Pharmacy Practice
Department of Pharmacy Services
Henry Ford Hospital, and
Wayne State University
Detroit, MI 48202

Darwin E. Zaske, Pharm.D.

Director, Pharmaceutical Services
St. Paul-Ramsey Medical Center
  and
Professor, College of Pharmacy
University of Minnesota
St. Paul, MN 55101

Editorial Review Board

Burke A. Cunha, M.D.

Chief, Infectious Diseases
Division and Associate Professor of Medicine
Winthrop University Hospital
Mineola, Long Island, NY 11501

Richard O. Day, M.D.

Clinical Pharmacologist
St. Vincent's Hospital
Department of Clinical Pharmacology
Darlinghurst, New South Wales 2010
Australia

Courtney Fletcher, Pharm.D.

Assistant Professor
Department of Pharmacy Practice
University of Minnesota
College of Pharmacy
Minneapolis, MN 55455

John G. Gambertoglio, Pharm.D.

Professor of Pharmacy
University of California School of Pharmacy
Division of Clinical Pharmacy
San Francisco, CA 94143

Milo Gibaldi, Ph.D.

Professor of Pharmaceutical Sciences
School of Pharmacy
Warren G. Magnuson Health Sciences Center
University of Washington
Seattle, WA 98195

David J. Greenblatt, M.D.

Professor of Psychiatry and Medicine
New England Medical Center Hospital
Division of Clinical Pharmacology
Boston, MA 02111

Mary A. Gutierrez, Pharm.D.

School of Pharmacy
University of Southern California
Los Angeles, CA 90033

Leslie Hendeles, Pharm.D.

Professor, Pharmacy and Pediatrics
College of Pharmacy
University of Florida
Gainesville, FL 32610

Julie Johnson, Pharm.D.

Assistant Professor
Department of Clinical Pharmacy
College of Pharmacy
University of Tennessee, Memphis
Memphis, TN 38163

Werner Kalow, M.D.

Professor
Department of Pharmacology
University of Toronto
Toronto, Ontario
Canada M5S 1A8

Terrence A. Killilea, Pharm.D.

Department of Pharmacy
Sacred Heart Medical Center
Eugene, OR 97401

Patricia D. Kroboth, Ph.D.

Department of Pharmacy and Therapeutics
University of Pittsburgh
Pittsburgh, PA 15261

Michael Oellerich, M.D.

Professor of Clinical Chemistry, and
Director of the Department of Clinical Chemistry
Georg–August–Universitat Gottingen
D–3400 Gottingen
Germany

William Z. Potter, M.D., Ph.D.

Chief, Section of Clinical Pharmacology
Clinical Neuroscience Branch
National Institute of Mental Health
Bethesda, MD 20892

Michael D. Reed, Pharm.D.

Associate Professor
Division of Pediatric Pharmacology/Critical Care
University of Virginia Health Science Center
Charlottesville, VA 22908

Keith A. Rodvold, Pharm.D.

Associate Professor
Department of Pharmacy Practice
Clinical Research Laboratory
University of Illinois at Chicago
Chicago, IL 60612

Philip Walson, M.D.

Professor and Chief
Clinical Pharmacology/Toxicology
Children's Hospital
Columbus, OH 43205

Lloyd R. Whitfield, Pharm.D.

Senior Research Associate
Parke Davis Research Division
Ann Arbor, MI 48106

Samuel Vozeh, M.D.

Medical Division
Intercantonal Office for the Control of Medicaments
IKS
Bern 3012
Switzerland

Contents

Notice to Reader

D rug therapy information is constantly evolving. Our ever–changing knowledge and experience with drugs and the continual development of new drugs necessitates changes in treatment and drug therapy. The editors, authors, and the publisher of this work have made every effort to ensure the information provided herein was accurate at the time of publication. *It remains the responsibility of every practitioner to evaluate the appropriateness of a particular opinion or therapy in the context of the actual clinical situation and with due consideration of any new developments in the field.* Although the authors have been careful to recommend dosages that are in agreement with current standards and responsible literature, we recommend the student or practitioner consult several appropriate information sources when dealing with new and unfamiliar drugs.

Preface to Third Edition

The third edition of *Applied Pharmacokinetics: Principles of Therapeutic Drug Monitoring* has been developed to retain the goals of our previous editions: to provide a rigorous yet practical text on the application of pharmacokinetic methods, pharmacodynamic principles, and relevant pharmacotherapeutic data to optimize drug therapy for individual patients.

All chapters have been extensively updated or completely rewritten, and six new chapters have been added on topics not addressed in previous editions. The 28 chapters repeated from the second edition are provided with data and concepts evolved over the past six years blended with selected material of earlier importance. New chapter topics include: Pharmacodynamics, Pharmacogenetics, Pharmacokinetic Considerations in the Obese, Dietary Influences on Drug Disposition, Zidovudine, Corticosteroids, and a Commentary on Dual Individualization of Antibiotics. Revisions and new contributions were developed by a cadre of authors whose insight and diligence will be evident. The third edition contains contributions from several new chapter authors, as well as the invaluable contributions of our new Assistant Editor, Dr. Mary Relling. As with previous editions, each chapter was reviewed by members of the Editorial Review Board to improve lucidity, balance, and accuracy.

To permit the addition of new chapters without expanding the overall size of the text, all chapter authors were asked to focus the content of each chapter on those principles and concepts which represent the most important and salient issues for the subject being covered, thereby further distinguishing the content of *Applied Pharmacokinetics* from texts covering other topics related the the optimal use of medications in patients. Each of the twenty chapters on specific drugs has been organized in a consistent format, with major subheadings of Clinical Pharmacokinetics, Pharmacodynamics, Clinical Application of Pharmacokinetic Data, Analytical Methods, and a Prospectus. It is hoped that the use of a consistent format, the addition of new introductory and drug chapters, and the added focus on pharmacokinetic and pharmacodynamic principles, will make the third edition easier to use by students, practitioners, and educators, while being more comprehensive than our previous editions.

We are sincerely appreciative of the dedication, enthusiasm, and cooperation of our many authors and reviewers, and the encouraging feedback we have received from our readers over the last ten years.

William E. Evans
Jerome J. Schentag
William J. Jusko

Applied Pharmacokinetics —A Prospectus

Gerhard Levy

During the last 30 years enormous advances have been made in the development of sensitive and specific methods for the determination of drug and drug metabolite concentrations in biologic fluids; in the mathematical description of the changes of these concentrations as a function of time after drug administration; and in the use of mathematical formulations and computers to predict the concentration-time profiles of drugs during chronic drug administration from knowledge obtained in single dose studies. It had also been established that the intensity of the pharmacologic effects of many drugs is related, directly or indirectly, to their concentration and/or to the concentration of their metabolite(s) in plasma. This has led to the determination of usual therapeutic plasma concentration ranges of such drugs and to an awareness that these concentration ranges can serve as an intermediate therapeutic target for the individualization of drug dosage.

Many genetic characteristics and environmental factors, including diet and concomitant use of other drugs, and physiologic variables such as age, gender, body composition, disease and pregnancy can affect the disposition of drugs and, therefore, can modify the relationship between dose and the drug concentration versus time profile in plasma and tissues. The dose-concentration relationship is also affected by incomplete absorption of the drug due to inadequate bioavailability of a particular dosage form, presystemic biotransformation of certain drugs administered by routes other than intravenous, and possible malabsorption secondary to pathologic conditions affecting the gastrointestinal tract. Another very important problem is poor compliance, either by the patient or by the medical personnel responsible for drug administration to patients. For all of these reasons, there is usually a much better relationship between drug concentration in plasma and the intensity of pharmacologic effects than there is between dose (or dosing rate) and these effects.

Individual adjustment of drug dosage on the basis of a targeted drug concentration in plasma may prevent or minimize adverse effects due to inadvertent overdosage and it may facilitate and increase the effectiveness of therapy, particularly in the case of drugs used to prevent pathologic episodes such as epileptic seizures, by providing an alternative to the titration of dosage on the basis of therapeutic response or toxic effects. Moreover, therapeutic response is often difficult to assess in individual patients, particularly when the condition of the patient is unstable. Individualization of drug dosage based on therapeutic response becomes even more difficult if the patient receives several drugs with similar indications.

These considerations have led to the extensive use of therapeutic drug concentration ("blood level") monitoring and to the development and rapid growth of a new discipline, clinical pharmacokinetics. Simply stated, clinical pharmacokinetics is a health sciences discipline that deals with the application of pharmacokinetics to optimize the pharmacotherapeutic management of individual patients. Pharmacokinetics itself is a biologic science concerned with the characterization and mathematical description of the absorption, distribution, metabolism and excretion of medicinal agents, their metabolites, and other substances of biologic interest. It includes consideration of the relationship of these processes to the time course of pharmacologic effects. Clinical pharmacokinetics is definitely an applied science—therefore the title of this book—and cannot be practiced in isolation (i.e., without consideration of the pathophysiologic status, therapeutic environment, and even the personality of the patient). The functions of a comprehensive clinical pharmacokinetics service were outlined in 1974 at the first symposium devoted to this subject:[1]

1. Initial design of drug dosage regimens (dose, dosing interval, route, dosage form) for individual patients upon request of the attending physician, based upon the generally available knowledge of the pharmacokinetics of the drug, the intended purpose of the medication, the disease(s) or tentative diagnosis and such variables as age, sex, body weight or surface area (or lean body mass), race or other indicator of possible pharmacogenetic influence (e.g., family history, tests of acetylator status), renal function, plasma albumin concentration, hematocrit, preceding and/or concomitant use of other drugs, urine pH, and blood electrolytes, where applicable.

2. Refinement and re-adjustment of dosage regimens, where necessary, based usually on serial monitoring of drug concentrations in plasma or other fluids, but sometimes on direct assessment of clinical response or on indirect assessment of response (e.g., on the basis of changes in certain biochemical parameters).

3. Pharmacokinetic diagnostic work-ups to help determine the reasons for a quantitatively unusual response (usually lack of therapeutic effect or pronounced adverse effects) to a drug. Such diagnostic work-up, if carried out properly by a qualified individual, should lead to the detection of lack of compliance by the patient, bioavailability problems, medication errors, drug interactions, unusual distribution and elimination kinetics, or certain pharmacogenetic effects including unusual receptor site sensitivity.

4. Consultation and follow-up in special situations such as assessment of need for intermittent dosage adjustment for patients on hemodialysis or peritoneal dialysis, and the management of acute drug intoxications.

5. Retrospective assessment of potential or suspected therapeutic mishaps or mismanagement (clinical conferences, post-mortems).

6. Educational activities to help assure that drugs are used safely and effectively.

Research, including an assessment of cost-benefit aspects of clinical pharmacokinetic services for individual drugs under various conditions, discovery of bioavailability problems and as yet unrecognized drug interactions, pharmacokinetic measurements to enlarge the data base (e.g., half-life, total and renal clearance, apparent volume of distribution) for a particular drug, and definition of parameters which may be useful in the design of individualized dosage regimens.

The application of clinical pharmacokinetic principles to the individualization and optimization of drug dosing regimens is a rational process. It begins with a clear formulation of the therapeutic problem (in the form of questions such as: Why does this patient not respond to a population-average drug dosing regimen? What is the most appropriate drug dosing regimen for this elderly patient with renal failure?), leading to a provisional decision (the dosage adjustment to be made or the initial dosage regimen to be used), followed by an assessment of the outcome of that decision (drug concentration in plasma and therapeutic response). If necessary, the drug regimen must be modified or other actions must be taken. This rational process usually requires a review of the patient's chart (for drug history and pathophysiologic information, an understanding of what the therapist wishes to accomplish, and adequate knowledge of the clinical pharmacokinetic characteristics of the drug). It should be obvious, therefore, that determination of one or more drug-in-plasma concentrations is only a small -albeit important—part of the rational application of clinical pharmacokinetics to drug therapy. More important is the professional competence of the individual who has to determine when, what, and how to monitor, and who must interpret the results and recommend appropriate action to the physician responsible for the patient's therapeutic management. This book is devoted to that individual—the clinical pharmacokineticist—and to those pharmacists and physicians who share our view that drug dosage must be individualized and that this should be done, whenever possible, by objective means.

As the term indicates, clinical pharmacokinetics focuses primarily on the pharmacokinetic aspects of the individualized optimization of drug dosage. However, this represents only one side of the coin. Research in the area of clinical pharmacodynamics (drug concentration-pharmacologic effect relationships) is making considerable progress; assessment of the time course of drug action in relation to drug and/or drug metabolite concentrations has become feasible for different types of therapeutic agents. In the course of such studies it has become evident that there can be appreciable interindividual differences in pharmacodynamics, differences of one or even two orders of magnitude! As we learn more about the role of age, gender, underlying diseases, and other individual characteristics as determinants of the relationship between drug concentration and pharmacologic activity, it will become possible to make reasonable predictions and to combine this information with our pharmacokinetic data base. The chapter by Schentag and his colleagues on dual individualization of antibiotics represents one aspect of this emerging capability. The newly added chapter on pharmacodynamics by Lalonde will introduce the reader to pharmacodynamic models and concepts.

Irrespective of the drug or class of drugs under consideration, clinical pharmacokinetic assessments and decisions will have to be based on certain general principles that constitute the framework of the discipline. That is reflected by the organization of this book. The first several chapters are concerned with such broadly applicable subjects as general principles of applied pharmacokinetics, the collection of pharmacokinetic data and their analysis, the role of population pharmacokinetics in individualizing drug dosage, pharmacodynamics, the influence of hepatic and renal dysfunction and age on pharmacokinetics, and the practical implications of drug-protein binding. The increased emphasis on individual determinants of pharmacokinetics is reflected by new chapters on the role of obesity, diet and heredity. The subsequent chapters are detailed expositions of the clinical pharmacokinetics of individual drugs; the kinetics of their absorption, distribution, metabolism and excretion; the usual therapeutic concentration range, as well as the relationships between concentration and pharmacologic effects and (if known) factors affecting these relationships; the application of the available information concerning the pharmacokinetic characteristics of the drug to the individualization of therapy; available analytical methods, including the advantages and shortcomings of different methods; and an outline of a rational approach to the optimization of drug dosage, including the design of the initial regimen and subsequent adjustments of dosage.

On a personal note, many of the contributors of this book are present or former colleagues, collaborators and former students who are leading investigators and/or outstanding practitioners of clinical pharmacokinetics. Their efforts have produced a book that I find invaluable as a teacher of clinical pharmacokinetics. My students view it as the bible of the discipline. If the book helps to make the reader a more effective clinical pharmacist, clinical pharmacologist, physician or other health care professional, then the authors of *Applied Pharmacokinetics* will feel amply rewarded.

REFERENCES

1. Levy, G. An orientation to clinical pharmacokinetics. In: Levy, G., ed. Clinical Pharmacokinetics—A Symposium. Washington: Am. Pharm. Assoc., 1974; 1-9.

Chapter 1

General Principles of Applied Pharmacokinetics

William E. Evans

The concept of "applied pharmacokinetics" has evolved considerably during the last two decades as a logical clinical extension of pharmacokinetic and pharmacodynamic research. Although research continues to further refine the mathematical approaches, drug analysis techniques, and physiological basis of pharmacokinetics, it has now become common for pharmacokinetic principles to be routinely used to assess and optimize drug therapy of individual patients. There are many published examples of how this process can be beneficial, and most of these studies are discussed in detail in the following chapters. Despite the strong theoretical basis for applied pharmacokinetics and the intuitively obvious rationale for its value, the process is not always straightforward and may have considerable limitations under certain circumstances. Recognition of where limitations may exist should lead to more appropriate application of pharmacokinetic principles, as well as help direct areas of future research. This chapter will attempt to identify various elements of applied pharmacokinetics which may have substantial effects on therapeutic drug monitoring and individualization of drug therapy. These general considerations should serve as a framework for evaluation and application of data presented in subsequent chapters.

WHAT IS "APPLIED PHARMACOKINETICS"?

Applied pharmacokinetics, as defined for this text, is the process of using drug concentrations, pharmacokinetic principles, and pharmacodynamic criteria to optimize drug therapy in individual patients. Other names referring to essentially the same process include "therapeutic drug monitoring" and "clinical pharmacokinetics." Exclusive use of either of these two terms has been avoided here because "therapeutic drug monitoring" could describe a much broader process not necessarily involving drug concentrations or pharmacokinetics and "clinical pharmaco-kinetics" has been commonly used to describe various types of human pharmaco-kinetic research which may not involve patients or the individualization of drug therapy. Although this may be a relatively trivial issue, it is a potential source of confusion among practitioners, academicians, and students.

Regardless of the terminology, the end goal is the same: optimization of drug therapy for individual patients. With some drugs, optimization is accomplished primarily by minimizing the probability of toxicity, while with other drugs, benefits are achieved by increasing the probability of the desired therapeutic effects. To accomplish either of these two end points (i.e., reduce toxicity without compromising efficacy or increase efficacy without unacceptable toxicity) is an appropriate justification for applied pharmacokinetics. It follows, therefore, that drugs which do not produce toxicity at dosages or serum concentrations close to those required for therapeutic effects will not usually require serum concentration monitoring. For such drugs, it is common to use dosages high enough to ensure "therapeutic concentrations" in essentially all patients, since toxicity is of little concern. An exception to this practice might arise when noncompliance or mal-absorption is suspected or when the cost of a drug is so great that therapy with the minimum effective dosage is advantageous. Usually, concentrations of drugs with high toxic:therapeutic concentration ratios (e.g., penicillins, benzodiazepines) are not routinely monitored, and simple, reliable assays are generally not commer-cially available.

Conversely, drugs which frequently produce toxicity at dosages close to those required for therapeutic effects are the drugs most commonly monitored and for which commercial assays are usually available. With such drugs, the "target" serum concentration range is usually narrow, necessitating relatively precise selection of an appropriate dosage schedule.

THERAPEUTIC RANGE

The concept of a "therapeutic range" for serum concentrations of drugs is commonly misunderstood. Unfortunately, many inexperienced users of therapeu-tic drug concentration monitoring assume that the therapeutic range for most drugs has been well-defined from carefully controlled clinical trials. Another common misconception is that concentrations in the therapeutic range will result in the desired clinical response. By developing a better appreciation of the general definition of a "therapeutic range" and then more closely evaluating the basis for therapeutic ranges of individual drugs, one can develop a more rational approach to using drug concentrations in clinical practice. In general, a "therapeutic range" should never be considered in absolute terms, since it represents no more than a combination of probability charts. In other words, a "therapeutic range" is a range of drug concentrations within which the probability of the desired clinical response is relatively high and the probability of unacceptable toxicity is relatively low. This concept is depicted graphically in Figure 1-1 for a hypothetical drug. As can be seen, the probability of the desired therapeutic effect is very low (i.e., less than 5%) when drug concentrations are low (i.e., less than 5 mg/L), as is the probability of toxicity. This conclusion seems reasonable, but it should be noticed that there is a small possibility of either the desired response or toxicity, even in the absence of a measurable drug concentration. Such would be expected in a large study, assuming that some patients will recover spontaneously without any drug therapy and that some will develop an adverse effect which is unrelated but coincidental with drug administration. More importantly, as drug concentrations increase between about 5 and 20 mg/L, the probability of response increases from less than 20% to about 75%, and then plateaus. Over the same concentration range, the probability of toxicity increases more slowly, from less than 5% to only about 10%, and then begins to increase more rapidly as concentrations exceed 20 mg/L.

Thus, for a given patient, if one were given such data from a large, well-controlled study of comparable patients, what "therapeutic range" would one use? If 10 mg/L were selected as the lower end of the range, then the minimum probability of response would be about 50%. If 20 mg/L were chosen as the upper end of the therapeutic range, then the maximum probability of response would be about 75%. Over this same concentration range, the probability of unacceptable toxicity would remain less than about 10%.

In this hypothetical example, the potential benefits of achieving a drug concentration in the "therapeutic range" are clear, since below this range the probability of response is considerably less, and above the range there is a considerable increase in the probability of toxicity without any appreciable increase in response. However, it should be clear from this example that patients with concentrations below the "therapeutic range" may respond (5% to 50% chance), while those in the upper end of the range may fail to respond (25% chance). Likewise, toxicity may occur in those patients within the therapeutic range (less than 10% chance) or may be absent in those exceeding the upper end of the range.

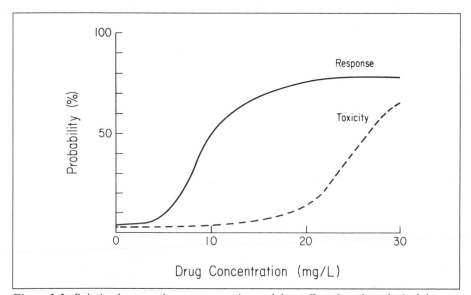

Figure 1-1. *Relation between drug concentration and drug effects for a hypothetical drug.*

For comparison, Figure 1-2, Panel A, shows a hypothetical response-toxicity probability chart for a drug with essentially no toxicity at concentrations associated with the greatest probability of response. Such would be the case for drugs with high toxic:therapeutic ratios. Figure 1-2, Panel B, depicts a similar plot for a hypothetical drug which also has a relatively high toxic:therapeutic ratio, but which clearly produces toxicity in a large percentage of patients at concentrations above 60 mg/L. As mentioned previously, for drugs with plots like Figure 1-2, Panel A, there is little reason to routinely monitor serum concentrations and individualize therapy. One would simply select an average dosage which reliably produces concentrations of about 40 mg/L. A similar approach would be reasonable for drugs depicted by Figure 1-2, Panel B, although there would be greater reason to monitor such drugs, especially if their pharmacokinetics are highly variable and/or their toxicity is potentially serious.

Unfortunately, concentration-effect charts such as those shown in Figures 1-1 and 1-2, based on large numbers of prospectively studied patients, do not exist for many drugs. Moreover, with most drugs there are discrete subpopulations (because of disease, age, concurrent therapy, etc.) for whom concentration-effect relationships differ from the norm. The process of selecting the most appropriate dosage regimen to achieve concentrations in a relatively narrow range may be complicated by unpredictable intra- and interpatient variability in the drug's pharmacokinetics. A sophisticated application of pharmacokinetic principles, incorporating prior and subsequent measures of drug concentration and effects, can improve the quality of one's predictions. Guidelines to this end are addressed in the following chapters.

Although a single "best" approach to using drug concentrations does not exist for every drug, it is imperative to realize that without a systematic approach to therapeutic drug concentration monitoring, drug concentrations may be uninterpretable, unhelpful, and potentially harmful. It thus becomes essential to recognize the key elements of applied pharmacokinetics and develop strategies to perform and use them most effectively.

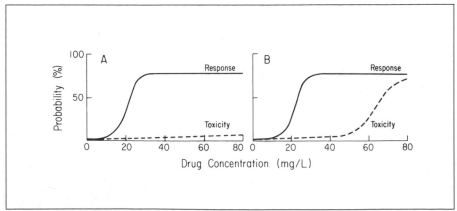

Figure 1-2. *Relation between drug concentration and drug effects for a hypothetical drug. Panel A: Hypothetical drug with essentially no toxicity at concentrations yielding maximum probability of response. Panel B: Hypothetical drug with increasing probability of toxicity as concentrations increase above concentrations needed for maximum probability of response.*

A MULTIFACTORAL MULTIDISCIPLINARY PROCESS

There are numerous drug, host, logistical, and analytical variables which influence the interpretation of drug concentration data: time, route, and dose of drug given, time blood (urine, CSF) samples are obtained, handling and storage conditions of samples, precision and accuracy of the analytical method, validity of pharmacokinetic models and assumptions, concurrent drug therapy, and the individual patient's disease and biological tolerance to drug therapy. As summarized in Figure 1-3, many different professionals are involved with the various elements of drug concentration monitoring, which is a truly multidisciplinary process. Since failure to properly carry out any one of these components can severely affect the usefulness of monitoring drug concentrations, an organized approach to the overall process is critical.

Important factors relevant to specific drugs are addressed in the individual drug chapters which follow. However, there is no single structure which ensures a

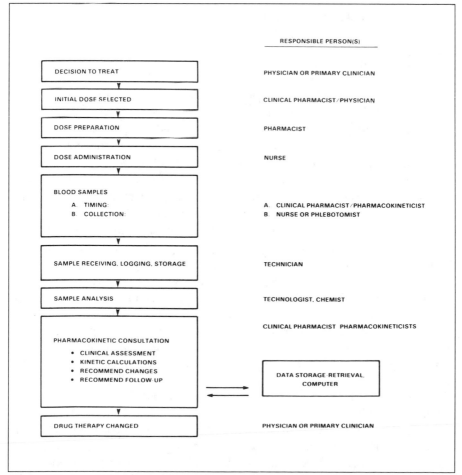

Figure 1-3. A multidisciplinary approach to individualizing drug therapy.

well-coordinated process for each drug, since the organizational structure will have to accommodate the specific needs of each institution. The organizational structure may even differ within a single institution, depending on the location of patients, special collection procedures for selected drugs, and the expertise and interest of medical, pharmacy, nursing, and clinical chemistry personnel. Regardless of the specific organizational structure selected, it should function in a manner that facilitates optimal performance of the individual component, and it should routinely monitor the various procedures to document their quality. Although some of the variables affecting drug concentration monitoring can be controlled or adjusted for (e.g., the accurate preparation and administration of drug doses), others are difficult or impossible to know or control (e.g., individual differences in biological response to drugs). These latter variables, which obviously have a major influence on individual responsiveness to drug therapy, are why drug concentrations are only intermediate therapeutic objectives and will not replace clinical response as the ultimate measure of success of drug therapy.

IS THERE A RATIONALE FOR APPLIED PHARMACOKINETICS?

Given the rather large number of events which may have an impact on therapeutic drug concentration monitoring, one might question whether it is ever of great value, particularly outside the strict controls of a research environment. Although the answer is probably different for each drug or drug class, intuitive logic suggests that drug concentration monitoring should be quite helpful for drugs with low toxic:therapeutic ratios and unpredictably variable pharmacokinetics. If one monitors and controls only the amount (i.e., dosage) of drug given to individual patients, variability in drug absorption, distribution, and elimination will influence the actual systemic exposure to the drug. By monitoring concentrations of drug that are attained in individual patients, one can modify therapy to adjust for variability in these pharmacokinetic processes. Thus, an appropriately obtained and measured concentration more directly reflects the amount of drug actually delivered than does simply the dose given. For example, one patient given 300 mg of phenytoin by mouth each day might absorb 90% of the dose, whereas a second patient might absorb 20%. All else being equal, the latter patient would have substantially lower and probably "subtherapeutic" phenytoin serum concentrations, despite having received the same dosage. Monitoring drug therapy based only on dose taken would indicate similar drug exposure (and response) in these two patients, while monitoring phenytoin serum concentrations would reveal substantial differences in drug exposure and forecast probable differences in clinical outcome. However, it must be recognized that drug concentrations in serum are generally not equivalent to drug concentrations at the site of action; it is simply assumed that they are in equilibrium with drug concentrations at the receptor and that there is a better correlation between serum concentration and drug effects than between the dose prescribed and drug effects. These relationships have been defined more clearly for some drugs than others, as detailed in the individual chapters. Chapter 2 addresses important issues related to the collection and analysis of pharmacokinetic data, Chapters 3 and 4 discuss sophisticated methods for characterizing pharmacokinetic and pharmacodynamic relationships, and the individual chapters address these issues as they pertain to individual drugs. For each drug, one should look closely at the definition of its "therapeutic range," paying particular attention to the types of studies, patients, diseases, and measures of drug effects which provide the basis for each therapeutic range. Within each of the individual drug chapters, the authors have critically evaluated the pharmaco-dynamic data which provide the basis for the individual therapeutic ranges. When reading this material, one should look closely at how the studies were designed (e.g., were they prospective, well-controlled, randomized?), the type of patient population studied (e.g., did the patients have the same disease, concurrent therapy, and age as the individual patient being treated?), and the methods used to measure drug concentrations and effects (e.g., was the endpoint of response objective, and was the therapeutic range based on an analytical method comparable in accuracy and precision to the one you are using?). By answering these types of questions, one can more closely determine the extent to which the published "therapeutic range" can be applied in specific clinical situations.

PROVIDING CONSULTATIONS

There are several good approaches to providing pharmacokinetic consultations, depending on the circumstances involved. Consults may be relatively informal verbal recommendations in conjunction with a written laboratory report of the drug concentration. Conversely, many programs provide a formal written consult which is a permanent part of the medical record. Although the latter approach is usually not feasible or necessary for all drug concentrations, exclusive use of the informal approach is also undesirable. Based on the general considerations previously addressed in this chapter and the specific issues covered in subsequent chapters, it should be obvious that simply comparing a laboratory value to a published "therapeutic range" (the "rubber stamp" approach) is inappropriate. Even when the multidisciplinary approach to dose preparation, drug administration, sample collection, and drug analysis is well organized and of high quality, one must interpret drug concentrations in light of patient-specific variables (e.g., disease status, concurrent therapy). When consultation is provided in a formal manner, inclusion of selected drug and patient-specific information is recommended. This includes the following:

- a brief statement of the problem leading to measurement of drug concentrations
- a summary of subjective and objective criteria influencing drug disposition and effects
- an assessment of prior and present pharmacokinetic data
- recommendations for possible changes in drug therapy and follow-up evaluations

One must also remain cognizant of the "therapeutic range concept" when providing consultations and always recognize that drug concentrations are only intermediate therapeutic objectives. Such an approach will be most likely to lead to more rational use of applied pharmacokinetics and the greatest benefit to individual patients.

Chapter 2

Guidelines for Collection and Analysis of Pharmacokinetic Data

William J. Jusko

Efforts in both theoretical and applied pharmacokinetics over the past decades have emphasized the utilization of the principles of **physiological pharmacokinetics** and the use of **noncompartmental** approaches to analysis of drug disposition data. Physiological pharmacokinetics involves the deployment of pharmacokinetic models and equations based on anatomical constructions and functions, such as tissue masses, blood flow, organ metabolism and clearance, specific drug input rates and sites, and processes of partitioning, binding, and transport. While the complete applications of physiologic systems analysis may require extensive models,[1] even the simplest of pharmacokinetic treatments should have a physiologic basis for interpretation. Noncompartmental techniques in pharmacokinetics can serve in this regard. This term applies to curve analysis methods of data treatment which do not require a specific model and which yield the prime pharmacokinetic parameters, such as systemic clearance (CL) and steady-state volume of distribution (V_{ss}), which summarize the major elimination and distribution properties.

This chapter is intended to provide an overview of major components of experimentally applied pharmacokinetics. A summary is provided of the most relevant concepts, models, equations, and caveats which may be useful in the design, analysis, and interpretation of pharmacokinetic studies. References are provided for more complete details of the assumptions, derivations, and applications of these guidelines and relationships. This material may be helpful as a checklist in designing animal and/or human experiments in pharmacokinetics and in reviewing drug disposition reports; with greater elaboration, it has served as a basis for a graduate course in physiological pharmacokinetics.

CONTEXT OF PHARMACOKINETICS

A pharmacokinetic analysis must be made in context of, be consistent with, and explain the array of basic data regarding the properties and disposition character-istics of the drug.

The tasks of model and equation selection and interpretation of data require a fundamental appreciation and integration of principles of physiology, pharmacol-ogy, biochemistry, physicochemistry, analytical methodology, mathematics, and statistics. Pharmacokinetics has derived from these disciplines, and the relevant aspects of many of these areas must be considered in reaching any conclusions regarding a particular set of data. The physicochemical properties of a drug such as chemical form (salt, ester, complex), stability, partition coefficient, pKa, and molecular weight can affect drug absorption, distribution, and clearance. A drug disposition profile must be correlated with studies of structure-activity, disposition in alternative species, perfused organ experiments, tissue or microsomal metabo-lism, tissue drug residues, disease-state effects, and pharmacology and toxicology. For example, a much larger LD_{50} for oral doses of a drug compared with parenteral administration may be indicative of either poor gastrointestinal absorption (low aqueous solubility?) or a substantial first-pass effect. Drug metabolism pathways may differ between species, but the biotransformation rate (V_{max} and K_m) of microsomes, homogenates, or perfused organs can often be applied directly to whole-body disposition rates and often correlate between species.[1-3]

In general, the pharmacokinetic model and analysis should either conform to, or account for, the known properties and accumulated data related to the drug. One set of disposition data may misrepresent the characteristics of the drug because of any one or combination of reasons. Experienced judgment is usually required in the final interpretation of any experimental findings and analysis.

ARRAY OF BASIC DATA

Pharmacokinetic studies often serve to answer specific questions about the properties of a drug. For example, a limited experimental protocol can easily resolve the question of how renal impairment affects the systemic clearance of an antibiotic. In the total design and implementation of pharmacokinetic studies, an **ideal** and **complete** array of experimental data should include a number of considerations:

A. *The dosage form should be pre-analyzed.* All calculations stem from knowledge of the exact dose given [e.g., CL = dose / AUC (area under the plasma concentration-time curve)]. Most commercial dosage forms are inexact, and content uniformity should be examined. Vials or ampules of injectables typically contain some overage and require analysis or aliquoting for administration of a precise dose. Solid dosage forms are required to yield an average of the stated quantity of drug with limited variability, but both injectable and solid forms may be inaccurate for pharmacokinetic purposes. Manninen and Koriionen[4] provide an excellent example of both the variability and lack of stated quantity of digoxin in many commercial tablets. One product contained a range of 39% to 189% of the stated 0.25 mg dose of digoxin, while the most uniform product, Lanoxin, exhibited a range of about 95% to 106% for one batch of drug. To evaluate the potential uncertainty of the dose of drug used in disposition studies, it may be necessary to collect and analyze replicate doses of the product used. Poorly soluble and highly potent drugs are of most concern regarding erratic formulation.

B. *Accuracy in administration of the dose should be confirmed.* All doses should be timed exactly for starting time and duration of administration. For ease in subsequent calculations, pharmacokinetic equations can be used to correct data from short-term infusion studies to the intercepts expected after bolus injection. The particular materials used in drug administration may cause loss of drug. In one of the most dramatic examples, MacKichan et al.[5] found immediate loss of about 50% of a dose of intravenous diazepam by adsorption during passage through the plastic tubing of an infusion set. Inline filtration can also significantly reduce the potency of drugs administered intravenously.[6]

C. *Attention to methods and sites of blood collection is needed.* Ideally, blood samples should be collected by direct venipuncture in clean glass tubes without anticoagulant. Otherwise, the presence of possible artifacts should be tested. In the absence of any *in vitro* artifacts, serum and plasma concentrations are usually identical, and these terms are commonly used interchangeably. However, there are several reasons why they may not be identical. For example, the presence of heparin can result in increased free fatty acid concentrations, causing altered plasma-protein binding.[7] Also, the type of blood collection tube or anticoagulant may be a factor.[8] If protein binding is temperature dependent, it may be necessary to centrifuge the blood sample at 37 °C to avoid changes in red cell-plasma distribution of some compounds.[9] These problems primarily pertain to weak bases, such as propranolol and imipramine, for which binding to α_1 acid glyco-protein is appreciable and displacement alters plasma-red cell drug distribution.

Plasma or serum protein binding and red cell partitioning should be measured at 37 °C over the expected range of plasma drug concentrations. Both rate and degree of binding and uptake are theoretically important. This information may be especially needed for interpretation or normalization of nonlinear disposition patterns.

Sometimes the site of blood collection and the presence of a tourniquet can alter the composition of the blood sample: serum proteins, calcium, and magnesium concentrations rise by 5% to 13% during venous stasis.[10]

One of the major assumptions employed in most pharmacokinetic studies is that venous blood collected from one site adequately reflects circulating arterial blood concentrations. For practical purposes, venous blood samples are usually collected. The pharmacokinetic analysis may need to be somewhat qualified, because arterial and capillary blood concentrations may differ markedly from venous blood concentrations of many drugs.[11] The AUC of arterial versus venous blood is expected to be identical for a non-clearing organ, and thus the principal difference expected is in distribution volumes. Physiologically, organ uptake of drugs occurs from the arterial blood, and clearance organ models are based on arterial-venous extraction principles.

    D. *Serum (or blood) concentration data following **intravenous** injection (bolus or infusion) provides partial characterization of drug disposition properties.* Accurate assessment of volumes of distribution, distribution clearance (CL_D), and systemic clearance (CL) can best be attained with intravenous washout data.

    E. *Serum (or blood) concentration data following **oral** doses of the drug in solution and common dosage forms provides additional pharmacokinetic parameters related to absorption and intrinsic clearance.* The doses (or resultant serum or blood concentrations of drug) should be comparable to those from the intravenous dose. These data permit assessment of either oral clearance (CL_{oral}) or bioavailability (F), and of the mean absorption time (MAT). If relevant, other routes of administration should be studied. For these, the FDA guidelines for bioavailability studies should be consulted.[12]

    F. *Three dosage levels (both oral and intravenous) should be administered* to span the usual therapeutic range of the drug to permit assessment of possible dose-dependence (nonlinearity) in absorption, distribution, and elimination.

    G. *Urinary excretion rates of drug (as a function of time, dose and route of administration) should be measured to accompany the above studies.* Urinary excretion is often a major route of drug elimination, and analyses permit quantitation of renal clearance (CL_R). Collection of other excreta or body fluids (feces, bile, milk, saliva) may permit determination of other relevant elimination or distributional pathways.

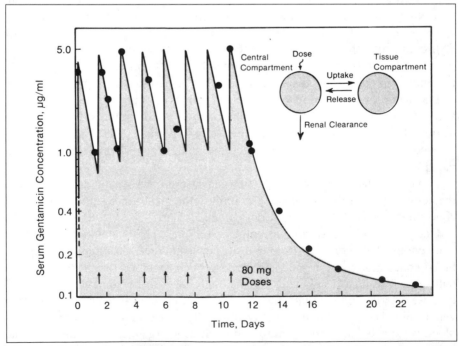

Figure 2-1. *Plasma concentration-time profile for gentamicin disposition during multiple dosing in a patient showing the prolonged terminal phase caused by strong tissue binding. These data were characterized with a two-compartment model (inset) which included prediction of drug remaining in the body at the time of death of the patients. Data from reference 15.*

H. *Many drug metabolites are either pharmacologically active or otherwise of pharmacokinetic interest.* Phase I products such as hydroxylated or demethylated metabolites are most commonly either active or toxic.[13] Their measurement will allow evaluation of AUC and mean residence time (MRT) and perhaps permit quantitation of metabolite formation and disposition clearances.

I. *Multiple-dose and steady-state experiments are necessary if therapeutic use of the drug relies on steady-state concentrations.* The duration of multiple-dosing in relation to the terminal half-life is crucial for ascertaining applicability to steady-state conditions. Comparative single- and multiple-dose studies permit further assessment of linearity and/or allow determination of chronic or time-dependent drug effects, such as enzyme induction,[14] unusual accumulation,[15] or drug-induced alterations in disposition. For example, aminoglycoside uptake into tissues is extremely slow and difficult to assess from single-dose studies. Multiple-dose washout measures (see Figure 2-1) led to observation of a slow disposition phase for gentamicin which was the result of tissue accumulation and release.[16]

J. *Tissue analyses add reality and specificity to drug distribution characteristics.* Comprehensive studies in animals permit detection of unusual tissue affinities while generating partition coefficients (K_{pi}) for individual tissues (V_{ti}). This can lead to complete physiologic models for the drug in each species studied.[1,2] Autopsy or biopsy studies in man may extend or complement pharmacokinetic

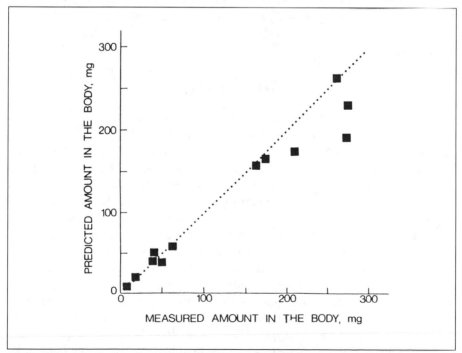

Figure 2-2. *Correlation of gentamicin accumulation in the body determined by pharmacokinetic analysis of serum concentration data (see Figure 2-1) and by direct analysis of body tissues obtained at autopsy from the same patients who were evaluated pharmacokinetically before death. Dotted line indicates correlation. Data from references 15 and 16.*

expectations. This approach was found to be extremely helpful (see Figure 2-2) in confirming the strong tissue binding of gentamicin in man which was anticipated on the basis of serum concentration profiles (see Figure 2-1).[16]

K. *Suitable drug disposition studies in patients with various diseases and ages or given secondary drugs form the basis of clinical pharmacokinetics.* Perturbations in organ function, blood flow, or response will often alter drug disposition in a way that may warrant quantitative characterization. General principles may not always apply, and each drug needs individualized study. For example, while hepatic dysfunction may diminish the rate of oxidation of many drugs, some compounds, such as oxazepam and lorazepam, are predominantly metabolized by glucuronide conjugation, a process largely unaffected by liver diseases such as cirrhosis.[17] Each disease state may require evaluation of direct effects on pharmacokinetic processes such as changes in renal clearance caused by kidney disease. However, indirect changes also require attention, such as the effects on both distribution and clearance caused by altered plasma protein binding.[18] Finally, commonly encountered patient factors such as smoking habit[19] and obesity may cause unusual changes in drug disposition and require specific study and notation in patient surveys.

L. *Many questions of drug disposition can be resolved from selected, carefully designed studies, and alternative types of information may be sufficient to validate various assumptions and reduce experimental procedures.* The investigator's obligation is to adequately assess the literature, to avoid unwarranted assumptions, and to seek experimental strategies that would resolve a proposed hypothesis.

A comprehensive overview of pharmacokinetic needs in drug development has been constructed by Balant et al.[20]

DRUG ASSAYS

Certainty of specificity, sensitivity, and accuracy in measurement of drugs and their metabolites is a *sine qua non* in pharmacokinetics and deserves considerable attention. Guidelines for quality assurance in laboratory analyses have been concisely summarized by the American Chemical Society.[21] It is now commonplace to report the linearity, the coefficient of variation of the assay at low and high drug concentrations, the minimum level of detection, and the procedures used to assure specificity and stability, especially in the presence of metabolites, secondary drugs, and in specimens from diseased patients. Microbiological assays are notoriously unreliable with problems due to other antibiotics and active metabolites. An extreme case of metabolite inclusion is in the use of radioisotopic tracers; total radioisotope counts generally yield total drug and metabolite activity and possibly the products of radiolysis. Separation of parent drug and individual metabolites is required for specificity. Microbiologic, enzymatic, and radioimmunoassays are often of uncertain specificity, and matrix effects may require preparation of standards in each patient's pretreatment plasma. Most drug companies provide analytical-grade samples of their drugs (and sometimes metabolites) to qualified investigators upon written request.

Sample Handling

Coupled with assay reliability is concern for the stability of drug in biological specimens, even in the frozen state. Ampicillin is unusual in that it is less stable frozen than when refrigerated.[22] Some drug esters, such as hetacillin (a prodrug of ampicillin), continue hydrolyzing in blood and during the bioassay. Penicillamine is unstable in the presence of plasma proteins, and immediate deproteination after blood collection avoids loss of reduced penicillamine before analysis.[23] Cyclosporine is best assayed in EDTA rather than heparinized blood as the latter yields red cell aggregates that increase assay variability.[94] Measurement of drug stability in blood will reveal whether hydrolysis can occur in blood or whether exposure to other body organs is required. Additional concerns in handling samples from a pharmacokinetic study include labeling and record-keeping procedures and documentation of storage conditions.

Sample Timing

Appropriate pharmacokinetic evaluation requires properly timed specimens. The simplest and least ambiguous experiment is the determination of systemic plasma clearance during continuous infusion at steady state:

$$CL = \frac{k_o}{C_{ss}}$$

(Eq. 2-1)

where k_o is the infusion rate and C_{ss} is the steady-state plasma or serum concentration. For this equation to apply, the infusion period must be sufficiently long (about five terminal disposition half-lives) to allow steady state to be attained. Alternatively, a loading dose or short-term infusion may be administered to more rapidly achieve equilibrium.[24]

Practical and cost-effective methods are available for designing optimal sampling strategies for kinetic experiments where the number of specimens is limited,[25] such as in the clinic. Optimal designs largely depend on the likely "true" model parameter values, the structure of the model, and the measurement error. A sequential approach has been advocated with pilot studies and a sampling schedule which distributes time points over the major phases of drug disposition as the first step. Subsequent experiments can then resolve a specific hypothesis.

A common and severe problem in applied pharmacokinetics is the inadequate or incomplete measurement of drug washout from the system, either because of premature termination of sample collection or because of analytical limitations. The "true" terminal disposition phase must be examined in order for most aspects of data treatment and interpretation to be accurate. For example, the early distributive phase of aminoglycoside disposition measured by bioassay had long been accepted as the only phase, yet more sensitive radioimmunoassays, lengthier sample collection, and evaluation of multiple-dose washout revealed the slower phase of prolonged drug release from tissues (see Figure 2-1).

The two summary physiologic parameters in pharmacokinetics, namely systemic clearance and steady-state volume of distribution, can be most easily calculated by use of the area under the plasma concentration-time curve (AUC) and the area under the moment curve (AUMC). Both area values require extrapolation of plasma concentrations to time infinity, and the AUMC is, in particular, prone to exaggerated error from an inaccurate terminal slope.[26] If analytical or ethical constraints limit blood sample availability, extended saliva or urine collection may aid in defining the terminal disposition slope while adding one or two other pharmacokinetic parameters to the analysis. Urine may be particularly useful in this regard (if renal clearance is linear), as the sample volume is large and urine concentrations often exceed plasma values by one or more orders of magnitude.

The "midpoint" (C_{av}) is generally the most desirable time to collect blood samples to match an excretion interval in order to assess a time-dependent clearance process:

$$\text{Clearance} = \frac{\text{Excretion Rate}}{C_{av}} = \frac{\text{Amount Excreted}}{\text{AUC}} \qquad \text{(Eq. 2-2)}$$

The arithmetic mean time is acceptable for slow processes, but errors will be incurred if the kinetic process produces rapid changes in plasma concentrations.[27] It is common to miss an early exponential phase of drug disposition because of infrequent blood sampling. For a polyexponential curve with intercepts C_i and slopes λ_i the total AUC is:

$$\text{AUC} = \Sigma \left(\frac{C_i}{\lambda_i} \right) \qquad \text{(Eq. 2-3)}$$

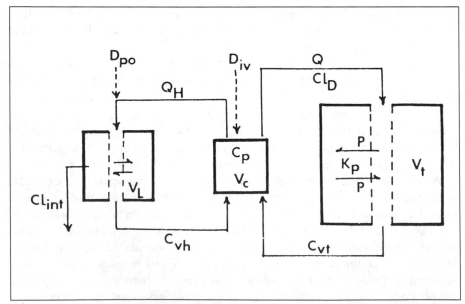

Figure 2-3. *Basic physiologic pharmacokinetic model for drug distribution and elimination. (Symbols are defined in the text.) The clearance organ is pharmacokinetically perceived as separate from other compartments for drugs with high intrinsic clearances (CL_{int}) allowing characterization of the first-pass input.*

If the initial distributive phase is missing (area $= C_1 / \lambda_1$), then the error incurred in calculation of a clearance parameter (CL = dose / AUC) is

$$\% \text{ of CL error} = \frac{100 \left(\dfrac{C_i}{\lambda_i} \right)}{AUC} \qquad \text{(Eq. 2-4)}$$

BASIC PHYSIOLOGIC PARAMETERS

The evolution of complete physiologic models[1] and clearance concepts applied to perfused organ systems,[28,29] with the restrictions incurred by the limited *in vivo* visibility offered by most blood or plasma drug disposition profiles, has led to the employment of partial physiologic models for description of pharmacokinetic data. One such model is shown in Figure 2-3. Its construction and use should be viewed with some conceptual flexibility, and this material will apply to linear processes unless stated otherwise.

Volumes

The drug in blood or plasma (C_p) is considered to be part of the central compartment (V_c). The minimum value of V_c is plasma volume (V_p), but, either because drug diffuses rapidly out of plasma or the number of early time data are limited, the V_c value often exceeds V_p.

Drug which is located outside of V_p or V_c is, of course, present in tissues. The apparent volume of the tissue compartment (V_T) has two basic determinants: physiologic weight or volume of each tissue (V_{ti}) and partition or distribution factors (K_{pi}). In analysis of plasma concentration-time profiles, tissues must commonly be clustered together (including the clearing organs) thus:

$$V_T = \Sigma K_{pi} \cdot V_{ti} \qquad \text{(Eq. 2-5)}$$

This equation leads to definition of one of the primary pharmacokinetic parameters with a physiologic basis, volume of distribution at steady state (V_{ss}):

$$V_{ss} = V_c + V_T \qquad \text{(Eq. 2-6)}$$

Table 2-1. *Physiological Determinants of Drug Partition or Distribution Ratios between Tissues and Plasma*

Active transport	Plasma protein binding
Donnon ion effect	Tissue binding
pH differences	Lipid partitioning

If plasma and tissue binding are the sole determinants of nonhomogeneous distribution of drug in the body, then one definition of V_{ss} is

$$V_{ss} = V_p + \frac{f_{up}}{f_{ut}} \cdot V_T$$

(Eq. 2-7)

where f_{up} and f_{ut} are the fractions of drug unbound in plasma and tissue.[30] Other factors may also contribute to the apparent partition coefficient of drugs between tissues and plasma (see Table 2-1). Since, by definition, V_p and ΣV_{ti} comprise total body weight (TBW),

$$TBW = V_p + \Sigma V_{ti}$$

(Eq. 2-8)

then the quotient of

$$K_D = \frac{V_{ss}}{TBW}$$

(Eq. 2-9)

defines the distribution coefficient (K_D), a physicochemical and physiological measure of the average tissue:plasma ratio of the drug throughout the body. Approximate values of K_D and the primary rationalization of the size of K_D are

Table 2-2. *Distribution Coefficients (K_D) for Various Drugs and Probable Physiologic (Physicochemical) Cause*

Drug	$K_D = \dfrac{V_{ss}}{TBW}$	Explanation/indication
Indocyanine Green	0.06	Strong binding to plasma proteins and limited extravascular permeability.
Inulin	0.25	Distribution limited to plasma and interstitial fluid owing to large molecular weight (5500) and lipid insolubility.
Ampicillin	0.25	Limited intracellular distribution owing to poor lipid solubility (common to penicillins).
Theophylline	0.5	Moderate plasma binding and distribution primarily into total body water.
Antipyrine	0.6	Slight plasma binding and fairly uniform distribution into total body water.
Gentamicin	1.1	Strong tissue binding (common to aminoglycosides).
Tetracycline	1.6	Strong tissue binding to calcium in bone.
Diazepam	1.7	Appreciable lipid partitioning.
Digoxin	8.0	Strong binding to Na/K transport ATPase in cell membranes.
Imipramine	10.0	Strong tissue binding (common to weak bases).

provided in Table 2-2 for several common drugs. Normalization of V_{ss} for TBW is thus of value for generating the K_D and for making interindividual and interspecies[2] comparisons of this parameter.

One qualification of V_{ss} is needed. Drug equilibration between plasma and tissue of a clearing organ is affected by blood flow (Q_H) and intrinsic clearance (CL_{int}).[31] For hepatic tissue, this yields the following relationship between the true partition coefficient (K_{ph}) and the lower, apparent value which would be experimentally measured at steady state K_{ph}^{exp}:

$$K_{ph} = K_{ph}^{exp}\left(1 + \frac{CL_{int}}{Q_H}\right)$$

(Eq. 2-10)

Distribution Clearance

The least developed and appreciated element of the basic pharmacokinetic properties of drugs is the distribution clearance (CL_D) or intercompartmental clearance. This term reflects the flow or permeability property of drugs between plasma and tissue spaces. The simplest assumption made in constructing a generalized model is that distribution clearance is equal in both directions in and out of tissues.

Renkin has characterized distribution clearance in terms of transcapillary movement of small molecular weight substances.[32] The model proposed is depicted in Figure 2-4. Drug transfer from blood to tissues is represented by flow

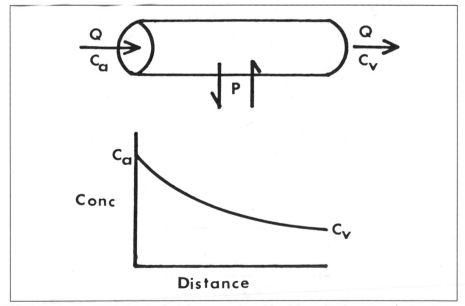

Figure 2-4. *Model for distribution clearance where blood flow (Q) along the cylindrical tube and capillary permeability (P) are the primary determinants of drug loss from arterial blood (C_a). Drug concentration in the tube will decline monoexponentially according to distance (length) along the tube emerging at the venous concentration (C_v).*

down a cylindrical tube (Q) with permeability (P) determined by diffusion across the capillary. Distribution clearance is thus defined by flow and permeability according to the following relationship:

$$CL_D = Q\left(1 - e^{-P/Q}\right)$$ (Eq. 2-11)

Compounds with high tissue permeability will exhibit a limiting CL_D of Q, while those with low permeability are limited by P. These concepts have been applied by Stec and Atkinson[33] to a multicompartment model of procainamide and NAPA disposition and used to predict the extent of hemodynamic changes caused by hemodialysis. The flow or permeability coefficient can be calculated for drugs exhibiting polyexponential disposition and is of more fundamental value than intercompartmental rate constants.

Hepatic Clearance

The model shown in Figure 2-3 represents the common situation where drug must pass through a specific organ such as the liver or kidney for elimination. It does not apply to enzymatic hydrolysis in blood. This type of model reflects the dual role of blood flow (Q) and either biotransformation (V_{max}, K_m) or renal filtration (GFR) and transport (T_{max}, T_m) on removal of drug from the body and allows for some effects of route of administration (e.g., first-pass).

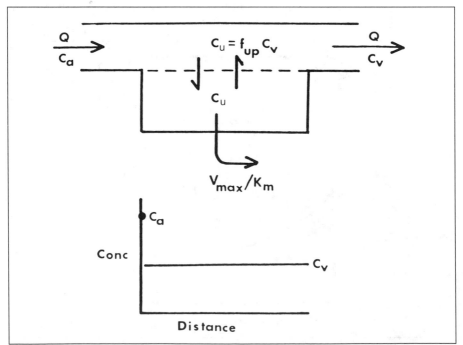

Figure 2-5. *The "well-stirred" or "jar" model for hepatic uptake and metabolism (V_{max}/K_m) of drug where instantaneous venous and hepatic equilibration of unbound (C_u) drug is assumed. Inflow and outflow (Q) are assumed to be identical.*

Two types of clearing organ models are commonly used for hepatic elimination: The "Jar" or Venous Equilibrium Model[28] (see Figure 2-5) and the "Tube" Model[34] (see Figure 2-6). Both include blood flow for systemic drug access to the organ and, as shown in the figures, assume that free or unbound drug (f_{up}) in plasma equilibrates with free drug in the tissue available to enzymes. The Jar Model assumes that drug in arterial blood (C_a) entering the clearing organ instantaneously equilibrates with that in the venous blood (C_v). The Tube Model assumes that a drug concentration gradient exists down the tube, with enzymes acting upon declining perfusate concentrations.

The Jar Model yields the following relationship for hepatic clearance:

$$CL_H = \frac{Q_H \cdot f_{up} \cdot CLu_{int}}{Q_H + f_{up} \cdot CLu_{int}} = Q_H \cdot E_H \qquad \text{(Eq. 2-12)}$$

where intrinsic clearance is the ratio of V_{max} / K_m for linear biotransformation and E_H is the extraction ratio.

The corresponding equation for CL_H described by the Tube Model is

$$CL_H = Q_H\left(1 - e^{-f_{up} \cdot CLu_{int}/Q_H}\right) = Q_H \cdot E_H \qquad \text{(Eq. 2-13)}$$

Figure 2-7 depicts the dual effects of blood flow and intrinsic clearance on hepatic clearance for the two clearance organ models. Both models predict a lower CL_H limit of $f_{up}\, CLu_{int}$ (or CL_{int} in the absence of protein binding considerations)

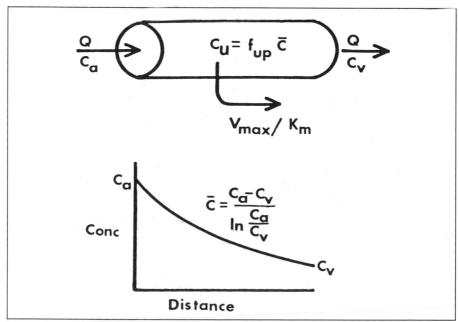

Figure 2-6. *The "tube" or "parallel tube" model for hepatic uptake and metabolism V_{max} / K_m of drug where venous concentrations (C_v) decline monoexponentially as flow (Q) carries drug past homogeneously distributed sites of biotransformation. The log-mean concentration ($\bar{C}$) in the tube is indicated.*

and an upper value of Q_H. Thus, CL_H of low clearance drugs is essentially equal to the product of intrinsic clearance and the fraction unbound in plasma.[35] The maximum hepatic clearance will be organ blood flow. As seen by the shape of the surfaces in Figure 2-7, the two models diverge somewhat in characterizing drugs with intermediate to high clearance. The Jar Model has had most extensive use in physiological pharmacokinetics.[1] A new unifying model of hepatic elimination, the dispersion model, has been shown to be consistent with and explain the functioning of all existing models of disposition by the liver; however, the equations are too complex for direct application and are best used in their simplified forms.[36]

The organ clearance models provide definitions for two types of general clearance terms. **Systemic clearance** (CL) reflects any situation where drug is administered without its initially passing through the clearing organ. Intravenous, intramuscular, buccal, and subcutaneous injection of drugs yields plasma concentration-time data governed by systemic clearance, e.g.,

$$CL = \frac{D_{iv}}{AUC_{iv}} = Q \cdot E_H$$

(Eq. 2-14)

The systemic clearance is equal to the sum of all organ clearance processes:

$$CL = CL_H + CL_R + CL_{other}$$

(Eq. 2-15)

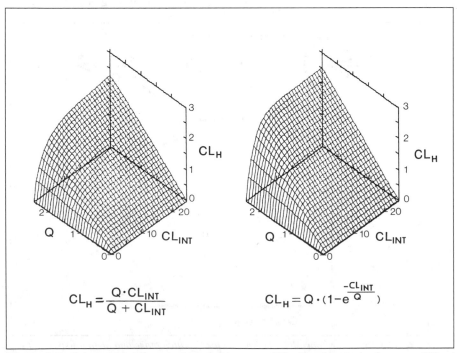

Figure 2-7. *Relationships between hepatic clearance (CL_H) and intrinsic clearance (CL_{int}) and hepatic blood flow (Q_H) for the Jar (LHS) and Tube (RHS) models. The equations are shown without the protein binding factor (see Equations 2-12 and 2-13).*

where the upper limit in removal of drug from the body can be perceived as the sum of each organ blood flow. For drugs subject to enzymatic degradation in blood, the upper limit of CL is, of course, V_{max} / K_m for this biotransformation process.

The **intrinsic clearance** is a related, complementary term which reflects the maximum metabolic or transport capability of the clearing organ. It can be measured by directly introducing the drug into the circulation feeding the clearing organ. Oral, intraperitoneal, and, in part, rectal doses place the drug directly into the liver via the mesenteric vein. If the drug is fully absorbed from the administration site (F = 1) and undergoes biotransformation entirely by the liver, then

$$\frac{F \cdot D_{po}}{AUC_{po}} = CL_{oral}$$
(Eq. 2-16)

and

$$\frac{F \cdot D_{po}}{f_{up} \cdot AUC_{po}} = CLu_{int} = \frac{V_{max}}{K_m}$$
(Eq. 2-17)

where CL_{oral}, or oral dose clearance, provides the intrinsic clearance uncorrected for protein binding (f_{up}). The V_{max} / K_m values from *in vitro* drug metabolizing systems can be used to predict reasonable values of E_H for perfused organ disposition of various drugs. These data are presented in Table 2-3 and demonstrate that both the Jar and Tube models allow reasonable prediction of E_H for several drugs.

The role of plasma protein binding in affecting organ clearance is only partly accounted for by the f_{up} term in Equations 2-12 and 2-13. Experimental data for the relationship of E_H to f_{up} according to Equation 2-12 are depicted in Figure 2-8.[37] For compounds with low intrinsic clearance such as warfarin, the E_H and CL_H are linearly dependent on f_{up}.[35] This phenomenon has been termed "restrictive clearance." High-clearance compounds such as propranolol allow total hepatic extraction with $E_H \rightarrow 1$ or $CL_H \rightarrow Q_H$ when CL_{int} is very high (nonrestrictive clearance). A

Table 2-3. *Comparison of Hepatic Extraction Ratios Predicted from In Vitro Drug Metabolism Data and Observed in Liver Perfusion Studies[a]*

Drug	In Vitro V_{max}/K_m mL/(min) (gm liver)	Observed	Jar model predicted	Tube model predicted
		Extraction ratio		
Alprenolol	23.5	> 0.90	0.92	0.99
Propranolol	10.0	> 0.90	0.83	0.99
Lidocaine	8.21	> 0.90	0.80	0.98
Phenytoin	1.99	0.53	0.50	0.63
Hexobarbital	1.60	0.33	0.44	0.54
Carbamazepine	0.11	0.04	0.05	0.05
Antipyrine	0.08	0.01	0.04	0.04

[a] From reference 2 and calculated from part of Eq. 2-13.

compound like phenytoin is intermediate in behavior in the perfused rat liver system. What must occur in reality for "nonrestrictive" compounds is that the rate of dissociation of the drug protein complex must be relatively rapid in relation to the transit time of drug through the organ. The models require a more complex form to mathematically account for this kinetic process,[38] and development of more fundamental principles related to the role of protein binding in organ drug uptake remains of interest. Similar complications pertain to the role of red cell uptake and release of drugs in relation to organ transit time.[39] In general, the liver appears to be capable of extracting drugs from both plasma and red cells, whereas the kidney has access only to drugs in plasma.

Renal Clearance

A second clearing process can be added to the model shown in Figure 2-3 to represent renal clearance (which is always a type of systemic clearance in whole-body disposition studies). One relationship which defines many of the common factors affecting renal clearance (CL_R) is

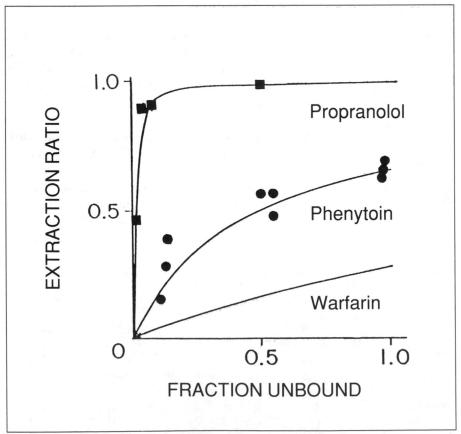

Figure 2-8. *Effect of plasma protein binding on hepatic extraction of drugs with low (warfarin), intermediate (phenytoin), and high (propranolol) intrinsic clearance values. Adapted from reference 37.*

$$CL_R = (Q_{RP})\,(E) = \left(f_{up}\,GFR + \frac{Q_{RP} \cdot f_{up} \cdot CL_{int}^R}{Q_{RP} + f_{up} \cdot CL_{int}^R} \right)(1 - R_F) \qquad \text{(Eq. 2-18)}$$

where Q_{RP} is the effective renal plasma flow, GFR is the glomerular filtration rate, R_F is the fraction of drug reabsorbed in the tubules, and CL_{int}^R is the intrinsic renal clearance, which under linear conditions is governed by the T_{max}/T_m for the active transport process.[40]

Renal clearance is commonly calculated using Equation 2-2. Tucker[41] offers a concise review of practical and theoretical concepts pertaining to measurement and interpretation of renal clearance.

Absorption

Two properties of drugs exhibiting an absorption profile can be considered as primary pharmacokinetic parameters. These are the systemic availability (FF*) and the mean absorption time (MAT). The systemic availability represents the net fraction of the dose reaching the blood or plasma following possible losses from incomplete release from the dosage form, destruction in the gastrointestinal tract (F), and first-pass metabolism (F*):

$$F^* = 1 - \frac{f_{up} \cdot CLu_{int}}{Q_{II}} \qquad \text{(Eq. 2-19)}$$

The oral:IV AUC ratio indicates systemic availability:

$$FF^* = \frac{D_{iv} \cdot AUC_{po}}{D_{po} \cdot AUC_{iv}} \qquad \text{(Eq. 2-20)}$$

A noncompartmental parameter for characterizing absorption rate is the MAT.[26] As indicated by its name, this parameter represents the average duration of time that drug molecules persist in the dosage form and GI tract. Drug absorption rate constants (k_a) are usually the least secure of conventionally calculated pharmacokinetic parameters, because of the complications incurred by incomplete release of drug from the dosage form, instability in GI contents (k_d), irregular absorption, lag times (t_{lag}), mixed zero-order (k_o) and other dissolution rates, effects of changing GI motility and contents, GI blood flow effects, first-pass effect, blurred exponential terms in equations, inadequate blood sampling, and poor model specificity.[42] The MAT provides a quantitative parameter which basically summarizes how long, on average, drug molecules remain unabsorbed. It is calculated as follows for a low-clearance drug:

$$MAT = MRT_{oral} - MRT_{iv} - t_{lag} \qquad \text{(Eq. 2-21)}$$

where the measured residence times of oral (MRT_{oral}) and IV (MRT_{iv}) doses of drugs can be obtained from their AUMC / AUC ratios (to be described), and t_{lag} is the lag-time before absorption begins. The calculation is more complicated for high-clearance drugs.

As indicated from Equation 2-21 and the models shown in Figure 2-9, a useful feature of the mean residence time (MRT) is its additivity of catenary components. A basic property that allows calculations of MAT is that the disposition portion ($MRT_{iv} = V_{ss} / CL$) of an infusion or oral dose can be separated from the total MRT as shown.

TIME- AND DOSE-AVERAGE PARAMETERS

IV Disposition

The initial goal of any drug disposition study, and the minimum requirement in pharmacokinetic data analysis, is the generation of four to six primary parameters with physiologic basis. The purpose of this section is to present the common noncompartmental equations that may be applied in curve analyses. The relationships generally assume that clearance occurs directly from plasma and that the system is linear and stationary or time-invariant. They allow for preliminary analysis of drug disposition data before deciding whether a specific model is needed

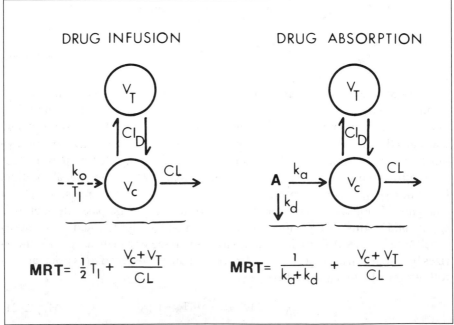

Figure 2-9. *Two-compartment pharmacokinetic models depicting central (V_c) and tissue (V_T) compartments, intercompartmental (CL_D) and plasma (CL) clearances, and additivity of residence times (MRT) for infusion (rate = k_o, duration = T_I) and absorption (amount = A, input = k_a, degradation = k_d) processes with plasma disposition (V_{ss} / CL).*[26]

and may serve to summarize the major disposition properties of the drug. Primary benefits of this approach are its relative simplicity and the reasonable degree of stability of the generated parameters.

The starting point in the analysis should involve curve-fitting the data as polyexponentials to characterize the SHAM properties of a curve: [43,44]

S: Slopes $(\lambda_i: \lambda_1, \lambda_2... \lambda_z)$
H: Heights $(C_i: C_1, C_2... C_z)$ (Intercepts)
A: Area $(AUC = \Sigma(C_i / \lambda_i))$
M: Moment $[AUMC = \Sigma(Ci / \lambda_i^2)]$

These characteristics for an IV dose and biexponential disposition function are shown in Figure 2-10. From these values, the data yield systemic plasma or blood clearance,

$$CL = \frac{D_{iv}}{AUC}$$

(Eq. 2-22)

and volume of distribution at steady state,[46,47]

$$V_{ss} = D_{iv} \cdot \frac{AUMC}{AUC^2} = CL \cdot MRT_{iv}$$

(Eq. 2-23)

The mean residence time (MRT_{iv}) of an IV bolus dose is determined by:

$$MRT_{iv} = \frac{AUMC}{AUC} = \frac{\Sigma\left(\frac{C_i}{\lambda_i^2}\right)}{\Sigma\left(\frac{C_i}{\lambda_i}\right)}$$

(Eq. 2-24)

The mean transit time of a monoexponential function can also be viewed as the time point where 63.2% of the total AUC is attained or 63.2% of the IV dose is eliminated.

The above equations apply regardless of the number of exponential terms and are appropriate for any "n-compartment mammillary model with linear clearance only from plasma." This is the extent to which they may be termed "model-independent."

The presence of multiple exponential phases in an IV disposition profile allows the partial assignment of a model, as two additional parameters can be calculated:

The volume of the central compartment (V_c),

$$V_c = \frac{D_{iv}}{C_p^o} = \frac{D_{iv}}{\Sigma C_i}$$

(Eq. 2-25)

and distribution clearance,[95]

$$CL_D = D_{iv} \left[\frac{\Sigma (\lambda_i C_i)}{(\Sigma C_i)^2} - \frac{1}{AUC} \right]$$

(Eq. 2-26)

Thus, SHAM analysis allows direct calculation of the two to four primary parameters commonly associated with the mammillary compartmental model: CL and V_{ss} and often V_c and CL_D. Other clearance terms can be added if drug excretion by specific pathways is measured (see Equation 2-2).

The simplest methods of estimating the AUC and AUMC (see Equation 2-24) are by curve-stripping using graphical methods such as residuals (see Figure 2-10) or computer-based techniques which sequentially pare the slowest exponential phases from the overall curve. More efficient procedures involve nonlinear least-squares regression to obtain C_i and λ_i values as will be described further.

Oral Dose Disposition

The addition of drug disposition data (AUC_{po}) following oral doses (D_o) yields apparent oral clearance (CL_{oral}, Equation 2-16), systemic availability (FF*, Equation 2-20) and mean absorption time (MAT, Equation 2-21). Until the contribu-

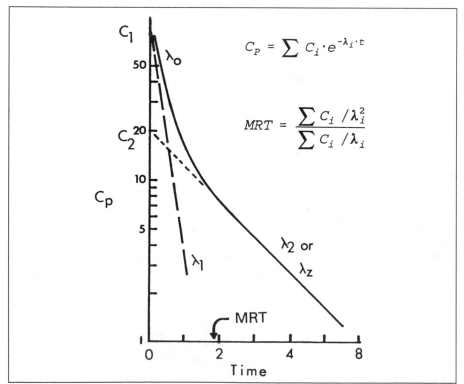

$$C_p = \sum C_i \cdot e^{-\lambda_i \cdot t}$$

$$MRT = \frac{\sum C_i / \lambda_i^2}{\sum C_i / \lambda_i}$$

Figure 2-10. *Log-linear intravenous drug disposition curve showing the biexponential decline in plasma concentrations (C_p) as a function of time (t). The SHAM properties include Slopes (λ_1 and λ_2 or λ_z), Heights (C_1 and C_2), Area ($\Sigma C_i / \lambda_i$), and Moment ($\Sigma C_i / \lambda_i^2$).*

tions of either incomplete absorption (F) or the first-pass effect (F*) can be quantitated, it is preferable to consider the possibility of both factors compromising the overall systemic availability of the drug.

The AUMC and MRT are determined by both the input and dispositional rate processes of the system (Figure 2-9). Additional equations have been derived for noncompartmental determination V_{ss} for any mode of drug administration.[45]

The AUC and AUMC can be generated by numerical integration to facilitate data analysis when the shape of the plasma concentration-time curve is irregular, as often occurs following oral doses (see Figure 2-11):

$$\text{AUC} = \int_0^T C_p \cdot dt + \frac{C_p^*}{\lambda_z}$$

(Eq. 2-27)

and

$$\text{AUMC} = \int_0^T t \cdot C_p \cdot dt + \frac{T \cdot C_p^*}{\lambda_z} + \frac{C_p^*}{\lambda_z^2}$$

(Eq. 2-28)

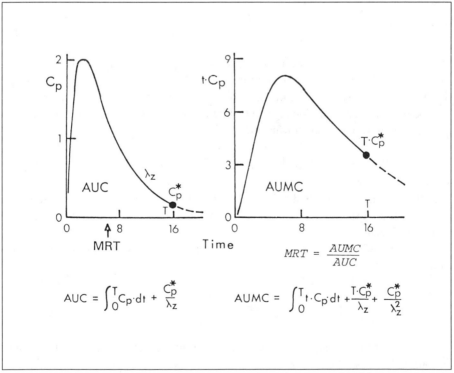

Figure 2-11. *Graphical depiction of the Area (AUC) and Moment (AUMC) properties of a pharmacokinetic disposition (C_p versus t) curve. The last measured plasma concentration C_p^* at t = T is extrapolated to time infinity using the terminal slope (λ_z) of the log-linear disposition curve. The mean residence time (MRT) is indicated on the AUC curve and in relation to the AUMC. Note the larger portion of the AUMC curve requiring extrapolation, compared to that of the AUC curve.*

where λ_2 is the terminal slope of the curve and C_p^* and T are the last measured C_p and time values.[46] The quotient terms provide extrapolations of each function to time infinity. Numerical integration is commonly carried out either by linear or log trapezoidal, LaGrange, or Spline methods to generate both the AUC and AUMC values.[48,49]

Multiple Doses and Infusions

For linear pharmacokinetic systems, the time-average parameters can be extrapolated to steady-state situations. Steady-state plasma concentrations C_{ss} are determined by four factors:[50]

$$C_{ss} = \frac{F \cdot D_o}{CL \cdot \tau}$$ (Eq. 2-29)

where D_o is either the oral or intravenous dose, CL applies as the respective oral or systemic clearance, and τ is the dosing interval. Distribution parameters obviously do not influence steady-state conditions. If $F = 1$, CL can be calculated from:

$$CL = \frac{D_o / \tau}{C_{ss}} = \frac{D_o}{AUC_{ss}}$$ (Eq. 2-30)

where AUC_{ss} is the AUC over one dosing interval at steady state. This equation is identical to Equation 2-1 when the drug is given by IV infusion. It should be noted that the $AUC_{iv} = AUC_{ss}$ if the kinetics of the drug are linear and stationary.

The noncompartmental approach can be employed to generate V_{ss} from multiple-dose data. It has been shown[51] that:

$$AUMC_{IV} \Big|_0^\infty = AUMC_{ss} \Big|_0^\tau + \tau \cdot AUC_{ss} \Big|_\tau^\infty$$ (Eq. 2-31)

which essentially converts the AUMC from multiple- to single-dose conditions, thus allowing use of calculation methods described above to obtain V_{ss} (see Equation 2-23).

Another useful equation allows V_{ss} to be generated during constant-rate infusion of drug:[52]

$$V_{ss} = \frac{k_o \cdot T - CL \cdot AUC_0^T}{C_{ss}}$$ (Eq. 2-32)

where k_o is the infusion rate, T is the duration of infusion, and CL is obtained using Equation 2-1.

Drug Absorption Rate

The MAT provides a time-average measure of absorption rate and is useful when more specific input constants cannot be obtained. A new method of assessing drug absorption rates, called the Area Function method, has been developed.[53] When drug is dosed orally (po) and IV, the absorption rate can be initially calculated from:

$$\text{Absorption Rate} = \frac{C_{po}(t)}{F \cdot AUC_{iv}^{0 \to t}}$$

(Eq. 2-33)

where t represents any time during the absorption phase. After plotting Absorption Rate versus time to identify the nature of the input process, more specific equations can be used to obtain k_o or k_a.

Deconvolution methods form a noncompartmental approach to assessing the type and rate of drug input to the systemic circulation.[54] These methods compare oral and IV pharmacokinetic profiles and use the latter to separate the input from the disposition elements of the oral curve. High clearance drugs cannot be evaluated because the IV disposition curve does not reflect the intrinsic clearance pathway which effects removal of part of an oral dose of drug. Deconvolution is usually sensitive to irregularities in the data which can produce a cascading error effect.

The basic Wagner-Nelson method, while specific for a one-compartment model, has had extensive use in assessing drug absorption.[55] This method has been extended to multiple-dose regimens.[56] The following equation pertains:

$$\frac{A_T}{V} = C_n + k_{el} \int_0^T C_n \cdot dt - C_n^0$$

(Eq. 2-34)

where A_T is the amount of drug absorbed from time zero, V is the volume of distribution, k_{el} is the one-compartment elimination rate constant (CL / V), C_n is the drug concentration over the $O \leq T \leq \tau$ dosing interval, and C_n^0 is C_n at time zero. Thus the usual Wagner-Nelson calculation can be performed with subtraction of the C_n value from the preceding terms in Equation 2-34. Multiple-dosing conditions may require extended sample collection after the last dose to obtain an accurate value of k_{el} or λ_z. The fraction absorbed cannot be calculated if absorption continues from earlier doses, or if steady state has not been achieved. Since the method is graphical and commonly used without full certainty regarding confounding factors such as nonlinearity and obfuscated exponential terms, it is advisable to reapply the absorption rate process to the data by simulation to confirm the validity of the approach.

PHARMACOKINETIC MODELS

Deployment of specific compartmental physiologic models should be with sound biopharmaceutical and physiologic justification. Ideally, the initial phase of developing a study should include assignment of a suitable model to the system, the design of the system and the optimization of the data collection phase, followed by resolution of the experimental question or hypothesis tested. This obviates a subsequent search for an appropriate model in the midst of assessing whether suitable data have been collected.

Several factors can be considered in either prospective or retrospective assignment of a pharmacokinetic model to typical drug disposition data. First, the number of exponential terms in decline of plasma drug concentrations is not a direct indication of a specific model.[57,58] Drug disposition usually occurs with each portion of a curve comprised of mixed absorption, distributive, mixing, volume, clearance, and recycling elements which can vary among subjects and with dose and time.[57-59] The visibility of an exponential phase depends partly on the route and speed of drug administration and the intensity and length of blood sampling. Thus, bolus IV doses are usually preferred in pharmacokinetics, because they improve determination of the distributive phase of disposition. Slopes, intercepts, and shapes of any curves are seldom unique.

If a model is justified, there would be loss of information about the drug disposition system if the pharmacokinetic analysis was limited to the time-average, noncompartmental parameters. The use of a specific model most often occurs for characterizing time- or concentration-dependent processes, for assessing drug input rates, for making multiple-dose analyses and extrapolations, and for directly seeking primary parameters by nonlinear least-squares curve fitting. Most importantly, a specific model may add parameters of physiological or biochemical interest and allow testing of hypotheses regarding mechanisms of drug disposition or effects.

The development and testing of specific models requires an extensive array of physiologic and mathematical considerations which have been addressed in many monographs[60] and textbooks.[44,61,62] Only some general principles are presented here.

The number of parameters (NP) which can be calculated for a given compartmental or physiologic model is dependent on the following:

EX: the number of exponentials visible in the plasma disposition pattern
PE: the number of elimination or excretory pathways suitably measured
TS: the number of tissue spaces or binding proteins analyzed
NL: the number of visible nonlinear features in the data, according to

$$NP = 2EX + PE + 2TS + NL \qquad \text{(Eq. 2-35)}$$

provided that accurate and sufficient data are obtained. The 2EX segment is omitted if **all** tissues and fluid spaces of the body are analyzed in a full physiological assessment.

Examples of the application of Equation 2-35 can be given. The biexponential decline in plasma drug concentrations (EX = 2) after intravenous drug injection together with urinary excretion data (PE = 1) as depicted for ampicillin in Figure 2-12 yields NP = 5. These comprise either the SHAM values (C_1, λ_1, C_2, λ_2, and CL_R) or the parameters of the two-compartment model (CL, V_c, CL_D, V_{ss}, and CL_R).[63] Tissue and plasma analyses as a function of time allow calculation of CL_{di}

and K_{pi} for each specific tissue space. Each nonlinear condition may permit calculation of one additional parameter (both V_{max} and K_m instead of their ratio of V_{max} / K_m or CL_{int}).

In general, the most physiologically meaningful pharmacokinetic parameters are those derived by simultaneous measurement of both the substrate concentration and the velocity, product, or outcome of a clearance, distribution, or pharmacodynamic function. This is most easily accomplished for a process such as renal clearance (substrate = plasma concentration; velocity = excretion rate) and reduces or obviates the "black box" nature of the model.

At least three major classes of models are commonly applied in pharmacokinetic analysis of drug disposition data. Their major features and application rationales will be outlined.

Multiple-Compartment Mammillary Models

The primary model used in analysis of multi-exponential disposition data is the "two-compartment open model with clearance from the central compartment" (see Figure 2-9). This model was popularized by Riegelman et al.[64] who invoked a "tissue cluster" concept in explaining why the body acts as though the blood and highly perfused lean tissues (heart, lung, liver, kidneys, brain) often cluster as a "central compartment" and the more slowly perfused tissues (muscle, skin, fat, bone) behave as the "tissue compartment." The alternative explanation for non-homogeneous distribution pertains to drug access to body fluid and solid spaces, as the plasma-interstitial-fluid interface is highly permeable, whereas, cell and other membranes limit drug access to cell water and body solids in general accordance with the pH-partition hypothesis. Reality is an amalgam of the two ideas which is reflected kinetically in the features of distributional clearance (see Equation 2-1 and Figure 2-4) and V_{ss} relationships (see Equation 2-7).

The two-compartment open model, while it is an oversimplification of physiological compartments, has had extensive use because it is the most tractable to parameter resolution, has functioned effectively in describing the apparent pharmacokinetics of numerous drugs (e.g., gentamicin, Figures 2-1 and 2-2; ampicillin, Figure 2-12), and suffices to allow characterization of drug disposition in the absence of more specific information regarding an appropriate model.

The methods for calculating the primary parameters of the two-compartment model are identical to those already listed for the time and dose-average values: CL (Equation 2-22), V_{ss} (Equation 2-23), V_c (Equation 2-25), and CL_D (Equation 2-26). The parameter V_T can be obtained by difference ($V_{ss} - V_c$, Equation 2-6). The noncompartmental parameters obtained by SHAM analysis are equivalent to those of the multicompartment mammillary model **under the conditions that the system is linear and clearance occurs from the plasma compartment.** The CL and V_{ss} are "model-independent" only in the sense that they apply to this mammillary scheme with any number of peripheral compartments with no eliminating clearances.[47,65,66]

The classic approach to evolving parameters of the two-compartment open model is the generation of V_c and three rate constants (k_{12}, k_{21}, k_{el}).[60] These parameters can, in turn, be converted to volume and clearance terms. However, in construction and characterization of these models, the volume and clearance values are preferable in quantitation of the fundamental properties of drugs, as they are kinetically more stable, easily estimated, and reflective of basic physiologic processes. Rate constants are ambiguous **ratio** terms. Most commonly, for example, for a two-compartment systemic clearance model (see Figure 2-9) they are as follows:

$$k_{el} = \frac{CL}{V_c}$$

(Eq. 2-36)

$$k_{12} = \frac{CL_D}{V_c}$$

(Eq. 2-37)

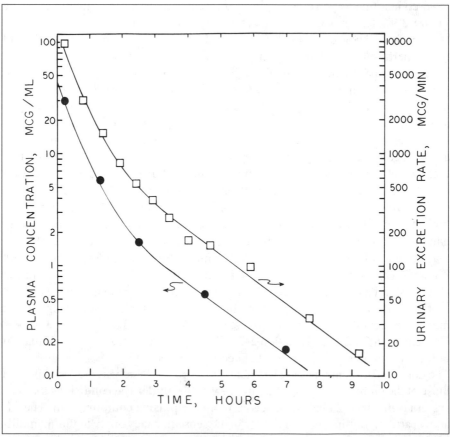

Figure 2-12. *Plasma concentrations (C_p) and urinary excretion rates (dAu / dt) of ampicillin as a function of time after IV injection of 570 mg into a 75 kg male subject. The data were fitted with two functions simultaneously ($C_p = C_1 \times e^{\lambda_1 \tau} + C_2 \times e^{\lambda_2 \tau}$ and $dAu / dt = CL_R \times C_p$), yielding five parameters: $C_1 = 42.0\ \mu g/mL$, $\lambda_1 = 2.28\ hr^{-1}$, $C_2 = 5.5\ \mu g/mL$, $\lambda_2 = 0.517\ hr^{-1}$, and $CL_R = 298\ mL/min$.*

$$k_{21} = \frac{CL_D}{V_T}$$

(Eq. 2-38)

Rate constants, therefore, are dependent variables which do not quantitate individual processes, as they depict the ratio of two primarily independent variables. Similarly, slope values (λ_i) and half-lives $(t\frac{1}{2}_z)$ are complex functions of distribution and clearance and may not adequately reflect the individual elements of a system. Again, for the two-compartment systemic clearance model, the multiple determinants of λ_i slopes can be assessed from: [61]

$$\lambda_1^+, \lambda_2^- = \frac{-b \pm (b^2 - 4c)^{\frac{1}{2}}}{2}$$

(Eq. 2-39)

where

$$-b = \frac{CL}{V_c} + \frac{CL_D}{V_c} + \frac{CL_D}{V_T}$$

(Eq. 2-40)

and

$$c = \frac{CL \cdot CL_D}{V_c \cdot V_T}$$

(Eq. 2-41)

It can be pointed out that the λ_2 or λ_z approaches a limiting value of CL / V_{ss} for low-clearance drugs.

The employment of multicompartment models has also led to introduction of a sampling time- and clearance-dependent volume of distribution parameter, $V_{D\beta}$ or V_{area}. This parameter is calculated from

$$V_{D\beta} = \frac{F \cdot D_o}{AUC \cdot \lambda_z}$$

(Eq. 2-42)

and represents a proportionality factor between plasma concentrations and amount of drug in the body during the terminal or λ_z phase of disposition (A_z). As shown in Table 2-4, it is affected by elimination, and it changes as clearance is altered.[67] A slower clearance allows more time for drug equilibration between plasma and tissues and creates a smaller $V_{D\beta}$. It can be noted that the lower limit of $V_{D\beta}$ is:

$$\lim_{CL \to 0} V_{D\beta} = V_{ss}$$

(Eq. 2-43)

and thus $V_{D\beta}$ has value in representing V_{ss} for low-clearance drugs as well as estimating A_z. Smaller $V_{D\beta}$ values than normal are often observed in patients with renal failure, because of the reduced CL and CL_R. This is a consequence of the CL-dependent time of equilibration between plasma and tissue. Thus, V_{ss} is preferred in separating the effects of changes in elimination from those of distribution.

Organ Clearance Models

A second general class of models requires use of a specific clearing organ (see Figure 2-3) as opposed to considering elimination directly from the plasma compartment (see Figure 2-9). This configuration is more physiologic and applies to most high-clearance drugs for which generalized enzymatic or chemical hydrolysis does not occur. The model in Figure 2-3 is the simplest of this class of models, as either multiple clearing organs (e.g., kidney, liver, lung) or multiple peripheral compartments would add increased complexity.

The application of organ clearance models requires dual IV and direct (oral) administration routes and subsequently allows for quantitation of first-pass effects. It creates the differential concepts of systemic clearance (see Equation 2-14) when an IV dose is administered versus intrinsic clearance (see Equation 2-17) when the dose directly enters the clearing organ. These models reduce to the mammillary plasma clearance model for low-clearance drugs, as $CL \rightarrow CL_{int}$ and no route-dependent changes in elimination occur. Parameters such as V_{ss} calculated using noncompartmental methods do not strictly apply to organ clearance models, but may approximate the "true" values.[68] For example, IV and oral doses (with extremely rapid absorption) in the model in Figure 2-3 yield the following residence times when measuring the AUMC:AUC ratio of plasma concentration-time curves:

$$MRT_{iv} = \frac{V_c + V_T}{CL} + \frac{F^* \cdot V_L}{CL_{int}}$$

(Eq. 2-44)

and

$$MRT_{po} = \frac{V_c + V_T}{CL} + \frac{V_L}{CL_{int}}$$

(Eq. 2-45)

Thus, systems with either small values of V_L / CL_{int} or low values of CL_{int} allow $MRT_{iv} \rightarrow V_{ss} / CL$ and can be used to estimate V_{ss} by the usual noncompartmental approach (Equation 2-24). For intermediate situations, the system requires a complex analysis using equations analogous to a three-compartment model with elimination from a peripheral compartment in order to obtain the major kinetic parameters other than elimination clearances.[69]

Table 2-4. *Effect of Changing Systemic Clearance on Values of $V_{D\beta}$ and V_{ss}* [67,a]

CL (L/hr)	$V_{D\beta}$ (L)	V_{ss} (L)	$\lambda_{z_{-1}}$ (hr)
0.12	20.0	20.0	0.006
1.2	20.3	20.0	0.059
12.0	24.0	20.0	0.500
120.0	89.2	20.0	1.345

[a] Parameters maintained constant: $V_c = 12$ L; $V_T = 8$ L; $CL_D = 12$ L/hr

---

A Special Note

Perhaps the most common source of confusion in the introductory facets of pharmacokinetics is the recognition of variables or parameters which are largely "independent" and have a primary physiological basis versus those which are "dependent" and represent a combination of factors. Summary parameters such as CL (or more specifically CLu_{int} and CL_R) and V_{ss} are close to being independent and physiologically based, as CL directly reflects elimination mechanisms and V_{ss} directly indicates equilibrium distribution mechanisms. Perturbation of either mechanism typically produces a direct alteration in the value of the indicative parameter without affecting the other. When properly calculated, CL and V_{ss} can be considered separate and noninteracting parameters. The other extreme pertains to dependent variables such as $t\frac{1}{2}$. For monoexponential data, it is well recognized that $t\frac{1}{2} = 0.693 \times V_{ss} / CL$, an equation structure that portrays the appropriate relationship between the variables and shows that $t\frac{1}{2}$ will increase as either V_{ss} is enlarged or CL is reduced. A frequently misinterpreted relationship is $CL = k_{el}V_{ss}$, an equation that simply allows CL to be calculated from k_{el} (or $0.693 / t\frac{1}{2}$) and V_{ss}, but one which should not be viewed as indicative of the determinants of CL. Analogously, we can write $CL = D_0 / AUC$, which is a method of calculation, not a definition or a function for CL. Just as $t\frac{1}{2}$ is comprised of a mix of more fundamental distributive and elimination parameters, the same can be said of factors such as most rate constants, all slope and most intercept values of plasma concentration-time curves, and the $V_{D\beta}$ value. Hayton[96] has provided an instructive pictorial method of denoting such relationships between variables. A continued goal in the summarization of data and in the development of specific pharmacokinetic models should be the extraction of parameters which have a fundamental biochemical and physiologic basis, and for which individual mechanisms can be discerned without contamination either by other mechanisms or by artifacts and nonlinearities in the system.

Reversible Models

A third general category of common models is necessary to account for phenomena such as reversible metabolism and enterohepatic cycling. The role of reversible metabolism in drug disposition is gaining increased appreciation, as compounds such as sulindac, spironolactone, dapsone, some sulfonamides, vitamin K, various corticosteroids, and some sex steroids have metabolites which can revert in part to the parent drug.[70] In addition, the acyl glucuronide metabolites of some drugs are labile and can reform the original compound. The process may be overlooked unless metabolite is administered directly or its stability is assessed in various body fluids.

The basic model for reversible metabolism is depicted in Figure 2-13. Resolution of the clearance parameters for elimination of drug (CL_{10}) and metabolite (CL_{20}) and the interconversion clearances (CL_{12}, CL_{21}) requires direct administration of a dose of drug (D_0) into its volume (V_1) and a dose of metabolite (M_0) into its volume (V_2). Equations for calculation of the clearances are as follows:[70]

$$CL_{10} = \frac{AUC_2^M \cdot D_0 - AUC_2^D \cdot M_0}{AUC_1^D \cdot AUC_2^M - AUC_2^D \cdot AUC_1^M} \qquad \text{(Eq. 2-46)}$$

$$CL_{20} = \frac{AUC_1^D \cdot M_0 - AUC_1^M \cdot D_0}{AUC_1^D \cdot AUC_2^M - AUC_2^D \cdot AUC_1^M} \qquad \text{(Eq. 2-47)}$$

$$CL_{12} = \frac{M_0 \cdot AUC_2^D}{AUC_1^D \cdot AUC_2^M - AUC_2^D \cdot AUC_1^M} \qquad \text{(Eq. 2-48)}$$

$$CL_{21} = \frac{D_0 \cdot AUC_1^M}{AUC_1^D \cdot AUC_2^M - AUC_2^D \cdot AUC_1^M} \qquad \text{(Eq. 2-49)}$$

where D_0 and M_0 are the administered doses of drug and metabolite, and AUC_i^x refers to the AUC of the superscripted species in the subscripted compartments.

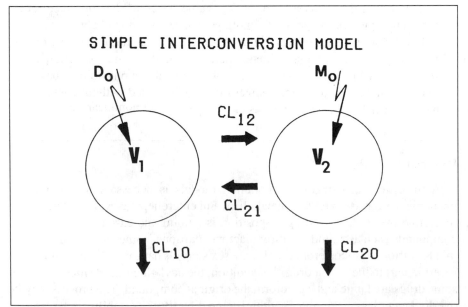

Figure 2-13. *Model for drug disposition where drug-metabolite interconversion (CL_{12}, CL_{21}) occurs. Elimination by all other pathways is depicted for drug (CL_{10}) and metabolite (CL_{20}). Volumes of distribution of drug (V_1) and metabolite (V_2) are also shown.*

An example of experimental data is shown for methylprednisolone-methyl-prednisone interconversion in Figure 2-14.[70] One special characteristic of the model and these data are the multi-exponential disposition curves of both compounds, which, if observed individually, would appear consistent with a conventional multicompartment model. All of the curves attain a pseudo-equilibrium where the terminal slopes decline in parallel. This is expected for a linear, reversible system. The same model could be applied to enterohepatic cycling, although such processes often produce irregularly shaped curves.

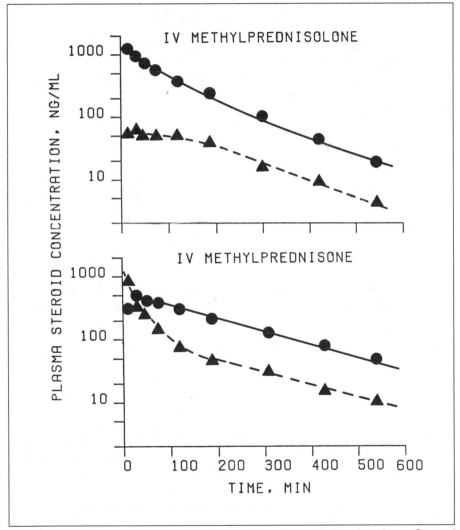

Figure 2-14. *Plasma concentration-time profiles for methylprednisolone (●) and methylprednisone (▲) after intravenous administration of each compound to a rabbit. Each compound is formed from the other. Application of the model shown in Figure 2-13 (Equations 2-46 to 2-49) to data from ten rabbits yields clearance values of $CL_{10} = 6.26$, $CL_{12} = 4.98$, $CL_{20} = 14.5$, and $CL_{21} = 28.9$ mL/min/kg.[71]*

If no peripheral compartments exist, V_1 and V_2 can be calculated from D_0 / C_p^o and M_0 / C_M^o. Moment analysis allows calculations of V_{ss} values[70] and equations that provide all residence, interconversion, and distributional parameters of the reversible model are available.[71]

Evolving in pharmacokinetics is the application of area moment analysis to more complex models.[68,71] Just as an AUC value can be applied to calculation of various types of clearance values (e.g., Equations 2-44 through 2-47), the AUMC can be of analogous value in generating volume terms for specific distributional models.

DRUG METABOLITES

Measurement of drug metabolite concentrations in plasma, or of excretion rates with time, adds additional power and complexity in characterizing disposition of the primary drug. It aids in discerning the properties of the drug if the fraction of the dose which is metabolized (f_m) can be quantitated. The metabolic clearance, in turn, can be obtained in a manner analogous to that for renal clearance because of the additivity feature of clearance terms:

$$CL_m = f_m \cdot CL \qquad \text{(Eq. 2-50)}$$

The AUC of metabolite relates to the dose of drug according to commonly expected dose-clearance principles:

$$AUC_{(m)} = \frac{f_m \cdot D_0}{CL_{(m)}} \qquad \text{(Eq. 2-51)}$$

where $CL_{(m)}$ represents the dispositional clearance of the metabolite. Of additional value is the relationship of $AUC_{(m)}$ to the AUC of the parent drug:

$$\text{Area ratio} = \frac{AUC_{(m)}}{AUC} = \frac{CL_m}{CL_{(m)}} \qquad \text{(Eq. 2-52)}$$

as this ratio (as does $C_{(m)} / C_{ss}$) depicts the $\dfrac{\text{formation}}{\text{disposition}}$ rates of the metabolite.

These are the major dose-AUC features of drug metabolite kinetics. Houston[72] has elaborated other characteristics of drug metabolite properties which are relevant for both the plasma and organ clearance models of drug disposition. The pattern of formation of drug metabolites can be of value in discerning whether formation or disposition kinetics and whether first-pass concepts apply.

A noncompartmental method[97] of calculating the elimination constant of a metabolite (k_{met}) is:

$$k_{met} = \frac{C_m \cdot t}{\left(\dfrac{AUC_{(m)}}{AUC}\right) AUC^{0 \to t} - AUC_{(m)}^{0 \to t}} \qquad \text{(Eq. 2-53)}$$

NONLINEAR PHARMACOKINETICS

Moment analysis yields pharmacokinetic parameters which are dose- and time-average values. They may adequately represent the average properties of the drug, but will have limited application to nonlinear drug disposition at other doses, as a function of time, as a function of plasma or blood concentrations, and in multiple-dosing situations. A similar effect may result from use of a specific model or equation in which linear functions fit the data but are used inappropriately. Kinetic analysis allowing parameters to vary as a function of time or plasma concentrations may sometimes be feasible to evaluate whether nonlinearity exists. For example, serial renal clearances can be assessed to determine whether saturable tubular secretion or reabsorption of drug occurs. Common sources of nonlinearity are listed in Table 2-5.

The Michaelis-Menten function,[73]

$$\text{Velocity} = \frac{V_{max} \cdot C_p}{K_m + C_p} \quad \text{or} \quad \frac{T_{max} \cdot C_p}{T_m + C_p} \qquad \text{(Eq. 2-54)}$$

Table 2-5. *Mechanisms of Nonlinear Drug Disposition*[74–76]

Process and mechanism	Examples
Gastrointestinal absorption	
Saturable transport	Riboflavin, penicillins
Intestinal metabolism	Salicylamide
Biotransformation	
Saturable metabolism	Phenytoin, salicylate
Product inhibition	Phenytoin (rats)
Co-substrate depletion	Acetaminophen
Plasma protein binding	Prednisolone, disopyramide
Renal excretion	
Glomerular filtration/	
protein binding	Naproxen
Tubular secretion	Para-aminohippuric acid, mezlocillin
Tublar reabsorption	Riboflavin, cephapirin
Biliary excretion	
Biliary secretion	Iodipamide, BSP
Enterohepatic cycling	Cimetidine, isotretinoin
Tissue distribution	
Plasma protein binding	Prednisolone, ceftriaxone
Hepatic uptake	Indocyanine green
CSF transport	Benzylpenicillins
Cellular uptake	Methicillin (rabbit)
Tissue binding	Methylene blue

is highly useful for processes in which limited enzyme capacity exists. This function is usually evident in data as a nonlinear relationship between the dependent variable and the substrate concentration similar to the shape of the curves in Figure 2-8. Linearity is expected at very low substrate concentrations ($K_m > C_p$).

The presence of nonlinear kinetics in some aspect of drug disposition may be determined in several ways. The primary methods are to assess velocity versus substrate concentration directly or to determine pharmacokinetic parameters over several dosage levels. The Michaelis-Menten decline in phenytoin or salicylate plasma concentrations readily reveals its characteristic nonlinearity at sufficiently high doses, but lower doses and the presence of mixed absorptive, distributive, and elimination exponentials may obfuscate the occurrence of nonlinearity. Theophylline[77] and mezlocillin[78] provide examples in which the use of plasma concentration-time data at a single dosage level do not allow mixed nonlinear functions to be discerned.

Techniques for discerning nonlinearity include the following:

A. Lack of superposition (dividing all C_p values by dose) indicates occurrence of some type of dose-dependence, but further evaluation of the parameters is needed to determine the cause of nonlinearity.

B. An AUC disproportionate to dose indicates that either FF* (oral doses) or clearance (systemic or oral) is nonlinear.

C. An AUMC or MRT change with dose indicates that absorption rate, V_{ss}, or clearance (CL or CL_{oral}) is nonlinear. Caution, however, is needed in the application of moment analysis when clearance is nonlinear.[98]

D. Direct calculation of CL, CL_{oral}, V_c, V_{ss}, CL_D, FF*, and MAT (if feasible) at several dose levels is needed to evaluate whether nonlinearity exists in any of these parameters. Significant and consistent changes must occur in relation to dose, and thus three dose levels are helpful. For a Michaelis-Menten process, these doses should produce maximum C_p values which are both below and above the K_m value.

E. Nonlinearity may or may not alter $t\frac{1}{2}$, λ_z, the fractional excretory composition of drug metabolites, or the amount excreted unchanged in urine. However, changes in one or more of these parameters often indicate the presence of nonlinearity.

F. The dosage input rate will alter the AUC and other parameters derived from the AUC of a nonlinear drug. The calculation of FF* = AUC_{PO} / AUC_{iv} is distorted for drugs with nonlinear clearance.[79]

The accurate characterization of the pharmacokinetics of a drug in the presence of a nonlinear absorption or disposition process requires the utilization of a specific model with one or more nonlinear mechanisms assigned at suitable sites. Gengo et al.[76] provide an instructive approach to blending noncompartmental and specific nonlinear modeling methods to characterize the saturable tissue distribution of methicillin in the rabbit.

CURVE FITTING

Both a noncompartmental analysis and data characterization with a specific pharmacokinetic model share the basic need of adequate curve-fitting of experimental data to appropriate equations. The slopes and intercepts which underlie the SHAM approach and the specific parameters which can be generated when using a formulated model will depend on assay factors, the number and placement of experimental points, the completeness of data collection, the nonlinearity of the function, initial estimates, data transformation, the computer algorithms, and other aspects already described here and elsewhere.[80]

Several curve-fitting programs are in frequent use; NONLIN is the most common.[81] These are typically iterative procedures based on approximation of nonlinear mathematic functions with partial linear Taylor series estimates. Each program must be used extensively with diverse equations and types of data for the user to gain familiarity with the reliability and range of applications. However, some general guidelines can be recommended for appropriate use of nonlinear least-squares regression computer programs:

A. Multiple functions (plasma concentrations, urinary excretion rates) for each dosage level and sampled compartment should be employed simultaneously when possible to allow all measured data to influence the analysis and to generate a minimal number of parameters common to all disposition data for the drug (see Figure 2-12). This necessitates the use of weighting or data normalization to prevent the functions with larger numerical values from dominating the least-squares fitting process.

B. When data are fitted to a specific model, equations should be provided to allow iterative fitting of the primary pharmacokinetic parameters (e.g., V_c, V_{ss}, CL_D, and CL for the two-compartment model). This eliminates the necessity for further computations, allows the structure of the model to directly influence the curve-fitting process, and generates confidence intervals or other variance estimates for the primary parameters.

C. Weighting functions are usually necessary to offset the non-Gaussian distribution of error in pharmacokinetic data and thereby prevent large numbers from overwhelming the least-squares criteria.[82] For example, the data in Figure 2-12 show a 400-fold range of plasma concentrations, and the weighting function used was essentially $1/Y_i$. However, the method of extended least-squares nonlinear regression appears to accommodate the need for weighting by allowing the incorporation of a general parametric variance model.[83]

D. Reasonable initial parameter estimates should be obtained using SHAM analysis, curve stripping, or preliminary evaluation of the data. The initial estimates may bias the fitting, and this bias requires consideration.[80] Many computer programs permit assignment of minimum and maximum parameter values. Physiological constraints such as plasma volume for V_c and cardiac output or organ blood flow for distribution clearance or systemic clearance may be helpful in limiting the parameter range in complex models.

E. The absence of systematic deviations between the measured data and fitted curves is one of the most important criteria for a suitable least-squares fit.[84] This criterion pertains to all functions; such deviations in one or more functions may be indicative of nonlinearity, an inappropriate predictor equation, or an improper least-squares fitting. Inspection of graphs of all measured and fitted pharmacokinetic data is most useful (see Figure 2-12) in this regard.

F. Coefficients of determination (r^2) or correlation (r) are usually very high, even for unsuitable curve fittings. That they are high is not, alone, a good criterion.

G. Small, reasonable, or explainable (lack of pertinent data) standard deviations should be expected for the individual fitting parameters. These alone are very poor guides to the adequacy of fit.

H. The iterative procedure should attain satisfactory convergence rather than reaching a specified upper limit in number of iterations.

Both the **initial** and the **final** step in consideration of the appropriateness of data fitting is whether the model is suitable. One must consider the nature of the drug and biological system as well as pharmacokinetic and statistical factors. A starting point is to observe **parsimony** (i.e., to employ the simplest model which explains the major features of the system). A final step is to consider procedures such as an F-test for nested models, or the Akaike and Schwarz criteria, which aid in picking the model with the fewest number of parameters that best fit the data.[58]

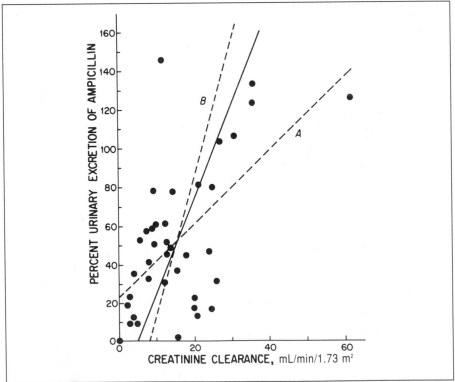

Figure 2-15. *Relationship between percent urinary excretion of ampicillin (Y) and normalized creatinine clearance (X) in a group of infants. Data are from Kaplan et al.*[88] *Lines A and B show the results of regressing variable Y on X and X on Y, respectively, while the solid line shows the results of the perpendicular least-squares regression method.*[89] *The last method comes nearest to depicting the true relationship, which, physiologically, should have a zero intercept and the same mean as the other lines.*

PARAMETER NORMALIZATION

Pharmacokinetic parameters related to volume or clearance should be normalized to standard body size. Most physiologic flow and clearance functions can be correlated among species in parallel with body surface area, and the most logical expression of clearance appears[2,85] to be L/hr/1.73 m^2. Adolph's data[86] suggest that organ sizes and body space sizes are closely proportional to total body weight. Thus, volumes expressed as L/kg seem appropriate and thereby directly yield the distribution coefficient K_D (see Equation 2-10 and Table 2-2). The question of whether to normalize pharmacokinetic parameters according to surface area or body weight is difficult to resolve in humans alone. Humans show greatest changes or differences in body size in neonatal and infant ages; at this time developmental effects complicate this type of correlation. Normalization is most important for averaging data from individuals of markedly different sizes.

STATISTICAL CONSIDERATIONS

The design, analysis, and interpretation of pharmacokinetic data require many logical uses of statistics to assure a lack of bias in the arrangement of studies, to use curve fitting, and to employ standard tests to assess possible significant differences between treatments. Several important points are special to consideration of pharmacokinetic data.

Before an experiment, the number of subjects or animals needed to discern an effect or lack thereof can be estimated using an appropriate statistical method of "determination of the power of the test."[87] For a bioavailability study, this method usually predicts the need for far more subjects than most investigators are willing to include. Pharmacokinetic studies of this nature involve intensive human and analytical work, and multiple blood sampling points form the basis of each AUC value. Based on extensive experience and ethical concerns, use of 10 to 18 subjects has become common for many types of crossover drug disposition studies.

Multiple dose levels and routes of drug administration in groups of subjects or animals often entail use of a balanced crossover design to randomize or equalize drug or sequence effects on the subjects.[87] A well-planned study facilitates the later statistical analysis considerably.

Averaging data often distorts pharmacokinetic parameters. The arithmetic mean can be used when averaging normally distributed data. This has the advantage of yielding interpretable standard deviations and facilitating subsequent statistical tests. Unfortunately, pharmacokinetic data often follow a log-normal distribution for which either the geometric mean or the median may yield the best measure of the central tendency of the data. These values are awkward or impossible to employ in statistical tests and necessitate nonparametric methods of data analysis.

Correlation and least-squares regression analyses are often performed to assess interrelationships between pharmacokinetic parameters. A frequent problem arises when both variables contain experimental error—for example, when assessing drug excretion or clearance versus creatinine clearance (see Figure 2-15). This does not affect a correlation analysis, but the ordinary least-squares regression entails the requirement that one variable (the abscissa value) contain no error. Appropriate techniques exist for "fitting straight lines when both variables are subject to error." Riggs et al.[89] indicate that no one method is universally appropriate; however, the writer prefers the "weighted perpendicular method" as a first-choice procedure for many types of pharmacokinetic data in which the error is reasonably proportional to the variance of parameters in each dimension.

ETHICAL FACTORS

Part of any study design includes a clear and reasonably detailed protocol to standardize all elements of the investigation and to make certain that all collabo-

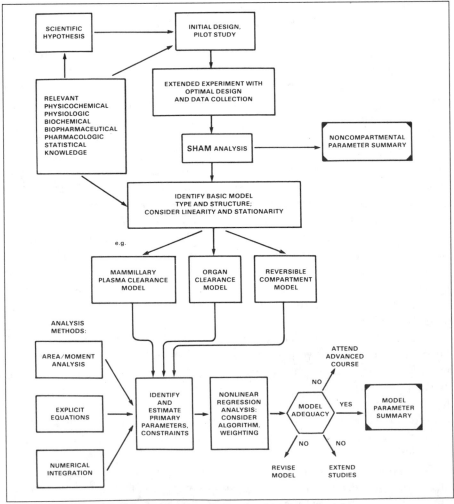

Figure 2-16. *Flow chart for application of pharmacokinetic methodology.*

rators and assistants follow proper directions. These protocols usually serve a dual purpose in grant applications and for submission to Committees on Human Research.

Guidelines exist for use of animals[90] and human subjects[91] in pharmacological experimentation. Common sense must also prevail. Well-planned experiments and expert use of pharmacokinetic methods can aid considerably in minimizing the degree of risk to which patients or volunteers are exposed. Further evolution of principles of physiological pharmacokinetics and "animal scale-up" methods will add greater meaningfulness to data from *in vitro* and animal studies and may eventually lead to the need for only confirmatory experiments in man.

PROSPECTUS

A distillation of the basic philosophy and implementation of applied pharmacokinetics as outlined in this chapter is presented in Figure 2-16. Major features of this pharmacokinetic profile and review include the initial reliance on a broad array of basic information especially regarding the properties of the drug and physiologic system and careful preparation including awareness of potential artifacts, formulation of an experimental hypothesis, collection of pilot data, and optimal design of an extensive study. Expertise in pharmacokinetics is particularly needed in recognizing and evolving an appropriate and parsimonious model and in utilizing mathematical and computer methods for construction and testing of the model. Noncompartmental methods are advantageous in their ease and consistency of application and can either suffice in summarizing major features of the system or serve as parameter estimates in evolution of a more comprehensive and structurally accurate model of the system. Major trends in pharmacokinetics in the 1980s were the development of noncompartmental methods and in the utilization of parameters and models which pertain to physiological reality. We have gained increased clarity regarding the limitations of moment analysis[53,98] and better recognition of when specific models are most relevant in pharmacokinetics. Areas of growth in the field in the 1990s will include applications of systems analysis,[92] use of noninvasive techniques such as PET scanning,[93] evolution of dispositional concepts for peptides and proteins, and the development of pharmacodynamic models which bear greater relevance to real biochemical, physiological, and pharmacologic events.

ACKNOWLEDGMENTS

The skilled secretarial assistance of Ms. Nancy L. Clark is appreciated. Supported in part by Grant 24211 from the National Institutes of General Medical Sciences, NIH. Special thanks are due for the feedback from the pharmaceutics graduate students in my Advanced Pharmacokinetics course, PHC 608, for whom this material was developed.

REFERENCES

1. Gerlowski LE, Jain RK. Physiologically based pharmacokinetic modeling: Principles and applications. J Pharm Sci. 1983;72:1103–1127.
2. Boxenbaum H. Interspecies scaling, allometry, physiologic time, and the ground plan of pharmacokinetics. J Pharmacokinet Biopharm. 1982;10:201–227.
3. Rane A, Wilkinson GR, Shand DG. Prediction of hepatic extraction rate from *in vitro* measurement of intrinsic clearance. J Pharmacol Exp Ther. 1977;200:420–424.
4. Manninen V, Koriionen A. Inequal digoxin tablets. Lancet. 1973;2:1268.
5. MacKichan J, Duffner PK, Cohen ME. Adsorption of diazepam to plastic tubing. N Eng J Med. 1979;301:332–333.
6. Butler LD, Munson JM, DeLuca PP. Effect of inline filtration on the potency of low-dose drugs, Am J Hosp Pharm. 1980;37:935–941.
7. Giacomini KM, Swezey SE, Giacomini JC et al. Administration of heparin causes *in vitro* release of non-esterified fatty acids in human plasma. Life Sciences. 1980;27:771–780.
8. Cotham RH, Shand D. Spuriously low plasma propranolol concentrations resulting from blood collection methods. Clin Pharmacol Ther. 1975;18:535–538.
9. Tamura A, Sugimoto K, Sato T, Fujii T. The effects of hematocrit, plasma protien concentration and temperature of drug-containing blood *in vitro* on the concentrations of the drug in the plasma. J Pharm Pharmacol. 1990;42:577–580.
10. McNair P, Nielsen SL, Christiansen C et al. Gross errors made by routine blood sampling from two sites using a tourniquet applied at different positions. Clin Chim Acta. 1979;98:113–118.
11. Chiou WL, Lam G, Chen M-L et al. Arterial-venous plasma concentration differences of six drugs in the dog and rabbit after intravenous administration. Res Commun Chem Pathol Pharmacol. 1981;32:27–39.
12. Food and Drug Administration. Bioequivalence requirements and *in vivo* bioavailability procedures. Federal Register. 1977;42:1623–1653.
13. Sutfin TA, Jusko WJ. Compendium of Active Drug Metabolities. In: Rawling MD, Wilkinson GR, eds. Clinical Pharmacology and Therapeutics: Drug Metabolism and Disposition. Kent:Butterworth and Co.;1985;2:91–159.
14. Levy RH, Dumain M. Time-dependent kinetics VI: Direct relationship between equations for drug levels during induction and those involving constant clearance. J Pharm Sci. 1979;68:934–936.
15. Schentag JJ, Jusko WJ, Plaut ME et al. Tissue persistence of gentamicin in man. JAMA. 1977;238:327–329.
16. Schentag JJ, Jusko WJ, Vance JW et al. Gentamicin disposition and tissue accumulation on multiple dosing. J Pharmacokinet Biopharm. 1977;5:559–577.
17. Kraus JW, Desmond PV, Marshall JP et al. Effects of aging and liver disease on disposition of lorazepam. Clin Pharmacol Ther. 1978;24:411–419.
18. Jusko WJ, Gretch M. Plasma and tissue protein binding of drugs in pharmacokinetics. Drug Metab Rev. 1976;5:43–140.
19. Jusko WJ. Role of tobacco smoking in pharmacokinetics. J Pharmacokinet Biopharm. 1980;6:7–39.
20. Balant LP, Roseboom H, Gundert-Remy UM. Pharmacokinetic criteria for drug research and development. Advances Drug Res. 1990;19:1–138.
21. American Chemical Society. Guidelines for data acquisition and data quality evaluation in environmental chemistry. Anal Chem. 1980;52:2242–2249.
22. Savello DR, Shangraw RF. Stability of sodium ampicillin solutions in the frozen and liquid states. Am J Hosp Pharm. 1971;28:754–759.
23. Bergstom RF, Kay DR, Wagner JG. The *in vitro* loss of penicillamine in plasma, albumin solutions, and whole blood: Implications for pharmacokinetic studies of penicillamine. Life Sci. 1980;27:189–198.
24. Wagner JG. A safe method for rapidly achieving plasma concentration plateaus. Clin Pharmacol Ther. 1974;16:691–700.
25. DiStefano JJ. Optimized blood sampling protocols and sequential design of kinetic experiments. Am J Physiol. 1981;240:R259–265.

26. Yamaoka K, Nakagawa T, Uno T. Statistical moments in pharmacokinetics. J Pharmacokinet Biopharm. 1978;6:547–558.

27. Martin BK. Drug urinary exeretion data—some aspects concerning the interpretation. Br J Pharmacol Chemother. 1967;29;181–193.

28. Rowland M, Benet LZ, Graham G. Clearance concepts in pharmacokinetics. J Pharmacokinet Biopharm. 1973;1:123–136.

29. Wilkinson GR, Shand DG. A physiologic approach to hepatic drug clearance. Clin Pharmacol Ther. 1975;18:377–390.

30. Gillette JR. Factors affecting drug metabolism. Ann NY Acad Sci. 1971;1979:43–66.

31. Chen H-SG, Gross JF. Estimation of tissue-to-plasma partition coefficients used in physiological pharmacokinetic models. J Pharmacokinet Biopharm. 1979;7:117–125.

32. Renkin EM. Effects of blood flow on diffusion kinetics in isolated, perfused hindlegs of cats: A double circulation hypothesis. Am J Physiol. 1955;183:125–136.

33. Stec GP, Atkinson AJ. Analysis of the contributions of permeability and flow to intercompartmental clearance. J Pharmacokinet Biopharm. 1981;9:167–180.

34. Bass L. Current models of hepatic elimination. Gasteroenterology. 1979;76:1504–1505.

35. Levy G, Yacobi A. Effect of plasma protein binding on elimination of warfarin. J Pharm Sci. 1974;63:805–806.

36. Roberts MS and Rowland M. Hepatic elimination—dispersion model. J Pharm Sci. 1985;74:585–587.

37. Shand DG, Cotham RH, Wilkinson GR. Perfusion-limited effects of plasma drug binding on hepatic drug extraction. Life Sci. 1976;19:125–130.

38. Jansen JA. Influence of plasma protein binding kinetics on hepatic clearance assessed from a "Tube" model and a "Well-Stirred" model. J Pharmacokinet Biopharm. 1981;9:15–26.

39. Perl W. Red cell permeability effect on the mean transit time of an indicator transported through an organ by red cells and plasma. Circ Res. 1975;36:352–357.

40. Levy G. Effect of plasma protein binding on renal clearance of drugs. J Pharm Sci. 1980;69:483.

41. Tucker GT. Measurement of the renal clearance of drugs. Br J Clin Pharmacol. 1981;12:761–770.

42. Perrier D, Gibaldi M. Calculation of absorption rate constants for drugs with incomplete availability. J Pharm Sci. 1973;62:225.

43. Caprani 0, Sveinsdottir E, Lassen N. SHAM, A method for biexponential curve resolution using initial slope, height, area, and moment of the experimental decay type curve. J Theor Biol. 1975;52:299–315.

44. Lassen NA, Perl W. Tracer Kinetic Methods in Medical Physiology. New York, NY:Raven Press;1979.

45. Perrier D. Mayersohn M. Noncompartmental determination of the steady-state volume of distribution for any mode of administration. J Pharm Sci. 1982;71:372–373.

46. Oppenheimer JH, Schwartz HL, Surks MI. Determination of common parameters of iodothyronine metabolism and distribution in man by noncompartmental analysis. J Clin Endocrinol Metab. 1975;41:319–324,1172–1173.

47. Benet LZ, Galeazzi RL. Noncompartmental determination of the steady-state volume of distribution. J Pharm Sci. 1979;68:1071–1074.

48. Yeh KC, Kwan KC. A comparison of numerical integrating algorithms by trapezoidal, LaGrange, and Spline approximation. J Pharmacokinet Biopharm. 1978;6:79–98.

49. Rocci ML, Jusko WJ. LAGRAN program for area and moments in pharmacokinetic analysis. Comput Programs Biomed. 1983;16:203–216.

50. Wagner JG, Northam JI, Alway CD et al. Blood levels of drug at the equilibrium state after multiple dosing. Nature. 1965;207:1301–1302.

51. Smith IL, Schentag JJ. Noncompartmental determination of the steady-state volume of distribution during multiple dosing. J Pharm Sci. 1984;73:281–282.

52. Kowarski CR, Kowarski AA. Simplified method for estimating volume of distribution at steady state. J Pharm Sci. 1980;69:1222–1223.

53. Cheng H, Jusko WJ. The area function method for assessing the drug absorption rate in linear systems with zero-order input. Pharmaceut Res. 1989;6:133–139.

54. Simon W. Mathematical Techniques for Biology and Medicine. Cambridge, MA:The MIT Press;1977.

55. Wagner JG, Nelson E. Percent absorbed time plots derived from blood level and or urinary excretion data. J Pharm Sci. 1963;52:610–611.

56. Wagner JG. Modified Wagner-Nelson absorption equations for multiple-dose regimens. J Pharm Sci. 1983;72:578–579.

57. Wagner JG. Linear pharmacokinetic models and vanishing exponential terms: Implications in pharmacokinetics. J Pharmacokinet Biopharm. 1976;4:395–425.

58. Landaw EM, DiStefano JJ III. Multiexponential, multicompartmental, and noncompartmental modeling. II. Data analysis and statistical considerations. Am J Physiol. 1984;246:R651–465.

59. Chiou W. Potential pitfalls in the conventional pharmacokinetic studies: Effects of the initial mixing of drug in blood and the pulmonary first-pass elimination. J Pharmacokinet Biopharm. 1979;7:527–536.

60. Benet LZ. General treatment of linear mammillary models with elimination from any compartment as used in pharmacokinetics. J Pharm Sci. 1972;61:536–541.

61. Gibaldi M, Perrier D. Pharmacokinetics. 2nd ed. New York,NY:Marcel Dekker;1982.

62. Wagner G. Fundamentals of Clinical Pharmacokinetics. Hamilton,IL:Drug Intelligence Publications;1975.

63. Jusko WJ, Lewis GP. Comparison of ampicillin and hetacillin pharmacokinetics in man. J Pharm Sci. 1973;62:69–76.

64. Riegelman S, Loo JCK, Rowland M. Shortcomings in pharmacokinetic analysis by conceiving the body to exhibit properties of a single compartment. J Pharm Sci. 1968;57:117–123.

65. Wagner JG. Linear pharmacokinetic equations allowing direct calculation of many needed pharmacokinetic parameters from the coefficients and exponents of polyexponential equations which have been fitted to the data. J Pharmacokinet Biopharm. 1976;4:443–467.

66. DiStefano JJ III. Noncompartmental vs. compartmental analysis: Some bases for choice. Am J Physiol. 1982;243:R1–6.

67. Jusko WJ, Gibaldi M. Effects of change in elimination on various parameters of the two-compartment open model. J Pharm Sci. 1972;61:1270–1273.

68. Sutfin TA, Ph.D. Thesis. State University of New York at Buffalo. 1984.

69. Nagashima R, Levy G, O'Reilly RA. Comparative pharmacokinetics of coumarin anticoagulants IV. Application of a three-compartment model to the analysis of the dose-dependent kinetics of bis hydroxycoumarin elimination. J Pharm Sci. 1968;57:1888–1895.

70. Ebling WF, Szefler SJ, Jusko WJ. Methylprednisolone disposition in rabbits. Analysis, prodrug conversion, reversible metabolism, and comparison with man. Drug Metab Dispos. 1985;13;296–301.

71. Cheng H and Jusko WJ. Mean interconversion times and distribution rate parameters for drugs undergoing reversible metabolism. Pharmaceut Res. 1990;7:1003–1010.

72. Houston JB. Drug metabolite kinetics. Pharmacol Ther. 1982;15:521–552.

73. Michaelis L, Menten ML. Die kinetik der invertinwirkung. Biochem Z. 1913;49:333–369.

74. Levy G. Dose dependent effects in pharmacokinetics. In: Tedeschi DH, Tedeschi RE, eds. Importance of Fundamental Principles in Drug Evaluation. New York:Raven Press;1968.

75. Van Rossum JM, van Lingen G, Burgers JPT. Dose-dependent pharmacokinetics. Pharmacol Ther. 1983;21:77–99.

76. Gengo FM, Schentag JJ, Jusko WJ. Pharmacokinetics of capacity-limited tissue distribution of methicillin in rabbits. J Pharm Sci. 1984;73:867–731.

77. Tang-Liu DD-S, Williams RL, Riegelman S. Nonlinear theophylline elimination. Clin Pharmacol Ther. 1982;31:358–369.

78. Mangione A, Boudinot FD, Schultz RM et al. Dose-dependent pharmacokinetics of mezlocillin in relation to renal impairment. Antimicrob Agents Chemother. 1982;21:428–435.

79. Jusko WJ, Koup JR, Alvan G. Nonlinear assessment of phenytoin bioavailability. J Pharmacokinet Biopharm. 1976;4:327–336.

80. Metzler CM. Estimation of pharmacokinetic parameters: Statistical considerations. Pharmacol Ther. 1981;13:543–556.

81. Metzler CM, Elfring GL, McEwen AJ. A package of computer programs for pharmacokinetic modeling. Biometrics. 1974;30:562.
82. Daniel C, Wood FS. Fitting Equations to Data. New York,NY:Wiley-Interscience;1971.
83. Peck CC, Beal SL, Sheiner LB et al. Extended least-squares nonlinear regression: A possible solution to the "Choice of Weights" problem in analysis of individual pharmacokinetic data. J Pharmacokinet Biopharm. 1984;12:545–558.
84. Boxenbaum HG, Riegelman S, Elashoff RM. Statistical estimations in pharmacokinetics. J Pharmacokinet Biopharm. 1974;2:123–148.
85. Weiss M, Sziegoleit W, Forster W. Dependence of pharmacokinetic parameters on the body weight. Intl J Clin Pharmacol. 1977;15:572–75.
86. Adolph EF. Quantitative relations in the physiological constitutions of mammals. Science. 1949;109:579–585.
87. Westlake WJ. The design and analysis of comparative blood-level trials. In: Swarbrick J, ed. Dosage Form Design and Bioavailability. Philadelphia:Lea and Febiger;1973:149–179.
88. Kaplan JM, McCracken GH, Horton LJ et al. Pharmacologic studies in neonates given large does of ampicillin. J Pediatr. 1974;84:571–577.
89. Riggs DS, Guarnieri JA, Addelman S. Fitting straight lines when both variables are subject to error. Life Sci. 1978;22:1305–1360.
90. National Institutes of Health. Guide for the Care and Use of Laboratory Animals. Rockville, MD:Dept. of Health, Education, and Welfare;1978.
91. Food and Drug Administration. Obligations of clinical investigators of regulated articles. Federal Register. 1978;43:35210–35229.
92. Veng-Pedersen. Linear and nonlinear system approaches in pharmacokinetics: How much do they have to offer? I. General considerations. J Pharmacokinet Biopharm. 1988;16:413–472.
93. Blomqvist G, Pauli S, Farde L et al. Maps of receptor binding parameters in the human brain—a kinetic analysis of PET measurements. Eur J Nucl Med. 1990;16:257–265.
94. Potter JM and Self H. Cyclosporin A: Variation in whole blood levels related to *in vitro* anticoagulant usage. Ther Drug Monitoring. 1986;8:122–125.
95. Veng-Pedersen P and Gillespie WR. Single pass mean residence time in peripheral tissues: A distribution parameter intrinsic to the tissue affinity of a drug. J Pharm Sci. 1986;75:1119–1126.
96. Hayton WL. Symbol-and-arrow diagrams in teaching pharmacokinetics. Amer J Pharm Educ. 1990;54:290–292.
97. Cheng H and Jusko WJ. An area function method for calculating the apparent elimination rate constant of a metabolite. J Pharmacokinet Biopharm. 1989;17:125–130.
98. Cheng H and Jusko WJ. Mean residence time concepts for pharmacokinetic systems with nonlinear drug elimination described by the Michaelis-Menten Equation. Pharmaceut Res. 1988;5:156–164.

Chapter 3

Analysis of Pharmacokinetic Data for Individualizing Drug Dosage Regimens

Carl C. Peck, David Z. D'Argenio, and John H. Rodman

Applied pharmacokinetics is a challenging clinical discipline with a strong theoretical framework for application to patient care. Continued developments in this area, along with the widespread availability of drug assays, have facilitated the transfer of information gained from the experimental studies of drug absorption, distribution, metabolism, and elimination to clinical strategies for improving the precision of therapeutic decisions in the individual patient. This chapter in the prior edition of this text reviewed important earlier work in applied pharmacokinetics. While retaining discussion of introductory concepts, this revision expands on some of the more recent developments in pharmacokinetic data analysis with selected illustrative examples relevant to optimizing therapeutic drug regimens.

The increasing number of clinically useful drugs suitable for therapeutic drug monitoring is reflected by the growing number of chapters with each new edition of this textbook. Drug assay technology has now progressed to the degree that, given the clinical need, a practical analytical procedure can usually be developed. The prerequisites for the usefulness of drug concentrations in routine patient care include a narrow therapeutic range, significant consequences associated with therapeutic failure or toxicity, wide interpatient pharmacokinetic variability, and the demonstrated utility of drug concentration monitoring as an intermediate endpoint to guide therapeutic decisions.

To be clinically useful, applied pharmacokinetics requires the ability to establish a kinetic model descriptive of the time course of drug concentrations and a definable relationship between drug concentrations and therapeutic effects. The pharmacokinetic model is integral to the process of selecting an initial dosage regimen, modifying the regimen and establishing relationships between patient characteristics (e.g., weight, renal function) and pharmacokinetic parameters. Ideally, the model used would reflect the physiological disposition of the drug.[1] However, extensive data and computational requirements make physiological models untenable for routine clinical use. Compartmental models have been most commonly used and a substantial literature is available to guide their application.[2,3] Noncompartmental data analysis is appropriate for selected problems[4-7] but poorly suited for dynamic, clinical data[8] without an extensive sampling scheme.[9] For clinical applications and the approaches discussed here, compartment models are most often appropriate.

A relationship between a drug's concentration in blood and its therapeutic effect can be derived from kinetic and drug receptor considerations consistent with many therapeutic agents.[10] Explicit pharmacodynamic modeling approaches incorporating a measured effect are described in Chapter 4: Pharmacodynamics. Most frequently relationships between drug concentrations and response are determined empirically, rather than from an explicit effect model (see Figure 3-1). Although some work has been done outlining relative-risk guidelines[11-16] to allow specifying goals that incorporate quantitative efficacy and toxicity relationships, existing information is remarkably sparse.

It should be noted that pharmacokinetic models commonly used for dosage regimen optimization utilize drug concentrations in blood which do not necessarily reflect drug concentration (or amount) at the site of drug effect at all times following administration. Further, even when blood concentrations correspond to drug effect or site concentrations, host factors may confound measurement of the response. For example, the response of heart rate to a concentration of propranolol

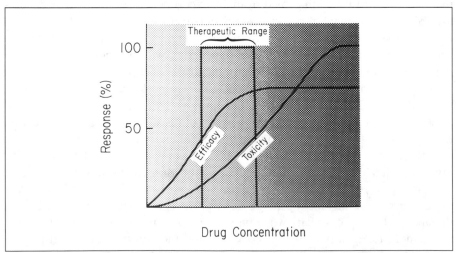

Figure 3-1. *Therapeutic ranges for measured drug concentration are commonly expressed as absolute values (i.e., digoxin therapeutic range equals 0.5–2.0 ng/mL). A more appropriate and informative definition of concentration-response relationships defines the likelihood of efficacy and toxicity for a given concentration. Note that the asymptote for toxicity approaches 100% since, if given large enough doses, all patients will demonstrate adverse effects. In contrast, the asymptote for efficacy seldom approaches 100% and often may be only 20% to 30% (e.g., anticancer drugs).*

is strongly influenced by the status of endogenous adrenergic activity. Additional confounding factors include the presence of unmeasured active metabolites, the influence of concomitant disease, imprecise measurements of response (e.g., effect of digitalis on heart failure), timing of blood samples in relation to timing of drug administration, concurrent or prior drug use, and time differentials between peak concentrations and peak responses. Despite these limitations, relatively simple pharmacokinetic models can be a useful basis for more precise drug therapy.[17-20] The assumption here is that a relationship exists which allows the use of drug concentration(s) as an *intermediate* endpoint for managing therapy.

DEVELOPING A QUANTITATIVE FRAMEWORK FOR INDIVIDUALIZING DOSAGE REGIMENS

Individualizing dosage regimens is comprised of discrete but interrelated components which then allow the use of measured drug concentration(s) to achieve a target endpoint. The process of modifying the input (i.e., dose regimen) to achieve the target (e.g., drug concentration) is a problem that can be cast in the general context of adaptive control. Figure 3-2 represents a schematic approach

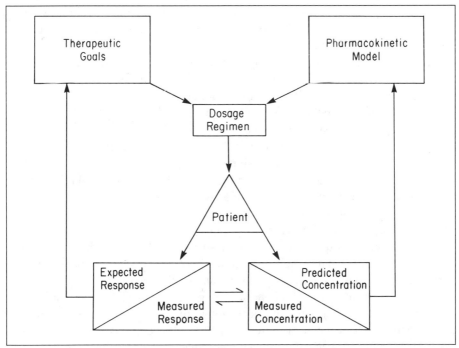

Figure 3-2. The process of adaptive control for applied pharmacokinetics begins with selection of an initial dosage regimen based on 1) therapeutic goals determined by known drug concentration-clinical response relationships (see Figure 3-1) and the patient's clinical status and 2) a pharmacokinetic model relating patient characteristics to pharmacokinetic parameters. Dosage regimen revision includes adjusting the parameter estimates for the pharmacokinetic model based on measured drug concentrations and in relation to the therapeutic goals and the patient's clinical response.

that highlights the components and interaction of the adaptive control process applied to pharmacokinetics. The principles of control theory widely applied in engineering have been reviewed for their potential for improving control of drug therapy.[21,22] While there is a growing number of studies demonstrating clinical benefit from applied pharmacokinetics,[15,23–28] further advances in applied pharmacokinetics will draw on the important concepts of control theory. To provide a link between these concepts and applied pharmacokinetics, it is useful to review some basic terminology.

Control strategies in drug therapy are commonly present in empirical form in clinical practice and are often formalized as rules and nomograms.[11,17,29–31] For example, doses are adjusted to body size for pediatric patients[32] and for creatinine clearance in patients with renal failure.[17] In control theory this would be referred to as open loop control because the algorithms are based on *a priori* (e.g., population) assumptions for drug disposition parameters. When measured responses (e.g., drug concentrations, blood pressure, prothrombin time) are available, the process can be made *adaptive* (for the individual) and this is defined as open loop *feedback* control. In clinical therapeutics this is often accomplished intuitively. However, for adaptive control to be implemented in a reproducible fashion, a formal structure must be invoked making the process more complex. The challenge for applied pharmacokinetics is to develop, refine, and evaluate strategies within the quantitative framework of adaptive control which measurably improve the precision of drug therapy. The improved precision must be such that the increased complexity is offset by improved patient outcome. The following elements are required for implementation of adaptive control:

1) a pharmacokinetic (structural) model
2) a variance model for (random residual) variation in data
3) a population model for intersubject variability
4) a model for relationships between patient characteristics and the pharmacokinetic model parameters

Each of these components will be introduced and then estimation methods for a population of subjects and the individual will be described. The emphasis on estimation reflects the major recent advances in clinically useful methods. Innovative approaches for the estimation of population pharmacokinetic parameters[33–36] provided the impetus for the development of population based methods for the individual,[37–39] most notably the Bayesian methods. Open loop feedback methods are now finding increased acceptance for routine clinical use.[28,40–54]

The control problem in drug therapy is generally posed as estimating the parameters for an appropriate pharmacokinetic model and then determining the dose to achieve a target concentration. Implicit in this approach is the separation principle for estimation and control. This pharmacokinetic approach is defined as *deterministic* open loop feedback (OLF)[55,56] in control theory and is illustrated by the method described by Sawchuk and Zaske[20] which has proven extremely useful for drugs such as the aminoglycoside antibiotics.[24,43,53]

An important, but potentially limiting, assumption arising from the separation of estimation and control is that the parameters of the model are deterministic, or estimated without error, when in practice there is inevitable uncertainty. When the model is simple, the data are accurate and precise, and the estimation method is reliable, the deterministic OLF control strategy has the distinct advantages of being familiar and widely implemented in the form of clinically used computer software.[22,38,44,57,58] The use of Bayesian estimation, rather than least squares, has demonstrated improved precision for deterministic OLF control.[21,22,24,28] However, when there is substantial error in the estimates of parameters, consideration of the randomly variable, or stochastic, character of the parameters can be important in reliably determining the most appropriate dosage regimen. *Stochastic* OLF control strategies have been described[26,59–62] but have yet to be tested clinically.

A further refinement in control strategies is stochastic *closed loop* control.[56] Stochastic closed loop control explicitly acknowledges the potential of obtaining additional data, as well as the random variability present in the model and the response. The control strategy (i.e., dosage regimen) is then determined with the composite objectives of improving the estimates for the model parameters as well as achieving the target. Such an approach is particularly suited for serial steps of data acquisition and dose adjustments for complex or poorly specified models. This rigorous but computationally challenging approach has the intriguing characteristic of "learning" about the model, but it has not yet been fully implemented in a clinically useful form. It is the potential for the control strategy to actively learn about the system that distinguishes closed loop from open loop methods. Current control strategies are largely of the deterministic OLF class and the remainder of this discussion will be limited to that context.

Defining the Pharmacokinetic Model

Conventional pharmacokinetic models have usually been presented in the form of integrated equations (closed form solutions) for specific inputs (e.g., bolus, constant rate infusion) and compartmental models (e.g., one-compartment model). With the advent of powerful numerical algorithms, it is now easier and less restrictive to employ more general mathematical notation.[2,63] This notation is becoming commonplace and relatively uniform and will be briefly introduced here. More detailed presentations are presented by investigators responsible for introducing the state variable representation for dynamic systems into pharmacokinetics and, more importantly, introducing major innovations in modeling and data analysis of drug disposition and effects.[35,64–67]

The expected response (e.g., drug concentration) in an individual subject can be described as:

$$y_{ij} = f(\phi_j, x_{ij}) + \varepsilon_{ij} \qquad \text{(Eq. 3-1)}$$

where y_{ij} is the ith measurement in the jth individual, $\emptyset_j$ is the appropriate set of pharmacokinetic model parameters (e.g., V_d, CL) for individual j, and x_{ij} includes information such as doses and times for the ith measurement in the jth individual. The function f may be implicitly defined, for example, from the solution of differential equations. The power of this notational approach is that we can now use complex structures, such as Michaelis-Menten models and parent-metabolite models, with irregular multiple dose regimens and sampling times. Moreover, this approach has facilitated the important notion that the individual subject arises from a population.

Accommodating Random Variability in the Data

The measured value can never be determined without errors such as assay variability, requiring introduction of a term (ε_{ij}) to explicitly recognize this "noise" in the data. By rearranging Equation 3-1, the variability is now expressed as an independent variable.

$$\varepsilon_{ij} = y_{ij} - f(\phi_j, x_{ij})$$ (Eq. 3-2)

For example, when a pharmacokinetic model is fitted to a series of drug concentrations, the residuals (measured-predicted values) represent this variability. The residual variance of the error, ε_{ij}, can be empirically modelled in a manner similar to the use of a pharmacokinetic model for the drug. It is common to assume that the variance of ε_{ij} is a function of the *predicted* drug concentration.[34,35,56] One representative model for the variance is

$$\text{Var}(\varepsilon_{ij}) = a \cdot (f(\phi_j, x_{ij}))^b$$ (Eq. 3-3)

where a and b represent proportional and exponential parameters respectively, that attempt to account for the random residual variability not accommodated by the pharmacokinetic model. There are several important implications for expanding the model structure to explicitly account for variability. Importantly, it acknowledges that the variability in the measurement is unknown and arises from a variety of sources (assay variability, doses, times, incorrect pharmacokinetic model). Second, the variability parameters a and b can be estimated *at the same time* as the pharmacokinetic parameters (e.g., clearance and half-life). One estimation approach that takes advantage of the complete pharmacostatistical (i.e., structural and variance) model is extended least squares.[68]

Population Variability

The most relevant source of variability in pharmacokinetic experiments arises from differences between patients. To reflect the intersubject variability, the pharmacokinetic parameter(s), $\varnothing_j$, must be described as arising from a population. This can be written as

$$\phi_j = \theta + \eta_j$$ (Eq. 3-4)

where θ are population average parameters and η_j are the differences of the individual from the population parameter averages. We can now consider a model given by

$$y_{ij} = f_{ij}(\theta + \eta_j) + \varepsilon_{ij}$$ (Eq. 3-5)

The full mathematical development of the pharmacostatistical model requires additional details, in particular with respect to the distributional characteristics of the population.[35] However, this concept of defining the pharmacokinetic parameters for the individual as the sum of the population average and plus or minus the difference attributable to the individual[34] is central to the methods that have led to the use of population pharmacokinetic estimation.

Interaction of Observation and Intersubject Variability: An Example

The observational error present in all clinical and experimental pharmacokinetic data is of importance primarily because of its potential to confound a reliable estimate of differences between subjects. The interaction of these sources of variability is not entirely intuitive and is further complicated by the nonlinear relationship between drug concentrations and parameters. To provide some insight into the pharmacostatistical model developed above, a computer simulation will be used to illustrate several important points. For convenience we will assume that the only two sources of variability are observation error and differences among subjects, or population variability. Real data and additional variability arising from model misspecification would add further uncertainty.

The pattern and relative magnitude of interindividual variability and the random residual error are based on studies with teniposide (VM26), an investigational anticancer drug.[50] For the simulation, two doses of 200 mg/m² were given over four hours at 0 and 24 hours, assuming a two-compartment linear model. The four parameters of the two-compartment model were defined as arising from independent log normal distributions such that the mean clearance was 0.964 L/m²/hr with a coefficient of variation of (CV) 35%. The solid line in each panel of Figure 3-3 represents the drug concentration profile for the *average (mean) pharmacokinetic parameters*. The boxes and error bars represent mean concentrations and one standard deviation, for the 200 mg/m² dose at selected times when 500 simulations (i.e., studies) are done including different known sources of variability.

When only observation error is considered (Panel A), the variability corresponds to repeated studies of the same subject. If the data are known without error and the simulated variability arises only from randomly selecting model parameters from the population, the results correspond to the real differences from studying different subjects (Panel B) and being able to determine the model parameters without error. Panel C combines the observation (e.g., measurement) error with the true population, or intersubject, variability. The population estimation problem is to reliably determine the variability reflected in Panel B when confounded by measurement error (e.g., Panel A). This information can then be incorporated into the estimation method for the individual.[36,37]

In Panel A the variability would be attributable to random factors such as assay error, recording wrong times, and errors in dose preparation and has a cumulative CV of 25% in this simulation and remains constant over time. Note that the variability of the normally distributed observation error is proportional to the

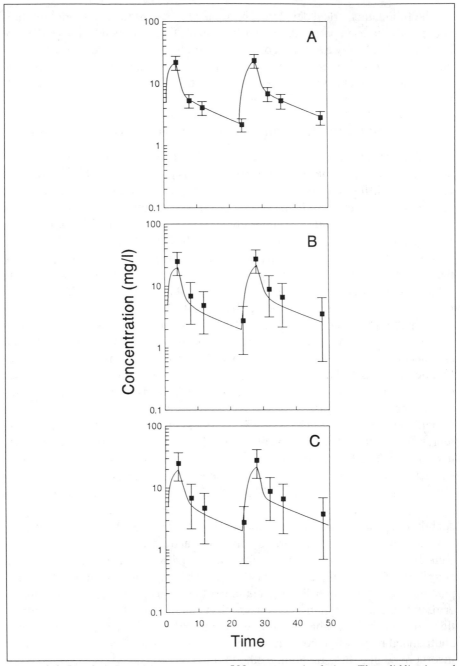

Figure 3-3. *Panels A, B, and C each represent 500 computer simulations. The solid line in each panel is a simulation of average pharmacokinetic parameters for a two-compartment model describing teniposide, an anticancer drug, when 200 mg/m² is given as a four-hour infusion at time 0 and 24 hours. The ■ are the mean observations and the error bars represent 1 standard deviation when the following sources of variability are introduced: Panel A—observation (e.g., assay) error only with a 25% CV; Panel B—population (e.g., intersubject) variability only, with parameters yielding a clearance with a 35% CV; Panel C—a combination of both observation and population variability. See text and Table 3-1.*

predicted value, and thus the absolute value is greater at higher concentrations; the average (shown by boxes) of the repeated studies falls on the predicted line for the mean model parameters.

In Panel B, the variability in observed concentrations shown by the error bars, represents the true population variability arising from studying a large number of subjects but not confounded by observation error (i.e., Panel A). In contrast to Panel A, the coefficient of variation of the observed concentration varies with time. Furthermore, the average concentrations for the population do not fall on the solid line predicted from the mean parameters. This is a consequence of the nonlinear (exponential) relationship between the elimination and distribution parameters and the time course of drug concentrations. A practical implication of this important concept is that pharmacokinetic parameters should never be determined from averaged data. This has been referred to as the "naive pooled data" method[35] and unfortunately is still occasionally used.

Panel C combines the observation error (Panel A) and the population variability (Panel B). Table 3-1 compares measurements taken at selected times during the study to illustrate the influence of the source of variability on the model response as reflected in drug concentrations. By comparing the coefficient of variation for the observation and population variability alone with that for the combined variability, it is clear the result is substantially less than additive. For the four-hour concentration, the observation variability yields the expected CV of 25%. The 35% CV for clearance (intersubject variability) produces a 40% CV for the four-hour concentration. However, when both sources of variability are combined, the CV for the four-hour concentration rises only to 49%. At the subsequent times of 12 and 48 hours, the combined variability is only slightly greater than that arising from population variability alone. As shown in rows two and three of Table 3-1, the variability in concentrations is a function of when they are measured relative to the dose. Thus the information content of drug concentrations regarding population variability is dependent on when they are obtained (see discussion of Selection of Sampling Times).

The population estimation problem is to appropriately account for the random residual error, illustrated here as observation error, to correctly estimate the true intersubject variability. The difference between the response of the mean model

Table 3-1. *Simulation Study of Pharmacokinetic Variability*

	CV% of observed concentrations at selected times		
Source of variability[a]	**4 hr**	**12 hr**	**48 hr**
Observation variability	25	25	25
Population variability	40	66	76
Combined variability	49	74	82

[a] Each row represents 500 simulations for normally distributed variability in the measurement with a CV of 25%, then population variability only with a CV of 35% for elimination clearance, and then finally a simulation combining both observation (e.g., measurement) and population (e.g., intersubject) variability. The times correspond to a subset of the data in Figure 3-3.

parameters (the solid line) and the mean response of the population (the boxes in Panels B and C of Figure 3-3) is a problem which has not been fully resolved with currently used estimation methods as discussed elsewhere in this chapter.

Incorporating Patient Characteristics into Pharmacokinetic Models

Once a pharmacokinetic model is selected, it is useful to establish functional relationships between pharmacokinetic parameters and patient characteristics. Volume of distribution is commonly referenced to body weight, and drug elimination or clearance may be a function of creatinine clearance. The use of patient characteristics as indicator variables[33] can be formally cast into the pharmacokinetic model and adds significant flexibility to individualizing therapy. This also offers the potential for testing the appropriateness of the proposed relationships.

Developing a pharmacokinetic parameter which can be predicted from a patient characteristic is illustrated by the common practice of referencing renal drug clearance to creatinine clearance. The total clearance (CL_T) of a drug eliminated by both renal and nonrenal routes can be written as:

$$CL_T = CL_R + CL_{NR} \qquad \text{(Eq. 3-6)}$$

where CL_R = renal clearance and CL_{NR} = nonrenal clearance. CL_R can then be related to creatinine clearance (CL_{cr}) as follows:

$$CL_R = \alpha \cdot CL_{cr} \qquad \text{(Eq. 3-7)}$$

where α is a regression parameter that defines the linear relationship between the patient characteristic (CL_{cr}) and the pharmacokinetic parameter (CL_R). The functional relationship between CL_T and CL_R accommodating differences in CL_{cr} between or within patient(s) is:

$$CL_T = \alpha \cdot CL_{cr} + CL_{NR} \qquad \text{(Eq. 3-8)}$$

In a population study, CL_T and CL_{cr} are determined for each of a group of patients with varying values of CL_{cr}. This enables the statistical estimation of the regression parameters α and CL_{NR}, which define the slope (α) and intercept (CL_{NR}) of a linear relationship between CL_T and CL_{cr} for any value of creatinine clearance. A graphical summary of this relationship is shown in Figure 3-4. This regression relationship then allows the population-based prediction of drug clearance for initial therapy in patients with varying values of CL_{cr} and can accommodate changes in renal function for an individual patient.

The aminoglycoside antibiotics are an example of renally eliminated drugs for which this general approach is useful. Population studies of the CL_T of gentamicin (CL_{gent}) and CL_{cr}[26,44,53] define specific regression relationships in the form of Equation 3-8 above. For example:

$$CL_{gent}(\text{mL/min/kg}) = 0.9 \cdot CL_{cr} + 0.06 \qquad \text{(Eq. 3-9)}$$

allows CL_{gent} to be adjusted for differing CL_{cr} (mL/min/kg) using α equal to 0.9 and CL_{NR} equal to 0.06 for gentamicin. When gentamicin concentrations are measured in a particular patient, the regression parameter (α) and CL_{NR} may be estimated rather than CL_{gent}, and the revised estimates can then be used to modify the dosage regimen based on subsequent changes in CL_{cr} without waiting for drug concentrations to be repeated.

The entire model now constructed is often referred to as the pharmacostatistical model. The key elements include a pharmacokinetic model, a model for random residual error (ε_{ij}), a referencing of the individual pharmacokinetic parameters to the population values, and the direct incorporation of patient variables (e.g., renal function and clearance) to allow adjustment of pharmacokinetic parameters for patient characteristics.

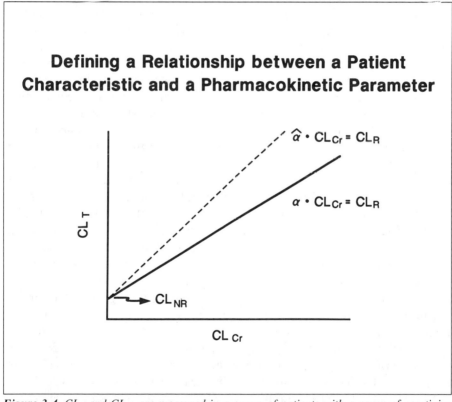

Defining a Relationship between a Patient Characteristic and a Pharmacokinetic Parameter

Figure 3-4. CL_T and CL_{Cr} are measured in a group of patients with a range of creatinine clearances. The regression of parameters α (slope) and CL_{NR} (intercept) define the average population relationship between CL_{Cr} and CT_T. An individualized estimate of this relationship may be obtained by comparing a patient's drug concentration response with that predicted by the population parameters. If drug concentrations are measured in a patient with CL_R that is greater than the population average, a revised value for α ($\hat{\alpha}$) is estimated to adjust the relationship between CL_{Cr} and CL_T for that patient. If drug concentrations are measured at only one value of CL_{Cr}, CL_{NR} would be fixed and only α would be revised. CL_T = total drug clearance, CL_{NR} = nonrenal clearance, CL_R = renal drug clearance, α = regression parameter (slope), CL_{Cr} = creatinine clearance.

POPULATION PHARMACOKINETICS AND THE INDIVIDUAL

The clinical use of pharmacokinetic methods to individualize drug therapy is initiated with the aid of population pharmacokinetic data. If absolutely no prior information on a drug's disposition were available, then its initial use in a patient would constitute an entirely new experiment, the consequences of which would be unpredictable. Only after a complete **individual pharmacokinetic** experiment (see Chapter 2: Guidelines for Collection and Analysis of Pharmacokinetic Data) in the patient had been completed would the pharmacokinetics of a drug in that patient be available to determine a dosage regimen. However, for clinical applications, population pharmacokinetic information from prior studies provides the basis for determining the initial drug regimen (i.e., open loop control). Thereafter, measured drug concentrations taken from the patient early in the course of therapy enables one to estimate patient-specific pharmacokinetic parameters to further refine the dosage regimen (i.e., adaptive control). However, when this is done using least squares regression, illustrated by the method commonly used for aminoglycosides,[20] the population data can no longer be used. A theoretically sound and empirically attractive alternative is to interpret the data from the individual in concert with the population information using Bayes theorem.[37]

There are two requirements for integrating population data with the individual data: 1) a relevant population pharmacokinetic database, and 2) a framework for linking the individual patient to the population. **Population pharmacokinetics** entails the summarization of pharmacokinetic studies in groups of individuals and the establishment of relationships between individual patient characteristics and pharmacokinetic parameters. Studies of drug disposition in a number of individuals generally reveal that the essential pharmacokinetic parameters (e.g., bioavailability, volume of distribution, clearance) lie within a restricted range of values. This is especially true if the study group is homogeneous with regard to individual characteristics that influence drug disposition, such as might be observed in a group of healthy volunteers. A value for each pharmacokinetic parameter which typifies the group may be identified. The representative value, no matter how it is estimated, is termed the **population-typical value** for the parameter (θ). Current methods of population pharmacokinetic analysis usually use the *mean* (average) as the population-typical value.[38]

Of equal importance, however, is the extent to which the pharmacokinetic values for an individual in the study group differ from the population-typical value. Independent of its method of estimation, this measure of interindividual deviation is termed the **population-variability value** for the parameter (η_j). Current population pharmacokinetic analysis methods[33] entail calculation of the **standard deviation** as the population variability value (see Equations 3-4 and 3-5).

Implicit, therefore, in population pharmacokinetic studies is the estimation of population-typical (e.g., mean) and population-variability (e.g., standard deviation) values for each pharmacokinetic parameter. The population mean and standard deviation thus summarize the **population distribution** of pharmacokinetic parameters. The mean and standard deviation for a "normal" distribution may be interpreted parametrically[65,66] (i.e., the mean is located in the center of the normal distribution and ± one standard deviation accounts for 68% of population values). If the parameter distribution is skewed, the natural log (ln) of the parameter will often transform the distribution to a normal curve. Figure 3-5 illustrates relationships between normal and log-normal distributions of the pharmacokinetic parameter, clearance. A lack of normality in the population distribution may impact upon the appropriateness of using a parameter in a Bayesian forecasting technique, which is sensitive to the form of the distribution for the calculation of individualized parameter values.[26,69,70]

Population pharmacokinetics should be studied in a heterogeneous group of individuals exhibiting a range of values of patient characteristics which are thought to influence drug disposition, such as in a group of patients with varying weights, ages, and degrees of renal dysfunction who are receiving a drug for therapy. This is done deliberately to establish relationships between individual patient characteristics and population pharmacokinetic parameter distributions (see Figure 3-6, Panels A and C). The relationships discovered may be **categorically quantitative** as in the observation that smokers (an individual characteristic) tend to have typical

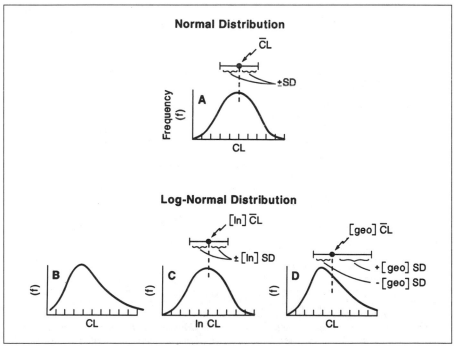

Figure 3-5. *Histograms illustrating normal and log-normal distributions of the pharmacokinetic parameter, clearance (CL). In the normal case (Histogram A), the CL values are symmetrically distributed about the mean value, CL with a constant standard deviation = SD. When the CL values are skewed to the right (Histogram B), the distribution of the natural logarithms of the CL values may be log-normally distributed (Histogram C) with mean, [ln], and standard deviation, ± [ln]SD. When transformed back to non-logarithm value (Histogram D), by taking the anti-logarithms of [ln]CL and [ln]SD, the geometric mean clearance, [geo]CL = (exp([ln]CL)), lies to the right of the mode, and the geometric standard deviations, [geo]SD, above and below the mode, are unequal; the positive [geo]SD (=[geo]CL × (exp([ln]SD) – 1)) being greater than the negative [geo]SD(=[geo]CL × (1 – exp(–[ln]SD))).*

theophylline clearance values about 50% to 60% higher than those of nonsmokers (see Figure 3-6, Panel B).[29] Alternatively, a *continuous quantitative* relationship may be discerned as in the linear relationship between creatinine clearance and aminoglycoside clearance values discussed above and illustrated in Figure 3-6, Panels C and D. It is important to consider the reduction in the population-variability value which is accounted for by the relationship. For example, compare the range of CL values for all patients (see Figure 3-6, Panel A) with the smaller ranges

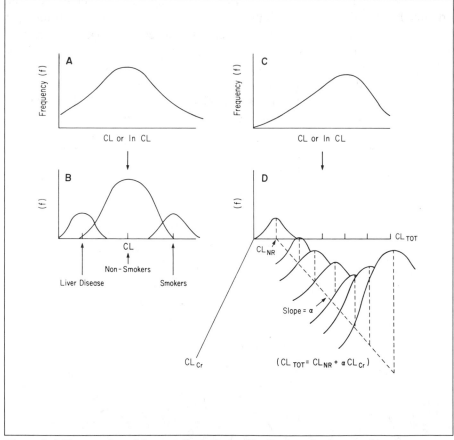

Figure 3-6. *The mapping of the overall population distribution of a pharmacokinetic parameter (CL) into component subpopulations in relation to categorically quantitative (Panels A and B) and continuously quantitative (Panels C and D) individual patient characteristics. Panels A and B depict a broad overall population distribution for clearances of a drug such as theophylline, which is then refined into subpopulations by sorting clearances by smoking and liver disease status, as depicted in Panel B. Panel C depicts a leftward skewed overall population distribution for clearances of a drug such as gentamicin when examined independent of renal function. Panel D is refined into a continuous subpopulation by relating drug clearance (CL_{TOT}) to creatinine clearance (CL_{cr}). In Panel D, the dotted lines indicate the location of the midpoint of the* **continuous** *relationship between the patient characteristic (CL_{cr}) and the pharmacokinetic parameter (CL_{TOT}). In both cases, it can be seen that subpopulations differ in the location and spread of typical values (e.g., means), which should improve both accuracy and precision of* **a priori** *parameter value assignments when applied appropriately to individual patients in the context of Bayesian estimation.*

for the subpopulations in Figure 3-6, Panel B. Typically, this variability will be lower in magnitude than the interindividual variability of the parameter when the related patient characteristic is not taken into account. When these relationships are used to predict a patient's pharmacokinetic responses, the reduced interindividual variability should translate into improved prediction.

METHODS OF DETERMINING POPULATION PHARMACOKINETICS

Two-Stage Method, the Traditional Approach

The traditional method of determining population pharmacokinetics consists of undertaking intensive experimental studies of a drug in a small number of individual subjects. Each patient's data are then analyzed by curve-stripping, log-linear regression, or least-squares nonlinear regression, for estimating individual pharmacokinetic parameters by fitting a pharmacokinetic model to the data. Alternatively, certain pharmacokinetic parameters (e.g., steady-state distribution volume, clearance, extent of bioavailability) may be estimated using noncompartmental techniques. In any case, the end result of Stage 1 is a collection of individual estimates of pharmacokinetic parameters. In Stage 2a, the parameters are summarized by calculating the mean and standard deviation. These may be taken as estimates of the population-typical and population-variability values. In Stage 2b, relationships between patient characteristics and the estimated pharmacokinetic parameters are established by categorization or regression techniques.

The traditional approach is illustrated by the studies of Koup et al. on the population pharmacokinetics of digoxin.[71,72] In Stage 1, digoxin was given intravenously to eight healthy volunteers and then measured in 12 blood and six urine samples collected over two and six days, respectively. A similar protocol was carried out in six patients with renal failure. Stage 1 and Stage 2a analyses resulted in the reported population pharmacokinetic values shown in Table 3-2. Linear regression analysis of digoxin clearances on creatinine clearances carried out in Stage 2b yield a predictive relationship which can be used for open loop control. However, these population pharmacokinetic values are representative of only the few healthy individuals and renal failure patients studied, and may not be repre-

Table 3-2. *Results of a Two Stage Analysis of Digoxin Data*[a, b, c]

Parameter	Units	Normal subjects (n = 8)	Renal failure patients (n = 5)
V_d	L/1.73 m^2	570 (25%)	328 (38%)
CL	mL/min/1.73 m^2	190 (29%)	49 (36%)

[a] V = Volume of distribution (L/1.73 m^2 body surface area); CL = Clearance (mL/min/1.73 m^2 body surface area); CL_{cr} = Clearance of creatinine (mL/min/1.73 m^2 body surface area).
[b] From the results in the normal and renal failure subjects, the following regression relationship was constructed: $CL_{Digoxin} = 36 + 1.1 \, (CL_{cr})$. However, the small number of subjects studied provides a limited basis for extrapolation to other patients.
[c] From Koup et al.[71,72] Mean (coefficient of variation).

sentative of all patients receiving digoxin for the treatment of congestive heart failure. The apparently linear relationship between creatinine and digoxin clearances affords an insight into the renal handling of the drug, but this was derived from only a few individuals who represented the extremes of renal function.

The two-stage method enjoys several positive features. Weighted nonlinear least-squares regression is a familiar technique which is understood by most pharmacokineticists. When applied properly, it has proven to be a reliable method of estimating pharmacokinetic parameters in experimental studies. The computer routines for performing the two-stage method are available on a variety of computers ranging from mainframes to microcomputers. When sufficient data are available in each individual to obtain statistically precise estimates of individual pharmacokinetic parameters and a large number of individuals are included in the analysis, Stage 2a and 2b analyses of data provide reasonable, but potentially upwardly biased, estimates of population pharmacokinetic parameter distributions.

Several drawbacks are inherent in the two-stage method of population pharmacokinetic analysis. Accurate and precise Stage 1 estimates of individual pharmacokinetic parameters require multiple, appropriately-timed blood samples within costly, contrived experiments.[73,74] These are most easily applied to groups of healthy volunteers and are often impossible to perform in large numbers of patients undergoing routine therapy. The method fails when the number of samples per patient is insufficient to independently estimate the individual's pharmacokinetics. The latter is a serious drawback, since the most pertinent population pharmacokinetic information is likely to arise from patients actually undergoing therapy. Constraints upon the number and timing of blood samples from seriously ill patients often preclude the use of the two-stage method. Thus the population pharmacokinetic information from the two-stage method often comes mainly from studies of healthy individuals or small numbers of patients who often inadequately represent those undergoing routine therapy. Therefore, information generated by the two-stage method constitutes a limited foundation upon which to base strategies for drug regimen design or pharmacokinetic adaptive control.

Mixed Effects Modeling

Mixed effects modeling for nonlinear systems is a technique of population pharmacokinetic estimation developed specifically to rectify some drawbacks inherent in the two-stage approach.[33,35] Mixed effects modeling allows direct estimation of population pharmacokinetic parameters in a single stage of analysis applied simultaneously to data from many individuals. In this method, an individual's pharmacokinetic parameters are not directly determined. Rather, a generalized form of least-squares regression, known as extended least squares, is used to estimate fixed-effects and random-effects parameters. Fixed-effects parameters include the population-typical values (means) as well as the coefficients of regression relationships between individual patient characteristics and population-typical values for the pharmacokinetic parameters (e.g., "α" in Equation 3-8). Random-effects parameters are the population-variability values (standard deviations) representing interindividual deviation from fixed-effects parameter estimates after population relationships and residual random error have been taken into account. Thus, in contrast to the two-stage method, the variability among individuals and the variability arising from observation error are both estimated which permits a less biased estimate of true variability in the population.

A powerful feature of the mixed effects modeling technique is the ability to accommodate patient pharmacokinetic data as it arises in the course of routine clinical therapy. Such data are typically sparse and obtained at less structured times. For example, only one or two drug concentrations, drawn at convenient but known times, from a sufficient number of patients, may provide a suitable database for mixed effects modeling. Sheiner et al.[33] introduced this method by describing its application to the estimation of the population pharmacokinetics of digoxin from data in 141 patients receiving the drug orally or intravenously. Five hundred eighty-six serum concentrations and 46 urine digoxin determinations constituted the pharmacokinetic database. The average number of serum digoxin measurements per patient was four, but a sizable number of patients were represented by only one or two digoxin concentrations. Fixed-effects parameters included the extent of oral bioavailability and linear coefficients relating creatinine clearance separately to digoxin distribution volume and clearance. Random-effects parameters estimated included the population standard deviation (creatinine clearance adjusted) for digoxin distribution volume and clearance, as well as the residual random error. Partial results of the analysis appear in Table 3-3 and, when compared with Koup's two-stage derived estimates in Table 3-2, demonstrate substantial differences for the estimates of population variability values (% CV). The fixed- and random-effects parameter estimates, derived from 141 patients, are representative of a sizable pool of patients who receive the drug as therapy, since the patient sample included inpatients and outpatients receiving digoxin for acute and nonacute conditions. This constitutes an extensive, patient-derived database on which to base patient digoxin regimens and predictions of serum digoxin concentrations in other patients.

The strengths of mixed-effects modeling include the ability to accommodate actual clinical data from large populations receiving routine therapy, enhancing

Table 3-3. *Mixed-Effects Modeling of Digoxin Data[a]*

Parameter	Units	CV%
F = 0.6		30
$V_d = 3.84 + 3.12 \cdot (CL_{cr})$	4 kg	34
$CL = 0.02 + 0.06 \cdot (CL_{cr})$	4 hr/kg	34
Residual Error		25

[a] F = Extent of bioavailability (± % CV); V_d = Volume of distribution (L/kg ± % CV); CL = Clearance (L/hr/kg ± % CV); CL_{cr} = Clearance of creatinine (L/hr/kg).
[b] The results of the mixed effects modeling analysis yield regression relationships similar to the Two-Stage Analysis (see Table 3-2) but are based on a much larger, presumably more representative, population and provide an explicit estimate of the residual error not accounted for in the former approach.
[c] From Sheiner et al.[33]

the relevance of the parameter estimates for incorporation into techniques of clinical pharmacokinetic forecasting, and offering statistical advantages over the traditional two-stage method. Limitations to the current use of mixed effects modeling are related to implementation and a necessary approximation to accommodate the nonlinear parameters of pharmacokinetic models. The method is unfamiliar to many pharmacokineticists, and its theoretical statistical basis is complex. Building the population pharmacostatistical model requires familiarity with variance models in addition to knowledge of standard pharmacokinetic modeling. In addition, effective use of this method requires knowledge of parametric statistical hypothesis-testing concepts to guide the analysis toward adequate choice of models. Few computer programs are available to implement mixed effects modeling for population pharmacokinetic analysis. The most well-known program, NONMEM, utilizes an estimation approach referred to as the first-order method,[83] is extensively documented, and can run on appropriately configured mainframe and microcomputers. Cumulative experience with the application of this method to real and simulated pharmacokinetic data is mounting,[75–81] but it is minimal compared to experience with the two-stage method.[82]

A recent comparison of the first-order method and the two-stage method for an intensive pharmacokinetic study revealed a bias in the first-order method estimates for the population mean for both patient data and in a simulation study.[80] There was substantially less bias from a two-stage maximum likelihood estimation approach. However, the estimates for intersubject and random residual error from the first order method were generally less biased than the two-stage method. These results are in contrast to an earlier simulation study based on smaller number of replications and a different study design.[84] Further work will undoubtedly improve these currently available population estimation approaches. The nonparametric maximum likelihood approach[36] has a strong theoretical framework and has been applied to gentamicin,[26] cyclosporine,[85] and zidovudine.[86] However, the lack of generally available software has limited a more extensive evaluation of this intriguing alternative for population estimation.

ADAPTIVE CONTROL OF INDIVIDUAL PATIENT DOSAGE REGIMENS

An individual patient's pharmacokinetic (drug concentration) response to a dosage regimen will frequently differ substantially from the target (drug concentration) response when the dosage regimen is based upon typical pharmacokinetic parameter values of a population of which the patient is apparently a member. Such differences are clinically important when subtherapeutic or potentially toxic drug concentrations are frequent or interfere with effective therapy. The frequency of excursions outside the therapeutic range may be predicted in advance from knowledge of the population distribution of pharmacokinetic parameters. Suppose that the population standard deviation of digoxin clearance is 50% of the mean value even after body size and renal function are taken into account. The variability in average steady-state digoxin concentrations in patients whose dosage regimens are based upon the population mean clearance can be expected to vary at least as much. Consequently, for a target level of 1.25 ng/mL, 25% or more of patients will need adjustments in their digoxin dosage to ensure concentrations within a therapeutic range of 0.5 to 2 ng/mL. Moreover, unappreciated patient-specific influences on drug disposition (e.g., undiagnosed diseases or concurrent therapy affecting drug distribution or elimination) may invalidate the initial assignment of population-based average pharmacokinetic parameters to a given patient. Thus, individualized estimates of patient pharmacokinetic parameters obtained by analyzing the drug concentration response directly in the patient should translate to improved patient outcome over that obtained with population average doses.

Least-Squares (LS) Methods

As discussed in Chapter 2: Guidelines for Collection and Analysis of Pharmacokinetic Data, pharmacokinetic parameter estimates may be obtained from a formal pharmacokinetic experiment using least squares (LS) estimation or "fitting" of the pharmacokinetic model to the data (e.g., drug concentrations in urine and/or blood). Least-squares methods, under certain statistical assumptions, can be derived from a more general estimation method known as maximum likelihood.[64,82] Least-squares has proven useful for selected clinical pharmacokinetic applications[20,22,53] and, more importantly, provides a basis for understanding newer methods.[61]

An LS analysis involves a computer search for parameter values of the pharmacokinetic model which minimizes an objective function (OBJ) defined as:

$$OBJ = \sum_{i=1}^{n} \frac{(C_i - \hat{C}_i)^2}{\sigma_i^2}$$

(Eq. 3-10)

where C_i and $\hat{C}_i$ denote the observed and predicted drug concentrations, and σ_i are the standard deviations from the random error model for $i = 1$ to n available drug concentrations. Thus, the LS computer search selects parameter values for the pharmacokinetic model that yield estimates, $\hat{C}_i$, which most closely correspond to the measured concentrations. The σ_i can either be entered in the fitting procedure as "known" values or estimated automatically in the procedure under explicit assumptions about the functional form of the random error model.[34,68] The need to weight observations with the appropriate σ_i stems from the varying absolute error for different values of concentration measured. For example, if an assay has a constant coefficient of variation of 10% and values of 1 to 10 units are measured (see Figure 3-7), the absolute error would range from 0.1 (i.e., 10% of 1) to 1 (i.e., 10% of 10) units. To minimize the sum of the squared residuals, $(C_i - \hat{C}_i)^2$, a reliable estimate for the variance (σ_i^2) is critical to obtaining meaningful parameter estimates.

Certain inherent assumptions and characteristics of the LS method limit its appropriateness for estimating individualized pharmacokinetic parameters in patients. Importantly, the LS method derives **all** of its information regarding the values of the pharmacokinetic parameters **entirely from the patient's drug concentration data alone**. Thus, any prior knowledge regarding the patient's pharmacokinetic values which the clinician may have from patient characteristics and population pharmacokinetic data are excluded from the LS analysis. It requires multiple, well-timed ("information-rich") drug concentrations to provide accurate and precise estimates of the parameters. The minimum number of measurements for least squares is determined by the number of parameters in the model. For example, the one-compartment model commonly used for aminoglycosides and theophylline has two parameters (e.g., volume and elimination rate or clearance) and LS requires a minimum of three measurements for statistically valid parameter estimates. The noise, or variability, in the observations (e.g., due to assay error, administration error) requires additional measurements for adequate precision. However, clinical realities generally preclude obtaining the desired number of drug concentrations at informative times.

The LS method can be modified to accommodate fewer available drug concentrations by fixing one (or more) parameters at assumed values, or defining a proportional relationship between clearance and observations obtained at a fixed time, leaving fewer parameters for individualized estimation.[87–90] Inherent in this approach, however, is either an assumption of limited variability of the fixed parameter(s) and/or a very optimistic estimate of the precision of the observations. Further, when this approach is applied in one- or certain two-sample schemes, the analysis interprets the predicted drug concentration to be exactly equal to the measured concentration, an assumption which runs contrary to our knowledge of

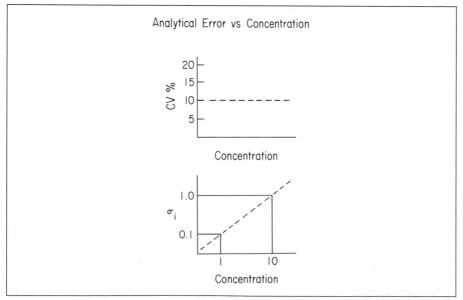

Figure 3-7. *The weighting for drug concentrations using least-squares estimation procedures is a major determinant of pharmacokinetic parameter estimates. A commonly employed weighing function assumes the coefficient of variation (CV%) to be constant (upper panel) for all drug concentrations. Thus, the standard deviation (lower panel) will be proportional to the drug concentration.*

clinical data. Some modified LS methods require restrictive clinical paradigms such as extensive blood sampling following a "test dose"[91] or at presumed steady state.[92] Despite these limitations, the LS method has been successfully employed in various forms to estimate individualized patient pharmacokinetic parameters for digoxin,[22] aminoglycosides,[43] lidocaine,[40] and other drugs.[31]

Bayesian Methods

A common sense approach to obtaining individualized estimates of the pharmacokinetic parameters for a particular patient might go as follows: 1) initiate targeted therapy, using population-based parameter values adjusted for patient characteristics (e.g., weight, serum creatinine); when possible, use parameters from a patient population similar to that of the patient; 2) measure drug concentrations at informative times and compare with expected values; and 3) cautiously make individualized pharmacokinetic parameter estimates which take into account both a) the expected drug concentrations and their variability (based upon the average parameter values and variability in the population) and b) the measured drug concentrations and their expected variability (due to the measurement and other sources of random variability). Steps 2) and 3) can be repeated, if necessary, until the patient's drug concentration and clinical responses are clinically acceptable (see Figure 3-2). The appeal of this approach, in contrast to the intuitive or least-squares approaches, which either rely entirely on prior expectations or depend solely upon measured drug concentrations, is that it mimics human thinking. That is, the result of any clinical test is or should be interpreted by clinicians in light of both their *a priori* expectations and knowledge of the variability of the test itself.[42]

The "common sense" approach described above can be implemented by applying Bayes' theorem to the problem of estimating individual pharmacokinetic parameters as follows:

$$\text{prob}(P|C) = \frac{\text{prob}(P) \cdot \text{prob}(C|P)}{\text{prob}(C)} \qquad \text{(Eq. 3-11)}$$

where prob (P|C) is the probability distribution of the patient's pharmacokinetic parameters (P) taking into account the measured drug concentrations (C), the probability of the patient's parameters within the assumed population parameter distribution [prob (P)], and the probability of measured concentrations [prob (C|P)] in the context of the pharmacokinetic model, random (measurement) errors, and the unconditional probability distribution of the observed levels [prob (C)]. When the population distributions of pharmacokinetic parameters are approximately Gaussian (i.e., normally distributed), application of the method of maximum-likelihood estimation to the above expression of Bayes' theorem results in the following objective function:

$$\text{OBJ}_{\text{Bayes}} = \sum_{j=1}^{P} \frac{(P_j - \hat{P}_j)^2}{\sigma_{P_j}^2} + \sum_{i=1}^{n} \frac{(C_i - \hat{C}_i)^2}{\sigma_i^2} \qquad \text{(Eq. 3-12)}$$

where P_j and $\hat{P}_j$ denote the population and (the estimate of the) individual's $j = 1$ to p pharmacokinetic parameters respectively, σ_{P_j} are the population parameter standard deviations, and C_i, $\hat{C}_i$, n, and σ_i are as defined for Equation 3-10. If the parameters in the population are log-normally distributed, the above objective function remains valid if the natural logarithms of P_j (geometric mean), $\hat{P}_{jj}$, and geometric population standard deviations are substituted for P_j, $\hat{P}_j$, and σ_{pj}. Minimization of the Bayesian objective function results in estimates of pharmacokinetic parameters unique to the patient which take into the account measured and predicted drug concentrations, along with information on measurement error and the typical variability values of pharmacokinetic parameters in the population.

It is important to note that taken together, the above pharmacokinetic Bayes' theorem and Bayesian objective function encompass all of the usual methods for estimating individual patient's pharmacokinetic parameters, assuming independent and normally distributed population parameters. When no drug concentrations are available in a patient (e.g., before starting therapy), the usual basis for assigning parameter values is to assume population average values. Since there are no concentrations, Bayes' theorem reduces to: prob (P), the maximum likelihood estimates of which are the average population parameter values. Only the first summation term remains in the Bayes' objective function, the minimum value of which is again the set of average population pharmacokinetic parameters. If drug concentrations are available, but no population-based prior expectations are admitted, Bayes' theorem reduces to: prob (C|P), the maximum likelihood estimate of which is the set of patient pharmacokinetic parameters that minimizes the least squares objective function. When both prior expectations are admitted and drug concentrations are available, the complete Bayesian method is expressed. This interpretation of the generality of the Bayesian approach is instructive in evaluating the assets and limitations of the various methods for estimating individual patient pharmacokinetics. Figure 3-8 and its legend provide a representative example of the manner in which these methods use drug concentration data for individualizing pharmacokinetic estimates.

SELECTION OF SAMPLING TIMES FOR MEASURED DRUG CONCENTRATIONS

The ability to successfully individualize a patient's dosage regimen using either of the methods discussed above, depends in part on the amount of pharmacokinetic information contained in the patient's measured drug concentrations. Accordingly, the blood sampling schedule to be used in monitoring the patient should be designed to maximize this information, subject to clinical constraints (e.g., number of samples, sampling interval) and any other therapeutic objectives (e.g., qualitative patient monitoring). Selection of a pharmacokinetically informative blood sampling schedule for the purpose of individualizing drug therapy can be posed as a problem in the statistical design of experiments. Quantitative experiment design methods have been proposed for several pharmacokinetic modeling problems, including model discrimination,[93] noncompartmental estimation of AUC and

MRT,[94,95] and kinetic model parameter estimation.[96–100] For the latter problem, several clinical studies have also been conducted to evaluate the estimation performance of formally designed sampling schedules.[101,102] For the purpose of individualizing a patient's therapy, it is reasonable to design the blood sampling schedule to precisely estimate the unknown pharmacokinetic model parameters.

A statistical framework for the design of experiments for nonlinear parameter estimation was first proposed by Box and Lucas in 1959,[103] and referred to as D-optimal experiment design. Since then, a number of extensions to this method have been proposed that are relevant to the problem of pharmacokinetic sample schedule design. An especially thorough review of experiment design for param-

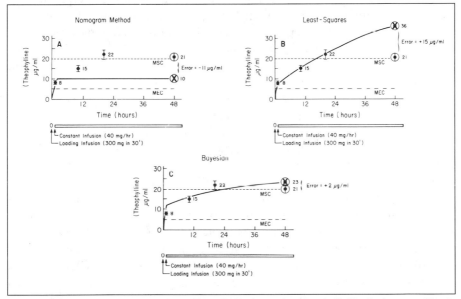

Figure 3-8. *Illustrative comparison of methods for estimating individual pharmacokinetic parameters for the purpose of predicting a future drug concentration. Theophylline therapy is instituted in a patient with the following characteristics: age 30 years, smoker, possible liver disease, lean body weight 60 kg; true (but unknown) theophylline distribution volume (V_d) 0.6 L/kg and clearance (CL) 0.034 L/kg/hr. The target theophylline concentration is 10 μg/mL, (denoted by X) between the Minimum Effective Concentration (MEC = 5 μg/mL) and the Maximum Safe Concentration (MSC = 20 μg/mL). Population-based estimates for V_d (0.5 L/kg) and CL (0.067 L/kg/hr.)[31] dictate the 30-minute loading infusion (300 mg) followed by a constant infusion of 40 mg/hr. Three plasma theophylline concentrations drawn at 0.5, 10, and 20 hours after onset of therapy are reported to be 8, 15, and 22 μg/mL, respectively, while a fourth concentration to be predicted by the various methods is 21 μg/mL at 48 hours with no change in therapy. The Nomogram Method cannot take the three early concentrations into account, persistently predicts the fourth concentration to be 10 μg/mL, yielding an error of –11 μg/mL. The Least-Squares Method, which bases its prediction solely on information extracted from the three available concentrations, overpredicts the fourth level by 15 μg/mL. The Bayesian method, which takes into account the **a priori** population estimates of CL (0.064 and 15% measurement error), predicts the fourth concentration with clinically acceptable error (± 2 μg/mL). This case illustrates the protective effect of incorporation of **a priori** expectations into the Bayesian prediction method, when the data available for feedback are scanty and potentially misleading when analyzed using least squares methods. See text for further discussion of comparative performance of the methods.*

eter estimation has been written by Walter and Pronzato.[104] The discussion to follow will briefly review the conceptual basis of the D-optimal experiment design approach and it's application to sample schedule design for use in individualizing drug therapy (see Endrenyi[99] for a more complete discussion).

The rationale behind the D-optimal design approach is to select sample times (or more generally any design variables) which will lead to model parameter estimates with the smallest possible joint confidence region. For the special case of a pharmacokinetic model with one unknown parameter and constant error variance, the D-optimal design minimizes an approximation to the variance of the unknown parameter. This is equivalent to sampling at the time when a change in the model parameter produces the largest change in the measured output (time of maximum sensitivity). The sensitivity interpretation allows for the following intuitive explanation of the replicated nature of D-optimal sampling schedules; if there is a single time of maximum sensitivity (minimum variance), then all the available observations should be obtained at that time. The D-optimal design method depends critically on correctly specifying the following:

- the structure of the kinetic model;
- the model inputs (i.e., the dosage regimen);
- the variance of the additive measurement error;
- prior values for the unknown model parameters.

A change in any of the above will in general change the D-optimal sampling, schedule and, in some cases, the influence will be dramatic.

Despite these assumptions, this quantitative approach to experiment design can provide valuable guidance for designing informative therapeutic drug monitoring sampling strategies as the following example involving the individualization of intravenous continuous infusion theophylline therapy serves to illustrate. The theoretical variance associated with the theophylline clearance (CL) estimated using two measured concentrations, depends on the time interval between the two observations.[105,106] With the first observation fixed at 1.0 hour post loading dose, the D-optimal sampling analysis indicates that the variance of the estimated CL falls dramatically as the time interval between the two observations is increased from 0.3 elimination half-life to one half-life; further increases in the sampling interval produce only modest reductions in the variance of the CL estimate. These theoretical results were confirmed in a population simulation study in which individual dosage adjustments were determined to achieve a steady-state theophylline concentration (C_{ss}) of 15 µg/mL. When using a sampling interval of 0.3 half-lives, the actual values for C_{ss} were in the interval of 8 to 30 µg/mL for 95% of the simulated subjects. With the time interval between samples increased to equal the mean population half-life, the 95% concentration interval was 12 to 21 µg/mL, indicating a clinically important improvement in achieving the target concentration in the patient population.

This example demonstrates the benefits of using a quantitative sample schedule analysis to guide the design of a therapeutic drug monitoring strategy. General-purpose software is available to perform the required computations.[98,107,108] Combining the results from such an analysis with population simulation studies of a candidate therapeutic protocol can provide information on prediction errors expected from the clinical implementation of the proposed feedback control process, thereby leading to better strategies for individualizing drug therapy.

Recent work on techniques for the design of nonlinear parameter estimation experiments have focused on formally including more complete prior parameter information to provide design resistance ("robustness") to the inaccuracy of parameter estimation.[104] Several proposed approaches involve maximizing the expected value, over a prior parameter distribution, of some function of the Fisher information matrix.[109,110] Other parameter robust design strategies are based on the efficiency of a design relative to local D-optimal designs (D-efficiency), and are calculated to either maximize the expected D-efficiency or maximize the minimum D-efficiency over some admissible parameter domain.[111,112] Further evaluation of these approaches on representative pharmacokinetic examples are needed, as well as general software that implements these computationally intensive experiment design methods.

PERFORMANCE OF PHARMACOKINETICALLY BASED DOSING METHODS

Performance of dosing methods may be judged on a pharmacokinetic, pharmacodynamic, or clinical cost/benefit basis. Pharmacokinetic performance measures include accuracy and precision of drug concentration prediction or achievement; pharmacodynamic performance comprises forecasting and achievement of pharmacologic or clinical outcomes; and cost/benefit performance embraces appraisal of economic as well as qualitative sociologic values. Two important contributions to the establishment of objective standards for measuring predictive performance and cost/benefit utilities are the papers of Sheiner and Beal[113] and Bootman et al.[23] Since Burton et al.[24] have reviewed comparative pharmacokinetic and cost/benefit performance of various dosing methods, and Schumacher and Barr[42] have summarized reports of pharmacokinetic performance studies using Bayesian dosing methods, we will illustrate comparative performance by citing a few representative reports.

Accuracy and precision of prediction and achievement of target drug concentrations are often assessed by tabulating the mean error (ME), mean absolute error (MAE), and root mean squared prediction error (RMSE).[113] While population-based dosing algorithms may, in some instances, appear to be accurate (ME not significantly different from zero) when applied to a group of patients, individual prediction errors contribute to large values for precision relative to the drug's therapeutic range. Examples of this include reports of algorithmic prediction of concentrations of digoxin: RMSE = 0.6, 0.64 ng/mL,[13,16] MAE = 0.45 ng/mL;[28] lidocaine: RMSE = 0.9, 1.1, and 1.6 µg/mL;[16,27,114] and theophylline: RMSE = 13.2, 7.8 µg/mL.[16,115] Bayesian prediction and dosing methods using measured drug concentrations to individualize pharmacokinetic estimates usually improve prediction precision. For comparison with the above, the following have been reported for digoxin: RMSE = 0.35, 0.36, and 0.30, 0.24 ng/mL (one or two digoxin concentrations, respectively);[16,28] lidocaine: RMSE 0.7, 0.55, 0.9 µg/mL;[16,114,116] theophylline: RMSE = 2.3, 1.2 µg/mL,[16,117] MAE = 1.1 µg/mL.[117]

Two studies of the impact of dosing methods of theophylline on clinical outcome in asthmatic patients serve to illustrate assessments of pharmacodynamic performance. Mungall et al.[12] reported fewer adverse reactions (16% versus 50%) and shorter intensive care unit (7 versus 12 days) or hospital (15 versus 22 days) stays in patients whose theophylline regimens were individualized pharmaco-kinetically compared to "empirically" derived dosages. Vozeh et al.[21] demonstrated that pharmacokinetically individualized regimens improved clinical outcome when drug concentrations fell within the therapeutic range. Comparing two patient groups achieving average theophylline concentrations of 9.7 and 19 µg/mL, respectively, they showed a 50% improvement in pulmonary function and a 50% reduction in duration of intravenous therapy in the group with higher concentrations.

Comparable demonstrations of the efficacy of pharmacokinetically based amino-glycoside dosing methods, especially those utilizing blood concentrations for forecasting and controlling pharmacokinetic outcomes have been reported. Moreover, a sophisticated cost/benefit analysis has been reported for aminoglycoside therapy using a formal econometric model.[23] In this investigation, direct benefits in dollar values of individualized gentamicin therapy in burn patients included lengths of hospital stay and of infection, number of septic episodes, number of adverse drug reactions, as well as various related hospitalization and treatment costs. This report served not just to demonstrate an $8.70 savings for every $1.00 spent on pharmacokinetic services, but also to demonstrate the use of a credible econometric model for investigating cost/benefit outcomes of dosing methods.

Such evidence of benefit from applied pharmacokinetics is leading to expansion into new therapeutic areas (such as oncology)[118] with inclusion of pharmacody-namic endpoints,[119] study design to assess therapeutic response,[120] and Phase I-II clinical trials.[50,121,122] Large prospective clinical trials[123] are being undertaken to compare these innovative approaches to conventional therapeutic methods that rely on average doses and clinical judgment. In addition, adaptive control of dosage regimens (in the context of randomized concentration-controlled clinical trials) has been proposed as an alternative to traditional placebo or dose-controlled trials.[124]

Quantitative strategies for optimizing drug regimens in patients are now feasible in the context of routine patient care. Such strategies are becoming more widely used and offer substantial potential for improving patient outcomes. Additional clinical research will provide more sophisticated and powerful pharmacokinetic tools, but these will have to be carefully examined to determine which method is most appropriate for a given therapeutic situation. Selecting the "best" dose is a necessary but not sufficient condition for a successful therapeutic outcome. However, applied pharmacokinetic strategies that recognize and control for intra- and intersubject variability in drug disposition, have now been demonstrated to be feasible and clinically useful for drugs with narrow therapeutic indices.

REFERENCES

1. Gerlowski L, Jain R. Physiologically based pharmacokinetic modeling: principles and applications. J Pharm Sci. 1983;10:1103–126.
2. Godfrey K. Compartmental models and their application. New York: Academic Press; 1983.
3. Jacquez J. Compartmental Analysis in Biology and Medicine. Amsterdam: Elsevier Publishing; 1972.
4. Yamaoko K et al. Statistical moments in pharmacokinetics. J Pharmacokin Biopharm. 1978;6:547.
5. Benet L, Galeazzi R. Non-compartmental determination of the steady-state volume of distribution. J Pharm Sci. 1979;8:1071–74.
6. Riegelman S, Collier P. The application of statistical moment theory to ther evaluation of *in vivo* dissolution time and absorption time. J Pharmacokin Biopharm. 1980;8:509.
7. Chow AT, Jusko WJ. Application of moment analysis to nonlinear drug disposition described by the Michaelis Menten equation. Pharm Res. 1987;4:59.
8. DiStefano JJ. Non-compartmental vs. compartmental analysis: some basis for choice. Am J Physiol. 1982;243:R1–R6.
9. Grevel J et al. Area-under-the-curve monitoring of cyclosporine therapy: performance of different assay methods and their target concentrations. Ther Drug Monit. 1990;12:8.
10. Holford NHG, Sheiner LB. Understanding the dose-effect relationship: clinical application of pharmacokinetic-pharmacodynamic models. Clin Pharmacokin. 1981;6:429.
11. Jelliffe R. An improved method of digoxin therapy. Ann Intern Med. 1968;4:703-17.
12. Mungall D et al. Individualizing theophylline therapy: the impact of clinical pharmacokinctics on patient outcomes. Ther Drug Monit. 1983;5:95–101.
13. Ried LD et al. Therapeutic drug monitoring reduces toxic drug reactions: a meta-Analysis. Ther Drug Monit. 1990;12:72.
14. Richens A, Dunlop A. Serum phenytoin levels in management of epilepsy. Lancet. 1975;9:247–48.
15. Schumacher GE, Barr JT. Making serum drug levels more meaningful. Ther Drug Monit. 1989;11:580.
16. Whiting B et al. Clinical pharmacokinetics: a comprehensive system for therapeutic drug monitoring and prescribing. Br Med J. 1984;288:641.
17. Hull J, Sarubbi F. Gentamicin serum concentrations: pharmacokinetic predictions. Ann Intern Med. 1976;85:183–89.
18. Peck C et al. Computer-assisted digoxin therapy. N Engl J Med. 1973;9:441–46.
19. Peck CC et al. Clinical pharmacodynamics of theophylline. J Allergy Clin Immunol. 1985;76:292–97.
20. Sawchuk R et al. Kinetic model for gentamicin dosing with the use of individual patient parameters. Clin Pharmacol Ther. 1977;21:362–69.
21. Vozeh S, Steimer JL. Feedback control methods for drug dosage optimization. Clin Pharmacokin. 1985;10:457–76.
22. Jelliffe RW. Open-loop feedback control of serum drug concentrations: pharmacokinetic approaches to drug therapy. Medical Instr. 1983;17:267.
23. Bootman J et al. Individualizing gentamicin dosage regimens in burn patients with gram-negative septicemia: a cost-benefit analysis. J Pharm Sci. 1979;3:267–72.
24. Burton ME et al. Comparison of drug dosing methods. Clin Pharmacokin. 1985;10:1–37.
25. Jelliffe R, Buell J, Kalaba R. Reduction of digitalis toxicity by computer-assisted glycoside dosage regimens. Ann Intern Med. 1972;77:891–906.
26. Mallet A et al. Handling covariates in population pharmacokinetics with an application to gentamicin. Biomed Meas Infor Contr. 1988;2:673–83.
27. Rodman J et al. Clinical studies with computer-assisted initial lidocaine therapy. Arch Intern Med. 1984;144:703–9.
28. Sheiner L et al. Improved computer-assisted digoxin therapy: a method using feedback of measured serum digoxin concentrations. Ann Intern Med. 1975;82:619-27.
29. Jusko WJ et al. Factors affecting theophylline clearances. J Pharm Sci. 1979;68:1358–366.
30. Ludden T et al. Individualization of phenytoin dosage regimens. Clin Pharmacol Ther. 1977;21:287–93.

31. Peck CC. Bedside clinical pharmacokinetics: simple techniques for individualizing drug therapy. Rockville, MD: Pharmacometrics Press; 1985.

32. Crom WR et al. Pharmacokinetics of anticancer drugs in children. Clin Pharmacokin. 1987;12:168.

33. Sheiner LB et al. Estimation of population characteristics of pharmacokinetic parameters from routine clinical data. J Pharmacokin Biopharm. 1977;5:445–79.

34. Sheiner LB. Modeling pharmacokinetic/pharmacodynamic variability. In: Rowland M et al., eds. Variability in Drug Therapy. New York: Raven Press; 1985;51–64.

35. Steimer JL et al. Estimating interindividual pharmacokinetic variability. In Variability in Drug Therapy, M Rowland et al., eds. New York: Raven Press; 1985;65–111.

36. Mallet A. A maximum likelihood estimation method or random coefficient regression models. Biometrika. 1986;73:645–56.

37. Sheiner LB et al. Forecasting individual pharmacokinetics. Clin Pharmacol Ther. 1979;26:294–305.

38. Sheiner LB, Beal SL. Bayesian individualization of pharmacokinetics: simple implementation and comparison with non-Bayesian methods. J Pharm Sci. 1982;71:1344.

39. Katz D et al. Bayesian approach to the analysis of nonlinear models: implementation and evaluation. Biometrics. 1981;37:137–42.

40. Jelliffe R et al. A time-shared computer program for adaptive control of lidocaine therapy using an optimal strategy for obtaining serum concentrations. Comp Applic Med Care. 1980;3:975–81.

41. Murphy MG et al. An evaluation of Bayesian microcomputer predictions of theophylline concentrations in newborn infants. Ther Drug Monit. 1990;12:47.

42. Schumacher GE, Barr JT. Bayesian approaches in pharmacokinetic decision making. Clin Pharm. 1984;3:525–29.

43. Burton ME et al. Accuracy of Bayesian and Sawchuk-Zaske dosing methods for gentamicin. Clin Pharm. 1986;5:143.

44. Burton ME et al. A Bayesian feedback method of aminoglycoside dosing. Clin Pharmacol Ther. 1985;35:349.

45. Burton ME et al. Evaluation of a Bayesian method for predicting vancomycin dosing. Drug Int Clin Pharm. 1989;23:294.

46. Serre-Deveauvais F et al. Bayesian estimation of cyclosporine clearance in bone marrow graft. Ther Drug Monit. 1990;12:16.

47. Chrystyn H. Validation of the use of Bayesian analysis in the optimization of gentamicin therapy from the commencement of dosing. Drug Int Clin Pharm. 1988;22:49.

48. Kelman AW, Whiting B. A Bayesian approach to the utility of drug therapy. Biomed Meas Inform Contr. 1988;2:170.

49. Pryka RD et al. Individualizing vancomycin dosage regimens: one versus two compartment Bayesian models. Ther Drug Monit. 1989;11:450.

50. Rodman JH et al. Pharmacokinetics of continuous infusion methotrexate and teniposide in pediatric cancer patients. Cancer Res. 1990;50:4267.

51. Vozeh S et al. Computer-assisted drug assay interpretation based on Bayesian estimation of individual pharmacokinetics: application to lidocaine. Ther Drug Monit. 1985;7:66.

52. Zantvoort FA et al. Evaluation of a microcomputer program for parameter optimisation in clinical pharmacokinetics: gentamicin and tobramycin. Br J Clin Pharmacol. 1987;24:511.

53. Hurst AK et al. A comparison of different methods for predicting serum gentamicin concentrations in surgical patients with perforated and gangrenous appendicitis. Clin Pharm. 1987;6:234.

54. Rodman JH et al. Pharmacokinetics and clinical response of NAPA during multiple dosing. Clin Pharmacol Ther. 1982;32:378.

55. Schumitzky A et al. Stochastic control of pharmacokinetic systems. Comp Applic Med Care. 1983;7:222–25.

56. Schumitzky A. Stochastic control of pharmacokinetic systems. In: Maronde RF ed. Clinical Pharmacology and Therapeutics. New York: Springer Verlaag; 1986;13.

57. Peck C et al. A microcomputer drug (theophylline) dosing program which assists and teaches physicians. Comp Appl Med Care. 1980;4:988–94.

58. Sheiner L et al. Modeling of individual pharmacokinetics for computer-aided drug dosage. Comput Biomed Res. 1972;5:441–59.

59. Gaillot J et al. *A priori* lithium dosage regimen using population characteristics of pharmaco-kinetic parameters. J Pharmacokin Biopharm. 1979;7:579.

60. Richter O, Teinhardt. Methods for evaluating optimal dosage regimens and their application to theophylline. Int J Clin Pharmacol. 1982;20:564

61. D'Argenio DZ, Katz D. Application of stochastic control methods the problem of individual-izing intravenous theophylline therapy. Biomed Meas Inform Contr. 1988;2:115.

62. Katz D, D'Argenio DZ. Implementation and evaluation of control strategies for individualizing dosage regimens, with application to the aminoglycoside antibiotics. J Pharmacokin Biopharm. 1986;14:523.

63. van Rossum JM. Systems dynamics in clinical pharmacokinetics. An introduction. Clin Phar-macokin. 1989;17:27.

64. Sheiner LB. Analysis of pharmacokinetic data using parametric models-1: regression models. J Pharmacokin Biopharm. 1984;1:93–117.

65. Sheiner LB. Analysis of pharmacokinetic data using parametric models. II. Point estimates of an individuals parameters. J Pharmacokin Biopharm. 1985;13:514.

66. Sheiner LB. Analysis of pharmacokinetic data using parametric models. III. Hypothesis tests and confidence intervals. J Pharmacokin Biopharm. 1986;14:539.

67. D'Argenio DZ, Schumitzky A. A program package for simulation and parameter estimation in pharmacokinetic systems. Comput Prog Biomed. 1979;9:115.

68. Peck CC et al. Extended least squares nonlinear regression: a possible solution to the "choice of weights" problem in analysis of individual pharmacokinetic data. J Pharmacokinet Biopharm. 1984;12:545–58.

69. Vozeh S, Steiner C. Estimates of the population pharmacokinetic parameters and performance of Bayesian feedback: a sensitivity analysis. J Pharmacokin Biopharm. 1987;15:511.

70. Peck CC, Chen BC. Importance of assumptions in Bayesian pharmacokinetic control of drug therapy. Clin Pharm Ther. 1985;37:220.

71. Koup JR et al. Pharmacokinetics of digoxin in normal subjects after intravenous bolus and infusion doses. J Pharmacokinet Biopharm. 1975;3:181–92.

72. Koup JR et al. Digoxin pharmacokinetics: role of renal failure in dosage regimen design. Clin Pharmacol Ther. 1975;18:9–21.

73. Myhill J. Investigation of the effect of data error in the analysis of biological tracer data from three compartment systems. J Theor Biol. 1968;23:218–31.

74. Westlake W. Problems associated with analysis of pharmacokinetic models. J Pharm Sci. 1971;6:882–85.

75. Driscoll MS et al. Evaluation theophylline pharmacokinetics in a pediatric population using mixed effects models. J Pharmacokin Biopharm. 1989;17:141.

76. Grasela TH et al. An evaluation of population pharmacokinetics in therapeutic trials. Part I. Comparison of methodologies. Clin Pharmacol Ther. 1986;39:605.

77. Grasela TH et al. An evaluation of population pharmacokinetics in therapeutic trials. Part II. Detection of a drug-drug interaction. Clin Pharmacol Ther. 1987;42:433.

78. Antal EJ et al. An evaluation of population pharmacokinetics in therapeutic trial. Part III. Prospective data collection versus retrospective data assembly. Clin Pharmacol Ther. 1989;46:552.

79. Graves DA, Chang I. Application of NONMEM to routine bioavailability data. J Pharmacokin Biopharm. 1990;18:145.

80. Rodman JH, Silverstein K. Comparison of two stage and first order methods for estimation of population pharmacokinetic parameters. Clin Pharmacol Ther. 1990;47:151.

81. Vozeh S et al. Evaluation of population (NONMEM) pharmacokinetic parameter estimates. J Pharmacokin Biopharm. 1990;18:161.

82. D'Argenio DZ, Maneval DM. Estimation approaches for modeling sparse data systems. In: IFAC Symposium: Modeling and Control in Biomedical Systems. Venice, Italy. 1988;61.

83. Beal SL. Population pharmacokinetic data and parameter estimation based on their first two statistical moments. Drug Metab Rev. 1984;15:173.

84. Sheiner LB, Beal SL. Evaluation of methods for estimating population pharmacokinetic parameters II. Biexponential model and experimental pharmacokinetic data. J Pharmacokin Biopharm. 1981;8:635–51.

85. Mallet A et al. Nonparametric maximum likelihood estimation for population pharmacokinetics. An application to cyclosporine. J Pharmacokin Biopharm. 1988;16:311–27.

86. Mentre F et al. Population kinetics of AZT in AIDS patients. Europ J Clin Pharmacol. 1989;36:230.

87. Slattery JT. Single-point maintenance dose prediction: role of interindividual differences in clearance and volume of distribution in choice of sampling time. J Pharm Sci. 1981;70:1174–176.

88. Bahn MM, Landaw EM. A minimax approach to the single-point method of drug dosing. J Pharmacokin Biopharm. 1987;15:255.

89. Loft S et al. Metronidazole clearance: a one-sample method and influencing factors. Clin Pharmacol Ther. 1988;43:420.

90. Ratain MJ, Vogelzang NJ. Limited sampling model for vinblastine pharmacokinetics. Cancer Treat Rep. 1987;71:935.

91. Kerr IG et al. Test dose for predicting high dose methotrexate infusions. Clin Pharmacol Ther. 1982;33:44–51.

92. Ritschel W. The one-point method as a clinical tool to calculate and/or adjust dosage regimens. Drug Dev Indust Pharm. 1977;3:547–53.

93. Lacey L, Dunne A. The design of pharmacokinetic experiments for model discrimination. J Pharmacokinet Biopharm. 1984;12:351–65.

94. Katz D, D'Argenio DZ. Experimental design for estimating integrals by numerical quadrature, with application to pharmacokinetic studies. Biometrics. 1983;39:621–28.

95. D'Argenio DZ, Katz D. Sampling strategies for noncompartmental estimation of mean residence time. J Pharmacokin Biopharm. 1983;11:435–46.

96. Westlake WJ. Use of statistical methods in evaluation of *in vivo* performance of dosage forms. J Pharm Sci. 1973;62:1579–589.

97. DiStefano III JJ. Optimized blood sampling protocols and sequential design of kinetic experiments. Am J Physiol. 1981;9:259–65.

98. D'Argenio DZ. Optimal sampling times for pharmacokinetic experiments. J Pharmacokin Biopharm. 1981;9:739–56.

99. Endrenyi L. Design of experiments for estimating enzyme and pharmacokinetic parameters. In: Kinetic Data Analysis. New York: Plenum Press; 1980;137-67.

100. Landaw EM. Optimal multicompartmental sampling designs for parameter estimation: practical aspects of the identification problem. Math Comp Simulat. 1982;24:525–30.

101. Drusano GL et al. An evaluation of optimal sampling strategy and adaptive study design. Clin Pharmacol Ther. 1988;44:232–38.

102. Drusano GL et al. A prospective evaluation of optimal sampling theory in the determination of the steady-state pharmacokinetics of piperacillin in febrile neutropenic cancer patients. Clin Pharmacol Ther. 1989;45:635–41.

103. Box GEP, Lucas HL. Design of experiments in nonlinear situations. Biometrika. 1959;46:77–90.

104. Walter E, Pronzato L. Qualitative and quantitative experiment design for phenomenological models—a survey. Automatica. 1990;26:195–213.

105. D'Argenio DZ, Khakmahd K. Adaptive control of theophylline therapy, importance of blood sampling times. J Pharmacokin Biopharm. 1983;11(5):547–59.

106. Peck CC, Chen BC. Influence of sampling times of drug levels in Bayesian pharmacokinetic control of drug therapy. Clin Pharmacol Ther. 1985;37:220.

107. DiStefano III JJ. Algorithms, software and sequential optimal sampling schedule designs for pharmacokinetic and physiologic experiments. Math Comput Simulat. 1982;24:531–34.

108. Vila JP. New algorithmic and software tools for D-optimal design computation in nonlinear regression. COMPSTAT, Physica, Heidelberg. 1988;409–14.

109. Walter E, Pronzato L. Optimal experiment design for nonlinear models subject to large prior parameter uncertainties. Am J Physiol. 253;530–34.

110. D'Argenio DZ. Incorporating prior parameter uncertainty in the design of sampling schedules for pharmacokinetic parameter estimation experiments. Math Biosciences. 1990;99:105–18.

111. Suverkrup R. Optimization of sampling schedules for pharmacokinetic data analysis and evaluation techniques. Bolzer G, Van Rossum UTM, eds. Stuttgart: Gustav Fischer Verlag. 1982;174–90.

112. Landaw EM. Optimal design for individual parameter estimation in pharmacokinetics. Description, Estimation, and Control. In: Variability in Drug Therapy. Rowland M, et al., eds. New York: Raven Press. 1985;187–200.

113. Sheiner LB, Beal SL. Some suggestions for measuring predictive performance. J Pharmacokinet Biopharm. 1981;9:503–12.

114. Vozeh S et al. Accurate prediction of lidocaine individual dosage requirements. Clin Pharmacol Ther. 1983;33:212.

115. Vozeh S et al. Accurate prediction of theophylline serum concentrations using a rapid estimation of theophylline clearance. Clin Pharmacol Ther. 1980;27:291.

116. Lenert LA et al. Lidocaine forecaster: a two-compartment Bayesian patient pharmacokinetic computer program. Clin Pharmacol Ther. 1982;31:242.

117. Lenert L et al. Bayesian pharmacokinetic forecasting as a research tool. Clin Pharmacol Ther. 1983;33:201.

118. Moore MJ, Erlichman C. Therapeutic drug monitoring in oncology. Clin Pharmacokin. 1987;13:205.

119. Evans WE, Relling MV. Clinical pharmacokinetics-pharmacodynamics of anticancer drugs in children. Clin Pharmacokin. 1989;16:327.

120. Sheiner LB et al. Study designs for dose ranging. Clin Pharmacol Ther. 1989;46:63.

121. Ratain MJ et al. Adaptive control of etoposide administration: impact of interpatient pharmacodynamic variability. Clin Pharmacol Ther. 1989;45:226.

122. Conley BA et al. Phase I trial using adaptive control of hexamethylene bisacetamide(NSC 95580). Cancer Res. 1989;49:3436.

123. Evans WE et al. Individualized chemotherapy: pharmacokinetic dose adjustments of pulse therapy for childhood acute lymphocytic leukemia. Clin Pharmacol Ther. 1990;47:151.

124. Peck CC. The randomized concentration controlled clinical trial: an information rich alternative to the randomized placebo controlled clinical trial. Clin Pharmacol Ther. 1990;47:148.

Chapter 4

Pharmacodynamics

Richard L. Lalonde

S ome confusion exists over the use of the term pharmacodynamics because there is no clearly accepted definition. It is relevant to first look at the Greek roots of the word itself. "Pharmakon" is translated as drug, whereas "dynamikos" means power. If pharmacokinetics is the movement (i.e., kinetics) of drugs, then pharmacodynamics in its most common usage, is the action (i.e., "power") of drugs. More specifically, pharmacodynamics has been defined as the study of the biological effects resulting from the interaction between drugs and biological systems.[1] Figure 4-1 is a simplistic illustration of how pharmacokinetics and pharmacodynamics determine the observed pharmacologic effects of a drug. This figure also demonstrates the limitation of standard pharmacokinetic investigations which stop short of assessing the actual consequences or effects (efficacy/toxicity) of the observed plasma drug concentrations. Since the late 1970s, there has been an increased emphasis on combining pharmacokinetics and pharmacodynamics in the clinical evaluation of drugs. This has resulted in a large increase in the body of knowledge on the relationshp between pharmacokinetics and pharmacodynamics. Proposals for the development of randomized concentration-controlled trials, as opposed to the more traditional randomized dose-controlled trials, are other examples of the increased emphasis given to the pharmacokinetic-pharmacodynamic relationship in the evaluation of drugs.[82]

Figure 4-1 also illustrates why pharmacokinetics and pharmacodynamics are often linked. The relationship between drug dose and biological fluid concentra-

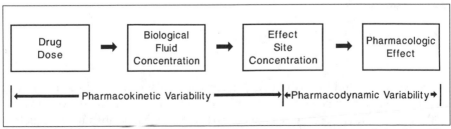

Figure 4-1. Pharmacokinetics and pharmacodynamics as determinants of the dose-effect relationship.

tion is most useful when it also is linked to a pharmacologic effect that is associated with a particular concentration. Similarly, the pharmacologic response by itself does not provide information about some very important determinants of that response (e.g., dose, drug concentration in plasma or at the site of action). This chapter focuses on the evaluation of concentration-effect relationship (pharmaco-dynamics) and the advantages of linking this information to pharmacokinetic principles.

The relationship between drug concentration and pharmacologic response depends on the mechanism by which a drug exerts its effect. Some drugs exert a direct reversible effect which is often mediated through binding with a specific receptor (beta blockers, neuromuscular blocking agents). For these drugs, there should be a direct relationship between the time course of drug concentrations and pharmacologic effect. For certain other drugs, the effect is indirect. The best example is warfarin which blocks the synthesis of vitamin K-dependent clotting factors but has no effect on the degradation of these same factors. In this case, drug concentration may be related to clotting factor synthesis but only indirectly related to the ultimate therapeutic effect.[2] Although most pharmacologic effects are reversible, certain drugs have an irreversible effect. The best examples are bactericidal antibiotics and antineoplastic agents, both of which cause cell death after being irreversibly incorporated into specific cellular biochemical processes. Because more data are available on those drugs that exert a direct and reversible effect, greater emphasis will be put on this type of drug action in this chapter.

RECEPTOR THEORY AS A BASIS FOR PHARMACODYNAMICS

The most useful models to describe the relationship between drug dose or plasma concentrations and pharmacologic response can be derived from the law of mass action. Pharmacologic response can be assumed to reflect the combination of drug molecules with receptors. Let R represent the concentration of available or unoccupied receptors, C the concentration of drug in the receptor "compart-ment," and RC the concentration of receptor-drug complex. If drug binding to the receptor is reversible as shown below:

$$R + C \xrightarrow{\ k_1\ } RC \xrightarrow{\ k_2\ } R + C \qquad \text{(Eq. 4-1)}$$

then at equilibrium:

$$\frac{(R)\,(C)}{RC} = \frac{k_2}{k_1} = K_d \qquad \text{(Eq. 4-2)}$$

where K_d is the equilibrium dissociation constant of the receptor-drug complex. If R_T equals the total concentration of receptors, then $R_T = R + RC$. If we solve for R, the concentration of receptors not bound to any drug, and substitute in Equation 4-2, we obtain the following:

$$\frac{(R_T - RC)\,(C)}{RC} = K_d \qquad \text{(Eq. 4-3)}$$

which can be rearranged to give Equation 4-4.

$$\frac{RC}{R_T} = \frac{C}{K_d + C} \qquad \text{(Eq. 4-4)}$$

If it is assumed that the extent of pharmacologic response (E) is proportional to the concentration of receptors that are occupied, then E and RC can be related by an arbitrary constant α, so that $E = \alpha \times RC$. Similarly, if the maximal response (E_{max}) occurs when all receptors are occupied, then E_{max} will be related to R_T by the same arbitrary constant, so that $E_{max} = \alpha \times R_T$. Substitution of these values of RC and R_T into the left side of Equation 4-4 yields:

$$\frac{E}{E_{max}} = \frac{C}{K_d + C} \qquad \text{(Eq. 4-5)}$$

and

$$E = \frac{(E_{max})\,(C)}{K_d + C} \qquad \text{(Eq. 4-6)}$$

Furthermore, if n drug molecules bind to each receptor site, then Equation 4-6 will be modified as follows:

$$E = \frac{(E_{max})\,(C^n)}{K_d + C^n} \qquad \text{(Eq. 4-7)}$$

where K_d is the dissociation constant for the interaction of n molecules with a receptor. It must be emphasized that certain assumptions are made in the derivation and usual application of Equations 4-6 and 4-7. First, response is assumed to be proportional to the concentration of receptors that are occupied at a particular time ("receptor occupancy theory"). Although this assumption appears logical, maximum response can be produced in certain biological systems without total receptor occupancy. In addition, it is assumed that a negligible amount of drug is bound to the receptor relative to the total amount of drug (C_T) so that the concentration of drug not bound to the receptor (C), as used in the above equations, is approximated by C_T. The response at equilibrium is also assumed to be independent of time (i.e., no development of tolerance or sensitization). The hyperbolic function described by Equation 4-6 is very useful to describe the dose/concentration-effect relationship for numerous systems. It is intuitively appealing because the function predicts no effect in the absence of drug and a maximum effect as the dose or concentration approaches infinity. The more general Equation 4-7 has also been widely used, often without any specific knowledge of the number of molecules that bind to a specific receptor (i.e., value of n).

Similar equations and models have been used to describe a variety of biochemical processes (e.g., protein binding, enzyme kinetics). The classic Michaelis-Menten equation, which relates the rate of a chemical reaction to the concentration of substrate, the maximum velocity (V_{max}) and the Michaelis constant (K_m), is in the form of Equation 4-6. The same relationship is used to describe the rate of elimination of drugs like phenytoin which exhibit saturable hepatic metabolism. The equation is also analogous to the Langmuir adsorption isotherm which is used to describe the adsorption of gases to solid surfaces.[3] Similarly, the association of oxygen and hemoglobin was described by Hill[4] in 1910 using the following equation:

$$\% \text{ saturation of hemoglobin} = \frac{(100)\,(K)\,(C^n)}{1 + (K)\,(C^n)} \qquad \text{(Eq. 4-8)}$$

where C is oxygen tension, K and n are parameters of the model, and 100 represents the maximum saturation when the latter is expressed as a percentage. Equation 4-8 can be rearranged to the form of Equation 4-7 (K in Equation 4-8 is equivalent to $1/K_d$ in Equation 4-7) and is often called the Hill equation. It is noteworthy that Hill used Equation 4-8 empirically without necessarily attributing any particular significance to the parameters K and n.

Clark is generally recognized as the first investigator to have used pharmacodynamic models, based on the concept of drug-receptor interactions, to evaluate the effects of drugs.[5] He evaluated the effects of acetylcholine on isolated frog muscles and used yet another rearrangement of Equation 4-7 to describe the relationship between drug concentration (C) and pharmacologic response (E) expressed as a percentage of the maximum effect:

$$\frac{E}{100 - E} = (K)\,(C^n) \qquad \text{(Eq. 4-9)}$$

where K and n are model parameters and 100 is the maximum effect (K in Equation 4-9 is equivalent to $1/K_d$ in Equation 4-7). Based on his results, Clark proposed that this particular effect of acetylcholine was mediated by a reversible monomolecular interaction with a drug receptor. Interestingly, he also commented on the limitations of a simple log-linear model (see Pharmacodynamic Models: Logarithmic Models) to describe the concentration-effect relationship at very low or very high drug concentrations.

Based on the above discussion, it should be apparent that many pharmacodynamic concepts and principles have their roots in a rather broad range of scientific endeavors. The mathematical relationships are relatively simple and can be derived by application of principles that have been widely recognized for several decades.[6,7]

PHARMACODYNAMIC MODELS

Models are typically used to help provide a simplified description of the observations in an experiment and possibly make predictions for future experiments. In many ways, the use of pharmacodynamic models to assess concentration-effect relationships *in vivo* is an extension of the same principles that investigators have used for several decades with *in vitro* data (see above). Traditionally, pharmacodynamic models relate *effect site* concentrations and pharmacologic response. Whenever plasma or other tissue concentrations are used in pharmacodynamic models, there is an inherent assumption that these concentrations are in equilibrium with those at the effect site. This may be difficult to validate when dealing with clinical data and may necessitate the use of more complex pharmacodynamic models that are linked to pharmacokinetic models (see below). The most widely used pharmacodynamic models are described briefly below.[1,8–10]

Fixed-Effect Model

The simplest model relates drug concentration to a pharmacologic effect that is either present or absent (e.g., relapse of leukemia, seizures). Alternatively, the fixed response could be a specific measure of effect such as a ventricular rate less than 100 beats per minute in patients with atrial fibrillation. In either case, there is no assumption about the shape of the concentration-effect relationship except that pharmacologic response is present above a certain concentration and absent below it. Because this threshold concentration will vary among patients, the fraction of patients that respond at a particular concentration will be a function of the threshold concentration distribution in the population.[1] The cumulative response rate in the population, as a function of concentration, will have a sigmoid shape. However, the basis for this sigmoidal relationship (i.e., statistical distribution of threshold concentration in the population) is different from that of the sigmoid E_{max} model described below which is based on receptor-drug interaction in each subject. The cumulative response rate can be compared to the cumulative adverse effect or toxicity rate of a drug in order to obtain a measure of the therapeutic index (e.g., concentration that produces toxicity in 50% of patients divided by the concentration that produces a desired response in 50% of patients).

Sigmoid E_{max} Model

The Hill equation, rearranged in the form of Equation 4-7, has been proposed as a useful model to describe the *in vivo* relationship between dose/concentration and continuous pharmacologic effect for many different drugs.[8] The equation can be reparameterized as follows:

$$E = \frac{(E_{max})\,(C^n)}{EC_{50}^n + C^n} \qquad \text{(Eq. 4-10)}$$

where C is the drug concentration and EC_{50} is the "effective" concentration that produces half of the maximum effect attributable to the drug (E_{max}). The only difference compared to Equation 4-7 is that the parameter K_d is replaced with EC_{50}^n. This latest version has been called the sigmoid E_{max} model and is conceptually simpler because it includes a parameter, EC_{50}, that is more relevant in clinical pharmacology.[1] Although Equation 4-10 can be derived based on receptor theory, one must be cautious in attributing any particular meaning to certain parameters when the model is applied to clinical pharmacodynamic data. Theoretically, n is an integer reflecting the number of molecules that bind to a specific drug receptor, but non-integer values can be obtained when analyzing specific data. For example, values of n of 2.3 to 20 for tocainide suppression of ventricular ectopic depolarizations probably cannot be taken to reflect the number of molecules that bind to any receptor.[11] There may not even be any convincing evidence that a particular drug exerts its pharmacologic effect through an interaction with a specific receptor. This should not detract from using the model which may still provide a very good and simple method to describe and/or predict pharmacologic response. Therefore, the sigmoid E_{max} model and other models must often be regarded as empirical mathematical functions that describe the shape of the concentration-effect relationship for a particular drug. In this context, n can be considered a parameter that determines the sigmoid shape of the relationship (see Figure 4-2). If n equals 1, a simple hyperbolic function will result (see Pharmacodynamic Models: E_{max} Model below). When n is greater than 1, the function becomes more sigmoid in shape with a steeper slope in its central region. Conversely, when n is less than 1, the curve is steeper at low concentrations but more shallow at higher concentrations.

Investigators should resist the temptation to use the sigmoid E_{max} model if a simpler model (see Equation 4-14) will be adequate to describe the observed data. If concentration-effect measurements are not made over a broad enough range, it

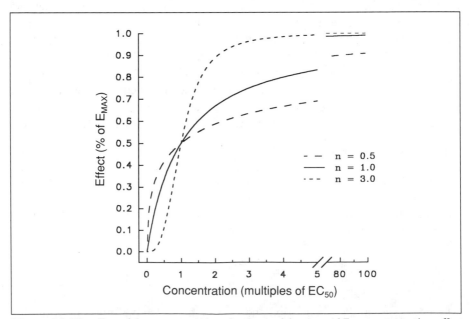

Figure 4-2. *The effect of the exponent (n) on the shape of the sigmoid E_{max} concentration-effect relationship. A hyperbolic function or E_{max} model is the result when n = 1.*

will be difficult or impossible to precisely estimate all three parameters of the model. This is particularly evident when, upon inspection of the data, there is little if any evidence that pharmacologic effects are approaching E_{max}. Similarly, whenever the experimental data do not allow the value of n to be identified precisely or its value is only slightly different from unity, then the simpler E_{max} model (see Equation 4-14 below) should probably be used. Optimal design theory should provide some valuable assistance in planning studies that will generate data from which meaningful (adequate precision and minimal bias) parameters can be estimated.[12]

As defined above, the sigmoid E_{max} model predicts that the effect will be zero when the concentration is zero. When evaluating certain responses (e.g., heart rate, blood pressure, PR interval) there is a baseline effect in the absence of drug which must be incorporated into the model. In such cases, the following modification can be used.

$$E = E_0 + \frac{(E_{max})\,(C^n)}{EC_{50}{}^n + C^n} \qquad \text{(Eq. 4-11)}$$

The only new parameter is E_0, which is the baseline effect measured in the absence of drug or preferably during placebo administration. If E_0 is known with much greater reliability than the effects measured during drug administration, then E_0 should not be estimated as a separate parameter, but the change in effect from baseline should be used.[1]

$$E - E_0 = \frac{(E_{max})\,(C^n)}{EC_{50}{}^n + C^n} \qquad \text{(Eq. 4-12)}$$

Alternatively, the percentage change instead of the absolute change from baseline could also be used. As discussed previously,[9] Equation 4-12 will avoid the paradox of estimating a value of E_0 which is significantly different from reliably known effects in the absence of drug. Colburn and Gibson[13] have discussed the potential problems that may arise when the baseline effect is due to the action of an endogenous agonist (see Pharmacodynamics of Drug Combinations).

In other cases, the effect of the drug may be the inhibition of a physiologic response such as the lowering of exercise heart rate with a beta blocker. In those circumstances, the sigmoid E_{max} equation is subtracted from the baseline effect.

$$E = E_0 - \frac{(E_{max})\,(C^n)}{EC_{50}{}^n + C^n} \qquad \text{(Eq. 4-13)}$$

When using Equation 4-13 some authors prefer to rename the EC_{50} as an inhibitory concentration or IC_{50}, but this is only semantically different. Another modification is to calculate the percentage inhibition from baseline or E_0. If the maximum effect is total inhibition of the baseline response (e.g., number of ventricular ectopic depolarizations with antiarrhythmic agents), then E_{max} and E_o will have the same value and there will be one less parameter in Equation 4-13. This approach has been used to model the antiarrhythmic effects of tocainide and cibenzoline.[11,14]

E_{max} Model

Just as Equation 4-7 can be reparameterized in terms of EC_{50} to give the sigmoid E_{max} model (Equation 4-10), Equation 4-6 can be expressed in terms of the same parameters to give the E_{max} model.

$$E = \frac{(E_{max})\,(C)}{EC_{50} + C}$$

(Eq. 4-14)

All parameters are the same as the sigmoid E_{max} model except that n equals 1 and is not estimated as a separate parameter. As discussed above, the E_{max} model can be given new parameters to evaluate data with a baseline effect, an absolute/relative change from baseline or inhibition of a baseline effect (Equations 4-11 to 4-13). Equation 4-14 is based on the interaction of a single drug molecule with a receptor site, but the same caution must be used in giving meaning to the parameters as that applied to the use of the sigmoid E_{max} model. The E_{max} model will describe a typical hyperbolic concentration-effect relationship with no effect in the absence of drug and a maximum effect (E_{max}) when concentrations approach infinity. These attributes of the E_{max} model may appear self evident or trivial, but they differentiate it from the log-linear model which historically has been the most commonly used model (see Equation 4-15).

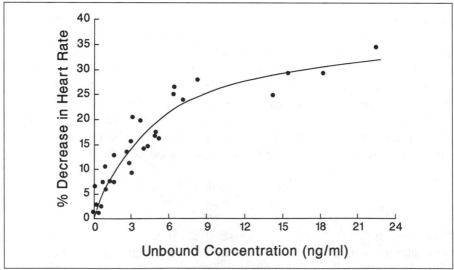

Figure 4-3. Relationship between unbound propranolol serum concentrations and the inhibition of tachycardia after a standard treadmill exercise in one subject. The solid line was obtained by nonlinear least-squares regression with the E_{max} model (reproduced with permission from reference 15).

The E_{max} model has been described as obeying the "law of diminishing returns" because of the smaller increments in pharmacologic response as concentrations increase (see Figure 4-2). This concept is also illustrated by the relationship between propranolol unbound serum concentrations and the percent inhibition of exercise heart rate (see Figure 4-3).[15] In this study of nine subjects, the mean E_{max} was 33.5% and reflects the adrenergic component of exercise-induced tachycardia. Based on the mean EC_{50} value of 1.7 ng/mL (18 ng/mL for total propranolol), 4/5 of E_{max} will be achieved at unbound concentrations of 6.8 ng/mL or total concentrations of 72 ng/mL. Relatively little additional beta blockade is produced if concentrations are increased further. Conversely at concentrations well below the EC_{50}, there is a near linear relationship between effect and concentrations. This is the basis for the linear model which can be considered as a submodel of the E_{max} model (see below). It is noteworthy that the E_{max} model, like the Michaelis-Menten equation, can be expressed in several different linear forms (direct linear plot, double reciprocal or Lineweaver-Burk method, Eadie-Hofstee plot, etc.), but that nonlinear regression using Equation 4-14 should provide the best estimates of E_{max} and EC_{50}.[16]

Logarithmic Models

In his classic paper, Clark[5] described the advantages of the logarithmic transformation of Equation 4-9 (analogous to Equations 4-7, 4-8, and 4-10 or the sigmoid E_{max} model) to give the following relationship:

$$\log \frac{E}{E_{max} - E} = \log K + (n)(\log C)$$

(Eq. 4-15)

where all parameters are as previously defined (note that E_{max} is used instead of 100 in Equation 4-9; therefore E is no longer expressed in terms of a percentage and K is equivalent to $1/K_d$ in Equation 4-7). This allows all parameters of the Hill equation or sigmoid E_{max} model to be determined by simple graphical methods or linear regression. However, a different and empirical log-linear model has traditionally been used by pharmacologists for the past several decades. This method relates the logarithm of the concentration to the effect (not the logarithm) as follows:

$$E = (S)(\log C) + A$$

(Eq. 4-16)

where A is a constant with no clear biological significance, S is a slope parameter, E and C are the same as defined for previous models. The log-linear method (Equation 4-16) will effectively compress the scale of the abscissa and facilitate graphical representation of the wide range of concentrations typically used with *in vitro* or animal studies. The major advantage of the log-linear model, however, is that it will tend to linearize the typical E_{max} or sigmoid E_{max} concentration-effect relationship when the observed effects range from 20% to 80% of the maximum response. In the past, this was particularly useful to scientists because such results could then be analyzed by simple linear regression and allowed the comparison of slopes and concentration (or dose) ratios to assess relative potency and competitive inhibition. However, linearization of data with the log-linear model is no longer such an advantage since the development of nonlinear regression methods and the widespread availability of such software for microcomputers.

Several inherent disadvantages to the log-linear model are evident upon inspection of Equation 4-16. First, pharmacologic effect cannot be predicted when the concentration is zero because of the logarithmic function. Second, there is no maximum effect predicted at very high concentrations. The absence of a maximum effect goes against some widely accepted principles of pharmacodynamics (see above). For example, competitive and noncompetitive inhibitors of a certain pharmacologic response are often differentiated based on their effects on maximum response. Finally, if an apparent maximum effect is not clearly determined by the observations, then it is difficult or impossible to conclude that specific parts of the data fall between 20% and 80% of the maximum effect. These limitations notwithstanding, the log-linear model has been used successfully by numerous investigators to describe *in vivo* pharmacodynamic data including the now classic study of the time course of anticoagulation effect of warfarin by Nagashima et al.[2]

Despite the widespread use of the log-linear model in the past, there appears to be little biological basis for such a transformation of the concentration data. Although it has been stated that the range from 20% to 80% of maximum effect is often very important, one must question the use of a model that cannot be applied to data that describe a significant portion of the concentration-effect relationship. Observations will likely deviate from the predictions of the log-linear model at concentrations well below or well above the EC_{50} and lead to errors in predicting the time course of pharmacologic effect, as was reported with the beta-blocking actions of bopindolol.[17] Consequently, the E_{max} or sigmoid E_{max} models, which can describe the whole concentration-effect relationship, should be used whenever possible.

Linear Model

When concentrations are small relative to the EC_{50}, the E_{max} model will collapse into a linear model of the form

$$E = (S)(C) \qquad\qquad (Eq.\ 4\text{-}17)$$

where S is a slope parameter which will approach the value of E_{max}/EC_{50}. At these low concentrations, E_{max} and EC_{50} cannot be determined independently but the ratio or slope can be determined. This situation is analogous to the case in pharmacokinetics where a drug may exhibit Michaelis-Menten kinetics at higher concentrations but near linear kinetics when concentrations are significantly less than the Michaelis constant, K_m. Figure 4-3 illustrates how the hyperbolic function of the E_{max} model is approximately linear at low concentrations. The linear model will predict no effect when concentrations are zero, but its major limitation is that it cannot predict a maximum effect. Like the E_{max} and sigmoid E_{max} models, the linear model can be modified to evaluate data with a baseline effect [E = (S)(C) + E_o], an absolute/relative change from baseline [E – E_o = (S)(C)] or inhibition of a baseline effect [E = E_o – (S)(C)] as described in Equations 4-11 to 4-13.

KINETICS OF PHARMACOLOGIC RESPONSE: THE LINK BETWEEN PHARMACODYNAMICS AND PHARMACOKINETICS

Direct Link Independent of a Pharmacokinetic Model

The pharmacodynamic models described above relate drug concentration at the *"effect site"* to pharmacologic response. When evaluating pharmacodynamic data *in vivo*, investigators often make the assumption that drug concentrations measured in plasma (or other tissue) are in equilibrium with those at the "effect site." It should be emphasized that it is not necessary to assume that plasma concentrations are equivalent to "effect site" concentrations but that they are in direct proportion to the "effect site" concentrations. In such studies, plasma concentrations have to be determined at the same time as the measurement of pharmacologic effect. The propranolol concentration-effect data in Figure 4-3 are an example of this approach and are therefore independent of any assumptions concerning pharmacokinetic models (see below for description of other nonparametric methods). Concentrations that are measured in other tissues or biological fluids may also be directly related to drug effect. Thus, Galeazzi et al.[18] found that saliva concentrations of procainamide were better than plasma concentrations in predicting the time course of QT interval prolongation. These results indicated that the equilibration time between plasma and saliva was similar to that between plasma and procainamide's "effect site." Consequently, saliva concentrations could be considered to be in equilibrium with the "effect site" concentrations of procainamide.

Direct Link to the Central Compartment of a Pharmacokinetic Model

Another approach is to link pharmacokinetic and pharmacodynamic models to allow a description of the time course of pharmacologic response. The simplest method is to relate pharmacologic effects to the central compartment concentrations in the pharmacokinetic model. Therefore, the C term in the various pharmacodynamic models is replaced by the equation that describes the (plasma) concentration-time profile for the drug. The use of a pharmacokinetic model will eliminate the need to measure concentration and effect at the same time since the predicted concentration can be used. Levy[19,20] was probably the first to use these principles to describe the time course of pharmacologic effect. He used a one-compartment pharmacokinetic model with first-order elimination and the log-linear pharmacodynamic model to demonstrate that pharmacologic effects would decline as a linear function of time. This principle can actually be extended to the terminal log-linear phase of drug disposition for any drug. Levy supported his theoretical arguments with observations on the time course of muscle strength after tubocurarine administration. However, these predictions will hold only for that range of pharmacologic effect where there is a linear relationship between the logarithm of the concentration and effect (about 20% to 80% of E_{max}). As indicated above, these predictions will be in error at concentrations which lead to responses that are above or below this range.[17]

A more complete description of the time course of pharmacologic effect is achieved if the pharmacokinetic model is linked to the E_{max} or sigmoid E_{max} model. Obviously, such an approach assumes that these models provide a good description of the concentration-effect relationship. Integration of these principles can help explain the relatively common observation of a discrepancy between the time course of plasma concentrations and pharmacologic effects. Over 20 years ago, Wagner did extensive simulations on the time course of pharmacologic response using the sigmoid E_{max} model and simple pharmacokinetic models.[8] A similar approach was used to relate plasma concentrations during the terminal elimination phase (first-order) and the decline in pharmacologic effect based on the E_{max} model (see Figure 4-4). In order to make the figure more generally applicable, concentrations are in multiples of EC_{50}, time is in terms of half-life and the effect is expressed as a percentage of E_{max}. Two important points are obvious upon inspection of Figure 4-4. First, there is a clear discrepancy between the rate of decline of concentrations and the rate of decline of pharmacologic effect. Second, the rate

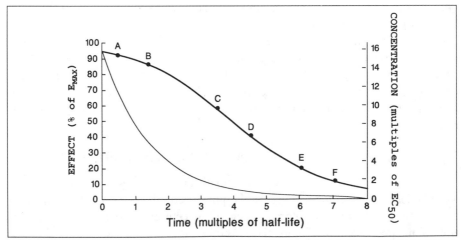

Figure 4-4. *Simulated time course of pharmacologic effect based on the E_{max} model (thick line). The simulation was done assuming first-order decline in drug concentration (thin line) and no delay in observed effect. The initial concentration is $16 \times EC_{50}$ and the time axis is in terms of the drug's elimination half-life. There is one half-life between points A and B, C and D, as well as E and F. At concentrations far exceeding the EC_{50}, a 50% decrease in concentration leads only to a small change in effect from 92.4% (A) to 85.8% (B) of E_{max}. It will take four half-lives for the initial effect to decline by one-half, thus emphasizing how the "apparent pharmacodynamic half-life" is much longer than the "pharmacokinetic half-life." At concentrations approximating the EC_{50}, the effect declines as a linear function of time, from 58.6% (C) to 41.4% (D) of E_{max}. More than 1.7 half-lives are still necessary for the effect to decline by one-half. Finally, at concentrations below $0.25 \times EC_{50}$, the effect declines from 20.0% (E) to 11.1% (F) of E_{max} and approximates the first-order rate of decline in concentration (reproduced with permission from reference 15).*

of decline of effect is not constant but varies depending on the concentration range. Despite a steady first-order decline in concentrations, pharmacologic effect is relatively constant when concentrations are well above the EC_{50}. In terms of receptor theory, we can state that there is enough drug to occupy most receptors even if the concentration is reduced by one-half. Within the range from 80% of E_{max} ($4 \times EC_{50}$) to 20% of E_{max} ($0.25 \times EC_{50}$), pharmacologic effect will decline as a linear function of time, as predicted by Levy.[19] At concentrations well below the EC_{50}, there is a nearly linear relationship between concentration and effect (see linear model above); consequently, pharmacologic response declines in parallel (first-order) with the same half-life as drug concentrations. Therefore, there is no single parameter that can describe, for example, a "pharmacodynamic half-life" of a particular drug because the rate of decline in pharmacologic effect varies based on the concentration. Actually, the term half-life is applicable only for a first-order process which, for pharmacologic response, occurs only when concentrations are very small relative to the EC_{50}.

The integration of pharmacokinetic and pharmacodynamic principles can be used to explain some interesting clinical observations. Propranolol, for example, can maintain its cardiac beta-blocking effect for a time period that greatly exceeds its half-life[21] because typical plasma concentrations often exceed the EC_{50}.[15] A similar explanation was used to account for the persistence of cardiac beta-blockade for more than 48 hours after a dose of bopindolol despite the drug's four-hour half-life.[17] In this particular example, the effect persisted long after the drug could no longer be measured in plasma.

Equilibration Delays and Links to Other Compartments

Under certain circumstances, the link or relationship between plasma drug concentration and pharmacologic effect may not be a direct one. This can be evaluated by plotting the plasma concentration-effect data and connecting the points in time sequence. Figure 4-5A is an example of counterclockwise hysteresis that can occur with certain pharmacodynamic data. The term hysteresis is used to mean "late" in the sense that a particular concentration, late after a dose, will produce a greater effect compared to the same concentration measured earlier. A counterclockwise hysteresis may indicate increased sensitivity (e.g., up-regulation of receptors) or formation of an active metabolite if the ratio of metabolite to parent drug increases with time. However, another common occurrence is a delay in equilibration between plasma concentrations and the concentrations at the "effect site." Such a delay can be avoided if the concentration-effect relationship is evaluated under steady-state conditions (e.g., continuous intravenous infusions at several different rates), but these studies are much more difficult to conduct in humans. Another approach is to account for the delay observed in nonsteady-state experiments using one of the two general methods described below.

Tissue Compartment

If a drug exhibits multicompartment characteristics for its disposition, then pharmacologic effect could be related to the estimated peripheral or "tissue" compartment amount or concentration[22] instead of the central compartment concentration. Thus, the delay in equilibration between the central and peripheral compartments of the pharmacokinetic model could explain the hysteresis shown in Figure 4-5A. Wagner[23] was apparently the first to propose this approach when he demonstrated that the effects of lysergic acid diethylamide (LSD) on mental performance were more closely related to the predicted peripheral compartment concentrations than to plasma concentrations. A linear pharmacodynamic model and a two-compartment pharmacokinetic model were used and clearly illustrated that while plasma concentrations were decreasing shortly after the intravenous dose, the peripheral compartment concentrations and effects were increasing.

A more clinically relevant example is the inotropic effect of digoxin. Many clinicians are familiar with the multicompartment characteristics of digoxin and the usual delay in its onset of action. Reuning et al.[24] used a two-compartment model to describe digoxin kinetics and showed that the inotropic effect (measured using systolic time intervals) related more closely to concentrations in the tissue compartment than to those in plasma. Subsequently, Kramer et al.[25] used a

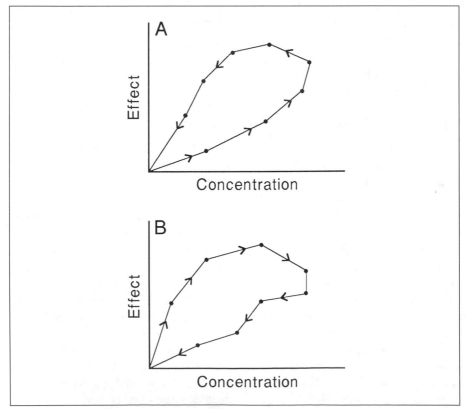

Figure 4-5. *Concentration-effect relationship with the observations connected in time sequence. The upper panel (A) is an example of counterclockwise hysteresis which may be caused by several factors including an equilibration delay between the sampling and effect compartments. The lower panel (B) shows a clockwise hysteresis or proteresis which is characteristic of tolerance but may also be caused by other factors (see text).*

three-compartment pharmacokinetic model to demonstrate that concentrations in the deeper peripheral compartment were even better predictors of digoxin's effect on systolic time intervals.

There are some drawbacks to the use of peripheral compartment concentrations to describe concentration-effect relationships. Figure 4-6 shows how the time course of pharmacologic effect may be out of phase with the drug concentrations in each compartment of the pharmacokinetic model.[26] Actually, there is no reason to assume that the "effect site" concentrations must have the same time course as any pharmacokinetic compartment that is identified from measurement of plasma concentrations. If the pharmacologic "effect site" receives only a small amount of drug, then there will be no measurable effect on drug disposition in plasma or the particular pharmacokinetic model necessary to describe drug disposition. Therefore, it is probably a coincidence if the "effect site" happens to have a similar time course of drug concentration as a particular "peripheral compartment" which represents a type of weighted average of several different tissues/organs. Another limitation is the large degree of error often involved in the estimation of the amount of drug in a peripheral compartment of a multicompartmental model.[27] Finally, a peripheral compartment approach can only be used for multicompartmental drugs, despite the fact that equilibration delays can occur with drugs that exhibit apparent one-compartment characteristics.[28]

Effect Compartment

A totally different approach is to use the time course of pharmacologic effect itself to estimate the rate of movement into the effect site. This concept is illustrated in Figure 4-7. If plasma concentrations are suddenly increased from zero to a value C and maintained at that level, then the pharmacologic effect will progressively

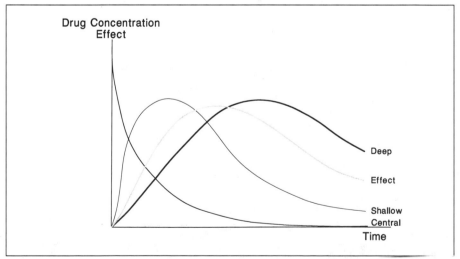

Figure 4-6. *Time course of pharmacologic effect and drug concentrations in the various compartments of a three-compartment pharmacokinetic model. The pharmacologic response is not in phase with drug concentration in any compartment (reproduced with permission from reference 26).*

increase based on the rate of drug accumulation at the effect site. Furthermore, if drug entry and exit from the "effect site" are determined by separate first-order rate constants, then the rate of onset of effect up to the asymptotic value (E_c) will be determined by the rate constant describing drug loss from the effect site. This situation is analogous to a continuous intravenous drug infusion where the time to reach steady state is determined by the elimination rate constant. Therefore, the time required to reach 50% of E_c is the half-time of effect equilibration and is calculated as $\ln2/k_{e0}$, where k_{e0} is the rate constant for drug loss from the effect site. A similar approach was first used by Forrester et al.[29] to describe the onset of pharmacologic effect after intravenous administration of various digitalis glycosides. These investigators reported equilibration half-times of 23 minutes for digoxin and almost one hour for digitoxin; however, they neglected the fact that plasma drug concentrations were not constant but decreasing after the intravenous bolus.

Sheiner et al.[30] have developed a method to estimate the half-time for effect equilibration when plasma concentrations are not constant. Based on the concepts developed by Segre[31] and Hull et al.,[32] these investigators proposed a model (see Figure 4-8) to describe the time course of muscle paralysis with d-tubocurarine. The exact form of the pharmacokinetic model is irrelevant as long as it adequately describes the central compartment concentrations. The central compartment of the pharmacokinetic model is linked to a hypothetical effect compartment by a rate constant, k_{1e}. However, it is assumed that k_{1e} is very small relative to any other rate constant in the pharmacokinetic model, and consequently a negligible amount of drug enters the effect compartment relative to the amount of drug in the other compartments. Because the amount of drug that enters the effect compartment is negligible, the amount returning to the central compartment is inconsequential and

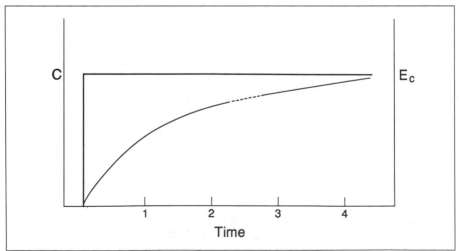

Figure 4-7. *Time course of effect (dashed line) when plasma drug concentration (solid line) is suddenly increased and maintained at C and there is an equilibration delay controlled by a first-order rate constant (see Figure 4-8). Pharmacologic effect reaches an asymptotic value of E_c once there is equilibrium between C and the effect site concentration (reproduced with permission from reference 1).*

can be taken outside rather than back into the system. Therefore, the effect compartment does not alter the plasma concentration-time curve, and an additional exponential term is not necessary in the pharmacokinetic model. Under these assumptions, the value of k_{1e} is unimportant, whereas the rate constant k_{e0} will characterize the equilibration time between plasma concentrations and pharmacologic effect. Based on this approach, equations can be developed to describe the time course of drug concentration in the effect compartment for various pharmacokinetic models.[10] For example, the equation for a one-compartment model with bolus input is as follows:

$$\frac{C_e}{k_p} = \left[\frac{(D)\,(k_{e0})}{(V_d)\,(k_{e0} - k_{el})}\right]\left[e^{-(k_{el})\,(t)} - e^{-(k_{e0})\,(t)}\right] \qquad \text{(Eq. 4-18)}$$

where D is the dose, V_d the volume of distribution, k_{el} is the elimination rate constant, C_e is the theoretical effect compartment concentration, k_p is a proportionality constant between plasma and "effect site" concentrations at equilibrium, so that the ratio $C_e{:}k_p$ is then in terms of equivalent plasma concentrations. The right side of Equation 4-18 is substituted for concentration (C) in the various pharmacodynamic models described above (see Equations 4-10 to 4-17). The pharmacodynamic models can then be used, with the pharmacologic effect-time data as input, to estimate the usual model parameters (e.g., EC_{50} and E_{max} for the E_{max} model) as well as the new parameter k_{e0}. Because Equation 4-18 and the various equations developed by Holford and Sheiner[10] give estimates of the effect compartment concentrations in terms of equivalent plasma concentrations, the EC'_{50} estimated with E_{max} type models will be in terms of equivalent plasma concentra-

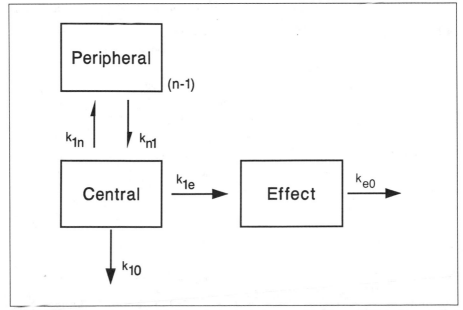

Figure 4-8. *Schematic representation of a typical pharmacokinetic model linked to an effect compartment (based on the model from reference 30).*

tions and thus more relevant. It should be emphasized that this "equivalent" plasma concentration is often discussed as though it is the actual effect compartment concentration.

With the use of a suitable nonlinear regression method, a pharmacokinetic model can first be fitted to the plasma concentration-time data, and then these parameters used as constants for the pharmacodynamic model to estimate the remaining parameters. Alternatively, both the pharmacokinetic and pharmacodynamic models can be fitted simultaneously. In either case, the result will be a description of the concentration-effect relationship that accounts for the delay or equilibration between plasma concentrations and the effect site. This approach has been used successfully to describe the time course of pharmacologic effect of several drugs including d-tubocurarine,[30] disopyramide,[33] quinidine,[34] digoxin,[26] terbutaline,[35,36] theophylline,[37] verapamil,[38] nizatidine,[39] thiopental,[40] fentanyl,[41] alfentanil,[41] ergotamine,[28] vecuronium,[42] and N-acetylprocainamide[43] (see Table 4-1).

The magnitude of k_{e0} will depend on many factors such as perfusion of the effect site, rate of drug diffusion from capillaries to the effect site, blood-tissue partition coefficient of the drug, rate of drug-receptor association and dissociation, and time course of the subsequent pharmacologic response. Thus, Stanski et al.[44] reported that halothane decreased the k_{e0} for d-tubocurarine muscle paralysis and attributed this effect to a halothane-induced reduction in muscle perfusion. Examination of Equation 4-18 will reveal that whenever k_{e0} is much larger than k_{el} (or any other exponent in the case of multicompartment models), the time course of "effect site"

Table 4-1. *Equilibration Half-Times Determined using the Effect Compartment Method.*[30]

Drug	Equilibration half-time (min)	Pharmacologic effect[a]	References
d-Tubocurarine	4	Muscle paralysis	30
Disopyramide	2	QT prolongation	33
Quinidine	8	QT prolongation	34
Digoxin	214	LVET shortening	26
Terbutaline	7.5	FEV$_1$	35
Terbutaline	11.5	Hypokalemia	36
Theophylline	11	FEV$_1$	37
Verapamil	2	PR prolongation	38
Nizatidine	83	Gastric pH	39
Thiopental	1.2 (arterial blood)	Spectral edge	40
Fentanyl	6.4	Spectral edge	41
Alfentanil	1.1	Spectral edge	41
Ergotamine	594	Vasoconstriction	28
Vecuronium	4	Muscle paralysis	42
N-acetylprocainamide	6.4	QT prolongation	43

[a] QT and PR refer to the electrocardiographic intervals; LVET = Left ventricular ejection time; FEV$_1$ = Forced expiratory volume in one second; spectral edge refers to the spectral edge frequency of the electroencephalogram.

concentrations will exactly parallel the concentrations in plasma. In other words, equilibration time will be very short, there will be no hysteresis due to equilibration delays, and plasma concentrations can be used with the various pharmacodynamic models. Furthermore, if k_{e0} is the same as the rate constant from a peripheral compartment to the central compartment (k_{n1} in Figure 4-8), then the effect compartment concentrations will exactly parallel those in the peripheral compartment. Therefore, the use of a "tissue compartment" concentration to predict pharmacologic effects, as discussed in the previous section, is only appropriate when k_{e0} happens to be equal or nearly equal to a particular k_{n1}. Another version of this approach is to link the effect compartment to a peripheral compartment instead of the central compartment. This particular variation was discussed extensively by Colburn[45] and compared to the more commonly used model in Figure 4-8.

A major advantage of the effect-compartment method is that nonsteady-state data can be used. As discussed previously, the various pharmacodynamic models (see Equations 4-10 to 4-17) assume that there is an equilibrium between the concentrations that are measured (usually in plasma) and the corresponding concentrations at the "effect site." This assumption is not required with the effect compartment approach because the onset of pharmacologic effect itself is used to estimate the concentration at the "effect site." Otherwise, the only way to assure this equilibrium is to evaluate the concentration-effect relationship at steady state. However, many if not most studies are conducted after single-dose administration. If there is evidence of a delay between plasma concentrations and pharmacologic effect (counterclockwise hysteresis, see Figure 4-5), some investigators have suggested using only those points after the peak effect is attained (i.e., those from the descending limb of the concentration-effect curve).[46] In order to critically compare these methods, Schwartz et al.[38] evaluated PR interval prolongation after a single intravenous dose and during a continuous (steady-state) intravenous infusion of verapamil in the same subjects. When these investigators used only the concentration-effect data that were collected after the peak plasma concentration, it was quite apparent that the results were different from those obtained at steady state during the continuous infusion. Both the shape of the concentration-effect relationship and the pharmacodynamic model parameters were different. Conversely, the results using the effect compartment method with the single-dose data were similar to those obtained under steady-state conditions. This study highlights the fact that analysis of nonsteady-state data, even if restricted to "descending limb" data, can lead to misleading results. Furthermore, it demonstrates that the effect-compartment approach can be used to evaluate the "true" steady-state concentration-effect relationship with single-dose data.

Nonparametric Pharmacodynamic Models

The effect compartment method described above involves the use of three models linked in series. A pharmacokinetic model relates dose to plasma concentrations; a link model relates plasma concentrations to the "effect site" concentrations; and a pharmacodynamic model relates the "effect site" concentrations to the pharmacologic effect. Specific assumptions are made about the structure of these models which may or may not reflect physiologic reality. Therefore a nonparametric approach, which makes fewer assumptions, has been suggested for the analysis of pharmacodynamic data.[47] This method estimates the value of k_{e0} that will "collapse" the two limbs of the hysteresis loop in the concentration-effect relationship but without specifying a pharmacodynamic model. Therefore, the "true" effect site concentration-response relationship can be evaluated even with nonsteady-state data. The method was subsequently extended to include a nonparametric approach for both the pharmacokinetic and pharmacodynamic data.[48] Nevertheless, specific assumptions are still necessary regarding the "link model" between plasma and "effect site." These nonparametric or semiparametric methods will not allow the investigator to make the type of predictions that can be made with the various parametric models, but they may help initially to describe the "effect site" concentration-response relationship and consequently assist in the selection of an appropriate pharmacodynamic model without having to first make assumptions about its structure.[38]

Duration and Extent of Pharmacologic Effect

Duration of effect implies that there is a specific level of pharmacologic response that is of particular interest (e.g., 90% inhibition of ventricular ectopic depolarizations). If the plasma concentration (after equilibration) that produces this effect is known, then the duration of action can be predicted simply based on the pharmacokinetic model and will be independent of any pharmacodynamic model. When drug disposition after intravenous administration can be described by a one-compartment model, the time to reach a certain minimum concentration will be determined by the dose (or initial drug concentration) and the half-life. In this case, the duration of action of a particular drug will be proportional to the logarithm of the intravenous dose (or the concentration immediately after the dose). Thus, increasing the dose is a relatively inefficient method to extend the duration of action of a drug. However, if a second intravenous dose, equal to the initial dose, is administered immediately when pharmacologic response disappears (at the threshold concentration), then the observed response is likely to be more intense and prolonged than after the initial dose. This is a simple consequence of the higher concentrations achieved because the second dose is superimposed on the remaining drug in the body when the threshold concentration is reached.[49] Relative to this second dose, a further increase in duration or extent of effect will not occur if a third dose is administered at the threshold concentration.

The situation is different for drugs with two-compartment characteristics or when the "effect site" concentrations do not parallel those in plasma. For example, Gibaldi et al.[50] demonstrated that the time to recovery of muscle strength after d-tubocurarine increased when subsequent doses were administered at the same threshold level of muscle strength. In the multicompartment case, the duration of effect is not a simple function of the dose but also depends on the distribution characteristics of the drug and the "depth" of the "effect site."[51,52]

With appropriate pharmacokinetic and pharmacodynamic models, the complete time course of pharmacologic response and duration of effect can be predicted for any drug regimen. The concepts used above to illustrate the rate of decline in pharmacologic response (see Figure 4-4) can be extended to the dosage regimens used in the clinical setting. Based on the E_{max} and one-compartment models, Wagner[8] calculated the area under the effect-time curve (AUC_e) as a measure of the total pharmacologic response over 24 hours and then evaluated how AUC_e was affected by changing the dosing interval. He demonstrated that the AUC_e over 24 hours progressively increased as the same total daily dose was administered over progressively shorter dosing intervals. The largest increase in AUC_e occurred when the dosing interval was decreased from 24 hours to 12 hours, with smaller increases occurring as the dosing interval was further decreased to six or three hours. The results are predictable based on Equation 4-14 and the continuously decreasing slope of the E_{max} model as concentrations increase (see Figure 4-2). The greater fluctuations associated with once-daily administration will lead to higher peak concentrations, but these will not produce proportionately higher pharmacologic effects. Therefore, the increased pharmacologic response at the higher concentrations will not fully compensate for the decreased response at the lower concentrations, and there will be a net decrease in AUC_e over 24 hours with once-daily administration. The extent of the increase in AUC_e with shorter dosing intervals will depend on the EC_{50} relative to the observed concentrations. When concentrations are above the EC_{50}, the increase in AUC_e will be less than when the concentrations are below the EC_{50} because of the change in the slope of the concentration-effect relationship (see Figure 4-2). A similar argument can be used to explain why the AUC_e for propranolol inhibition of exercise-induced tachycardia produced by sustained-release capsules and immediate-release tablets did not differ statistically despite a twofold lower bioavailability of the sustained-release product.[21] Furthermore, Wagner[8] demonstrated that the increase in AUC_e with shorter dosing intervals was relatively greater for drugs with short half-lives (see Figure 4-9). These results were used to explain the greater overall diuretic effects of chlorothiazide when administered in divided doses compared to a single daily dose.[53]

PHARMACODYNAMICS OF DRUG COMBINATIONS

The pharmacologic effect of drug combinations was extensively reviewed by Ariens and Simonis in 1964.[6,7] If two drugs act at different sites to produce a similar pharmacologic effect (e.g., antihypertensive agents with central and peripheral mechanisms of action), then the overall pharmacologic response can be described as the sum of two functions such as the E_{max} or sigmoid E_{max} models (Equation 4-10 or 4-14). In this case, each drug has its own pharmacodynamic parameters (E_{max}, EC_{50}) which are best determined after administration of the individual agents. Synergism or antagonism will be evident if pharmacologic response to the drug combination is different from that predicted by the simple addition of the individual concentration-effect relationships.

Many drugs act at the same type of receptors and consequently will compete for access to those receptors. Just as the interaction between a drug molecule and a receptor was used as the basis to develop Equations 4-1 to 4-6 and the E_{max} model (Equation 4-14), the following relationship can be developed if two different drug molecules competitively bind with a common receptor:[6]

$$E_{A+B} = \frac{(E_{max_A})(C_A)}{\left[(EC_{50_A})\left(1 + \frac{C_B}{EC_{50_B}}\right) + C_A\right]} + \frac{(E_{max_B})(C_B)}{\left[(EC_{50_B})\left(1 + \frac{C_A}{EC_{50_A}}\right) + C_B\right]} \quad \text{(Eq. 4-19)}$$

where the subscripts A and B refer to the two different drugs, E_{A+B} is the combined effect of the two drugs and the remaining parameters are as defined previously. The above relationship will describe the combined effects of two agonists when their pharmacologic responses are mediated through a single receptor (e.g., iso-

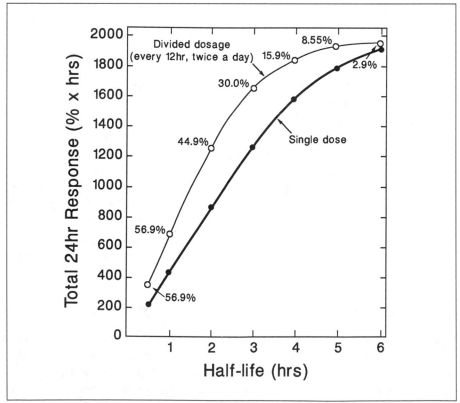

Figure 4-9. *Simulated total 24-hour pharmacologic response (area under the effect-time curve) as a function of drug elimination half-life. Relationships are shown for a single daily dose and for the same total daily dose administered in equally divided doses everyr 12 hours. The numbers indicate the percentage increase in total 24-hour response with the divided dosage over the single dose. Simulations were done with the E_{max} model ($E_{max} = 100\%$), a one-compartment model with bolus intravenous administration, and a peak concentration of $19 \times EC_{50}$ after the single dose thus producing a response of 95% at that time (reproduced with permission from reference 8).*

proterenol and epinephrine with β-adrenoceptors). Equation 4-19 can also be modified if more than one molecule of each drug binds to each receptor or more than two drugs competitively bind to the same receptor.[1] If E_{maxB} is significantly less than E_{maxA}, then drug B is said to be a partial agonist. When this occurs, E_{A+B} may be greater or less than the effect of each drug alone depending on the concentrations of the two agents.[54] Similarly, drug B may have no intrinsic activity when it binds to the receptor ($E_{max} = 0$) and will be considered a competitive antagonist. In such a case, Equation 4-19 will simplify to the following relationship.

$$E_{A+B} = \frac{(E_{max_A})(C_A)}{\left[(EC_{50_A})\left(1 + \frac{C_B}{EC_{50_B}}\right) + C_A\right]}$$

(Eq. 4-20)

Compared to the E_{max} model (Equation 4-14), the net effect of antagonist B is to cause a shift in the agonist A concentration-effect relationship and increase the apparent agonist EC_{50} value because EC_{50A} is multiplied by the term $(1 + C_B/EC_{50B})$. Therefore, low antagonist concentrations relative to its EC_{50} will cause little change in the agonist concentration-effect relationship. The effect of the antagonist will become more apparent as its concentrations approach or exceed its EC_{50}. The maximum effect of the agonist is not affected by the antagonist (when C_A is very large, $E_{A+B} = E_{maxA}$) which is a characteristic of competitive antagonism.

Pharmacodynamic studies are often confounded by the presence of endogenous agonists. The best clinical example is the effect of beta blockers in the presence of variable concentrations of catecholamines. For example, Wellstein et al.[55] demonstrated that the propranolol EC_{50} for inhibition of effort-induced tachycardia was dependent on the level of exercise. Thus at higher exercise levels, the apparent EC_{50} increased two- to threefold presumably because of the higher concentrations of endogenous agonist(s) at the effect site compared to lower effort levels. The situation is analogous to that described for Equation 4-20 in the previous paragraph, except that now the effect of the antagonist is altered by the presence of an agonist. Interestingly, these authors also demonstrated that the propranolol EC_{50} at low effort levels was similar to the β-receptor dissociation constant determined *in vitro*. This should occur if the concentration of agonist at the effect site is much less than its EC_{50}.[55] Jonkers et al.[56] combined a model analogous to Equation 4-20 with the effect-compartment method discussed above in order to describe the hypokalemic response to terbutaline and its inhibition by beta blockers. Because the terbutaline-induced hypokalemic response is thought to be mediated by β_2-adrenoceptors, the investigators were able to demonstrate that the *in vivo* potency of oxprenolol was greater (lower EC_{50}) than that of the β_1-selective agent metoprolol.

If the concentration of agonist is adjusted to produce the *same* pharmacologic response both in the presence and absence of antagonist, then Equation 4-20 greatly simplifies to the following:

$$\frac{C_A^*}{C_A} - 1 = \frac{C_B}{EC_{50_B}}$$

(Eq. 4-21)

where C_A^* is the concentration of agonist in the presence of antagonist and C_A is the concentration of agonist in the absence of antagonist. The ratio on the left side of Equation 4-21 is often called the concentration ratio, or dose ratio if only doses are known. Based on Equation 4-21, the EC_{50} of the antagonist can be determined if the concentration of antagonist is known, even without knowledge of the EC_{50} of the agonist. The assumption is that the concentrations measured (e.g., plasma) are in equilibrium with those at the effect site. This very useful relationship has been used in clinical studies to determine the EC_{50} of beta blockers with isoproterenol as the agonist[57] and subsequently to evaluate the effects of age, stereoselective disposition, and protein binding on the sensitivity (i.e., EC_{50}) to propranolol.[58–60] Although the combined effects of β agonists and antagonists have been commonly studied in clinical pharmacodynamic investigations, the above principles will apply to any drug combinations that act through a common receptor.

TOLERANCE AND SENSITIZATION

The various methods described thus far assume that the "effect site" concentration-effect relationship does not vary over time (i.e., the pharmacodynamic parameters are constant). Therefore, the effect compartment method assumes that the counterclockwise hysteresis loop (see Figure 4-5A) is due only to an equilibration delay between plasma and effect site, and that a certain "effect site" concentration will lead to the same pharmacologic effect at any time after the dose. However, there are numerous pharmacologic examples where this assumption is clearly erroneous. Tolerance, defined as a decrease in pharmacologic response after exposure to a drug, has been demonstrated with nicotine,[61] cocaine,[62] and the benzodiazepines,[63] to name a few examples. This type of functional tolerance is differentiated from metabolic tolerance due to auto-induction of drug metabolism. Tolerance will lead to clockwise hysteresis, or proteresis,[64] in the concentration-effect data as shown in Figure 4-5B. Proteresis also can occur if an inhibitory metabolite is produced and there is an increase in the metabolite to parent drug ratio over time, or when the "effect site" equilibrates with arterial blood drug concentrations faster than does the concentration at the sampling site (e.g., forearm venous blood).[65]

Generally, tolerance can result from a down-regulation of receptors (decreased number), a decreased affinity between the drug and receptor, a decrease in receptor-generated response despite drug-receptor binding, or even the presence of autoregulatory reflexes that may counteract the primary effect of a drug. Depending on the mechanism, tolerance can develop acutely (minutes to hours) or chronically (days to weeks). Several different methods have been proposed to describe the development of tolerance with modification of some of the models described above.[61,62,66,67] For example, the E_{max} model can be reparameterized to include a time-dependent exponential decrease in E_{max} (i.e., $E_{max} \times e^{-kt}$, down-regulation of receptors), increase in EC_{50} (i.e., $EC_{50} \times e^{kt}$, decreased affinity), where k is a constant that governs the rate of development of tolerance and t is time of exposure to the drug. Chow et al.[62] used a similar modification of a linear model to describe the development of tolerance to the chronotropic effects of cocaine. A disadvantage of these modifications is that it predicts that drug effect will disappear entirely if drug administration is maintained long enough. Another approach is to have an exponential increase in EC_{50} to a new higher value as shown below,

$$E = \frac{(E_{max})\,(C^n)}{\left[EC_{50_x} + (EC_{50_y})\,(1 - e^{-kt})\right]^n + C^n} \qquad \text{(Eq. 4-22)}$$

where EC_{50X} is the baseline value, EC_{50Y} is the maximum increase in EC_{50} that can occur so that $EC_{50X} + EC_{50Y}$ equals the maximum value of EC_{50} with full tolerance; the remaining symbols are the same as defined previously. In this case, the concentration-effect curve is only shifted to the right, and a higher dose would be required to produce the same response. A model similar to Equation 4-22 was used by Kroboth et al.[63] to describe the development of tolerance to alprazolam.

A more versatile method was proposed by Porchet et al.[61] to describe the development of acute tolerance to the effects of nicotine on heart rate. These investigators postulated the generation of a hypothetical substance (e.g., metabo-

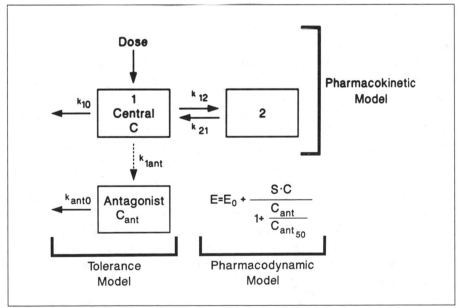

Figure 4-10. *Representation of the pharmacokinetic-pharmacodynamic model proposed for nicotine tolerance. The different k symbols represent the intercompartmental and elimination rate constants, C is the concentration of the agonist, S is the slope of the linear relationship between effect and agonist concentration, C_{ant} is the concentration of the hypothetical antagonist, C_{ant50} is a parameter which determines the extent of tolerance at various concentrations of C_{ant}, E is the effect, and E_0 is the baseline effect (reproduced with permission from reference 61).*

lite of nicotine) that acts as a noncompetitive antagonist of the effects of nicotine (see Figure 4-10). The antagonist is assumed to arise as a first-order process driven by the concentration of the agonist (nicotine) and is eliminated by another first-order process (k_{ant0}) which will determine the rate of appearance and disappearance of tolerance. As with the effect compartment model discussed above, the antagonist concentrations are scaled in terms of equivalent nicotine plasma concentrations at steady state. A linear pharmacodynamic model was used (see Figure 4-10) and included the parameter C_{ant50} which quantified the extent of tolerance at specific concentrations of the hypothetical antagonist. Furthermore, the concentration of antagonist (actually, the "force" driving the tolerance) was assumed to be directly proportional to the past exposures to the antagonist, but it was also exponentially decreased over time after discontinuation of the agonist (i.e., nicotine). This method has an important advantage over the other tolerance models described above. Tolerance development is not simply a function of time; rather, it is dependent on the intensity (concentration, time) of drug exposure and also the time since drug exposure stopped (for the decrease in tolerance). Although the approach assumed the production of a noncompetitive antagonist which is consistent with receptor down-regulation, the linear model shown in Figure 4-10 can also be derived based on the production of a competitive antagonist. Porchet et al.[61] used this model to demonstrate that the half-life of tolerance development to the chronotropic effects of nicotine was 35 minutes. The model not only correctly predicted the development of tolerance but also the decrease in tolerance when the interval between drug exposure was extended. A similar approach was also used by Boyd et al.[68] to account for the apparent tolerance to the PR interval prolongation caused by diltiazem.

Sensitization, defined as an increase in pharmacologic response with time at the same "effect site" concentration, can occur when there is an up-regulation of receptors. When sensitization occurs quickly, a counterclockwise hysteresis in the concentration-effect data will be evident (see Figure 4-5A) although, as discussed above, there are several other possible explanations for such hysteresis. Up-regulation of receptors can occur when the negative feedback provided by the constant presence of agonist(s) is removed. Examples include surgical denervation and when receptors are blocked by antagonists for an extended period. The best clinical example would be the up-regulation of β-adrenoceptors and increase in adenylate cyclase activity after chronic administration of beta blockers which result in hypersensitivity to catecholamines after sudden withdrawal of the antagonist.[69,70]

Lima et al.[71] have proposed a method to describe the time course of adrenergic responsiveness both during and after sudden withdrawal of propranolol. The investigators proposed that up-regulation of β-adrenoceptors could be described by the following relationship:

$$fr = \left(\frac{B_{max}{}' - B_{max}}{B_{max}} \right) \left(1 - e^{-k_d T} \right) \left(e^{-k_d t} \right)$$

(Eq. 4-23)

where fr is the fractional increase in β-adrenoceptor density, B_{max} is the baseline β-adrenoceptor density, $B_{max}{}'$ is the maximum β-adrenoceptor density or the sum of B_{max} and the antagonist-induced increase in receptor density, k_d is the rate of disappearance of the up-regulated receptors, T is the duration of time the subjects were receiving the β-antagonist and t is the time since discontinuation of the β-antagonist. The rate constant k_d, estimated to be 0.462 days^{-1} based on the work of Aarons et al.,[70] determines the rate of increase and decrease in β-adrenoceptor density during and after treatment with beta blockers. Equation 4-23 was linked to a linear pharmacodynamic model to predict the increase in heart rate with isoproterenol. The pharmacodynamic model also included a slope adjustment for the variable concentration of antagonist, analogous to the equation in Figure 4-10. Therefore, the integrated approach could be used to describe the isoproterenol-induced increase in heart rate during and following β-antagonist administration. The model correctly predicted peak chronotropic hypersensitivity to isoproterenol 48 hours after abrupt withdrawal of propranolol. Furthermore, the model demonstrated that the time course of hypersensitivity was dependent on the differences in the rates of decline of propranolol (or other antagonist) concentrations and β-adrenoceptor density.

PHYSIOLOGICAL PHARMACODYNAMIC MODELS

The information discussed up to this point pertains mainly to drugs which exert reversible and direct effects. However, more "physiological" approaches have been proposed to describe the time course of pharmacologic response for drugs that exert indirect or irreversible effects. In order to adequately describe the effects of such drugs, specific physiological processes (e.g., synthesis of clotting factors, cell cycles) have to be included. This is necessary because the ultimate response may be the net result of several different processes, only one of which is affected by the drug. An excellent example is the work of Nichols et al.[72] with the pharmacodynamics of prednisolone in the rat. In this case, prednisolone plasma concentrations are related to the eventual pharmacologic effect (hepatic tyrosine aminotransferase activity) through a series of steps meant to account for the receptor and gene-mediated mechanism of steroid action. Simpler approaches were also used in humans to describe the more "direct" suppressive effects of methylprednisolone on whole blood histamine (basophil) concentrations and the circadian variation in cortisol plasma concentrations.[73,83] In addition, the above methods have been extended to study the effects of steroids on other cell types, such as T-helper lymphocytes.[84]

Indirect Effects

Warfarin and other coumarin anticoagulants provide the best examples of drugs that act indirectly. The hypoprothrombinemic effect is determined by both synthesis and degradation of the clotting factors, yet these drugs will only affect synthesis. Drug concentrations may be related to clotting factor synthesis but only indirectly related to the ultimate therapeutic effect. Thus, peak plasma concentrations of warfarin occur within a few hours after an oral dose, but the maximum hypoprothrombinemic effect will not be evident for a few days. Nagashima et al.[2]

developed a method that estimated the time course of prothrombin complex activity (PCA) as a function of its rate of degradation and synthesis. The rate of PCA degradation was calculated from its first order rate of decline (half-life = 13.8 hours) when synthesis is totally inhibited by warfarin. A log-linear pharmacodynamic model was used to relate warfarin concentrations to the fractional inhibition of the pre-drug PCA synthesis rate. Integration of these two processes with the (first-order) rate of elimination of warfarin from plasma after a single oral dose, provided a very good description of the observed time course of PCA. The method accurately predicted the PCA decrease over the first two days and the subsequent increase when warfarin concentrations had decreased sufficiently. The same approach was used later to determine that enzyme induction produced by heptabarbital decreased the anticoagulant effects of warfarin by increasing its rate of elimination and not by altering the warfarin plasma concentration-PCA synthesis rate relationship.[74] The same investigators also showed that phenylbutazone shifted the warfarin total (bound + unbound) concentration-effect relationship to the left by displacing warfarin from plasma proteins.[75]

Irreversible Effects

Unlike the examples discussed so far, certain antibiotics and antineoplastic agents cause irreversible effects (i.e., cell death) after they are incorporated into a specific cellular biochemical process. For antineoplastic agents, it is useful to separate pharmacologic response for cell- cycle-specific agents and for nonphase-

Table 4-2. General Considerations in the Planning of Pharmacodynamic Studies

- Is the pharmacologic effect direct, reversible, indirect, irreversible?

- Selection of a pharmacologic response which is clinically relevant.

- Validation of the measurement of pharmacologic response and drug concentration.

- Number of subjects to provide adequate statistical power.

- Optimal design and sampling strategy based on pilot study, including variability in pharmacokinetics and pharmacodynamics.

- Time dependence of pharmacologic effect (e.g., tolerance, diurnal variation, sensitization).

- Equilibration delays between sampling and effect compartments for non-steady-state investigations.

- Baseline and/or placebo effects and how to account for them.

- Presence of endogenous agonist(s).

- Presence of drug metabolite(s) which may be pharmacologically active.

- Selection of a suitable and parsimonious pharmacodynamic model (either empirical or preferably based on the mechanism of action of the drug).

- Optimal parameter estimation for an individual or population, statistical inference, model predictions.

specific agents. Two different methods have been proposed by Jusko[76,77] to relate antineoplastic drug concentrations and tumor cell response for these two drug categories. These models were slightly modified by Gibaldi and Perrier[78] and are actually similar to the model proposed in Figure 4-8, with the exception that the effect compartment includes variables to account for tumor cell number, tumor cell turnover and the number of cells in a specific cycle which may be sensitive to a drug effect.

The clinical response to antineoplastic agents is obviously difficult to quantitate and, if it can be done, there are usually significant limitations on the number of response measures that can be obtained in individual subjects. Despite these limitations, there is growing evidence to support the relationship between drug concentration and certain desirable and undesirable pharmacologic effects. Examples include the relationship between area under the plasma concentration-time curve (AUC) of ultrafiltrable platinum and platelet count,[79] the AUC of menogoril and white blood cell count,[80] as well as methotrexate plasma concentration and the likelihood of remission in children with acute lymphocytic leukemia.[81] The relationship between plasma concentrations of antibacterial agents and clinical response will be discussed in Chapters 14 to 17.

PROSPECTUS

The discipline of pharmacodynamics has evolved over centuries from a crude description of the link between dose and response to a sophisticated study of the mathematical relationships between precisely quantitated pharmacologic effects and drug concentrations. The planning of pharmacodynamic studies requires particular attention to the numerous confounding variables which may affect the results of clinical investigations. Initial steps in these investigations usually involve collection of preliminary data, development of a specific hypothesis and a pilot study. Then some or all of the factors in Table 4-2 should be considered in the design of the actual investigation. Once scientifically valid pharmacodynamic data have been collected and analyzed, this information is most useful if coupled with clinical pharmacokinetic principles so that the time course of therapeutic response can be characterized and the optimal dosage regimens can be designed. Randomized concentration-controlled trials and the newer designs proposed for dose-ranging studies are examples of the potential advantages to be gained from a better understanding of the relationship between pharmacokinetics and pharmacodynamics.[82,85,86] Thus, the benefits may extend from the care of a single patient to all phases of drug development.[87]

REFERENCES

1. Holford NHG, Sheiner LB. Pharmacokinetic and pharmacodynamic modeling *in vivo*. CRC Crit Rev Bioeng. 1981;5:273–322.
2. Nagashima R, et al. Kinetics of pharmacologic response in man: the anticoagulant action of warfarin. Clin Pharmacol Ther. 1969;10:22–35.
3. Langmuir I. The adsorption of gases on plane surfaces of glass, mica and platinum. J Am Chem Soc. 1918;40:1361–403.

4. Hill AV. The possible effects of the aggregation of the molecules of hemoglobin on its dissociation curves. J Physiol. 1910;40:iv–vii.

5. Clark AJ. The reaction between acetylcholine and muscle cells. J Physiol. 1926;61:530–46.

6. Ariens EJ, Simonis AM. A molecular basis of drug action. J Pharm Pharmacol. 1964;16:137–57.

7. Ariens EJ, Simonis AM. A molecular basis for drug action. The interaction of one or more drugs with different receptors. J Pharm Pharmacol. 1964;16:289–312.

8. Wagner JG. Kinetics of pharmacologic response. J Theor Biol. 1968;20:173–201.

9. Holford NHG, Sheiner LB. Kinetics of pharmacologic response. Pharmacol Ther. 1982;16:141–66.

10. Holford NHG, Sheiner LB. Understanding the dose-effect relationship: clinical application of pharmacokinetic-pharmacodynamic models. Clin Pharmacokinet. 1981;6:429–53.

11. Meffin PJ et al. Response optimization of drug dosage: antiarrhythmic studies with tocainide. Clin Pharmacol Ther. 1977;22:42–57.

12. D'Argenio DZ. Optimal sampling times for pharmacokinetic experiments. J Pharmacokinet Biopharm. 1981;9:739–56.

13. Colburn WA, Gibson DM. Endogenous agonists and pharmacokinetic/pharmacodynamic modeling of baseline effects. In: Kroboth PD, Smith RM, Juhl RP, eds. Pharmacokinetics and pharmacodynamics: Current problems, potential solutions. Cincinnati: Harvey Whitney Books;1988:167–84.

14. Holazo AA et al. Pharmacokinetic and pharmacodynamic modeling of cibenzoline plasma concentrations and antiarrhythmic effect. J Clin Pharmacol. 1986;26:336–45.

15. Lalonde RL et al. Propranolol pharmacodynamic modeling using unbound and total concentrations in healthy volunteers. J Pharmacokinet Biopharm. 1987;15:569–82.

16. Mullen PW, Foster RW. Comparative evaluation of six techniques for determining the Michaelis-Menten parameters relating phenytoin dose and steady-state serum concentrations. J Pharm Pharmacol. 1979;31:100–104.

17. Platzer R et al. Simultaneous modeling of bopindolol kinetics and dynamics. Clin Pharmacol Ther. 1984;36:5–13.

18. Galeazzi RL et al. Relationship between the pharmacokinetics and pharmacodynamics of procainamide. Clin Pharmacol Ther. 1976;20:278–89.

19. Levy G. Relationship between rate of elimination of tubocurarine and rate of decline of its pharmacological activity. Br J Anaesth. 1964;36:694–95.

20. Levy G. Kinetics of pharmacologic response. Clin Pharmacol Ther. 1966;7:362–72.

21. Lalonde RL et al. Pharmacokinetics and pharmacodynamics of propranolol after single doses and at steady state. Eur J Clin Pharmacol. 1987;33:315–18.

22. Benet LZ. General treatment of linear mammillary models with elimination from any compartment as used in pharmacokinetics. J Pharm Sci. 1972;61:536–41.

23. Wagner JG et al. Correlation of performance test scores with tissue concentration of lysergic acid diethylamide in human subjects. Clin Pharmacol Ther. 1968;9:635–38.

24. Reuning RH et al. Role of pharmacokinetics in drug dosage adjustment. I: Pharmacological effect kinetics and apparent volume of distribution of digoxin. J Clin Pharmacol. 1973;13:127–41.

25. Kramer WG, et al. Pharmacokinetics of digoxin: relationship between response intensity and predicted compartmental drug levels in man. J Pharmacokinet Biopharm. 1979;7:47–61.

26. Kelman AW, Whiting B. Modeling of drug response in individual subjects. J Pharmacokinet Biopharm. 1980;8:115–30.

27. Westlake WJ. Problems associated with analysis of pharmacokinetic models. J Pharm Sci. 1971;60:882–85.

28. Tfelt-Hansen P, Paalzow L. Intramuscular ergotamine: plasma levels and dynamic activity. Clin Pharmacol Ther. 1985;37:29–35.

29. Forrester W et al. The onset and magnitude of the contractile response to commonly used digitalis glycosides in normal subjects. Circulation 1974;49:517–21.

30. Sheiner LB et al. Simultaneous modeling of pharmacokinetics and pharmacodynamics: application to d-tubocurarine. Clin Pharmacol Ther. 1979;25:358–71.

31. Segre G. Kinetics of interaction between drugs and biological systems. Il Farmaco. 1968;23:906–18.

32. Hull C et al. A pharmacodynamic model for pancuronium. Br J Anaesth. 1978;50:1113–123.
33. Whiting B et al. Quantitative analysis of the disopyramide concentration-response relationship. Br J Clin Pharmacol. 1980;9:67–75.
34. Holford NHG et al. The effect of quinidine and its metabolites on the electrocardiogram and systolic time intervals: concentration-effect relationships. Br J Clin Pharmacol. 1981;11:187–95.
35. Oosterhuis B et al. Pharmacokinetic-pharmacodynamic modeling of terbutaline bronchodilation in asthma. Clin Pharmacol Ther. 1986;40:469–75.
36. Jonkers R et al. Beta-2-adrenoceptor-mediated hypokalemia and its abolishment by oxprenolol. Clin Pharmacol Ther. 1987;42:627–33.
37. Whiting B et al. Modeling theophylline response in individual patients with chronic bronchitis. Br J Clin Pharmacol. 1981;12:481.
38. Schwartz JB et al. Pharmacodynamic modeling of verapamil under steady-state and nonsteady-state conditions. J Pharmacol Exp Ther. 1989;251:1032–38.
39. Cunningham F et al. Pharmacokinetic/pharmacodynamic modeling for nizatidine effect on basal gastric acid output. Clin Pharmacol Ther. 1989;45:141. Abstract.
40. Stanski DR et al. Pharmacodynamic modeling of thiopental anesthesia. J Pharmacokinet Biopharm. 1984;12:223–40.
41. Scott JC et al. EEG quantitation of narcotic effect: the comparative pharmacodynamics of fentanyl and alfentanil. Anesthesiology 1985;62:234–41.
42. Fisher DM et al. Vecuronium kinetics and dynamics in anesthetized infants and children. Clin Pharmacol Ther. 1985;37:402–406.
43. Piergies AA et al. Effect kinetics of N-acetylprocainamide-induced QT interval prolongation. Clin Pharmacol Ther. 1987;42:107–112.
44. Stanski DR et al. Pharmacokinetics and pharmacodynamics of d-tubocurarine during nitrous oxide-narcotic and halothane anesthesia in man. Anesthesiology 1979;51:235–41.
45. Colburn WA. Simultaneous pharmacokinetic and pharmacodynamic modeling. J Pharmacokinet Biopharm. 1981;9:367–88.
46. Abernethy DR et al. Verapamil pharmacodynamics and disposition in young and elderly hypertensive patients. Ann Intern Med. 1986;105:329–36.
47. Fuseau E, Sheiner LB. Simultaneous modeling of pharmacokinetics and pharmacodynamics with a nonparametric pharmacodynamic model. Clin Pharmacol Ther. 1984;35:733–41.
48. Unadkat JD et al. Simultaneous modeling of pharmacokinetics and pharmacodynamics with nonparametric kinetic and dynamic models. Clin Pharmacol Ther. 1986;40:86–93.
49. Levy G. Apparent potentiating effect of a second dose of a drug. Nature 1965;206:517.
50. Gibaldi M et al. Kinetics of the elimination and neuromuscular blocking activity of d-tubocurarine in man. Anesthesiology 1972;36:213–18.
51. Gibaldi M, Levy G. Dose-dependent decline of pharmacologic effects of drugs with linear pharmacokinetic characteristics. J Pharm Sci. 1972;61:567.
52. Gibaldi M et al. Drug distribution and pharmacologic response. Clin Pharmacol Ther. 1971;12:734.
53. Murphy J et al. The effect of dosage regimen on the diuretic efficacy of chlorothiazide. J Pharmacol Exp Ther. 1961;134:286–90.
54. Oosterhuis B, van Boxtel CJ. Kinetics of drug effects in man. Ther Drug Monit. 1988;10:121–32.
55. Wellstein A et al. Receptor binding of propranolol is the missing link between plasma concentration kinetics and effect-time course in man. Eur J Clin Pharmacol. 1985;29:131–147.
56. Jonkers R et al. A nonsteady-state agonist antagonist interaction model using plasma potassium concentrations to quantify the beta-2 selectivity of beta blockers. J Pharmacol Exp Ther. 1989;249:297–302.
57. Cleveland CR et al. A standardized isoproterenol sensitivity test. The effects of sinus arrhythmia, atropine and propranolol. Arch Intern Med. 1972;130:47 52.
58. McDevitt DG et al. Plasma binding and the affinity of propranolol for a beta receptor in man. Clin Pharmacol Ther. 1976;20:152–57.

59. Vestal RE et al. Reduced beta-adrenoceptor sensitivity in the elderly. Clin Pharmacol Ther. 1979;26:181–86.

60. Tenero DM, et al. Altered beta-adrenergic sensitivity and protein binding to l-propranolol in the elderly. J Cardiovasc Pharmacol 1990;16:702–7.

61. Porchet HC et al. Pharmacodynamic modeling of tolerance: application to nicotine. J Pharmacol Exp Ther. 1988;244:231–36.

62. Chow MJ et al. Kinetics of cocaine distribution, elimination, and chronotropic effects. Clin Pharmacol Ther. 1985;38:318–24.

63. Kroboth PD, Smith RB, Erb RJ. Tolerance to EEG and psychomotor effects after alprazolam intravenous bolus or continuous infusion. Clin Pharmacol Ther. 1988;43:270–77.

64. Girard P, Boissel JP. Clockwise hysteresis or proteresis. J Pharmacokinet Biopharm. 1989;17:401–402.

65. Porchet HC et al. Apparent tolerance to the acute effect of nicotine results in part from distribution kinetics. J Clin Invest. 1988;244:231–36.

66. Smith RB, Kroboth PD. Alprazolam: Development of a pharmacodynamic tolerance model. In: Kroboth PD, Smith RM, Juhl RP, eds. Pharmacokinetics and pharmacodynamics: Current problems, potential solutions. Cincinnati: Harvey Whitney Books;1988:75–89.

67. Hammarlund MM et al. Acute tolerance to the furosemide diuresis in humans: Pharmacokinetic-pharmacodynamic modeling. J Pharmacol Exp Ther. 1985;223:447–53.

68. Boyd RA et al. The pharmacokinetics and pharmacodynamics of diltiazem and its metabolites in healthy adults after a single oral dose. Clin Pharmacol Ther. 1989;46:408–19.

69. van den Meiracker AH et al. Hemodynamic and beta-adrenergic receptor adaptation during long-term beta-adrenoceptor blockade. Circulation 1989;80:903–14.

70. Aarons RD et al. Elevation of beta-adrenergic receptor density in human lymphocytes after propranolol administration. J Clin Invest. 1980;65:949–57.

71. Lima JJ et al. Drug- or hormone-induced adaptation: model of adrenergic hypersensitivity. J Pharmacokinet Biopharm. 1989;17:347–64.

72. Nichols AI et al. Second generation model for prednisolone pharmacodynamics in the rat. J Pharmacokinet Biopharm. 1989;17:209–27.

73. Kong AN et al. Pharmacokinetics and pharmacodynamic modeling of direct suppression effects of methylprednisolone and blood histamine in human subjects. Clin Pharmacol Ther. 1989;46:616–28.

74. Levy G et al. Pharmacokinetic analysis of the effect of barbiturate on the anticoagulant action of warfarin in man. Clin Pharmacol Ther. 1970;11:372–77.

75. O'Reilly RA, Levy G. Pharmacokinetic analysis of potentiating effect of phenylbutazone on anticoagulating action of warfarin in man. J Pharm Sci. 1970;59:1258–261.

76. Jusko WJ. Pharmacodynamics of chemotherapeutic effects: dose-time-response relationships for phase-nonspecific agents. J Pharm Sci. 1971;60:892.

77. Jusko WJ. A pharmacodynamic model for cell-cycle-specific chemotherapeutic agents. J Pharmacokinet Biopharm. 1973;1:175.

78. Gibaldi M, Perrier D. Pharmacokinetics, 2nd edition. New York: Marcel Dekker Inc;1982:254–65.

79. Egorin MJ et al. Prospective validation of a pharmacologically based dosing scheme for carboplatin. Cancer Res. 1985;45:6502–506.

80. Egorin MJ et al. Human pharmacokinetics, excretion, and metabolism of the anthracycline antibiotic menogaril and their correlation with clinical toxicities. Cancer Res. 1986;46:1513–520.

81. Evans WE et al. Clinical pharmacodynamics of high-dose methotrexate in acute lymphocytic leukemia. N Engl J Med. 1986;314:471–77.

82. Sanathanan LP, Peck CC. The randomized concentration-controlled trial: An evaluation of its sample size efficiency. Controlled Clinical Trials. 1991;12:780–94.

83. Wald JA et al. Two-compartment basophil cell trafficking model for methylprednisolone pharmacodynamics. J Pharmacokinet Biopharm. 1991;19:521–36.

84. Dunn TE et al. Pharmacokinetics and pharmacodynamics of methylprednisolone in obese and non-obese men. Clin Pharmacol Ther. 1991;50:536–49.

85. Sheiner LB et al. Study designs for dose-ranging. Clin Pharmacol Ther. 1989;46:63–77.

86. Sambol NC, Sheiner LB. Population dose versus response of betaxolol and atenolol: A comparison of potency and variability. Clin Pharmacol Ther. 1991;49:24–31.

87. Kroboth PD et al. Pharmacodynamic modeling: Application to new drug development. Clin Pharmacokinet. 1991;20:91–8.

Chapter 5

Influence of Protein Binding and Use of Unbound (Free) Drug Concentrations

Janis J. MacKichan

Total drug concentrations in blood or plasma are often used as a guide to adjusting drug doses despite the fact that free or unbound drug concentrations are more closely correlated to drug effect.[1–4,201,202] This is because it is easier to measure the total concentration and because the ratio of free to total drug concentration in blood is usually constant within and between individuals. For some drugs, however, the relationship between free and total drug concentration is extremely variable among patients, or it may be altered by disease or drug interactions. While free drug concentration monitoring might be more appropriate in these situations, the technology to do this is not widely available. Thus, one must be able to predict the effects of altered protein binding on drug effect.

This chapter reviews the following aspects of drug-protein binding: 1) the determinants of protein binding and examples of clinical situations associated with altered plasma protein binding; 2) the effects of altered plasma and tissue protein binding on the pharmacokinetics of a drug using the concepts of restrictive and nonrestrictive drug clearance; 3) the advantages and disadvantages of the most commonly used methods to determine plasma protein binding; and 4) the utility of monitoring free drug concentrations in clinical settings. With this information, the clinician should be able to anticipate situations in which altered plasma protein binding is likely to occur, recognize situations for which free concentration monitoring is appropriate, be able to appropriately interpret total concentration measurements, and predict the need for dosage regimen adjustments.

DETERMINATION OF PROTEIN BINDING PARAMETERS

The reversible binding of a drug to macromolecules, such as proteins, obeys the law of mass action:

$$[D] + [P] \;\; \underset{k_2}{\overset{k_1}{\rightleftharpoons}} \;\; [DP]$$

where [D], [P], and [DP] are the molar concentrations of unbound drug, unoccupied protein, and drug-protein complex, respectively, and k_1 and k_2 are rate constants for the forward and reverse reactions, respectively. The equilibrium association constant for this reaction (K_A) is defined as k_1/k_2 and provides an index of the affinity between the binding site and ligand. The inverse of the association constant ($1/K_A$) is the equilibrium dissociation constant (K_D) for the drug-protein complex. The total concentration of binding sites in a given system is the sum of unoccupied ([P]) and occupied ([DP]) binding sites. This total concentration of sites is referred to as the capacity constant (N) and has units of sites/L. Since a given protein molecule can have several equivalent and independent binding sites

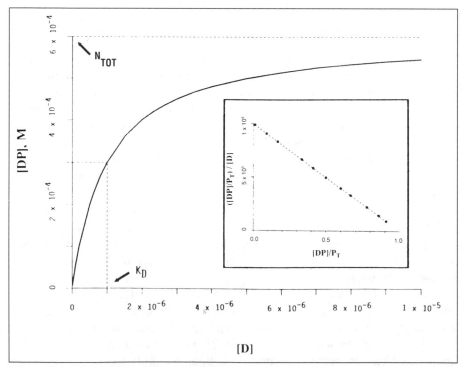

Figure 5-1. *Effect of increasing unbound drug concentration ([D]) on the concentration of bound drug/occupied protein ([DP]). N_{TOT} = Concentration of binding sites; K_D = [D] at which bound drug or [DP] is equal to $N_{TOT}/2$. The inset shows a Scatchard plot for the same data, where P_T is the concentration of occupied and unoccupied protein.*

(meaning that they have the same affinities for the drug and the binding to one site does not affect binding to another), the capacity constant represents the product of the number of sites per mole of protein and the molar concentration of protein.

The concentration of bound drug in a protein solution can be expressed as a function of the capacity constant, dissociation constant, and unbound drug concentration according to the following equation:

$$[DP] = \sum \frac{N_{TOTi} \, [D]}{K_{Di} + [D]}$$

(Eq. 5-1)

where i refers to the number of different classes of binding sites. A plot of [DP] on the y-axis versus [D] on the x-axis for a single class of binding sites gives a plot as shown in Figure 5-1. As unbound drug concentration is increased, the concentration of bound sites increases until [DP] becomes constant and equal to the maximum number of sites, N_{TOT}. Equation 5-1 predicts that this occurs when $[D] > K_D$. The dissociation constant, K_D, is analogous to the Michaelis constant (K_m) described for enzymatic metabolism. As seen in Figure 5-1, the K_D represents the concentration of unbound drug at which exactly one-half of the sites are occupied $([DP] = N_{TOT}/2)$.

Several linear transformations of Equation 5-1 can be used to determine the dissociation and capacity constants that define a particular drug-protein interaction. When there is one class of equivalent and independent binding sites, the plots based on these equations (Scatchard plot, double reciprocal plot, and Woolf plot) are linear. When there are two or more classes of binding sites, these three plots are theoretically curved. Of these, the Scatchard plot is most sensitive in detecting curvature. The Scatchard equation for a single class of binding sites is:

$$\frac{\frac{[DP]}{P_T}}{[D]} = N \cdot K_A - \left(\frac{[DP]}{P_T} \cdot K_A \right)$$

(Eq. 5-2)

where $[P_T]$ is the molar concentration of protein (occupied plus unoccupied) and N is the number of sites per mole of protein. A plot of $([DP]/[P_T] \div [D])$ on the y-axis versus $[DP]/[P_T]$ on the x-axis (Scatchard plot) gives a slope of $-K_A$ and a y-intercept of $N \times K_A$. Such a plot is illustrated in the inset of Figure 5-1. The Rosenthal plot,[5] also known as a modified Scatchard plot, is more useful in situations where protein concentration is not known. In that case, a plot of [DP]/[D] against [DP] gives a slope of $-K_A$ and a y-intercept of $N \times K_A$. Although the number of sites per mole of protein cannot be determined using the Rosenthal plot, knowledge of the concentration of binding sites is just as useful for the purpose of simulations.

A typical experiment used to determine binding constants involves measuring the percent of drug bound in protein solutions or sera containing a wide range of drug concentrations. The [D] and [DP] corresponding to each concentration are calculated, then a Rosenthal or Scatchard plot is used to determine the number of binding site classes. As an example, the curvilinear shape of the Rosenthal plot shown in Figure 5-2 for carbamazepine in serum provided evidence that carbamazepine either binds to two or more classes of sites on albumin (the principal binding protein) or that it binds to sites on one or more proteins in addition to albumin.[6] The capacity and affinity constants characterizing each class of binding sites are estimated graphically and used as initial estimates in a nonlinear least squares program such as MACMOL or NONLIN.[7,8] By fitting the appropriate equation to the measured data (i.e., percentage binding, [DP], [D]), refined estimates of the binding constants can be determined.

The following rearrangement of Equation 5-1 describes the determinants of the unbound plasma fraction (f_{up}) for a drug that binds to a single class of binding sites in plasma:

$$f_{up} = \frac{[D]}{[D] + [DP]} = \frac{K_D + [D]}{N_{TOT} + [D] + K_D} \qquad \text{(Eq. 5-3)}$$

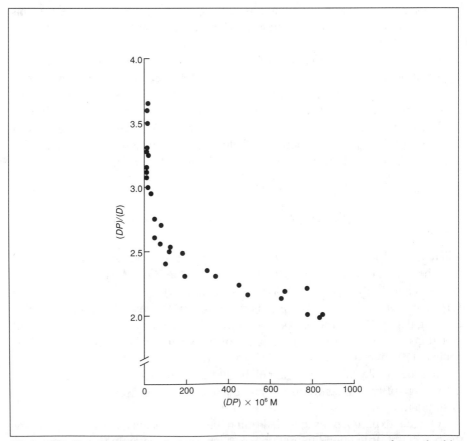

Figure 5-2. *Curvilinear Rosenthal plot for carbamazepine binding to serum from a healthy subject. Subsequent experiments of carbamazepine binding to individual serum proteins indicated that the binding constants associated with the steep and shallow slopes of the plot corresponded to α_1-acid glycoprotein (AAG) and albumin, respectively (reproduced with permission from reference 6).*

The equation expressing the unbound fraction for a drug that binds to two classes of binding sites (for example, one that binds to both albumin and AAG) is:

$$f_{up} = \cfrac{1}{1 + \cfrac{N_{TOT_1}}{K_{D1} + [D]} + \cfrac{N_{TOT_2}}{K_{D2} + [D]}}$$

(Eq. 5-4)

These equations predict that the unbound fraction of drug in a protein solution is determined not only by the binding capacity (N_{TOT}) and "strength" of binding (K_A or $1/K_D$) by each protein, but by the equilibrium unbound drug concentration, [D]. They are therefore useful in simulating how each of these parameters will affect f_{up} in a variety of situations. It should also be evident from the above equations that at low free drug concentrations (i.e., when [D] < K_D), the unbound fraction of drug will be independent of changes in drug concentration.

THE DRUG BINDING PROTEINS

Human plasma contains over 60 proteins.[9] Of these, three proteins account for the binding of most drugs. Albumin, which comprises approximately 60% of total plasma protein,[10] fully accounts for the plasma binding of most anionic drugs and many endogenous anions.[11] Many cationic and neutral drugs bind appreciably to α_1-acid glycoprotein (AAG) and/or lipoproteins in addition to albumin.[12] Other proteins, such as transcortin, thyroid binding globulin, and certain antibodies have specific affinities for a small number of drugs.[11,13]

Important characteristics of albumin, AAG, and lipoproteins have been reviewed by others,[9–11,14–17] and are summarized in Table 5-1. Selected acid, basic, and neutral drugs which are more than 70% bound in plasma following therapeutic doses are listed in Table 5-2, along with their principal binding proteins.[11,12,15,17–23]

Table 5-1. *Characteristics of the Drug Binding Proteins*[9–11,14,15,203]

	Albumin	AAG	Lipoproteins
Molecular weight	66,300	40,000	200,000–10,000,000
Normal serum concentrations (mg/100 mL)	3500–5500	55–140	VLDL-cholesterol: <40 HDL-cholesterol: >35 LDL-cholesterol: 70–205
Biosynthesis site(s)	Liver	Liver	Liver, intestinal mucosa
Catabolism site(s)	Liver, kidney, spleen, lymph nodes	Liver	Liver, kidney, intestine
Half-life	19 days	5.5 days	up to 6 days
Distribution	40% intravascular; 60% extravascular (interstitial)		

DRUGS THAT BIND PREDOMINANTLY TO ALBUMIN

While most acid drugs bind principally to albumin, some basic drugs such as the benzodiazepines also bind mainly to albumin. Albumin is a single peptide chain of about 580 amino acid residues.[9] Genetic variants of albumin have been reported, but they are restricted to only a small number of individuals. The primary physiologic roles of albumin in plasma are to maintain colloid osmotic pressure in the vascular system and to transport fatty acids and bilirubin.[9] Albumin is not confined to plasma, but is continuously filtered at a relatively slow rate into interstitial fluid and then returned to plasma at the same rate via the thoracic duct.[22] Albumin-bound drug is therefore found not only in plasma, which contains 40% of albumin in the body, but also in extravascular interstitial fluid, which contains the remaining 60%.[22]

Two primary "high affinity" drug binding sites or areas have been defined on human albumin.[16] The warfarin binding area (site I) is shared by several other drugs including phenylbutazone, sulfonamides, phenytoin, and valproic acid, while the benzodiazepine binding area (site II) is shared by some of the semi-synthetic penicillins, probenecid, and medium chain fatty acids. Several drugs, including naproxen, tolbutamide, and indomethecin, bind to both sites. Two additional binding areas on albumin (digitoxin and tamoxifen sites) have also been proposed. The presumption of preformed, specific binding sites on albumin is

Table 5-2. *Predominant Binding Proteins of Drugs >70% Bound to Plasma Proteins* [a,11,12,15,17–23, 201, 202]

Albumin	Albumin and AAG	Albumin and Lipoproteins	Albumin, AAG, and Lipoproteins
Ceftriaxone (A)	Alprenolol (B)	Cyclosporine (N)[b]	Amitriptylline (B)
Clindamycin (A)	Carbamazepine (N)	Probucol (N)[b]	Bupivicaine (B)
Clofibrate (A)	Disopyramide (B)[b]		Chlorpromazine (B)
Dexamethasone (N)	Erythromycin (B)		Diltiazem (B)
Diazepam (B)	Lidocaine (B)		Imipramine (B)
Diazoxide (A)	Meperidine (B)		Nortriptyline (B)
Dicloxacillin (A)	Methadone (B)		Perazine (B)
Digitoxin (N)	Verapamil (B)		Propranolol (B)
Etoposide (N)			Quinidine (B)
Ibuprofen (A)			
Indomethacin (A)			
Nafcillin (A)			
Naproxen (A)			
Oxacillin (A)			
Phenylbutazone (A)			
Phenytoin (A)			
Probenecid (A)			
Salicylic acid (A)			
Sulfisoxazole (A)			
Teniposide (N)			
Thiopental (A)			
Tolbutamide (A)			
Valproic acid (A)			
Warfarin (A)			

[a]   A = Acid; B = Base; N = Neutral.
[b]   Albumin is minor binding protein.

helpful in order to predict the likelihood of drug-drug displacement interactions. Recent studies, however, suggest that the sites are not preformed. Rather, these "sites" may be formed by conformational changes in albumin that occur during the drug-binding process itself.[20] Thus, the prediction of drug displacement interactions should also consider the allosteric effects that the binding of one drug can have on this very flexible protein molecule thereby affecting the binding of other drugs.[16]

Albumin Binding Capacity

Alterations in albumin concentrations in plasma occur as a result of altered synthesis, loss, or a shift of albumin from the intravascular to extravascular spaces.[11,22] The most common alteration, hypoalbuminemia, is associated with a wide variety of pathological and physiological conditions[11,18,22,24–27] as summarized in Table 5-3. For many albumin-bound drugs, this decrease in binding capacity results in significant increases in the unbound fraction of drug in plasma (Equation 5-3). The unbound plasma fractions of several highly bound drugs have been correlated to albumin concentration in plasma, as shown in Figure 5-3 for phenytoin in nephrotic syndrome.[28] Hypcralbuminemia is unusual, as shown in Table 5-3.

Albumin Affinity

Altered affinity of albumin for drugs can occur as a result of drug- or disease-induced changes in the structure of the albumin molecule, drug-induced allosteric changes in the binding site(s), or direct displacement by exogenous or endogenous inhibitors.[11,22,29,30] Competitive displacement is the most common cause of a

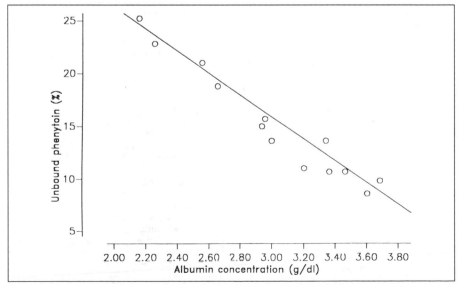

Figure 5-3. *Unbound percentage of phenytoin in serum of patients with nephrotic syndrome as a function of serum albumin concentration (data from Figure 1 of reference 28).*

Table 5-3. *Pathologic/Physiologic Conditions Associated with Altered Protein Concentrations*[11,12,15,18,22–27,204]

↓ plasma protein concentration	↑ plasma protein concentration
ALBUMIN	

↓ plasma protein concentration	↑ plasma protein concentration
Acute febrile infections	Dehydration
Acute viral hepatitis	Gynecologic syndrome
Acute pancreatitis	Optic neuritis/retinitis
Advanced age[a]	Psychosis
Analbuminemia[a]	Unspecified neuroses
Burn injury[a]	
Cancer[a]	
Cirrhosis[a]	
Cystic fibrosis	
Hyperthyroidism	
Malabsorption	
Malnutrition	
Neonates/young infants	
Nephrotic syndrome[a]	
Pregnancy[a]	
Prolonged bed-rest	
Protein-losing nephropathy	
Renal failure	
Rheumatoid arthritis	
Stress	
Surgery[a]	
Trauma injury[a]	

AAG

↓ plasma protein concentration	↑ plasma protein concentration
Advanced age	Acute myocardial infarction[a]
Cirrhosis[a]	Administration of some enzyme inducers[a]
Neonates/young infants	Advanced age
Nephrotic syndrome	Burn injury[a]
Oral contraceptives	Cancer[a]
Pregnancy	Chronic pain syndrome
Severe liver disease	Inflammatory disease[a]
	Pneumonia
	Renal transplantation
	Surgery[a]
	Trauma injury[a]

LIPOPROTEINS

↓ plasma protein concentration	↑ plasma protein concentration
Familial deficiencies[a]	Alcoholism
Hyperthyroidism	Antihypertensive drugs
Low cholesterol diet	Biliary obstruction
	Diabetes mellitus
	Familial hyperlipoproteinemia[a]
	Gout
	High cholesterol diet
	Hypothyroidism
	Liver disease
	Nephrotic syndrome
	Pancreatitis
	Phenytoin or cyclosporine administration
	Pregnancy
	Renal failure

[a] Conditions likely to be associated with major changes.

decreased apparent affinity of albumin for drugs and may result in an increase in the unbound fraction of drug in plasma (Equation 5-3). Under conditions of competitive displacement, the apparent dissociation constant (K_{Dapp}) for the displaced drug is determined by:

$$K_{Dapp} = K_D \left(1 + \frac{[I]}{K_I} \right)$$

(Eq. 5-5)

where [I] is the unbound concentration of the inhibitor in plasma, and K_I is the dissociation constant for the binding of the inhibitor to the same protein site.[20] For significant displacement to occur, the following criteria must be satisfied:[30] 1) the displaced drug must be highly bound; 2) the displacer and displaced drugs must share a common binding site (if competitive) or a common protein (if noncompetitive); 3) the binding sites must be limited in number such that the summed molar concentrations of the displaced and displacer approach the binding capacity (N_{TOT}); and 4) the free concentration of the displacer ([I]) must be higher than that of the displaced drug and/or the binding affinity for the displacer ($1/K_I$) must be higher than that for the displaced drug. Salicylate and sulfonamides, which have relatively high binding affinities for sites on albumin and achieve high concentrations in plasma following therapeutic doses, are examples of drugs that displace other drugs from albumin sites. Free fatty acids and bilirubin are examples of endogenous substances that bind to albumin with high affinities and can accumulate to relatively high concentrations in plasma. Under these conditions, they may displace certain drugs from albumin binding sites.[11,19,22]

Special note must be made of the possibility that drug enantiomers may displace one another from albumin binding sites. Many of the nonsteroidal anti-inflammatory drugs are administered as racemic mixtures. If one enantiomer has a higher affinity for binding and is present at higher concentrations, it can theoretically displace the other enantiomer. The higher oral clearance and distribution volume of R-ibuprofen in the presence of S-ibuprofen as compared to these values when R-ibuprofen is administered alone was proposed to be the result of R-ibuprofen displacement by the S-enantiomer.[31]

Concentration-Dependent Binding to Albumin

The percentage binding of a drug is independent of drug concentration as long as the molar unbound concentration ([D]) is well below the dissociation constants characterizing the drug-protein interactions, as seen in Equations 5-3 and 5-4. Concentration-dependent binding following therapeutic doses is therefore most likely to occur for drugs that bind with high affinity to albumin sites and for which therapeutic drug concentrations are relatively high (i.e., in the mg/L range). Examples of such drugs are valproic acid[32] (K_D for high affinity site: 5×10^{-5} M; therapeutic range of free concentrations: 0.7 to 2×10^{-4} M), salicylic acid[11] (K_D for high affinity site: 1×10^{-5} M; therapeutic range of free concentrations: 3 to 7×10^{-5} M), and several other nonsteroidal anti-inflammatory drugs.[20] Increases in the unbound plasma fractions of these drugs are seen with increases in therapeutic dose-rates.[20,26,33-35] Warfarin, which also binds to a high affinity site on albumin, does not show concentration-dependent binding following therapeutic doses because of its much lower free concentrations. Concentration-dependent binding is also reported for thiopental and diazoxide. When given by rapid intravenous injection, thiopental may achieve peak concentrations as high as 150 mg/L,[36] while peak concentrations of diazoxide are as high as 200 mg/L.[37] In the case of diazoxide, the decreased protein binding associated with rapid administration is a proposed advantage to obtaining maximal hypotensive response.[37]

DRUGS THAT BIND TO AAG

α_1-acid glycoprotein (orosomucoid) is now known to be a major binding protein for many basic drugs.[12] AAG also binds some acid[38,39] and neutral drugs,[6,40] but to a lesser extent. AAG is an α_1-globulin protein that is smaller than albumin (see Table 5-1) and is characterized by its high carbohydrate content.[9] In contrast to the homogeneity of albumin, polymorphic forms of AAG are normally found in human plasma.[17] At least four different polymorphic patterns and three different genetic variants have been reported, and there is evidence that these are genetically transmitted.[17,41] The biologic roles of AAG in plasma are still undefined. AAG is one of a group of proteins known as acute phase reactants.[9] Because increases in the plasma levels of these proteins are seen in a variety of apparently unrelated diseases and in states of inflammation or injury [12,18,22,24–27] (see Table 5-3), it is speculated that AAG may be required as an aid to cell proliferation.[14] Numerous other roles have also been proposed. The drug binding site on AAG is believed to be located on the polypeptide chain, rather than on the carbohydrate units, and may be shared by both acids and bases.[38,42] While a single binding site was reported for lidocaine in a pure AAG solution, two sites were reported when albumin was also present.[43] This was presumed to be the result of a conformational change in AAG caused by albumin.[43]

AAG Binding Capacity

Although decreases in plasma AAG concentrations occur in some situations, an increase in AAG binding capacity is most commonly observed in patients. As much as four- to fivefold increases in AAG concentrations are seen in a wide variety of conditions characterized by physiologic trauma or stress (see Table 5-3).[24] For drugs that are highly bound to AAG, an increase in capacity will significantly decrease the unbound plasma fraction. Examples include quinidine after surgery,[44] imipramine in cardiac patients,[45] propranolol,[46] lidocaine,[47] and disopyramide[48] after acute myocardial infarction, and propranolol and chlorpromazine in Crohn's disease.[49] Interpatient variability in the unbound plasma fractions of a number of drugs (e.g., alprenolol,[50] carbamazepine,[51] disopyramide,[48] imipramine,[50] lidocaine,[52] methadone,[53] and propranolol) are related to AAG concentrations in plasma.[54] Figure 5-4 shows an example of the relationship between unbound percentage of lidocaine in serum and serum AAG concentrations in patients with and without cancer.[55] Relative concentrations of the different AAG variants differ depending on disease states.[41,42,56] Since these variants also differ in their affinities for certain drugs,[56] correlations of total AAG concentration with unbound drug fraction in patients with a variety of disease states may be extremely variable.

AAG Affinity

For drugs that bind to both AAG and albumin, the affinity for AAG is generally higher than the affinity for albumin. For that reason and because of the lower concentrations of AAG in plasma relative to albumin, AAG is referred to as a "low capacity, high affinity" protein, while albumin is a "high capacity, low affinity" protein. Altered affinity of drug binding to AAG is most often caused by displacement by other drugs (usually bases) that also bind to AAG. Whether this displacement results in a significant increase in the unbound fraction in plasma depends on how much AAG accounts for the total binding in plasma.[30] Equation 5-4 predicts that for a drug binding to two proteins, the fraction bound is determined by the individual binding constants for both proteins. While the criteria for significant displacement may hold for drugs in a pure AAG solution (in particular that [I] + [D] approaches the molar concentration of AAG), the presence of high-capacity albumin in plasma tends to buffer any displacement effect. This is why significant displacement interactions involving basic drugs that bind appreciably to both albumin and AAG are uncommon. Simulations based on Equations 5-3 and 5-4 and the binding constants for carbamazepine[6] and lidocaine[57] illustrate this concept. A twofold decrease in the apparent K_A for carbamazepine binding to

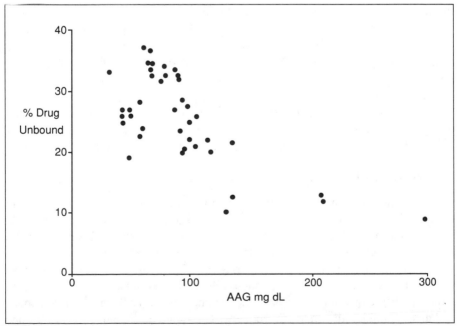

Figure 5-4. *Unbound percentage of lidocaine in serum as a function of serum AAG concentration in patients with cancer (●) and control patients (○) (reproduced with permission from reference 55).*

AAG (as might be caused by the presence of a displacer) results in a 31% increase in the unbound fraction of carbamazepine in a pure AAG solution, but only a 12% increase in plasma. On the other hand, a twofold decrease in the apparent K_A for lidocaine binding to AAG results in a 45% increase in the unbound fraction in a pure AAG solution, as compared to a 37% increase in plasma. In the case of lidocaine, a greater proportion of total binding in plasma is accounted for by AAG; thus, the buffering effect of albumin is minimized. For drugs like lidocaine, significant increases in unbound *plasma* fractions may occur if displacing drugs are present in sufficiently high concentration. For example, the unbound serum fraction of lidocaine is significantly increased by "therapeutic" bupivicaine concentrations of 3 to 4 mg/L.[57,58] Disopyramide is almost exclusively bound to AAG; however, no significant displacement interactions have been reported. This is probably because of the very high affinity of AAG for disopyramide.[4]

The displacement of drugs from AAG in plasma could become important in patients who have both elevated AAG concentrations and hypoalbuminemia. This pattern might be observed in patients with cancer, rheumatoid arthritis, severe burn injury, or after surgery (see Table 5-3). Since a smaller proportion of total drug binding is accounted for by albumin in this situation, its buffering effects on AAG displacement should be minimized. Studies showing minimal displacement using plasma from healthy volunteers must therefore be cautiously extrapolated to patients.

The enantiomers of disopyramide displace one another from AAG binding sites. This is shown by the lower affinity constants and higher unbound serum fractions of each enantiomer that exist when both are present in contrast to those that exist when each enantiomer is evaluated alone.[59] Our studies have shown dramatic displacement of S-verapamil from AAG by R-verapamil. The magnitude of this displacement was minimal in studies of serum, however, presumably because albumin was present. (MacKichan and Earle, unpublished data.) The absence of an enantiomer-enantiomer protein binding interaction in serum was confirmed in *in vivo* studies.[60]

Altered affinity of AAG for drugs may also occur as a result of conformational changes. The ability of nonesterified free fatty acids to increase the affinity of AAG for bupivicaine and etidocaine may be attributed to this effect.[61]

Concentration-Dependent Binding to AAG

As with albumin, the likelihood of concentration-dependent binding following therapeutic doses of drugs that bind to AAG is highest when unbound concentrations in plasma approach or exceed the dissociation constant (K_D) defining the AAG-drug interaction. Thus, those drugs with the highest affinities for AAG as well as relatively high therapeutic ranges (i.e., in the mg/L range) are likely to demonstrate concentration-dependent binding. The simulations in Figure 5-5, which are based on binding constants determined for carbamazepine,[6] lidocaine,[57] and disopyramide,[4] illustrate this concept. The range of unbound concentrations observed following therapeutic doses is roughly the same for the three drugs: 5×10^{-7} to 1.5×10^{-5} M. The affinity constants characterizing the drug-AAG interactions differ markedly, however. The affinity constant is highest for disopyramide (1×10^6 M^{-1}), next highest for lidocaine (1.3×10^5 M^{-1}), and lowest for carbamazepine (1.2×10^4 M^{-1}). As seen from Figure 5-5, there is pronounced concentration-dependence for disopyramide over the entire range of concentrations seen following therapeutic doses, while concentration-dependence for lidocaine is most evident at the high end of this concentration range. These simulations are consistent with the pronounced concentration-dependent binding for disopyramide observed in patients following therapeutic doses[4,62] and the concentration-dependent binding observed for lidocaine at the upper end of the therapeutic range[63,64] and following an overdose.[65] Carbamazepine binding is constant over the entire concentration range, as has been shown experimentally.[6]

Although the affinity constant describing the interaction between propranolol and AAG is similar in magnitude to that describing the lidocaine-AAG interaction, concentration-dependent binding of propranolol has not been reported. This is because of the very low unbound concentrations of propranolol observed following therapeutic doses. The concentration-dependent binding of prednisolone observed at very low unbound concentrations[66] can be explained by its binding to transcortin, which has an exceptionally high affinity for steroids and is present at quite low concentrations in plasma ($\approx 6 \times 10^{-7}$ M).

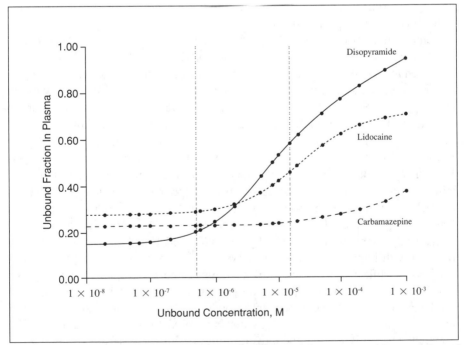

Figure 5-5. *Simulations of the effect of increasing unbound drug concentration on unbound plasma fraction for three drugs: carbamazepine ($K_D = 8.3 \times 10^{-5}$), lidocaine ($K_D = 7.7 \times 10^{-6}$), and disopyramide ($K_D = 1 \times 10^{-6}$). The vertical lines represent the concentration range of unbound drug associated with therapeutic doses of the three drugs.*

DRUGS THAT BIND TO LIPOPROTEINS

The lipoproteins are an extremely heterogeneous group of proteins that have a wide range of molecular weights and lipid contents ranging from 40% to 95%.[67] They are classified into four groups: chylomicrons, very low density lipoproteins (VLDL), low density lipoproteins (LDL), and high density lipoproteins (HDL). The VLDLs are the major carriers of triglycerides, while cholesterol is the major lipid associated with LDL and HDL.[15,67] Measurements of serum cholesterol or triglycerides provide an indirect measure of the concentrations of these lipoproteins. Although plasma concentrations of lipoproteins are relatively low (see Table 5-1), they can account for as much as 95% of total drug binding in plasma (e.g., probucol).[15] Neutral and basic lipophilic drugs most commonly bind to lipoproteins; some acid drugs may bind to a lesser extent.[15]

Many drugs that "bind" to lipoproteins are thought to actually partition into the lipid core of the protein instead of associating with a specific site.[12,68] Although the liposolubilization process is reversible, it appears to be "nonsaturable" over the drug concentration ranges usually used to determine drug binding parameters. Drugs which are believed to interact with lipoproteins by liposolubilization include probucol, cyclosporine, propranolol, pindolol, digoxin, digitoxin, and tetracycline.[12,15,69,203] Quinidine and several of the tricyclic antidepressants are among the drugs that exhibit "saturable" binding to lipoproteins and therefore are believed to bind to specific sites.[12,15]

Lipoprotein concentrations vary extensively within the normal population.[12,15] In addition, elevated serum concentrations of cholesterol and triglycerides are observed in a variety of disease states, in genetic or acquired disorders of lipoprotein metabolism, and even in patients taking certain drugs such as phenytoin or cyclosporine (see Table 5-3).[70,204] Correlations between unbound drug fractions in plasma and lipoprotein, cholesterol or triglyceride concentrations would therefore be expected for drugs that bind significantly to lipoproteins. The following findings support this. Unbound fractions of amitriptyline, imipramine, nortriptyline, and cyclosporine correlated inversely with concentrations of various lipoproteins in serum.[12,15,71] The unbound fraction of cyclosporine, which binds preferentially to HDL,[71] correlated with serum cholesterol concentrations,[72] while the unbound fraction of quinidine, which binds preferentially to VLDL,[73] correlated with serum triglyceride concentrations.[74] Finally, the unbound fractions of imipramine in patients with hyperlipoproteinemia were lower than those measured in normal subjects,[75] while unbound fractions of bupivicaine in fetal plasma were high relative to maternal plasma, presumably due to the lower HDL concentrations in fetal plasma.[76] Lipoprotein concentration is not always the best predictor of unbound plasma fractions of drugs that also bind to AAG and albumin. The apparent insensitivity of unbound quinidine fractions in serum to changes in lipoprotein concentrations[77] may be explained by the more important contribution of AAG to the total binding of quinidine.

Because liposolubilization is probably the major mechanism for drug association with the lipoproteins, competition between drugs for specific sites is not likely to occur. The lack of interaction between imipramine and propranolol for the "binding" to different lipoprotein fractions is consistent with this.[15] Likewise, concentration-dependent "binding" to lipoproteins is not expected following therapeutic doses. While even a partitioning process is theoretically saturable, the concentrations required for this are probably quite high.

ALTERED DRUG BINDING

Physiologic Conditions Associated With Altered Binding

Extremes of Age. The plasma protein binding of many albumin- and AAG-bound drugs is significantly lower in neonates than in healthy adults (see Table 5-4). There are several possible reasons for the decreased binding: 1) lower albumin and AAG concentrations; 2) persistence of fetal albumin, which may show a lower binding affinity for some drugs; 3) high concentrations of bilirubin and free fatty acids, which can displace drugs from albumin binding sites; and 4) unique interactions between albumin and globulins that may alter albumin binding affinity.[78 82] Modest decreases in albumin concentration in the elderly[83] probably account for the slightly lower plasma binding of drugs like diazepam,[84,85] phenylbutazone,[86] salicylate,[86] and valproic acid.[87] In contrast, consistent increases in the plasma binding of AAG-bound drugs occur with advancing age.[83] While AAG concentrations may be as much as twofold higher in the elderly, some of this effect may be attributable to the presence of inflammatory disease in this group.[83] In healthy elderly subjects, the average unbound fraction of lidocaine was only 9% lower than that observed in young subjects and was associated with AAG concentrations that were 16% higher.[85]

Pregnancy. Reduced plasma protein binding of several albumin-bound drugs occurs during pregnancy, particularly during the third trimester. Seventy to eighty percent increases in the unbound fractions of salicylate[20,88] and sulfisoxazole[88] have been reported, while moderate increases have been reported for phenytoin (25% to 30% increase),[88–90] diazepam (40% to 60% increase),[88,89] and valproic acid (50% increase).[89] Only a 10% increase in the unbound fraction of

Table 5-4. *Drugs Showing Decreased Plasma Binding in Neonates*

Albumin-bound drugs		AAG-bound drugs	
Drug	% free in plasma neonate/adult	Drug	% free in plasma neonate/adult
Carbamazepine[78]	32/27	Bupivicaine[76]	10–100/2–25
Chloramphenicol[79]	54/34	Desipramine[79]	35/17
Diazepam[81]	32/12	Imipramine[81]	26/12
Nafcillin[81]	38/26	Lidocaine[82]	69/32
Nitrofurantoin[79]	38/26	Morphine[79]	69/58
Phenobarbital[79]	68/49	Promethazine[79]	30/17
Phenylbutazone[81]	13/3	Propranolol[82]	43/15
Phenytoin[79]	26/14		
Salicylic acid[79]	9/4		
Sulfamethoxydiazine[79]	20/10		
Theophylline[80]	64/50		
Thiopental[79]	13/7		

dexamethasone was observed,[88] and little to no effect was observed for carbamazepine.[90] Lower albumin concentrations, higher concentrations of free fatty
acids (especially during labor), and the possible presence of other binding inhibitors are likely responsible for the lower binding of these drugs.[25,88–90] Unbound
fractions of AAG-bound drugs such as bupivicaine,[91] propranolol,[82] and lidocaine[82]
are reported to increase by 35% to 80% in late pregnancy. In the case of lidocaine
and propranolol, correlations between AAG concentration and plasma binding
suggest that lower AAG concentrations are likely to be responsible for the
decreased binding.[82] Normalization of AAG and free fatty acid concentrations
occurs within a few days of delivery, while normal levels of albumin are attained
within one month.[90]

Gender, Smoking, Obesity, Nutritional Status, and Surgery. Slightly higher
unbound fractions of chlordiazepoxide, diazepam, imipramine, and nitrazepam
have been reported in nonpregnant females as compared to males.[25,92,93] In the case
of diazepam, the 14% higher average unbound fraction in females was accounted
for by the slightly lower albumin and AAG concentrations in this group.[93] No
differences in the binding of lidocaine were seen between males and females.[93]
Smoking was associated with increased plasma binding of lidocaine in one study
(unbound fraction of 0.26 versus 0.31 in nonsmokers) and was suggested to be
due to higher AAG concentrations in this population.[64] Another study showed no
effect of smoking on albumin, AAG, free fatty acid concentrations, or on the
plasma binding of lidocaine and diazepam.[85] AAG concentrations in obese female
subjects were shown to be twice those in females of normal body weight and were
associated with a 30% lower plasma unbound fraction of propranolol.[94] Albumin
concentrations were normal in the obese subjects thus accounting for the normal
binding of phenytoin and only slight decrease in diazepam binding.[94] AAG
concentrations in undernourished or hospitalized patients were 30% to 40% higher
than unhospitalized subjects and were associated with a reduction in the free
fraction of propranolol of approximately 30%.[95] The lower albumin concentrations
and higher AAG concentrations associated with the post-operative condition (see
Table 5-3) are the most likely explanations for the 100% to 150% higher unbound
plasma fractions of albumin-bound phenytoin in these patients[96,97] and the 30% to
40% reductions in unbound plasma fractions of quinidine[44] and propranolol.[98] The
almost fourfold higher unbound plasma fraction of ceftriaxone in patients undergoing open heart surgery as compared to healthy subjects is due to a combination
of low plasma albumin and high free fatty acid concentrations.[99,23]

Diurnal Variations. Variations in plasma unbound fractions throughout the
day occur for several drugs, and for albumin-bound drugs are often temporally
related to food intake. Free fatty acid concentrations are highest in the fasting state
and reduced after meals[100] which likely explains the 18% reduction in plasma
unbound fraction of diazepam[100] observed after meals. In addition to meal-related
changes in free fatty acid concentrations, concentration-dependent binding of
valproic acid contributes to the marked fluctuations in unbound fraction observed
during the day in epileptic patients.[101,102] Diurnal variations in plasma concentra-

tions of AAG have also been reported, with coefficients of variation within subjects during a 24-hour period ranging from 6% to 50%.[103] Fluctuations in the binding of AAG-bound drugs should be anticipated as well.

Pathologic Conditions Associated With Altered Binding

Altered plasma protein binding as a consequence of disease can be the result of altered protein concentrations, qualitative changes in the protein molecules, or displacement by accumulated endogenous substances. A list of drugs and the disease states associated with altered plasma protein binding is presented in Table 5-5.[12,18,20,22,25,27,104–108]

Renal Disease. Several mechanisms have been proposed to explain the decreased binding of many albumin-bound drugs in chronic renal failure and uremia (see Table 5-5). These include: 1) a change in the primary structure of albumin which either occurs during synthesis or as a consequence of prolonged exposure to high cyanate levels, or 2) displacement by endogenous inhibitors that accumulate in renal failure.[29,106] Although there is strong evidence for both mechanisms, endogenous inhibitors are believed to account for most of the decreased binding.[106] Renal transplantation appears to normalize the binding somewhat, while hemodialysis has little effect.[106] A 30% reduction in the average unbound plasma fraction of lidocaine was seen in patients with uremia and in patients who had undergone kidney transplant operations and was accounted for by elevated plasma concentrations of AAG.[109] Higher AAG concentrations occur in patients with chronic renal failure who also have superimposed inflammatory disease as compared to patients with uncomplicated renal disease.[49] This probably accounts for the 20% to 40% lower unbound plasma fractions of chlorpromazine and propranolol observed in the former group. The unbound percentages of phenytoin and clofibrate are reportedly 90% and 200% higher, respectively, in patients with nephrotic syndrome as compared to normals.[28] Since nephrotic syndrome appears to be the only disease state in which hypoalbuminemia alone accounts for the decreased binding of drugs,[28] decreased binding of other albumin-bound drugs in nephrotic syndrome should also be anticipated.

Liver Disease. Because of the variety of hepatic diseases, altered drug binding in liver disease is difficult to predict. While decreased binding is reported for some drugs (see Table 5-5), no changes are reported for others.[12] Mechanisms for decreased drug binding in patients with liver disease include: 1) decreased albumin and AAG concentrations due to either a decreased rate of synthesis or loss of protein from plasma to interstitial compartments; 2) the accumulation of endogenous inhibitors such as bilirubin; and 3) possible qualitative changes in the albumin molecule.[20,25,108] Chronic conditions, such as cirrhosis, are more likely to be associated with altered drug binding than acute conditions such as viral hepatitis.[26] The average unbound fractions of albumin-bound diazepam and tolbutamide were 65% to 75% higher in chronic alcoholics compared to controls,[110] while unbound fractions of AAG-bound erythromycin were two to four times higher in patients with severe cirrhosis compared to controls.[111] The unbound fractions of diazepam and tolbutamide were highly correlated to albumin concentrations, while the

Table 5-5.   *Diseases Associated with Altered Plasma Protein Binding of Drugs* [12,18,20,22,24,27,104–108]

Disease	Drug examples	
	↓ binding	↑ binding
Acute myocardial infarction		Disopyramide Imipramine Lidocaine Propranolol
Burn injury	Diazepam Phenytoin Valproic acid	Imipramine
Cancer	Tolbutamide	Lidocaine Methadone Propranolol
Cystic fibrosis	Theophylline	
Diabetes mellitus	Cyclosporine Diazepam Sulfisoxazole	
Hyperlipoproteinemia		Fentanyl Imipramine
Inflammatory disease/injury[a]		Chlorpromazine (A, C) Lidocaine (T) Propranolol (C)
Liver Disease[b]	Chlordiazepoxide (C, VH) Diazepam (C) Erythromycin (C) Lorazepam (C, VH) Morphine Phenylbutazone (C) Phenytoin (C,VH) Propranolol (C) Quinidine (C) Tolbutamide (C,VH) Verapamil	
Nephrotic syndrome	Clofibrate Diazepam Phenytoin	
Renal failure	Cephalosporins Chloramphenicol Dicloxacillin Diazepam Diazoxide Diflunisal Digitoxin Furosemide Midazolam Naproxen Penicillin G Phenylbutazone Phenytoin Salicylic acid Sulfonamides Triamterene Warfarin	Chlorpromazine[c] Propranolol[c] Lidocaine

Table 5-5. *Diseases Associated with Altered Plasma Protein Binding of Drugs*[12,18,20,22,24,27,104–108] *(cont.)*

| Disease | Drug examples | |
	↓ binding	↑ binding
Thyroid disease		
Hyperthyroid	Propranolol	
	Warfarin	
Hypothyroid		Propranolol

[a] A = Arthritis; C = Crohn's disease; T = Trauma injury.
[b] C = Cirrhosis; VH = Viral hepatitis.
[c] Associated with inflammatory disease.

unbound fraction of erythromycin correlated with AAG concentrations. The higher unbound fractions of phenytoin in patients with hepatitis or cirrhosis (15.9% as compared to 10.6% for controls) did not correlate with albumin concentration but did correlate with plasma bilirubin concentration.[112]

Acute Myocardial Infarction. The plasma binding of several cationic drugs (see Table 5-5) is higher in patients diagnosed with acute myocardial infarction.[45-48] AAG concentrations increased by 50% to 250% within five days after infarction and returned to normal within 75 days.[45,47] The implications of this increase in binding may be especially important for drugs like lidocaine and propranolol which are used to prevent life-threatening arrhythmias in these patients.

Cancer and Severe Burn Injury. Cancer and severe burn injury are associated with increased concentrations of AAG and decreased concentrations of albumin in plasma.[53-55,113] Twenty to thirty percent decreases in the unbound plasma fractions of AAG-bound drugs such as lidocaine,[55] methadone,[53] propranolol,[55] and imipramine[113] have been reported in these patients, while increased unbound fractions of albumin-bound drugs such as tolbutamide (30% increase),[55] diazepam (180% increase),[113] and phenytoin (150% increase)[114] have been shown. The affinity of lidocaine for the presumed AAG binding site was higher in cancer patients as compared to normals.[55] An unusual AAG variant pattern in cancer may explain this phenomenon.[115]

Diabetes Mellitus. The decreased plasma binding of sulfisoxazole in diabetics is explained by *in vivo* glycosylation of albumin, a consequence of prolonged exposure to high serum glucose levels.[116,117] In contrast, the decreased plasma binding of diazepam is proposed to be caused by high concentrations of free fatty acid displacers, not by glycosylation.[116,117] The slightly higher unbound plasma fraction of cyclosporine in diabetics after renal transplant relative to post-transplant non-diabetics was explained by the lower lipoprotein and albumin concentrations in the diabetics.[71]

Thyroid Disease. Hyperthyroidism is associated with decreased concentrations of all drug-binding proteins and increased concentrations of free fatty acids in plasma. Twenty percent to thirty percent increases in the unbound plasma fractions of warfarin and propranolol, respectively, have been reported in hyper-thyroid patients.[118] The effects of hypothyroidism, which is associated with in-creased protein concentrations and lower free fatty acids, may not be as predictable.[118]

Cystic Fibrosis. There are few reports of altered plasma binding of drugs in cystic fibrosis patients despite the well-documented occurrence of hypoalbumine-mia in this group.[105] Of the drugs studied, the unbound fraction in the plasma of cystic fibrosis patients compared to controls was significantly higher (30%) only for theophylline. While the unbound plasma fraction of dicloxacillin was normal in the majority of cystic fibrosis patients, some had unbound fractions that were grossly elevated.[119] Thus, while decreased plasma protein binding should always be anticipated in cystic fibrosis patients, it may not always be evident.

Conditions Associated with Elevated AAG and Lipoprotein Concentra-tions. Increased lidocaine binding was reported in trauma patients, and this was associated with a progressive rise in AAG concentrations over three weeks.[52] The average unbound fraction of lidocaine was 0.28 when AAG concentrations were at a minimum and 0.15 when AAG concentrations were at a peak.[52] Unbound plasma fractions of propranolol and chlorpromazine were between 30% and 40% lower in patients with Crohn's disease and inflammatory arthritis.[49] We observed a lower affinity constant for disopyramide binding to AAG in patients with arthritis but not in those with Crohn's disease and attribute this to either the presence of a binding inhibitor or to a change in the variant composition of AAG (MacKichan and Lima, unpublished data). Hyperlipoproteinemia was associated with 20% to 30% decreases in the unbound plasma fractions of imipramine and fentanyl.[75,120] The 25% decrease in the mean unbound plasma fraction of cyclosporine im-mediately before an acute kidney transplant rejection episode may also be caused by high lipoprotein concentrations during this time.[71]

Drug-Induced Alterations in Binding

One drug can alter the binding of another drug by: 1) displacing it from its binding sites and hence altering the apparent affinity; 2) changing the protein conformation and thus altering true binding affinity; or 3) causing a change in protein concentration in plasma.

Drug displacement is the most common mechanism for drug-induced alter-ations in drug binding. Reports of displacement are more common for drugs that are bound predominantly to a single protein with high affinity, as described previously. Thus, examples of drug displacement are more common for drugs that are highly bound only to albumin as compared to drugs that bind to AAG with high affinity and to albumin with low affinity. Examples of drug displacement interactions involving albumin-bound drugs are provided in Table 5-6.[30] Examples of displacement interactions that involve AAG-bound drugs include verapamil displacement by its metabolites[60,121] and lidocaine displacement by bupivicaine.[58]

High-dose acetylsalicylic acid can alter drug binding by altering albumin binding site conformation. Aspirin acetylates a lysine residue in the peptide A region of albumin[122] and thus is likely to affect only those drugs binding in that region. The binding of phenylbutazone and acetriazoate (a contrast medium) was enhanced during aspirin therapy, while the binding of flufenamic acid was reduced.[122,123]

Certain drugs can also alter the concentrations of drug binding proteins in plasma. AAG concentrations in plasma were approximately 60% higher in patients taking phenytoin[124,125] and 23% higher in patients taking carbamazepine.[125] Higher AAG concentrations were also observed in patients taking amitriptyline.[126] The finding of increased lidocaine binding in patients taking antiepileptic drugs is consistent with these findings.[124] Increased concentrations of certain lipoprotein fractions have also been reported following treatment with phenytoin, phenobarbital and cyclosporine.[70,127,204] While a link between enzyme induction and AAG synthesis has been proposed, enzyme induction caused by rifampicin was not associated with an increase in plasma AAG concentrations.[128] Albumin and AAG concentrations are reduced in women taking estrogen/progesterone oral contraceptive therapy.[93] The unbound fractions of diazepam and lidocaine were 10% to 20% higher in women taking oral contraceptives compared to those who were not.[93]

Altered Protein Binding Due to *In Vitro* Artifact

Artifactually high unbound fractions of drugs in plasma have been associated with the use of certain blood collection devices, the use of heparin, the method of sample storage, or the sample source itself. Early studies of the binding of basic drugs in blood samples collected using Vacutainers showed unusually high and variable unbound fractions.[12,129,130] This was attributed to displacement of basic drugs from AAG binding sites by a plasticizer in the stopper.[130] Although the stopper has since been reformulated, blood contact with any plastic device should be considered a possible source of error when unusually low binding measurements are observed.

Heparin, even at the low doses used to flush indwelling cannulae, reduced the plasma binding of several drugs, including phenytoin, propranolol, lidocaine, diazepam, quinidine, and verapamil.[131,132] This effect was originally attributed to heparin-induced release of lipoprotein lipase which was presumed to cause large increases in the *in vivo* levels of free fatty acid displacers of albumin-bound drugs. For most drugs, this effect is now believed to be an *in vitro* artifact caused by the continued activity of the lipase enzyme and accumulation of fatty acids in the blood collection tube.[132,133] For these drugs, addition of a lipoprotein lipase inhibitor to the blood sample upon collection may eliminate the artifact.[132] Not all heparin effects appear to be artifact mediated by free fatty acids (e.g., diazepam).[134] If there is a direct effect of heparin on the *in vivo* binding of drugs, it will be most obvious in situations that require high doses of heparin, such as coronary by-pass surgery and hemodialysis.

Prolonged storage and higher temperatures were associated with *in vitro* increases in the unbound fractions of valproic acid.[135] The effect occurred in both serum and heparinized plasma and was highly correlated to free fatty acid concentration. Overestimates of valproic acid unbound fractions by as much as

160% were seen when plasma or serum was incubated at 37 °C for 24 hours.[135] Methods requiring minimal incubation times are therefore recommended when unbound fractions of this drug are to be determined.

Anticoagulants or storage containers may also affect drug binding measurements. The unbound fractions of phenytoin and meperidine were 80% higher in citrated plasma than in serum or heparinized plasma.[136] The mean unbound fraction of disopyramide was 20% higher in pooled blood bank plasma than in fresh drug-free serum at the same post-dialysis total drug concentration.[4] The restoration of normal disopyramide binding by charcoal treatment of the blood bank plasma led investigators to conclude that binding inhibitors (probably plasticizers in the bags) were responsible.[4]

Finally, contamination of apparently pure proteins with other proteins can lead to inaccurate conclusions regarding the predominant binding proteins of drugs. Early studies of disopyramide are suspected of having overestimated the contribution of albumin to total plasma binding because of AAG-contaminated commercial albumin lots.[137] The use of defatted serum albumin can also lead to inappropriate conclusions of high binding values for acid drugs because normal levels of circulating inhibitors such as free fatty acids are absent.[138] Lipophilic contamination of an isolated AAG preparation was believed to account for the lower binding capacity and affinity of bupivicaine in a pure AAG solution as compared to those parameters measured in serum.[139]

PHARMACOKINETIC CONSEQUENCES OF ALTERED PLASMA AND TISSUE PROTEIN BINDING

Determinants of Drug Concentration-Time Profiles

The pharmacokinetic parameters of clearance (CL), steady-state volume of distribution (V_{ss}), and elimination half-life (t½) can be influenced by changes in plasma and/or tissue protein binding. This will lead to changes in the concentration-time profiles for total and/or unbound drug during chronic drug intake and thus necessitate either a dosage regimen adjustment and/or cautious interpretation of the total drug concentration measurement. [The reader should note that pharmacokinetic parameters should ideally be based on blood rather than plasma concentrations. While the fraction of drug unbound in blood (f_{ub}) is not the same as the unbound fraction in plasma (f_{up}) for most drugs, unbound blood concentrations will always be the same as unbound plasma concentrations since: $f_{up} \cdot C_p = f_{ub} \cdot C_b$. Thus, plasma binding and plasma concentrations, which are most commonly measured, will always provide an accurate estimate of unbound blood concentration. The use of plasma-related parameters can sometimes lead to inaccurate estimates of organ extraction ratios and intrinsic clearances, however.[140] In these situations, the ratio of blood to plasma concentrations (B:P) must be used to convert plasma parameters to blood parameters as follows: $f_{ub} = f_{up}/B{:}P$; $C_b = C_p \cdot B{:}P$.] The average steady-state plasma drug concentration ($C_{av,ss}$) achieved during chronic dosing is determined by the administered dose-rate, (D/τ), bioavailable fraction (F), and plasma clearance according to:

$$C_{av,ss} = F \cdot \frac{\frac{D}{\tau}}{CL} \qquad \text{(Eq. 5-6)}$$

The average unbound drug concentration in plasma at steady state is more important in determining drug response, particularly in situations of unusual plasma protein binding, and is determined by:

$$C_u = f_{up} \cdot C_{av,ss} \qquad \text{(Eq. 5-7)}$$

The degree of fluctuation in the concentration-time profile (peak-to-trough ratio, P:T) during a dosing interval can also be important and is determined by the rate of drug input and the drug's elimination half-life (t½) relative to the chosen dosing interval. The influence of half-life on P:T can be seen by:

$$P:T \approx e^{(0.693)\left(\frac{\tau}{t^{1/2}}\right)} \qquad \text{(Eq. 5-8)}$$

where t½, assuming that $V_\beta \approx V_{ss}$,[141] is determined by:

$$t^{1/2} \approx \frac{V_{ss}}{CL} \cdot 0.693 \qquad \text{(Eq. 5-9)}$$

From the above, it is evident that changes in C_u that occur as a consequence of altered plasma binding may require an adjustment in the drug dose-rate, while a change in degree of fluctuation may require a change in the dosing interval.

Volume of Distribution

Both tissue and plasma protein binding will influence the apparent volume of distribution of a drug according to the following relationship:[142–145]

$$V_{ss} = V_p + \left(\frac{f_{up}}{f_{ut}}\right)V_t \qquad \text{(Eq. 5-10)}$$

where f_{up} is the unbound fraction of drug in plasma, f_{ut} is the unbound fraction of drug in "tissue," and V_p is plasma volume (0.07 L/kg).[144] For lipophilic drugs that penetrate cells, "tissue" volume (V_t) is equal to total body water minus plasma volume (approximately 0.6 L/kg). For polar drugs that cannot penetrate cells, such as the aminoglycosides, V_t is extracellular fluid minus plasma volume (approximately 0.13 L/kg).[144] A more complex relationship for V_{ss} which includes a term for the intravascular-extravascular distribution of binding proteins has also been proposed.[146]

The magnitude of drug binding in plasma versus that in tissue is the primary determinant of the apparent volume of distribution for a drug. For example, amiodarone, digoxin, and the tricyclic antidepressants have very large distribution volumes because they are much more highly bound to proteins in tissues than to proteins in plasma.[147] On the other hand, the small distribution volumes of warfarin, valproic acid, and the penicillins are attributable to high plasma binding relative to tissue binding.[147]

The determinants of drug binding in tissue are the same as those for plasma binding: protein concentration in tissue, affinity of tissue protein for drug, and unbound drug concentration. Unfortunately, tissue binding is difficult to measure because it is invasive and because there are various degrees of binding to a variety of proteins in different tissues. An estimate of overall tissue binding in the body (f_{ut}) can be made, however, by use of Equation 5-10 when V_{ss} and f_{up} are known and anatomic volumes are assumed.[144] This method was used to conclude that the f_{ut} of tolbutamide in patients with acute viral hepatitis increases in parallel with f_{up}, thus explaining why the V_{ss} of tolbutamide is unaltered.[144] The demonstration of altered phenytoin binding in the plasma of uremic and nephrotic syndrome patients without a change in tissue binding[28,144] reinforces the notion that there is no *a priori* reason to suspect that changes in plasma binding will be paralleled by changes in tissue binding. Other examples of altered tissue binding include tissue displacement of digoxin by quinidine[148] and decreased tissue binding of digoxin in uremia.[149] Since plasma binding of digoxin is unaffected, the distribution volume of digoxin is decreased in both cases.

Increased distribution volumes are most often the result of increased unbound fractions in plasma. Examples include propranolol in chronic stable liver disease, phenytoin in uremia and nephrotic syndrome, diazepam and phenytoin in liver disease, and many drugs in neonates.[80,149] Increased volumes of distribution may also be caused by shifts of albumin-bound drug from the vascular to interstitial spaces, as noted for ceftriaxone during open heart surgery.[99] Decreased volumes of distribution caused by increased binding in plasma would be expected for drugs that bind to AAG in cases of trauma.

An unusual effect of increased plasma binding on distribution volume has been reported for cyclosporine[150] which binds predominantly to lipoproteins in plasma. High-fat meals, which consist mainly of VLDL and chylomicrons, were associated with increased plasma binding of cyclosporine and an increased rather than decreased distribution volume. This was attributed to the fact that, unlike the other drug-binding proteins, lipoproteins are rapidly cleared from blood into adipose tissue. Theoretically, the cyclosporine-lipoprotein complex was also carried into adipose tissue thus increasing the tissue binding of this drug.[150]

Clearance

Restrictive versus Nonrestrictive Clearance Models. Gillette[142] conceptualized the notion of "restrictive" and "nonrestrictive" clearance in relation to the degree of protein binding in plasma or blood. This concept helps to predict the effects of altered protein binding on blood or plasma clearance and hence, on total and free drug concentrations. A drug is said to undergo restrictive clearance if the extraction efficiency (E) by an eliminating organ is less than or equal to the unbound fraction of drug measured in the venous circulation (f_{ub}). Extraction of drug by the organ—and consequently clearance—is considered to be limited by protein binding in this case and hence, is altered by changes in f_{ub}.[143,145,151] On the other hand, nonrestrictive clearance is observed when E is greater than the measured unbound fraction. In this case, protein binding does not appear to protect the drug from elimination and, in fact, may be viewed as a delivery system for elimination.[143,145,151]

Rowland et al.[152] and Wilkinson and Shand[143] used the simple venous equilibrium model of organ clearance to quantitatively account for the effects of altered blood flow, intrinsic clearance, and blood protein binding on hepatic clearance and the first-pass metabolism of drugs. Other models of hepatic clearance have also been developed including the undistributed and distributed sinusoidal models as well as the dispersion model.[153] These models all make the following assumptions, explicitly or implicitly, with respect to blood protein binding: 1) that only unbound drug can traverse membranes; and 2) that the fraction of drug available for metabolism in the liver is the same as the unbound fraction of drug that is measured in the systemic circulation (f_{ub}). These assumptions are used to justify calculating intrinsic clearance of free drug (CLu_{int} or V_{max}/K_m) by dividing the measured intrinsic clearance of total drug by the measured unbound fraction in blood. While these assumptions may be valid for restrictively cleared drugs,[153] there is growing evidence that the fraction of drug available for metabolism may not be limited to the unbound fraction of drug measured in blood[154] as described below.

There is evidence that AAG-drug and lipoprotein-drug complexes can be directly taken up into hepatocytes by endocytotic mechanisms.[15,150,155] The fact that nonrestrictive clearance by the liver appears to occur only for drugs that bind to AAG and possibly lipoproteins, makes this "receptor-mediated endocytosis" theory a plausible mechanism for nonrestrictive behavior. Restrictive versus nonrestrictive clearance can also be explained on the basis of the rate of drug dissociation from protein during its passage through the eliminating organ.[156] Accordingly, an "albumin-receptor model" was proposed to account for the high extraction of certain very highly albumin-bound substrates.[157,158] This model suggests that association of the albumin-drug complex with a special receptor on the hepatocyte surface results in a conformational change in the albumin molecule and an increased rate of dissociation of drug from albumin.[157] Rapid dissociation of the drug-protein complex was also proposed to explain the nonrestrictive elimination behavior of the basic drug d-tubocurarine in a rat liver perfusion model, in which four- to sixfold increases in drug binding had no effect on d-tubocurarine clearance.[155]

It thus appears that the assumptions of the traditional hepatic clearance models may not be appropriate for drugs that are nonrestrictively cleared. This could explain the large differences in predictions among the models for the effects of altered binding on unbound concentrations of highly extracted drugs, especially when they are given orally.[153] In this chapter, a "modified" venous equilibrium model is used to predict the effects of altered blood protein binding on blood clearance:

$$CL = \frac{Q \cdot (CLu_{int} \cdot f_{avail})}{Q + (CLu_{int} \cdot f_{avail})}$$

(Eq. 5-11)

Equation 5-11 says that the clearance of drug by an eliminating organ depends on the fraction of drug in blood that is available for elimination (f_{avail}), organ blood flow (Q), and intrinsic clearance (CLu_{int}), which reflects either enzyme activity or renal tubular secretion activity. In the case of a restrictively cleared drug ($E \leq f_{ub}$), f_{ub} and f_{avail} are presumed to be equal, so that changes in f_{ub} will affect blood clearance. For nonrestrictively cleared drugs ($E > f_{ub}$), f_{avail} is greater than f_{ub} (in fact it is somewhere between f_{ub} and E) because the drug is rapidly dissociated from protein or there is direct uptake of the drug-protein complex. The unbound fraction of drug in blood is therefore not rate-limiting and changes in f_{ub} will have no effect on f_{avail}. Drug clearance will therefore be unaffected by changes in blood or plasma protein binding.

Unfortunately, the validity and applicability of this and the other models of nonrestrictive clearance are difficult to confirm experimentally. Data from studies using isolated perfused rat livers may be problematic because of the very high intrinsic clearances of drugs by the rat liver compared to the human liver. Also, there are no experimental data in humans regarding the effects of altered plasma protein binding on clearance and first-pass metabolism. Diseases that result in altered binding are often also associated with alterations in organ blood flows or intrinsic clearances, thus making it difficult to attribute a particular effect to a change in protein binding only. While a protein binding displacement interaction would provide an ideal experimental situation, most nonrestrictively cleared drugs are bound to AAG and displacement usually will not result in a measurable increase in f_{up} or f_{ub} because albumin and lipoproteins also bind the drug. Despite these difficulties, the data by Kornhauser et al.[159] suggest that clearance and bioavailability of propranolol are independent of f_{up}, which is consistent with the "modified" venous equilibrium model.

Restrictive Clearance. For drugs that are inefficiently extracted by an elimination organ, such that $[(CLu_{int})(f_{avail})] < Q$, and for which $E \leq f_{ub}$ (restrictive clearance: $f_{avail} = f_{ub}$), Equation 5-11 simplifies to:

$$CL \approx CLu_{int} \cdot f_{ub} \qquad \text{(Eq. 5-12)}$$

Because the drug is restrictively cleared, changes in f_{ub} will result in proportional changes in blood clearance for very low extraction drugs and less than proportional effects for drugs with higher intrinsic clearances.[160] An example of the dependence of plasma clearance on f_{up} is illustrated in Figure 5-6 for phenytoin in patients with nephrotic syndrome.[28] Other drugs that are restrictively cleared by the liver include diazepam, tolbutamide, phenylbutazone, warfarin, valproic acid,[108] disopyramide,[4] quinidine,[161] and ibuprofen.[31] Disopyramide[4] and quinidine[161] also are reported to be restrictively cleared by renal tubular secretion.

The average steady-state unbound drug concentration in plasma for a poorly extracted, restrictively-cleared drug is determined only by the bioavailable fraction (which is determined primarily by the extent of absorption) and intrinsic organ clearance:

$$C_u \approx \frac{F \cdot \dfrac{D}{\tau}}{CLu_{int}}$$ (Eq. 5-13)

Thus, changes in blood or plasma protein binding will have no effect on unbound drug concentrations provided there is no effect on intrinsic clearance via enzyme induction or inhibition, liver disease, or inhibition of renal tubular secretion. While dose-rate changes should not be required as a consequence of altered binding, cautious interpretation of total drug concentration will always be necessary.

It is important to recognize that a sudden increase in f_{up}, such as that which might occur when a displacer is administered, will cause a transient rise in unbound drug concentration. As shown in Figure 5-7, unbound drug concentration will rise immediately after displacement and eventually return to the predisplacement average value once a new steady state has been reached. The unbound concentration immediately after displacement will be highest for drugs with small volumes of distribution and will decline most slowly for drugs with long elimination half-lives.[30,145] Because drugs with small volumes rarely have long half-lives, clinically-important transient rises in free concentration are seen with only a few drugs such as warfarin.[30,145]

The effect that altered plasma and/or tissue protein binding has on the elimination half-life of a restrictively-cleared drug depends on the drug's volume of

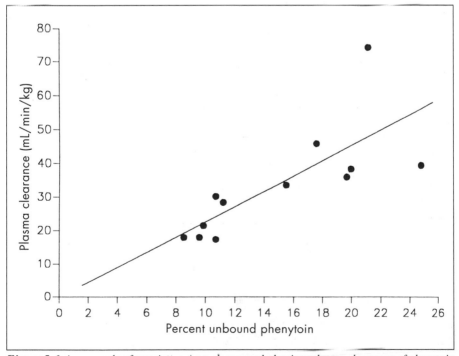

Figure 5-6. *An example of restrictive drug clearance behavior: plasma clearance of phenytoin as a function of the unbound percentage of phenytoin in plasma (data from Figure 2 of reference 28).*

distribution.[141] Most drugs have moderate to large V_{ss} values (i.e., >0.4 L/kg). For these drugs, V_p in Equation 5-10 contributes little to V_{ss}, and half-life is determined by:

$$t\tfrac{1}{2} \approx 0.693 \left(\frac{V_t}{CLu_{int} \cdot f_{ut}} \right)$$

(Eq. 5-14)

Altered plasma binding will therefore have little effect on the half-lives of restrictively-cleared drugs such as diazepam and phenytoin.[145] For a smaller number of drugs, V_{ss} values are less than 0.4 L/kg; for them, $t\tfrac{1}{2}$ is affected by changes in plasma and tissue binding according to:

$$t\tfrac{1}{2} \approx 0.693 \left(\frac{V_p}{CLu_{int} \cdot f_{up}} + \frac{V_t}{CLu_{int} \cdot f_{ut}} \right)$$

(Eq. 5-15)

The effect of altered plasma binding on the half-life of a warfarin-like drug (small V_{ss}) is illustrated in Figure 5-8a. Displacement of this drug from plasma proteins does not affect the average unbound concentration once a new steady state is reached, but the peak-to-trough ratio is slightly higher because of the shorter half-life. As expected for all restrictively cleared drugs, the average total concentration is lower during concurrent administration of the displacer.

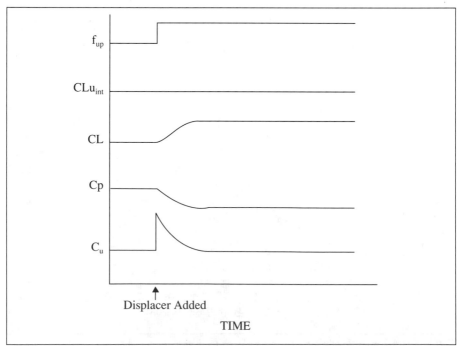

Figure 5-7. *Time course of changes in unbound drug fraction (f_{up}), total (Cp) and unbound drug concentrations (C_u) for a displaced drug that is restrictively cleared.*

Nonrestrictive Clearance. For drugs that are efficiently extracted by an eliminating organ [$(CLu_{int} \times f_{avail}) > Q$] and nonrestrictively cleared ($E > f_{ub}$), clearance will be determined primarily by organ blood flow, less influenced by intrinsic clearance, and independent of changes in f_{ub} or f_{up}. The lack of dependence of propranolol clearance on f_{up} is illustrated in Figure 5-9 which is based on the data of Kornhauser et al.[159,162] The bioavailable fraction of an oral dose will be low due to first-pass metabolism and will also be independent of changes in blood or plasma protein binding. Thus, altered plasma binding should not affect the average total drug concentrations of nonrestrictively cleared drugs given orally or intravenously.[145] Examples of other drugs that are nonrestrictively cleared include morphine, meperidine, lidocaine,[108] verapamil,[60] and the tricyclic antidepressants,[26] while those nonrestrictively cleared by renal tubular secretion include some of the penicillins and acetazolamide.[30]

Since unbound drug concentration is determined by the product of total plasma concentration and f_{up}, a change in f_{up} will cause a proportional change in unbound drug concentration and, presumably, in response. Thus, in contrast to restrictively cleared drugs, changes in oral or intravenous dose-rates of nonrestrictively-cleared drugs might be required in situations where f_{up} is altered. In addition, monitoring total (bound plus unbound) drug concentrations in this situation may be misleading since a change in response may be seen without a change in total drug concentration.

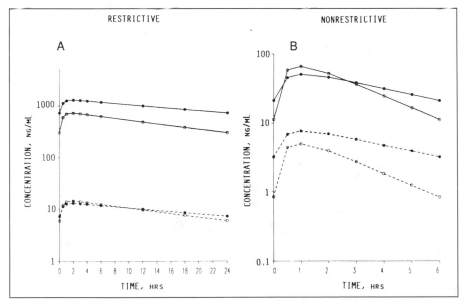

Figure 5-8. *a) Effect of plasma protein displacement on simulated steady-state concentration-time profiles of a restrictively cleared drug with a small volume of distribution. Upper curves are total drug concentration; lower curves are unbound drug concentration.* ● = *before displacement;* ○ = *after displacement. b) Effect of increased plasma protein binding on the simulated steady-state concentration-time profiles of a nonrestrictively cleared drug. Upper curves are total drug concentration; lower curves are unbound drug concentration.* ● = *normal binding;* ○ = *increased binding.*

The elimination half-lives of nonrestrictively cleared drugs are influenced by both plasma and tissue binding changes according to:

$$t\frac{1}{2} \approx 0.693 \left[V_p + \left(\frac{f_{up}}{f_{ut}} \right) V_t \right]$$

(Eq. 5-16)

Thus, decreased binding in plasma will increase the V_{ss} and prolong the half-life, while increased plasma binding will shorten the half-life. This effect is illustrated in Figure 5-8b for a propranolol-like drug given orally. A lower unbound drug fraction in plasma results in a lower average unbound drug concentration and a higher degree of fluctuation during the dosing interval due to the shorter half-life. The average total concentration in this simulation is unaffected by the change in plasma binding. For drugs with very small volumes of distribution like the penicillins, the effects of altered plasma and tissue protein binding on elimination half-life will be minimal.

Clinical Examples

Restrictively-Cleared Drugs. Displacement of restrictively-cleared drugs from plasma proteins will theoretically result in lower total drug concentrations in plasma but no change in average unbound concentrations as long as the displacing drug does not alter intrinsic clearance. Examples of such "pure" displacement interactions are phenytoin displacement by salicylate and tolbutamide and warfa-

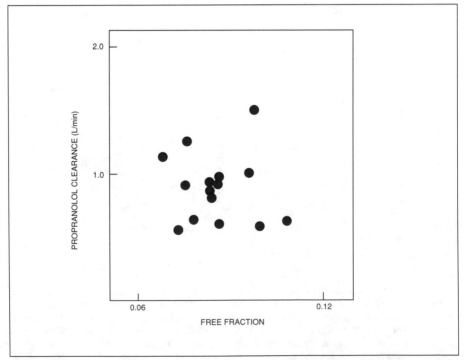

Figure 5-9. *An example of nonrestrictive clearance behavior: propranolol clearance is independent of the unbound fraction in plasma (reproduced with permission from reference 162).*

rin displacement by trichloroacetic acid, a metabolite of chloral hydrate.[30] While dosage adjustments are not required for phenytoin in the above examples, temporary but significant elevations in unbound warfarin concentrations may necessitate a temporary dose-rate reduction for warfarin.[30,145] This is because of warfarin's very small volume of distribution (0.1 L/kg), long elimination half-life (37 hours), and narrow therapeutic index. As shown in Table 5-6, drug displacement interactions often involve a simultaneous decrease in the intrinsic clearance of the displaced drug. Clinically important examples include phenytoin displacement by valproic acid and warfarin displacement by phenylbutazone.[30] In all cases, sustained reductions in dose-rate may be required because of the displacer's effect on intrinsic clearance, not because of its effects on protein binding.

The implications of concentration-dependent binding for restrictively-cleared drugs is best illustrated by disopyramide. Figure 5-10 shows the effect of increasing disopyramide dose-rate on average total and free disopyramide concentrations in serum.[4] Unbound drug concentration increases in proportion to the increase in dose-rate of disopyramide. Because of the progressive rise in unbound fraction with dose-rate, however, the clearance of this restrictively cleared drug also increases. Therefore, total concentrations increase less than proportionally. Because total serum disopyramide concentrations are misleading, clinicians are advised to rely on unbound disopyramide concentrations, if available, or to rely solely on the patient's clinical response.[163] A more complex situation is observed for salicylic acid which undergoes concentration-dependent metabolism in addition to concentration-dependent plasma binding.[20,34] Increases in salicylate dose-rates result in greater-than-proportional increases in free salicylate concentrations, but total concentrations do not reflect this because of the progressive increase in f_{up}.[34] Because salicylate concentrations are not routinely monitored, however, this situation is not as likely to mislead the clinician.

Drugs that are restrictively cleared and bind to AAG are likely to show higher total concentrations in conditions associated with higher AAG concentrations. If

Table 5-6. *In-vivo Displacement as a Cause of Increased Unbound Fractions in Plasma*[30]

Displaced drug	Displacer	Displaced drug	Displacer
Carbamazepine	Valproic acid[a]	Phenytoin	Salicylic acid Tolbutamide Phenylbutazone[a] Valproic acid[a]
Ceftriaxone	Probenecid[a]	Tolbutamide	Sulfadimethoxine
Diazepam	Valproic acid[a]	Valproic acid	Salicylic acid[a]
Methotrexate	Salicylic acid[a] Probenecid[a] Sulfisoxazole[a]	Warfarin	Trichloroacetic acid[b] Diflunisal Phenylbutazone[a]

[a] These drugs also known to inhibit renal tubular secretion activity or hepatic metabolism of displaced drugs.
[b] Metabolite of chloral hydrate.

there is no effect on intrinsic clearance, no effect on unbound drug concentration should be anticipated. Examples include disopyramide after myocardial infarction[48] and quinidine after surgery.[44]

Nonrestrictively-Cleared Drugs. Higher AAG concentrations following acute myocardial infarction cause a decrease in the unbound plasma fractions of propranolol and lidocaine.[46,47] In the case of intravenous or oral propranolol, higher dose-rates may be required to achieve the desired level of protection as long as liver blood flow and the intrinsic clearance of propranolol are not impaired. There is some evidence that higher-than-normal dose-rates of propranolol are required to exert a protective effect in both threatened and established infarction.[46] In contrast, normal infusion rates of lidocaine should be used in myocardial infarction patients because total lidocaine concentrations may rise progressively during prolonged infusion; the simultaneous rise in plasma binding of lidocaine means that unbound lidocaine concentrations do not significantly change during this period.[47] While it is tempting to speculate that the decreased clearance of lidocaine is caused by the increased plasma protein binding, this explanation would be inconsistent with the nonrestrictive clearance behavior of lidocaine as established in single-dose studies. The decreased lidocaine clearance is more likely caused by a decrease in liver blood flow or a decrease in the drug's hepatic intrinsic clearance.

The apparent resistance to oral propranolol in a small group of patients was attributed to higher plasma binding.[164] Those patients defined as resistant (requiring 480 to 1280 mg/day) had an average unbound fraction in plasma of approximately 5% while the average unbound fraction among propranolol responsive

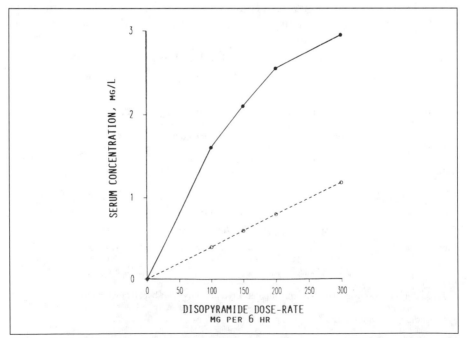

Figure 5-10. *The effect of increasing disopyramide dose-rate on total (●) and free (○) disopyramide average steady-state serum concentrations (based on data from reference 4).*

patients (those requiring 40 to 400 mg/day) was approximately 18%.[164] Thus, differences in plasma protein binding of nonrestrictively-cleared drugs may account for higher oral dose-rates needed by certain patients. This is in contrast to restrictively-cleared, low-extraction drugs for which dose-rate requirements depend only on intrinsic clearance.

In vivo displacement of several penicillins by aspirin or sulfonamides was reported by Kunin.[30,165] While the unbound fractions of the penicillins increased by as much as 88%, there was no change in total penicillin concentrations. An increase in unbound concentrations was observed, however.[165] Although such displacement interactions are not likely to be of clinical concern due to the wide therapeutic indices of these drugs, they illustrate nonrestrictive clearance behavior.

METHODS FOR MEASURING UNBOUND CONCENTRATIONS IN PLASMA

The advantages and disadvantages of methods used to measure drug-protein binding have been extensively reviewed.[20,25,166–168] The methods which are most likely to be used in a clinical laboratory include equilibrium dialysis, ultrafiltration, and possibly, ultracentrifugation.[168] Because it is difficult to simulate *in vivo* conditions, these methods must be carefully chosen and extensively evaluated before it can be concluded that they reflect *in vivo* unbound fractions or concentrations. All of the methods may be performed using radiolabeled drugs, but radiochemical purity must be high for accurate measurements, especially for drugs that are highly bound.[169]

Equilibrium Dialysis

Equilibrium dialysis has long been considered the reference method against which other methods are compared. Separation of the bound and free drug in plasma or protein solution is accomplished by placing a semipermeable membrane between two chambers: one containing the plasma and drug, and the other containing a physiologic buffer. At equilibrium, the unbound drug concentration is equal on both sides of the membrane, and the unbound fraction corresponding to that post-dialysis plasma concentration is determined by the ratio of drug concentration in buffer ([D]) to that in plasma ([D] + [DP]). Dialysis temperature is easily controlled by immersing the cells in a temperature-controlled water bath.

Equilibrium dialysis may not be appropriate for all drugs. Some dialysis devices require prolonged dialysis times (often up to 24 hours) which can lead to increases in pH[170] and increased fatty acid concentrations due to lipolysis.[171] This has led to artifactual measures of unbound plasma fractions for drugs that show pH dependent binding (e.g., propranolol, imipramine, quinidine,[25] and lidocaine)[57] and those for which fatty acids serve as displacing agents, such as valproic acid.[135,171] Prolonged dialysis times can also lead to significant shifts in volume between plasma and buffer.[172] This can be avoided by adding dextran to the buffer, or it may be corrected for after measuring the magnitude of volume shift.[172,173] Dialysis time can be significantly shortened in many cases by devices that provide better mixing of the cell contents and/or by the use of high permeability membranes.[171] The dialysis time for valproic acid was shortened to 45 minutes using this approach,[171] and problems associated with plasma lipolysis were thus avoided. Another method for reducing dialysis time is by use of a kinetic dialysis method[174] which requires the use of radiolabeled drug. The principle of this method is that the rate of exchange of labeled drug across a membrane separating two cells containing identical plasma samples is proportional to the unbound fraction of drug in those samples. Since dialysis begins under equilibrium conditions, dialysis times as short as 30 minutes can be used.[174]

Another problem associated with equilibrium dialysis is the possibility of drug adsorption to the membrane and/or the device itself. Most devices are made of Teflon or plastic, to which lipophilic compounds may bind.[168] Theoretically, adsorption should not be a problem for most drugs as long as sufficient time is given for equilibrium to be attained and as long as the unbound fraction is determined by measuring drug concentrations on both sides of the membrane. For extremely hydrophobic drugs, however, adsorption to the device and membrane can occur to such an extent that drug concentrations on the buffer side are difficult to measure.[175,176] This leads to inaccurate and imprecise determinations of f_{up}. In many cases, attempts to "saturate" the adsorption sites by pretreatment with solutions of high drug concentration are unsuccessful. Adsorption of the very lipophilic drug, cyclosporine, to the dialysis device was avoided by use of specially designed steel dialysis chambers.[71]

Conventional equilibrium dialysis is not ideal for drugs that exhibit concentration-dependent binding following therapeutic doses. Because dialysis involves the passage of free drug into a second volume of drug-free buffer, the post-dialysis concentration of drug on the plasma side of the membrane is lower than the pre-dialysis concentration. The unbound fraction thus determined corresponds only to the post-dialysis concentration and is an underestimate of the actual unbound fraction *in vivo*. To determine the unbound fraction corresponding to the pre-dialysis sample, a calibration curve must be established for each patient, as was done for disopyramide.[4,62] Additional corrections are needed when there is adsorption of drug to the membrane and/or device.[167,177] The kinetic dialysis method discussed previously[174] might be preferable to the conventional dialysis approach. Since this method involves placing equivalent plasma samples on both sides of the membrane, the dilutional effects of buffer are avoided.

The Donnan effect is widely cited as a disadvantage of equilibrium dialysis. The error caused by this effect, however, is most significant for drugs that are highly ionized and not highly bound.[25,156,167] Use of a buffer with a high ionic strength or use of plasma ultrafiltrate in place of buffer will generally overcome this problem. Protein leakage into the buffer can obviously cause an overestimation of unbound fraction, especially for very highly bound drugs. For this reason, it is recommended that protein concentrations in buffer be routinely measured.[167]

Ultrafiltration

Because ultrafiltration is the simplest and quickest of all protein binding methods, it is most likely to be used for routine measurements of unbound drug concentration in a clinical laboratory. Plasma water containing unbound drug is forced through a membrane either by applying positive pressure to the plasma side of the membrane, or negative pressure to the ultrafiltrate side. Several commercial systems that utilize centrifugation as the means of generating a pressure gradient have been developed. For all of these procedures, measurement of drug concentration in the ultrafiltrate provides a direct measure of free drug concentration in plasma. The unbound fraction is determined as the ratio of ultrafiltrate concentration to pre-filtered plasma concentration. Because ultrafiltration does not have the dilutional effects of equilibrium dialysis, it holds a special advantage for drugs exhibiting concentration-dependent binding following therapeutic doses.

Ultrafiltration shares with equilibrium dialysis the potential of drug adsorption to the device and/or membrane. This has limited the utility of ultrafiltration for routine measurements of several basic, lipophilic compounds.[178-180] In contrast to equilibrium dialysis, adsorption to the ultrafiltration device or membrane will always lead to underestimates of free drug concentration, and hence, of unbound drug fraction in plasma. While pre-saturation of the membrane appeared to overcome this problem in one case,[179] the recent availability of membranes that minimize adsorption is a more reliable solution to this problem.[91,181] Another potential problem of ultrafiltration can also lead to underestimation of the unbound drug concentration. The "sieve effect," in which water molecules are preferentially filtered over drug molecules, is believed to be worse for high molecular weight compounds and when high filtration pressures are used.[25,168] This error can be minimized using low filtration pressures and membranes with sufficiently large pore diameters and selectivity.[167,168] If centrifugation is used, a low speed of 1000 to 2000 g (gravitational force) is generally recommended; protein accumulation on the membrane can be minimized by use of a fixed-angle centrifuge rotor.[25]

Other problems of ultrafiltration pertain to drugs that show temperature- or pH-dependent binding. If centrifugation is being used, a temperature-controlled centrifuge is necessary to overcome the heat generated by the motor.[25] It should be recognized, however, that most temperature-controlled ultrafiltrations are done at 25 °C. This may account for the observed differences in unbound fractions of some drugs when they are measured by both ultrafiltration and equilibrium dialysis, which is often performed at 37 °C. Changes in pH can be controlled by tightly capping centrifuge devices to prevent CO_2 loss or by centrifuging samples in a microchamber filled with 5% CO_2.[205]

The volume of collected ultrafiltrate was previously felt to be an important determinant of the accuracy of free drug concentration measurements, but it is now regarded as less important.[167] Ultrafiltrate volumes as high as 40% of the plasma volume may be collected without concern of disrupting the protein binding equilibrium in the retentate.[25]

Ultracentrifugation

Ultracentrifugation is less likely to be used in a clinical laboratory, but it may be essential to accurately determine the unbound fractions of very hydrophobic compounds such as cyclosporine.[176] Because this method does not involve the introduction of a membrane, plastic device, or aqueous buffer, the adsorption of these very lipophilic compounds is not a problem. The method is based on the differential sedimentation rates of solutes based on their molecular weights. Centrifugation of plasma at very high speeds for long periods of time (i.e., 24 hours at 100,000 g) will result in albumin and AAG-bound drug at the bottom of the tube, free drug molecules near the center, and lipoprotein-bound drug at the top. By sampling the center portion and assuring it to be protein-free, a measure of unbound drug concentration is obtained. Although adsorption of drug to the tube is a potential problem, the binding of many drugs to nitrocellulose tubes is minimal;[168] there was no binding of the very hydrophobic cyclosporine to poly-allomer tubes.[176]

One possible problem with ultracentrifugation is co-sedimentation of free drug with protein-bound drug which will lead to underestimates of free drug concentration; this problem will be most serious for high molecular weight drugs (>300).[168] The slightly lower unbound fraction of phenytoin obtained by ultracentrifugation compared to those measured by ultrafiltration and equilibrium dialysis was attributed to this sedimentation effect.[206] Preliminary studies can be done using protein-free solutions with the same viscosity as serum to determine the influence of drug sedimentation on the calculation of unbound fraction.[176,206] There is also a possibility that protein binding equilibrium might be disturbed during centrifugation; methods for detecting this phenomenon have been described.[206] Finally, the major disadvantages of ultracentrifugation are the availability and cost of high-speed, temperature-controlled centrifuges, the long centrifugation time, and the requirement for relatively large plasma volumes. Although these seem to be major limitations, ultracentrifugation may be the only reliable method for measurement of free concentrations of very hydrophobic compounds.

In Vivo Methods

Drug concentrations in "natural ultrafiltrates of plasma" such as saliva, tears, or cerebrospinal fluid may be equivalent to unbound drug concentrations in plasma for certain drugs.[18] Saliva concentrations of carbamazepine and phenytoin provide reliable estimates of their corresponding free concentrations in plasma,[182–184] while saliva concentrations of valproic acid do not.[183] This can be explained by the fact that the ionized fraction of valproic acid changes with normal changes in saliva pH, while phenytoin and carbamazepine are essentially unionized over the entire range of saliva pH.[18] The degree of drug partitioning into red blood cells has also been used as a reflection of unbound drug fractions in plasma. The erythrocyte partitioning method has been used to measure unbound fractions of imipramine, amitriptyline, quinidine, lidocaine, and propranolol, and has compared favorably with equilibrium dialysis.[178] Although tedious, this method avoids prolonged dialysis times and extensive adsorption to membranes and devices. As an example, this approach was used successfully to measure unbound plasma fractions of the very hydrophobic drug amiodarone, for which equilibrium dialysis and ultrafiltration had been unsuccessful because of extensive membrane/device adsorption.[175] For the same reasons, we found this method to be the only acceptable means of measuring the unbound fraction of a hydrophobic insecticide in human plasma. (Novak and MacKichan, unpublished data.)

UTILITY OF FREE DRUG CONCENTRATIONS IN THERAPEUTIC DRUG MONITORING

Monitoring free drug concentrations is not necessary as long as the more easily measured total concentration provides a consistent and accurate reflection of the free concentration. This only occurs, however, if the unbound fraction is the same within and among all patients. If there is concentration-dependent binding following therapeutic doses, or if the unbound plasma fraction of a drug is significantly different from the norm in certain patients, free and total drug concentrations will be "dissociated."[107] In these situations, the direct measurement of free concentration may provide more meaningful information as long as the therapeutic range of free concentrations has been established. Drugs that are highly bound in plasma are most likely to show wide variations among patients in the unbound plasma fraction and are therefore the most likely candidates for free concentration monitoring.

Drugs for which total concentration monitoring is routinely performed and for which free concentration monitoring has been proposed are listed in Table 5-7, along with the criteria that support the utility of free concentrations.[18,195,196] On a theoretical basis, disopyramide and valproic acid present the most convincing cases for routine monitoring of free drug concentration because of their concentration-dependent binding following therapeutic doses. In the case of valproic acid, however, there is no evidence that free concentration correlates better with response or signs of toxicity than total concentration.[18] This may be because many of the effects of valproic acid do not appear to be strongly dependent on concentration, and because of the confounding presence of active metabolites.[18] The case for routine monitoring of free concentrations is stronger for disopyramide,[163] but should be further restricted to measurement of the active enantiomer.[181] In general, most investigators agree that routine free concentration monitoring of the drugs in Table 5-7 is not warranted. Rather, this practice should be limited to certain patients:[18,195,196] 1) those with diseases likely to be associated with altered plasma protein binding; 2) those taking drugs that are likely to displace the drug of interest from plasma protein binding sites; and 3) those who show an unexpected drug response at a given total drug concentration. The utility of this selective approach to monitoring free concentrations has been most widely established for phenytoin.[197–199,206]

Another consideration for the utility of free concentration monitoring is more practical in nature. Accuracy and precision of the free concentration or free fraction measurement must be assured before it can be considered as a better predictor of

Table 5-7. *Criteria for Utility of Free Concentration Monitoring*

Drug	Variable f_{up}	Evidence for better correlation of response to free versus total	Free therapeutic range established
Carbamazepine	Among patients	Limited evidence, based on a case report[185] and study of intermittent side effects.[186]	Upper limit 1.7 mg/L;[186] possible contribution from active metabolite.
Phenytoin	Among patients	Direct evidence based on study of toxic symptoms[1] and case reports;[187,188,206] indirect evidence based on side effects in hypoalbuminemic and renal failure patients.[115,189]	Upper limit 1.5 mg/L;[1] upper limit 2.1 mg/L.[206]
Valproic acid	Among patients; within patients	No evidence.[181]	Not established; possible contributions from active metabolites.
Disopyramide	Among patients; within patients	Yes, based on ECG changes in animals[190] and humans.[4,191,192]	Lower limit for active S (+) enantiomer, 0.6 mg/L.[181]
Lidocaine	Among patients; within patients at high doses	Limited evidence, based on symptoms of toxicity.[193]	Not established.
Quinidine	Among patients	Limited evidence, based on acute ECG changes.[194]	Not established.

response than total concentration.[200] Because of the many factors that can affect the measurement of an unbound plasma concentration in a given laboratory (e.g., temperature, choice of anticoagulant, storage conditions), strict attention to details of the technique seems to be more important than for total concentration measurements.[200] In addition, a laboratory that only occasionally determines free concentrations may be more likely to introduce error. Because of these concerns about quality control for free drug concentration measurements, some investigators suggest that they be used only as a last resort.[200] Instead, total concentration measurements are recommended even in situations in which altered plasma binding is expected (e.g., phenytoin in nephrotic syndrome). In such a situation, the effect of altered plasma binding on total and free drug concentration can be predicted, as discussed below.

CLINICAL GUIDELINES FOR SUSPECTED ALTERATIONS IN PLASMA PROTEIN BINDING

It is critical that the clinician be able to predict how unusual plasma protein binding can affect a patient's response to any drug, whether its concentrations are routinely monitored or not. If total concentrations of a drug are not routinely monitored, the clinician need only be concerned with how altered plasma binding will affect response and hence, dosage regimen requirements. If total concentrations are routinely monitored, and if free concentration measurements are not desired or are unavailable, the clinician must also be able to properly interpret the total concentration measurement. Approaches to these situations are discussed below.

Dosage Regimen Adjustments

The goal here is to predict how altered binding will affect the unbound concentration and hence, the response of the drug in question. This approach assumes that there is a good relationship between unbound concentration and response and requires a knowledge of how the drug's clearance will be influenced by changes in plasma protein binding [i.e., whether clearance is sensitive to changes in binding (restrictive) or insensitive (nonrestrictive)]. For drugs cleared predominantly by the liver, nonrestrictive behavior is evident if normal hepatic blood clearance divided by the normal unbound fraction in blood is greater than normal hepatic blood flow (1.2 to 1.5 L/min). Alternatively, the hepatic extraction ratio can be estimated by dividing hepatic blood clearance by hepatic blood flow and comparing this to the unbound fraction in blood as previously described. An $E > f_{ub}$ will imply nonrestrictive behavior, while an $E \leq f_{ub}$ implies restrictive behavior. In the case of drugs cleared by the kidneys, nonrestrictive secretion clearance occurs if the renal plasma clearance divided by the unbound plasma fraction (the "corrected renal clearance") gives a value higher than normal renal plasma flow (i.e., 700 mL/min). If a drug is also efficiently reabsorbed, the corrected renal clearance value may be lower than renal plasma flow despite its nonrestrictive behavior. Additional experimental evidence of the influence of protein binding on renal clearance will be needed in that case.

Once the clearance behavior of the drug has been determined, the direction and magnitude of a change in f_{ub} or f_{up} should be estimated based on information from the literature. The effect of this alteration on $C_{av,ss}$ and C_u can then be anticipated based on the principles of restrictive and nonrestrictive clearance behavior described previously. As an example, a normal dose-rate of diazepam (restrictively cleared) in a patient with hypoalbuminemia (increased f_{up}) is predicted to provide a normal unbound concentration and hence, a normal response as long as there is no evidence for impaired metabolism. In contrast, the dose-rate of diazepam may need to be reduced in a patient with severe liver disease because the intrinsic clearance for diazepam is decreased. As another example, a higher-than-normal dose-rate of amitriptyline (nonrestrictively cleared) may be required for a patient with elevated concentrations of AAG. In this case, the f_{up} is predicted to be lower, which should result in lower unbound concentrations of this drug.

Interpretation of Total Drug Concentration

If a total drug concentration measurement is available, the unbound concentration can be estimated by determining the direction and probable degree of alteration in the patient's unbound plasma fraction (as determined from the literature). For example, the f_{up} of phenytoin in neonates is approximately twice that in adults.[79] If the total drug concentration in a neonate is 6.5 mg/L, the unbound concentration can be estimated to be 1.3 mg/L by assuming that f_{up} is 0.2 (see Equation 5-7). The estimated unbound concentration should then be compared to an estimated therapeutic range of unbound plasma concentrations. This range is determined by multiplying the therapeutic range of total concentrations by the "normal" unbound plasma fraction in adult patients. Thus, the therapeutic range of free phenytoin concentrations is estimated as 10% of 10 to 20 mg/L, or 1 to 2 mg/L. [Note: The therapeutic range of free drug concentrations must be estimated because complete ranges have not been determined directly (see Table 5-7). For drugs showing variable unbound fractions among patients, this estimated range is undoubtedly wider than the actual range and should be interpreted with caution.] By comparing the estimated unbound concentration with the estimated therapeutic range of free phenytoin concentrations in the context of the clinical picture, one can determine whether a dose-rate adjustment is needed. In this particular case, it is important to recognize that an apparently "sub-therapeutic" total concentration of phenytoin is appropriate for a neonate. Even if only the direction of change in f_{up} is known, the clinician has an improved ability to interpret the measured total drug concentration.

In summary, changes in plasma protein binding do not always mean that dose-rate adjustments are needed. However, total drug concentrations must be evaluated with care because misinterpretation may lead to important clinical consequences. Anytime there is a suspected change in plasma protein binding, the total drug concentration will not reflect the same level of activity as in a patient with normal binding. Use of these guidelines will certainly increase the utility of total drug concentration measurements.

NOTE TO READER

The following abbreviations differ from or are not included in the Glossary because they are specific to this chapter:

K_D = Dissociation constant; N_{TOT} = Capacity constant.

K_I = Dissociation constant for the binding of a competitive inhibitor to protein; D/τ = Dose rate

REFERENCES

1. Booker HE, Darcey B. Serum concentrations of free diphenylhydantoin and their relationship to clinical intoxication. Epilepsia. 1973;14:177.
2. Kunin CM et al. Influence of binding on the pharmacologic activity of antibiotics. Ann NY Acad Sci. 1973;226:214.
3. McDevitt DG et al. Plasma binding and the affinity of propranolol for a beta receptor in man. Clin Pharmacol Ther. 1976;20:152.
4. Lima JJ et al. Concentration-dependence of disopyramide binding to plasma protein and its influence on kinetics and dynamics. J Pharmacol Exp Ther. 1981;219:741.
5. Rosenthal HE. A graphical method for the determination and presentation of binding parameters in a complex system. Anal Biochem. 1967;20:525.
6. MacKichan JJ, Zola EM. Determinants of carbamazepine and carbamazepine 10,11-epoxide binding to serum protein, albumin, and α_1-acid glycoprotein. Br J Clin Pharmacol. 1984;18:487.
7. Priore RL, Rosenthal HE. A statistical method for estimation of binding parameters in a complex system. Anal Biochem. 1976;70:231.
8. Metzler GM et al. A user's manual for NONLIN and associated programs. Kalamazoo, MI: The Upjohn Co. 1974.
9. Putnam FW. Alpha, beta, gamma, omega. The roster of the plasma proteins. In: Putnam FW, ed. The Plasma Proteins. New York: Academic Press;1975;57–131.
10. Peters T Jr. Serum albumin. In: Putnam FW, ed. The Plasma Proteins. New York: Academic Press; 1975;133–81.
11. Jusko WJ, Gretch M. Plasma and tissue protein binding of drugs in pharmacokinetics. Drug Metab Rev. 1983;14:427.
12. Piafsky KM. Disease-induced changes in the plasma binding of basic drugs. Clin Pharmacokinet. 1980;5:246.
13. Ochs HR, Smith TW. Reversal of advanced digitoxin toxicity and modification of pharmacokinetics by specific antibodies and Fab fragments. J Clin Invest. 1977;60:1303.
14. Schmid K. α_1-acid glycoprotein. In: Putnam FW, ed. The Plasma Proteins. New York: Academic Press;1975;183–228.
15. Lemaire M et al. Lipoprotein binding of drugs. In: Reidenberg MM, Erill S, eds. Drug-Protein Binding. New York: Praeger Publishers;1986;93–108.
16. Sjöholm I. The specificity of drug binding sites on human serum albumin. In: Reidenberg MM, Erill S, eds. Drug-Protein Binding. New York: Praeger Publishers;1986;36–45.
17. Lunde PKM et al. Inflammation and α1-acid glycoprotein: effect on drug binding. In: Reidenberg MM, Erill S, eds. Drug-Protein Binding. New York: Praeger Publishers;1986;201–19.
18. Svensson CK et al. Free drug concentration monitoring in clinical practice. Rationale and current status. Clin Pharmacokinet. 1986;11:450.
19. Vallner JJ. Binding of drugs by albumin and plasma protein. J Pharm Sci. 1977;66:447.

20. Lin JH et al. Protein binding as a primary determinant of the clinical pharmacokinetic properties of non-steroidal anti-inflammatory drugs. Clin Pharmacokinet. 1987;12:402.

21. Kwong TC et al. Lipoprotein and protein binding of the calcium channel blocker diltiazem. Proc Soc Exp Biol Med. 1985;178:313.

22. Tillement JP et al. Diseases and drug protein binding. Clin Pharmacokinet. 1978;3:144.

23. Jungbluth GL et al. Factors affecting ceftriaxone plasma protein binding during open heart surgery. J Pharm Sci. 1989;78:807.

24. Wilkinson GR. Plasma and tissue binding considerations in drug disposition. Drug Metab Rev. 1983;14:427.

25. Kwong TC. Free drug measurements: methodology and clinical significance. Clin Chim Acta. 1985;151:193.

26. Tozer TN. Implications of altered plasma protein binding in disease states. In: Benet LZ et al, eds. Pharmacokinetic Basis for Drug Treatment. New York: Raven Press;1984;173–93.

27. Wandell M, Wilcox-Thole WL. Protein binding and free drug concentrations. In: Mungall D, ed. Applied Clinical Pharmacokinetics. New York: Raven Press; 1983;17-48.

28. Gugler R, Azarnoff DL. Drug protein binding and the nephrotic syndrome. Clin Pharmacokinet. 1976;1:25.

29. Calvo R et al. Effects of carbamylation on plasma proteins and competitive displacers on drug binding in uremia. Pharmacology. 1982;24:248.

30. MacKichan JJ. Protein binding displacement interactions. Fact or fiction? Clin Pharmacokinet. 1989;16:65.

31. Lee EJD et al. Stereoselective disposition of ibuprofen enantiomers in man. Br J Clin Pharmacol. 1985;19:669.

32. Patel IH, Levy RH. Valproic acid binding to human serum albumin and determination of free fraction in the presence of anticonvulsants and free fatty acids. Epilepsia. 1979;20:85.

33. Bowdle TA et al. Valproic acid dosage and plasma protein binding and clearance. Clin Pharmacol Ther. 1980;28:486.

34. Furst DE et al. Salicylate clearance, the resultant of protein binding and metabolism. Clin Pharmacol Ther. 1979;26:380.

35. Runkle R et al. Nonlinear plasma level response to high doses of naproxen. Clin Pharmacol Ther. 1974;15:261.

36. Morgan DJ et al. Pharmacokinetics and plasma binding of thiopental. I: Studies in surgical patients. Anesthesiology. 1981;54:468.

37. Pearson RM. Pharmacokinetics and response to diazoxide in renal failure. Clin Pharmacokinet. 1977;2:198.

38. Urien S et al. Evidence for binding of certain acidic drugs to α_1-acid glycoprotein. Biochem Pharmacol. 1982;31:3687.

39. Urien S et al. Role of α_1-acid glycoprotein, albumin, and nonesterified fatty acids in serum binding of apazone and warfarin. Clin Pharmacol Ther. 1986;39:683.

40. Milsap RL, Jusko WJ. Binding of prednisolone to α_1-acid glycoprotein. J Steroid Biochem. 1983;18:191.

41. Tinguely D et al. Interindividual differences in the binding of antidepressives to plasma proteins: the role of the variants of α_1-acid glycoprotein. Eur J Clin Pharmacol. 1985;27:661.

42. Fraeyman NF et al. α_1-acid glycoprotein concentration and molecular heterogeneity: relationship to oxprenolol binding in serum from healthy volunteers and patients with lung carcinoma or cirrhosis. Br J Clin Pharmacol. 1988;25:733.

43. Holtzman JL. The study of drug-protein interactions by spin labeling. In: Reidenberg MM, Erill S, eds. Drug-Protein Binding. New York: Praeger Publishers;1986;46–69.

44. Fremstad D et al. Increased plasma binding of quinidine after surgery: a preliminary report. Eur J Clin Pharmacol. 1976;10:441.

45. Freilich DI, Giardina EV. Imipramine binding to α_1-acid glycoprotein in normal subjects and cardiac patients. Clin Pharmacol Ther. 1984;35:670.

46. Routledge PA et al. Increased plasma propranolol binding in myocardial infarction. Br J Clin Pharmacol. 1980;9:438. Letter.

47. Routledge PA et al. Relationship between α_1-acid glycoprotein and lidocaine disposition in myocardial infarction. Clin Pharmacol Ther. 1981;30:154.

48. David BM et al. Prolonged variability in plasma protein binding of disopyramide after acute myocardial infarction. Br J Clin Pharmacol. 1983;15:435.

49. Piafsky KM et al. Increased plasma protein binding of propranolol and chlorpromazine mediated by disease-induced elevations of plasma α_1-acid glycoprotein. N Engl J Med. 1978;299:1435.

50. Piafsky KM, Borga O. Plasma protein binding of basic drugs. II: Importance of α_1-acid glycoprotein for interindividual variation. Clin Pharmacol Ther. 1977;22:545.

51. Baruzzi A et al. Altered serum protein binding of carbamazepine in disease states associated with an increased α_1-acid glycoprotein concentration. Eur J Clin Pharmacol. 1986;31:85.

52. Edwards DJ et al. α_1-acid glycoprotein concentration and protein binding in trauma. Clin Pharmacol Ther. 1982;31:62.

53. Abramson FP. Methadone plasma protein binding: alterations in cancer and displacement from α_1-acid glycoprotein. Clin Pharmacol Ther. 1982;32:652.

54. Abramson FP et al. Effects of cancer and its treatments on plasma concentration of α_1-acid glycoprotein and propranolol binding. Clin Pharmacol Ther. 1982;32:659.

55. Jackson PR et al. Altered plasma drug binding in cancer: role of α_1-acid glycoprotein and albumin. Clin Pharmacol Ther. 1982;32:295.

56. Pederson LE et al. Quantitative and qualitative binding characteristics of disopyramide in serum from patients with decreased renal and hepatic function. Br J Clin Pharmacol. 1987;23:41.

57. McNamara PJ et al. Factors influencing serum protein binding of lidocaine in humans. Anesth Analg. 1981;60:395.

58. Goolkasian DL et al. Displacement of lidocaine from serum α_1-acid glycoprotein binding sites by basic drugs. Eur J Clin Pharmacol. 1983;25:413.

59. Lima JJ. Interaction of disopyramide enantiomers for sites on plasma protein. Life Sci. 1987;41:2807.

60. Gross AS et al. Stereoselective protein binding of verapamil enantiomers. Biochem Pharmacol. 1988; 37:4623.

61. Coyle DE et al. The effect of nonesterified fatty acids and progesterone on bupivicaine protein binding. Clin Pharmacol Ther. 1986;39:559.

62. Meffin PJ et al. Role of concentration-dependent plasma protein binding on disopyramide disposition. J Pharmacokinet Biopharm. 1979;7:29.

63. Tucker GT et al. Binding of anilide-type local anesthetics in human plasma. I: Relationships between binding, physicochemical properties, and anesthetic activity. Anesthesiology. 1970;33:287.

64. McNamara PJ et al. Effect of smoking on binding of lidocaine to human serum proteins. J Pharm Sci. 1980;69:749.

65. Armstrong DK et al. Clinical response and total and unbound plasma concentrations after lidocaine overdose. Ther Drug Monit. 1988;10:499.

66. Jusko WJ, Rose JQ. Monitoring prednisone and prednisolone. Ther Drug Monit. 1980;2:169.

67. Scanu AM et al. Serum lipoproteins. In: Putnam FW, ed. The Plasma Proteins. New York: Academic Press;1975;317–91.

68. Rudman D et al. Transport of drugs, hormones and fatty acids in lipemic serum. J Pharmacol Exp Ther. 1972;180:797.

69. Lemaire M, Tillement JP. Role of lipoproteins and erythrocytes in the *in vitro* binding and distribution of cyclosporin A in the blood. J Pharm Pharmacol. 1982;34:715.

70. Nikkilä EA et al. Increase of serum high-density lipoprotein in phenytoin users. Br Med J. 1978;2:99.

71. Lindholm A, Henricsson S. Intra- and interindividual variability in the free fraction of cyclosporine in plasma in recipients of renal transplants. Ther Drug Monit. 1989;11:623.

72. Legg B et al. A model to account for the variation in cyclosporin binding to plasma lipids in transplant patients. Ther Drug Monit. 1988;10:20.

73. Nilsen OG. Serum albumin and lipoproteins as the quinidine binding molecules in normal human sera. Biochem Pharmacol. 1976;25:1007.

74. Nilsen OG et al. Binding of quinidine in sera with different levels of triglycerides, cholesterol, and orosomucoid protein. Biochem Pharmacol. 1978;27:871.

75. Danon A, Chen Z. Binding of imipramine to plasma proteins: effect of hyperlipoproteinemia. Clin Pharmacol Ther. 1979;25:316.

76. Mather LE, Thomas J. Bupivicaine binding to plasma protein fractions. J Pharm Pharmacol. 1978;30:653.

77. Edwards DJ et al. Factors affecting quinidine protein binding in humans. J Pharm Sci. 1984;73:1264.

78. Kuhnz W. et al. Protein binding of carbamazepine and its epoxide in maternal and fetal plasma at delivery: comparison to other anticonvulsants. Dev Pharmacol Ther. 1984;7:61.

79. Kurz H et al. Differences in the binding of drugs to plasma proteins from newborn and adult man. I. Eur J Clin Pharmacol. 1977;11:463.

80. Besunder JB et al. Principles of drug biodisposition in the neonate. A critical evaluation of the pharmacokinetic-pharmacodynamic interface (Part I). Clin Pharmacokinet. 1988;14:189.

81. Morselli PL. Clinical pharmacokinetics in neonates. Clin Pharmacokinet. 1976;1:81.

82. Wood M, Wood AJJ. Changes in plasma drug binding and α_1-acid glycoprotein in mother and newborn infant. Clin Pharmacol Ther. 1980;29:522.

83. Kelly JG, O'Malley K. Drug-protein binding in old age. In: Reidenberg MM, Erill S, eds. Drug-Protein Binding. New York: Praeger Publishers; 1986;163–71.

84. Greenblatt DJ et al. Diazepam disposition determinants. Clin Pharmacol Ther. 1980;27:301.

85. Davis D et al. The effects of age and smoking on the plasma protein binding of lignocaine and diazepam. Br J Clin Pharmacol. 1985;19:261.

86. Wallace S et al. Factors affecting drug binding in plasma of elderly patients. Br J Clin Pharmacol. 1976;3:327.

87. Perucca E et al. Pharmacokinetics of valproic acid in the elderly. Br J Clin Pharmacol. 1984;17:665.

88. Dean M et al. Serum protein binding of drugs during and after pregnancy in humans. Clin Pharmacol Ther. 1980;28:253.

89. Perucca E et al. Altered drug binding to serum proteins in pregnant women: therapeutic relevance. J R Soc Med. 1981;74:422.

90. Bardy AH et al. Protein binding of antiepileptic drugs during pregnancy, labor and puerperium. Ther Drug Monit. 1990;12:40.

91. Denson DD et al. Bupivicaine protein binding in the term parturient: effects of lactic acidosis. Clin Pharmacol Ther. 1984;35:702.

92. Wilson K. Sex-related differences in drug disposition in man. Clin Pharmacokinet. 1984;9:189.

93. Routledge PA et al. Sex-related differences in the plasma protein binding of lignocaine and diazepam. Br J Clin Pharmacol. 1981;11:245.

94. Benedek IH et al. Serum α_1-acid glycoprotein and the binding of drugs in obesity. Br J Clin Pharmacol. 1983;16:751.

95. Jagadeesan V, Krishnaswamy K. Drug binding in the undernourished: a study of the binding of propranolol to α_1-acid glycoprotein. Eur J Clin Pharmacol. 1985;27:657.

96. Elfstrom J. Drug pharmacokinetics in the post-operative period. Clin Pharmacokinet. 1979;4:16.

97. Elfstrom J. Plasma protein binding of phenytoin after cholecystectomy and neurosurgical operations. Acta Neurol Scand. 55;1977:455.

98. Feely J et al. Influence of surgery on plasma propranolol levels and protein binding. Clin Pharmacol Ther. 1980;28:759.

99. Jungbluth GL et al. Ceftriaxone disposition in open-heart surgery patients. Antimicrob Agents Chemother. 1989;33:850.

100. Naranjo CA et al. Fatty acids modulation of meal-induced variations in diazepam free fraction. Br J Clin Pharmacol. 1980;10:308. Letter.

101. Riva R et al. Valproic acid free fraction in epileptic children under chronic monotherapy. Ther Drug Monit. 1983;5:191.

102. Riva R et al. Diurnal fluctuations in free and total plasma concentrations of valproic acid at steady state in epileptic patients. Ther Drug Monit. 1983;5:191.

103. Yost RL, Devane CL. Diurnal variation of α_1-acid glycoprotein concentration in normal volunteers. J Pharm Sci. 1985;74:777.

104. Vinik HR et al. The pharmacokinetics of midazolam in chronic renal failure patients. Anesthesiology. 1983;59:390.

105. Prandota J. Clinical pharmacology of antibiotics and other drugs in cystic fibrosis. Drugs 1988;35:542.

106. Reidenberg MM, Drayer DE. Alteration of drug-protein binding in renal disease. Clin Pharmacokinet. 1984;9(Suppl.1):18.

107. Levy RH, Moreland TA. Rationale for monitoring free drug levels. Clin Pharmacokinet. 1984;9(Suppl.1):1.

108. Blaschke TF. Protein binding and kinetics of drugs in liver diseases. Clin Pharmacokinet. 1977;2:32.

109. Grossman SH et al. Diazepam and lidocaine plasma protein binding in renal disease. Clin Pharmacol Ther. 1982;31:350.

110. Thiessen JJ et al. Plasma protein binding of diazepam and tolbutamide in chronic alcoholics. J Clin Pharmacol. 1976;16:345.

111. Barre J et al. Decreased α_1-acid glycoprotein in liver cirrhosis: consequences for drug protein binding. Br J Clin Pharmacol. 1984;18:652. Letter.

112. Hooper WD et al. Plasma protein binding of diphenylhydantoin: Effects of sex hormones, renal and hepatic disease. Clin Pharmacol Ther. 1973;15:276.

113. Martyn JAJ et al. Plasma protein binding of drugs after severe burn injury. Clin Pharmacol Ther. 1984;35:535.

114. Bowdle TA et al. Phenytoin pharmacokinetics in burned rats and plasma protein binding of phenytoin in burned patients. J Pharmacol Exp Ther. 1980;213:97.

115. Rudman D et al. An abnormal orosomucoid in the plasma of patients with neoplastic disease. Cancer Res. 1972;32:1951.

116. Ruiz-Cabello F, Erill S. Abnormal serum protein binding of acidic drugs in diabetes mellitus. Clin Pharmacol Ther. 1984;36:691.

117. Erill S, Calva R. Post-translational changes of albumin as a cause of altered drug-plasma protein binding. In: Reidenberg MM, Erill S, eds. Drug-Protein Binding. New York: Praeger Publishers; 1986;220–32.

118. Feely J et al. Altered plasma protein binding of drugs in thyroid disease. Clin Pharmacokinet. 1981;6:298.

119. Jusko WJ et al. Enhanced renal excretion of dicloxacillin in patients with cystic fibrosis. Pediatrics. 1975;56:1038.

120. Bower S. Plasma protein binding of fentanyl: the effect of hyperlipoproteinemia and chronic renal failure. J Pharm Pharmacol. 1982;34:102.

121. Yong C et al. Factors affecting the plasma protein binding of verapamil and norverapamil in man. Res Commun Chem Pathol Pharmacol. 1980;30:329.

122. Pinckard RN et al. The influence of acetylsalicylic acid on the binding of acetrizoate to human albumin. Ann NY Acad Sci. 1973;226:341.

123. Chignell CF, Starkweather DK. Optical studies of drug-protein complexes. V: The interaction of phenylbutazone, flufenamic acid, and dicoumarol with acetylsalicylic acid-treated human serum albumin. Mol Pharmacol. 1971;7:229.

124. Routledge PA et al. Lignocaine disposition in blood in epilepsy. Br J Clin Pharmacol. 1981;12:663.

125. Tiula E et al. Antiepileptic drugs and α_1-acid glycoprotein. N Engl J Med. 1982;307:1148. Letter.

126. Baumann P et al. Increase of α_1-acid glycoprotein after treatment with amitriptyline. Br J Clin Pharmacol. 1982;14:102.

127. Durrington PN. Effect of phenobarbitone on plasma apolipoprotein B and plasma high-density lipoprotein cholesterol in normal subjects. Clin Sci. 1979;56:501.

128. Feely J et al. Enzyme induction with rifampicin; lipoproteins and drug binding to α_1-acid glycoprotein. Br J Clin Pharmacol. 1983;16:195.

129. Cotham RH, Shand D. Spuriously low plasma propranolol concentrations resulting from blood collection methods. Clin Pharmacol Ther. 1975;18:535.

130. Borga O et al. Plasma protein binding of basic drugs. I: Selective displacement from α_1-acid glycoprotein by tris (2-butoxyethyl) phosphate. Clin Pharmacol Ther. 1977;22:539.

131. Wood M et al. Altered binding due to the use of indwelling heparinized cannulas (heparin lock) for sampling. Clin Pharmacol Ther. 1979;25:103.

132. Brown JE et al. The artifactual nature of heparin-induced drug protein-binding alterations. Clin Pharmacol Ther. 1981;30:636.

133. Giacomini KM et al. Administration of heparin causes in vitro release of non-esterified fatty acids in human plasma. Life Sci. 1980;27:771.

134. Naranjo CA et al. Non-fatty acid-modulated variations in drug binding due to heparin. Clin Pharmacol Ther. 1982;31:746.

135. Albani F et al. Free fraction of valproic acid: In vitro time-dependent increase and correlation with free fatty acid concentration in human plasma and serum. Epilepsia. 1983;24:65.

136. Jackson AJ et al. Human blood preservation: effect on in vitro protein binding. J Pharm Sci. 1981;70:1168.

137. Lima JJ, Salzer LB. Contamination of albumin by α_1-acid glycoprotein. Biochem Pharmacol. 1981;30:2633.

138. Sjöholm I et al. Protein binding of drugs in uremic and normal serum: the role of endogenous binding inhibitors. Biochem Pharmacol. 1976;25:1205.

139. Denson D et al. α_1-acid glycoprotein and albumin in human serum bupivicaine binding. Clin Pharmacol Ther. 1984;35:409.

140. Gibaldi M, Perrier D. Pharmacokinetics, 2nd ed. New York: Marcel Dekker, Inc.;1982;351.

141. Gibaldi M et al. Effect of plasma protein and tissue binding on the biologic half-life of drugs. Clin Pharmacol Ther. 1978;24:1.

142. Gillette JR. Overview of drug-protein binding. Ann N Y Acad Sci. 1973;226:6.

143. Wilkinson GR, Shand DG. A physiological approach to hepatic clearance. Clin Pharmacol Ther. 1975;18:377.

144. Gibaldi M, McNamara PJ. Apparent volumes of distribution and drug binding to plasma proteins and tissues. Eur J Clin Pharmacol. 1978;13:373.

145. MacKichan JJ. Pharmacokinetic consequences of drug displacement from blood and tissue proteins. Clin Pharmacokinet. 1984;9(Suppl.1):32.

146. Oie S, Tozer TN. Effect of altered plasma protein binding on apparent volume of distribution. J Pharm Sci. 1979;68:1203. Letter.

147. Benet LZ, Massoud N. Pharmacokinetics. In: Benet LZ et al, eds. Pharmacokinetic Basis for Drug Treatment. New York: Raven Press; 1984;1–28.

148. D'Arcy PF, McElnay JC. Drug interactions involving the displacement of drugs from plasma protein and tissue binding sites. Pharmacol Ther. 1982;17:211.

149. Klotz U. Pathophysiological and disease-induced changes in drug distribution volume: pharmacokinetic implications. Clin Pharmacokinet. 1976;1:204.

150. Gupta SK, Benet LZ. High-fat meals increase the clearance of cyclosporine. Pharm Res. 1990;7:46.

151. Evans GH, Shand DG. Disposition of propranolol VI. Independent variation in steady-state circulating drug concentrations and half-life as a result of plasma drug binding in man. Clin Pharmacol Ther. 1973;14:494.

152. Rowland M et al. Clearance concepts in pharmacokinetics. J Pharmacokinet Biopharm. 1973;1:123.

153. Morgan DJ, Smallwood RA. Clinical significance of pharmacokinetic models of hepatic elimination. Clin Pharmacokinet. 1990;18:61.

154. Wilkinson GR. Plasma binding and hepatic drug elimination. In: Reidenberg MM, Erill S, eds. Drug-Protein Binding. New York: Praeger Publishers;1986;220–32.

155. Meijer DKF, van der Sluijs P. Covalent and noncovalent protein binding of drugs: implications for hepatic clearance, storage, and cell-specific drug delivery. Pharm Res. 1989;6:105.

156. Jansen JA. Influence of plasma protein binding kinetics on hepatic clearance assessed from a "tube" model and a "well-stirred" model. J Pharmacokinet Biopharm. 1981;9:15.

157. Weisiger RA. Dissociation from albumin: A potentially rate-limiting step in the clearance of substances by the liver. Proc Natl Acad Sci. 1985;82:1563.

158. Morgan DJ et al. Modeling of substrate elimination by the liver: has the albumin receptor model superseded the well-stirred model? Hepatology. 1985;5:1231.

159. Kornhauser DM et al. Biological determinants of propranolol disposition in man. Clin Pharmacol Ther. 1978;23:165.

160. Shand DG et al. Perfusion-limited effects of plasma drug binding on hepatic drug extraction. Life Sci. 1976;19:125.

161. MacKichan JJ et al. Effect of cimetidine on quinidine bioavailability. Biopharm Drug Dispos. 1989;10:121.

162. Gibaldi M, Perrier D. Pharmacokinetics, 2nd ed. New York: Marcel Dekker;1982:328.

163. Lima JJ. Disopyramide. In: Evans WE et al, eds. Applied Pharmacokinetics, 2nd ed. Spokane, WA: Applied Therapeutics, Inc;1986;1210–253.

164. Steinberg SF, Bilezikian JP. Total and free propranolol levels in sensitive and resistant patients. Clin Pharmacol Ther. 1983;33:162.

165. Kunin CM. Clinical pharmacology of the new penicillins. II: Effect of drugs which interfere with binding to serum proteins. Clin Pharmacol Ther. 1966;7:180–88.

166. Chignell CF. Protein binding. In: Garret ER, Hirtz JL, eds. Drug Fate and Metabolism. Methods and Techniques, Vol 1. New York: Marcel Dekker;1977;187–228.

167. Bowers WF et al. Ultrafiltration versus equilibrium dialysis for determination of free fraction. Clin Pharmacokinet. 1984;9(Suppl.1):49.

168. Kurz H. Methodological problems in drug-binding studies. In: Reidenberg MM, Erill S, eds. Drug-Protein Binding. New York: Praeger Publishers;1986;70–92.

169. Bjornssen TD et al. Importance of radiochemical purity of radiolabelled drugs used for determining plasma protein binding of drugs. J Pharm Sci. 1981;70:1372.

170. Brors O, Jacobsen S. pH lability in serum during equilibrium dialysis. Br J Clin Pharmacol. 1985;20:85.

171. Riva R et al. Determination of unbound valproic acid concentration in plasma by equilibrium dialysis and gas-liquid chromatography: methodological aspects and observations in epileptic patients. Ther Drug Monit. 1982;4:341.

172. Lima JJ et al. Influence of volume shifts on drug binding during equilibrium dialysis: correction and attenuation. J Pharmacokinet Biopharm. 1983;11:483.

173. Tozer TN et al. Volume shifts and protein binding estimates using equilibrium dialysis: application to prednisolone binding in humans. J Pharm Sci. 1983;72:1442.

174. Pedersen AO et al. Laurate binding to human serum albumin. Multiple binding equilibria investigated by a dialysis exchange method. Eur J Biochem. 1986;154:545.

175. Veronese ME et al. Plasma protein binding of amiodarone in a patient population: measurement by erythrocyte partitioning and a novel glass-binding method. Br J Clin Pharmacol. 1988;26:721.

176. Legg B, Rowland M. Cyclosporin: measurement of fraction unbound in plasma. J Pharm Pharmacol. 1987;39:599.

177. Behm HL, Wagner JG. Errors in interpretation of data from equilibrium dialysis protein binding experiments. Res Commun Chem Pathol Pharmacol. 1979;26:145.

178. Trung AHN et al. Comparison of the erythrocyte partitioning method with two classical methods for estimating free drug fraction in plasma. Biopharm Drug Dispos. 1984;5:281.

179. Hinderling PG et al. Protein binding and erythrocyte partitioning of disopyramide and its monodealkylated metabolite. J Pharm Sci. 1974;63:1684.

180. Parsons DL, Fan HF. Loss of propranolol during ultrafiltration in plasma protein binding studies. Res Commun Chem Pathol Pharmacol. 1986;54:405.

181. Lima JJ et al. Antiarrhythmic activity and unbound concentrations of disopyramide enantiomers in patients. Ther Drug Monit. 1990;12:23.

182. MacKichan JJ et al. Salivary concentrations and plasma protein binding of carbamazepine and carbamazepine 10,ll-epoxide in epileptic patients. Br J Clin Pharmacol. 1981;12:31.

183. Knott C, Reynolds F. The place of saliva in antiepileptic drug monitoring. Ther Drug Monit. 1984;6:35.

184. Bachmann K et al. Monitoring phenytoin in salivary and plasma ultrafiltrates of pediatric patients. Ther Drug Monit. 1983;5:325.

185. Wheeler SD et al. Drug-induced down-beat nystagmus. Ann Neurol. 1982;12:227.

186. Riva R et al. Diurnal fluctuations in free and total plasma concentrations of carbamazepine at steady-state and correlation with intermittent side effects in epileptic patients. Epilepsia. 1984;25:476.

187. Blum MR et al. Altered protein binding of diphenylhydantoin in uremic plasma. N Engl J Med. 1972;286:109.

188. Odar-Cederlöf I et al. Abnormal pharmacokinetics of phenytoin in a patient with uremia. Lancet. 1970;2:831.

189. Boston Collaborative Drug Surveillance Program: Diphenylhydantoin side effects and serum albumin levels. Clin Pharmacol Ther. 1973;14:529.

190. Huang J-D, Öie S. Effect of altered disopyramide binding on its pharmacologic response in rabbits. J Pharmacol Exp Ther. 1982;223:469.

191. Chiang W-T et al. Kinetics and dynamics of disopyramide and its dealkylated metabolite in healthy subjects. Clin Pharmacol Ther. 1985;38:37.

192. Thibonnier M et al. Pharmacokinetic-pharmacodynamic analysis of unbound disopyramide directly measured in serial plasma samples in man. J Pharmacokinet Biopharm. 1984;12:559.

193. Pieper JA et al. Lidocaine toxicity: effects of total versus free lidocaine concentrations. Circulation. 1980;62(Suppl.3):111.

194. Woo E, Greenblatt DJ. Pharmacokinetic and clinical implications of quinidine-protein binding. J Pharm Sci. 1979;68:466.

195. Perucca E. Free level monitoring of antiepileptic drugs. Clinical usefulness and case studies. Clin Pharmacokinet. 1984;9(Suppl.1):71.

196. Woosley RL et al. Potential applications of free drug level monitoring in cardiovascular therapy. Clin Pharmacokinet. 1984;9(Suppl 1):79.

197. Rimmer EM et al. Should we routinely measure free plasma phenytoin concentration? Br J Clin Pharmacol. 1984;17:99.

198. Theodore WH et al. The clinical value of free phenytoin levels. Ann Neurol. 1985;18:90.

199. Baird-Lambert J et al. Identifying patients who might benefit from free phenytoin monitoring. Ther Drug Monit. 1987;9:134.

200. Theodore WH. Should we measure free antiepileptic drug levels? Clin Neuropharmacol. 1987;10:26.

201. Evans WE et al. Differences in teniposide diposition and pharmacodynamics in patients with newly diagnosed and relapsed acute lymphocytic leukemia. J Pharmacol Exp Ther. 1992;260:71.

202. Stewart CF et al. Relation of systemic exposure to unbound etoposide and hematologic toxicity. Clin Pharmacol Ther. 1991;50:385.

203. Hughes TA et al. Plasma distribution of cyclosporine within lipoproteins and "*in vitro*" transfer between very-low density lipoproteins, low-density lipoproteins, and high-density lipoproteins. Ther Drug Monit. 1991;13:289.

204. Ballantyne CM et al. Effects of cyclosporine therapy on plasma lipoprotein levels. JAMA. 1989;262:53.

205. Ha HR et al. Measurement of free lidocaine serum concentration by equilibrium dialysis and ultrafiltration techniques: The influence of pH and heparin. Clin Pharmacokinet. 1984;9(Suppl.1):96.

206. Oëllerich M. Müller-Vahl H. The EMIT® FreeLevel™ ultrafiltration technique compared with equilibrium dialysis and ultracentrifugation to determine protein binding of phenytoin. Clin Pharmacokinet. 1984;9(Suppl.1):61.

Chapter 6

Influence of Liver Function on Drug Disposition

Kim L.R. Brouwer, George E. Dukes, and J. Robert Powell

The liver is the principle organ of xenobiotic metabolism and a major organ of elimination. Consequently, it determines the disposition of many drugs and other foreign substances. Because of this central role that the liver assumes in the disposition of drugs, many factors that contribute to the inter- and intrapatient variability in drug disposition tend to be hepatic in origin. This chapter will focus on those factors that determine the liver's influence on drug disposition (patient characteristics, liver diseases, and concomitant drug administration) and when to anticipate that the alterations in drug disposition are of such magnitude that dosage adjustments will be necessary to maintain the desired effects of drug therapy. To fully understand these factors, one must understand the fundamental pharmacokinetic principles of drug disposition and the underlying determinants of hepatic drug clearance.

BASIC CONCEPTS

Hepatic Physiology

As an eliminating organ, the liver is uniquely situated to receive a dual blood supply (approximately 1.5 L/min in healthy adults) from the hepatic artery (approximately 25%) and portal vein (approximately 75%) (see Figure 6-1). This vasculature diverges into hepatic arterioles and portal venules which supply hepatic sinusoids with highly oxygenated arterial blood and nutrient-rich venous blood. Each sinusoid drains into a central vein that empties into the hepatic veins and, ultimately, into the vena cava. Hepatic sinusoids are modified capillaries lined with endothelial and Kupffer (phagocytic) cells in a discontinuous matrix. Intercellular gaps (fenestrae) between endothelial cells lining the sinusoids permit plasma, plasma proteins, and endogenous and exogenous substances in plasma (including both protein bound and unbound drug molecules) to move freely into the space of Disse and to have direct contact with the microvilli of hepatocytes. Red blood cells are too large to pass through the fenestrae and cannot reach the space of Disse. The parenchymal cells (hepatocytes), in which the majority of drug metabolizing activity resides, are arranged in a three-dimensional framework; each hepatocyte has direct contact with the space of Disse, adjacent hepatocytes, and the bile canaliculi. This structural arrangement facilitates rapid exchange of drugs and metabolites between plasma and hepatocytes, and between hepatocytes and bile. The movement of drugs and metabolites across the sinusoidal membrane of the hepatocyte may be influenced by hepatic blood flow, the extent of protein binding (since only unbound drug is believed to be available for transfer) and the mechanism of transfer. It is generally assumed that drug molecules and resulting metabolites readily diffuse into and out of the hepatocyte. While this may be the case for lipophilic substances, polar compounds may not cross the lipid domain of the hepatic sinusoidal membrane as readily, and carrier-mediated transport processes may be required to facilitate entry and exit.[2] For example, indocyanine green (ICG), an organic anion dye used to measure liver blood flow, is transported into hepatocytes (hepatic uptake) by an energy-dependent, saturable process.[3]

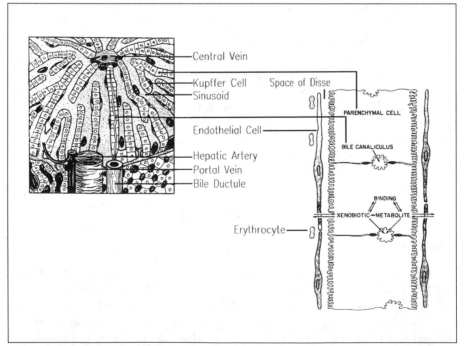

Figure 6-1. *Diagram depicting the basic structure of a liver lobule. Blood flows from the hepatic artery and portal vein into hepatic sinusoids which drain into a central vein. The sinusoids are lined with endothelial cells and Kupffer cells. Intercellular gaps (fenestrae) permit plasma constituents to gain access to the space of Disse and microvilli of the hepatocyte. Bile flows in the opposite direction of blood flow through bile canaliculi toward the bile ductules (adapted with permission from reference 1).*

Additionally, excretion of drugs and their respective metabolites into bile also is assumed to be carrier-mediated. Disease- or drug-induced changes in hepatic transport systems may alter significantly the disposition and hepatic clearance of drugs.

Numerous pathophysiologic changes occur in the liver during hepatic disease that may influence drug disposition. For example, the development of cirrhosis begins with initial hepatocellular damage that produces inflammation; dead or necrotic cells are removed by phagocytosis. In response to the insult, fibroblasts secrete collagen to help maintain the integrity of the liver architecture while the damaged or dead cells are repaired or replaced. As the disease progresses, collagen fibrils accumulate in the sinusoidal space, including the space of Disse, producing bands of connective scar tissue characteristic of cirrhosis. Finally, a basement membrane devoid of microvilli forms along the sinusoidal surface of the hepatocyte. The collagen barrier between hepatocyte and sinusoid, in conjunction with alterations in the sinusoidal membrane of the hepatocyte (e.g., loss of microvilli), may interfere significantly with the exchange of oxygen, nutrients, and plasma constituents, including drugs and metabolites, between blood and hepatocytes. In an effort to compensate for hepatocellular damage, hepatocytes regenerate, resulting in clustered formations that increase in size and eventually form liver nodules. The distorted liver architecture increases vascular resistance, thus increasing portal venous pressure and promoting the development of extrahepatic and intrahepatic shunts. Hepatocyte loss and fibrosis also facilitate the formation of intrahepatic shunts. Blood flowing through these shunts may bypass functioning hepatocytes and pass directly from the portal tracts into the central veins. On average, 70% of mesenteric and 95% of splanchnic blood flow may undergo extrahepatic shunting in patients with alcoholic liver disease who are bleeding from esophageal varices;[4] intrahepatic portosystemic shunting has been reported to range from 4% to 66% of total hepatic flow.[5] The net result of pathophysiologic alterations in the liver during hepatic disease is that a drug may be less accessible to functional hepatocytes containing the enzyme systems responsible for drug metabolism.

Drug Metabolism

The chemical reactions involved in drug biotransformations are facilitated by enzymes. In general, lipophilic drug molecules are converted into water-soluble metabolites which are ionized at physiological pH and are excreted readily, usually by the kidneys. Biotransformation reactions are divided into two categories. *Phase I* (nonsynthetic/functionalization) biotransformation includes oxidation [the addition of a functional group (e.g., hydroxyl) to the parent compound or deletion of an alkyl group (e.g., N-demethylation)], reduction, and hydrolysis reactions. *Phase II* (synthetic/conjugation) biotransformation links a parent drug molecule or product of Phase I metabolism with an endogenous substrate such as glucuronic acid, sulfate, or glycine. Methylation and acetylation are other clinically important conjugation reactions. However, these latter routes of metabolism usually do not enhance water solubility. Most drugs are biotransformed by enzyme systems located within the hepatocyte, although extrahepatic metabolism plays an important role in the disposition of some drugs and will be addressed in a subsequent section of this chapter. Localization, as well as the capacity, of enzyme systems involved in hepatic drug metabolism may influence which metabolic pathways remain functional during hepatic disease.

Hepatic Drug Metabolism. *Oxidation.* The microsomal mixed-function oxidase system, located in the smooth endoplasmic reticulum of the hepatocyte, is quantitatively the most important enzyme system responsible for drug oxidation and some reduction reactions. This system consists of two enzymes (cytochrome P450 and NADPH-dependent cytochrome P450 reductase) and requires nicotinamide adenine dinucleotide phosphate (NADPH) and molecular oxygen to function. Cytochrome P450, a heme-containing protein that reacts with carbon monoxide to yield a complex with a UV absorbance maximum at 450 nm, is embedded primarily in the phospholipid bilayer of the smooth endoplasmic reticulum, with a portion exposed to the cytosol (see Figure 6-2). The reductase is a flavoprotein located primarily on the surface of the membrane, but in close proximity to cytochrome P450. In the oxidized state, cytochrome P450 combines with an endogenous or exogenous substrate (e.g., drug molecule) to form a complex which then undergoes reduction by cytochrome P450 reductase. Molecular oxygen, an electron, and two hydrogen ions combine with the reduced cytochrome P450-drug complex, resulting in release of the oxidized drug, re-oxidation of cytochrome P450, and production of water.

Multiple forms (isozymes) of cytochrome P450 have been identified in various animal species, including humans. Each P450 is encoded by a separate gene. P450 genes are classified according to families and subfamilies based on the degree of similarity in amino acid sequence of the isozymes which they encode. Genes which encode proteins that are less than 40% similar in amino acid sequence belong to different families, designated by roman numerals.[6] At the present time, eight different families are known in humans (I, II, III, IV, XI, XVII, XIX, XXI). The drug-metabolizing P450s belong to families I through IV.[7] Genes that encode P450 enzymes that are 70% or more similar are classified in the same subfamily. Subfamilies are designated by capital letters (A, B, C, etc.). The individual

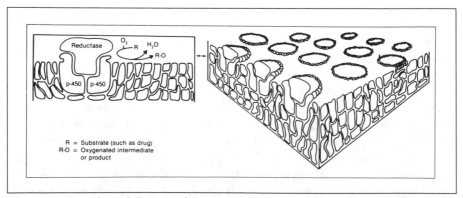

Figure 6-2. *Hypothetical diagram of the relationship between the cytochrome P450 isozymes embedded within the lipid bilayer of the endoplasmic reticulum and the flavoprotein reductases (adapted with permission from reference 311).*

gene is designated by an Arabic numeral. Human cytochrome P450 isozymes known to oxidize clinically used drugs are listed in Table 6-1. As shown, many clinically useful drugs have been identified as substrates for the P450IA, P450IIC, P450IID, and P450IIIA subfamilies, although the specific P450 responsible for the oxidation of numerous other drugs in humans remains to be identified. Present evidence suggests that the total number of P450 isozymes in humans may range from 20 to 200.[8] Isozymes of cytochrome P450 vary in metabolic activity toward a given substrate and exhibit varying degrees of substrate specificity, which may overlap. Differences in genetic composition and exposure to enzyme-inducing agents may influence the pattern of activity of these isozymes.

Studies in rats indicate that cytochrome P450 enzyme systems are localized predominantly in pericentral hepatocytes (those located close to the central vein) and are not distributed evenly throughout all hepatocytes within the liver.[9,10] Alterations in cytochrome P450 may occur under hypoxic conditions,[11] and the cytochrome P450 content of human liver microsomes is decreased by approximately 50% in cirrhosis.[12] Thus, Phase I biotransformation may be impaired in various types of hepatic disease, particularly in patients with cirrhosis and chronic liver disease. For example, the total clearance of diazepam and chlordiazepoxide, initially metabolized by Phase I biotransformation, is significantly reduced in cirrhotics as compared to controls.[13,14]

Conjugation. The majority of drugs that undergo Phase II biotransformation are conjugated with glucuronic acid. The formation of uridine diphosphate glucu-

Table 6-1. *Human Cytochrome P450 Isozymes Known to Oxidize Clinically Used Drugs[f]*

Gene designation			
P450IA2	**P450IIC9**	**P450IID6**	**P450IIIA4**
Phenacetin	N-desmethyldiazepam[b]	Amitriptyline[c]	Cyclosporine A
Caffeine[a]	Diazepam[b]	Codeine[d]	Erythromycin
	Hexobarbital	Debrisoquine	Lidocaine[e]
	Mephenytoin	Desipramine	Midazolam
	Methylphenobarbital[b]	Dextromethorphan	Nifedipine
	Alprenolol	Encainide	Quinidine
		Flecainide[c]	Triazolam
		Imipramine[c]	
		Metoprolol	
		Nortriptyline[c]	
		Perhexiline[c]	
		Perphenazine[c]	
		Propranolol[d]	
		Sparteine	
		Thioridazine[c]	
		Timolol[c]	

[a] 3–demethylation pathway.
[b] *In vivo* studies have established the relationship between metabolism and the mephenytoin oxidation polymorphism.
[c] Metabolism of drug *in vivo* controlled by the sparteine/debrisoquine oxidation polymorphism.
[d] P450IID6 catalyses a minor pathway.
[e] Formation of monoethylglicinexylidide.
[f] Adapted with permission from reference 7.

ronic acid (UDPGA), the cofactor necessary for UDP-glucuronyltransferase enzymes to form glucuronide conjugates of drugs, requires a carbohydrate source, energy, and an NAD^+-dependent dehydrogenation. Glucuronidation is a low-affinity, high-capacity pathway, and activity is frequently preserved in various types of liver disease, even when mixed-function oxidase activity has been impaired.[15] For example, in contrast to diazepam and chlordiazepoxide, the clearance of oxazepam, which is only glucuronidated, is not decreased in patients with cirrhosis.[16] However, more recent investigations have indicated that glucuronidation of some substrates may be impaired significantly in hepatic disease. The formation clearance of the glucuronide conjugate of zidovudine was decreased more than sixfold in patients with cirrhosis.[17] The conjugation of 3-hydroxy-antipyrine,[18] zomepirac,[19] and morphine[20] also was impaired significantly in patients with cirrhosis. Multiple forms of human UDP-glucuronyltransferases, the heterogeneous distribution of enzyme systems within the liver, and heterogeneity in the routes of metabolism of some drugs also may play an important role in disease-associated or drug-induced alterations in hepatic metabolism. Results of studies in rats suggest that glucuronidation activity is distributed uniformly throughout the liver lobule, while sulfation decreases from periportal to pericentral regions.[21,10]

In contrast to glucuronidation, sulfation is a high-affinity, low-capacity system. Two moles of adenosine triphosphate (ATP) are required to form one mole of adenosine 3'-phosphate 5'-phosphosulfate, the cofactor necessary for sulphotransferase enzymes to transfer inorganic sulfate to drug molecules. The nonlinear pharmacokinetics of phenolic drugs undergoing sulfate conjugation, such as acetaminophen, has been attributed, in part, to the limited availability and consequent depletion of inorganic sulfate.[22]

The activity of enzyme systems involved in hepatic drug metabolism may be enhanced or impaired by endogenous as well as exogenous substances (e.g., environmental contaminants and drugs). Enzyme induction refers to a relative increase in the number of molecules of the enzyme system, resulting in an increase in the rate of metabolism. The available evidence indicates that increased mixed-function oxidase activity is due to an increase in enzyme protein synthesis as opposed to either a decrease in the enzyme degradation rate or an allosteric change in the enzyme molecule.[23] Traditionally, two general types of inducing agents have been studied: the phenobarbital type and the polycyclic aromatic hydrocarbon type. The ability to measure numerous isozymes of cytochrome P450 has led to the hypothesis that each inducing agent may produce a specific pattern of isozyme synthesis rates, resulting in different isozyme steady-state concentrations and different relative induction patterns, regardless of the classification of the inducing agent.[24]

Inhibition of drug metabolizing enzyme systems may be due to either direct or indirect interactions between the inhibitor and the enzyme. The mechanism of inhibition may be an important consideration in determining both the specificity of an inhibitor and the time-course of metabolic inhibition. Enzyme induction and inhibition will be discussed in greater detail in a subsequent section of this chapter.

Extrahepatic Drug Metabolism. Numerous routes of extrahepatic drug metabolism exist[25] and may be altered, either directly or indirectly, by hepatic disease or hepatic-associated drug interactions. The *kidney* contains many of the drug metabolizing enzymes found in the liver and is an important site of metabolism and activation of some xenobiotics. A recent evaluation of morphine pharmacokinetics in patients indicated that morphine total body clearance exceeded hepatic clearance by 38%.[26] Since no gut wall metabolism of morphine occurred, the authors concluded that the kidney is an important site of morphine metabolism in humans.

Drug metabolism in the *gastrointestinal tract* is mediated by either intestinal bacteria in the gut contents or enzyme systems located in the epithelial cells of the gut wall. Cytochrome P450-dependent mixed-function oxidases, esterases, and conjugation systems for acetylation, sulfation, methylation, and glucuronidation have been identified in the gut wall in experimental animals and man; these enzyme systems, which may be induced or inhibited, play an important role in the presystemic metabolism of drugs.[27] Ethinyloestradiol undergoes significant presystemic metabolism in the gut wall of humans.[28]

In some cases, the human *lung* contributes to drug clearance. For example, approximately 75% of an intravenous bolus dose of propranolol was removed on first passage through the pulmonary vasculature in patients who had not previously taken the drug.[29] Compared to the liver, lung tissue possesses much lower activities of drug metabolizing enzymes. The local formation of toxic and/or reactive metabolites within the lung appears to be the mechanism of pulmonary toxicity associated with many exogenous substances.

Human *skin* contains a variety of drug metabolizing enzymes, including cytochrome P450 mixed-function oxidases, reductases, esterases, glutathione S-transferases, and glucuronyltransferases. Steroidal compounds such as hydrocortisone and testosterone are metabolized by human skin.[30]

Other important extrahepatic metabolic organs include the *blood* and *brain*. The effect of hepatic disease on extrahepatic drug metabolism has not been investigated extensively.

Hepatic Excretion

The importance of the liver as an excretory organ is overlooked frequently, in part because attention is usually focused on hepatic biotransformation. However, some drug molecules taken up by the hepatocyte are not metabolized prior to excretion by the liver. For example, indocyanine green is highly extracted by the liver and excreted unchanged into bile.[31] In order to be eliminated from the liver, unchanged drug (as well as derived metabolites) must cross either the hepatic sinusoidal membrane of the hepatocyte and return to the sinusoidal blood as it flows toward the central vein, or be transported across the canalicular membrane of the hepatocyte into bile. The biliary transport of drugs is similar to active secretion in the kidneys and may be inhibited competitively. The potential for disease-associated or drug-induced alterations in hepatic excretion may be significant. For example, ornidazole clearance is decreased significantly and its two major hydroxylated metabolites accumulate in plasma in patients with hepatitis, noncholestatic cirrhosis, and extrahepatic cholestasis.[32] Although hepatic disease usually results in decreased metabolite concentrations subsequent to impaired metabolism, accumulation of metabolites may occur if the route of excretion (either conjugation or biliary secretion) is impaired by progression of the disease.

Pharmacokinetic Principles

Hepatic Extraction Ratio (E_H). The liver may remove a drug from 1) the systemic circulation on each pass through the liver and 2) the splanchnic blood supply (via the portal system) on the drug's "first-pass" through the liver before it reaches the systemic circulation. The efficiency of drug removal by the liver may be described by the E_H, calculated from hepatic inflow (C_a, mixed portal venous and hepatic arterial) and outflow (C_v, hepatic venous) drug concentrations:

$$E_H = \frac{C_a - C_v}{C_a}$$

(Eq. 6-1)

If the liver is not capable of removing drug from the circulation, $C_v = C_a$, and the extraction ratio is zero. In contrast, if the liver is maximally efficient at removing drug on a single pass through the organ, $C_v = 0$, and the extraction ratio equals one. It is important to recognize that the hepatic extraction ratio is a measure of the efficiency of the removal process and is not related to the extent of metabolism. Many drugs (e.g., phenytoin, diazepam, valproic acid) are metabolized extensively or completely by the liver, yet exhibit a low hepatic extraction ratio. It is useful to think of hepatic drug extraction as a measure of the organ's effectiveness in extracting the drug from blood as it perfuses through the hepatic sinusoids.

Bioavailability (F^*). Following oral drug administration, the fraction of the absorbed dose which reaches the systemic circulation (F^*), thus escaping hepatic elimination on its "first-pass" through the liver, is related to the hepatic extraction ratio:

$$F^* = 1 - E_H$$

(Eq. 6-2)

This equation assumes that all splanchnic blood flows through the liver. The fraction of the absorbed dose that reaches the systemic circulation will approximate 1.0 for drugs that are not extracted efficiently by the liver. Alterations in presystemic elimination associated with hepatic disease or drug interactions will be relatively insignificant for these poorly extracted compounds (i.e., a 50% decrease in E_H from 0.1 to 0.05 will increase F^* from 0.9 to 0.95; the percent of the absorbed dose that reaches the systemic circulation increases only 5.6%). However, if a drug is extracted efficiently by the liver, only a small fraction of the absorbed dose reaches the systemic circulation. Hepatic disease or drug-induced alterations in "first-pass" extraction may alter significantly the systemic availability of these types of drugs (i.e., a 10% decrease in E_H from 0.9 to 0.8 will increase F^* from 0.1 to 0.2; the percent of the absorbed dose that reaches the systemic circulation increases 100%).

Hepatic Intrinsic Clearance. Factors that influence the hepatic extraction of a drug include hepatic blood flow, protein binding, and the metabolic activity (or other rate-limiting processes) involved in hepatic elimination. The hepatic intrinsic clearance of unbound drug in the liver ($CL_{u_{int}}$) represents the maximal ability of hepatocytes to irreversibly remove drug from liver water when blood flow, protein binding and translocation to the site of metabolism or elimination are not rate-limiting. Thus, $CL_{u_{int}}$ will be $\geq CL_H$. The hepatic intrinsic clearance of unbound drug is frequently related to metabolic activity, which usually is assumed to be the rate-limiting step in hepatic elimination.

$$CL_{u_{int}} = \Sigma \, \frac{V_{max,i}}{K_{m,i} + C_{u,L}}$$

(Eq. 6-3)

where $V_{max,i}$ is the maximum rate of the reaction, $K_{m,i}$ is the substrate-enzyme affinity constant for the ith enzyme, and $C_{u,L}$ is the concentration of unbound drug at the enzyme site in the liver. While it is assumed generally that dissociation of drug from protein binding sites and diffusion (or transport of some substrates) across the sinusoidal membrane from blood into the hepatocyte occurs much more rapidly than metabolic clearance, these generalizations may not be correct in all cases.[33,34]

Hepatic Clearance (CL_H). Defined as the volume of blood from which drug is removed completely by the liver per unit time, CL_H is a function of hepatic blood flow (Q_H) and the extraction efficiency of the liver for the drug (E_H):

$$CL_H = Q_H \cdot E_H$$

(Eq. 6-4)

Based on these relationships, CL_H can range from zero (when the liver is incapable of removing the drug: $E_H = 0$) to Q_H (when the liver extracts all of the drug presented to it: $E_H = 1$). However, CL_H can never exceed hepatic blood flow because maximal E_H is 100%. It should be noted that total hepatic clearance is equal to systemic clearance only when the drug is completely cleared by the liver following intravenous administration.

Currently, our understanding of hepatic drug disposition is relatively simplistic, in part because of our inability to sample drug concentrations at the site of elimination within the hepatocyte. Numerous mathematical models have been developed to describe the complex relationships between hepatic clearance and the three primary determinants of hepatic drug elimination: hepatic blood flow, the fraction of unbound drug in the blood (f_{ub}), and the hepatic intrinsic clearance of unbound drug.[35] The kinetic model of hepatic drug clearance that is employed most frequently in clinical pharmacokinetic applications is the "venous equilibrium" or "well-stirred" model, which relates hepatic clearance to $CL_{u_{int}}$ and f_{ub} as follows:

$$CL_H = Q_H \cdot \frac{f_{ub} \cdot CL_{u_{int}}}{Q_H + f_{ub} \cdot CL_{u_{int}}}$$

(Eq. 6-5)

This model assumes the liver is a single, well-stirred compartment where unbound drug concentrations in emergent hepatic venous blood are in equilibrium with unbound concentrations of drug in the liver.[36-38] A second model, the "undistributed sinusoidal model" or "parallel-tube model," has been used to describe the hepatic elimination of some drugs in patients. In this latter model, the hepatic sinusoids are viewed as a set of parallel tubes; drug concentrations decrease exponentially along the tubes; and the average concentration of drug within the liver is calculated as the logarithmic average of the hepatic inflow and outflow concentrations.[38,39] The equation relating total hepatic clearance to its principal determinants for this model is:

$$CL_H = [Q_H] \left[1 - e^{-\left(f_{ub} \cdot \frac{CL_{u_{int}}}{Q_H} \right)} \right] \qquad \text{(Eq. 6-6)}$$

These models are useful to quantitatively predict and/or explain the effects that disease or drug-induced alterations in hepatic blood flow, drug protein binding, and/or hepatic intrinsic clearance of unbound drug have on the hepatic clearance of drugs.[36] The influence of these changes on total and unbound drug concentrations must be considered by the clinician in order to assess whether or not a dosage adjustment is necessary. Although total drug concentrations are assayed routinely, pharmacological effect usually correlates better with unbound than with total plasma drug concentrations.[40] To simplify these pharmacokinetic relationships for clinical applications, drugs are classified based on their hepatic extraction ratio (see Table 6-2).

Low Extraction Ratio (E_H <0.3). When total hepatic intrinsic clearance ($f_{ub} \times CL_{u_{int}}$) is small relative to liver blood flow (<650 mL/min), Equations 6-5 and 6-6 consistently predict that hepatic clearance will approximate $f_{ub} \times CL_{u_{int}}$ ($CL_H \approx f_{ub} \times CL_{u_{int}}$). If the drug is not bound extensively to plasma proteins (f_{ub} >0.5), the hepatic clearance after intravenous or oral administration will depend primarily on the hepatic intrinsic clearance of unbound drug. In contrast, if the drug is highly protein bound, hepatic clearance will depend on the extent of protein binding as well as the hepatic intrinsic clearance of unbound drug. Dosage adjustments for low extraction ratio drugs administered either intravenously or orally would be necessary only when hepatic disease or drug interactions alter the hepatic intrinsic clearance of unbound drug (e.g., enzyme induction or inhibition). Although alterations in protein binding would change total drug concentrations, unbound drug concentrations should remain constant since hepatic clearance of unbound drug remains unchanged. This is a particularly important concept because clinicians frequently assume that alterations in total drug concentrations necessitate a dosage adjustment. As noted, if unbound drug concentrations remain unchanged, a dosage adjustment may not be warranted. Changes in liver blood flow would not be expected to alter significantly total or unbound concentrations of a low extraction ratio drug because the hepatic clearance of these compounds is not rate-limited by liver blood flow.

High Extraction Ratio (E_H >0.7). When total hepatic intrinsic clearance ($f_{ub} \times CL_{u_{int}}$) is large relative to liver blood flow (>3500 mL/min), Equations 6-5 and 6-6 consistently predict that hepatic clearance approximates Q_H. Since the liver can extract these drugs as rapidly as they are presented to the organ, hepatic clearance is rate-limited by liver blood flow. Thus, drugs that are extracted efficiently by the liver are sensitive to changes in liver blood flow.

1) *Intravenous Administration.* Dosage adjustments for high extraction ratio drugs administered intravenously may be necessary when disease or drug-induced alterations in hepatic blood flow occur. Alterations in protein binding do not change total hepatic clearance for drugs that exhibit a high extraction ratio ($CL_H \approx Q_H$), but would be expected to change the hepatic clearance of unbound drug and alter unbound drug concentrations. A dosage adjustment may be necessary to maintain the same unbound drug concentrations, even though total drug concentrations remain constant. This is another particularly important concept because clinicians frequently assume that dosage adjustments are unnecessary as long as total drug concentrations remain constant. Changes in the hepatic intrinsic clearance of unbound drug would not be expected to alter significantly total or unbound concentrations of a high extraction ratio drug after intravenous administration because the hepatic clearance of these compounds is rate-limited by liver blood flow.

2) *Oral Administration.* A significant first-pass effect following oral administration is clinically important only for drugs that are efficiently extracted by the liver, where only a small fraction of the absorbed dose reaches the systemic circulation. As previously discussed, a small change in the first-pass extraction of efficiently extracted drugs may alter systemic availability markedly. Traditionally, based on the venous equilibrium model (Equation 6-5), it has been assumed that only changes in the hepatic intrinsic clearance of unbound drug alter unbound drug concentrations of an efficiently extracted drug following oral administration (a change in $CL_{u_{int}}$ will alter F* but not CL_H). Alterations in protein binding would be expected to change total, but not unbound, drug concentrations. Any changes in liver blood flow that alter hepatic clearance would be offset by a change in systemic availability of equal magnitude. Therefore, assuming no extra-

Table 6-2. *Drugs Exhibiting Greater than 20% Decrease in Clearance in Chronic Liver Disease[172,173]*

High extraction ($E_H > 0.7$)	Low extraction ($E_H < 0.3$)
Encainide	Antipyrine
Lidocaine	Caffeine
Meperidine	Chloramphenicol
Metoprolol	Chlordiazepoxide
Pentazocine	Diazepam
Propranolol	Erythromycin
Tocainide	Hexobarbital
Verapamil	Metronidazole
	Theophylline

hepatic route of elimination, unbound drug concentrations should be independent of changes in protein binding or liver blood flow following oral administration of drugs with a high hepatic extraction. However, an important difference in the predictions between the venous equilibrium and undistributed sinusoidal models is noted in this case. The undistributed sinusoidal model (see Equation 6-6) predicts that unbound drug concentrations would be sensitive to changes in protein binding and liver blood flow in addition to alterations in the hepatic intrinsic clearance of unbound drug. Unbound drug concentrations would be predicted to decrease as Q_H decreases or f_{ub} increases. The clinical implications of differences in predictions between these two pharmacokinetic models of hepatic elimination have been reviewed.[41]

Intermediate Extraction Ratio (0.3 $\leq E_H \leq 0.7$). A few drugs exhibit intermediate extraction ratios, although most drugs appear to have either a low ($E_H < 0.3$) or high ($E_H > 0.7$) hepatic extraction. Disease- or drug-induced alterations in hepatic blood flow and/or the hepatic intrinsic clearance of unbound drug may alter significantly the unbound concentration of drugs that exhibit intermediate hepatic extraction following intravenous administration. Following oral administration, unbound concentrations of such drugs are sensitive to changes in the hepatic intrinsic clearance of unbound drug, and also may be affected by alterations in hepatic blood flow and/or drug protein binding. Clearly, an understanding of these fundamental pharmacokinetic principles related to hepatic drug clearance is essential for proper therapeutic drug monitoring.

Volume of Distribution (V_d). In addition to CL_H and F^*, V_d is a primary pharmacokinetic parameter that may be affected by hepatic disease or drug-associated alterations in physiologic variables. V_d subsequent to tissue pseudo-equilibrium is dependent upon the fraction of unbound drug in blood and tissue (f_{ut}):

$$V_d = V_B + V_T \cdot \left(\frac{f_{ub}}{f_{ut}}\right)$$

(Eq. 6-7)

where V_B and V_T represent the true blood and tissue water volumes, respectively.[36,42] Based on Equation 6-7, V_d would increase linearly with f_{ub} as long as tissue binding was unaffected. However, the distribution volume of unbound drug (V_d/f_{ub}) would not be altered significantly by changes in f_{ub} unless extravascular distribution is negligible, in which case an increase in f_{ub} will result in a decrease in the distribution volume of unbound drug.[43] If the disease- or drug-associated alteration also perturbs tissue binding, V_d may or may not be affected depending on the relative magnitude of change in f_{ub} and f_{ut}.

Half-Life ($t\frac{1}{2}$). The elimination half-life of a drug, an important pharmacokinetic parameter in clinical practice, is a value derived from, and dependent on, the clearance (CL) and V_d of the drug:

$$t\frac{1}{2} = \frac{0.693 \cdot V_d}{CL}$$

(Eq. 6-8)

Frequently, clinicians erroneously use $t^{1/2}$ as an index of hepatic clearance, or measure of hepatic function. Equation 6-8 clearly shows that the elimination half-life will vary indirectly as clearance changes only when the volume of distribution remains constant. As previously stated, hepatic disease or drug-associated alterations in physiologic variables frequently cause a change in the volume of distribution. Indiscriminate use of $t^{1/2}$ as a measure of CL under such conditions will yield incorrect conclusions. For example, if the effect of a drug interaction on V_d and CL were quantitatively similar, $t^{1/2}$ would remain unchanged; important alterations in V_d and CL would be overlooked if only $t^{1/2}$ was measured. In all cases, the primary pharmacokinetic parameters, CL and V_d, should be measured directly to assess whether hepatic disease or drug-associated alterations significantly influence drug disposition.

LIVER FUNCTION ASSESSMENT

The liver is responsible for a number of physiologic processes besides the metabolism of endogenous and exogenous substances. These processes include plasma protein synthesis, glucose homeostasis, lipid and lipoprotein synthesis, vitamin storage, clotting factor synthesis, and bile acid synthesis and secretion. In addition, the liver is an important organ of the reticuloendothelial system. Hepatic disease constitutes a group of acute and chronic inflammatory, degenerative, and neoplastic disorders. These disorders vary in their pathology and, therefore, each disease should not be assumed to affect each of the hepatic physiologic functions in the same way as other hepatic diseases. Even within the same type of liver disease, inter- and intrapatient variability in the quantitative dysfunction of each hepatic physiologic process occurs due to variable pathologic changes (e.g., amount of hepatocyte damage and/or degree of portosystemic shunting). No single test can be used to assess the overall function of the liver due to the number and variety of hepatic physiologic processes. A test which reflects one hepatic process may not accurately reflect other hepatic functions. For example, the liver's ability to secrete bile does not correlate with its capacity to metabolize xenobiotics by the cytochrome P450 system. Because we are unable to simply and accurately predict the degree of hepatic dysfunction, it is difficult to precisely alter drug dosages in individual patients with liver disease.

Biochemical Markers

Individual Tests. The "liver function" tests routinely employed in the clinical evaluation of patients with liver disease are biochemical measurements of individual hepatic functions (e.g., serum albumin reflects protein synthetic capacity) or evidence of pathologic conditions (e.g., serum aminotransferase elevation signifies hepatocyte damage). If abnormal, these tests indicate that the particular physiologic process is malfunctioning or that a pathologic process is occurring, but they do not necessarily reflect the degree of liver dysfunction. Potential qualitative pharmacokinetic alterations can be predicted from these individual liver function tests, although the degree of those alterations is difficult to determine. For example, if a patient has an elevated prothrombin time (without a vitamin K deficiency) it may be assumed that the liver's ability to synthesize protein (in this case, the vitamin K dependent clotting factors—II, VII, IX, and X) is impaired secondary to some functional defect in the hepatocyte. An extrapolation is often made from this information that there also may be qualitative defects in other hepatocyte functions, including drug metabolism. Unfortunately, the sensitivity and specificity of these tests are low and do not allow quantitative assessment of the degree of dysfunction. Although these tests lack sufficient discrimination to be consistent predictors of impaired drug metabolism, they do indicate the potential for qualitative pharmacokinetic changes (see Table 6-3).

Patterns of Test Abnormalities. Collectively, the pattern of the liver test abnormalities is useful as an indication of the type of hepatic disease, the time course of the disease, and as a crude marker of the severity of hepatic dysfunction. Large increases in serum alkaline phosphatase and conjugated (direct) bilirubin concentrations along with normal prothrombin time and serum transaminase concentrations indicate cholestasis. The higher the elevations, the more severe the obstruction. It follows that the clearance of drugs eliminated via the bile may be decreased in this situation.[32] Patients with hepatocyte damage sufficient to cause decreased drug metabolism will generally have a serum albumin concentration less than 3.0 to 3.5 gm/dL and impaired prothrombin activity (less than 80% of normal).[44]

Classification Schemes. The best way to estimate the severity of hepatic impairment is through classification schemes that use a combination of clinical

Table 6-3. *Potential Pharmacokinetic Alterations Predicted by Abnormal Biochemical Measurements of Hepatic Function*

Biochemical measurement	Physiologic/ pathologic alteration	Potential pharmacokinetic alteration	Problems in interpretation
Prothrombin time	Acute ↓ protein synthesis	↓ metabolism	Low vitamin K
Serum albumin	Chronic ↓ protein synthesis	↓ metabolism; ↓ protein binding; ↑ V_d	Poor nutrition
Serum bilirubin Conjugated (direct)	Cholestasis	↓ biliary elimination of drugs	Prolonged elevations despite return of normal function
Unconjugated (indirect)	Hepatocyte dysfunction or ↓ extraction from blood	↓ metabolism	Hemolysis
Serum alkaline phosphatase	Cholestasis	↓ biliary elimination of drugs	↑ production
Serum amino-transferase [Alanine (ALT)] [Aspartate (AST)]	Hepatocyte damage	↓ metabolism	Normal in chronic disease. High elevations in acute disease may not reflect hepatic malfunction.

assessments and biochemical measurements. The most widely accepted of these severity scales are the Child-Turcotte classification[45] and the Pugh's modification of Child's classification (see Table 6-4).[46] Child's scale identifies three levels of hepatic dysfunction (A, B, or C), from mildly to severely impaired. Pugh's modification of Child's system adds other indices (prothrombin time) and assigns points for increasing degrees of abnormality of each index; the total score indicates the degree of liver disease severity. These classification schemes are useful in following an individual patient's disease course and in comparing patient groups, but they still lack the sensitivity to quantitate the specific ability of the liver to metabolize individual drugs.

Model Substrate Markers

Definition and Characteristics. An alternative to endogenous biochemical markers is to use exogenously administered model substrates to measure the liver's ability to metabolize drugs. The ideal model substrate would be nontoxic and pharmacologically inert; could be given intravenously or would be 100% orally available in all patient populations; would be predominantly hepatically metabolized to products that could be easily and reproducibly measured in biological fluids; would not be highly protein bound; and would be inexpensive and readily available.[47] In addition, these models should be sufficiently sensitive to detect impaired hepatic drug elimination, and specific enough to predict alterations in the disposition of other drugs. Although many compounds have been proposed as good markers of hepatic function,[48] all have limitations.

Limitations. The major limitation to the use of model compounds is the multiplicity of processes involved in the hepatic clearance of drugs. Within the

Table 6-4. Severity Classification Schemes for Liver Disease

CHILD-TURCOTTE CLASSIFICATION[45]			
	Grade A	Grade B	Grade C
Bilirubin (mg/dL)	< 2.0	2.0–3.0	> 3.0
Albumin (gm/dL)	> 3.5	3.0–3.5	< 3.0
Ascites	none	easily controlled	poorly controlled
Neurological disorder	none	minimal	advanced
Nutrition	excellent	good	poor

PUGH'S MODIFICATION OF CHILD'S CLASSIFICATION[46, a]			
	1 Point	2 Points	3 Points
Encephalopathy (grade)	none	1 or 2	3 or 4
Ascites	absent	slight	moderate
Bilirubin (mg/dL)	1–2	2–3	> 3
Albumin (gm/dL)	> 3.5	2.8–3.5	< 2.8
Prothrombin time (sec > control)	1–4	4–10	> 10

[a] 5–6 Total Points = Mild dysfunction; 7–9 = Moderate dysfunction; > 9 = Severe dysfunction.

cytochrome P450 superfamily, each cytochrome P450 enzyme family/subfamily has substrates that are uniquely metabolized by that one system. Therefore, the degree of clearance of a model substrate will reflect changes in the content or function of one or more P450 enzyme families/subfamilies specifically involved in the metabolism of that particular model substrate and may have little utility in predicting changes in other P450 enzyme families. For example, the clearance of antipyrine to its 3-methylhydroxy metabolite, significantly correlates with benzo-[*a*]pyrene activity, but not with 7-ethoxycoumarin 0-deethylase activity.[49] Abnormalities in the clearance of antipyrine to this metabolite will reflect the activity of the former enzyme system and not the latter. Conversely, utilizing markers that have known metabolic pathways should provide useful information about the metabolism of other compounds that utilize the same enzyme system. This would include the use of substrates such as dextromethorphan to predict the ability of an individual to metabolize drugs via the cytochrome P450 IID6 isozyme (debrisoquine hydroxylase).[50] A broader picture of liver function may be obtained when several model substrates with different metabolic pathways are evaluated within the same individual.[47,51]

The model substrates that have been studied have been chosen because they are highly extracted compounds and, therefore, good indicators of liver blood flow [i.e., indocyanine green (ICG), lidocaine, galactose] or poorly extracted compounds whose clearance reflects the metabolic capacity of the liver (antipyrine, aminopyrine). The most studied model compounds are antipyrine, ^{14}C-aminopyrine, and ICG.

Antipyrine has been extensively used to investigate the effect of disease states on drug metabolism, as well as the effect of other drugs or environmental factors on hepatic metabolism. Antipyrine is a pyrazolone derivative that is widely used in Europe as an antipyretic, analgesic, and anti-inflammatory agent. Its therapeutic use in the United States was discontinued after agranulocytosis was associated with aminopyrine, another pyrazolone derivative. Antipyrine possesses many of the qualities of an ideal model substrate in that it is well tolerated, it is almost completely absorbed after oral administration, it is not bound to serum proteins to any great extent, its volume of distribution is equal to total body water, and it is mainly eliminated via hepatic metabolism (2% to 5% excreted unchanged in urine).[52] Additionally, it is easily and reliably measured in saliva.[53] Since antipyrine is a poorly extracted compound, its clearance is independent of liver blood flow.[54] The three major metabolites (N-demethyl, 4-hydroxy, and 3-methylhydroxy) are each formed via different cytochrome P450 enzymatic pathways.[55] This multiple pathway metabolism suggests that antipyrine should be a "broad spectrum" model substrate of hepatic metabolism.

Antipyrine clearance decreases significantly in patients with chronic liver disease and less so in those with acute hepatitis, cholestastis, or compensated cirrhosis.[56,58] Decreases in antipyrine clearance correlate significantly with abnormalities in serum albumin and prothrombin time,[57] but failed to predict complications of cirrhosis (ascites, portal hypertension, or encephalopathy) or mortality.[56] *In vivo* antipyrine clearance correlates significantly with the histologic severity of hepatocyte necrosis,[59] as well as with the amount of hepatocyte cytochrome P450 content.[60] In contrast to these findings, measurement of the *in vivo* clearance of antipyrine does not appear to be sensitive enough to be able to predict the *in vitro* activity of selective cytochrome P450 isozymes.[49,61] Drugs whose clearance correlates well with that of antipyrine include: lidocaine,[62] acetaminophen,[62] propranolol,[63] ICG,[63] diazepam,[64] aminopyrine,[64] and galactose.[83]

[14]C-Aminopyrine (^{14}C-dimethyl amino-antipyrine) is N-demethylated by the cytochrome P450 enzyme system. Metabolism of this compound produces $^{14}CO_2$ which is expired in the breath and can be quantified. The amount of $^{14}CO_2$ expired during a two-hour period after oral administration of the marker discriminates between patients with chronic hepatocellular damage and normals.[65] The aminopyrine breath test also correlates with short-term prognosis and mortality from alcoholic hepatitis,[66] fulminant liver failure,[67] and nonalcoholic cirrhosis.[68] However, its use as a predictor of survival was only as good as the Child-Turcotte classification.[69] The aminopyrine breath test appears to be more specific than antipyrine for hepatocellular dysfunction, since antipyrine's clearance is significantly decreased in cholestasis while aminopyrine's elimination remains unaltered.[64] The aminopyrine breath test may be useful in following the progression of disease or serially monitoring the efficacy of treatment for individual patients.[66]

Indocyanine green (ICG) is a tricarbocyanine dye that undergoes extensive hepatic extraction (70% to 90%),[70] is not taken up in the peripheral tissue, and is eliminated unchanged in the bile (97%) with no enterohepatic recycling.[71] Therefore, its elimination depends on its rate of delivery to the liver (Q) and the ability of the liver to extract it from the blood (CL_{int}). If extraction remains constant, the clearance of ICG reflects "apparent" hepatic blood flow. ICG clearance has been correlated significantly with liver blood flow as measured by electromagnetic flow meters;[72] however, ICG hepatic uptake is decreased in cirrhotic patients indicating that impaired elimination of ICG is not totally reflective of decreased hepatic blood flow.[73]

The clearance of ICG appears to be a good measure of the severity of chronic liver disease and its prognosis.[56,74,75] Changes in the disposition of ICG correlate significantly with abnormal prothrombin time and serum bilirubin concentrations, but not with the Child-Turcotte classification.[75] ICG clearance also predicts the presence of ascites, portal hypertension, encephalopathy, and mortality due to cirrhosis.[56] Unfortunately, many methodologic problems may affect the determination of ICG clearance (posture, activity, food intake, time of day) resulting in high inter- and intrapatient variability.[76]

Other model compounds that have been examined for their ability to predict quantitative defects in hepatic metabolism involving cytochrome P450 include: lidocaine (clearance of parent compound,[77] formation of monoethylglycinexylidide,[78] binding to α_1-acid glycoprotein[79]), ^{14}C-phenacetin,[80] caffeine,[81,82] galactose,[83] ^{14}C-galactose,[84] sorbitol,[85] d-propranolol,[63] and ^{14}C-diazepam.[64] In addition, model compounds such as lorazepam[51] and acetaminophen[62] have been proposed to estimate an individual's ability to conjugate substrates.

PATIENT FACTORS INFLUENCING HEPATIC CLEARANCE

Hormones

In animals there is abundant information on the complexity of hormonal regulation of metabolism. While there is far less information on this topic in humans, it is likely that physiologic and pathologic changes in hormones at least partially explain intra- and interpatient differences in metabolic clearance.

Thyroid. Hyperthyroidism increases the clearance of several drugs which are eliminated from the body by various routes of hepatic metabolism (antipyrine,[86,87] theophylline,[88] propranolol,[89] propylthiouracil,[86] methimazole).[86] In the thyrotoxic state, drug clearance is 25% higher for intravenous theophylline[88] and 42% higher for oral propranolol.[89] In hypothyroidism, metabolic drug clearance decreases to a similar extent.[86] In euthyroid patients being treated with theophylline for bronchial obstruction, there is a positive correlation between thyroxine serum concentration (T_4) and total body theophylline clearance.[88] In contrast, total body theophylline clearance did not correlate with tri-iodothyronine (T_3) or reverse T_3 serum concentrations.[90]

Drug metabolism studies in the rat present a more complex influence of the thyroid gland on hepatic metabolism.[91,92] Thyroidectomy produces substrate- and gender-dependent effects on drug metabolism, some of which are reversed by T_4. There appears to be an optimal thyroxine concentration for maintaining maximal drug metabolic capacity. An apparent anomaly is that both hypo- and hyperthyroidism reduce hepatic microsomal enzyme activity in the rat.

In patient care, a possible dosage change should be anticipated when thyroid status changes from either hypo- or hyperthyroid to euthyroid or vice versa. Variation in thyroid function in euthyroid patients does not appear to have a clinically significant effect on metabolic drug clearance.

Pituitary. The anterior pituitary gland is an important regulator of xenobiotic metabolism in rats, primarily by regulating the hormones released by other organs. Aside from the influence of thyroid and sex hormones which are discussed elsewhere, administration of human growth hormone to deficient children increases the amobarbital elimination half-life twofold and decreases the theophylline half-life by 50%.[93] In rats, growth hormone administration decreases hepatic mixed function oxidase activity[94] while decreasing liver size.

Pancreas. The effect of diabetes on hepatic drug metabolism is complicated by different forms of the disease and the chronic diabetic complication of degenerative hepatic changes. The most thorough studies conducted in large diabetic groups[95] found the antipyrine elimination half-life was prolonged about 50% in insulin-dependent diabetes (Type 1) compared to healthy controls but was either unchanged or slightly decreased in elderly, non-insulin-dependent diabetes (Type 2). Cytochrome P450 content and arylhydrocarbon hydroxylase activity were both increased in Type 1 diabetes (compared to healthy controls) and were both decreased in Type 2 diabetes. The same investigators found that drug metabolism (i.e., hepatic cytochrome P450 content, antipyrine clearance) in patients with Type 2 diabetes correlated better with histologic liver changes (fatty liver, inflammation, cirrhosis) than the severity of the disease. It appears that antipyrine clearance is more variable in diabetics due to different disease types and the coexistence of hepatic abnormalities. Other human studies found an increased antipyrine metabolic rate in insulin-treated diabetics,[96,97] decreased phenacetin elimination,[98] and no change in tolbutamide elimination rate.[99]

In animal models, the metabolic effects of the diabetic state are primarily associated with androgen-responsive enzymes. Drug-induced diabetes decreases androgen levels,[100] and androgen replacement partially reverses the diabetic metabolic effect.[101]

Gonads. This section will focus on the effects of exogenous androgens, estrogens and progestogens on drug metabolism.

Androgens. Testosterone given to human males for three weeks decreases the antipyrine elimination half-life by 29%.[102] This apparent induction is contrasted to increased oxyphenylbutazone blood levels with androgen administration.[103] This limited experience probably reflects the infrequency of legitimate androgen use in humans.

Estrogens and Progestogens. The combination estrogen and progestogen oral contraceptives have been shown both to inhibit and induce drug metabolism. Six months treatment with 30 μg ethinylestradiol and 500 μg norgestrol was associated with a 17% increase in liver volume and a 21% decrease in antipyrine clearance. Within one month after hormone dosing was stopped, the antipyrine clearance returned to pretreatment values.[104] Low dose oral contraceptives also inhibit antipyrine elimination.[105] The pattern of antipyrine and metabolites in the urine does not change.[105]

There is a clear tendency for oral contraceptives to inhibit the metabolism or decrease the clearance of drugs which are primarily eliminated by Phase I oxidation reactions. Other drugs with decreased elimination in the presence of oral contraceptives include aminopyrine,[106] a variety of benzodiazepines (chlordiazepoxide,[107] diazepam,[108] alprazolam,[109] triazolam,[109] nitrazepam),[110] caffeine,[111] imipramine,[112] and phenylbutazone.[113] The oral clearance for a number of these drugs is decreased about 40% (e.g., caffeine, diazepam, imipramine). Oral contraceptives abolish the usual mid-menstrual cycle increase in the rate of methaqualone metabolism within one month of starting hormone treatment.[114]

Oral contraceptives also increase the clearance of some drugs which are primarily eliminated by glucuronidation. These include acetaminophen,[115] clofibric acid,[116] diflunisal,[117] lorazepam,[118] oxazepam,[118] and temazepam.[109] Increases in the oral clearance were large, ranging from 53% for diflunisal to 273% for lorazepam.

The impaired oxidative metabolism associated with oral contraceptives is attributed primarily to the estrogenic component, which decreases hepatic cytochrome P450 content.[119] The mechanism by which oral contraceptives induce conjugation is not known. The molecular mechanisms for hormone action are complex, rapidly evolving, and not well understood.[120]

Gender

Apart from the hormone differences between males and females, hormone levels change acutely during the menstrual cycle and with increasing age (menarche to menopause) in women. In asking the simple question, "Is drug metabolism or clearance different in males versus females?" the need to control for these time-related variables would seem obvious. However, since the majority of studies addressing the effect of gender on drug metabolism have not been synchronized with the menstrual cycle phase, it is difficult to determine the magnitude and significance of gender effects.

In 1984, this topic was reviewed and the following reported. Males and females have similar elimination characteristics for aminopyrine, antipyrine, bupropion, cimetidine, and lorazepam.[121] Women eliminate diazepam, desmethyldiazepam, oxazepam, and temazepam more slowly than men.[121] Acetaminophen[122,123] and clofibric acid[116] are both eliminated primarily by conjugation and are eliminated more rapidly in females. Salicylate elimination is not gender dependent.[124]

Propranolol and ethanol are more recent examples of drugs for which large gender differences were found in their metabolic clearance.[125,126] Both studies employed an adequate number of subjects and standardized dosing according to the menstrual cycle. Propranolol oral clearance was decreased 40% in women. The fractional propranolol metabolic clearance in women was decreased 34% for glucuronidation and 58% for side chain oxidation, while ring oxidation was not different from that in males.[125] The hepatic first-pass effect is markedly lower in both nonalcoholic and alcoholic women than their male counterparts.[126] The absolute bioavailability of ethanol following a 0.3 gm/kg ethanol dose is 60.9% and 74.2% in nonalcoholic and alcoholic men, respectively, versus 91% and 97% in nonalcoholic and alcoholic females.[126] First-pass ethanol metabolism correlated with gastric alcohol dehydrogenase activity measured by endoscopic gastric biopsies. Gender differences in the metabolism of isosorbide dinitrate also have been reported. Isosorbide dinitrate is rapidly metabolized in blood by the erythrocyte to isosorbide mononitrate. The disappearance half-life in blood is 90.6 minutes for males and 161.4 minutes for females.[127]

The influence of the menstrual cycle on drug metabolism is not consistent.[121] For example, whereas Nayak et al.[128] found antipyrine clearance to be lowest on day 5 of the cycle (30% and 24% lower than days 15 and 21), Riester et al. [129] reported almost no change during the cycle. In the Nayak study, antipyrine clearance in males is similar to females on day 5, but not on days 15 and 21 of the menstrual cycle. A marked and convincing decrease in methaqualone metabolism was reported on day 1 versus 15 of the cycle.[130] No change in acetaminophen clearance could be detected during the menstrual cycle.[131]

Pregnancy

Pregnancy is associated with a number of physiologic changes which have pharmacokinetic consequences. As pregnancy evolves, there is an increase in total body water and an increase in the glomerular filtration rate, a decrease in serum albumin, and a change in hormone balance. While oversimplified, the V_d and renal clearance of drugs tend to increase and oxidative metabolic clearance tends to decrease.[132] The optimal design of pharmacokinetic studies to investigate the effects of pregnancy is to follow patients serially throughout pregnancy to term and continue in the same patients following term until the nonpregnant baseline is re-established. Studies should define plasma protein binding, intrinsic renal and nonrenal clearance of the parent drug (unbound), and metabolite profiles.

Alterations in clearance have been reported for a few drugs during pregnancy. As an example of a drug eliminated primarily by renal excretion, ampicillin[133] total clearance increases by 50% to 100% by the last trimester. The increase in phenytoin oral clearance during pregnancy is due in part to a decrease in plasma protein binding.[134,135] Oral phenobarbital clearance does not appear to change during pregnancy.[134] Caffeine oral clearance progressively decreases in each trimester to a maximal value at term of 30% of the nonpregnant control.[136] Alternatively, theophylline total and unbound clearance did not change during the third trimester due to a decrease in unbound nonrenal clearance which was offset by an increase in renal clearance.[137] Since theophylline and caffeine have similar pharmacokinetic and metabolic characteristics, it is difficult to resolve this apparent discrepancy. Following delivery, pharmacokinetic values return to near normal values within days to weeks.

Race

Genetic factors influence not only personal characteristics such as race, height, and disease predilection, but also the rate of drug metabolism.[138,139] While this topic is covered in detail in Chapter 7: Genetic Polymorphisms of Drug Metabolism, it is important to recognize here that there is an association between race and the rate of drug acetylation and oxidation. However, the therapeutic complexity of heredity extends well beyond drug metabolism. For example, the propranolol dosage in China is substantially lower than in the United States.[140] Even though subjects of Chinese descent (compared to Caucasian) metabolize propranolol more rapidly[140,141] and have a higher free fraction in plasma due to lower α_1-acid glycoprotein plasma concentration,[142] there appears to be a separate and greater pharmacodynamic difference in sensitivity.[140] Generally, knowledge of race alone will be a poor predictor of drug metabolism rate.

Food

While food is a complex mixture of macro- and micronutrients, total energy consumption and protein appear to be the two most important components which regulate drug metabolism in humans. These effects are described most easily by classification as either chronic or acute phenomena. Chronic food effects include dietary abnormalities or malnutrition which can lead to weight loss or weight gain. Acute food effects refer to the dietary components of a single meal influencing presystemic drug metabolic clearance.

Chronic Effects. Antipyrine clearance is decreased about 33% in children suffering from *chronic malnutrition* compared to normal age- and gender-matched children.[143] Nutritional rehabilitation for two to four weeks in children increases antipyrine clearance by 40%.[143,144] The antipyrine metabolite profile does not change;[144] glucuronidation is also decreased in malnutrition.[144,145]

In *obesity*, the clearance of highly metabolized drugs does not present a clear pattern of alteration. While antipyrine clearance is decreased, theophylline and diazepam clearances are not different, and acetaminophen clearance is increased in obese versus control adults.[146] See Chapter 11: Special Pharmacokinetic Considerations in the Obese for a more detailed discussion of the influence of obesity on pharmacokinetics.

Various clinical studies indicate that protein and total energy intake (*calories*) are the most important macronutrient influences on drug metabolism. Americans generally consume about 2500 calories daily which is composed of about 15% protein, 50% carbohydrate, and 35% fat. A marked reduction in the total caloric intake by 50% or more for two to three weeks decreases antipyrine clearance by 23%[147] and theophylline clearance by 28%.[148,149] Both studies used the same macronutrient percentages with the normal and low calorie diets.

Protein is the principal dietary macronutrient which regulates antipyrine[147,148] and theophylline[148,150] clearance. Compared to the home diet and employing isocaloric diets, theophylline clearance increased 26% with a high-protein diet (44% protein) and decreased 21% with a low-protein diet (5% protein).[150] Using an isocaloric diet of 3000 calories, antipyrine clearance decreased 32% when the dietary protein content decreased from 15% to 5%.[147] A high-protein diet increased the clearance of orally administered theophylline by 32% and oral propranolol by 74%.[151] A high-carbohydrate diet did not affect either. Both drugs were given in the fasting state to avoid a more direct food effect. High clearance drugs administered orally may be more sensitive to dietary factors influencing metabolism. Dietary fat or carbohydrate content do not regulate either theophylline or antipyrine clearance.[152] In obese people, starvation did not change antipyrine or tolbutamide elimination.[153] Changes in metabolic clearance associated with caloric and protein intake may be different in obese subjects. In animals, protein content in the diet correlates with cytochrome P450 content in liver.[154,155] Restriction of dietary protein protects the liver from metabolically activated hepatotoxins[156] and decreases the V_{max} for several markers of oxidative metabolism.[155]

Other dietary components have been shown to alter drug metabolism in humans. Consumption of charcoal broiled beef increases the metabolic rate of phenacetin,[157] antipyrine,[158] and theophylline.[158] Ingestion of vegetables of the Brassecea species (brussels sprouts, cabbage) increases the metabolism of phenacetin and caffeine.[159] Antipyrine elimination also may be enhanced by ascorbic acid[160] and zinc.[161]

Diet is probably one of the most important and least recognized factors contributing to inter- and intrasubject variation in human drug metabolism. When illness occurs, one of the most common symptoms is appetite loss. *Short-term protein calorie deprivation* during acute illness and subsequent refeeding should be expected to change the rate of metabolic oxidation. Indicators of nutritional status which should be considered include recent weight change, diet history, and serum pre-albumin. Dietary changes also are likely to influence induction and inhibition of drug metabolism. While a low protein-calorie diet decreased theophylline clearance 28% and cimetidine decreased theophylline clearance 23%, the combination of a low protein-calorie diet and cimetidine decreased theophylline clearance 49%.[149]

Acute Effects. Drug administration within three hours after feeding decreases the presystemic clearance and increases the bioavailability of some high clearance drugs (e.g., propranolol, metoprolol, labetalol, propafenone, hydralazine),[162,163] but not others (amitriptyline, nifedipine, verapamil, codeine, d-propoxyphene, aspirin).[162,164,165] Simultaneous drug administration with food decreases the first-pass metabolism of drugs selectively in a manner which cannot be predicted for a given drug. This phenomenon is interesting because of both the magnitude of effect and potential underlying mechanisms. Concomitant drug administration with food increases the mean area under the concentration-time curve for propranolol by 60% to 80%[166] and for propafenone by 120%.[163] However, in some individuals the percent increase was 200% for propranolol[167] and 638% for propafenone.[163]

Food, by a mechanism yet to be determined, inhibits the metabolism of these drugs during absorption. Conjugated propranolol was about 50% lower in serum when taken with food than in the fasting state.[167] The food effect is greater in people with a high intrinsic drug clearance.[163,167] "Slow" metabolizers of propafenone did not exhibit a food effect on presystemic clearance.[163] When propranolol is slowly released in the gastrointestinal tract (i.e., slow release formulation), food does not increase the bioavailability.[167] Until recently, most scientists believed this food effect on presystemic drug clearance was caused by a transient 20% to 50% increase in liver blood flow. Using posture (i.e., standing or sitting) to create similar changes in liver blood flow as those that occur with food, no change was detected upon propranolol oral absorption.[168] By deduction, it must be assumed that food directly and transiently inhibits the enzyme(s) associated with intrinsic metabolic clearance and/or alters plasma protein binding.

Food-induced decreases in presystemic clearance may be of such magnitude that they lead to undesirable variation in drug exposure in the patient. Patients taking affected drugs should be instructed to standardize the timing of drug administration with meals, recognizing that this food effect operates for about three hours.

Circadian Variation

While drug absorption is slowed at night, clinically significant changes in hepatic metabolism have not been found. Major problems in evaluating this literature are the lack of convincing metabolism information and drug administration by the oral route which can confound systemic clearance data if there are alterations in absorption.[169] Since liver blood flow is decreased 37% in standing as compared to the supine position,[170] there should be a predictable change in the systemic clearance of drugs with high hepatic extraction.

SPECIFIC LIVER DISEASES

Liver diseases vary significantly in their pathophysiology and, therefore, in how they affect the hepatic metabolism of drugs. In addition, the effect on drug disposition will vary depending on the severity of each disease. Although our ability to predict specific changes in drug disposition within individual patients with liver disease is somewhat limited, anticipation of the need to change drug doses should lead to enhanced monitoring of drug therapy in selected patients. Limited data are available on the effect of liver disease on the pharmacokinetics of specific drugs. Since these data are generally derived from small groups of patients with varying degrees of cirrhosis, one should be cautious in making extrapolations to patients with other forms of liver disease or to all degrees of severity. A comprehensive presentation of these data is beyond the scope of this chapter and the reader is referred to published listings for specifics.[171,172] The following discussion focuses on the major hepatic diseases and the type of alterations in drug disposition that can be expected in patients with these diseases.

Chronic Liver Disease

Chronic liver disease generally is secondary to chronic alcohol abuse or chronic viral hepatitis and is characterized by irreversible, chronic hepatocyte damage resulting in fibrosis, disruption of the normal hepatic vascular architecture (intra- and/or extrahepatic portosystemic shunts), and formation of nodules of regener- ated hepatocytes. The pathologic changes of this complex disorder result in an absolute decrease in hepatocyte function (50% decrease in cytochrome P450 content)[12] and/or shunting of blood (and, hence, substrate) away from optimally functioning hepatocytes. In general, chronic liver disease affects drug disposition more than any other form of liver disease; alterations in drug disposition increase with the severity of disease.

Clearance. The clearance of high extraction (E_H >0.7) and low extraction (E_H <0.3) drugs is most extensively influenced by this form of liver disease. Highly extracted drugs are more affected in patients exhibiting a high degree of porto- systemic shunting, and low extraction drugs are more sensitive to changes in intrinsic clearance (see Table 6-2).[172,173] The clearance of high extraction drugs appears to be more consistently decreased in chronic liver disease than that of low extraction drugs.[173] Generally, it is assumed that the clearance of drugs which undergo only conjugation is not altered significantly in patients with severe liver disorders, although this has been questioned.[17,19]

Bioavailability. The bioavailability of orally administered high extraction drugs in patients with chronic liver disease may be increased significantly second- ary to a decreased first-pass effect. This is particularly true in those patients who exhibit significant portosystemic shunting along with decreased intrinsic clearance (see Figure 6-3).[174] Oral dosing of high extraction drugs will result in high maximum plasma concentrations. This, combined with the abnormal clearance due to hepatic dysfunction, may produce an exaggerated and prolonged pharma- cologic effect with potential toxic consequences, particularly for drugs with a low therapeutic index. Drugs exhibiting large increases in bioavailability secondary to this phenomena include: lidocaine,[77] meperidine,[175] pentazocine,[175] propranolol,[176] labetalol,[177] salicylamide,[175] and nicardipine.[174]

Volume of Distribution. The volume of distribution of drugs, particularly those that are highly protein bound (>90%),[178] may be increased in patients with chronic liver disease who exhibit hypoalbuminemia[172] or ascites.[63,179] This increased volume of distribution will increase significantly the drug's half-life and the time required to reach steady state. An example of this pharmacokinetic change is verapamil. Not only does chronic liver disease cause a 50% decrease in verapamil clearance, but it also causes a significant increase in this drug's volume of distribution resulting in a greater than 300% increase in half-life (3.7 versus 14.2 hours).[180] This will extend the time to reach steady state as well as the time to eliminate the drug from 12 to 45 hours. This phenomena also occurs with lorazepam[181] and chloramphenicol.[182]

Renal Elimination. Hepatorenal syndrome is a complication of severe chronic liver disease and is characterized by decreased renal blood flow and glomerular filtration despite normally functioning kidneys. In the presence of this complication, the renal elimination of drugs may be impaired. For example, bumetanide is partially metabolized by the liver and partially eliminated unchanged via the kidneys. In renal insufficiency, bumetanide's total clearance is decreased, although its nonrenal clearance is increased. In hepatically impaired patients, both the renal and nonrenal clearances are decreased.[183]

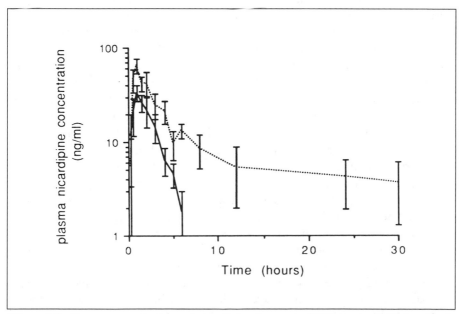

Figure 6-3. *Plasma concentrations of nicardipine (mean ± SEM) in nine patients with abnormal antipyrine clearance and in eight volunteers with normal liver function. Solid line, control subjects; broken line, patients with liver disease. Area under the curve for patients with liver disease was five times that of controls (432 ± 80 versus 97 ± 12 µg/mL × hr) (adapted with permission from reference 174).*

Acute Hepatitis

Acute hepatitis is an inflammatory condition of the liver that is caused by viruses or hepatotoxins. The acute inflammatory changes in the hepatocyte are generally mild and transient, although they can be chronic (chronic active hepatitis) and severe, resulting in cirrhosis or death. Changes in drug disposition tend to be less in acute hepatitis than in chronic liver disease.[184] The functional consequences of the disease upon drug disposition are determined by the extent as opposed to the cause of the injury. The few studies that have been conducted in patients with acute hepatitis indicate that the changes observed in drug disposition are variable and are related to the extent of damage incurred; patients with mild disease may have no alterations, while those with severe disease may have significant alterations. As the acute disease resolves, drug disposition returns to normal and may do so before normalization of the biochemical liver function tests.[185] Patients who develop chronic active hepatitis will exhibit decreases in hepatic drug clearance.[186]

INDUCTION AND INHIBITION OF DRUG METABOLISM

An extensive and growing body of literature confronts the practitioner interested in drug interactions related to the induction and inhibition of drug metabolism. Our ability to detect interactions associated with induction and inhibition of drug metabolizing enzymes has improved significantly in recent years due, in part, to the increased analytical nature of patient care and the widespread availability of drug assays in biological fluids. Furthermore, we have become more aware of the potential clinical significance of drug-induced alterations in drug metabolism. For example, induction of drug metabolism has been linked to therapeutic failures (e.g., pregnancy in oral contraceptive users), disease progression (e.g., asthma, arrhythmias, heart failure), and hepatotoxicity in humans. Inducers such as phenobarbital act as potent tumor promoters in animal models. In humans, it remains unclear whether enzyme induction increases the risk of cancer formation through bioactivation of procarcinogens or reduces this risk via detoxification of carcinogens. Enzyme inhibition may result in excessive blood concentrations of drugs and lead to undesirable side effects (e.g., hemorrhage following warfarin therapy; nausea or arrhythmias associated with digoxin overdose) or toxicity (e.g., seizures, sedation, death) due to the affected drug. The ultimate clinical importance of these interactions depends on the therapeutic index of the affected drug, the magnitude of inhibition or induction, and the patient's clinical status at the time of the drug interaction. Thus, it is important for the clinician to understand the underlying concepts of drug interactions related to enzyme induction and inhibition. With this knowledge, drug interactions for currently marketed as well as investigational drugs can be anticipated, and dosage regimens can be adjusted accordingly to prevent undesirable outcomes.

Induction and inhibition of drug metabolism are usually important only during transition periods when the inducer or inhibitor is started, stopped or when the dosage is changed. The magnitude and time course of interaction are important characteristics to remember, since they determine if and when an action should be taken. It may be useful to remember that the magnitude of the clearance change resulting from the interaction usually has to exceed the intrapatient clearance variation before the interaction is likely to be detected. For example, since the intrapatient variation in theophylline clearance is 15% after controlling for known factors which alter clearance,[187] the clearance resulting from induction or inhibition must exceed this amount (e.g., 25%) to be recognizable.

Pharmacokinetic Considerations

The pharmacokinetic concepts of clearance and hepatic drug metabolism are fundamental to understanding the clinical implications of induction and inhibition of drug metabolism (see Equation 6-5).[36] Enzyme induction usually increases the amount of enzyme in the liver resulting in an increase in the rate of drug metabolism (V_{max}); according to Equation 6-3, $CL_{u_{int}}$ subsequently increases. In contrast, inhibition of drug metabolism results in a decrease in $CL_{u_{int}}$. Inhibition may be due to competitive interactions (two chemicals compete for the same enzyme) resulting in an increase in K_m, or noncompetitive inhibition resulting in a decrease in V_{max}.

It also is important to recognize the relationship between the percent change in clearance produced by an inducer or inhibitor of drug metabolism and the resultant change in the average steady-state plasma drug concentration. Average steady-state plasma drug concentrations (C_{ss}) are inversely related to total body drug clearance (CL_T):

$$\overline{C_{ss}} = \frac{FF^* \cdot D}{CL_T \cdot \tau}$$

(Eq. 6-9)

Induction or inhibition of drug metabolism usually results in less than a 50% change in drug clearance. If drug clearance increases from 10 to 15 L/hr (a 50% increase) due to enzyme induction, $\overline{C_{ss}}$ will decrease 33%, assuming FF^* (systemic availability), D, and τ remain constant. In contrast, if drug clearance decreases from 10 to 5 L/hr (a 50% decrease) due to enzyme inhibition, $\overline{C_{ss}}$ will increase twofold (100% increase). Thus, enzyme inhibition may result in a more pronounced change in average steady-state concentrations compared to enzyme induction.

The magnitude of effect (i.e., change in drug plasma concentration) from induction or inhibition is dependent upon several factors including the fraction of clearance which is due to metabolism, the hepatic extraction ratio, and the route of administration of the affected drug. Obviously, the clearance of a drug which is totally eliminated by the affected enzyme system will change to a greater extent than a drug which is 90% eliminated by other pathways. Drugs that exhibit low hepatic extraction ratios, administered by either the intravenous or oral routes, are susceptible to large clearance changes from inducers or inhibitors that alter the hepatic intrinsic clearance of unbound drug (see Figure 6-4). At the other extreme, drugs that exhibit a high hepatic extraction ratio are most affected by induction or inhibition of drug metabolism when the affected drug is administered orally. Induction or inhibition of metabolism will change the plasma drug concentration of orally administered drugs to the same extent (assuming equal changes in

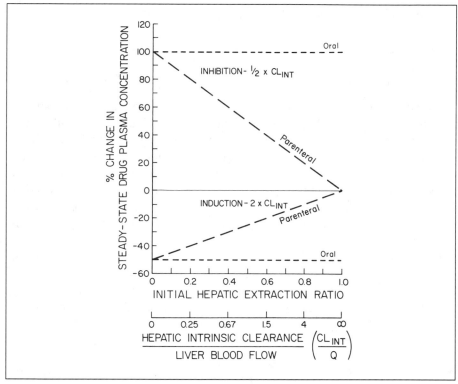

Figure 6-4. *The change in steady-state drug plasma concentrations due to inhibition (upper panel) or induction (lower panel) of metabolism is dependent upon the initial hepatic extraction ratio (prior to inhibition or induction) and the route of administration of the affected drug. This figure is constructed based on the following assumptions: total body drug clearance equals hepatic clearance; intrinsic clearance is decreased 50% for inhibition and increased 100% for induction; the inducer or inhibitor does not change liver blood flow; the drug is not protein bound ($f_{ub} = 1$). To use the figure, place a straight edge perpendicular to the x axis at the initial hepatic extraction ratio of a given drug. If the initial hepatic extraction ratio is 0.8, then a 50% decrease in CL_{int} will result in a 20% increase in C_{ss} when the drug is injected, and a 100% increase in C_{ss} when the drug is given orally. These calculations are presented in Table 6-5.*

CL_{int} (equivalent to $f_{ub} \times CL_{u_{int}}$) is expressed in terms of Q_H which is set to unity for ease of calculation. Under baseline conditions, when CL_{int}/Q_H is 4, the extraction ratio is $4/(1+4) = 0.8$ and the hepatic clearance is 1×0.8. The bioavailability is 1.0 when the drug is injected and $1 - E_H = 0.2$ when administered orally. In the presence of enzyme inhibition, CL_{int} is reduced by 50% so that CL_{int}/Q_H is 2. The remaining calculations are the same as above. The change in C_{ss} assumes there is no change in dose or dosage interval before and after the inhibitor is administered. For the same drug with induction ($2 \times CL_{int}$), the ratio of CL_{int}/Q_H is 8 and there is a 10% decrease in C_{ss} when the drug is injected, and a 50% decrease in C_{ss} when it is taken orally. The impact of inhibition and induction on a low extraction drug can be viewed by moving the straight edge to 0.2 extraction ratio. For low extraction drugs, there is less difference between the two routes of administration.

Table 6-5.

Baseline conditions	Parenteral	Oral
CL_{int}/Q_H (where Q_H = unity or 1)	4	4
$E_H = \dfrac{CL_{int}}{Q_H + CL_{int}}$	0.8	0.8
$CL_H = Q_H \cdot E_H$	0.8	0.8
$F^* = 1 \cdot E_H$	1	0.2
Enzyme inhibition		
CL_{int}/Q_H (where CL_{int} = ½ Baseline CL_{int})	2	2
E_H	0.67	0.67
CL_H	0.67	0.67
F^*	1	0.33
% Change C_{ss} = $\left[\dfrac{\dfrac{F^*}{CL_H\ Inhib} - \dfrac{F^*}{CL_H\ Base}}{\dfrac{F^*}{CL_H\ Base}} \right] \times 100$	+20%	+100%

intrinsic clearance) regardless of the hepatic extraction ratio. However, when drugs are administered by the parenteral route, the influence of induction or inhibition decreases as the hepatic extraction ratio approaches one.

Induction

Induction of drug metabolism is a relatively recently recognized phenomenon. While induction was first described in 1940,[188] it was not until the early 1950s that the importance of enzyme induction became recognized in xenobiotic metabolism and carcinogenesis.[189–191] Since then, there have been hundreds of chemicals recognized which can induce the mixed-function oxidase system. Inducing chemicals in animals are structurally diverse and seem to share only one common characteristic: lipophilicity. Earlier literature emphasized two general types of inducing agents: "phenobarbital-like" inducers (e.g., phenobarbital, phenytoin) and "polycyclic aromatic hydrocarbon-like" inducers (e.g., cigarette smoke, charcoal-broiled beef, omeprazole). Three additional major inducer categories are recognized currently: pregnenolone-16α-carbonitrile (PCN)/glucocorticoids (e.g., dexamethasone, rifampin, erythromycin), ethanol (e.g., ethanol, isoniazid), and peroxisome proliferators (e.g., clofibrate, phthalates used in plasticizers).[192,193] The varied mechanisms of P450 induction by these diverse agents have been reviewed.[192]

Mechanisms. Enzyme inducers can increase hepatic drug clearance by increasing the hepatic extraction ratio and/or increasing functional hepatic blood flow (see Equation 6-4). In rats, phenobarbital and other enzyme inducers increase cytochrome P450 content in liver.[194,195] Phenobarbital increases liver weight in a dose-dependent manner.[196] Female rats are less sensitive to phenobarbital induction than males.[196,197] Phenobarbital (but not 3-methylcholanthrene or 3,4-benzpyrene) increases ICG clearance (an index of hepatic blood flow) in proportion to the 33% increase in hepatic mass.[198] In monkeys, phenobarbital also increases hepatic blood flow by 30%.[199] While this increase was due in part to a 21% increase in cardiac output, portal venous flow increased to a greater extent than hepatic arterial flow.

In humans, the most complete investigations on the effects of phenobarbital-like enzyme inducers have been conducted in epileptic patients (see Figure 6-5).[200–202] In a study by Pirttiaho et al.,[202] all patients had undergone liver biopsy because of suspicion of liver disease. Cytochrome P450 content was measured from the biopsy material; liver size and liver blood flow were estimated by injecting radiolabelled technetium sulfur colloid, which is, presumably, completely extracted by the liver; antipyrine clearance was measured as an overall *in vivo* index of cytochrome P450 activity. Compared to patients with normal liver architecture, patients receiving anticonvulsants had 52% larger absolute hepatic size which was still 29% larger after correcting for body weight. Absolute liver blood flow was 40% greater in epileptics than nonepileptics. However, when liver blood flow was corrected for liver size, there was no difference. That is, liver blood flow increases in proportion to liver size in patients on anticonvulsants. Total hepatic cytochrome P450 content (P450 concentration × hepatic size) was increased 135% in epileptics; this change explains a 173% increase in antipyrine

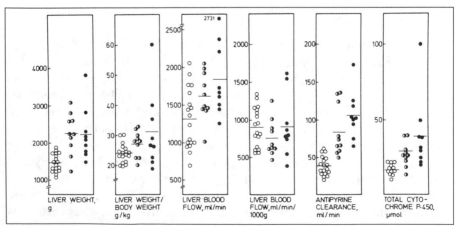

Figure 6-5. *Liver size, blood flow, and indices of hepatic drug metabolism (antipyrine systemic clearance, total cytochrome P450 liver content) in control subjects (open circles), epileptics with altered liver parenchyma by biopsy (semi-closed circles) and epileptics with normal liver biopsy (closed circles). Note that none of the control subjects were taking enzyme-inducing drugs, whereas all epileptics were taking phenytoin, carbamazepine, or phenobarbital in varying combinations from 2 to 15 years (adapted with permission from reference 202).*

clearance. Patients who were receiving anticonvulsants, but who had altered liver parenchyma ranging from fatty accumulation to cirrhosis, generally had values for the above measurements which were intermediate between those of the control subjects and epileptic patients with normal liver biopsy. Previous studies indicated that patients with cirrhosis or hepatitis had both lower baseline hepatic cytochrome P450 concentrations and lower antipyrine clearances than patients with a normal biopsy.[203] They confirmed that even though patients with an abnormal liver biopsy are inducible with anticonvulsants, the degree of induction, as measured by cytochrome P450 content and antipyrine clearance, was only one-half that of patients with normal livers. When interpreting these data, it is assumed that epilepsy does not, *per se*, alter hepatic function. Patients from these studies were not categorized according to smoking status.

The above studies, which described induction differences *between* patients (i.e., anticonvulsant-treated versus untreated patients), are not entirely consistent with a report which evaluated the *within* subject changes in ten healthy adults administered phenobarbital 180 mg/day for three weeks.[204] Phenobarbital increased antipyrine clearance (+ 90%) but did not change either liver size (+ 3%) or the index of hepatic blood flow, ICG clearance (+ 16%). In contrast, Rutledge et al.[205] reported a 32% increase in apparent hepatic blood flow in seven healthy volunteers following administration of phenobarbital 100 mg/day for three weeks. In this study, liver blood flow was estimated from administration of intravenous and oral verapamil, on separate occasions, in a crossover fashion. The discrepancies between these studies could be due to differences in measurement methods, treatment period for the inducing agent, and/or patient population (e.g., changes in posture which may alter liver blood flow).

Cytochrome P450IA, formerly called cytochrome P448, is induced by inhaled cigarette smoke in humans. Whereas it has been recognized widely that cigarette smoking increases the oxidation of numerous substrates in humans *in vivo*, including phenacetin,[206] it has been more difficult to demonstrate such an effect *in vitro* with human liver microsomes. In man, significant increases in cytochrome P450 concentration or aryl hydrocarbon hydroxylase activity have not been observed in smokers compared to nonsmokers.[207,208] Recently however, Sesardic et al.[209] used both immunological and metabolic methods to identify a major hepatic form of cytochrome P450 induced by cigarette smoking in man. Immunoreactive P450 content and phenacetin O-deethylase activity were 3.5- and 4-fold higher, respectively, in smokers compared to nonsmokers. Smoking[210] and rifampin[211] do not alter the disposition of markers for hepatic blood flow in adults.

Omeprazole recently has been identified as the first pharmacological agent to induce human cytochrome P450IA.[212] Cytochrome P450IA is responsible for the conversion of procarcinogens to reactive metabolites that cause chemical carcinogenesis and/or mutagenesis.[213] Interestingly, omeprazole is a known inhibitor of several cytochrome-P450-mediated monooxygenase reactions and reduces the clearance of diazepam and phenytoin in humans.[214]

Conjugating Phase II enzymes also consist of families of isoenzymes which are inducible based on animal and limited human data.[215] For example, phenobarbital increases the clearance of chloramphenicol,[216] which is predominately glucuronidated in humans. Glucuronidation of acetaminophen[217] and oxazepam[218] was increased in heavy smokers (20 to 40 cigarettes per day). Induction by polycyclic aromatic hydrocarbon-type inducers (e.g., cigarette smoke) appears to be weak in human liver since acetaminophen glucuronidation is not increased significantly in moderate smokers (10 to 20 cigarettes per day).[219]

Clinical Consequences of Induction. The most likely clinical manifestation arising from induction of drug metabolism is an exacerbation of the treated disease due to diminished efficacy of the induced drug. When the inducing agent is discontinued, failure to decrease the dosage of the induced drug may result in drug toxicity. Since induction may expose the patient to greater quantities of drug metabolites, the pharmacologic profile of the induced drug may change. Table 6-6 summarizes reported clinical problems resulting from induction of drug metabolism. The most frequently reported problem was the loss of drug efficacy, which usually was rectified by increasing the dose of the induced drug. However, drug toxicity and altered drug activity also have been reported. The reported problems range in severity. In some instances, it only resulted in a temporary inconvenience; in others, the interaction had a major impact on the patient (e.g., pregnancy, death). The frequency of adverse reactions resulting from enzyme induction is not known. However, from the list of reported manifestations, it is clear that the problems can be serious, and these usually can be avoided if enzyme induction is anticipated.

Comparison of Inducing Agents. Although numerous enzyme inducing agents have been described in humans (see Table 6-7), this review focuses on the experience with phenobarbital, rifampin, and smoking. These agents predominate in the clinical literature on this topic, and they differ in a number of fundamental aspects: clinical indication, duration and extent of exposure, chemical purity, chemical structure, elimination half-life, pattern of induction, and alteration of liver blood flow.

Phenobarbital is primarily used as an anticonvulsant, rifampin as an antibiotic, and smoking as a social habit. Phenobarbital is usually administered on a chronic basis, rifampin is used for a limited period, and smokers may vary in their cigarette

Table 6–6. *Reported Clinical Manifestations of Induction of Drug Metabolism*[222]

Induced drug	Inducer	Manifestations
Acetaminophen	Various	Acetaminophen overdose; enhanced toxicity
Corticosteroids		
Cortisone	Rifampin	Addison's disease; difficult control
Methylprednisolone	Rifampin	Kidney allograft; diminished function/survival
	Phenobarbital	Kidney allograft; diminished function/survival
Prednisone	Phenobarbital	Asthma; difficult control
Prednisolone	Rifampin	Asthma; difficult control
		Nephrotic syndrome; treatment failure
	Phenobarbital	Rheumatoid arthritis; worsening symptoms
Digitoxin	Rifampin	Congestive heart failure; worsening
Digoxin	Rifampin	Congestive heart failure; worsening
Methadone	Rifampin	Narcotic withdrawl
Oral contraceptives	Rifampin	Menstrual irregularities; pregnancy
	Phenobarbital	Menstrual irregularities; pregnancy
Quinidine	Rifampin	Cardiac arrhythmia; worsening
Warfarin	Barbiturates	Bleeding and death upon discontinuation of inducer

use (heavy versus moderate). Phenobarbital and rifampin are chemically pure, whereas smoke composition is very heterogeneous. Phenobarbital, rifampin and smoke constituents vary significantly in chemical structure. In adults, phenobarbital has a three to five day half-life, versus only two to four hours for rifampin. The pattern of isoenzyme induction is markedly different for phenobarbital versus polycyclic hydrocarbons from smoke. Liver blood flow increases only with phenobarbital administration.

The influences of these inducing agents on the clearance of other drugs are summarized in Table 6-8 for phenobarbital, Table 6-9 for rifampin, and Table 6-10 for smoking. Drugs listed in the tables are limited to those for which changes in clearance or elimination half-life could be estimated. When there were several studies of the same interaction, in each case the study was selected which demonstrated the central tendency. Oral or systemic clearance changes were calculated from reported data.

The change in mean clearance for a particular drug can be projected to an expected change in mean drug plasma concentration by making the direct calculation (Equation 6-9). It is important to recognize that variability in drug clearance appears to be similar in the noninduced and induced states.[220] Inducibility is related to initial liver size.[220] This finding is in opposition to the earlier suggestion that patients who metabolize drugs more slowly will demonstrate a greater change from induction than rapid metabolizers.[221] Population drug clearance estimates are calculated as follows:

$$CL_T \text{ (induced)} = CL_T \text{ (uninduced)} \cdot \left(1 + \frac{\%CL \text{ change}}{100} \right) \qquad \text{(Eq. 6-10)}$$

Examples of changes in drug clearance following enzyme induction are listed in Tables 6-8 to 6-10. There are several considerations which should be recognized when examining these tables. While rifampin and smoking were studied in subjects who were either healthy or had no other characteristic known to alter drug metabolism, phenobarbital studies have been conducted commonly in patients characterized as receiving enzyme-inducing anticonvulsant drugs (i.e., phenobarbital, phenytoin, carbamazepine) alone or in combination. Studies conducted in epileptic patients (often using matched healthy volunteer controls) are designated

Table 6-7. Inducers of Drug Metabolism in Humans

Aminoglutethimide	Glutethimide	Phenylbutazone[a]
Aminopyrine	Griseofulvin	Phenytoin[a]
Amobarbital	Industrial chemicals (e.g., paint,	Protein in diet
Antipyrine	herbicides)	Rifampin[a]
Ascorbic Acid	Insecticides (e.g., DDT, Endrin)	Secobarbital
Brussels sprouts	Mandrax	Smoke
Carbamazepine[a]	Meprobamate	Spironolactone
Charcoal broiled beef	Methaqualone	Testosterone
Chloral hydrate	Omeprazole	Theobromine
Chlorimipramine	Pentobarbital	Theophylline
Ethanol	Phenobarbital[a]	Warfarin

[a] Most potent inducers in humans.

as such in Table 6-8, since the phenobarbital dose may have been larger, administered for a longer time, and given with other drugs which can alter drug metabolic activity. In most of the volunteer studies, phenobarbital was administered for a minimum of ten days. In most instances, phenobarbital induces phenytoin metabolism, although changes in phenytoin V_{max} or K_m have not been reported. Phenobarbital-induced increases in the apparent oral clearance of phenytoin range from 17% to 256%.[222] It appears that the greatest discrepancy between results occurs from relatively uncontrolled studies in outpatients. Most of the rifampin studies in Table 6-9 were conducted using a 600 mg daily dose for one week. The large change in the clearance for most of the studied drugs is very striking in contrast to those observed with phenobarbital and smoking. Smoking studies (see Table 6-10) are not crossover in nature. Since it is impossible to accurately characterize these subjects according to the actual dose and duration of exposure to polycyclic aromatic hydrocarbon inducing agent(s), it is likely that the induction effect of smoking is more variable and less predictable than that of phenobarbital or rifampin.

Smokers and nonsmokers appear to be equally susceptible to enzyme induction by phenobarbital, based on a study of the pharmacokinetics and metabolism of disopyramide in two relatively young, age-matched populations.[223] Enzyme induc-

Table 6–8. Effect of Phenobarbital (Pb)[a] on Drug Elimination [222]

Drug	Patients	Volunteers	Clearance change (%)
		Route of administration	
Acetaminophen	PO[bc]		69
	IV[bc]		44
Antipyrine		PO	56
	PO[bc]		89
Carbamazepine	PO		100
Chloramphenicol	IV[c]		76
Cimetidine		PO	16
		IV	18
Clonazepam		PO	24
Dexamethasone	IV		87
Doxycycline	IV		t½ ↓ 27%
Ethanol[e]	IV		26 (estimated)
Fenoprofen		IV	30 Pb 60 mg/dL
		IV	58 Pb 240 mg/dL
Lidocaine	PO[bc]		180
Meperidine		IM	24
Methylprednisolone		IV	85
Phenytoin	PO[bc]		56
Prednisolone	IV[bc]		37
Quinidine		PO	191
Timolol		PO	31[d]
Theophylline		IV	34
Verapamil[205]		IV	90
		PO	401
Vitamin K		PO	−20[d]
Warfarin		PO	t½ ↓ 46%

[a] Phenobarbital dose is 60–100 mg/day unless stated otherwise.
[b] Epileptic patient studies include phenobarbital and/or other anticonvulsant drugs.
[c] Not a crossover study.
[d] Not statistically significant.
[e] Apparent clearance, since drug exhibits saturable elimination.

Table 6–9. *Effect of Rifampin on Drug Elimination* [222]

Drug	Route of administration	Clearance change (%)
Antipyrine	PO	85
Clofibrate	PO	53
Diazepam	IV	305
Digitoxin	PO	t½ ↓ 45%
Disopyramide	PO	146
Ethinylestradiol	PO	72
Hexobarbital	IV	200
Methadone	PO	111 (estimated)
Metoprolol	PO	49
Mexiletine	PO	51
Norethisterone	PO	73
Prednisolone	PO	49
Propranolol	PO	169
Quinidine	PO	496
	IV	271
Rifampin	PO	t½ ↓ 49%
Theophylline	PO	25
Tolbutamide	IV	124
Warfarin	PO	132
	IV	136

tion may be partially additive as shown in patients taking combinations of antiepileptic drugs.[224] The degree of enzyme induction and the effects of adding or withdrawing inducing agents will vary with the potency of each drug as an inducer of the hepatic mixed-function oxidase system.

Dose-Dependency. Ample data in animals and limited data in humans indicate that barbiturate enzyme induction is a dose-dependent phenomenon.[225,226] In humans, dose-dependent enzyme induction by phenobarbital may not be obvious because the range of prescribed phenobarbital doses is narrow. Phenobarbital doses of 7.5 and 15 mg daily for four weeks have been reported to increase the mean antipyrine clearance by 10% and 15%, respectively, in a group of eight healthy nonsmoking volunteers.[227] Although the concept of a dose threshold for phenobarbital above which enzyme induction occurs is an oversimplification, it has been suggested that clinically significant drug interactions due to enzyme induction are unlikely at phenobarbital doses less than 15 mg/day.[227]

Rifampin increases antipyrine clearance by 59% at a 600 mg/day rifampin dose and by 125% at a 1200 mg/day dose.[228] However, a dose-dependent (600, 900, 1200 mg) effect of rifampin on propranolol oral clearance cannot be demonstrated.[229] There is not a significant correlation between the frequency of smoking[230] or serum thiocyanate concentrations[231] and changes in antipyrine or phenytoin clearances, respectively.

Time Course. Induction can be detected within about six to seven days after starting phenobarbital[232,233] and within two days after starting rifampin[234] (see Figure 6-6). When phenobarbital is administered without a loading dose, the maximum effect on the warfarin plasma concentration occurs within 14 to 21 days.[232] The maximum effect of rifampin occurs within four days for warfarin[234] (see Figure 6-6), eight days for antipyrine,[235] and ten days for propranolol.[236] It is clear from Figure 6-6 that the time to maximum change in prothrombin time occurs four to five days after warfarin achieves a new steady state. The time course of induction following exposure to smoke has not been reported.

After the inducer is discontinued, return to the noninduced state follows a time-course similar to induction. Following discontinuation of phenobarbital, it takes about four weeks to reach the approximate noninduced state. Even four weeks after discontinuation of phenobarbital, theophylline clearance was statistically higher than the pre-phenobarbital clearance.[237] Upon stopping rifampin, propranolol oral clearance decreases on the first day[229] and returns to pre-rifampin levels by 20 days.[236] When smokers stop smoking, a decrease in induction can be detected within two weeks for warfarin[238] and two months for antipyrine.[239] However, it appears to take a longer time for theophylline clearance to decrease.[240,241]

Attenuating Factors. The ability to induce drug metabolism decreases as the age of the subject increases.[210,230,242] Drug metabolism in elderly subjects (greater than 60 to 65 years) is not induced by smoking[210,230] or dichloralphenazone[242] as it is in younger subjects. While the same observation has been made in rats,[243,244] the explanation is not known. Rifampin induces drug metabolism in patients with cirrhosis[245] or cholestasis;[246] however, induction from smoking appears to be diminished or absent in patients with cirrhosis or hepatitis.[247] While epileptic

Table 6-10. *Effect of Smoking on Drug Elimination*[222]

Drug [a,b]	Route of administration	Clearance change (%)
Antipyrine	IV/young (18–39)	30
	middle (40–59)	35
	old (60–92)	6[c]
	all ages (18–92)	31
Caffeine	PO	65
Chlordiazepoxide	IV	13.7[c]
Codeine	PO	14[c]
Desmethyldiazepam	PO	175
Dexamethasone	IV	18[c]
Diflunisal[250]	PO	35[c]
Ethinylestradiol	PO	−9.7
Imipramine	PO	81
Lidocaine	PO	68
Lorazepam	IV	23
Nortriptyline	PO	12.9[c]
	PO	74
Oxazepam	PO	61
Phenacetin	PO	466
Phenytoin	IV	−3.4[c]
Pindolol	PO	−7.9[c]
Prednisolone	IV	−3.6[c]
Prednisone	PO	7.4[c]
Theophylline	PO	57.5
Warfarin	PO	13

[a] Other drugs induced by smoking for which pharmacokinetic estimates are not available: nicotine, pentazocine, propranolol.
[b] Other drugs not induced by smoking for which pharmacokinetic estimates are not available: diazepam, glucaric acid, meperidine.
[c] Not statistically significant.

patients receiving anticonvulsants who are shown by biopsy to have altered liver architecture do demonstrate induction, the magnitude of change is less than that observed in epileptic patients who have normal biopsies.[200,202]

Other Characteristics. Enzyme induction may alter the synthesis or elimination of endogenous or exogenous compounds; these effects may be of direct therapeutic importance or may alter drug distribution. In dogs[248] and epileptic humans,[249] anticonvulsant drugs (i.e., phenobarbital, phenytoin, carbamazepine) may increase serum α_1-acid glycoprotein (AAG) concentrations. In one study in epileptic patients, this protein concentration increased about 60%, which could result in a marked reduction in the unbound fraction of drug. However, the effect of enzyme inducers on serum AAG concentrations in humans remains to be clarified, as Kapil et al.[223] demonstrated that phenobarbital, 100 mg for three weeks, had no effect on serum AAG concentrations or disopyramide free fraction. AAG is the principal plasma binding protein for propranolol, lidocaine, and many other basic drugs. A decrease in the unbound drug fraction in plasma may result in alterations in the apparent volume of distribution and/or drug clearance. From a clinical perspective, any given drug plasma concentration will reflect less pharmacologic activity when the fraction of unbound drug decreases. Plasma protein binding of lidocaine has been noted to be 19% higher in smokers than in

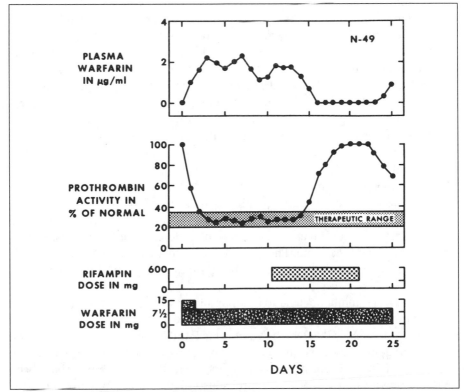

Figure 6-6. *Plasma warfarin concentration and one-stage prothrombin activity in a healthy adult who received a constant warfarin dose followed by warfarin plus rifampin 600 mg/day (adapted from reference 234).*

nonsmokers.[251] However, rifampin treatment for three weeks did not alter propranolol protein binding.[229] Rifampin treatment of tuberculosis for an average of five months also did not increase AAG plasma concentrations or lidocaine plasma protein binding.[252] Anticonvulsant administration also is associated with an increase in sex hormone binding globulin.[253]

Anticonvulsants, [254] but not rifampin,[255] increase plasma high-density lipoprotein cholesterol concentrations and decrease serum triglyceride concentrations. Epileptic patients, who responded to enzyme-inducing drug therapy (e.g., phenytoin, phenobarbital, and/or carbamazepine) with an increase in liver size, had a serum cholesterol distribution profile typical of subjects with a low risk of coronary heart disease.[256]

Inhibition of Metabolism

Mechanisms. Drug metabolizing enzymes can be inhibited competitively or noncompetitively. In competitive inhibition, the inhibitor acts as an alternate substrate for the enzyme. In the case of noncompetitive inhibition, the inhibitor inactivates the enzyme but substrate binding remains normal. Indirect inhibition of the metabolic rate occurs through alteration of the physiologic environment or a decrease in enzyme protein synthesis (e.g., malnutrition, hormone imbalance). The mechanism of inhibition may be an important consideration in determining the specificity of an inhibitor and the time course of interaction. If the inhibitor acts directly through an enzyme system which is fundamental to the metabolism of numerous drugs (e.g., cytochrome P450, glucuronyltransferase), then it is likely that the metabolic inhibition may have broad implications. Alternatively, if the inhibited enzyme has a narrow spectrum of activity (e.g., xanthine oxidase), then it is less likely that many drugs will be affected. Upon starting or stopping inhibitor administration, direct-acting reversible inhibitors should be expected to have a rapid onset and decay of inhibition. However, if the inhibitor decreases enzyme synthesis, then the onset and decay of inhibition might be slower.

Numerous drugs inhibit the metabolism of a substrate after acute administration, but induce enzymes after chronic administration; a prime example is ethanol. This phenomenon also may explain the reports that phenobarbital inhibits, induces, or has no effect on phenytoin elimination. Inhibition of drug metabolism also may be stereospecific. For example, coadministration of phenylbutazone and racemic warfarin results in an enhancement of anticoagulation; yet, plasma warfarin levels remain the same. Phenylbutazone increases the clearance of the R isomer, but inhibits the clearance of the S isomer, which is five times more potent.[257]

Like inducers, inhibitors tend to be lipophilic. Most drugs inhibit metabolism by inhibiting the hepatic mixed-function oxidase system. This is primarily a reflection of the major role which cytochrome P450 has in the biotransformation of a multitude of drugs, and the lack of substrate specificity of the cytochrome P450 system. The mechanisms by which cytochrome P450 are inhibited have been reviewed previously.[258,259] However, drugs also may inhibit nonmicrosomal systems. For example, disulfiram inhibits the nonmicrosomal enzyme, aldehyde dehydrogenase, which is involved in the conversion of ethanol to acetic acid;

disulfiram also is known to inhibit metabolism of antipyrine,[260] warfarin,[261] and phenytoin[262] which are all metabolized by the microsomal oxidase system. Allopurinol inhibits xanthine oxidase, which is a nonmicrosomal enzyme involved in the metabolism of mercaptopurine. Allopurinol also inhibits the cytochrome P450 metabolism of dicumarol,[263] and theophylline at a 600 mg/day allopurinol dose.[264] Monoamine oxidase inhibitors irreversibly bind to hepatic nonmicrosomal monoamine oxidases and inhibit the metabolism of tyramine. Therefore, inhibition of nonmicrosomal enzymes is as significant as inhibition of microsomal enzymes, although not as common, because of the large number of exogenous (e.g., drug) and endogenous (e.g., hormones) substrates metabolized by the cytochrome P450 enzymes.

Clinical Consequences of Inhibition. The most frequently reported clinical manifestation of inhibition of metabolism is toxicity of the inhibited drug. Table 6-11 lists those reports which have described toxicity resulting from inhibition. The toxicities range from mild clinical problems (e.g., decreased sleep latency) to severe adverse events (e.g., hemorrhage) and death. Therefore, inhibition of drug metabolism can lead to serious consequences for the individual patient. Inhibition potentially could result in decreased efficacy of a drug whose pharmacologic action resides in its metabolites (e.g., cyclophosphamide). Metabolic pathways may be differentially inhibited, which could result in variation in the pharmacologic action of the drug. Inhibition could be of benefit in preventing the formation of toxic metabolites, as in the case of acetaminophen overdose. The problems resulting from enzyme inhibition usually can be avoided if inhibition is anticipated.

Comparison of Inhibitors. Drugs listed in Table 6-12 have been reported to inhibit the metabolism of other drugs in humans. Chloramphenicol and the quinolone antibiotics are important inhibitors of drug metabolism from a therapeutic standpoint. Chloramphenicol inhibits cytochrome P450 in a noncompetitive manner and may also impair enzyme synthesis. Little is known about the mechanisms of inhibition of the quinolone antibiotics and why some fluoroquinolones are more potent inhibitors of drug metabolism. For example, enoxacin and pipemidic acid in humans decrease theophylline clearance by approximately 50%; ciprofloxacin and pefloxacin decrease theophylline clearance by approximately 25%.[265] In contrast, ofloxacin, norfloxacin, and nalidixic acid appear to have little influence on theophylline clearance. Enoxacin also has been reported to reduce significantly the clearance of caffeine,[265] R-warfarin,[266] and antipyrine[267] in healthy male volunteers, but has no significant effect on chlorpropamide[267] or phenytoin disposition.[268]

The following review will focus on the inhibitory characteristics of three representative drugs: cimetidine, ethanol, and disulfiram. Cimetidine reversibly inhibits cytochrome P450 in either a competitive or noncompetitive manner, and its characteristics as an inhibitor have been reviewed.[304] Acute ethanol administration inhibits microsomal oxidation indirectly through its metabolite, acetaldehyde, which depletes NADPH. At very high concentrations, ethanol may be a direct competitive inhibitor of the cytochrome P450 component of the microsomal system. Ethanol inhibits Phase II biotransformation (i.e., conjugation) by inhibiting UDP glucuronic acid synthesis. Disulfiram inhibits a number of enzymes, including alcohol dehydrogenase, dopamine β-hydroxylase, xanthine oxidase, and cytochrome P450. Disulfiram and its metabolite, diethyldithiocarbamate, are thought to inhibit cytochrome P450 by binding to its cysteinic sulfhydryl groups. The majority of clinical information on enzyme inhibition relates to cimetidine; little information is available regarding the inhibitory effects of ethanol and disulfiram. However, they are included in this discussion to highlight seven different features of inhibitors: clinical indication, prevalence, exposure, chemical structure, mechanism of inhibition, intrinsic pharmacologic activity and metabolites.

Cimetidine is used primarily as an anti-ulcer agent, disulfiram as an alcohol abuse deterrent, and ethanol as a social adjuvant. Cimetidine is one of the most frequently prescribed drugs, and ethanol is perhaps the most frequently used drug. Ethanol inhibits drug metabolism after acute administration, but induces drug metabolism after chronic exposure.[269-271] Cimetidine and disulfiram inhibit metabolism after both acute and chronic administration.[272-274] Cimetidine, ethanol, and disulfiram differ significantly in chemical structure. Ethanol inhibits Phase II biotransformations as well as Phase I.[275] Cimetidine inhibits only Phase I reactions.[274] Acute ethanol ingestion exerts an additive pharmacologic effect, as well as an inhibitory pharmacokinetic effect on benzodiazepines.[276,277] The metabolite, acetaldehyde, generated from ethanol oxidation, may be involved in the inhibition

Table 6–11. *Reported Manifestations of Inhibition of Drug Metabolism*[222]

Inhibited drug	Inhibitor	Manifestations
Tolbutamide	Chloramphenicol	Severe hypoglycemia
	Sulfisoxazole	Severe hypoglycemia
Phenytoin	Chloramphenicol	Nystagmus, lethargy
	Cimetidine	"Clinically toxic"
	Isoniazid	Nystagmus, ataxia, seizures
	Thioridazine	Nystagmus, ataxia, seizures
BCNU	Cimetidine	Leukopenia, thrombocytopenia, neutropenia
Diazepam	Cimetidine	↓ sleep latency
	Ethanol	
		Enhanced sedation
Chlordiazepoxide	Ethanol	Sedation
Theophylline	Cimetidine	Seizures, atrial fibrillation, hypotension, death
Warfarin	Cimetidine	Hemorrhage
	Disulfiram	Hemorrhage
	Metronidazole	Bruising
	Oxyphenylbutazone	Hematuria
	Phenylbutazone	Hemorrhage
	Sulfinpyrazone	Hemorrhage
Carbamazepine	Isoniazid	Confusion, lethargy, ataxia
Phenobarbital	Valproic Acid	Sedation, lethargy

of cytochrome P450, and not ethanol itself.[278,279] Both disulfiram and its metabolite, diethyldithiocarbamate, inhibit cytochrome P450.[280] However, only cimetidine, not its primary metabolite cimetidine sulfoxide, inhibits metabolism.[281]

Table 6-13 depicts the effect of cimetidine on the clearance of numerous low and high hepatic extraction drugs. Drugs listed are limited to those for which changes in clearance could be estimated. When several studies of the same interaction were noted, the reported changes in clearance indicate the central tendency. Cimetidine decreases both the systemic and oral clearance of low extraction drugs to the same extent; this is consistent with the relationship depicted in Figure 6-4. The oral clearance of high hepatic extraction drugs tends to decrease 30% to 50% after cimetidine administration, whereas systemic clearance generally decreases only 15% to 30%. A third point to note is that the oral clearance of high extraction drugs is reduced to a similar degree as the systemic clearance of low hepatic extraction drugs in the presence of cimetidine, as projected in Figure 6-4.

The elimination of drugs may be affected by ethanol in different ways. Chronic alcoholism is known to lead to cirrhosis, hypoalbuminemia, nutritional deficiencies, altered blood flow, and other pathological conditions, all of which may exert an effect on the elimination of a particular drug, depending on the characteristics of the drug and the extent and degree of the pathology. However, chronic and acute administration of ethanol in the absence of liver disease is known to influence the elimination of drugs. In general, chronic alcohol intake increases the rate of microsomal metabolism, whereas acute ethanol administration inhibits hepatic microsomal enzymes. Therefore, in the context of metabolic inhibition, it is the acute administration of ethanol which is of interest.

Ethanol given as a single doses or acutely throughout blood sampling, in healthy adults has been reported to decrease the systemic clearance of chlordiazepoxide (37%),[283] diazepam (24%),[284] and lorazepam (18%),[275] and increase the half-life of tolbutamide.[285] Ethanol had no effect on the oral or systemic clearance of chlormethiazole.[286] Ethanol administration patterns and quantity varied considerably among the studies. Blood alcohol concentration was determined in only a few studies.

Disulfiram has been reported to decrease the clearance of antipyrine (38%),[260] diazepam (41%),[287] chlordiazepoxide (54%),[287] phenytoin (34%),[262] and warfarin (21%).[288] Disulfiram generally was given as a single dose in most studies. By

Table 6-12. *Inhibitors of Drug Metabolism in Humans*

Allopurinol	Ketoconazole	Propranolol
Amitriptyline	L-dopa	Quinolone antibiotics
Chloramphenicol	Methyldopa	Sulfinpyrazone
Cimetidine	Metoprolol	Sulphaphenazole
Delta-9-tetrahydrocannabinol	Metronidazole	Thiabendazole
Dicoumarol	Monoamine oxidase inhibitors	Thioridazine
Disulfiram	Nadolol	Trimethoprim-sulfamethoxazole
Erythromycin	Omeprazole	Troleandomycin
Ethanol	Oral contraceptives	Valproic acid
Isoniazid	Phenylbutazone	

comparing the drugs which have been studied after cimetidine, ethanol, and disulfiram administration, it is apparent that the clearance of these inhibited drugs is decreased to approximately the same extent by all three inhibitors.

Dose Dependency. The dose of inhibitor may affect the degree of inhibition of a given drug. For example, cimetidine exhibits dose-dependent decreases in metabolic inhibition over a 300 to 1600 mg/day dose range for a number of

Table 6-13. Effect of Cimetidine on Drug Elimination[222]

Drug	Route of administration	Clearance change (%)
Low Hepatic Extraction Drugs		
Antipyrine	PO	−22
	IV	−23
Benzodiazepines		
Alprazolam	PO	−37
Chlordiazepoxide	IV	−57
Diazepam	PO	−33
	IV	−43
Caffeine	PO	−28
Metronidazole	IV	−29
Phenytoin	PO	−37
	IV	−12
Quinidine[282]	PO	−27
	IV	−36
Theophylline	PO	−31
	IV	−31
Warfarin	PO	−26
High Hepatic Extraction Drugs		
5−Fluorouracil	IV	−28
Imipramine	PO	−46
	IV	−40
Labetalol	PO	−40
	IV	− 8[a]
Lidocaine	PO	−42
	IV	−21
Metoprolol	PO	−38
Morphine	IV	−10[a]
Propranolol	PO	−38
	IV	−21
Verapamil	PO	−39[a]
	IV	19[a]

[a] Not statistically significant.

drugs.[289–292] Antipyrine clearance is decreased by 17%, 24%, and 34% after cimetidine 400, 800, and 1600 mg/day.[290] It should be noted that while the clearance of antipyrine is cimetidine-dose-dependent, it is not dose-proportional (i.e., a twofold increase in cimetidine dose per day did not result in a twofold decrease in antipyrine clearance). Since competitive inhibition can be described as a dose-response relationship, maximal inhibition will occur at a given dose when the substrate (inhibited drug) concentration does not change further. Since cimetidine 2400 mg/day decreases theophylline clearance to a similar extent as 1200 mg/day (see Figure 6-7),[293] it may be that near maximal cimetidine inhibition occurs at the 1200 mg/day dose. Low doses of an inhibitor could be used to avoid or minimize the interaction if this dose also achieves the therapeutic endpoint.

The administration time of the inhibitor relative to that of the inhibited drug also may affect the degree of inhibition. Coadministration of an inhibitor after the absorption phase of an orally administered, high extraction drug such as propranolol would be expected to have little or no effect on propranolol's apparent oral clearance. Therefore, significant clinical interactions may be avoided in certain cases by changing the administration times of two drugs.

Time Course. The onset, time to maximum effect, and termination of inhibition depend upon the mechanism of inhibition and the drug inhibited. Generally, inhibition involving binding of the inhibitor to the enzyme is evident shortly after an effective concentration of the inhibitor is present. For example, chloramphen-

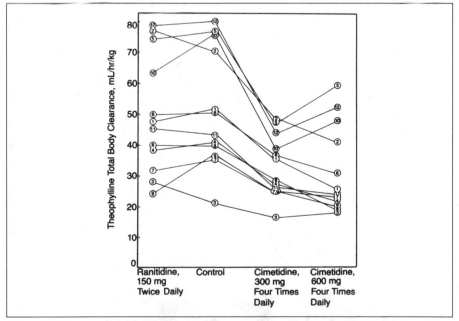

Figure 6-7. Comparison of the effect of two histamine H_2-antagonists, cimetidine and ranitidine, on theophylline clearance. While ranitidine does not change theophylline clearance, cimetidine consistently decreases clearance, although there is no difference in effect between the 1200 mg and 2400 mg/day cimetidine doses (adapted with permission from reference 293).

icol, ethanol, and cimetidine inhibit drug metabolism within 24 hours of a single dose. However, the inhibitory effect will be delayed if the inhibitor acts by decreasing the synthesis of the enzyme.

The time to maximum effect is dependent upon the dose or plasma concentration of the inhibitor, the time required for the inhibitory drug to achieve this concentration, and the time required for the inhibited drug to reach a new steady state. As shown in Figure 6-8, an immediate increase in serum phenytoin concentrations occurred after chloramphenicol administration, although the maximum serum phenytoin concentration was not seen for a few days.[294] Even though cimetidine exerts its maximal inhibitory effect within the first day of administration,[290] the maximum increase in theophylline concentrations is not seen for three days, since this is the time required for theophylline to reach a new steady state.[295]

In the same manner, termination of the effect of an inhibitor depends on the plasma concentration of the inhibitor, the elimination rate of the inhibitor, and the elimination rate of the inhibited drug. As shown in Figure 6-8, there is a time lag between discontinuation of chloramphenicol and a maximal decrease in serum phenytoin concentrations.[294] When the elimination half-life of the inhibitor is shorter than that of the inhibited drug, less time is required for serum concentra-

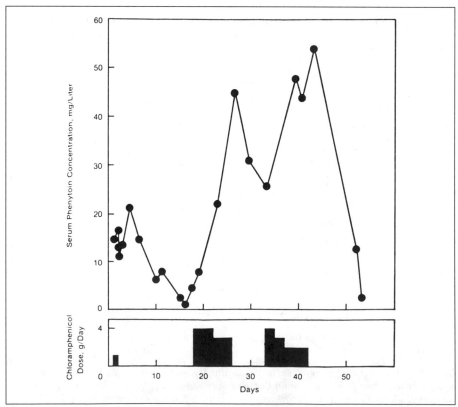

Figure 6-8. *Phenytoin serum concentrations in a patient who received a constant phenytoin dose (300 mg/day) until day 43 and intermittent administration of chloramphenicol (adapted from reference 294).*

tions of the inhibited drug to revert to a lower steady state after the inhibitor is stopped than is required to reach a new higher steady state upon starting the inhibitor. This is because the elimination half-life is decreased after discontinuation of an inhibitor, and, therefore, less time is required to reach a new steady state.

Integration of the onset, maximal effect and termination of inhibition and their clinical impact is depicted in Figure 6-9. Upon initiation of cimetidine, plasma warfarin concentrations and prothrombin times increase significantly; however, the maximal plasma warfarin concentration and prothrombin time are not seen for several days. A decrease in plasma warfarin concentrations and prothrombin time occurs immediately upon discontinuation of cimetidine, but these values do not return to baseline for several days.[296] The time course of cimetidine-induced metabolic inhibition has been evaluated for a number of other drugs.[289,290,297–299]

Attenuating Factors. *Patients.* Although the majority of inhibition studies involve healthy volunteers, inhibition of drug metabolism is known to occur in patients, as supported by case reports and controlled studies. Chloramphenicol inhibits the metabolism of tolbutamide in diabetics[300] and phenytoin in epileptics.[301,302] Disulfiram decreases the clearance of chlordiazepoxide to the same degree in normal volunteers and chronic alcoholics without serious liver disease.[287] Cimetidine decreases the clearance of theophylline in patients with chronic obstructive pulmonary disease by 33%[289] and 28%.[303] This decrease is of a similar magnitude to that found in healthy volunteers.[304] Therefore, studies with healthy volunteers are useful in indicating the effect an inhibitor will have on the clearance of a drug in patients. However, since patients may differ from volunteers in having a number of other characteristics which can affect drug clearance, it is likely that the effect may differ in variability and magnitude.

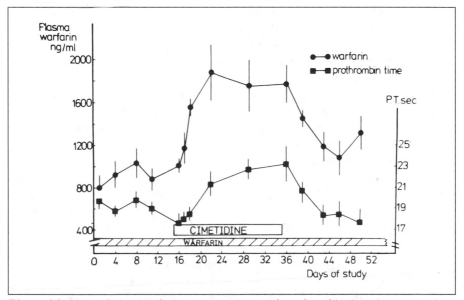

Figure 6-9. Mean plasma warfarin concentrations and prothrombin times in seven patients who received a constant anticoagulant dose of warfarin. Cimetidine (1000 mg/day) was added to the regimen on day 15 (adapted with permission from reference 296).

Age. Cimetidine decreased the clearance of antipyrine by 25% in young (21 to 26 years of age) and elderly (65 to 78 years of age) subjects,[290] and by 20% in children (6 to 13 years old).[305] While age does not alter cimetidine inhibition of antipyrine clearance, this does not preclude age-related differences for other substrates or other inhibitors with different mechanisms of action, as discussed in a subsequent chapter.

Enzyme Induction. Enzyme induction may increase a patient's sensitivity to inhibition of oxidative metabolism. For example, the mean decrease in antipyrine clearance after cimetidine administration was greater in subjects pretreated with the enzyme inducer, rifampin (44%), than in noninduced subjects (24%).[290] Cigarette smoking increases the clearance of theophylline in the absence of an inhibitor.[240] When cimetidine is administered to smokers, the clearance of theophylline decreases to a greater extent in those who had higher initial theophylline clearance values.[306] Consistent with this observation, theophylline clearance was reduced more in smokers (28%) than in nonsmokers (11%) after cimetidine.[307] However, enzyme induction may not increase the responsiveness to inhibition in all cases. For instance, caffeine clearance is increased by smoking; however, the clearance of caffeine was decreased to a greater degree when cimetidine was administered to nonsmokers (42%) as opposed to smokers (31%).[308]

Liver Disease. It is recognized that liver disease may adversely affect the elimination of drugs metabolized primarily by the liver. Likewise, pathophysiological alterations in the liver might be expected to change the sensitivity to inhibitors. Patients with chronic liver disease who demonstrate an impaired capacity for aminopyrine demethylation are twice as sensitive to the inhibitory effect of cimetidine as patients with normal liver function.[309] In another study, cimetidine decreased the clearance of antipyrine in patients without cirrhosis (26%), but not in those with cirrhosis.[310] However, in this nonrandomized study, the subjects with cirrhosis showed clinical signs of improvement in liver function after the antipyrine control period and before the cimetidine-antipyrine portion of the study. Therefore, the inhibitory effect of cimetidine in cirrhotic patients was not adequately assessed.

Specificity. Based on current information, the most thoroughly studied inducers (phenobarbital, rifampin, cigarette smoke) induce different cytochrome P450 isozymes. However, there does appear to be some overlap in substrate specificity. For example, as shown in Tables 6-8 to 6-10, phenobarbital, rifampin and cigarette smoke induce the metabolism of some of the same drugs, although at the clinically used dosages, rifampin generally produces a much greater change in drug clearance. Drugs which are induced by phenobarbital, rifampin, and cigarette smoke are generally inhibited by cimetidine. There is not enough experience with ethanol and disulfiram to discuss specificity.

DOSING CONSIDERATIONS

Patients with hepatic cirrhosis are about two to five times more prone to experience adverse drug reactions than patients without liver dysfunction,[312] and frequency correlates with the severity of liver dysfunction. This phenomenon probably can be attributed to pharmacodynamic and pharmacokinetic alterations in hepatic disease.

Remarkably little information is available on the pharmacodynamics of drugs in patients with hepatic dysfunction. Central nervous system sensitivity is increased for morphine,[313] chlorpromazine,[314] and diazepam.[315] Hepatic encephalopathy can be precipitated by sedatives, analgesics, and tranquilizers.[316] Yet, drug-induced hepatic encephalopathy in cirrhotic patients was caused by diuretics seven times more frequently than sedatives.[312] Pharmacodynamic studies of phenobarbital, ethanol, and theophylline in animals with experimentally-induced liver disease indicated that there were no appreciable differences from control animals with regard to gross central nervous system effects.[317,318]

Pharmacokinetic changes for specific drugs in liver disease are reviewed elsewhere.[172,173,319,320] Because there are no tests which accurately predict the clearance of unbound drugs in liver disease, dosing recommendations are, by necessity, broad and general. Even if antipyrine or ICG did reliably predict the clearance of a large number of drugs, it seems unlikely that these test drugs would be useful clinically. The poor predictive ability of any one test is due, in part, to the large number of variables which influence hepatic metabolism. In patients with chronic liver disease, the decreased clearance of oxidized drugs correlates best with a low serum albumin (<3.5 gm/dl), decreased prothrombin activity (<80% normal), and/or elevated serum bilirubin. Unfortunately, these laboratory changes may not always reflect decreased hepatic synthetic activity. Drugs which are metabolized primarily by conjugation are much less sensitive to hepatic dysfunction and may be preferred.

As a gross initial dosing guideline, patients with cirrhosis or chronic active hepatitis may start with one-half the usual dose of a drug if it is eliminated by oxidative metabolism. If the patient has signs of decompensation (ascites, encephalopathy, severe hypoalbuminemia), even lower doses may be used. Drugs that are metabolized extensively before reaching the systemic circulation may be completely absorbed as parent drug in cirrhotic patients. Similarly, the first-pass effect may not exist in patients with a portacaval shunt. Upward or downward dose adjustments should be based on therapeutic response or adverse effects. When using plasma or serum drug assays to guide dosing, remember that protein binding measurements may be useful if the drug is greater than 70% to 80% bound.

In the future, pharmacokinetic studies should characterize patients with hepatic dysfunction according to Child's classification or Pugh's modification (preferably the latter) to allow functional comparison of patients across studies. This may help relate pharmacokinetic alterations to disease severity. A greater effort should be made to evaluate the pharmacodynamics of drugs which are likely to be used in patients with hepatic dysfunction.

ACKNOWLEDGEMENT

We gratefully acknowledge the secretarial assistance of Renee M. Brinkhous.

REFERENCES

1. Klaassen CD, Watkins JB. Mechanisms of bile formation, hepatic uptake, and biliary excretion. Pharmacol Rev. 1984;36:1.
2. Meijer DK. Current concepts on hepatic transport of drugs. J Hepatol. 1987;4:259.
3. Scharschmidt BF et al. Hepatic organic anion uptake in the rat. J Clin Invest. 1975;56:1280.
4. Lebrec D et al. Splanchnic hemodynamics in cirrhotic patients with esophageal varices and gastrointestinal bleeding. Gastroenterology. 1976;70:1108.
5. Gross G, Perrier CV. Intra hepatic porta systemic shunting in cirrhotic patients. N Engl J Med. 1975;293:1046.
6. Nebert DW et al. The P450 superfamily: updated listing of all genes and recommended nomenclature for the chromosomal loci. DNA 1989;8:1.
7. Brosen K. Recent developments in hepatic drug oxidation. Clin Pharmacokinet. 1990;18:220.
8. Nelson DR, Strobel HW. Evolution of P450 proteins. Mol Biol Evol. 1987;4:572.
9. Pang KS, Gillette JR. Kinetics of metabolite formation and elimination in the perfused rat liver preparation: differences between the elimination of preformed acetaminophen and acetaminophen formed from phenacetin. J Pharmacol Exp Ther. 1978;207:178.
10. Pang KS, Terrell JA. Retrograde perfusion to probe the heterogeneous distribution of hepatic drug metabolizing enzymes in rats. J Pharmacol Exp Ther. 1981;216:339.
11. Jones DP. Hypoxia and drug metabolism. Biochem Pharmacol. 1981;30:1019.
12. Brodie MJ et al. Influence of liver disease and environmental factors on hepatic monooxygenase activity *in vitro*. Eur J Clin Pharmacol. 1981;20:39.
13. Klotz U et al. The effects of age and liver disease on the disposition and elimination of diazepam in adult man. J Clin Invest. 1975;55:347.
14. Roberts RK et al. Effects of age and parenchymal liver disease on the disposition and elimination of chlordiazepoxide. Gastroenterology. 1978;75:479.
15. Desmond PV et al. Preservation of glucuronidation in carbon tetrachloride-induced acute liver injury in the rat. Biochem Pharmacol. 1981;30:993.
16. Shull HJ et al. Normal disposition of oxazepam in acute viral hepatitis and cirrhosis. Ann Intern Med. 1976;84:420.
17. Taburet AM et al. Pharmacokinetics of zidovudine in patients with liver cirrhosis. Clin Pharmacol Ther. 1990;47:731.
18. Teunissen MWE et al. Antipyrine clearance and metabolite formation in patients with alcoholic cirrhosis. Br J Clin Pharmacol. 1984;18:707.
19. Witassek F et al. Abnormal glucuronidation of zomepirac in patients with cirrhosis of the liver. Hepatology. 1983;3:415.
20. Crotty B et al. Hepatic extraction of morphine is impaired in cirrhosis. Eur J Clin Pharmacol. 1989;36:501.
21. Dawson JR et al. Alteration of transit time and direction of flow to probe the heterogeneous distribution of conjugating activities for harmol in the perfused rat liver preparation. J Pharmacol Exp Ther. 1985;234:691.
22. Levy G. Sulfate conjugation in drug metabolism: role of inorganic sulfate. Fed Proc. 1986;45:2235.
23. Bresnick E. The molecular biology of the induction of the hepatic mixed function oxidases. Pharmacol Ther. 1978;2:319.
24. Nebert DW et al. Genetic mechanisms controlling the induction of polysubstrate monooxygenase (P-450) activities. Ann Rev Pharmacol Toxicol. 1981;21:431.
25. Rawlins MD. Extrahepatic drug metabolism. In: Wilkinson GR, Rawlins MD, eds. Drug Metabolism and Disposition: Considerations in Clinical Pharmacology. Lancaster: MTP Press, Ltd.; 1985:21–33.
26. Mazoit JX et al. Extrahepatic metabolism of morphine occurs in humans. Clin Pharmacol Ther. 1990;48:613.
27. George CF. Drug metabolism by the gastrointestinal mucosa. Clin Pharmacokinet. 1981;6:259.
28. Back DJ et al. The *in vitro* metabolism of ethinyloestradiol, levonorgestrel and mestranol by human jejunal mucosa. Br J Clin Pharmacol. 1980;9:281.

29. Geddes DM et al. First-pass uptake of ^{14}C-propranolol by the lung. Thorax 1979;34:810.

30. Barry BW. Properties that influence percutaneous absorption. In: Dermatological Formulations. New York: Marcel Dekker, Inc.; 1983:135–137.

31. Stoeckel K et al. Nonlinear pharmacokinetics of indocyanine green in the rabbit and rat. J Pharmacokinet Biopharm. 1980;8:483.

32. Taburet AM et al. Pharmacokinetics of ornidazole in patients with acute viral hepatitis, alcoholic cirrhosis, and extrahepatic cholestasis. Clin Pharmacol Ther. 1989;45:373.

33. Weisiger RA. Dissociation from albumin: a potentially rate-limiting step in the clearance of substances by the liver. Proc Natl Acad Sci (USA). 1985;82:1563.

34. deLannoy IAM, Pang KS. Presence of a diffusional barrier on metabolite kinetics: enalaprilat as a generated versus preformed metabolite. Drug Metab Dispos. 1986;14:513.

35. Wilkinson GR. Clearance approaches in pharmacology. Pharmacol Rev. 1987;39:1.

36. Wilkinson GR, Shand DG. A physiological approach to hepatic drug clearance. Clin Pharmacol Ther. 1975;18:377.

37. Gillette JR. Factors affecting drug metabolism. Ann NY Acad Sci. 1971;179:43.

38. Pang KS, Rowland M. Hepatic clearance of drugs. I. Theoretical considerations of a "well-stirred" model and a "parallel tube" model. Influence of hepatic blood flow, plasma and blood cell binding, and the hepatocellular enzymatic activity on hepatic drug clearance. J Pharmacokinet Biopharm. 1977;5:625.

39. Bass L et al. Enzymatic elimination of substrates flowing through the intact liver. J Theor Biol. 1976;61:393.

40. Svensson CK et al. Free drug concentration monitoring in clinical practice. Rationale and current status. Clin Pharmacokinet. 1986;11:450.

41. Morgan DJ, Smallwood RA. Clinical significance of pharmacokinetic models of hepatic elimination. Clin Pharmacokinet. 1990;18:61.

42. Gibaldi M, McNamara PJ. Apparent volumes of distribution and drug binding to plasma proteins and tissues. Eur J Clin Pharmacol. 1978;13:373.

43. Wilkinson GR. Plasma binding, distribution and elimination. In: Roe DA, Campbell TC, eds. Drugs and Nutrients: The Interactive Effects. New York: Marcel Dekker; 1984:21.

44. Wilkinson GR. Influence of Hepatic Disease on Pharmacokinetics. In: Applied Pharmacokinetics. WE Evans et al., eds. 2nd ed. Vancouver, Washington: Applied Therapeutics Inc.; 1986:116–138.

45. Child CG, Turcotte JG. Surgery and Portal Hypertension. In: The Liver and Portal Hypertension. CG Child, ed. Philadelphia: WB Saunders; 1964:1–85.

46. Pugh RNH et al. Transection of the oesophagus for bleeding oesophageal varices. Br J Surg. 1973;60:646.

47. Branch RA. Drugs as indicators of hepatic function. Hepatology. 1982;2:97.

48. Barstow L, Small RE. Liver function assessment by drug metabolism. Pharmacotherapy. 1990;10:280.

49. Wensing G et al. Antipyrine elimination and hepatic microsomal enzyme activity in patients with liver disease. Clin Pharmacol Ther. 1990;47:698.

50. Schmid B et al. Polymorphic dextromethorphan metabolism: co-segregation of oxidative O-demethylation with debrisoquin hydroxylation. Clin Pharmacol Ther. 1985; 38:618.

51. Crom WR et al. Simultaneous administration of multiple model substrates to assess hepatic drug clearance. Clin Pharmacol Ther. 1987;41:645.

52. Poulsen HE, Loft S. Antipyrine as a model drug to study hepatic drug-metabolizing capacity. J Hepatol. 1988;6:374.

53. Svensson CK. Is blood sampling for determination of antipyrine pharmacokinetics in healthy volunteers ethically justified? Clin Pharmacol Ther. 1988;44:365.

54. Danhof M, Breimer DD. Studies on the different metabolic pathways of antipyrine in man. I. Oral administration of 250, 500, and 1000 mg to healthy volunteers. Br J Clin Pharmacol. 1979;8:529.

55. Boobis AR et al. Comparison of the *in vivo* and *in vitro* rates of formation of the three main oxidative metabolites of antipyrine in man. Br J Clin Pharmacol. 1981;12:771.

56. Birnie GG et al. Antipyrine and indocyanine green kinetics in the prediction of the natural history of liver disease. Br J Clin Pharmacol. 1987;23:615P.

57. Branch RA et al. Determinants of serum antipyrine half-lives in patients with liver disease. Gut. 1973;14:569.

58. Farrell GC et al. Drug metabolism in liver disease. Identification of patients with impaired hepatic drug metabolism. Gastroenterology. 1978;75:580.

59. Sotaniemi EA et al. Measurement of hepatic drug-metabolizing enzyme activity in man. Comparison of three different assays. Eur J Clin Pharmac. 1980;17:267.

60. McPherson GAD et al. Antipyrine elimination as a dynamic test of hepatic functional integrity in obstructive jaundice. Gut. 1982;23:734.

61. Pelkonen RD et al. Coumarin 7-hydroxylase activity in human liver microsome: properties of the enzyme and interspecies comparisons. Br J Clin Pharmacol. 1985;19:59.

62. Forrest JAH et al. Antipyrine, paracetamol and lignocaine elimination in chronic liver disease. Br Med J. 1977;1:1384.

63. Branch RA et al. A study of factors influencing drug disposition in chronic liver disease using the model drug (+) propranolol. Br J Clin Pharmacol. 1976;3:243.

64. Hepner GW et al. Disposition of aminopyrine, antipyrine, diazepam and indocyanine green in patients with liver disease or on anticonvulsant drug therapy: diazepam breath test and correlations in drug elimination. J Lab Clin Med. 1977;90:440.

65. Hepner GW, Vesell ES. Aminopyrine disposition: studies on breath, saliva and urine of normal subjects and patients with liver disease. Clin Pharmacol Ther. 1976;20:654.

66. Schneider JF et al. Aminopyrine N-demethylation: a prognostic test of liver function in patients with alcoholic liver disease. Gastroenterology. 1980;79:1145.

67. Ramsoe K et al. Functioning liver mass in uncomplicated and fulminant acute hepatitis. Scand J Gastroent. 1980;15:65.

68. Irving CS et al. The aminopyrine breath test as a measure of liver function. J Lab Clin Med. 1982;100:356.

69. Henry DA et al. ^{14}C-aminopyrine breath analysis and conventional biochemical tests as predictors of survival in cirrhosis. Dig Dis Sci. 1985;30:813.

70. Wheeler HO et al. Hepatic uptake and biliary excretion of indocyanine green in the dog. Proc Soc Exp Biol Med. 1958;99:11.

71. Cherrick GR et al. Indocyanine green: observations on its physical properties, plasma decay, and hepatic extraction. J Clin Invest. 1960;39:592.

72. Nxumalo JL et al. Hepatic blood flow measurement. Arch Surg. 1978;113:169.

73. Kawasaki S et al. Pharmacokinetic study on the hepatic uptake of indocyanine green in cirrhotic patients. Am J Gastroenterol. 1985;80:801.

74. Branch RA et al. The clearance of antipyrine and indocyanine green in normal subjects and in patients with chronic liver disease. Clin Pharmacol Ther 1976;20:81.

75. Barbare JC et al. Intrinsic hepatic clearance and Child-Turcotte classification for assessment of liver function in cirrhosis. J Hepatol. 1985;1:253.

76. Bauer LA et al. Variability of indocyanine green pharmacokinetics in healthy adults. Clin Pharm. 1989;8:54.

77. Colli A et al. Disposition of a flow-limited drug (lidocaine) and a metabolic capacity-limited drug (theophylline) in liver cirrhosis. Clin Pharmacol Ther. 1988;44:642.

78. Oellerich M et al. Lidocaine metabolite formation as a measure of liver function in patients with cirrhosis. Ther Drug Monit. 1990;12:219.

79. Barry M et al. Severity of cirrhosis and the relationship of α_1-acid glycoprotein concentration to plasma protein binding of lidocaine. Clin Pharmacol Ther. 1990;47:366.

80. Breen KJ et al. τ^{14}C-phenacetin breath test to measure hepatic function in man. Hepatology. 1984;4:47.

81. Renner E et al. Caffeine: a model compound for measuring liver function. Hepatology. 1984;4:38.

82. Cheng WS et al. Dose-dependent pharmacokinetics of caffeine in humans: Relevance as a test of quantitative liver function. Clin Pharmacol Ther. 1990;47:516.

83. Kawasaki S et al. Hepatic clearances of antipyrine, indocyanine green, and galactose in normal subjects and in patients with chronic liver diseases. Clin Pharmacol Ther. 1988;44:217.

84. Caspary WF, Schaffer J. ^{14}C-D-galactose breath test for evaluation of liver function in patients with chronic liver disease. Digestion. 1978;17:410.

85. Zeeh J et al. Steady-state extrarenal sorbitol clearance as a measure of hepatic plasma flow. Gastroenterology. 1988;95:749.

86. Vesell ES et al. Altered plasma half-lives of antipyrine, propylthiouracil, and methimazole in thyroid dysfunction. Clin Pharmacol Ther. 1974;17:48.

87. Eichelbaum M et al. Influence of thyroid status on plasma half-life of antipyrine in man. N Engl J Med. 1974;290:1040.

88. Vozeh S et al. Influence of thyroid function on theophylline kinetics. Clin Pharmacol Ther. 1984;36:634.

89. Feely J et al. Increased clearance of propranolol in thyrotoxicosis. Ann Intern Med. 1981;94:472.

90. Williams PE et al. Determinants of free theophylline clearance in asthma. Br J Clin Pharmacol. 1987;24:655.

91. Rumbaugh RC et al. Dose dependent actions of thyroxine on hepatic drug metabolism in male and female rats. Biochem Pharmacol. 1978;27:2027.

92. Skett P, Weir A. Sex and substrate dependent effects of the thyroid gland on drug metabolism in the rat. Biochem Pharmacol. 1983;32:3115.

93. Redmond GP et al. Effect of growth hormone on human drug metabolism: time course and substrate specificity. Ped Pharmacol. 1989;1:63.

94. Wilson JT, Spelberg TC. Growth hormone and drug metabolism: acute effects on microsomal mixed-function oxidase activities in rat liver. Biochem J. 1976;154:433.

95. Sotaniemi EA et al. Hepatic microsomal enzyme activity in patients with non-insulin dependent diabetes mellitus (NIDDM) and its clinical significance. Acta Endocrinol. 1984;262(Suppl.):125.

96. Salmela PI et al. The evaluation of the drug-metabolizing capacity in patients with diabetes mellitus. Diabetes. 1980;29:788.

97. Daintith H et al. Influence of diabetes mellitus on drug metabolism in man. Int J Clin Pharmacol. 1976;13:55.

98. Dajani RM et al. A study on physiological disposition of acetophenetidin by the diabetic man. Comp Gen Pharmacol. 1974;5:1.

99. Ueda H et al. Disappearance rate of tolbutamide in normal subjects and in diabetes mellitus, liver cirrhosis, and renal disease. Diabetes. 1963;12:414.

100. Warren BL et al. Differential effects of diabetes on microsomal metabolism of various substrates. Biochem Pharmacol. 1983;32:327.

101. Skett P et al. The role of androgens in the effect of diabetes mellitus on hepatic drug metabolism in the male rat. Acta Endocrinol. 1984;107:506.

102. Johnsen SG et al. Enzyme induction by oral testosterone. Clin Pharmacol Ther. 1976;20:233.

103. Weiner M et al. Effects of steroids on disposition of oxyphenbutazone in man. Proc Soc Exp Biol Med. 1967;124:1170.

104. Homeida M et al. Effect of an oral contraceptive on hepatic size and antipyrine metabolism in premenopausal women. Clin Pharmacol Ther. 1978;24:228.

105. Teunissen MWE et al. Influence of sex and oral contraceptive steroids on antipyrine metabolite formation. Clin Pharmacol Ther. 1982;32:240.

106. Herz R et al. Inhibition of hepatic demethylation of aminopyrine by oral contraceptive steroids in humans. Eur J Clin Invest. 1978;8:27.

107. Roberts RK et al. Disposition of chlordiazepoxide: sex differences and effects of oral contraceptives. Clin Pharmacol Ther. 1979;25:826.

108. Abernethy DR et al. Impairment of diazepam metabolism by low-dose estrogen-containing oral contraceptive steroids. N Engl J Med. 1982;306:791.

109. Stoehr GP et al. Effect of oral contraceptives on triazolam, temazepam, alprazolam, and lorazepam kinetics. Clin Pharmacol Ther. 1984;36:683.

110. Jochemsen R et al. Influence of sex, menstrual cycle, and oral contraception on the disposition of nitrazepam. Br J Clin Pharmacol. 1982;13:319.

111. Padwardhan R et al. Impaired elimination of caffeine by oral contraceptive steroids. J Lab Clin Med. 1980;95:603.

112. Abernethy DR et al. Imipramine disposition in users of oral contraceptive steroids. Clin Pharmacol Ther. 1984;35:792.

113. O'Malley K et al. Impairment of human drug metabolism by oral contraceptive steroids. Clin Pharmacol Ther. 1972;13:552.

114. Oram M et al. The influence of oral contraceptives on the metabolism of methaqualone in man. Br J Clin Pharmacol. 1982;14:341.

115. Mitchell MC et al. Effects of oral contraceptive steroids on acetaminophen metabolism and elimination. Clin Pharmacol Ther. 1983;34:48.

116. Miners JO et al. Gender and oral contraceptive steroids as determinants of drug glucuronidation: effects on clofibric acid elimination. Br J Clin Pharmacol. 1984;18:240.

117. Macdonald JI et al. Sex-difference and the effects of smoking and oral contraceptive steroids on the kinetics of diflunisal. Eur J Clin Pharmacol. 1990;38:175.

118. Patwardhan RV et al. Differential effects of oral contraceptive steroids on the metabolism of benzodiazepines. Hepatology. 1983;3:248.

119. Tritapepe R et al. Effects of ethinyl estradiol on bile secretion and liver microsomal mixed function oxidase system in the mouse. Biochem Pharmacol. 1980;29:677.

120. Skett P. Biochemical basis of sex differences in drug metabolism. Pharmacal Ther. 1988;38:269.

121. Wilson K. Sex-related differences in drug disposition in man. Clin Pharmacokinet. 1984;9:189.

122. Miners JO et al. Influence of sex and oral contraceptive steroids on paracetamol metabolism. Br J Clin Pharmacol. 1983;16:503.

123. Wojcieki J et al. Comparative pharmacokinetics of paracetamol in men and women considering follicular and luteal phases. Arzneim-Forsch. 1979;29:350.

124. Montgomery PR et al. Salicylate metabolism: effects of age and sex in adults. Clin Pharmacol Ther. 1986;39:571.

125. Walle T et al. Pathway-selective sex differences in the metabolic clearance of propranolol in human subjects. Clin Pharmacol Ther. 1989;46:257.

126. Frezza M et al. High blood alcohol levels in women. N Engl J Med. 1990;322:95.

127. Bennett BM et al. Sex related differences in the metabolism of isosorbide dinitrate following incubation in human blood. Biochem Pharmacol. 1983;32:3729.

128. Nayak VK et al. Influence of menstrual cycle on antipyrine pharmacokinetics in healthy Indian female volunteers. Br J Clin Pharmacol. 1988;26:604.

129. Riester EF et al. Antipyrine metabolism during the menstrual cycle. Clin Pharmacol Ther. 1980;28:384.

130. Wilson K et al. The influence of the menstrual cycle on the metabolism and clearance of methaqualone. Br J Clin Pharmacol. 1982;14:333.

131. Somaja L, Thangam J. Salivary paracetamol elimination kinetics during the menstrual cycle. Br J Clin Pharmacol. 1987;23:348.

132. Cummings AJ. A survey of pharmacokinetic data from pregnant women. Clin Pharmacokinet. 1983;8:344.

133. Assael BM et al. Ampicillin kinetics in pregnancy. Br J Clin Pharmacol. 1979;8:286.

134. Dam M et al. Antiepileptic drugs: metabolism in pregnancy. Clin Pharmacokinet. 1979;4:53.

135. Dean M et al. Serum protein binding of drugs during and after pregnancy in humans. Clin Pharmacol Ther. 1980;28:253.

136. Aldridge A et al. The disposition of caffeine during and after pregnancy. Seminars Perinatology. 1981;5:310.

137. Frederiksen MC et al. Theophylline pharmacokinetics in pregnancy. Clin Pharmacol Ther. 1986;40:321.

138. Kalow W et al, eds. Ethnic Differences in Reactions to Drugs and Xenobiotics. New York: Alan R. Liss; 1986:21.

139. Clark DWJ. Genetically determined variability in acetylation and oxidation: Therapeutic implications. Drugs. 1985;29:342.

140. Zhou HH et al. Racial differences in drug response: altered sensitivity to and clearance of propranolol in men of Chinese descent as compared to American whites. N Engl J Med. 1989;320:565.

141. Zhou HH et al. Differences in stereoselective disposition of propranolol do not explain sensitivity differences between white and Chinese subjects: correlation between the clearance of (−) and (+) propranolol. Clin Pharmacol Ther. 1990;47:719.

142. Zhou HH et al. Differences in plasma binding of drugs between Caucasians and Chinese subjects. Clin Pharmacol Ther. 1990;48:10.

143. Narang RK et al. Pharmacokinetic study of antipyrine in malnourished children. Am J Clin Nutr. 1977;30:1979.

144. Buchanan N et al. Antipyrine metabolite formation in children in the acute phase of malnutrition and after recovery. Br J Clin Pharmacol. 1980;10:363.

145. Buchanan N et al. Antipyrine pharmacokinetics and D-glucaric acid excretion in kwashiorkor. Am J Clin Nutr. 1979;32:2439.

146. Abernethy DR, Greenblatt DJ. Pharmacokinetics of drugs in obesity. Clin Pharmacokinet. 1982; 7:108.

147. Krishnaswamy K et al. Dietary influences on the kinetics of antipyrine and aminopyrine in human subjects. Br J Clin Pharmacol. 1984;17:139.

148. Kappas A et al. Influence of dietary protein and carbohydrate on antipyrine and theophylline metabolism in man. Clin Pharmacol Ther. 1976;20:643.

149. Dean M, Powell JR. The effect of short-term protein-calorie deprivation on cimetidine inhibition of theophylline disposition. Drug Intell Clin Pharm. 1986;20:470. Abstract.

150. Juan D et al. Effects of dietary protein on theophylline pharmacokinetics and caffeine and aminopyrine breath tests. Clin Pharmacol Ther. 1986;40:187.

151. Fagan TC et al. Increased clearance of propranolol and theophylline by high-protein compared with high-carbohydrate diet. Clin Pharmacol Ther. 1987;41:402.

152. Anderson KE et al. Nutrition and oxidative drug metabolism in man. Relative influence of dietary lipids, carbohydrates, and protein. Clin Pharmacol Ther. 1979; 26:493.

153. Reidenberg MM, Vessell ES. Unaltered metabolism of antipyrine and tolbutamide in fasting man. Clin Pharmacol Ther. 1975;17:650.

154. Miranda CL, Webb RE. Effects of dietary protein quality on drug metabolism in the rat. J Nutr. 1973;103:1425.

155. Campbell TC, Hayes JR. The effect of quantity and quality of dietary protein on drug metabolism. Fed Proc. 1976;35:2470.

156. McLean AEM. Diet, DDT and the toxicity of drugs and chemicals. Fed Proc. 1977;36:1688.

157. Conney AH et al. Enhanced phenacetin metabolism in human subjects fed charcoal-broiled beef. Clin Pharmacol Ther. 1976;20:633.

158. Kappas A et al. Effect of charcoal-broiled beef on antipyrine and theophylline metabolism. Clin Pharmacol Ther. 1978;23:445.

159. Pantuck EJ et al. Simulatory effect of brussels sprouts and cabbage on human drug metabolism. Clin Pharmacol Ther. 1978;25:88.

160. Smithard DJ, Langman MJS. The effect of vitamin supplementation upon antipyrine metabolism in the elderly. Br J Clin Pharmacol. 1978;5:181.

161. Hartoma TR et al. Serum zinc and serum copper and indices of drug metabolism in alcoholics. Eur J Clin Pharmacol. 1977;12:147.

162. Melander A, McLean A. Influence of food intake on presystemic clearance of drugs. Clin Pharmacokinet. 1983;8:286.

163. Axelson JE et al. Food increases the bioavailability of propafenone. Br J Clin Pharmacol. 1987;23:735.

164. Challenor VF et al. Food and nifedipine pharmacokinetics. Br J Clin Pharmacol. 1987;23:248.

165. Woodcock BG et al. Effect of a high protein meal on the bioavailability of verapamil. Br J Clin Pharmacol. 1986;21:337.

166. Winstanley PA, Orme MLE. The effects of food on drug bioavailability. Br J Clin Pharmacol. 1989;28:621.

167. Liedholm H, Melander A. Concomitant food intake can increase the bioavailability of propranolol by transient inhibition of its presystemic primary conjugation. Clin Pharmacol Ther. 1986;40:29.

168. Modi MW et al. Influence of posture on hepatic perfusion and the presystemic biotransformation of propranolol: simulation of the food effect. Clin Pharmacol Ther. 1988;44:268.

169. Reinberg A, Smolensky MH. Circadian changes in drug dispositon in man. Clin Pharmacokinet. 1982;7:401.

170. Daneshmond TK et al. Physiological and pharmacological variability in estimated hepatic blood flow in man. Br J Clin Pharmacol. 1981;11:491.

171. Bass NM, Williams RL. Guide to drug dosage in hepatic disease. Clin Pharmacokinet. 1988;15:396.

172. Howden CW et al. Drug metabolism in liver disease. Pharmacol Ther. 1989;40:439.

173. Williams RL. Drug administration in hepatic disease. N Engl J Med. 1983;309:1616.

174. Razak TA et al. The effect of hepatic cirrhosis on the pharmacokinetics and blood pressure response to nicardipine. Clin Pharmacol Ther. 1990;47:463.

175. Neal EA et al. Enhanced bioavailability and decreased clearance of analgesics in patients with cirrhosis. Gastroenterology 1979;77:96.

176. Wood AJJ et al. The influence of cirrhosis on steady-state blood concentrations of unbound propranolol after oral administration. Clin Pharmacokinet. 1978;3:478.

177. Homeida M et al. Decreased first-pass metabolism of labetalol in chronic liver disease. Br J Med 1978;2:1048.

178. Blaschke TF. Protein binding and kinetics of drugs in liver diseases. Clin Pharmacokinet. 1977;2:32.

179. Lewis GP, Jusko WJ. Pharmacokinetics of ampicillin in cirrhosis. Clin Pharmacol Ther. 1975;18:475.

180. Somogyi A et al. Pharmacokinetics, bioavailability and ECG response of verapamil in patients with liver cirrhosis. Br J Clin Pharmacol. 1981;12:51.

181. Kraus JW et al. Effects of aging and liver disease on disposition of lorazepam. Clin Pharmacol Ther. 1978;24:411.

182. Azzollini F et al. Elimination of chloramphenicol and thiamphenicol in subjects with cirrhosis of the liver. Int J Clin Pharmacol Ther Toxical. 1972;6:130.

183. Marcantonio LA et al. The pharmacokinetics and pharmacodynamics of the diuretic bumetanide in hepatic and renal disease. Br J Clin Pharmacol. 1983;15:245.

184. Farrell GC et al. Drug metabolism in liver disease. Identification of patients with impaired hepatic drug metabolism. Gastroenterology. 1978;75:580.

185. Burnett DA et al. Altered elimination of antipyrine in patients with acute viral hepatitis. Gut. 1976;17:341.

186. Villeneuve JP et al. Drug disposition in patients with HBs Ag-positive chronic liver disease. Dig Dis Sci. 1987;32:710.

187. Powell JR et al. Theophylline disposition in acutely ill hospitalized patients. The effect of smoking, heart failure, severe airway obstruction, and pneumonia. Am Rev Respir Dis. 1978;118:229.

188. Longenecker HE et al. The effect of organic compounds upon vitamin C synthesis in the rat. J Biol Chem. 1940;135:497.

189. Richardson HL, Cunningham L. The inhibitory action of methylcholanthrene on rats fed the azo dye 3'-methyl-4-dimethylaminoazobenzene. Cancer Res. 1951;11:274.

190. Conney AH et al. The metabolism of methylated aminoazo dyes. V. Evidence for induction of enzyme synthesis in the rat by 3-methylcholanthrene. Cancer Res. 1956;16:450.

191. Remmer H, Merker HJ. Drug-induced changes in the liver endoplasmic reticulum: association with drug-metabolizing enzymes. Science. 1963;142:1657.

192. Okey AB. Enzyme induction in the cytochrome P-450 system. Pharmacol Ther. 1990;45:241.

193. Farrell GC, Murray M. Human cytochrome P-450 isoforms. Gastroenterology 1990;99:885.

194. Conney AH. Pharmacological implications of microsomal enzyme induction. Pharmacol Rev. 1967;19:317.

195. Gelehrter TD. Enzyme induction. N Engl J Med. 1976;294:522.

196. Yates MS et al. Differential effects of hepatic microsomal enzyme inducing agents on liver blood flow. Biochem Pharmacol. 1978;27:2617.

197. Kato R, Gilette JR. Sex differences in the effects of abnormal physiological states on the metabolism of drugs by rat liver microsomes. J Pharmacol Exp Ther. 1965;150:285.

198. McDevitt DG et al. Influence of phenobarbital on factors responsible for hepatic clearance of indocyanine green in the rat: relative contributions of induction and altered liver blood flow. Biochem Pharmacol. 1977;26:1247.

199. Branch RA et al. Increased clearance of antipyrine and d-propranolol after phenobarbital pretreatment in the monkey. J Clin Invest. 1974;53:1101.

200. Pirttiaho HI et al. Liver size and indices of drug metabolism in epileptics. Br J Clin Pharmacol. 1978;6:273.

201. Sotaniemi EA et al. Drug metabolism in epileptics: *in vivo* and *in vitro* correlations. Br J Clin Pharmacol. 1978;5:71.

202. Pirttiaho HI et al. Hepatic blood flow and drug metabolism in patients on enzyme-inducing anticonvulsants. Eur J Clin Pharmacol. 1982;22:441.

203. Sotaniemi EA et al. Measurement of hepatic drug-metabolizing enzyme activity in man: comparison of three different assays. Eur J Clin Pharmacol. 1980;17:267.

204. Roberts CJC et al. The relationship between liver volume, antipyrine clearance, and indocyanine green clearance before and after phenobarbitone administration in man. Br J Clin Pharmacol. 1976;3:907.

205. Rutledge DR et al. Effects of chronic phenobarbital on verapamil disposition in humans. J Pharmacol Exp Ther. 1988;246:7.

206. Pantuck EJ et al. Effect of cigarette smoking on phenacetin metabolism. Clin Pharmacol Ther. 1974;15:9.

207. Vahakangas K et al. Cigarette smoking and drug metabolism. Clin Pharmacol Ther. 1983;33:375.

208. Boobis AR et al. Monooxygenase activity of human liver in microsomal fractions of needle biopsy specimens. Br J Clin Pharmacol. 1980;9:11.

209. Sesardic D et al. A form of cytochrome P-450 in man, orthologous to form d in the rat, catalyses the o-deethylation of phenacetin and is inducible by cigarette smoking. Br J Clin Pharmacol. 1988;26:363.

210. Vestal RE, Wood AJJ. Influence of age and smoking on drug kinetics in man. Clin Pharmacokinet. 1980;5:309.

211. Breimer DD et al. Influence of rifampicin on drug metabolism: Differences between hexobarbital and antipyrine. Clin Pharmacol Ther. 1977;21:470.

212. Diaz D et al. Omeprazole is an aryl hydrocarbon-like inducer of human hepatic cytochrome P-450. Gastroenterology 1990;99:737.

213. Guengerich FP. Roles of cytochrome P-450 enzymes in chemical carcinogenesis and cancer chemotherapy. Cancer Res. 1988;48:2946.

214. Gugler R, Jensen JC. Omeprazole inhibits oxidative drug metabolism. Studies with diazepam and phenytoin *in vivo* and 7-ethoxycoumarin *in vitro*. Gastroenterology 1985;89:1235.

215. Bock KW et al. Induction and inhibition of conjugating enzymes with emphasis on UDP-glucuronyltransferases. Pharmacol Ther. 1987;33:23.

216. Krasinski K et al. Pharmacologic interactions among chloramphenicol, phenytoin, and phenobarbital. Pediatr Infect Dis. 1982;1:232.

217. Bock KW, Schirmer G. Species differences of glucuronidation and sulfation in relation to hepatocarcinogenesis. Arch Toxicol. 1987;10S:125.

218. Ochs HR et al. Disposition of oxazepam in relation to age, sex, and cigarette smoking. Klin Wochenschr. 1981;59:899.

219. Miners JO et al. Determinants of acetaminophen metabolism: effects of inducers and inhibitors of drug metabolism on acetaminophen's metabolic pathways. Clin Pharmacol Ther. 1984;35:480.

220. Branch RA, Shand DG. A re-evaluation of intersubject variation in enzyme induction in man. Clin Pharmacokinet. 1979;4:104.

221. Vesell ES, Page JG. Genetic control of the phenobarbital-induced shortening of plasma antipyrine half-lives in man. J Clin Invest. 1969;48:2202.

222. Powell JR, Cate EW. Induction and inhibition of drug metabolism. In: Evans WE et al, eds. Applied Pharmacokinetics. Vancouver, Washington: Applied Therapeutics Inc.; 1986:139–186.

223. Kapil RP et al. Disopyramide pharmacokinetics and metabolism: effect of inducers. Br J Clin Pharmacol. 1987;24:781.

224. Patsalos PN et al. Effect of the removal of individual antiepileptic drugs on antipyrine kinetics in patients taking polytherapy. Br J Clin Pharmacol. 1988;26:253.

225. Breckenridge A et al. Dose-dependent enzyme induction. Clin Pharmacol Ther. 1973;14:514.

226. Greim HA. An overview of the phenomena of enzyme induction and inhibition: Their relevance to drug action and drug interactions. In: Jenner P, Testa B, eds. Concepts in Drug Metabolism, Part B. New York:Marcel Dekker; 1981:240.

227. Price DE et al. The effect of low-dose phenobarbitone on three indices of hepatic microsomal enzyme induction. Br J Clin Pharmacol. 1986;22:744.

228. Ohnhaus EE, Park BK. Measurement of urinary 6-β-hydroxycortisol excretion as an *in vivo* parameter in the clinical assessment of the microsomal enzyme-inducing capacity of antipyrine, phenobarbitone, and rifampicin. Eur J Clin Pharmacol. 1979;15:139.

229. Herman RJ et al. Induction of propranolol metabolism by rifampicin. Br J Clin Pharmacol. 1983;16:565.

230. Vestal RE et al. Antipyrine metabolism in man: Influence of age, alcohol, caffeine, and smoking. Clin Pharmacol Ther. 1975;18:425.

231. Rose JQ et al. Phenytoin disposition in smokers and nonsmokers. Int J Clin Pharmacol. 1978;16:547.

232. Breckenridge AM, Orme MLE. Clinical implications of enzyme induction. Ann NY Acad Sci. 1971;179:421.

233. Dossing M et al. Time course of phenobarbital and cimetidine mediated changes in hepatic drug metabolism. Eur J Clin Pharmacol. 1983;25:215.

234. O'Reilly RA. Interaction of chronic daily warfarin therapy and rifampin. Ann Intern Med. 1974;81:337.

235. Ohnhaus EE et al. Enzyme-inducing drug combinations and their effects on liver microsomal enzyme activity in man. Eur J Clin Pharmacol. 1983;24:247.

236. Branch RA, Herman RJ. Enzyme induction and beta-adrenergic receptor blocking drugs. Br J Clin Pharmacol. 1984;17:77S.

237. Landay RA et al. Effect of phenobarbital on theophylline disposition. J Allergy Clin Immunol. 1978;62:27.

238. Bachmann K et al. Smoking and warfarin disposition. Clin Pharmacol Ther. 1979;25:309.

239. Hart P et al. Enhanced drug metabolism in cigarette smokers. Br Med J. 1976;2:147.

240. Powell JR et al. The influence of cigarette smoking and sex on theophylline disposition. Am Rev Respir Dis. 1977;116:17.

241. Hunt SN et al. Effect of smoking on theophylline disposition. Clin Pharmacol Ther. 1976;19:546.

242. Salem SAM et al. Reduced induction of drug metabolism in the elderly. Age Ageing. 1978;68–73.

243. Kato R, Takanaka A. Effect of phenobarbital on electron transport system, oxidation and reduction of drugs in liver microsomes of rats of different age. J Biochem (Tokyo). 1968;63:406.

244. Adelman RC. Impaired hormonal regulation of enzyme activity during aging. Fed Proc. 1975;34:179.

245. Zilly W et al. Stimulation of drug metabolism by rifampicin in patients with cirrhosis or cholestasis measured by increased hexobarbital and tolbutamide clearance. Eur J Clin Pharmacol. 1977;11:287.

246. Richter E et al. Disposition of hexobarbital in intra- and extrahepatic cholestasis in man and the influence of drug metabolism-inducing agents. Eur J Clin Pharmacol. 1980;17:197.

247. Farrell GC et al. Drug metabolism in liver disease. Identification of patients with impaired hepatic drug metabolism. Gastroenterology. 1978;75:580.

248. Bai SA, Abramson FP. Interactions of phenobarbital with propranolol in the dog. 1. Plasma protein binding. J Pharmacol Exp Ther. 1982;222:589.

249. Routledge PA et al. Lidocaine disposition in blood in epilepsy. Br J Clin Pharmacol. 1981;12:663.

250. Macdonald JI et al. Sex-difference and the effects of smoking and oral contraceptive steroids on the kinetics of diflunisal. Eur J Clin Pharmacol. 1990;38:175.

251. McNamara PJ et al. Effect of smoking on binding of lidocaine to human serum proteins. J Pharm Sci. 1980;69:749.

252. Feely J et al. Enzyme induction with rifampicin; lipoproteins and binding to α_1-acid glycoprotein. Br J Clin Pharmacol. 1983;16:195.

253. Black M et al. Effect of phenobarbitone on plasma ^{14}C-bilirubin clearance in patients with unconjugated hyperbilirubinemia. Clin Sci Mol Med. 1974;46:1.

254. Luoma PV et al. Plasma high-density lipoproteins and hepatic microsomal enzyme induction. Eur J Clin Pharmacol. 1982;23:275.

255. Acocella G et al. Serum concentrations and biliary of bilirubin excretion during short-term treatment with rifampicin. Tijdschrift voor Gastroenterol. 1973;16:186.

256. Luoma PV et al. Serum low-density lipoprotein and high-density lipoprotein cholesterol, and liver size in subjects on drugs inducing hepatic microsomal enzymes. Eur J Clin Pharmacol. 1985; 28:615.

257. Lewis RJ et al. Warfarin. Stereochemical aspects of its metabolism and the interaction with phenylbutazone. J Clin Invest. 1974;53:1607.

258. Netter KJ. Inhibition of oxidative drug metabolism in microsomes. Pharmacol Ther. 1980;10:515.

259. Testa B, Jenner P. Inhibitors of cytochrome P-450s and their mechanism of action. Drug Metab Rev. 1981;12:1.

260. Vesell ES et al. Impairment of drug metabolism by disulfiram in man. Clin Pharmacol Ther. 1971;12:785.

261. O'Reilly RA. Interaction of sodium warfarin and disulfiram (antabuse) in man. Ann Intern Med. 1973;78:73.

262. Svendsen TL et al. The influence of disulfiram on the half-life and metabolic clearance rate of diphenylhydantoin and tolbutamide in man. Eur J Clin Pharmacol. 1976;9:439.

263. Vesell ES et al. Impairment of drug metabolism in man by allopurinol and nortriptyline. N Engl J Med. 1970;283:1484.

264. Manfredi RL, Vesell ES. Inhibition of theophylline metabolism by long-term allopurinol administration. Clin Pharmacol Ther. 1981;29:224.

265. Edwards DJ et al. Inhibition of drug metabolism by quinolone antibiotics. Clin Pharmacokinet. 1988;15:194.

266. Toon S et al. Enoxacin-warfarin interaction: pharmacokinetic and stereochemical aspects. Clin Pharmacol Ther. 1987;42:33.

267. Logamann C, Ohnhaus EE. Enoxacin, a differential inhibitor of the microsomal liver enzyme system in men. Paper presented to 26th Interscience Conference on Antimicrobial Agents and Chemotherapy. New Orleans, LA: 1986.

268. Thomas D et al. A study to evaluate the potential pharmacokinetic interaction between oral enoxacin and oral phenytoin. Phar Res. 1986; 3:99S(#3).

269. Kalant H et al. Ethanol—a direct inducer of drug metabolism. Biochem Pharmacol. 1976;25:337.

270. Khanna JM et al. Effect of chronic ethanol treatment on metabolism of drugs *in vitro* and *in vivo*. Biochem Pharmacol. 1976;25:329.

271. Rubin E, Lieber CS. Hepatic microsomal enzymes in man and rat: induction and inhibition by ethanol. Science. 1968;162:690.

272. Zemaitis MA, Greene FE. Impairment of hepatic microsomal drug metabolism in the rat during daily disulfiram administration. Biochem Pharmacol. 1976;25:1355.

273. Honjo T, Netter KJ. Inhibition of drug demethylation by disulfiram *in vivo* and *in vitro*. Biochem Pharmacol. 1969;18:2681.

274. Knodell RG et al. Drug metabolism by rat and human hepatic microsomes in response to interaction with H_2-receptor antagonists. Gastroenterology. 1982;82:84.

275. Hoyumpa AM et al. Effect of short-term ethanol administration on lorazepam clearance. Hepatology. 1981;1:47.

276. Linnoila M, Hakkinen S. Effects of diazepam and codeine, alone and in combination with alcohol, on simulated driving. Clin Pharmacol Ther. 1974;15:368.

277. Palva ES, Linnoila M. Effect of active metabolites of chlordiazepoxide and diazepam, alone or in combination with alcohol, on psychomotor skills related to driving. Eur J Clin Pharmacol. 1978;13:345.

278. Thurman RG, Kauffman FC. Factors regulating drug metabolism in intact hepatocytes. Pharmacol Rev. 1979;31:229.

279. Reinke LA et al. Interactions between ethanol metabolism and mixed-function oxidation in perfused rat liver: Inhibition of p-nitroanisole o-demethylation. J Pharmacol Exp Ther. 1980;213:70.

280. Bertram B et al. Effects of disulfiram on mixed function oxidase system and trace element concentration in the liver of rats. Biochem Pharmacol. 1982;31:3613.

281. Speeg KV et al. Inhibition of microsomal drug metabolism by histamine H_2-receptor antagonists studied *in vivo* and *in vitro* in rodents. Gastroenterology. 1982;82:89.

282. MacKichan JJ et al. Effect of cimetidine on quinidine bioavailability. Biopharm Drug Dispos. 1989;10:121.

283. Desmond PV et al. Short-term ethanol administration impairs the elimination of chlordiazepoxide (Librium) in man. Eur J Clin Pharmacol. 1980;18:275.

284. Sellers EM et al. Intravenous diazepam and oral ethanol interaction. Clin Pharmacol Ther. 1980;28:638.

285. Carulli N et al. Alcohol-drugs interaction in man: alcohol and tolbutamide. Eur J Clin Invest. 1971;1:421.

286. Bury RW et al. The effect of ethanol administration on the disposition and elimination of chlormethiazole. Eur J Clin Pharmacol. 1983;24:383.

287. MacLeod SM et al. Interaction of disulfiram with benzodiazepines. Clin Pharmacol Ther. 1978;24:583.

288. O'Reilly RA. Interaction of sodium warfarin and disulfiram (antabuse) in man. Ann Intern Med. 1973;78:73.

289. Vestal RE et al. Cimetidine inhibits theophylline clearance in patients with chronic obstructive pulmonary disease: A study using stable isotope methodology during multiple oral dose administration. Br J Clin Pharmacol. 1983;15:411.

290. Feely J et al. Factors affecting the response to inhibition of drug metabolism by cimetidine-dose response and sensitivity of elderly and induced subjects. Br J Clin Pharmacol. 1984;17:77.

291. Bartle WR et al. Dose-dependent effect of cimetidine on phenytoin kinetics. Clin Pharmacol Ther. 1983;33:649.

292. Hetzel D et al. Cimetidine interaction with warfarin. Lancet. 1979;2:639.

293. Powell JR et al. Inhibition of theophylline clearance by cimetidine but not ranitidine. Arch Int Med. 1984;144:484.

294. Rose JQ et al. Intoxication caused by interaction of chloramphenicol and phenytoin. JAMA. 1977;237:2630.

295. Lalonde RL et al. The effects of cimetidine on theophylline pharmacokinetics at steady state. Chest. 1983;83:221.

296. Serlin MJ et al. Cimetidine: interaction with oral anticoagulants in man. Lancet. 1979;2:317.

297. Greenblatt DJ et al. Clinical importance of the interaction of diazepam and cimetidine. N Engl J Med. 1984;310:1639.

298. Patwardhan RV et al. Lack of tolerance and rapid recovery of cimetidine-inhibited chlordiazepoxide (Librium) elimination. Gastroenterology. 1981;81:547.

299. Reitberg DP et al. Alteration of theophylline clearance and half-life by cimetidine in normal volunteers. Ann Intern Med. 1981;95:582.

300. Brunova E et al. Interaction of tolbutamide and chloramphenicol in diabetic patients. Int J Clin Pharmacol. 1977;15:7.

301. Greenlaw CW. Chloramphenicol-phenytoin drug interaction. Drug Intell Clin Pharm. 1979;13:609.

302. Koup JR et al. Interaction of chloramphenicol with phenytoin and phenobarbital. Clin Pharmacol Ther. 1978;24:571.

303. Roberts RK et al. Cimetidine-theophylline interaction in patients with chronic obstructive airways disease. Med. J. Aust. 1984;140:279.

304. Powell JR, Donn KH. Histamine H_2-antagonist drug interactions in perspective: mechanistic concepts and clinical implications. Am J Med. 1984;77(Suppl 5B):57.

305. Bradbear RA et al. Cimetidine use in children with cystic fibrosis: inhibition of hepatic drug metabolism. J Pediatr. 1982;100:325.

306. Miners JO et al. Interaction between cimetidine and theophylline in smokers and non-smokers. Clin Exp Physiol Pharmacol. 1981;8:633.

307. Grygiel JJ et al. Differential effects of cimetidine on theophylline metabolic pathways. Eur J Clin Pharmacol. 1984;26:335.

308. May DC et al. Effects of cimetidine on caffeine disposition in smokers and nonsmokers. Clin Pharmacol Ther. 1982;31:656.

309. Rollinghoff W, Paumgartner G. Inhibition of drug metabolism by cimetidine in man: dependence on pretreatment microsomal liver function. Eur J Clin Invest. 1982;12:429.

310. Staiger C et al. The influence of cimetidine on antipyrine pharmacokinetics in patients with and without cirrhosis of the liver. Int J Clin Pharmacol Ther Toxicol. 1981;19:561.

311. Nebert DW et al. Genetic mechanisms controlling the induction of polysubstrate mono-oxygenase (P-450) activities. Ann Rev Pharmacol Toxicol. 1981;21:431.

312. Naranjo CA et al. An intensive drug monitoring study suggesting possible clinical irrelevance of impaired drug disposition in liver disease. Br J Clin Pharmacol. 1983; 15:451.

313. Laidlaw et al. Morphine tolerance in hepatic cirrhosis. Gastroenterology 1961; 40:389.

314. Maxwell JD et al. Plasma disappearance and cerebral effects of chlorpromazine in cirrhosis. Clin Sci. 1972; 43:143.

315. Branch RA et al. Intravenous administration of diazepam in patients with chronic liver disease. Gut. 1976;17:975.

316. Fessel JM, Conn HO. An analysis of causes and prevention of hepatic coma. Gastroenterology. 1972;62:191.

317. Danhof M et al. Kinetics of drug action in disease states. XII. effect of experimental liver diseases on the pharmacodynamics of phenobarbital and ethanol in rats. J Pharm Sci. 1985; 74:321.

318. Ramzan IM et al. Kinetics of drug action in disease states. XIX. effect of experimental liver disease on the neurotoxicity of theophylline in rats. J Pharmacol Exp Ther. 1987; 241:236.

319. Benet LZ, Williams RL. Design and optimization of dosage regimens: pharmacokinetic data. In: Gilman AG et al., eds. The Pharmacologic Basis of Therapeutics. New York: Pergamon Press; 1990:1650–1735.

320. Arns PA et al. Adjustment of medications in liver failure. In: Chernow B, ed. The Pharmacologic Approach to the Critically Ill Patient. Baltimore: Williams & Wilkins; 1988:85–111.

Chapter 7

Genetic Polymorphisms of Drug Metabolism

Mary V. Relling and William E. Evans

Many factors contribute to variability in drug metabolism among and within individuals. One of the most pronounced factors accounting for interindividual differences in metabolism and, thus, in the pharmacokinetics of certain drugs is genetically regulated polymorphic drug metabolism. That is, certain drug metabolizing activities exhibit a polymorphic distribution within a population, and the inheritance of that enzymatic activity is controlled at a single genetic locus. The broader topic of pharmacogenetics has been defined as the "attempt to understand the hereditary basis for two individuals . . . responding differently to drugs or other foreign chemicals."[1] Although both receptor-related and pharmacokinetic-related genetic factors are key influences on a patient's response to a given drug and/or metabolite, this chapter focuses on pharmacogenetics of drug metabolism related to polymorphisms of particular enzymes, given that these polymorphisms directly affect the pharmacokinetics of drugs. The reader is referred to other reviews for a discussion of other aspects of pharmacogenetics.[2-4]

This chapter focuses on three particular polymorphic enzymes: debrisoquin hydroxylase (CYP2D6), mephenytoin hydroxylase, and N-acetyltransferase, each of which has been the subject of recent reviews.[5-11] (Note: the nomenclature used in this chapter is that described by Nebert et al.[5] Previously, the IID6 protein and its cDNA were designated IID1. This enzyme is encoded by the CYP2D6 gene.) Polymorphisms of other enzymes, such as aldehyde dehydrogenase[12] (affecting ethanol's metabolite, acetaldehyde), thiopurine methyltransferase[13] (metabolizing mercaptopurine and azathioprine), and carbocysteine oxidation,[14] are also important for affected drugs but are beyond the scope of this review. The general principles underlying the biology and clinical pharmacokinetic and pharmacodynamic consequences of these particular polymorphisms should be applicable as other polymorphic enzymes are discovered and additional drugs are found to be polymorphic substrates.

DEBRISOQUIN-TYPE OXIDATION

Background, Inheritance, and Ethnic Differences

Debrisoquin is an antihypertensive agent which was found to exhibit a poly-morphism in both its hypotensive activity and pharmacokinetics by Dr. Robert Smith's group in 1977.[15] A small subset (3%) of subjects were termed "poor metabolizers" (PMs) in that they were deficient in their ability to oxidize, and thereby inactivate, debrisoquin to 4-hydroxydebrisoquin; they therefore suffered exaggerated pharmacologic response (prolonged low blood pressure) to doses of debrisoquin that the majority of the population (termed "extensive metabolizers" or EMs) tolerated without problems. These investigators also coined the term "metabolic ratio" to indicate the urinary concentration ratio of parent drug to the polymorphically formed metabolite in a timed urine collection. This ratio clearly divided the population into its two phenotypes (EMs and PMs), with the "anti-mode" being the metabolic ratio dividing the population into its two phenotypes. A typical frequency distribution for debrisoquin metabolic ratios is depicted in Figure 7-1.[16]

Family studies[15–18] have shown that the PM phenotype is inherited as an autosomal recessive trait; defective copies of both maternal and paternal genes are required for the PM phenotype (see Figure 7-2). Most clinical evidence to date indicates that heterozygous and homozygous EMs are not distinguishable on the basis of their metabolic ratio (see Figure 7-1);[16] however, this point is still

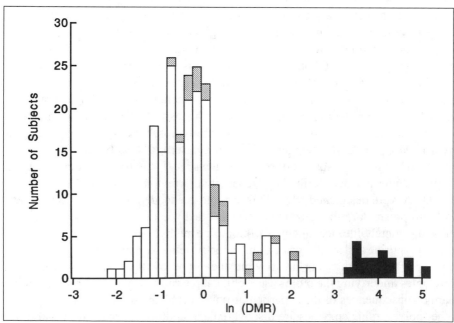

Figure 7-1. *Frequency distribution of the urinary metabolic ratio (MR) of debrisoquin to 4-hydroxydebrisoquin on a log scale among 225 Swedish subjects. Open bars indicate extensive metabolizers; closed bars indicate poor metabolizers; shaded bars indicate obligate heterozy-gotes (reproduced with permission, reference 16).*

somewhat controversial, and the assertion continues to be made by some that heterozygote EMs are likely to have higher ratios than homozygotes.[17,19] Cloning of the debrisoquin hydroxylase gene (CYP2D6) has helped to shed some light on this question.

Almost simultaneously with the British group, Eichelbaum and coworkers described a similar polymorphism for the oxytocic agent sparteine,[18] and showed that sparteine metabolism cosegregated with debrisoquin metabolism. The list of agents whose metabolism cosegregates with that of debrisoquin and sparteine has grown to over 25 (see Table 7-1). Potential substrates are identified either by systematic *in vitro* studies of competitive inhibitors of prototype debrisoquin hydroxylase reactions in human liver microsomes,[41,42] or by candidate substrates being chemically or pharmacologically similar to known substrates. There are several published studies of *in vitro* screenings for inhibitors. These studies have detected a large number of drugs that do not inhibit debrisoquin hydroxylase and, therefore must *not* be substrates *in vivo*.[41-44] These *in vitro* screenings are useful first steps in identifying and ruling out potential substrates for debrisoquin hydroxylase. When potential substrates are identified by competitive inhibition studies, further confirmatory studies are necessary. These should show that the human *in vivo* pharmacokinetics of the substrate cosegregate with those of a known substrate or that *in vitro* human microsomal kinetics for the candidate substrate are different in EM and PM livers, consistent with the prototype substrate.

Phenotyping studies have been performed in subjects of various ethnic origins to define the prevalence of the PM phenotype in different genetic groups.[45-50] In

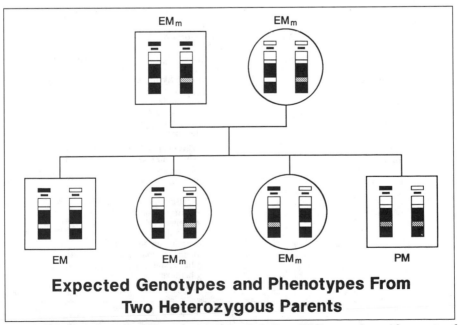

Expected Genotypes and Phenotypes From Two Heterozygous Parents

Figure 7-2. *Hypothetical pedigree for a poor metabolizer (PM) propositus with parents of extensive metabolizer (EM) phenotype. Their genotype is obligate heterozygote, and the expected probable distribution of genotypes and phenotypes in offspring is indicated.*

general, the prevalence for all groups studied has ranged between 2% and 10%, although in a few groups (Japanese, Panamanian Amerindians, Chinese) no or very few PMs have been identified.[49-51] It should be recognized that a sample size of 200 is required to distinguish between a 5% and 10% prevalence of the PM phenotype at about an 85% power, with an alpha equal to 0.05; therefore, many of the published studies have rather large confidence intervals about their estimates of the prevalence of PM phenotypes. In addition, a recent report which used both debrisoquin and codeine to determine phenotype in a group of Chinese, demonstrated the absence of a bimodal distribution of either of the substrates' metabolic ratios; it also revealed no PMs among Chinese when the antimode determined in European population studies was used.[52] Interestingly, using restriction fragment length polymorphism (RFLP) analysis of genomic DNA (see Molecular Basis), 7 of 21 Chinese subjects had RFLP patterns (i.e., 44/44 Kb and 44/11.5 Kb patterns) associated with the poor metabolizer phenotype in Caucasians, yet none were PMs by urinary metabolic ratios. However, different conclusions are reached if a different antimode is used to define PMs in the Chinese population. If a lower antimode were valid to separate Chinese EMs and PMs, the phenotype and RFLP analyses would be consistent with previously reported data.[53] Alternatively, if the frequency distribution of the metabolic ratios is not bimodal in the Chinese, it appears that RFLP patterns determined to identify the PM phenotype in one population cannot necessarily be extrapolated to an unrelated ethnic group. Hence, caution must be exercised when attempting to extrapolate data from one ethnic group to another because it may be necessary to establish reliable phenotyping and genotyping methods in each new population studied.

Table 7-1. *Substrates for Debrisoquin Hydroxylase*

Class	Reference	Class	Reference
Beta blockers		**Antiarrhythmics**	
bufuralol	20	propafenone	31
timolol	21	encainide	32
propranolol	22	N-propylajmaline	33
metoprolol	23	perhexiline	34
alprenolol	24	flecainide	35
Antidepressants		**Antihypertensives**	
amiflamine	25	debrisoquin	15
amitriptyline	26	guanoxan	34
nortriptyline	27	indoramin	36
clomipramine	28		
imipramine	21	**Miscellaneous**	
desipramine	29	dextromethorphan	37
		codeine	38
		metiamide	39
		methoxyamphetamine	34
		methoxphenamine	40
		phenacetin	34
		phenformin	34
		sparteine	18

Clinical Consequences for Affected Substrates

Before reviewing selected examples of clinical consequences of the debrisoquin polymorphism, it is worthwhile to note that if there are consequences for the PM phenotype, a relatively small percentage of the population will be affected. Initial Phase I pharmacokinetic studies of new drugs are often conducted in small groups of 8 to 12 subjects, so identification of the minority who comprise the PM phenotype is highly unlikely. For example, with a sample size of 10, there is a 60% chance that all of the subjects will be EMs. One needs a sample size of 60 to have 95% confidence that at least one subject will be a PM. Moreover, there has sometimes been a tendency to discount data obtained from rare "outliers" in such preliminary studies. Therefore, genetic polymorphisms of drug metabolism may go unrecognized until a new drug has been evaluated in several hundred subjects. In the future, awareness of genetic polymorphism of drug metabolism may change the way in which Phase I studies are interpreted and even conducted; examples in which oxidative phenotype determination has been incorporated in Phase I studies already exist.[54]

Not every possible clinical consequence of the debrisoquin hydroxylase polymorphism is reviewed in this chapter; however, most of the general principles underlying known clinical effects of genetic polymorphisms are addressed. There is additional information on tricyclic antidepressants and beta blocking agents in their respective chapters in this text, as well as several reviews on this subject.[46,55,56]

There are three general metabolic possibilities for debrisoquin hydroxylase polymorphism and drug metabolism. The enzyme may be responsible for in-activating the active moiety, it may form an active metabolite from an inactive precursor, or it may form an active metabolite from a compound which itself possesses pharmacologic activity. These three possibilities generally have greatest clinical importance when the affected pathway represents a major pathway in the elimination of the drug; there are several examples of substrates for debrisoquin hydroxylase which undergo substantial elimination by other enzymes or renal excretion.[22,24,57] One must bear in mind, however, that even in cases where the affected pathway is quantitatively minor (e.g., activation of codeine to morphine),[58] it may be qualitatively important for pharmacologic activity for that agent. Some examples are discussed below.

Antidepressants. For many drugs subject to the debrisoquin polymorphism, the relationship between pharmacologic effect and phenotype is complicated by the fact that both the parent drug and polymorphically formed metabolites elicit therapeutic and toxic effects. For instance, amitriptyline is demethylated to nor-triptyline, and both are hydroxylated. It has been suggested that all four compounds have antidepressant activity.[26] Hydroxylation of both compounds appears to be by debrisoquin hydroxylase, and it has been postulated that even demethylation cosegregates with debrisoquin phenotype in nonsmokers.[59] In smokers, induction of other cytochrome P450 enzymes presumably accounts for most of the demethylation. Most likely because of the confounding effects of pharmacologically active metabolites, there were no clinically significant differences in antidepressant effects in EMs versus PMs, although PMs had lower ratios of plasma hydroxylated metabolites to total amitriptyline plus nortriptyline.[26]

In contrast, the demethylation of imipramine to desipramine does not seem to be a pathway catalyzed by debrisoquin hydroxylase,[29,60] does not appear to be induced in smokers,[60] and has been shown not to be inhibited by the debrisoquin hydroxylase inhibitor, quinidine[61] (hydroxylation of imipramine was inhibited by quinidine). It has been suggested that, on average, PMs require smaller daily doses of imipramine (i.e., 50 mg) to achieve "therapeutic" plasma concentrations of imipramine plus desipramine, when compared to EMs (50 to 400 mg).[29] In fact, PMs have prolonged plasma concentrations of desipramine after IV doses of imipramine compared to EMs (terminal half-life of 125 versus 21.5 hours); in contrast, imipramine half-lives do not significantly differ (see Figure 7-3).[60] The fact that parent drug, imipramine, did not accumulate was hypothesized to be due to saturation of hydroxylation versus demethylation in EMs. PMs of desipramine have average apparent oral clearances almost ten times lower than EMs.[91] There is anecdotal evidence that PMs may have more CNS toxicity with nortriptyline (a monomethylated tricyclic) than EMs.[27] However, although the ratio of hydroxylated nortriptyline to nortriptyline correlated with the sparteine metabolic ratio, it has been suggested that the debrisoquin oxidative phenotype accounts for only 40% to 60% of the variability in nortriptyline plasma concentrations.[62] Moreover, activity of 10-hydroxynortriptyline in inhibiting norepinephrine uptake may complicate the clinical consequences for PMs taking nortriptyline.[59]

Beta-Adrenergic Blocking Agents. Beta-blockers serve as a paradigm for several principles governing the clinical importance of genetic polymorphism of drug metabolism. First, some metabolites which are formed by polymorphic enzymes are also formed by other P450s. Second, the quantitatively significant formation of other nonpolymorphically regulated metabolites diminishes the importance of genetic polymorphism for selected agents. Finally, the beta blockers exist as stereoisomers, and there is frequently stereoselective metabolism of the

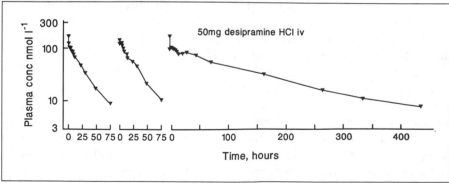

Figure 7-3. *Mean plasma concentrations of desipramine after an IV dose of desipramine in four rapid EMs (left), four slow EMs (middle), and three PMs for debrisoquine hydroxylase (reproduced with permission, reference 60).*

enantiomeric parent compounds by debrisoquin hydroxylase. Figure 7-4 summarizes the pharmacodynamic differences between EMs and PMs for four beta
blockers.[24]

Metoprolol metabolism to α-hydroxymetoprolol is catalyzed by debrisoquin
hydroxylase. This metabolite is reported to have beta-blocking activity equal to
one-tenth or less that of the parent compound.[63,64] Not surprisingly then, PMs
experience more pronounced beta-blockade from metoprolol than do EMs.[24] The
rather large difference in plasma concentration between EMs and PMs cannot be
entirely accounted for by α-hydroxylation, since this pathway only accounts for
about 10% of metoprolol elimination in EMs.[24] Using quinidine inhibition *in vitro*
to elucidate those reactions catalyzed by debrisoquin hydroxylase and/or other
enzymes,[65] it has been shown that the quantitatively more important reaction of
O-demethylation is partially catalyzed by debrisoquin hydroxylase. The biphasic
nature of this reaction *in vitro* with human liver microsomes also indicates the
involvement of more than one enzyme.[65] PMs stereoselectively O-demethylate
S(−)-metoprolol more quickly than R(+)-metoprolol. The picture in EMs is complicated because debrisoquin hydroxylase (IID6) appears to stereoselectively

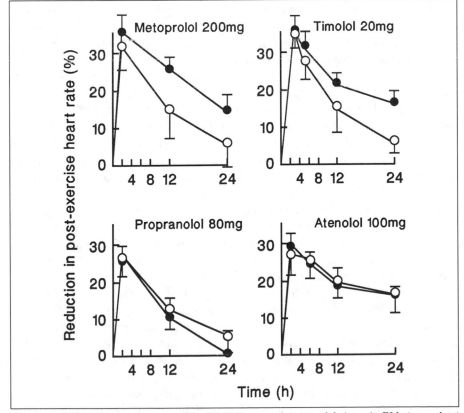

Figure 7-4. *Summary of pharmacodynamic differences between debrisoquin EMs (open dots)
and PMs (closed dots) for four beta-adrenergic blocking agents given orally. Number of
subjects: metoprolol six EMs, six PMs; timolol six EMs, four PMs; propranolol, seven EMs,
four PMs; and atenolol, six EMs, four PMs (reproduced with permission, reference 24).*

O-demethylate the R-isomer, the non-IID6 O-demethylating enzyme(s) is/are presumably also operative, and α-hydroxylation is nonstereoselective. Clinically, EMs tend to clear the R-enantiomer faster than the S-enantiomer.[66]

Timolol is administered as the S-isomer, so stereoselective metabolism is not a concern. The urinary concentration ratio of timolol to timolol ethanolamine corresponds best with the debrisoquin phenotype, although there is some overlap of this ratio in EMs versus PMs.[67] In addition, all timolol urinary metabolic ratios resulted in skewed unimodal rather than bimodal distributions in a population.[67] Although the exact pathways catalyzed by debrisoquin hydroxylase have not been elucidated, it is clear that PMs experience more beta-blockade from single doses than do EMs.[21] Such differences are not seen with atenolol, which is mostly renally excreted.[24]

Propranolol 4-hydroxylation is mediated by debrisoquin hydroxylase,[68] but it also undergoes substantial alternative metabolism by additional enzymes (including glucuronidation and side chain oxidation) in PM subjects; this results in nearly equivalent plasma concentration versus time profiles in EM and PM subjects.[22] The formation of naphthoxylactic acid by side chain oxidation correlates with the mephenytoin oxidative phenotype (see Mephenytoin),[68] as assessed by the urinary S:R mephenytoin ratio, with partial metabolic clearance to naphthoxylactic acid being 55% less in mephenytoin PMs. The fact that mephenytoin PMs are able to form significant quantities of naphthoxylactic acid indicates the involvement of one or more additional enzymes in this reaction.

The clinical implications of genetic polymorphism for beta-blocking agents have been reviewed,[24] and are also addressed in other chapters in this text.

Antiarrhythmics. *Encainide* is demethylated to two active metabolites, O-desmethyl encainide and 3-methoxydesmethyl encainide; both reactions appear to be mediated by debrisoquin hydroxylase.[32,69] All three compounds possess sodium channel blocking activities. Widening of the QRS interval on electrocardiogram is more prevalent in EMs than in PMs and has been correlated with plasma concentrations of O-desmethylencainide; however, antiarrhythmic efficacy has been demonstrated in both PMs and EMs.[70] It has been presumed that as long as adequate concentrations of either the parent drug, encainide, or demethylated metabolites are present,[45] antiarrhythmic efficacy is possible. The relative importance of the parent drug versus its metabolites as determinants of encainide's proarrhythmic effects remains to be clearly established.

Propafenone is a substrate for debrisoquin hydroxylase, with the affected metabolite being 5-hydroxypropafenone.[31,71] Both parent drug and metabolite have sodium channel-blocking effects; the parent drug (particularly the S-enantiomer) has more beta-blocking activity than does the metabolite. PMs have higher propafenone plasma concentrations; they are at higher risk of CNS side effects; they have less QRS widening at a given propafenone plasma concentration than EMs; and they are more likely to have greater beta-blockade effect than EMs because of increased concentrations of S-propafenone, although propafenone S:R ratios of parent drug are similar in EMs and PMs.[72]

Miscellaneous. The two initial prototype substrates (i.e., debrisoquin and sparteine) do not have active metabolites; therefore, enhanced drug effect is expected in PMs. Such effects include hypotension from debrisoquin[17] and blurred vision, headache, and dizziness from sparteine.[6] Conversely, PMs may be at risk for poor clinical response when the activity is primarily due to the affected metabolite. For instance, the failure of PMs to metabolize codeine to morphine results in lack of analgesic activity in these subjects.[38]

Inhibitors. Debrisoquin hydroxylase (IID6) is now known to be a specific form of cytochrome P450 which is absent in PMs (see Molecular Basis). Therefore, both "specific" IID6 inhibitors (e.g., quinidine) and relatively nonspecific inhibitors of P450 (e.g., cimetidine) may inhibit reactions catalyzed by debrisoquin hydroxylase. Moreover, any compound which is itself a substrate for this enzyme will inhibit the metabolism of another substrate for IID6, given that concentrations of the inhibitor are in the range of or exceed the Km of the reaction being inhibited. Much has been learned about these inhibitors from *in vitro* studies with human liver microsomes;[41–43] it can be assumed that compounds which do *not* inhibit debrisoquin *in vitro* at high concentrations will not inhibit debrisoquin hydroxylase *in vivo* and are not substrates for IID6. Conversely, compounds which are competitive inhibitors may or may not be substrates.

One compound which has proved very useful as a "specific" inhibitor of IID6 is quinidine, which competitively inhibits sparteine oxidation *in vitro* at a very low Ki of 60 nM.[41] (Ki is the dissociation constant of the enzyme-inhibitor complex.) However, quinidine itself is not a substrate for debrisoquin hydroxylase; in fact, quinidine 3-hydroxylation and N-oxidation appear to be catalyzed by the "nifedipine hydroxylase" P450 (IIIA4).[73] Therefore, quinidine's affinity is not absolutely specific for IID6, and at high enough concentrations, it theoretically also will inhibit the metabolism of substrates for IIIA4. However, it has potently and competitively inhibited every debrisoquin-hydroxylase-mediated reaction examined,[74,41,65,70,75] to the point that *in vivo* administration of even a single 250 mg dose of quinidine has resulted in "converting" EMs to PMs.[75] For example, when given a small dose of 50 mg every six hours before encainide, EMs developed pharmacokinetic and pharmacodynamic profiles similar to those of PMs, with a 90% decrease in the partial metabolic clearance to O-demethylated metabolites; encainide disposition in PMs was not affected.[70] Quinidine has also been useful in detecting the presence of more than one enzyme (i.e., more than just IID6) responsible for the formation of metabolite. Generally, a microsomal component with a low Km is inhibited by quinidine, while a component with a higher Km remains resistant to quinidine inhibition.[65,74]

Cimetidine is a nonspecific P450 inhibitor that decreases the clearance of desipramine by over 50% in EMs (mostly due to decreased 2-hydroxylation) without affecting the oral clearance or 2-hydroxylation in PMs.[91] Cimetidine also increased the debrisoquin urinary metabolic ratio in a group of EMs (although none were "converted" to PMs) and decreased the total, metabolic and renal clearance of sparteine in EMs as well as PMs.[76] The explanation for the reduction in clearance in PMs is partially ascribed to decreased renal clearance. These results are consistent with *in vitro* inhibition studies showing inhibition of sparteine oxidation[42] and desipramine hydroxylation in human liver microsomes.[77]

Inducers. Given that in at least some PMs IID6 is either deleted, or IID6 mutants result in mRNA splicing defects which are responsible for production of unstable, nonfunctional IID6 transcripts,[78] it seems unlikely that typical P450 enzyme inducers could increase production of IID6 cytochrome P450 in PMs, at least not by increasing transcription of the IID6 gene. However, there is evidence that debrisoquin hydroxylase is inducible in EMs. It should be acknowledged that the induction of other (non-IID6) cytochrome P450s capable of metabolizing a given substrate could affect the amount of parent compound and metabolite in urine, thus altering the metabolic ratio without affecting debrisoquin hydroxylase itself.

Rifampin. Eichelbaum et al. found that 1200 mg per day of rifampin for seven days significantly increased sparteine's apparent oral clearance from 7.5 to 9.5 mL/min/kg and its metabolic clearance from 6.2 to 8.5 mL/min/kg in EMs; it had no significant effect on either process in PMs.[79] Cumulative urinary excretion of sparteine, 2- and 5-dehydrosparteine, and the sum of all three compounds were significantly decreased after rifampin treatment in EMs; however, there was no significant change in the metabolic ratio. There were no significant effects in PMs.[79] Sparteine disposition was not affected by phenobarbital pretreatment in EMs (PMs not studied). Sparteine clearance was not induced in EMs or in PMs by eight days pretreatment with 100 mg per day of pentobarbital.[80]

The effects of rifampin 600 mg per day for 22 days on propranolol oral clearance, as well as on its metabolism to propranolol glucuronide, 4-hydroxy-propranolol and its glucuronide have also been studied.[81] Overall, propranolol oral clearance was increased about fourfold in both EMs and PMs, but the absolute increase in clearance in PMs was much smaller (758 versus 215 L/hr). The calculated "fractional clearances" to both 4-hydroxypropranolol and propranolol glucuronide increased after rifampin treatment, suggesting no selectivity in rifampin's effects. The mechanisms responsible for the enhanced overall clearance of propranolol did undergo a greater absolute induction in EMs than in PMs; the authors conclude that either debrisoquin hydroxylase or some coinherited P450 was induced more in EMs than PMs.

Taken together, these data indicate that debrisoquin hydroxylase is most likely not a phenobarbital-inducible P450, that it (or other enzymes with similar substrate specificity) appears to be induced by rifampin in EMs, and that its inducibility in PMs has not been clearly demonstrated.

Clinical Consequences Related to Other Disease States

It has been suggested that the prevalence of the debrisoquin oxidative pheno-type and/or metabolic ratio is associated with certain disease states. It is not known whether the phenotype is a cause or a result of these diseases or if the disease is merely casually associated with phenotype. An increased prevalence of debrisoquin EM phenotype (or the presence of very low metabolic ratios) has been associated with aggressive bladder cancer,[82] bronchial carcinoma in smokers,[47,113] and gastro-intestinal and liver carcinoma.[84] Conflicting results have been reported on the relationship between phenotype and bladder cancer.[85] The results of such disease-association studies are affected by the selection of subjects and controls and whether any multifactorial analysis has been performed to rule out confounding risk factors for development of cancer. A preponderance of the PM phenotype among subjects with non-drug-induced lupus erythematosus (21%) compared a group of healthy volunteers (8%), has also been reported,[50] although this was a small group (42 patients).

Phenotyping Methods

The objective for any phenotyping method is the assignment of the correct phenotypic trait for the polymorphism (i.e., one that if used in large family studies would result in correct phenotype assignments consistent with the mode of inheritance for all individuals). Thus, all new methods are compared with "gold standard" methods which have been validated with family studies, or they must themselves be independently validated. Determination of phenotype is generally by oral administration of a test drug (such as debrisoquin or sparteine); collection of urine for a defined period (4 to 24 hours); assay of a polymorphically formed metabolite and the parent drug; and calculation of a metabolic ratio (traditionally, the molar ratio of parent drug to metabolite has been used). Thus defined, EMs have the lowest metabolic ratios. The metabolic ratio discriminating EMs from PMs (i.e., the antimode) has been determined by visual inspection, probit analysis, and by various distribution analyses,[18,87] although probit analyses have recently been criticized.[88] Recently, the concurrent determination of debrisoquin-type phenotype (using dextromethorphan and a simple thin layer chromatography analytic technique) and mephenytoin phenotype (see Mephenytoin) has been reported.[89] As discussed by Kalow,[47] it is advisable to justify reliability and validity of phenotyping strategies in each new population studied. For instance, it is preferable that the amount of metabolite excreted in urine increases as the amount of parent drug decreases for a metabolic ratio to have maximal power to discriminate two phenotypes, and this inverse relationship should be present in each population studied.[47]

Although many early phenotyping studies were performed in normal, healthy volunteers who were taking no other drugs, many studies are now being performed in patients. It has thus become important to identify those environmental influences which may alter the measured metabolic ratio. Concurrent or prior use of agents known to be substrates for debrisoquin hydroxylase or known to bind to and competitively inhibit the P450 (without themselves being substrates) has resulted in spurious assignment of the PM phenotype. As discussed earlier, quinidine is the most impressive example of the latter type of inhibitor, and it has increased the metabolic ratio sufficiently to spuriously classify seven of seven EMs as PMs.[137] The higher the affinity of the inhibitor for IID6, the more likely it is to alter the metabolic ratio. For example, the concurrent use of dextromethorphan, a substrate that binds with high affinity, would be expected to spuriously alter the phenotype assessed using another IID6 substrate.[90] When both EMs and PMs are considered, genetic factors have remained the greatest contributor to interindividual variability, accounting for 79% of the variability in the debrisoquin metabolic ratio when examined in multivariate analyses (assuming there are no other concurrent factors known to potentially alter phenotype, such as quinidine use).[16] However, variability within a population of only EMs appears to be influenced by factors other than genetic variance (e.g., environmental), since heterozygous and homozygous EMs have overlapping metabolic ratios.[16]

An alternative method that could be used to determine hydroxylator status would be direct determination of the genotype, using the subject's genomic DNA and the molecular probes described below. This methodology does not rely upon drug administration and is unaffected by environmental influences. Unfortunately, in 97% of the cases, standard RFLP techniques and gene probes do not allow unambiguous assignment of phenotype using DNA alone.[92] However, allele specific amplification of normal (wild type) and mutant IID6 genes using polymerase chain reaction (PCR) technology, has recently been developed.[151] This new technique permits identification of over 95% of PMs using DNA obtained from leukocytes, although its utility has only been established in Caucasians.

Molecular Basis

The overall molecular basis of the debrisoquin polymorphism is depicted in Figure 7-5. Using specific antibodies raised against purified human liver debrisoquin hydroxylase cytochrome P450, the gene coding for debrisoquin hydroxylase (formerly identified as IID1,[93] now termed IID6),[5,94,95] has been cloned, sequenced, expressed in mammalian cells,[78] and mapped to chromosome 22.[93] It has been shown that the human liver in poor metabolizers has either none or only very small amounts of the enzyme expressed;[96] in a few cases, the defect in enzyme expression seems to be secondary to RNA splicing defects.[78] More than one mutation gives rise to the poor metabolizer phenotype.[78,95] In fact, two highly related genes, CYP2D7 and a pseudogene, CYP2D8, are located just upstream from CYP2D6 on chromosome 22.[95] It is not known whether the gene product of CYP2D7 can result in a functional debrisoquin hydroxylase enzyme, although this seems unlikely since the inheritance of the PM defect is clearly consistent with debrisoquin hydroxylase being under monogenic control. Moreover, it has been speculated that one of the variants described in mRNA from PM livers could have been transcripts of IID7 rather than IID6, while CYP2D8 would not appear to be capable of producing a functional protein because of multiple deletions and insertions in its exons.[95]

Although it is fairly simple to determine an individual's phenotype by administering a prototype substrate (such as debrisoquin or dextromethorphan) and collecting and analyzing the urine for the metabolic ratio, there are circumstances in which it would be extremely useful to be able to predict phenotype without having to administer a drug. For instance, many patients have a chronic need for medications which can bind to and inhibit debrisoquin hydroxylase activity; therefore, the constitutive level of IID6 activity in these patients cannot be determined. Also, oral drug administration and urine collections may not be feasible in all subjects (e.g., very young infants and those too ill to take oral medicines). Although it is not yet possible to uniformly predict phenotype based on an individual's DNA alone, using restriction fragment length polymorphism (RFLP) analysis, one can now unequivocally identify 25% of Caucasian PMs.[92] Genomic DNA can be easily extracted from as little as 20–30 mL of blood. After XbaI restriction enzyme (endonuclease) digestion, DNA is separated by size with agarose gel electrophoresis, transferred to a nylon membrane, and hybridized with a radiolabelled cDNA probe for IID6 (see Figure 7-6). With this enzyme, the 44 kb, 11.5 kb, and 16 + 9 kb bands are associated with nonfunctional mutant alleles of debrisoquin hydroxylase.[92,150] Therefore, individuals with only these polymorphic bands are clearly identified as PMs. However, this is the case in only 25% of PMs, or only 2.5% of the entire Caucasian population.

RFLP analysis has been useful in addressing the question of whether homozygote EM liver has intrinsically greater debrisoquin hydroxylase activity than does heterozygous liver.[97] This is a relevant question to pursue, since it has been claimed

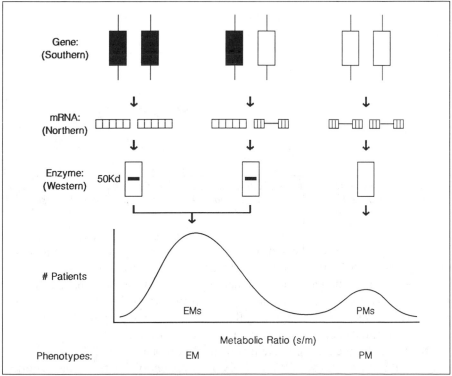

Figure 7-5. *Depiction of molecular basis of debrisoquin oxidative polymorphism. Those homozygous individuals with both maternal and paternal wild-type alleles (dark bars) or heterozygotes with only one wild-type allele produce normally spliced mRNA for debrisoquin hydroxylase. This gives rise to a functional enzyme, which can be detected on Western blot when immunoreacted with antibody against debrisoquin hydroxylase. Those who are homozygous or heterozygous for the wild-type allele have sufficient debrisoquin hydroxylase activity to confer the EM (extensive metabolizer) phenotype; presumably a number of environmental and/or genetic factors influence the numeric value of the urinary metabolic ratio (s:m or substrate:metabolite concentration) within the EM phenotype. Individuals homozygous for mutant alleles (open bars on right) produce only unstable or misspliced mRNA, which cannot give rise to a functional protein. No protein is detectable on Western blot, and the defect is manifested in the poor metabolizer (PM) phenotype with a very high metabolic ratio.*

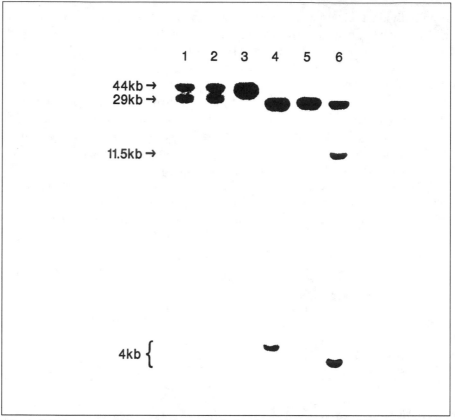

Figure 7-6. *Representative autoradiograph of a Southern blot of genomic DNA after digestion with the most informative restriction enzyme, XbaI. 44 Kb and 11.5 Kb bands are associated with mutant alleles in Caucasians.*

that homozygous EMs can be identified on the basis of very low metabolic ratios and are purported to be at increased risk for the development of lung carcinoma.[19,83] We have found that human liver from heterozygote EMs does not have different intrinsic activity compared to that of liver from predominantly homozygous EMs.[97] Therefore, it is not surprising that clinical phenotyping methods are not able to discriminate heterozygote from homozygote EMs.

Unfortunately, the high prevalence of the 29 kb band in both EMs and PMs precludes the definitive use of RFLP analysis as a phenotyping test in the majority of individuals. RFLP analysis remains useful in identifying some PMs and some heterozygotes and in defining the inheritance of maternal and paternal alleles for debrisoquin hydroxylase *within* families. The molecular biology of the debrisoquin hydroxylation defect is an area of active and ongoing research, which has recently yielded a PCR method for unequivocally identifying mutant IID6 alleles in Caucasians.[151] A comprehensive discussion of the molecular biology of cytochrome P450s is beyond the scope of this chapter, but has recently been extensively reviewed.[94]

N-ACETYLATION

Background, Inheritance, and Ethnic Differences

Polymorphic N-acetylation was discovered using isoniazid as the substrate probe. It was recognized in the 1950s that isoniazid serum concentrations obtained six hours after an oral dose exhibited substantial interindividual variability, resulting in a bimodal distribution of isoniazid concentrations.[98] Furthermore, it was shown that Japanese tended to have more subjects with very low isoniazid serum levels,[99] and this ethnic difference held up when American Caucasian and Japanese subjects were compared.[100] Shortly thereafter, a large study by Evans et al.[101] was published, using a spectrophotometric method for quantitating isoniazid in plasma. The study consisted of 483 subjects, including 53 families. Salient conclusions from these early studies are as follows:

- The tendency for high isoniazid concentrations (now known to be due to low N-acetyltransferase activity) is inherited as an autosomal recessive trait.[101]
- Although the groups had similar environments, Japanese Americans had a higher prevalence of rapid acetylators than Caucasian Americans (88% versus 56%).[100]
- Phenotype distribution did not differ between American whites and blacks or between males and females.[101]
- Extensive family studies identified 70 obligate heterozygote phenotype individuals and 55 fast acetylators of unknown genotype.[101] Because heterozygotes had higher isoniazid serum concentrations than the other group of fast acetylators, and because serum isoniazid concentrations were consistently higher in Caucasian fast acetylators than in Japanese fast acetylators[100] (a group which presumably had more homozygous fast genotypes), these data support a gene dosage effect for the allele controlling N-acetyltransferase expression. Whether heterozygote fast acetylators can be identified using clinical phenotyping methodologies (i.e., whether the population distribution is actually trimodal) has continued to be an area of research interest to the present day.
- Only certain "pharmacokinetic" parameters (i.e., the four- and six-hour post isoniazid serum concentrations, not the two-hour concentrations) yielded bimodal frequency distributions in these populations.[101] The fact that only certain pharmacokinetic parameters or metabolic ratios are able to divide a population into its polymorphic distribution and different phenotypes is relevant for a number of substrates used for acetylation phenotyping.[102,103]

It was not until a few years later that Evans and White showed that the polymorphism in isoniazid plasma concentrations was due to a genetic polymorphism in hepatic N-acetyltransferase activity and that acetylation of sulfamethazine and hydralazine cosegregated with isoniazid in humans.[11] Other compounds that are substrates for N-acetyltransferase are listed in Table 7-2, including a few agents that must undergo metabolic conversion prior to N-acetylation. They encompass many therapeutic drugs as well as a number of arylamines which have been shown to be carcinogenic (e.g., benzidine, 2-aminofluorene) and in fact may contribute to an increased risk of bladder cancer in slow acetylators.

Although the slow acetylator phenotype is inherited as an autosomal recessive trait, as mentioned previously, it is not clear whether heterozygotes have intermediate acetylator activity that lies between homozygous fast and slow acetylators. Even if one assumes that homozygous fast acetylators have higher N-acetyltransferase enzyme expression, the affinity of the probe substrate for N-acetyltransferase[a] and other pathways for the drug's elimination could affect the ability of a substrate to discriminate among the three genotypes. Heterozygotes usually have been classified as fast acetylator phenotypes. Several investigators who have found trimodal frequency distributions for acetylation indices have suggested that the three modes might indicate homozygous fast, heterozygous fast, and homozygous slow acetylator genotypes.[102,104,105] Family studies performed with isoniazid did indicate intermediate acetylation indices in obligate heterozygotes;[101] however, the frequency distribution did not divide the population into three modes. Moreover, studies reporting trimodal frequency distributions should yield percentages of homozygous fast, heterozygous fast, and homozygous slow genotypes that are consistent with genotype distribution predicted by the Hardy-Weinberg law. This law states that for a gene with only two alleles (F for fast and f for slow), with gene frequencies p and q = 1 − p, respectively, then the predicted genotype frequencies are p^2 (for FF, or homozygous fast acetylators), 2pq (for Ff, or heterozygotes), and q^2 (for ff, or slow acetylators). When q is known, as it is from the observed frequency of the slow acetylator phenotype, p can be calculated. For instance, with 50% slow acetylators, $q^2 = 0.5$, p = 0.29; therefore, $2 \times 0.71 \times 0.29$, or 42%, are predicted to be heterozygotes. In studies in which trimodal frequency distributions have been found, the reported modal frequency distributions have not always been consistent with that predicted by the Hardy-Weinberg theory.[102,104,105]

The prevalence of the slow acetylator phenotype differs among ethnic groups, as has been summarized previously.[106,107] In American and European Caucasian and American black groups, the prevalence of the slow acetylator phenotype is about 50%, while it has been consistently much lower in Japanese (about 10%) and Canadian Eskimo (5%) subjects, and as high as 80% to 90% in Egyptian and Moroccan groups.[9] Sunahara et al. studied isoniazid concentrations in over 2000 subjects falling into different racially homogeneous groups, and arranged them based on their north/south latitude.[104] They found a positive relationship between southern latitude and the prevalence of the slow acetylator phenotype for this

Table 7-2. *Substrates for N-Acetyltransferase*[9,11,104]

acebutolol[a]	dapsone	amrinone
p-Aminobenzoic acid[b]	sulfamethazine	procainamide
p-Aminosalicylic acid	sulfasalazine[a]	sulfadiazine
aminoglutethimide	isoniazid	sulfamerazine
caffeine[a]	nitrazepam[a]	hydralazine
clonazepam	phenelzine	sulfapyridine

[a] Requires metabolism prior to N-acetylation.

[b] Does not discriminate well between acetylator phenotypes.

Pacific region. A similar relationship between latitude and phenotype has not been as clear in Africa.[107] Recently, using isoniazid as a probe, the fast acetylator phenotype was reported to comprise 62% of 323 Nigerians studied.[108] These authors emphasize that a high prevalence of EMs in developing areas has implications for the use of intermittent isoniazid as antitubercular therapy.

In summary, there is great ethnic diversity in the expression of N-acetyltransferase activity, and there is (or was) most likely some relationship between geographic location and N-acetyltransferase activity. Given that very few populations now remain ethnically "pure" or geographically immobile, it is unlikely that an exact and stable relationship between location and acetylation activity can be established or should be expected.

Clinical Consequences

Several excellent reviews describe the clinical importance of the acetylation polymorphism.[9,107,109,110] Its clinical significance can be divided into two categories:

- implications for N-acetylated drug efficacy and/or toxicity
- disease states associated with acetylator phenotype

In general, the disposition of drugs undergoing polymorphic acetylation is not as dramatically different between the two phenotypes as it is for drugs subject to one of the polymorphisms affecting specific cytochrome P450s. However, the association of phenotype and disease is particularly relevant for N-acetyltransferase, given that there are several carcinogens known to be substrates for polymorphic N-acetyltransferase.[110,111]

Isoniazid provides a good example of drug toxicity and/or inefficacy. (Procainamide is discussed in Chapter 22 of this book.) Although neurotoxicity from isoniazid can largely be prevented by adequate pyridoxine supplementation, this adverse effect appears to be related to isoniazid concentrations and thus is more common in slow than in fast acetylators. Slow acetylators have been shown in some studies to be more likely to develop hepatotoxicity; however, the situation is complicated by the fact that presumed hepatotoxic metabolites, hydrazine and acetylhydrazine, may themselves be substrates for N-acetyltransferase.[112] It has recently been reported that slow acetylators excrete significantly more acetylhydrazine and hydrazine, and less of the nontoxic acetylisoniazid and diacetylhydrazine, than fast acetylators.[113] The differences between fast and slow acetylators do not appear to be large enough to influence isoniazid efficacy in the treatment of tuberculosis using standard schedules.[107] However, one year of once-weekly treatment regimens was less effective in eradicating bacteria in rapid versus slow acetylators.[107]

Sulfasalazine, a drug used to treat ulcerative colitis, rheumatoid arthritis, and Crohn's disease, is cleaved by gut bacteria to yield sulfapyridine and 5-aminosalicylic acid (the former is a substrate for N-acetyltransferase). Slow acetylators have been shown to have more side effects (nausea, headache, abdominal discomfort) than fast acetylators, and those who experienced side effects had higher sulfapyridine concentrations than those without side effects.[107] Moreover, the efficacy of this drug in the treatment of ulcerative colitis has also been related to serum sulfapyridine concentrations greater than 20 µg/mL. However, the efficacy of sulfasalazine in the treatment of rheumatoid arthritis is apparently not related to either acetylation phenotype or steady-state sulfapyridine concentrations.[114]

The development of a positive antinuclear antibody (ANA) test and clinical SLE have been associated with the use of several acetylated compounds, including procainamide and hydralazine. Given equal total doses of hydralazine, a greater percentage of slow acetylators developed positive ANA antibodies more rapidly and at a lower cumulative hydralazine dose than did rapid acetylators (see Figure 7-7). One-half of the slow acetylators were positive after hydralazine 50 gm. In contrast, one-half of the fast acetylators did not become positive until they had received a cumulative dose of hydralazine 200 gm.[115] Thereafter, there appeared to be a leveling off of ANA positivity, and in fact, some patients converted to a negative ANA titer. Therefore, it has been postulated that the main difference between phenotypes lies in the rate at which ANA positivity or SLE develops, with rapid acetylators developing ANA positivity more slowly (for hydralazine, 23 versus 15 months for fast versus slow acetylators, repectively; for procainamide, 7.3 versus 2.9 months).[116] Development of frank lupus is much more rare (1% to 3% after three years treatment) with hydralazine,[115] and there are conflicting data regarding the importance of acetylator phenotype and drug-induced lupus for this drug. Obviously, additional patient-specific factors other than acetylator phenotype must contribute to the development of lupus in individuals taking these medications.

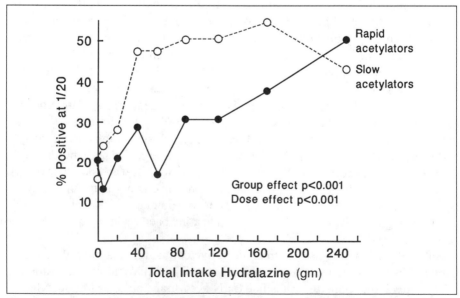

Figure 7-7. *Percentage of patients whose serum antinuclear antibody titer has converted to positive in fast versus slow acetylators, versus the total cumulative dose of hydralazine (reproduced with permission, reference 115).*

An interaction was reported when nitrazepam was begun in a slow acetylator who was stabilized on maximum recommended doses of the monoamine oxidase inhibitor (MAOI), phenelzine.[117] The patient developed classic symptoms of MAOI toxicity after ten days of maximum-dose nitrazepam. Although it has been controversial whether there are significant differences in nitrazepam plasma concentrations between acetylation phenotypes,[118] an awareness of such possible competitive acetylation reactions is warranted.

In evaluating the clinical importance of acetylator phenotype, it is important to consider that several carcinogenic compounds are known substrates for N-acetyltransferase. In 13 separate studies, the slow acetylator phenotype was associated with bladder cancer. On the basis of this association, it has been hypothesized that slow acetylators have less capacity to acetylate and thus detoxify arylamine carcinogens.[107] Human cancer has been linked to aromatic amine exposure in dye factories as early as the late 1800s.[110] In fact, in a study of 23 dye workers who had developed bladder cancer, only one was a fast acetylator.[106] It does not appear that the association can be explained by the possibility that slow acetylators survive longer with their disease. It should be mentioned that the fast acetylator phenotype has been associated with the development of other cancers (e.g., colorectal) and that the activation of carcinogens could be possible if polymorphic N-acetyltransferase were also responsible for N-hydroxylarylamine O acetyltransferase activity.[110] Studies of the tissue-specific degree of N- and O-acetyltransferase activity in human liver, bladder, and colon cell homogenates are ongoing.[111]

A number of genetic factors could predispose patients to drug toxicity. For example, sulfonamides can cause "idiosyncratic" reactions such as rash, blood dyscrasias, and nephritis.[119,120] In one study of six children who developed such toxicity, all were found to be slow acetylators. Obviously, not all slow acetylators develop idiosyncratic sulfonamide toxicities; thus, other mechanisms (e.g., the lack of glutathione transferase activity) have been postulated in slow acetylators who develop these reactions. Figure 7-8 shows how slow acetylators are more likely to have higher concentrations of parent sulfonamide. They are thus more likely to form hydroxylamine reactive metabolites that could covalently bind to proteins to form haptens. The latter could cause an immunologically-mediated response. If enzymes that detoxify the hydroxylamine metabolites, such as glutathione transferase, are concurrently present in low amounts, this may also contribute to "idiosyncratic" reactions in slow acetylators. The expression of these enzymes may also be genetically regulated.

Other clinical effects that might be associated with acetylator phenotype include isoniazid-induced hepatitis, spontaneous SLE, phenelzine adverse effects, colorectal carcinoma, and breast cancer.[9,107,121]

Phenotyping Methods

Several methods are used to determine acetylator phenotype, but none are commercially available. There is generally not as clear a separation between the two acetylator phenotypes as there is with either the debrisoquin or mephenytoin polymorphisms. It is not clear whether this is an artifact of the drug administration and sampling methods that have been developed or a reflection of the fact that more than one N-acetyltransferase may be involved in the metabolism of some substrates (see Molecular Basis). To be useful, a method should result in an unequivocal separation of fast and slow acetylators. Also, phenotypic assignments should be supported by family studies. Alternatively, an independent, previously validated method of phenotyping should give the same phenotype assignment as the method being tested. Early studies[100,101] which measured a single four- or six-hour isoniazid serum concentration following oral administration have been validated by family studies; thus, they remain the "gold standard" even though they do not use a "metabolic ratio." A variety of indices of sulfamethazine disposition have also been used as potential measures of acetylation (the apparent metabolic rate constant, terminal half-life, six-hour plasma ratio of acetylated to total sulfamethazine, and ratio of acetylated to total sulfamethazine in a six-hour urine collection or in the five- to six-hour urine collection). Simulations have shown that the six-hour plasma index is least sensitive to changes in nonmetabolic influences, such as renal clearance, distribution volume, and absorption variables, and is thus the most reliable.[103] It was the index least likely to "misphenotype" an individual given potential nongenetic influences. This is one of the few examples in which careful simulation studies have been performed to help evaluate the suitability of a phenotyping test. Others have studied the effects of urine pH and flow on renal clearance of sulfonamide metabolites;[122] sulfamethazine again discriminated well between fast and slow acetylators in this study. As substrates for phenotyping, both isoniazid and sulfamethazine have the disadvantage of causing adverse effects in rare individuals.

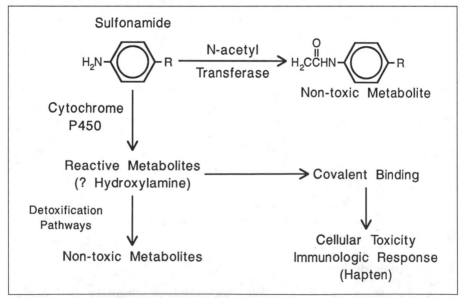

Figure 7-8. *Proposed pathway for sulfonamide metabolism and mechanism of formation of reactive metabolites which could contribute to adverse reactions. In this case, slow acetylators would be at higher risk to form reactive P450-mediated metabolites (reproduced with permission, reference 119).*

A newer phenotyping method using caffeine as a precursor to an acetylated derivative has now gained widespread use. Caffeine, a ubiquitous and safe compound, is metabolized to an intermediate which is either further oxidized to 1-methylxanthine (1X) or acetylated to 5-acetylamino-6-formylamino-3-methyluracil (AFMU). The urinary molar AFMU:1X ratio yields a bimodal (in some cases trimodal) frequency distribution, with phenotypic assignments that generally match those determined after sulfamethazine administration.[102,123–125] The test can be performed using a spot urine collection. The caffeine method does have some shortcomings:

- AFMU is unstable under alkaline conditions,[126] possibly even in the bladder.[127]
- Xanthine oxidase inhibitors may influence the metabolism of caffeine.[128]
- 1X may precipitate in an acidified urine.[127]

Nevertheless, this test has yielded reproducible phenotype assignments in several studies, and thus may represent one of the safest, most convenient methods of determining acetylator phenotype. Moreover, the molar AFMU/1X ratio determined in a group of individuals after caffeine ingestion correlated very well (r = 0.98) with the *in vitro* sulfamethazine activity determined in the cytosol of liver biopsies from those same individuals.[129] This lends additional credibility to this method of phenotyping. The use of procainamide, isoniazid, dapsone, hydralazine, and other sulfa drugs to determine acetylation phenotype has been reviewed elsewhere.[9,107]

The concurrent administration of another substrate for N-acetyltransferase with the phenotyping probe can result in spurious phenotype assignments in some instances. For example, sulfamethazine converted one fast acetylator to a slow acetylator when caffeine was used as the substrate probe.[125] Both isoniazid and sulfamethazine decreased the dapsone acetylation ratio and converted some fast phenotypes to slow ones, whereas hydralazine affected neither the dapsone nor the sulfamethazine acetylation indices.[130]

Molecular Basis

Unlike debrisoquin and mephenytoin hydroxylase, N-acetyltransferase is a cytosolic enzyme which comprises a very minor percentage of liver cytosol, even from high-activity human liver.[131] Although there is extrahepatic N-acetyltransferase activity, hepatic N-acetyltransferase appears to be predominantly responsible for the human polymorphism.[9] Two proteins (NAT-1 and NAT-2) of identical molecular masses have been partially purified from human liver,[131] and these proteins have differing affinities for the classic acetylation substrate, sulfamethazine. Using polyclonal rabbit antiserum raised against a purified preparation of human N-acetyltransferase, the immunodetectable amounts of both NAT-1 and NAT-2 were lower when sulfamethazine acetylating activity was low.[129] This suggests that the slow acetylator defect is due to reduced amounts of both active N-acetyltransferase enzymes. Given the clear Mendelian autosomal recessive nature of inheriting the slow acetylator phenotype, the expression of genes coding these two NAT enzymes must be coregulated or highly linked in man. The molecular basis for this polymorphism in humans has been partly unravelled: two genes for human arylamine N-acetyltransferase have recently been cloned using a cDNA for rabbit liver N-acetyltransferase, to which they have 82% homology.[132] Another group independently cloned three genes for N-acetyltransferase and functionally expressed them in mammalian cells.[133] Two of these cDNAs were closely related to the cDNAs cloned by Grant et al.,[132] one of which was essentially identical and should represent the wild-type gene. The activity of the three cDNAs expressed by Ohsako and Deguchi differed in their relative maximal acetylating activities toward several different substrates, but unfortunately, kinetic constants for the reactions were not determined.[133] It appears that one gene locus, termed NAT2[152] is responsible for encoding polymorphic N-acetyltransferases. Two forms of N-acetyltransferase (termed NAT2A and NAT2B),[152] perhaps representing two different protein products of the same gene transcript, are coregulated in human liver and are responsible for the polymorphic activity of the enzyme. A third protein, NAT1, is the protein product of the NAT1 gene locus and is less stable *in vitro*, and its activity appears to be independent of the polymorphism and may account for some of the "monomorphic" N-acetyltransferase activity, as well as some activity present in slow acetylators.[152] A method using RFLP analysis of genomic DNA and the O-7 cDNA probe has been reported to distinguish wild type alleles from two mutant variants;[153] however, given the high prevalence of fast acetylators among Japanese, the mutant forms described by Deguchi et al.[153] may not account for all of the mutations expected to be present in non-Japanese populations. The cloning of human N-acetyltransferase, as well as the elucidation of the molecular biology of all N-acetyltransferase enzymes in humans, should greatly improve our understanding of this polymorphism. It may also allow phenotyping (or genotyping) by methods that do not require substrate administration; these methods would not be subject to the environmental influences which affect currently available clinical phenotyping methods.

MEPHENYTOIN HYDROXYLATION

Background, Inheritance, and Ethnic Differences

The polymorphism of mephenytoin hydroxylation is distinct and independent from that affecting debrisoquin and its family of cosegregating drugs; the subject has recently been reviewed.[8,10] Mephenytoin is a hydantoin anticonvulsant that has been used clinically since 1945. It has remained distinct from its chemical congener, phenytoin, both because of a high incidence of adverse effects with chronic dosing and because of a different spectrum of activity.[8] Mephenytoin provides one of the most dramatic examples of stereoselective drug metabolism in humans. It is administered as the racemate of R- and S-isomers. Most humans are extensive metabolizers (EMs) and stereoselectively 4-hydroxylate S-mephenytoin to inactive 4-hydroxymephenytoin; this reaction is catalyzed by the cytochrome P450 mephenytoin hydroxylase (believed to be in the subfamily IIC).[94] Therefore, EMs have a low urinary S:R ratio of mephenytoin. In addition, both EMs and PMs

N-demethylate mephenytoin to nirvanol; this is not a stereoselective reaction. Nirvanol is an active metabolite which is itself hydroxylated very slowly by mephenytoin hydroxylase, with a half-life of at least several days.[134] Mephenytoin 4-hydroxylation and N-demethylation are mediated by separate cytochrome P450 enzymes.[135] In a study of the pharmacokinetics of mephenytoin, it was serendipitously found that one of the subjects had a defect in 4-hydroxylation of S-mephenytoin. Subsequently, two of the subject's brothers were found to share this defect, suggesting that it had a genetic basis.[136]

Küpfer and Preisig at the University of Berne conducted a population study[154] of mephenytoin (see Figure 7-9) and showed that the amount of 4-hydroxymephenytoin recovered in the urine (the "hydroxylation index") was bimodally distributed. The prevalence of poor metabolizers (PMs) was 5%. These investigators observed that the mephenytoin phenotype was independent of the debrisoquin hydroxylation defect and seemed to be inherited as a recessive trait.[136] It has since been shown that PMs are deficient in 4-hydroxylation of S-mephenytoin, although they are able to nonstereoselectively 4-hydroxylate a small amount of the drug.[138] Family studies identified obligate heterozygotes, and they were indistinguishable from homozygote EM subjects on the basis of their 4-hydroxylation index.[57,139] Population studies in Swiss, American, French, and Canadian Caucasians have

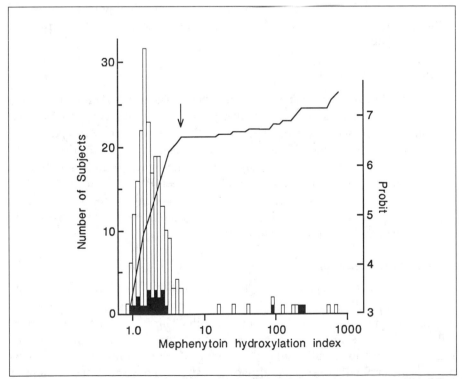

Figure 7-9. *Frequency distribution of the mephenytoin hydroxylation index on a log scale in 221 Swiss subjects. Solid bars indicate poor metabolizers of debrisoquin. The arrow indicates the antimode as determined by probit analysis (solid line) (reproduced with permission, reference 154).*

reconfirmed a 5% prevalence of the PM phenotype in these groups.[8,140] Interestingly, this frequency is higher (approximately 20%) in Japanese.[8,57] No PMs were found among 90 Panamanian Cuna Amerindians.[141]

Affected Agents

The number of agents whose metabolism is known to cosegregate with that of mephenytoin is relatively small. Sixty-four agents were screened as potential inhibitors of either mephenytoin or sparteine oxidation by human liver microsomes. The number of agents found to inhibit cytochrome P450 metabolism of mephenytoin was much smaller than for sparteine oxidation (24 versus 40, respectively),[42] and, as previously discussed, not all inhibitors were substrates. Two agents whose metabolism clearly cosegregates are mephobarbital[142] and S-nirvanol.[134] One propranolol oxidative pathway[68] and hexobarbital metabolism[143] also seem to cosegregate, although hexobarbital metabolism remains to be studied in a larger group of mephenytoin EMs and PMs. Tolbutamide was a suspected substrate for mephenytoin hydroxylase since it was found to cosegregate with mephenytoin in *in vitro* studies;[144] however, it did not cosegregate *in vivo*.[144] Furthermore, tolbutamide was found to be metabolized by two distinct P450s, IIC9 and IIC8, neither of which possessed S-mephenytoin hydroxylase activity.[145] Therefore, although careful clinical studies indicate a distinct polymorphism of a unique P450, no other widely used medication has yet been found to be primarily metabolized by mephenytoin hydroxylase.

Clinical Consequences

Poor metabolizers have increased somnolence and intellectual impairment after administration of mephenytoin, presumably because nirvanol concentrations accumulate to about twice those of EMs.[138] It is unknown whether the PM phenotype contributed to "idiosyncratic" hematologic toxicities described in the first 20 years of mephenytoin's use as an anticonvulsant. Certainly, leukopenia was reported in a larger percentage of patients than could have been PMs.[146] A relatively weak association of fast mephenytoin hydroxylation and nonaggressive bladder cancer which was independent of other risk factors (acetylation phenotype, smoking, and alcohol consumption) has been reported.[82]

Phenotyping Methods

Mephenytoin clinical phenotyping is accomplished by analysis of urine metabolites after the oral administration of a low dose. Almost all of the mephenytoin is metabolized to either 4-hydroxymephenytoin or nirvanol in EMs. Since most HPLC methods are not sufficiently sensitive to accurately measure mephenytoin, it is not possible to calculate a metabolic ratio of parent compound to the polymorphic metabolite.[8] Consequently, many investigators have made the assumption that the amount of urinary 4-hydroxymephenytoin recovered in a set interval (corrected for dose) represents a hydroxylation index. This index has divided the population into EMs and PMs. The disadvantage of this method is that it cannot discriminate noncomplying EMs from true PMs. However, one can combine mephenytoin with an independent substrate (e.g., debrisoquin) to determine if the substrate mixture has been taken.[147] This method was validated in a large population of subjects.[147] Others have used a sensitive stereoselective capillary gas chromatographic assay to measure the relative concentration of S:R mephenytoin in urine.[148] PMs should have an S:R ratio close to 1.0, since they have deficient S-mephenytoin hydroxylase activity and all other mephenytoin elimination pathways are nonstereoselective; EMs have ratios that are less than 0.8.[148] Some have suggested that it may be necessary to use a 24 to 32 hour urine collection to correctly assign a phenotype when the 0 to 8 hour urine produces an S:R ratio above 0.6. This is because the S:R ratio may decrease to its stable value over the first few hours of a urine collection in EMs, while it will remain high in PMs.[147,148]

Molecular Basis

The molecular basis of the mephenytoin hydroxylation defect in EMs and PMs remains unknown, although its biochemical characteristics in human liver have been well characterized.[135] Microsomes prepared from PM liver biopsies show a higher Km and lower V_{max} for 4-hydroxymephenytoin formation than do those from EMs. There is also a clear loss of stereoselectivity for the reaction (see Figure 7-10). Recently, a cDNA for a P450 with an N-terminal-deduced amino acid sequence quite similar to that of a purified mephenytoin hydroxylase P450, has

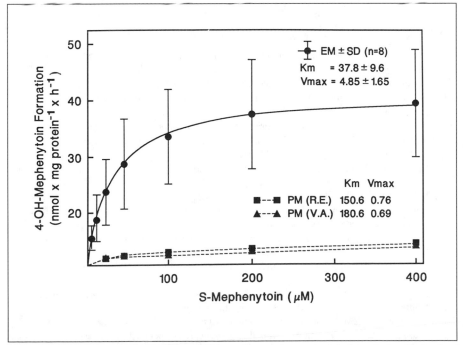

Figure 7-10. *Differences in both Km and Vmax for mephenytoin 4-hydroxylation determined in microsomes prepared from liver biopsies of EM versus PM subjects (reproduced with permission, reference 135).*

been functionally expressed in yeast and shown to possess S-mephenytoin hydroxylase activity.[149] Whether this P450 is the enzyme which is defective or missing in human PMs remains to be conclusively demonstrated. P450s with mephenytoin hydroxylase activity are in the CYP2C subfamily.[5,94,145,149]

PROSPECTUS

The three genetic polymorphisms for drug metabolism discussed in this chapter affect the disposition of over 40 medications, many of them widely used drugs. The effect is often dramatic, especially when the polymorphic enzyme is the major drug metabolizing enzyme for a particular agent. The elucidation of these polymorphisms explains the marked interindividual variability in disposition of the affected agents. In addition, we now have the phenotyping tools to *a priori* determine how an individual will metabolize medications which are substrates for one of these polymorphic enzymes. An awareness of genetic polymorphisms of drug metabolism is key to understanding the application of pharmacokinetic principles to these particular drugs. This is because the entire concept of "population" parameters must be modified to include at least two distinct subpopulations for these drugs. The area of genetic polymorphic drug metabolism is continuing to grow in scope as investigators continue to identify new substrates for known polymorphic enzymes, elucidate those factors that affect enzyme activity, unravel the genetic basis for these defects, and discover additional polymorphic drug metabolizing enzymes.

REFERENCES

1. Nebert DW. Possible clinical importance of genetic differences in drug metabolism. Br Med J. 1981;283:537.
2. Weinshilboum RM. Human pharmacogenetics, an introduction. Fed Proc. 1984;43:2295.
3. Kalow W et al. Ethnic Differences in Reactions to Drugs and Xenobiotics. New York:Alan R Liss, 1986.
4. Vesell ES. Genetic host factors: determinants of drug response. N Engl J Med. 1985;313:261.
5. Nebert DW et al. P450 Superfamily: updated listing of all genes and recommended nomenclature for the chromosomal loci. DNA 1989;8:1.
6. Eichelbaum M et al. The genetic polymorphism of sparteine metabolism. Xenobiotica. 1986;16:465.
7. Meyer UA et al. The molecular mechanisms of two common polymorphisms of drug oxidation-evidence for functional changes in cytochrome P450 isozymes catalysing bufuralol and mephenytoin oxidation. Xenobiotica. 1986;5:449.
8. Kalow W. The genetic defect of mephenytoin hydroxylation. Xenobiotica. 1986;16:379.
9. Weber WW, Hein DW. N-acetylation pharmacogenetics. Pharmacol Rev. 1985;37:25.
10. Wilkinson GR et al. Genetic polymorphism of S-mephenytoin hydroxylation. Pharmac Ther. 1989;43:53.
11. Evans DAP, White TA. Human acetylation polymorphism. J Lab Clin Med. 1964;63:395.
12. Kupfer A, Preisig R. Inherited defects of hepatic drug metabolism. Semin Liver Dis. 1983;3:341.
13. Weinshilboum RM. Human pharmacogenetics of methyl conjugation. Fed Proc. 1984;43:2303.
14. Waring RH et al. Polymorphic sulphoxidation of S-carboxymethyl-L-cysteine in man. Biochemical Pharm. 1982;31:3151.
15. Mahgoub A et al. Polymorphic hydroxylation of debrisoquine in man. Lancet. 1977;2:584.

16. Steiner E et al. A family study of genetic and environmental factors determining polymorphic hydroxylation of debrisoquin. Clin Pharmacol Ther. 1985;38:394.

17. Evans DAP et al. A family and population study of the genetic polymorphism of debrisoquine oxidation in a white British population. J Med Genet. 1980;17:102.

18. Eichelbaum M et al. Spannbrucker N, Steincke B, Dengler HJ. Defective N-oxidation of sparteine in man: a new pharmacogenetic defect. Eur J Clin Pharmacol. 1979;16:183.

19. Law MR et al. Debrisoquine metabolism and genetic predisposition to lung cancer. Br J Cancer. 1989;59:686.

20. Dayer P et al. Defective hydroxylation of bufuralol associated with side effects of the drug in poor metabolizers. Br J Clin Pharmacol. 1982;13:750.

21. McGourty JC et al. Pharmacokinetics and beta-blocking effects of timolol in poor and extensive metabolisers of debrisoquin. Clin Pharmacol Ther. 1985;38:409.

22. Raghuran TC et al. Polymorphic ability to metabolize propranolol alters 4-hydroxypropranolol levels but not beta-blockade. Clinical Pharmacol Ther. 1984;36:51.

23. Lennard MS et al. Oxidation phenotype—major determinant of metoprolol metabolism and response. N Engl J Med. 1982;307:1558.

24. Lennard MS et al. The polymorphic oxidation of beta-adrenoceptor antagonists. Clin Pharmacokinet. 1986;11:1.

25. Alvan G et al. Relationship of N-demethylation of amiflamine and its metabolite to debrisoquine hydroxylation polymorphism. Clin Pharmacol Ther. 1984;36:515.

26. Baumann P et al. Amitriptyline pharmacokinetics and clinical response. II. Metabolic polymorphism assessed by hydroxylation of debrisoquine and mephenytoin. Int Clin Psychopharm. 1986;1:102.

27. Bertilsson L et al. Slow hydroxylation of nortriptyline and concomitant poor debrisoquine hydroxylation: clinical implications. Lancet. 1981;1:560.

28. Balant-Gorgia AE et al. Importance of oxidative polymorphism and levomepromazine treatment on the steady-state blood concentrations of clomipramine and its major metabolites. Eur J Clin Pharmacol. 1986;31:449.

29. Brosen K et al. Steady-state concentrations of imipramine and its metabolites in relation to the sparteine/debrisoquine polymorphism. Eur J Clin Pharmacol. 1986;30:679.

30. Bertilsson L, Ålsberg-Wistedt A. The debrisoquine hydroxylation test predicts steady-state plasma levels of desipramine. Br J Clin Pharmacol. 1983;15:388.

31. Siddoway LA et al. Polymorphism of propafenone metabolism and disposition in man:clinical and pharmacokinetic consequences. Circulation. 1987;75:785.

32. Wang T et al. Influence of genetic polymorphism on the metabolism and disposition of encainide in man. J Pharmacol Exp Ther. 1984;228:605.

33. Zekorn C et al. Pharmacokinetics of N-propylajmaline in relation to polymorphic sparteine oxidation. Klin Wochenschr. 1985;63:1180.

34. Lennard MS et al. Protecting the poor metabolizer: clinical consequences of genetic polymorphism of drug oxidation. Pharmacy International. 1983;4:53.

35. Mikus G et al. The influence of the sparteine/debrisoquin phenotype on the disposition of flecainide. Clin Pharmacol Ther. 1989;45:562.

36. Pierce DM et al. The pharmacokinetics of indoramin and 6-hydroxyindoramin in poor and extensive hydroxylators of debrisoquine. Eur J Clin Pharmacol. 1987;33:59.

37. Küpfer A et al. Dextromethorphan as a safe probe for debrisoquine hydroxylation polymorphism. Lancet. 1984;2:517.

38. Desmeules J et al. Impact of genetic and environmental factors on codeine analgesia. Clin Pharmacol Ther. 1989;45:122.

39. Idle JR et al. Oxidation phenotype and metiamide metabolism. Br J Pharmacol. 1979;66:432P.

40. Roy SD et al. Metabolism of methoxyphenamine in extensive and poor metabolizers of debrisoquin. Clin Pharmacol Ther. 1985;38:128.

41. Otton SV et al. Competitive inhibition of sparteine oxidation in human liver by beta-adrenoceptor antagonists and other cardiovascular drugs. Life Sciences. 1984;34:73.

42. Inaba T et al. *In vitro* inhibition studies of two isozymes of human liver cytochrome P450, mephenytoin p-hydroxylase and sparteine monooxygenase. Drug Metab Dispos. 1985;13:443.

43. Fonne-Pfister R, Meyer UA. Xenobiotic and endobiotic inhibitors of cytochrome P450db1 function, the target of the debrisoquine/sparteine type polymorphism. Biochem Pharmacol. 1988;37:3829.

44. Relling MV et al. Anticancer drugs as inhibitors of two polymorphic cytochrome P450 enzymes, debrisoquin and mephenytoin hydroxylase, in human liver microsomes. Cancer Res 1989;49:68.

45. Benitez J et al. Debrisoquin oxidation polymorphism in a Spanish population. Clin Pharmacol Ther. 1988;44:74.

46. Horai Y, Ishizaki T. Pharmacogenetics and its clinical implications. II. Oxidation polymorphism. Ration Drug Ther. 1988;22:1.

47. Kalow W. Pharmacogenetics and anthropology. In: Lemberger L, Reidenberg M, eds. Proceedings of the Second World Conference on Clinical Pharmalogy and Therapeutics. Bethesda, MD: American Society for Pharmacology and Clinical Therapeutics; 1984:264–86.

48. Woolhouse NM. The debrisoquine/sparteine oxidation polymorphism: evidence of genetic heterogeneity among Ghanaians. In: Ethnic Differences in Reactions to Drugs and Xenobiotics. New York: Alan R Liss; 1986;189–206.

49. Nakamura K et al. Interethnic differences in genetic polymorphism of debrisoquine and mephenytoin hydroxylation between Japanese and Caucasian populations. Clin Pharmacol Ther. 1985;38:402.

50. Lou YC et al. Low frequency of slow debrisoquine hydroxylation in a native Chinese population. Lancet. 1987;2:852.

51. Arias TD et al. No evidence for the presence of poor metabolizers of sparteine in an Amerindian group: the Cunas of Panama. Br J Clin Pharmac. 1986;21:547.

52. Yue QY et al. Disassociation between debrisoquine hydroxylation phenotype and genotype among Chinese. Lancet. 1989;1:870.

53. Idle JR. Poor metabolisers of debrisoquine reveal their true colours. Lancet. 1989;2:1097.

54. Gleiter CH et al. Discovery of altered pharmacokinetics of CGP 15210 G in poor hydroxylators of debrisoquine during early drug development. Br J Clin Pharmacol. 1985;20:81.

55. Brosen K, Gram LF. Clinical significance of the sparteine/debrisoquine oxidation polymorphism. Eur J Clin Pharmacol. 1989;36:537.

56. Smith RL. Introduction: Xenobiotica. 1986;16:363.

57. Ward SA et al. S-mephenytoin 4-hydroxylase is inherited as an autosomal-recessive trait in Japanese families. Clin Pharmacol Ther. 1987;42:96.

58. Dayer P et al. Bioactivation of the narcotic drug codeine in human liver is mediated by the polymorphic monooxygenase catalyzing debrisoquine 4-hydroxylation. Biochem Biophys Res Comm. 1988;152:411.

59. Mellström B et al. E and Z-10 hydroxylation of nortriptyline:relationship to polymorphic debrisoquine hydroxylation. Clin Pharmacol Ther. 1981;30:189.

60. Brosen K, Gram LF. First-pass metabolism of imipramine and desipramine: impact of the sparteine oxidation phenotype. Clin Pharmacol Ther. 1988;43:400.

61. Brosen K, Gram LF. Quinidine inhibits the 2-hydroxylation of imipramine and desipramine but not the demethylation of imipramine. Eur J Clin Pharmacol. 1989;37:155.

62. Gram LF et al. Steady-state plasma levels of E- and Z-10-OH-nortriptyline in nortriptyline-treated patients: significance of concurrent medication and the sparteine oxidation phenotype. Ther Drug Monit. 1989;11:508.

63. Borg KO et al. Metabolism of metoprolol-(^{3}H) in man, the dog and the rate. Acta Pharmacol Toxicol. 1975;36(Suppl V):125.

64. Regardh DG et al. Plasma levels and beta-blocking effect of alpha-hydroxymetoprolol—metabolite of metoprolol—in the dog. J Pharmacokinet Biophys. 1979;7:471.

65. Otton SV et al. Use of quinidine inhibition to define the role of the sparteine/debrisoquine cytochrome P450 in metoprolol oxidation by human liver microsomes. J Pharm Exper Ther. 1988;247:242.

66. Lennard MS et al. Differential stereoselective of metoprolol in extensive and poor debrisoquine metabolisers. Clin Pharmacol Ther. 1983;34:732.

67. Lennard MS et al. Timolol metabolism and debrisoquine oxidation polymorphism: a population study. Br J Clin Pharmac. 1989;27:429.

68. Ward SA et al. Propranolol's metabolism is determined by both mephenytoin and debrisoquin hydroxylase activities. Clin Pharmacol Ther. 1989;45:72.

69. Woosley RL et al. Co-inheritance of the polymorphic metabolism of encainide and debrisoquin. Clin Pharmacol Ther. 1986;39:282.

70. Funck-Bretano C et al. Effect of low dose quinidine on encainide pharmacokinetics and pharmacodynamics. Influence of genetic polymorphism. J Pharmacol Exp Ther. 1989;249:134.

71. Lee JT et al. The role of genetically determined polymorphic drug metabolism in the beta-blockade produced by propafenone. N Engl J Med. 1990;322:1764.

72. Kroemer HK et al. Stereoselective disposition and pharmacologic activity of propafenone enantiomers. Circulation. 1989;79:1068.

73. Guengerich FP et al. Oxidation of quinidine by human liver cytochrome P450. Mol Pharmacol. 1986;30:287.

74. Broly F et al. Effect of quinidine on the dextromethorphan O-demethylase activity of microsomal fractions from human liver. Br J Clin Pharmacol. 1989;28:29.

75. Inaba T et al. Quinidine: potent inhibition of sparteine and debrisoquine oxidation *in vivo*. Br J Clin Pharmacol. 1986;22:199.

76. Philip PA et al. The influence of cimetidine on debrisoquine 4-hydroxylation in extensive metabolizers. Eur J Clin Pharmacol. 1989;36: 319.

77. Spina E, Koike Y. Differential effects of cimetidine and ranitidine on imipramine demethylation and desmethylimipramine hydroxylation by human liver microsomes. Eur J Clin Pharmacol. 1986;30:239.

78. Gonzalez FJ et al. Characterization of the common genetic defect in humans deficient in debrisoquine metabolism. Nature. 1988;331:442.

79. Eichelbaum M et al. The influence of enzyme induction on polymorphic sparteine oxidation. Br J Clin Pharmacol. 1986;22:49.

80. Schellens JHM et al. Influence of enzyme induction and inhibition on the oxidation of nifedipine, sparteine, mephenytoin and antipyrine in humans as assessed by a "cocktail" study design. J Pharmacol Exp Ther. 1989;249:638.

81. Shaheen O et al. Influence of debrisoquin phenotype on the inducibility of propranolol metabolism. Clin Pharmacol Ther. 1989;45:439.

82. Kaisary A et al. Genetic predisposition to bladder cancer: ability to hydroxylate debrisoquin and mephenytoin as risk factors. Cancer Res. 1987;47:5488.

83. Ayesh R et al. Metabolic oxidation phenotypes as markers for susceptibility to lung cancer. Nature. 1984;312:169.

84. Idle JR et al. Some observations on the oxidation phenotype status of Nigerian patients presenting with cancer. Cancer Lett. 1981;11:331.

85. Cartwright RA et al. Genetically determined debrisoqine oxidation capacity in bladder cancer. Carcinogenesis. 1984;5:1191.

86. Baer AN et al. Altered distribution of debrisoquine oxidation phenotypes in patients with systemic lupus erythematosus. Arthritis Rheum. 1986;29:843.

87. Henthorn TK et al. Assessment of the debrisoquin and dextromethorphan phenotyping tests by gaussian mixture distributions analysis. Clin Pharmacol Ther. 1989;45:328.

88. Jackson PR et al. Testing for bimodality in frequency distributions of data suggesting polymorphisms of drug metabolism: histograms and probit plots. Br J Clin Pharmacol. 1989;28:647.

89. Guttendorf RJ et al. Rapid screening for polymorphisms in dextromethorphan and mephenytoin metabolism. Br J Clin Pharmac. 1990; 29:373.

90. Dayer P et al. Dextromethorphan O-demethylation in liver microsomes as a prototype reaction to monitor cytochrome P450 db1 activity. Clin Pharmacol Ther. 1989;45:34.

91. Steiner E, Spina E. Differences in the inhibitory effect of cimetidine on desipramine metabolism between rapid and slow debrisoquin hydroxylators. Clin Pharmacol Ther. 1987;42:278–82.

92. Skoda RC et al. Two mutant alleles of the human cytochrome P450db1 gene associated with genetically deficient metabolism of debrisoquine and other drugs. Proc Natl Acad Sci. 1988;85:5240.

93. Gonzalez FJ et al. Human debrisoquine 4-hydroxylase (P450IID1): cDNA and deduced amino acid sequence and assignment of the CYP2D locus to chromosome 22. Genomics. 1988;2:174.

94. Gonzalez FJ. The molecular biology of cytochrome P450s. Pharmacol Rev. 1989;40:244.

95. Kimura S et al. The human debrisoquine 4-hydroxylase (CYP2D) locus: sequence and identification of the polymorphic CYP2D6 gene, a related gene, and a pseudogene. Am J Hum Genet. 1989;45:889.

96. Zanger UM et al. Absence of hepatic cytochrome P450bufI causes genetically deficient debrisoquin oxidation in man. Biochemistry. 1988;27:5447.

97. Evans WE et al. Debrisoquine-hydroxylase (P450db1) activity in human liver heterozygous for a mutant P450db1 allele. Clin Pharmacol Ther. 1989;45:181.

98. Mitchell RS, Bell JC. Clinical implications of isoniazid blood levels in pulmonary tuberculosis. N Engl J Med. 1957;257:1066.

99. Morse WC et al. Effect of oral PAS on biologically active isoniazid serum levels. Transcript of the 15th Conference on the Chemotherapy of Tuberculosis. VA Armed Forces, 1956;15:283.

100. Knight RA et al. Genetic factors influencing isoniazid blood levels in humans. Transcript of the Conference on Chemotherapy of Tuberculosis, Washington DC: Veterans Administration, 1959;18:52.

101. Evans DAP et al. Genetic control of isoniazid metabolism in man. Br Med J. 1960;2:485.

102. Grant DM et al. A simple test for acetylator phenotype using caffeine. Br J Clin Pharmacol. 1984;17:459.

103. du Souich P et al. Screening methods using sulfamethazine for determining acetylator phenotype. Clin Pharmacol Ther. 1979;26:757.

104. Sunahara S et al. Genetical and geographic studies on isoniazid inactivation. Science. 1961;134:1530.

104. Hamilton RA et al. Effect of the acetylator phenotype on amrinone pharmacokinetics. Clin Pharmacol Ther. 1986;40:615.

105. Chapron DJ et al. Kinetic discrimination of three sulfamethazine acetylation phenotypes. Clin Pharmacol Ther. 1980;27:104.

106. Evans DAP. Acetylation. In: Kalow W, Goedde HW, Agarwal DP, eds. Ethnic Differences in Reactions to Drugs and Xenobiotics. New York: Alan R Liss, 1986:209–42.

107. Evans DAP. N-acetyltransferase. Pharmacol Ther. 1989;42:157.

108. Odeigah PGC, Okunowo MA. High frequency of the rapid isoniazid acetylator phenotype in Lagos (Nigeria). Hum Hered. 1989;39:26.

109. Drayer D, Reidenberg MM. Clinical consequences of polymorphic acetylation of basic drugs. Clin Pharmacol Ther. 1977;22:251.

110. Hein DW. Acetylator genotype and arylamine-induced carcinogenesis. Biochim Biophys Acta. 1988;948:37.

111. Hein DW. Genetic polymorphism and cancer susceptibility: evidence concerning acetyltransferases and cancer of the urinary bladder. Bioessays. 1988;9:200.

112. Peretti E et al. Acetylation of acetylhydrazine, the toxic metabolite of isoniazid in humans. Inhibition by concomitant administration of isoniazid. J Pharmacol Exp Ther. 1987;243:686.

113. Peretti E et al. Increased urinary excretion of toxic hydrazino metabolites of isoniazid by slow acetylators. Effect of a slow-release preparation of isoniazid. Eur J Clin Pharmacol. 1987;33:283.

114. Astbury C, Taggart AJ. Acetylation, sulphasalazine and its effects. Br J Rheumatol. 1987;26:229.

115. Mansilla-Tinoco R et al. Hydralazine, antinuclear antibodies, and the lupus syndrome. Br Med J. 1982;284:936.

116. Woosley RL et al. Effect of acetylator phenotype on the rate at which procainamide induces antinuclear antibodies and the lupus syndrome. N Engl J Med. 1978;298:1157.

117. Harris AL, McIntyre N. Interaction of phenelzine and nitrazepam in a slow acetylator. Br J Clin Pharmacol. 1981;12:254.

118. Swift CG et al. Acetylator phenotype, nitrazepam plasma concentrations and residual effects. Br J Clin Pharmacol. 1980;9:312P.

119. Shear NH et al. Differences in metabolism of sulfonamides predisposing to idiosyncratic toxicity. Ann Intern Med. 1986;105:179.

120. Spielberg SP. *In vitro* assessment of pharmacogenetic susceptibility to toxic drug metabolites in humans. Fed Proc. 1984;43:2308.

121. Ilett KF et al. Acetylation phenotype in colorectal carcinoma. Cancer Res. 1987;47:1466.

122. Vree TB et al. Determination of the acetylator phenotype and pharmacokinetics of some sulphonamides in man. Clin Pharmacokinetics. 1980;5:274.

123. Grant DM et al. Variability in caffeine metabolism. Clin Pharmacol Ther. 1983;33:591.

124. Grant DM et al. Polymorphic N-acetylation of a caffeine metabolite. Clin Pharmacol Ther. 1983;33:355.

125. Rankin RB et al. Caffeine as a potential indicator for acetylator status. J Clin Pharm Ther. 1987;12:47.

126. Tang BK et al. Isolation and identification of 5-acetylamino-6-formylamino-3-methyluracil as a major metabolite of caffeine in man. Drug Metab Dispos. 1983;11:218.

127. Lorenzo B, Reidenberg MM. Potential artifacts in the use of caffeine to determine acetylation phenotype. Br J Clin Pharmacol. 1989;28:207.

128. Grant DM et al. Effect of allopurinol on caffeine disposition in man. Br J Clin Pharmacol. 1986;21:454.

129. Grant DM et al. Acetylation pharmacogenetics: the slow acetylator phenotype is caused by decreased or absent arylamine N-acetyltransferase in human liver. J Clin Invest. 1990;85:968.

130. Ahmad RA et al. Effects of concurrent administration of other substrates of N-acetyltransferase on dapsone acetylation. Br J Clin Pharmacol. 1981;12:83.

131. Grant DM et al. Evidence for two closely related isozymes of arylamine N acetyltransferase in human liver. FEBS Lett. 1989;244:203.

132. Blum M et al. Human arylamine N-acetyltransferase genes: isolation, chromosmal location, and functional expression. DNA and Cell Biology. 1990;9:193.

133. Ohsako S, Deguchi T. Cloning and expression of cDNAs for polymorphic and monomorphic arylamine N-acetyltransferases from human liver. J Biol Chem. 1989;265:4630.

134. Küpfer A et al. Stereoselective metabolism and pharmacogenetic control of 5-phenyl-5-methylhydantoin (Nirvanol) in humans. J Pharmacol Exp Ther. 1984;230:28.

135. Meier UT et al. Mephenytoin hydroxylation polymorphism: characterization of the enzymatic deficiency in liver microsomes of poor metabolizers phenotyped *in vivo*. Clin Pharmacol Ther. 1985;38:488.

136. Küpfer A et al. Family study of a genetically determined deficiency of mephenytoin hydroxylation in man. Pharmacologist. 1979;21:173.

137. Brinn R et al. Sparteine oxidation is practically abolished in quinidine-treated patients. Br J Clin Pharmacol. 1986;22:194.

138. Küpfer A et al. Mephenytoin hydroxylation deficiency: kinetics after repeated doses. Clin Pharmacol Ther. 1984;35:33.

139. Inaba T et al. Family studies of mephenytoin hydroxylation deficiency. Am J Hum Genet. 1986;38:768.

140. Jacqz E et al. Phenotyping polymorphic drug metabolism in the French Caucasian population. Eur J Clin Pharmacol. 1988;35:167.

141. Inaba T et al. Mephenytoin hydroxylation in the Cuna Amerindians of Panama. Br J Clin Pharmacol. 1988;25:75.

142. Küpfer A, Branch RA. Stereoselective mephobarbital hydroxylation cosegregates with mephenytoin hydroxylation. Clin Pharmacol Ther. 1985;38:414.

143. Knodell RG et al. Oxidative metabolism of hexobarbital in human liver: relationship to polymorphic S-mephenytoin 4-hydroxylation. J Pharmacol Exp Ther. 1988;245:845.

144. Knodell RG et al. Hepatic metabolism of tolbutamide: characterization of the form of cytochrome P450 involved in methyl hydroxylation and relationship to *in vivo* disposition. J Pharmacol Exper Ther. 1987;241:1112.

145. Relling MV et al. Tolbutamide and mephenytoin hydroxylation by human cytochrome P450s in the CYP2C subfamily. J Pharmacol Exper Ther. 1990;252:442.

146. Abbott JA, Schwab RS. Mesantoin in the treatment of epilepsy. N Engl J Med. 1954;250:197.

147. Sanz EJ et al. S-mephenytoin hydroxylation phenotypes in a Swedish population determined after coadministration with debrisoquin. Clin Pharmacol Ther. 1989;45:495.

148. Wedlund PJ et al. Mephenytoin hydroxylation deficiency in Caucasians: frequency of a new oxidative drug metabolism polymorphism. Clin Pharmacol Ther. 1984;36:773.

149. Yasumori T et al. Expression of a human P450IIC gene in yeast cells using galactose-inducible expression system. Mol Pharmacol. 1989;35:443.

150. Evans WE, Relling MV. XbaI 16+9 kb DNA restriction fragments identify a mutant allele for debrisoquin-hydroxylase: report of a family study. Mol Pharmacol. 1990;37:639–642.

151. Heim M, Meyer UA. Genotyping of poor metabolizers of debrisoquine by allele-specific PCR amplification. Lancet. 1990;336:529.

152. Grant DM et al. Monomorphic and polymorphic human arylamine N-acetyltransferases: a comparison of liver isozymes and expressed products of two cloned genes. Mol Pharmacol. 1991;39:184.

153. Deguchi T et al. Correlation between acetylation phenotypes and genotypes of polymorphic arylamine N-acetyltransferase in human liver. J Biol Chem. 1990;265:127–57.

154. Küpfer A, Preisig R. Pharmacogenetics of mephenytoin: a new drug hydroxylation polymorphism in man. Eur J Clin Pharmacol. 1984;26:753–57.

Chapter 8

Influence of Renal Function and Dialysis on Drug Disposition

Gary R. Matzke and Stephen P. Millikin

Progressive reductions in renal function as measured by creatinine clearance have been associated with alterations in the disposition of many drugs, and these changes are most evident in patients with end-stage renal disease (ESRD). Alterations in bioavailability, protein binding of acidic and basic drugs, distribution volume, and nonrenal clearance as well as reductions in renal clearance have been observed.

Thus, the design of an optimal therapeutic regimen for a patient with renal insufficiency requires integration of the degree and type of pharmacokinetic alterations of the agent which are associated with the patient's degree of renal insufficiency. This chapter summarizes the currently available methods for quantifying renal function and describes the etiology and progressive nature of renal insufficiency. The effect of various renal diseases on the absorption, distribution, metabolism, and excretion of drugs is discussed in depth. The effects of hemodialysis, hemofiltration, and peritoneal dialysis on drug disposition in the ESRD patient are conceptualized and methods to quantitate these are reviewed. Finally, practical approaches to the design of drug dosage regimens in patients with reduced renal function are presented.

INDICES OF RENAL FUNCTION

Glomerular Filtration Rate (GFR)

Drug clearance by the kidney (renal clearance) represents a composite of several processes which influence the movement of drugs between blood and urine: glomerular filtration, tubular secretion, and tubular reabsorption. Clinically, the glomerular filtration rate (GFR) can be approximated if the excretion rate of a freely filtered substance and its concentration in plasma are known:

$$GFR = \frac{(C_{ur})(Q_{ur})}{C_p}$$

(Eq. 8-1)

where C_{ur} and C_p are the concentration of the substance in urine and plasma, respectively, and Q_{ur} is the urine flow rate.

Although a number of substances could be used to quantify GFR, inulin has been the "freely filtered solute" of choice because its distribution is restricted to the plasma water (i.e., it is not bound to plasma proteins or tissues) and easily passes through the pores of the glomerulus (see Table 8-1). Furthermore, inulin is not secreted, reabsorbed, or metabolized in the renal tubules and is not eliminated by nonrenal routes.[1] This agent can be safely administered intravenously and is the preferred measure of GFR when an accurate measure is critical. The determination of inulin clearance is not, however, a clinically convenient procedure for several reasons. First, the supply of inulin is inconsistent and second, the procedure is complicated in that it requires the continuous intravenous infusion of inulin, the collection of a series of blood and urine samples at specified intervals, and a reliable assay for inulin measurement in both plasma and urine. Alternative methods of GFR measurement have been developed which utilize non-radioisotopic radiocontrast agents as the model solute (e.g., iothalamate,[2,3] diatrizoate meglumine).[4] Although radioactive marker solutes may also be used to measure glomerular filtration rate (e.g., ^{51}Cr–EDTA, 99^m–Tc DTPA,[125] or ^{131}I-diatrizoate, ^{125}I-iothalamate),[5,6] these substances are likely to become less commonly utilized as the analytical methods for the measurement of the nonradioactive solutes become more widely available.

Because serum creatinine (an easily measured endogenous substance) rises in proportion to the decline in GFR, the determination of creatinine clearance (CL_{cr}) is the predominant index of GFR utilized in clinical practice (see Figure 8-1). This measure is more convenient and inexpensive than the above-cited approaches but may be imprecise even under the best conditions. All of the following assumptions must be valid in order to consider a creatinine clearance an accurate estimate of GFR: 1) the daily anabolic production of creatine (the amino acid precursor of creatinine) in the liver is constant; 2) the daily anabolic conversion of creatine to

Table 8-1. *Relative Accuracy and Convenience with Which GFR Can be Quantified*

	Accuracy	Convenience
Inulin clearance	++++	+
Non-radioactive contrast agents	+++	++
Creatinine clearance	++	+++
Serum creatinine	+	++++

creatinine in striatal muscle is constant, and other nonconstant sources of creatinine production do not exist; 3) creatinine is filtered freely by the kidney and is not secreted or reabsorbed; 4) the measurement of creatinine in serum and urine is accurate; and 5) the urine collection is complete.

The synthesis of creatine from glycine, arginine, and methionine in the liver may not be constant in malnourished patients or in those with hepatic insufficiency.[7,8] Thus, the first assumption may not be valid, especially in the critically ill.

Several factors can compromise the validity of the second assumption as well. The production and release of creatinine from muscle is directly proportional to lean body weight (i.e., muscle mass).[9] Because lean body weight (total body weight minus the weight of all body fat) is difficult to estimate, ideal body weight (IBW) has been frequently utilized as the index of muscle mass.[10]

$$IBW_{males} \ (kg) = 50 + (2.3 \times \text{height in inches over 5 ft.}) \qquad \text{(Eq. 8-2)}$$

$$IBW_{females} \ (kg) = 45.5 + (2.3 \times \text{height in inches over 5 ft.}) \qquad \text{(Eq. 8-3)}$$

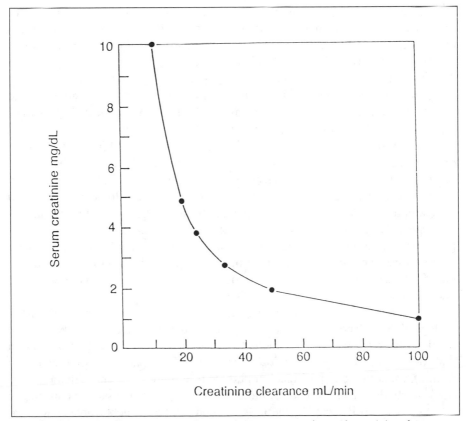

Figure 8-1. Relationship between serum creatinine concentration and creatinine clearance.

The interindividual variability in the relationship between ideal body weight and creatinine production, however, is large. This is because muscle mass constitutes a reduced fraction of ideal body weight in certain individuals; thus, urinary excretion of creatinine is relatively reduced in females;[11] neonates;[12] the elderly;[13] and in patients with cachexia,[14] muscular dystrophies, and other muscle-wasting conditions (paralysis,[15] Cushing syndrome).[16] In contrast, muscle mass constitutes a larger fraction of ideal body weight in athletes[1] and the obese.[17] This finding in obese patients is theoretically related to muscle hypertrophy associated with the excess fat burden. The rate of creatinine production/release also may not be constant in states of muscle destruction (e.g., rhabdomyolysis,[18] major burn, or trauma).[19] The administration of drugs may also change the metabolic production of creatinine in muscle (e.g., trimethoprim),[20] and finally, the dietary intake of cooked meat provides an exogenous source of creatinine which may confound interpretation of serum creatinine concentrations.[21]

Although a diurnal variability in creatinine production has been reported, production is generally considered to be relatively constant in relation to ideal body weight, gender, and age for healthy people.[22] The normal 24-hour excretion of creatinine in young males is 20 to 25 mg/kg ideal body weight; females excrete creatinine at a rate of 15 to 20 mg/kg ideal body weight/24 hours. Creatinine production falls by approximately 2 mg/kg/24 hours per decade in both males and females after age 20.[23] If patient parameters suggest that daily production of creatine and conversion to creatinine are constant, calculation of the total amount of creatinine excretion expected over a 24-hour period (using the figures above) can be used to verify whether a 24-hour urine collection is complete.

Creatinine, like inulin, is not extensively protein bound and is freely filtered at the glomerulus. However, unlike inulin, creatinine also undergoes active tubular secretion and thus is a less optimal measure of GFR.[24] When the GFR is greater than 15% to 20% of normal (approximately 30 mL/min for young males), CL_{cr} approximates GFR reasonably well. However, at lower GFRs, especially in disease states which primarily affect the glomeruli rather than the tubules (i.e., acute glomerulonephritis, hypertension), the contribution of tubular secretion may become significant, resulting in an overestimation of GFR. Nonrenal elimination of creatinine by gut metabolism may account for up to 50% of creatinine elimination in ESRD patients.[25] This would result in a lower-than-expected S_{cr} and an overestimation of the GFR. Additionally, several drugs which compete for tubular secretion with creatinine (e.g., trimethoprim,[20] cimetidine,[26] but not ranitidine)[27] may produce an elevated serum creatinine concentration; thus, the GFR would be underestimated.

Several diseases and drugs can interfere with the measurement of creatinine in biological fluids. The Jaffe enzymatic colorimetric method may be falsely elevated by high serum ketone concentrations (acetone or acetoacetic acid production in diabetic patients during ketoacidosis or in nondiabetic patients during extended fasting), ascorbic acid, phenolsulfonphthalein (a marker of renal tubular secretion), and barbiturates.[28,29] Each of these substances contributes to the chromogen in serum which is detected by the Jaffe method. Clinically achievable concentrations of cefoxitin, cefpirome, and ceforanide, but few other cephalosporins, cause false elevations of creatinine measurement which are proportionate to the serum concentration of the drug.[30,31]

The measurement of CL_{cr} is most accurately accomplished when the urine collection interval is 24 hours and serum creatinine is measured from a blood sample drawn at the midpoint of the collection period.[23,29,32] Urine collection periods as short as four to eight hours may provide a similar CL_{cr} value as a 24-hour collection if urine can be completely voided from the bladder before and at the end of these short collection intervals.[33,34] The over- or under-collection of urine for the assumed collection time period and degradation of creatinine in stored urine samples can dramatically alter the CL_{cr}, especially when urine is collected on an outpatient basis. Thus, a supervised collection in which the bladder is completely emptied before and at the end of the collection period and storage of the urine at 0 to 5 °C is preferred. The collection of urine for 24 hours is, however, not often reliable or convenient in any clinical setting because patients are not confined, compliant, or willing to collect all urine samples; the hospital staff is unable to supervise the collection; and the time required to measure CL_{cr} exceeds its clinical applicability. Recently, bioelectrical impedance, a noninvasive reproducible technique for measuring lean body mass used in conjunction with serum creatinine data, has been shown to provide a quick, accurate method for predicting CL_{cr} in some patient populations.[35,37]

Measurement of a serum creatinine concentration (unlike a 24-hour urine creatinine measurement) is routine, quick, and reliable. Thus, multiple methods for the estimation of CL_{cr} in adult and pediatric patients using the serum creatinine along with other routine clinical data such as patient age, gender, height, and weight have been developed and are widely utilized (see Table 8-2).[38–47]

Theoretically, the best method of estimating CL_{cr} should consider all factors that influence creatinine production and an estimate of nonrenal creatinine elimination. Since the method will be optimally applicable to patients with characteristics similar to those from whom the relationships were derived either broad populations should be studied or the method validated retrospectively for other populations. For example, the method of Cockcroft and Gault was derived from observations in approximately 200 adult male patients.[41] Their method estimates creatinine clearance for female patients by multiplying the value calculated for male patients by 0.85. This factor was extrapolated from theoretical and historical considerations but not from direct observation. The most significant limitation of the methods that rely on a single serum creatinine measurement (see Table 8-2) is that they require a steady-state serum creatinine value. As a rough guide, the serum creatinine can be considered to be at steady state if two values obtained within 24 hours vary by less than 10% to 15%.

The CL_{cr} of patients whose renal function is changing (e.g., patients with acute renal failure) can be estimated using three methods (see Table 8-3).[45–47] Since these methods do not assume that the serum creatinine is at steady state, they can be used when serum creatinine values are increasing or decreasing. With the Jeliffe and Jeliffe method, the most recent serum creatinine should be used in place of average serum creatinine when it is rising.[45] This will provide a lower estimate of

Table 8-2. Methods for Estimation of Creatinine Clearance from Serum Creatinine in Patients with Stable Renal Function

Reference	Units	Equations		Factors[a] not considered
		Males	Females	
ADULTS				
Mawer[38]	mL/min	$CL_{cr} = \dfrac{IBW\,[29.3 - 0.203\,(Age)][1 - 0.03(Scr)]}{14.4\,(Scr)}$	$CL_{cr} = \dfrac{IBW\,[25.3 - 0.175\,(Age)][1 - 0.03(Scr)]}{14.4\,(Scr)}$	1
Jellife[39]	mL/min/1.73 m²	$CL_{cr} = \dfrac{98 - 0.8\,(Age - 20)}{Scr}$	$CL_{cr} = $ male value × 0.90	1,2
Wagner[40]	mL/min	$\log CL_{cr} = 2.008 - 1.19 \log Scr$	$\log CL_{cr} = 1.888 - 1.20 \log Scr$	1,2,3
Cockroft and Gault[41]	mL/min	$CL_{cr} = \dfrac{(140 - Age)\,IBW}{72\,(Scr)}$	$CL_{cr} = $ male value × 0.85	1
Hull et al.[42]	mL/min/70 kg	$CL_{cr} = \dfrac{145 - Age}{Scr} - 3$	$CL_{cr} = $ male value × 0.85	1,2
CHILDREN				
Schwartz et al.[43,b]	mL/min/1.73 m²	$CL_{cr} = \dfrac{0.45\,(length\ in\ cm)}{Scr}$	—	1,2,4
Schwartz et al.[44,c]	mL/min/1.73 m²	$CL_{cr} = \dfrac{0.55\,(length\ in\ cm)}{Scr}$	—	1,2,3,4

[a] Factors: 1 = Nonrenal creatinine elimination; 2 = Ideal body weight; 3 = Age; 4 = Gender.
[b] Developed for neonates to infants 1 year of age.
[c] Developed for children 1 to 20 years of age.

Table 8–3. *Methods for Estimation of Creatinine Clearance from Serum Creatinine in Adult Patients with Unstable Renal Function*

Reference	Units	Equations	
		Males[a,b]	**Females**
Jellife and Jellife[45]	mL/min/1.73 m²	$E^{ss} = IBW [29.3 - 0.203 (Age)]$	$E^{ss} = IBW [25.1 - 0.175 (Age)]$
		$E^{ss}_{corr} = E^{ss} [1.035 - 0.0337 (Scr)]$	$E^{ss}_{corr} = E^{ss} [1.035 - 0.0337 (Scr)]$
		$E = E^{ss}_{corr} - \dfrac{[4\, IBW\, (Scr_2 - Scr_1)]}{\Delta t}$	$E = E^{ss}_{corr} - \dfrac{[4\, IBW\, (Scr_2 - Scr_1)]}{\Delta t}$
		$CL_{cr} = \dfrac{E}{14.4\,(Scr)}$	$CL_{cr} = \dfrac{E}{14.4\,(Scr)}$
Chiou et al.[46]	mL/min	$V_d = 0.6\,L\,(IBW)$	$V_d = 0.6\,L\,(IBW)$
		$CL_{cr} = \dfrac{2\,[28 - 0.2\,(Age)]}{(Scr_1 + Scr_2)} \times \dfrac{2\,[V_d\,(Scr_2 - Scr_1)]}{(Scr_1 + Scr_2)\,\Delta t} - [0.0286\,(V_d)]$	$CL_{cr} = \dfrac{2\,[22.4 - 0.16\,(Age)]}{(Scr_1 + Scr_2)} \times \dfrac{2\,[V_d\,(Scr_2 - Scr_1)]}{(Scr_1 + Scr_2)\,\Delta t} - [0.0286\,(V_d)]$
Brater[47]	mL/min/70 kg	$CL_{cr} = [293 - 2.03(Age)] \times [1.035 - 0.01685\,(Scr_1 + Scr_2)] + \dfrac{49\,(Scr_1 - Scr_2)\,/\,\Delta t}{Scr_1 + Scr_2}$	$CL_{cr} = $ male value $\times 0.86$

[a] E^{ss} = Steady-state urinary creatinine excretion rate.

[b] Δt = Time in days between the measurement of $Scr_1 + Scr_2$.

CL_{cr} and a more conservative estimate of a dosage adjustment in the face of declining renal function. The method of Chiou et al. utilizes creatinine production as a function of age alone and an assumed volume of distribution of 0.6 L/kg for all individuals to estimate CL_{cr}.[46] Although the volume of distribution for creatinine is not changed in patients with renal failure, the percent of total body weight which represents total body water is variable with respect to age, gender, and total body weight.[25] Thus, the ideal body weight of an individual patient should be utilized in this equation.

Estimation of CL_{cr} from serum creatinine values in dialyzed patients with severe renal insufficiency is difficult and imprecise. This is because the serum creatinine value which has been artificially lowered by dialysis does not reflect the functional capacity of the glomerulus. Up to seven days may be required after an acute dialysis procedure to once again reach steady-state conditions because the serum creatinine half-life may be extended to 42 hours.[48] If the serum creatinine value is changing during the interdialytic period, the methods of CL_{cr} estimation proposed for patients with unstable renal function may be applicable. The accuracy of these estimations, however, has not been thoroughly evaluated.

Quantitation of Tubular Function

Recent evidence suggests that the decline in renal tubular function may not parallel GFR in some disease states (see Indices of Renal Function: Excretion). Thus, the ability to characterize tubular secretory capacity may be clinically important, particularly for those drugs which have a narrow therapeutic index and for which active tubular secretion is a major elimination pathway (see Table 8-4). The net renal tubular secretion rate or clearance (CL_{sec}) of such a drug would be equal to the total renal clearance (CL_R) minus the filtration clearance, [GFR × the free fraction in plasma (f_{up})].

$$CL_{sec} = CL_R - (GFR)(f_{up}) \qquad \text{(Eq. 8-4)}$$

The CL_{sec} is determined in animals by infusing into the renal artery a standard marker for the anionic tubular secretion pathway [e.g., para-aminohippurate (PAH)][49] and/or a standard marker for the cationic pathway [e.g., tetraethylammonium bromide (TEAB)][50] along with a standard marker for glomerular filtration (e.g., GFR, inulin). Ideally, the marker used for each of the tubular secretion pathways should be completely extracted by the active tubular process in one pass through the vasculature of the kidney. In other words, the affinity of the transport system should be great and no tubular reabsorption should occur. If the plasma concentration of the secretory marker can be increased in a stepwise fashion, then the maximum tubular transport capacity for the pathway can be determined.[51,52]

The techniques used to characterize the renal tubular capacity in humans have been similar. A relatively innocuous marker of anionic renal tubular secretion (e.g., benzylpenicillin,[52] PAH,[53] or ceftizoxime)[54] or cationic tubular secretion (e.g., cimetidine,[55] ranitidine,[56] or procainamide)[57] is infused intravenously with a marker for glomerular filtration (e.g., inulin or iothalamate). Although benzyl-

Table 8-4. *Drugs Which Are Actively Secreted by Anionic and Cationic Transport*

ANIONS

acetazolamide	ceftazidime	nafcillin
amantadine	ceftizoxime	nitrofurantoin
ampicillin	cefuroxime	norfloxacin
bumetanide	cephalothin	para-aminohippurate
carbenicillin	cephapirin	penicillin G
cefamandole	cephradine	phenolsulfonphthalein
cefazolin	ciprofloxacin	phenylbutazone
cefmcnoxime	clofibrate	probenecid
cefmetazole	ethacrynic acid	thiazides
cefoperazone	folic acid	sulfamethoxazole
ceforanide	furosemide	sulfinpyrazone
cefotaxime	indomethacin	sulfisoxazole
cefotiam	methotrexate	zidovudine
cefoxitin	moxalactam	zomepirac

CATIONS

amiloride	n-acetyl procainamide (NAPA)	ranitidine
cimetidine	procainamide	triamterene
digoxin	quinidine	trimethoprim
morphine	quinine	vancomycin

penicillin[52] and phenolsulfonphthalein[58] have been used to establish the anionic tubular secretion capacity in various disease states, each undergoes tubular reabsorption to some degree and therefore underestimates CL_{sec}. Several maneuvers have been used to reduce the renal tubular reabsorption of these and other markers. These include enhancing tubular filtrate flow rate via infusion of intravenous fluids; ionizing the marker substrate within tubular filtrate by pH adjustment of the urine; and maintaining low to moderate concentrations of the marker substrate, which will minimize concentration-dependent transtubular passage.[59] The value of these methods outside of the context of clinical research is currently unclear. Identification of less innocuous markers (preferentially an endogenous solute) would greatly facilitate quantification of these two secretory pathways of renal excretion. For example, N-methylnicotinamide (NMN) is an endogenously released metabolite of niacin which is efficiently secreted by the cationic tubular pathway.[60–62] This substance would be ideal for routine, clinical tubular function studies should a rapid, automated assay technique be established.

ETIOLOGY AND PROGRESSION OF RENAL INSUFFICIENCY

The etiology of chronic renal insufficiency has changed over the last 20 to 30 years.[63] The proportion of ESRD cases attributable to diabetic nephropathy has increased dramatically while the proportion due to glomerulonephritis and tubule interstitial diseases has declined. Hypertension, however, remains one of the primary causes of ESRD despite the introduction of a multitude of new therapeutic alternatives. These changes in etiologies and the controversy regarding the intact nephron hypothesis may ultimately limit extrapolation of pharmacokinetic data from one renal failure population to another. (See Etiology and Progression of Renal Insufficiency: Influence of Renal Disease on Drug Excretion.)

Whatever the cause, renal insufficiency tends to become a progressive disease in which renal function declines over time to ESRD at a fairly constant rate once the serum creatinine exceeds 1.5 to 2.0 mg/dL.[64] Although the rate of decline in GFR can be estimated from a plot of the reciprocal of serum creatinine versus time,[63,64] several investigators have recently questioned its predictive utility.[24,65] Despite amelioration of the primary causative factor(s) or disease(s), renal function often continues to decline at a similar rate. This decline may be the result of the glomerular hemodynamic response to widespread renal injury. Fortunately, these hemodynamic changes can be reversed by restricting dietary protein intake, reducing systemic and glomerular capillary pressure, and/or by normalizing the abnormalities in lipid metabolism that invariably accompany renal disease.[64]

Influence of Renal Insufficiency on Drug Absorption

The oral absorption of drugs was once thought to be reduced in patients with renal insufficiency, especially those with end-stage renal disease.[66–68] This may have been more true in the past when patients were not dialyzed as aggressively as they are today. Then, higher levels of waste products such as urea nitrogen (BUN) may have altered gastric pH and induced edema of the gastrointestinal tract through local irritant properties. The continued administration of antacids to control the hyperphosphatemia (especially aluminum hydroxide) and other medications may have confounded previous bioavailability studies. Thus, any observed alteration in absorption must be interpreted in light of these factors.

Observation of a similar serum concentration-time profile [i.e., peak concentration, time to peak or area under the concentration-time curve (AUC)] after the oral administration of a drug to subjects with normal or impaired renal function does not necessarily mean that a similar fraction of the ingested drug was absorbed. This is because the peak concentration (C_{max}) of a drug after a single oral dose is determined by the following:

$$C_{max} = \frac{(D_M)\,(F)\left(\dfrac{K_a}{k_{el}}\right)^{\frac{k_{el}}{k_{el}-k_a}}}{V_d}$$

(Eq. 8-5)

where D_M is the maintenance dose, F is the bioavailability, k_a is the first-order absorption rate constant, k_{el} is the elimination rate constant, and V_d is the volume of distribution. Thus, C_{max} depends mainly on the ratio of k_a to k_{el}. If k_{el} is reduced much more than k_a, the expected peak concentration in renal failure may be the same as in normal subjects, even though F is decreased and V_d increased. Therefore, equivalent peak concentrations do not necessarily indicate equivalent F. Similarly, extremely disparate peak concentration values do not always indicate poor availability and may only represent slowed absorption, since the time to reach peak concentration (T_{max}) is also dependent upon k_a and k_{el}:

$$T_{max} = \frac{2.3}{k_a - k_{el}} \times \log \frac{k_a}{k_{el}} \qquad \text{(Eq. 8-6)}$$

Alterations in protein-binding, distribution volume, metabolism, and/or renal clearance (individually or combined) could mask the impact of renal disease on the oral absorption concentration-time curve. The optimal methodology to ascertain the effect of renal insufficiency on the bioavailability of a drug formulation is to compare the AUC to that of a reference standard in patients and healthy volunteers. Since the bioavailability of an intravenously administered drug is by definition 100%, comparison of any oral dosage form to the intravenous standard provides an index of the absolute bioavailability of the dosage form in the patient population.

$$F = \left(\frac{AUC_{po}}{AUC_{iv}}\right)\left(\frac{D_{iv}}{D_{po}}\right) \qquad \text{(Eq. 8-7)}$$

Although little quantitative information is available regarding the bioavailability of drugs in patients with renal disease, the bioavailability of three drugs has been reported to be diminished (see Table 8-5).[69–71] In fact, the bioavailability of the majority of drugs which have been evaluated in patients with renal insufficiency is either unchanged or increased.[72–78] The hypothesis which has been proposed to explain the observed increases in bioavailability is a reduced first-pass or presystemic metabolism of these drugs.[73,75–77]

Disparate observations with such structurally similar compounds as dihydrocodeine and codeine and the beta blockers may be due in part to the methodologic differences rather than differences in disease effect. For example, Barnes et al.[77] only administered dihydrocodeine orally to their subjects with normal (N) and impaired renal function (IRF) and noted a significant increase in the AUC [2.25 ± 0.39 (IRF) versus 1.32 ± 0.20 (N) mg × hr/L] (see Figure 8-2a). Guay et al.[72] administered codeine intravenously as well as orally in a crossover design to chronic hemodialysis patients (HD) and volunteers with normal renal function. They, like Barnes et al.[77] noted an increase in AUC after both the oral and

Table 8-5. *Bioavailability of Drugs in Patients with Renal Disease*

Decreased	Unchanged	Increased
d-xylose	cimetidine	bufuralol
furosemide	ciprofloxacin	dextropropoxyphene
pindolol	codeine	dihydrocodeine
	digoxin	oxprenolol
	labetalol	propranolol
	trimethoprim	tolamolol
	sulfamethoxazole	

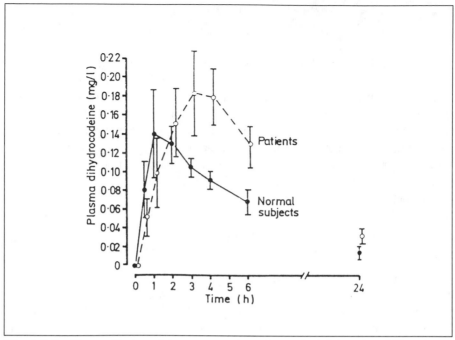

Figure 8-2a. *Plasma dihydrocodeine concentrations after oral administration of 60 mg (mean ± SEM) in patients with chronic renal failure (O) and subjects with normal renal function (●). Reprinted with permission from reference 77.*

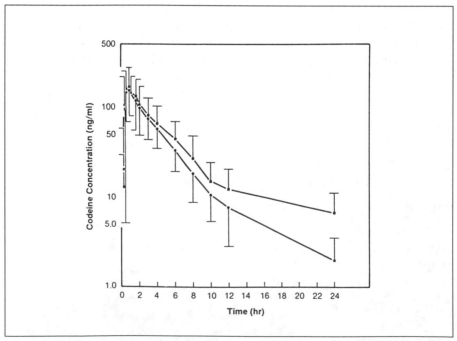

Figure 8-2b. *Plasma codeine concentrations (mean ± SD) after oral administration of 60 mg codeine sulfate in hemodialysis patients (■) and subjects with normal renal function (●). Reprinted with permission from reference 72.*

intravenous dose in the patients (see Figure 8-2b). However, the absolute bio-availability did not differ between the two groups [(80.5 ± 30.9 (N) versus 73.6 ± 32.3 (HD)].

Effect of Renal Insufficiency on Protein Binding and Volume of Distribution

The plasma protein-binding of acidic drugs (e.g., phenytoin, valproic acid, clofibrate, and salicylate) is markedly reduced in patients with severe renal insufficiency.[79] Unfortunately, for most agents, the degree of change in binding has not been evaluated in patients with mild to moderate renal insufficiency. Thus, the applicability of the reported data to many patients with renal dysfunction is unknown. The mechanism(s) for this reduced protein binding include decreased plasma albumin concentrations, accumulation of endogenous binding inhibitors, qualitative changes in the binding sites, and competition for binding by metabolites of the administered parent drug.[78,79]

Reduced protein binding generally results in an increase in the apparent distribution volume and for some compounds, an increase in total body clearance (see Table 8-6).[66,80,81] An increase in total body clearance is not necessarily indicative of a change in metabolism, however. For those drugs which demonstrate restrictive clearance [i.e., the total body clearance is directly proportional to the product of hepatic clearance (CL_H) and the free fraction in blood (f_{ub})], the increase in CL_T may be a direct consequence of the increased f_{ub}.

$$CL_T = CL_H \cdot f_{ub} \qquad \text{(Eq. 8-8)}$$

$$f_{ub} = \frac{f_{up} \cdot C_p}{C_b} \qquad \text{(Eq. 8-9)}$$

where f_{up} is the free fraction in plasma, C_p is the drug concentration in plasma, and C_b is the drug concentration in blood. In this situation, the average "free" concentration of the drug will not be altered providing there is no enzyme induction or inhibition, or competition with renal tubular secretion. However, an increase in f_{up} will result in an increase in distribution volume but no change in overall clearance for drugs that demonstrate nonrestrictive clearance behavior. This results in an increase in half-life and minimization of the fluctuation between peak and trough concentrations if the dose and dosing interval are unchanged.[82] (See Chapter 6: Influence of Liver Function on Drug Disposition for a more detailed discussion of restrictive and nonrestrictive clearance.)

Reduced protein binding is often accompanied by a decrease in total plasma or serum concentrations, and this may complicate the individualization of drug dosage regimens. The optimal solution to this problem is to monitor "free" or unbound drug concentrations; however, this procedure is not available in some clinical laboratories.[83] When "free" concentrations are unavailable, it is sometimes possible to equate the total drug concentration observed in a patient with renal failure to that which would be observed if the patient had normal renal function.[84] For example, in the case of phenytoin, the drug concentration that would be observed if a patient had normal renal function can be estimated as follows:

$$C_e = \frac{1}{1 + [(nKa)(p)]} (C_{pt})(10)$$

(Eq. 8-10)

Table 8-6. *The Effect of Renal Disease on Drug Distribution Volume*[66,80,81]

Drug	Volume of distribution (L/kg)	
	Normal	ESRD[a]
Increased		
amikacin	0.20	0.29
azlocillin	0.21	0.28
bretylium	3.58	4.48
cefazolin	0.13	0.16
cefonicid	0.11	0.14
cefoxitin	0.16	0.26
cefuroxime	0.20	0.26
clofibrate	0.14	0.24
cloxacillin	0.14	0.26
dicloxacillin	0.08	0.18
erythromycin	0.57	1.09
furosemide	0.11	0.18
gentamicin	0.20	0.29
isoniazid	0.60	0.80
minoxidil	2.60	4.90
phenytoin	0.64	1.40
sisomicin	0.19	0.25
sulfamethopyrazine	0.21	0.38
trimethoprim	1.36	1.83
vancomycin	0.64	0.85
Decreased		
chloramphenicol	0.87	0.60
digoxin	7.30	4.10
ethambutol	3.70	1.60
methicillin	0.45	0.30
pindolol	2.10	1.10
pipemidic acid	2.00	0.84
Unchanged		
cefamandole	0.13	0.16
cefmetazole	0.17	0.18
diazepam	2.80	2.10
disopyramide	0.60	0.57
5-flucytosine	0.58	0.59
guanadrel	10.7	11.8
lidocaine	1.30	1.20
nafcillin	1.10	0.80
n-acetylprocainamide	1.40	1.70
procainamide	1.90	1.70
pyridostigmine	1.10	1.00
quinidine	3.00	2.50
roxithromycin	0.44	0.43

[a] ESRD = End-stage renal disease.

where C_e is the equated concentration, C_{pt} is the patient's measured concentration, nKa is the protein binding parameter based on the patient's renal function, and p is the patient's serum albumin concentration.

Although far less data are available regarding the effect of renal insufficiency on the protein binding of basic drugs, some generalizations can be projected.[79] Haughey et al.[85] and Docci et al.[86] have demonstrated that the serum concentrations of α_1-acid glycoprotein (AAG) are significantly higher in dialysis patients than in patients with normal renal function or renal insufficiency. Furthermore, there is a relationship between the progressive loss and return of renal function and an increase and decrease, respectively, in AAG concentrations. These findings are clinically relevant since AAG is the principal plasma binding protein for several basic drugs (e.g., bepridil and disopyramide). Thus, an increase in AAG concentrations leads to an increase in the bound fraction. The effect of renal insufficiency on basic drugs which are bound to albumin as well as to AAG is more complex and a decrease or no change in the fraction bound has been the predominant finding.[66,68]

The apparent volume of distribution at steady state (V_{dss}) of a drug may be affected not only by changes in plasma protein binding but also by alterations in tissue binding:[87]

$$V_{dss} = V_b + \frac{(f_{ub})(V_t)}{f_{ut}}$$

(Eq. 8-11)

where V_b is blood volume, V_t is tissue volume, and f_{ut} is the unbound fraction of drug in tissue. The volume of distribution for several drugs is decreased in patients with end-stage renal disease and one of the proposed mechanisms for this change is an increase in f_{ut} (see Table 8-6). In fact, for some drugs, the relationship between the change in distribution volume and the degree of renal insufficiency CL_{cr} has been characterized. The relationship described by Jusko et al. for digoxin is an example of one of these clinically useful tools.[88]

$$V_{dss}\,(L) = 226 + \frac{298\,(CL_{cr}\ \text{in mL/min})}{29.1 + CL_{cr}}$$

(Eq. 8-12)

Drug Metabolism in Patients with Renal Insufficiency

Renal disease is generally thought to reduce only the renal clearance of drugs (i.e., the net elimination of unchanged drug by glomerular filtration and tubular secretion minus tubular reabsorption). However, it is now recognized that even if urinary excretion is not an important route of elimination for a particular drug, renal failure may affect the nonrenal clearance of the agent.[89–91]

Several investigators have demonstrated significant reductions in the activity of multiple microsomal enzymes in animals with acute as well as chronic renal failure.[92–96] Patterson et al.[92] recently observed a significant relationship between the degree of renal insufficiency and the degree of reduction in hepatic enzymatic activity. The decrease in total metabolic activity in intact animals with renal insufficiency may be due to the impairment of hepatic metabolic activity as well as the loss of renal metabolism. Since some drugs (e.g., acetaminophen, amino-pyrine, 7-ethoxycoumarin) are known to be metabolized by the kidney, the contribution of this metabolic activity may be significant.[95,97]

Recently, a factor present in the blood of rats with acute renal failure has been purported to be responsible for the reduced presystemic clearance (first-pass metabolism) of orally administered l-propranolol.[98] The metabolism of l-propran-olol was significantly lower in livers isolated from rats with acute renal failure when compared to livers from normal rats. Moreover, when livers from normal rats were cross-perfused with uremic blood, the extraction of l-propranolol was depressed to a level almost identical to that observed in livers isolated from rats with acute renal failure. These data suggest that the reduction in presystemic hepatic metabolism of l-propranolol in this animal model may be due to the presence of an inhibitory factor in uremic blood.

Despite these observations in experimental models of renal insufficiency, until recently there have been very few reports of alterations in the metabolic capacity (nonrenal clearance) of patients with renal insufficiency. In the mid 1970s, several investigations of antipyrine half-life and clearance (an index of hepatic mixed function oxidase activity) were conducted.[99-101] Although the data of Leichter et al.[99] were not analyzed statistically, they suggested that there was a marked reduction of the half-life of antipyrine in patients with renal insufficiency who were not undergoing dialysis relative to healthy normal volunteers. Maddocks et al.[100] used a more rigorous study design and concluded that the half-life of antipyrine was significantly shorter in patients with renal failure than in age-matched normal volunteers (7.3 $\pm$ 2.0 hours versus 13.2 $\pm$ 4.3 hours). How-ever, subsequent investigations by Harman et al.,[101] Teunissen et al.,[102] Awni et al.,[103] and Halstenson et al.[104] strongly contradict these early observations.

Teunissen et al.[102] were first to report the plasma concentration-time profiles of antipyrine metabolites in patients with chronic renal failure. The urinary recovery of antipyrine and metabolites was significantly reduced in these patients, with the primary reduction being in the formation of norantipyrine. This reduction in norantipyrine formation suggests that renal disease may preferentially affect the activity of different forms of cytochrome P450, in this case the isoenzymes responsible for N-demethylation.

Several clinical investigations during the last five to ten years have indicated that the disposition of some compounds is altered in patients with renal insufficiency, not only on the basis of a reduction in renal clearance but of nonrenal clearance as well (see Table 8-7). The reduction in nonrenal clearance parallels the decline in renal function for compounds that are metabolized by multiple routes, including deacetylation, hydroxylation, O-demethylation, N-demethylation, and sulfoxidation as well as glucuronidation. Although the degree of reduction in nonrenal clearance has generally been less than that of renal clearance, the absolute reductions have been significant, ranging from 17% to 71% of the nonrenal clearance observed in subjects with normal renal function.[68,90,91]

Many diseases may ultimately lead to the development of renal insufficiency. The most common causes of renal insufficiency in the United States are currently diabetes mellitus, glomerulonephritis, and hypertensive nephrosclerosis.[63] These three disease entities account for up to 60% of the patients who ultimately developed ESRD. The marked diversity which may have been represented in the patients with "renal insufficiency" who participated in clinical studies from which the data in Table 8-7 were derived complicates our interpretation of these data. The question might well be raised whether these are disease-state-specific effects or a reflection of renal insufficiency irrespective of the cause.

Currently, only limited data exist which address the potential for disease-state-specific effects on nonrenal clearance among patients with similar GFRs. In patients with Type II diabetes mellitus, a reduced total clearance of antipyrine as well as a prolongation in elimination half-life has been reported by some but not all investigators.[105] Data of Narang et al.[106] and Zysset et al.[107] suggest that antipyrine half-life and clearance, respectively, may be altered as much as 100%. Not only was the plasma clearance of antipyrine significantly reduced in the patients studied by Zysset et al. (by approximately 30% in the Type II diabetics),[107] but the urinary excretion of antipyrine and its metabolites was also decreased approximately 44%. Zysset et al.,[107] Aditham et al.,[108] and Matzke et al.[109] extended these observations to insulin-dependent diabetics (Type I). The results of their elegant investigations suggest that the clearance of antipyrine is increased by as much as 70% and the half-life is reduced from 12 to 13 hours in controls to 8 to 9 hours in Type I diabetics. The impact of diabetes on the elimination of drugs other than antipyrine has only received minimal attention. Tolbutamide and theophylline elimination have been reported to be unchanged in Type II pa-

Table 8-7. The Effect of Renal Disease on Non-Renal Clearance and Total Body Clearance

Drug	% change from normal clearance	
	Non-renal	Total body
acyclovir	−55	−90
aztreonam	−33	−74
bumetanide	+57	−33
captopril	−50	−65
cefmenoxime	−45	−83
cefmetazole	−80	−91
cefonicid	−62	−90
cefotaxime	−50	−71
cefotiam	−71	−91
ceftizoxime	−55	−90
cefsulodin	−52	−80
cetirizine	−17	−70
cimetidine	−62	−80
codeine	−17	−27
guanadrel	−83	−85
imipenem	−85	−77
metoclopramide	−66	−72
minoxidil	−46	−55
moxalactam	−63	−90
procainamide	60	−82
roxithromycin	−42	−48
verapamil	−54	−41

tients,[110,111] while the elimination of acetaminophen is reduced in Type II patients and unaltered in Type I patients.[112] These markedly different metabolic profiles in Type I and Type II diabetics suggest that the metabolism of drugs in patients with various etiologies of renal insufficiency may also be variable.

Influence of Renal Disease on Drug Excretion

Three processes comprise total renal drug excretion: glomerular filtration, tubular secretion, and tubular reabsorption (see Figure 8-3).[113] A drug's rate of filtration (Rf) is dependent on GFR, plasma concentration, and degree of protein binding.

$$Rf = (GFR)(C_p)(f_{up}) \qquad \text{(Eq. 8-13)}$$

Active tubular secretion of a drug, which may be through the anionic or cationic substrate-specific pathway, depends on the affinity of the tubular transport sites for the drug molecule, the capacity of the site to actively transport the molecules into the tubular lumen, and renal blood flow. Secretion can be so extensive that virtually all the drug in the blood is removed and must be operative if renal clearance (CL_R) exceeds $CL_{Filt.}$

$$CL_R = CL_{Filt} + \frac{R_s - R_r}{C_p} \qquad \text{(Eq. 8-14)}$$

where R_s is the rate of secretion, and R_r is the rate of reabsorption, and CL_{Filt} is Rf/C_p.

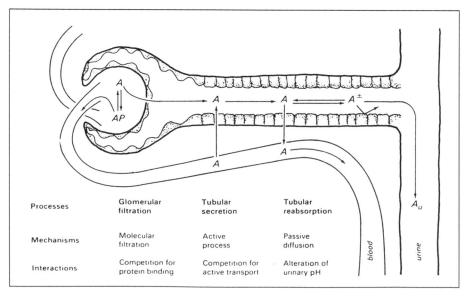

Processes	Glomerular filtration	Tubular secretion	Tubular reabsorption
Mechanisms	Molecular filtration	Active process	Passive diffusion
Interactions	Competition for protein binding	Competition for active transport	Alteration of urinary pH

Figure 8-3. Mechanisms of renal excretion of drugs and potential sites for drug interactions (reprinted with permission from reference 113).

The location of these transport sites in the tubules has been identified and their selectivity evaluated with several marker solutes. For more details on these processes, the reader is referred to the review by Kosoglou and Vlasses.[114] The passive tubular reabsorption of a drug is determined by its degree of lipophilicity, degree of ionization (pk_a and pH), and the urine flow rate. Reabsorption must occur if the CL_R is less than $CL_{Filt.}$ Highly lipid soluble drugs may be completely reabsorbed. The relative contribution of each of these processes to the renal excretion of any particular drug may vary greatly.

Many diseases which affect the kidney preferentially alter the normal histology of the glomeruli or tubules. However, according to the "Intact Nephron Hypothesis," the function of all segments of the remaining nephron are affected equally.[115,116] Thus, regardless of the relative contribution of these intrarenal pathways to drug excretion in the normal kidney, the rate of whole organ excretion in the diseased kidney has been purported to be quantifiable by a measure of GFR such as CL_{cr}.

Nevertheless, different diseases of the kidney may result in declines in glomerular and tubular function in a nonparallel manner.[62,117–120] Lin and Lin reported that two etiologically different models of acute renal failure in rats produced quantitatively different effects on glomerular filtration and tubular secretion by the anionic and the cationic pathway.[117] In both models of acute renal failure, secretion by the anionic pathway deteriorated faster than GFR. The decline in cationic secretion appeared to parallel the decrease in GFR in the glycerol-induced renal failure model, which produces a hemodynamically mediated renal ischemia. In contrast, the effect of uranyl nitrate (a direct nephrotoxin) on cationic secretion differed quantitatively from the decline in GFR. Gloff and Benet have recently confirmed these observations using the uranyl nitrate model.[118] Maiza and Daley-Yates reported further evidence of glomerular tubular imbalance in rats with proximal tubular necrosis, papillary necrosis, and glomerulonephritis.[62,119] The type of renal disease may thus be a major factor in determining the renal elimination of some drugs, and the Intact Nephron Hypothesis, at least in these animal models of renal insufficiency, appears to be invalid.

Dissimilar effects of various kidney diseases on tubular and glomerular function have also been observed in humans. Many of these studies used inulin clearance as a measure of GFR and the product of PAH clearance and renal extraction ratio as a measure of renal blood flow.[121–128] The clearance of PAH alone, however, may also be considered an index of tubular secretion by the anionic pathway. Linear regression analysis of these data for patient populations with four of the most common causes of renal insufficiency (diabetes mellitus, acute and chronic glomerulonephritis, and hypertension) appear in Figure 8-4. Good correlations between inulin and PAH clearance were obtained for each patient group. However, the degree of decline in anionic tubular secretion was greater than the decrease in GFR over the evaluated range of renal function. Furthermore, the difference in the ratios of the slopes of these relationships between diseases suggests that a particular disease state may markedly alter the relative contribution of net tubular secretion to total renal clearance.

The extent to which the total body clearance of a drug is changed in a patient with renal insufficiency depends on the fraction of the dose eliminated unchanged by the normal kidney, the intrarenal pathways for drug elimination, and the degree of functional impairment of each of these pathways. At present, pharmacokinetic analysis of new drug entities includes determination of the fraction of unchanged drug eliminated renally (see Table 8-8) and occasionally an estimation of the extent of renal tubular secretion. Clinical methods to determine an individual's net tubular clearance (total renal clearance minus filtration clearance) have been suggested and analyzed by Hori et al.[58] This procedure involves measuring the renal elimination of phenolsulfonphthalein, a high-capacity substrate of the anionic tubular secretory pathway. Although this method was validated prospectively by the original authors, no independent assessments of this test as an index of net tubular secretion have been reported.[129]

The renal clearance of a drug which is filtered and eliminated by renal tubular secretion can be affected in three ways by the administration of another substance.[130] Since tubular secretion is always accompanied by GFR, any compound that causes a change in GFR will also change the CL_R. Second, substances may alter the maximum tubular transport (T_M) of the secretory pathway through noncompetitive inhibition or degradation of transport carriers. However, the most common type of interaction at the level of the transport system is a competitive interaction between substances with an affinity for the same carrier. This interaction mechanism usually results in a concentration-dependent decrease in tubular clearance.

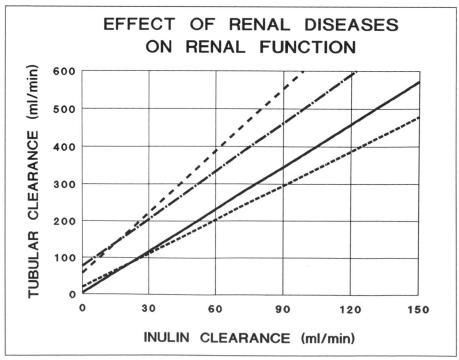

Figure 8-4. *Effect of diabetes mellitus (- - - -), acute (- - - -) and chronic (- • -) glomerulonephritis and hypertension (—) on GFR expressed as inulin clearance and net tubular clearance by the anionic pathway expressed as p-aminohippurate clearance.*

Clinically significant drug interactions involving renal transport mechanisms are common between organic cations and anions.[114,130-135] Although the distinct mechanisms of transport might suggest mutual exclusion between the two pathways, one of the remarkable characteristics of the anionic system is that it accepts chemically diverse compounds (see Table 8-4). These interactions may be clinically useful. For example, probenicid reduces the renal clearance of zidovudine and its glucuronidated metabolite,[136,137] and this may allow patients to take a reduced daily dose. However, toxic events also may be precipitated by this type of interaction. For example, concomitant administration of cimetidine with procainamide can decrease CL_R by up to 36% and has produced clinical toxicity.[114]

Drug Dosage Regimen Design in Renal Insufficiency

For a drug which is predominantly eliminated unchanged by the kidney, progressive reductions in CL_R and CL_T, but not necessarily in CL_{NR}, would be expected as renal function declines.

$$CL_T = CL_R + CL_{NR} \qquad \text{(Eq. 8-15)}$$

Indeed, changes in CL_R and CL_T have been correlated with CL_{cr} as the index of renal function by many investigators.[79,81,138] If there were no alteration in V_d or in CL_{NR}, then these relationships could be extrapolated to provide an index of k_{el} and the terminal elimination half-life:

$$CL_R = (\alpha)\,(CL_{cr}) \qquad \text{(Eq. 8-16)}$$

$$CL_T = (\alpha)\,(CL_{cr}) + CL_{NR} \qquad \text{(Eq. 8-17)}$$

$$k_{el} = \frac{CL_T}{V_d} = \frac{(\alpha)\,(CL_{cr})}{V_d} + \frac{CL_{NR}}{V_d} \qquad \text{(Eq. 8-18)}$$

$$k_{el} = \left(\frac{\alpha}{V_d}\right)(CL_{cr}) + k_{NR} \qquad \text{(Eq. 8-19)}$$

$$t\tfrac{1}{2} = \frac{0.693}{k_{el}} \qquad \text{(Eq. 8-20)}$$

The relationship in Equation 8-17 forms the basis of the dosing nomograms which were developed by Dettli and colleagues.[139-141] They utilized the projected change in k_{el} or CL_T along with the ratio (Q_o) of the k_{NR} or CL_{NR} to k_{el} and CL_T respectively from subjects with normal renal function ($CL_N = 100$ mL/min) as the basis for the calculation of their drug dosage adjustment factor (Q).

$$Q_o = \frac{k_{NR}}{k_{el}} = \frac{CL_{NR}}{CL_T}$$

(Eq. 8-21)

$$Q = Q_o + \left(\frac{\alpha}{k_{el}}\right)(CL_{cr})$$

(Eq. 8-22)

$$Q = Q_o + \left[\left(\frac{1 - Q_o}{CL_T}\right)(CL_{cr})\right]$$

(Eq. 8-23)

Tozer[142] and Welling et al.[143] expanded the applicability of these relationships by deriving individual approaches to predict the k_{el} or CL_T of a patient with renal insufficiency (i.e., k_{el}' and CL_T') from the fraction of unchanged drug eliminated renally unchanged in subjects with normal renal function (f_e) and the ratio of the patient's CL_{cr} to a presumed normal CL_{cr} of 120 mL/min/1.73 m^2 (KF). Welling and colleagues derived specific equations for 22 drugs, while Tozer proposed the following general equation:

$$Q = 1 - \left[(f_e)(1 - KF)\right]$$

(Eq. 8-24)

The elimination rate constant (k_{el}') and clearance CL_T') of a patient with renal insufficiency can thus be predicted once the value for the parameter in subjects with normal renal function is known:

$$k_{el}' = (k_{el})(Q)$$

(Eq. 8-25)

Table 8-8. *Select Drugs Grouped by Fraction of Dose Eliminated Unchanged in Urine*

75%–100%

acyclovir	cefazolin	flucytosine	netilmicin
amantadine	ceftazidime	ganciclovir	ofloxacin
amikacin	ceftizoxime	gentamicin	penicillin G
ampicillin	cefuroxime	lithium	ticarcillin
atenolol	cephalexin	methotrexate	tobramycin
bretylium	ethambutol	n-acetylprocainamide	vancomycin

50%–74%

aztreonam	cefoxitin	imipenem	piperacillin
captopril	ceftriaxone	mezlocillin	procainamide
cefotaxime	cimetidine	nadolol	ranitidine
cefotetan	digoxin	pindolol	trimethoprim

< 50%

amiodarone	clindamycin	isoniazid	norfloxacin
amphotericin B	corticosteroids	itraconazole	oxacillin
cefoperazone	enoxacin	ketoconazole	pentamidine
chloramphenicol	erythromycin	mezlocillin	sulfamethoxazole
ciprofloxacin	famotidine	nafcillin	zidovudine

$$CL_T' = (CL_T)(Q) \qquad \text{(Eq. 8-26)}$$

These general methods for estimating the kinetic parameters in a patient with renal insufficiency and/or projecting a new dosage regimen assume the following: 1) the elimination of the drug can be described by a first-order one-compartment model; 2) glomerular and tubular function decrease to the same extent in all renal diseases; 3) the bioavailability, protein binding, volume of distribution, and nonrenal clearance of the drug are not altered by renal insufficiency; 4) the metabolites of the drug are pharmacologically inactive and do not accumulate in the presence of renal insufficiency; and 5) the concentration/effect relationship of the drug is unchanged.

Tozer and Rowland modified the earlier method of Tozer to incorporate potential alterations in bioavailability and volume of distribution of unbound drug (V_{du}).[144] They also incorporated age and weight into the prediction of nonrenal clearance for the unbound drug fraction.

$$Q = \left(\frac{V_{du}}{V_{du}'}\right)\left(\frac{F}{F'}\right)\left[(KF)(f_e) + \left[(1 - f_e)\frac{(140 - age)(weight)^{0.7}}{1660}\right]\right]$$

Q = (distribution volume) (bioavailability) (renal clearance + nonrenal clearance)

$$\text{(Eq. 8-27)}$$

where V_{du}' and F′ are the volume of distribution for the unbound drug fraction and bioavailability in the patient with renal insufficiency. KF optimally would represent the ratio of unbound renal clearance of the drug in the patient with renal insufficiency (CL_{Ru}') and patients with normal renal function (CL_{Ru}). In most clinical situations, however, these two parameters will not be known and KF will be calculated as before (patient's CL_{cr} ÷ a normal CL_{cr} of 120 mL/min/1.73 m²). This more elegant approach still requires assumptions one, two, four, and five, which were operative with the earlier Tozer method. Furthermore, although the current adjustment of unbound nonrenal clearance considers age and weight, it still assumes that this value is not altered by the presence of renal insufficiency.

Although these methods are not ideal, they do permit a reasonable approach to continuous dose adjustment in the patient with renal failure. As such, they are clearly more optimal than the multiple guides to drug dosage in renal failure which propose the use of a fixed dose or dosage interval for patients with broad ranges of renal function.[145–147]

Once the kinetic parameters or the dosage adjustment factor(s) for the patient have been estimated, the dosage regimen must be modified to obtain the desired therapeutic serum concentration profile. If clinically significant relationships between peak and trough concentrations and efficacy or toxicity have been described, then the dosage regimen should be designed to attain and maintain these target values. If, however, no specific peak or trough concentrations are desired and particularly if a therapeutic serum concentration range has not been identified, then the goal of the adjusted dosage regimen may be to attain the same average steady-state concentration or a similar area under the serum concentration time-curve during the dosing interval observed in patients with normal renal function.[68] When a drug is administered by continuous intravenous infusion (where k_o = infusion rate), the desired goal is to maintain a specific average steady-state concentration (C_{ss}).

$$C_{ss} = \frac{k_o}{CL_T}$$

(Eq. 8-28)

In this case, the adjusted dosage regimen can be calculated as follows:

$$k_o' = (k_o)(Q)$$

(Eq. 8-29)

If no loading dose is administered, it will take four to five half-lives for the C_{ss} to be achieved. To achieve the desired C_{ss} more rapidly, a loading dose (D_L) may need to be administered. The desired D_L can be calculated if in addition to the C_{ss}, the V_d' (in L/kg) and the patient's total body weight (TBW) in kilograms are known:

$$D_L = (C_{ss})(V_d')(TBW)$$

(Eq. 8-30)

If the V_d' is significantly different from the V_d in patients with normal renal function, then the V_d' should be utilized in Equation 8-30. If not, V_d should provide a reasonable estimate of D_L (see Table 8-6 for V_d and V_d' data).

When a drug is administered intermittently, whether intravenously, orally, or by another nonparenteral route, the desired goal will guide the selection of the dosage adjustment method. If the goal is to maintain the same C_{ss} or AUC during the dosing interval, then one can either decrease the maintenance dose (D_M) or prolong the dosing interval (τ). Conversely, if a constant dosing interval is desired, the dose can be reduced to maintain the desired C_{ss}. The new dosing interval (τ') or maintenance dose (D_M') for the patient with renal insufficiency can be calculated as follows:

$$\tau' = \frac{\tau}{Q}$$

(Eq. 8-31)

$$D_M' = (D_M)(Q)$$

(Eq. 8-32)

Although both of these equations will achieve the same average C_{ss}, the resultant steady-state peak [($C\infty$) max] and trough [($C\infty$) min] concentrations will be markedly different (see Figure 8-5). The ($C\infty$) max and ($C\infty$) min concentrations following IV bolus (Equations 8-33 and 8-34) or intermittent infusion (Equations 8-35 and 8-36) administration where t_I is the duration of the infusion can be calculated as follows:

$$(C\infty)_{max} = \left(\frac{D_M}{V_d}\right)\left(\frac{1}{1 - e^{-k_{(el)(\tau)}}}\right)$$ (Eq. 8-33)

$$(C\infty)_{min} = (C\infty)_{max}\ (e^{-k_{(el)(\tau)}})$$ (Eq. 8-34)

$$(C\infty)_{max} = \frac{[k_o]\ [1 - e^{-k_{(el)(t_I)}}]}{[k_{el}]\ [V_d][1 - e^{-k_{(el)(\tau)}}]}$$ (Eq. 8-35)

$$(C\infty)_{min} = [C\infty]_{max}\ [e^{-k_{el}(\tau - t_I)}]$$ (Eq. 8-36)

If a specific $(C\infty)$ max or $(C\infty)$ min is desired, the τ' for the patient and the D_M can be calculated as follows if the drug can be described by a one-compartment linear model and administered by intermittent IV infusion.

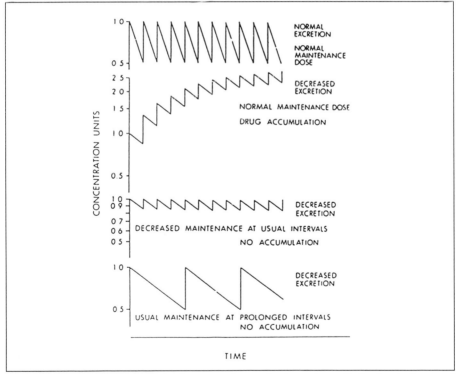

Figure 8-5. If no adjustment in the dosage regimen of a drug whose elimination is decreased in the presence of renal insufficiency is made, then the concentration of the drug in the body will increase. Acceptable concentrations can be achieved by administering a lower dose at the usual interval or by giving the same dose less frequently (reprinted with permission from reference 113).

$$\tau' = \left[\frac{1}{k_{el}'}\right] \ln \left(\frac{C\infty_{max}}{C\infty_{min}}\right) + t_I \tag{Eq. 8-37}$$

$$\frac{D_M'}{t_I} = \left[k_{el}' \, V_d' \, (C\infty)_{max}\right] \left[\frac{1 - e^{-k_{(el)'(\tau)'}}}{1 - e^{-k_{(el)'(\tau)'}}}\right] \tag{Eq. 8-38}$$

The above methods of dosage individualization are predominantly used in a setting where no serum concentration data are available to guide the therapeutic decision making process. These methods have been evaluated for several drugs, and generally, their use represents an improvement over empiric therapy; however, they are still associated with marked predictive error (see Table 8-9). The measurement of serum concentrations in individual patients with (fixed sampling approach) or without (individualized approach) the incorporation of historical population mean data is a more accurate way to attain a desired serum concentration-time profile in patients with renal insufficiency.[148] During the last decade, the use of Bayesian analysis has expanded greatly. This method incorporates population variance, mean data, and observed serum concentrations into the individualization formula. This approach yields a degree of accuracy similar to that of the individualized approach, but requires fewer serum concentration data points.[149-152] Although several Bayesian software programs are now available, the ultimate role of these programs in designing dosage regimens for patients with renal insufficiency and those on dialysis remains to be ascertained.

Table 8-9. *Drug Dosage Optimization Strategies[148]*

Methods	Description	Typical % error
Population means	Population-based *a priori* estimation of pharmacokinetic parameters using physical/functional information (age, weight, gender, CL_{cr}). No drug concentration data to assess individuals variability from population mean value.	50
Observed C_p	Multiple drug concentrations (usually ≤3) obtained at specific time points in order to individualize dosage regimen. Experiences represented by population-based methods not utilized to assess validity of observed data.	10–20
Population means + Observed C_p	Individual drug concentration data (often just one) obtained at a fixed sampling time after a standard dose. Additional data may be obtained to identify individual differences from population mean versus spurious initial concentration values. No assessment of true population outlier status possible.	20–30
Population means + Population variances + Observed C_p	Any number of drug concentrations (usually ≤2) obtained at various time points incorporated into population-based estimates of mean value and variance about mean value. Pharmacokinetic parameters determined by Bayesian technique to minimize error between predicted and observed data.	10–20

Table 8-10. *Clearance (CL) of Selected Drugs by Conventional Hemodialysis (HD) and Intermittent Peritoneal Dialysis (IPD) as Well as Total Body Clearance Patients with End-Stage Renal Disease (T)*

	CL_T (mL/min)	CL_{HD} (mL/min)	CL_{IPD}[a] (mL/min)
Penicillins			
amoxicillin	40	59–84	ND
ampicillin	30	30–154	ND
azlocillin	60	15	ND
mezlocillin	100	29	7.4
piperacillin	50	74	ND
ticarcillin	16	33	7.2
Cephalosporins			
cefaclor	90	75	ND
cephalexin	17	25	ND
cefixime	41	30	ND
cefazolin	5	25–45	ND
cefamandole	18	29	10.2
cefmetazole	7	86	ND
cefonicid	2	3.4	ND
cefoxitin	13	40	1.5
cefotaxime	100	14–40	ND
ceftazidime	11	27–50	8.5
ceftizoxime	12	45	ND
Aminoglycosides			
amikacin	4	30–36	6.7
gentamicin	4	24–47	12.5
netilmicin	5	38–65	ND
tobramycin	4	31–70	4.7
Miscellaneous anti-infectives			
acyclovir	29	82–100	ND
aztreonam	24	43	2.1
chloramphenicol	70–80	21–54	ND
ethambutol	295	62–86	ND
flucytosine	2–5	55–128	5–10
imipenem	56	84	ND
isoniazid	151	90	4.9
metronidazole	60–80	58–125	15.8
ribavirin	217	56–90	ND
sulfamethoxazole	25	21–84	1.2
trimethoprim	120	29–66	5.1
vancomycin	3–5	9–16	2.3–5
zidovudine	70–90	54–95	ND
Non-anti-infectives			
disopyramide	93	123	ND
ethosuximide	10	140	ND
lithium	20	150	ND
NAPA	200	41–97	ND
phenobarbital	9	25–60	ND
primidone	40	98	ND
procainamide	810	65	ND
theophylline	46	35–80	ND
valproic acid	10	23	ND

[a] ND = No data.

Effect of Dialysis on Pharmacokinetics

The effect of hemodialysis and peritoneal dialysis on the pharmacokinetics of many drugs was quantified in studies conducted in the 1960s, 1970s, and early 1980s (see Table 8-10). However, because several dramatic changes occurred in dialysis technology during the 1980s, the applicability of these data to current dialysis methods may be limited.[153-155] Rapid high-efficiency hemodialysis, high-flux dialysis, and hemodiafiltration represent the new wave in filter membrane and dialysate delivery technology. The most recent addition to the dialytic armamentarium has been the continuous renal replacement therapies (CRRT) which include slow continuous ultrafiltration (SCUF), continuous arteriovenous hemofiltration (CAVH), and continuous arteriovenous hemodialysis (CAVHD).[156,157] These CRRT techniques are primarily used to treat acute renal failure. Although continuous ambulatory peritoneal dialysis was introduced in the late 1970s, the number of patients treated with this dialysis modality has increased dramatically and now numbers over 30,000 worldwide.[158] This is now the predominant modality of peritoneal dialysis which is clinically utilized.

Hemodialysis

In order for a drug to be cleared from the systemic circulation by hemodialysis, it must move from the blood into the dialysate through the filter membrane.[159] This movement can be by passive diffusion (i.e., from an area of higher concentration to one of lower concentration) or by convection, which represents the simultaneous movement of plasma solute with ultrafiltered water. The diffusional contribution to drug clearance by dialysis can be expressed as a function of the total resistance to movement of drug in these three stages: 1) R_B or blood component resistance, 2) R_M or membrane resistance, and 3) R_D dialysate resistance.[157,159] These three factors plus blood flow rate through the dialyzer and dialyzer surface area can be utilized to quantitate the diffusional dialyzer clearance (CL_{HD}) of a given compound.

$$CL_{HD} = Q_b \left(1 - e^{\frac{-K_o SA}{Q_b}}\right)$$

(Eq. 8-39)

where K_o, the diffusional contribution to drug clearance, $= 1/(R_B + R_M + R_D)$; SA = surface area; and Q_b = blood flow rate. As a general rule, as the drug's molecular size increases, the effect of R_M becomes dominant, whereas at low molecular sizes, R_B and R_D are more important.

If convective transport is included in the dialysis treatment, the sieving coefficient (SC) as well as the diffusional component must be considered in the determination of dialyzer clearance.[156,157,160]

$$SC = \frac{2C_{uf}}{\dfrac{C_a}{1 - \theta} + \dfrac{C_v}{1 - \theta}}$$

(Eq. 8-40)

where C_{uf} = ultrafiltrate concentration; C_a = arterial concentration; C_v = venous concentration; and $\theta = 0.0107$ times the patient's total protein concentration. Thus, total hemodialyzer clearance would be the sum of the following:

$$CL_{HDTOT} = CL_{HD} + (SC)(Q_F) \qquad \text{(Eq. 8-41)}$$

where Q_F = ultrafiltrate flow rate.

The efficiency with which a drug is removed by hemodialysis or CRRT is also related to drug characteristics such as molecular size, water solubility, protein binding, and distribution volume.[85,159] Finally, dialysis membrane characteristics such as membrane type, membrane thickness and surface area, as well as the sieving coefficient for a given drug may also affect the dialyzer clearance of that compound.[155,161]

Molecular Size/Weight. Hemodialysis membranes have discrete pores of relatively uniform diameter that perforate the membrane. Alterations in the pore size and thickness can greatly alter the permeability of the membrane to solutes and water. Because conventional and second generation membranes have smaller pores than high-flux membranes, drug clearance decreases as molecular size/weight is increased.[159] Indeed, once molecular size/weight exceeds 500 daltons (D), conventional dialysis probably will not effectively remove the drug.[82] The clearance of small molecules (MW <500 D) by conventional hemodialysis membranes is primarily determined by blood and dialysate flow rates as well as by the membrane surface area. The clearance of larger molecules depends primarily on the membrane surface area. High-flux filters retain a drug clearance capacity that is similar to that of low molecular weight compounds for drugs that have molecular weights of 5000 D or greater.[159,162,163] Drug clearance by these filters remains dependent on blood and dialysate flow rates as well as on membrane surface area throughout this molecular size range.

The use of molecular size to predict the clearance of drugs by conventional dialysis is limited. Keller et al.[164] observed no significant relationship between dialyzability and the molecular size of 89 different drugs. These drugs, however, differed widely in several other key pharmacokinetic characteristics (e.g., protein binding and distribution volume) that can independently affect CL_{HD}. Furthermore, the dialysis membrane type and conditions were not reported in this tabulation.

Water Solubility. Drugs which are poorly soluble in water are likely to have a high resistance to transport into the aqueous dialysate. The transport of the drug into plasma water may further limit its movement across the dialysis membrane. This has been seen with low molecular weight compounds such as glutethimide as well as large compounds such as cyclosporine.

Protein Binding. The clearance of drugs by conventional hemodialysis is predominantly a passive diffusional process which is driven by the unbound concentration gradient between plasma water and dialysate. Therefore, as binding to plasma proteins increases, dialyzer clearance decreases. For example, oxacillin (with molecular size of 458 D) is 94% bound, and less than 5% is removed by conventional hemodialysis. In contrast, azlocillin which has essentially the same molecular size (461 D) is only 30% bound and up to 50% of the amount in the

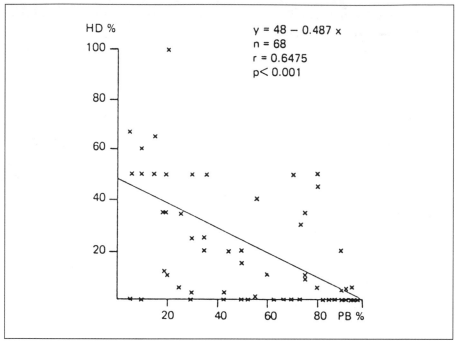

Figure 8-6a. *Linear regression between the dialyzability (HD%) and the percentage of plasma protein binding (PB%) of 89 drugs (reprinted with permission from reference 164).*

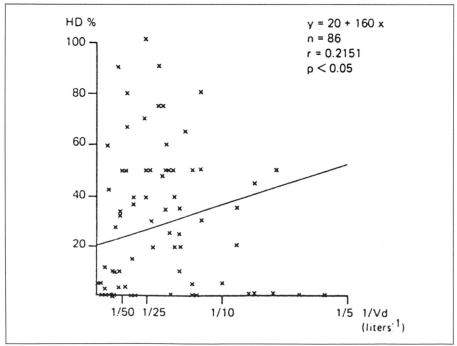

Figure 8-6b. *Linear regression between the dialyzability (HD%) and the reciprocal of volume of distribution ($1/V_d$) in liters of 89 drugs (reprinted with permission from reference 164).*

body may be eliminated during dialysis. Keller et al. have reported that the degree of protein binding correlates significantly with dialyzability[164] (see Figure 8-6a). However, multiple linear regression analysis indicates no correlation between dialyzability and other independent variables such as the distribution volume, molecular size, and protein binding.

Volume of Distribution. The impact of dialysis on the systemic removal of a drug will depend, in part, on the drug's volume of distribution[164] (see Figure 8-6b). If the dialyzer clearance of two drugs is similar (e.g., 50 mL/min during a four-hour hemodialysis treatment) then 12 L of the distribution volume will be cleared of drug. This would significantly impact clearance of a cephalosporin antibiotic which has a distribution volume of 10 to 30 L but would have little impact on the clearance of a tricyclic antidepressant which has a distribution volume of 800 to 1400 L.

Quantifying Hemodialysis Clearance

The effect of hemodialysis on drug disposition may be quantified in many ways.[68,165,166] Measuring the total body clearance and terminal elimination half-life of a drug on a non-dialysis day and on a dialysis day provides a complicated index of dialyzability. The measurements of CL_T and terminal elimination half-life in particular are likely to be affected by intrapatient variability in the disposition of the drug. Furthermore, changes in distribution volume may mask or exaggerate the degree of change in the terminal elimination half-life. Therefore, hemodialysis clearance has been primarily determined in the clinical setting with the following equation:

$$CL_{HD} = (Q)\left(\frac{C_a - C_v}{C_a}\right)$$

(Eq. 8-42)

where Q is the flow rate of blood or plasma through the dialysis filter, C_a is the concentration of the drug going into the filter (arterial side), and C_v is the concentration of the drug leaving the filter (venous side). Plasma (CL_{HDp}) or whole blood clearance (CL_{HDb}) can be calculated as follows:

$$CL_{HDp} = (Q_p)\left(\frac{C_{ap} - C_{vp}}{C_{ap}}\right)$$

(Eq. 8-43)

$$CL_{HDb} = (Q_b)\left(\frac{C_{ab} - C_{vb}}{C_{ab}}\right)$$

(Eq. 8-44)

where p and b represent plasma and blood, respectively. Finally, some have calculated a mixed hemodialysis clearance as:

$$CL_{HDm} = (Q_b)\left(\frac{C_{ap} - C_{vp}}{C_{ap}}\right)$$

(Eq. 8-45)

where CL_{HDm} is the combination of whole blood flow rate and plasma drug concentrations.

Calculations of clearance using Equation 8-45 assume that blood-water flow rate through the dialyzer is equal to whole-blood flow rate; solute concentration equilibrium, if any, exists between plasma and red blood cell water along the length of the dialyzer; and there is an absence of significant solute binding by plasma and red blood cell proteins. Unfortunately, concentration equilibrium between red blood cells and plasma may not exist along the length of the dialyzer, hemoglobin binding of solute is known to occur, and blood-water flow rate is not equal to whole blood flow rate. Thus, the use of this equation often overestimates the true CL_{HD}.[82,166]

Equations 8-43 to 8-45 depend upon an accurate estimation of blood flow through the dialysis filter. Blood flow is normally determined by pump revolutions per minute or bubble transit time. The use of calibrated pumps can be accurate if done carefully, but in the clinical setting where calibration may not be tightly controlled, errors of 30% to 40% may be encountered. For the bubble transit time, if it is assumed that the flow of the bubble is equal to the flow of blood, there may be a systematic overestimation of Q_b by about 7% at a flow of 100 mL/min, increasing to 16% at a flow of 400 mL/min.[167]

Drug concentrations are generally determined in plasma or serum. If a drug is present in red blood cells and equilibrates with plasma, plasma concentrations will underestimate the amount in whole blood, and use of Equation 8-43 may under-estimate the amount of drug removal by dialysis. For drugs present only in plasma, use of Equation 8-45 will overestimate drug removal by a factor equal to the hematocrit (HCT). While CL_{HDb} would therefore appear to be the method of choice for calculating dialysis clearance, this is usually not possible since drug concentrations are not generally measured in whole blood. Furthermore, CL_{HDb} is calculated using an entirely different data source (whole blood) than is CL_T; therefore, it is not directly comparable to CL_T. However, CL_{HDb} can be converted to CL_{HDp} if the partition coefficient (K_p) of the drug between red blood cells (RBC) and plasma is known:[166]

$$K_p = \frac{C_{RBC}}{C_p} \qquad \text{(Eq. 8-46)}$$

$$CL_{HDp} = [CL_{HDb}] [K_p HCT + (1 - HCT)] \qquad \text{(Eq. 8-47)}$$

Under conditions of ultrafiltration, movement of plasma water from blood to dialysate occurs. Therefore, unless the drug moves at the same rate, it will become concentrated in the venous sample and clearance will be underestimated as a result of the apparent increase in C_{vp}. If fluid is administered through the extracorporeal circuit, the drug concentration in the venous sample may be diluted and clearance will be overestimated. In these circumstances, simultaneous measurement of arterial and venous hematocrit or plasma protein concentration will allow for a partial correction of the venous concentration. An approximation of the venous concentration had ultrafiltration not taken place would be:

$$C_{\text{vp actual}} = (C_{\text{vp observed}})\left(1 - \frac{HCT_v - HCT_a}{HCT_v}\right) \quad \text{(Eq. 8-48)}$$

where HCT_v and HCT_a are the venous and arterial hematocrits, respectively.

Equations 8-43 to 8-45 are applicable to those situations where solute does not accumulate in the dialysate. Rarely, some dialysis centers may use recirculating dialysate delivery systems in which the removed substances accumulate in the hemodialysate fluid so that the concentration gradient is constantly decreasing. In these situations, removal of drug is expressed as shown in Equation 8-49 where C_{dial} is the concentration of the drug in the dialysate.

$$CL_{HD} = (Q_p)\left(\frac{C_{ap} - C_{vp}}{C_{ap} - C_{\text{dial}}}\right) \quad \text{(Eq. 8-49)}$$

If a drug is dialyzable, the concentration of drug which is present in the hemodialysate fluid should be able to be measured. The product of drug concentration in the hemodialysate (C_{dial}) and the total volume of hemodialysate fluid (V_{dial}) will thus yield the amount of drug removed from the patient (AR):

$$AR = (C_{\text{dial}})(V_{\text{dial}}) \quad \text{(Eq. 8-50)}$$

Hemodialysis clearance can be calculated as the quotient of the AR and the area under the plasma concentration-time curve during the hemodialysis procedure (AUC_p).

$$CL_{HD} = \frac{AR}{AUC_p} \quad \text{(Eq. 8-51)}$$

Alternatively, the CL_{HD} can be calculated by two other equations which utilize the measurement of drug concentrations in hemodialysate fluid and hemodialysate fluid flow rate (Q_{hd}). These equations are only valid for non-recirculating single-pass dialysate delivery systems.

$$CL_{HD} = \frac{(Q_{hd})(C_{\text{dial}})}{C_{a\,mid}} \quad \text{(Eq. 8-52)}$$

$$CL_{HD} = (Q_{hd})\left(\frac{AUC_{\text{dial}}}{AUC_p}\right) \quad \text{(Eq. 8-53)}$$

where $C_{a\,mid}$ is the arterial plasma concentration at the midpoint of the hemodialysate collection interval and AUC_{dial} is the area under the hemodialysate concentration-time curve during the dialysis period. These methods of clearance calculation are independent of blood-flow rate and are unaffected by ultrafiltration. For drugs present in plasma as well as red blood cell water, CL_{HD} calculated by Equations 8-51 to 8-53 may exceed the actual plasma flow rate if the drug is readily removed from the red blood cell. These three methods have been reported by Barbhaiya et al.[168] to yield similar estimates of CL_{HD} (see Table 8-11) of the cephalosporin, cefepime, which exceed the CL_{HD} calculated by Equation 8-43. This substantiates the desirability of basing CL_{HD} determinations on methods that employ drug measurement in the biologic fluid of interest (i.e., the hemodialysate). These data also confirm the recommendations of Gibson and others that these methods of CL_{HD} calculation should be the standard against which all other methods are compared.[82,165,166]

Types of Dialyzers

There are several types of hemodialysis filters available for the clinical treatment of patients with ESRD, acute renal failure, and/or drug intoxications. The selection of the optimal filter and the other components of the hemodialysis prescription will be determined by the patient's underlying status, the availability of technology, and the clinician's philosophy.

In the mid-1970s, there were only 56 filters available in three configurations: flat plate, coil, and hollow fiber.[153] The membrane utilized in all of these filters was made of regenerated cellulose. By the mid-1980s, significant changes had taken place in the dialysis filter arena. Several new second generation filter membrane materials were introduced including cellulose acetate and modified cellulose as well as the high-flux synthetic membranes: polyacrylonitrile (PAN), polysulfone, and polymethylmethacrylate (PMMA).[154] In addition, several modifications of the classic filter configurations were introduced and two new ones were introduced: hemofilters and combined hemodialysis/hemofilters.[153] As a result, there are now over 500 different types of dialysis filters available in the United States.[153,154,162,163] Thus, hemodialysis is no longer a generic procedure and evaluations of drug and toxin dialyzability must now include full disclosure of all the components of the dialysis prescription (e.g., filter characteristics, flow rates of blood and dialysate, ultrafiltration status).

Clinical investigations have confirmed the marked variance in dialyzability of selected drugs when different filter membranes and configurations are utilized. For example, the CL_{HD} of vancomycin (MW = 1400 D) was considered to be negligible until Matzke et al.,[169] Bastani et al.,[170] Lanese et al.,[171] and Torras et al.[172] documented up to a 15-fold variance in vancomycin's CL_{HD} which depended on

Table 8-11. *Comparison of Cefepime Hemodialysis Clearance Calculated Using Four Different Equations*

Subject	Eq. 8-43	Eq. 8-51	Eq. 8-52	Eq. 8-53
1	147.33	270.29	273.01	288.95
2	156.16	169.84	169.68	184.78
3	86.38	104.09	105.18	101.6
4	101.87	120.11	139.23	142.65
5	88.28	123.50	123.47	109.02
Mean	116.00	157.57	162.11	165.42
SD	33.32	67.60	66.36	76.48

the type of filter membrane utilized and its surface area. The clearance of vancomycin was approximately 9 mL/min with the cellulose and cuprophane membranes, 21 mL/min with the cellulose acetate membrane, and 31 to 60 mL/min with the polyacrylonitrile membrane, and ranged from 40 to 150 mL/min with the polysulfone membrane. These differences in dialysis are clinically significant because up to 50% of the vancomycin may be removed within four hours using the most efficient membranes (see Figure 8-7).

In vitro studies that characterize the clearance of low (e.g., urea) and high (e.g., vitamin B_{12}) molecular weight compounds at two or more blood flow rates by the various hemodialysis filters may be utilized to predict the *in vivo* dialysis clearance of drugs.[154,162,163] These data demonstrate marked variances between different filter membranes and configurations as well as between different manufacturers who utilize the same membrane and configuration. If the dialysis clearances (using a specific membrane) are known for the marker substance and a specific drug, this relationship can be used along with the projected *in vivo* clearance of the marker substance to predict the *in vivo* dialysis clearance of the specific drug by another membrane type.[139,168] Alternatively, the *in vivo* clearance may be predicted from *in vitro* experiments with the drug of interest by correcting for the degree of protein binding and for the hematocrit if the drug is only present in plasma.

$$CL_{in\ vivo} = CL_{in\ vitro}\ [(\%\ free)\ (1 - HCT)] \qquad (Eq.\ 8\text{-}54)$$

Redistribution Phenomenon After Hemodialysis

The quantification of CL_{HD} by the methods described above applies to drugs whose pharmacokinetic behavior can be adequately described using a one-com-

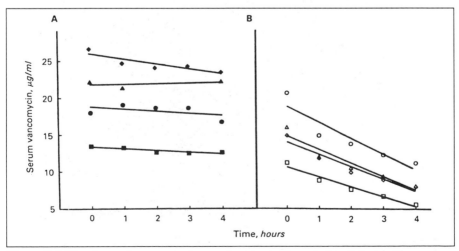

Figure 8-7. The change in vancomycin serum concentrations during dialysis with a conventional cuprophane (Travenol 12.11) filter (panel A) and high flux polysulfone (Fresenius F-80) filter (panel B). Individual symbols represent the same patient dialyzed on the two different filters (reprinted with permission from reference 171).

partment model. The rate of transport for drugs with multicompartmental pharma-cokinetics into and out of the central compartment, however, not only determines the rate of decline of the serum concentrations during the distributive phase, but also the effect of dialysis on the serum or plasma concentration-time profile.[82] A "rebound" in plasma concentrations can be expected after dialysis if the rate of transport of the drug from plasma during dialysis exceeded the rate of transport from the peripheral compartment(s) into the central compartment or if the tissue clearance is decreased during hemodialysis. The use of single pre- and post-dial-ysis serum concentrations may thus yield overestimates of the dialysis clearance (see Figure 8-8). To substantiate the effectiveness of hemodialysis, sufficient data must be presented to show that the post-dialysis serum concentration of the drug is sustained at a level significantly less than the pre-dialysis concentration.

Marked "rebounds" in the serum concentrations of endogenous substances such as potassium and urea[159] as well as several drugs (e.g., procainamide, n-acetyl pro-cainamide, cimetidine, vancomycin, gentamicin, tobramycin, and netilmicin) have been reported following hemodialysis/filtration with various filter types.[81,169,173–177] The degree of rebound and time to maximum increase in serum concentrations may differ among drugs of the same pharmacologic class. For example, the concentration of tobramycin and netilmicin increased by 7% and 29% respectively within ten minutes after dialysis while the maximum increase of 18.3% and 38.3% was observed at 1.7 and 1.9 hours, respectively.[176] A rebound in gentamicin serum concentrations one hour after dialysis of approximately 25.7% has also been observed.[177] Since post-dialysis administration of aminoglycosides and several

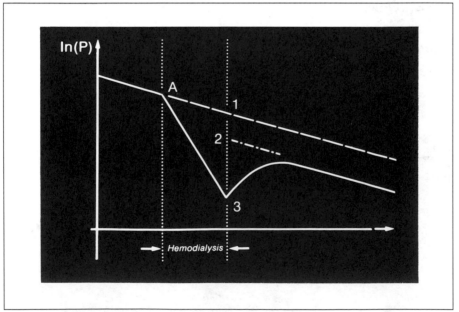

Figure 8-8. *The measured plasma concentrations before (A) and after hemodialysis (3) showing a rebound phenomenon. The net effect on drug plasma concentrations may be calculated from the extrapolated plasma concentration without dialysis (1) and the concentration back extrap-olated from the post rebound data (2) (adapted from reference 89).*

other drugs is a common practice, knowledge of the degree of rebound and its time course is critical in the interpretation of measured serum concentration data and the design of optimal dosage regimens (see Figure 8-9).

If a drug which demonstrates multicompartmental disposition is given intravenously just before or shortly after dialysis is begun, the percent of drug removed by hemodialysis may be greater than it would have been had dialysis been initiated after drug distribution was complete. When dialysis is begun immediately after the intravenous administration, more drug is present initially within the plasma compartment because insufficient time has been allowed for drug distribution. If dialysis decreases the intercompartmental clearance, even more drug will be trapped within the plasma compartment. The same should also occur if the drug is given during dialysis. Therefore, to more closely simulate the clinical situation, investigators should initiate dialysis after drug absorption and distribution processes are likely to be complete. Only in this way can one be certain that the amount of drug removed during the test period is meaningfully related to that which will be removed during normal clinical practice. The only case to be made for beginning dialysis before drug absorption and distribution are complete would be in the treatment of drug overdoses.

Peritoneal Dialysis

Intermittent peritoneal dialysis was developed in the 1920s and remained the primary mode of therapy until the "artificial kidney" was introduced in the 1940s and adequate vascular access techniques were developed in the 1960s. Peritoneal

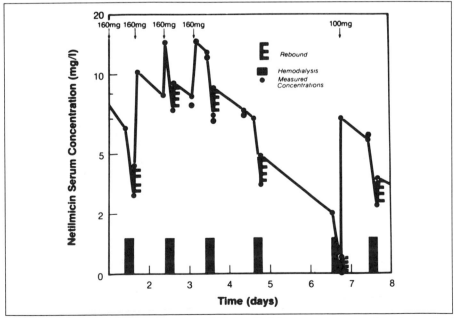

Figure 8-9. Predicted (■) and measured (●) netilmicin serum concentrations in a patient undergoing intermittent hemodialysis when the degree of post-dialysis rebound in serum concentration (E) is incorporated into the predictive model.

dialysis is as effective in treating patients with end stage renal failure as hemodialysis; however, its relative inefficiency (slower clearances for all solutes) and labor intensity caused it to lose favor as a mode of chronic dialytic therapy during the 1960s and 1970s. The clearance of only a few drugs has been evaluated in patients receiving intermittent peritoneal dialysis (see Table 8-12).

In contrast, **continuous ambulatory peritoneal dialysis (CAPD)** and **continuous cycling peritoneal dialysis (CCPD)** (introduced in the late 1970s) are considerably more attractive modes of dialysis, especially for selected patient populations, such as the elderly and those with unstable cardiac status.[158,178,179] Approximately 10,000 to 12,000 patients in the United States and over 35,000 worldwide are now receiving CAPD therapy. The impact of CAPD on the pharmacokinetics of many drugs, especially antibiotics and antifungal agents, has been extensively evaluated.[180–182]

The methods used to quantitate the CAPD clearance of drugs are generally analogous to those used for hemodialysis. The standard approach is to measure drug concentration in each bag of CAPD effluent fluid after oral or intravenous administration of the drug as well as the AUC_p during the same time interval.[182] The main difference with CAPD is that the sampling scheme may be prolonged since the therapy is continuous and the anticipated clearances are lower.

Two additional variables that should be evaluated are the bioavailability of a drug when it is administered intraperitoneally and the effect of peritonitis on systemic absorption and CL_{CAPD}. This is of particular importance for anti-infective agents which are commonly utilized intraperitoneally to treat peritonitis, the most common clinical problem in this patient population.[182] Although each CAPD patient is likely to experience one to two peritonitis episodes each year, only a few agents have been studied under these conditions.[183–196] For the majority of agents which have been evaluated, peritonitis increases both CL_{CAPD} and systemic absorption of intraperitoneally administered drug (see Table 8-12). Thus, characterization of drug disposition should optimally be carried out in the patient population with the disease for which the drug is indicated.

Continuous Renal Replacement Therapy

Although the concept of continuous renal replacement therapy (CRRT) dates back to the 1950s, these therapies were not widely used until the 1980s.[157] There are three basic forms of CRRT: slow continuous ultrafiltration (SCUF), continuous arteriovenous hemofiltration (CAVH), and continuous arteriovenous hemodialysis (CAVHD). Although the extracorporeal circuits of these therapies are similar, there are distinct and important differences. SCUF and CAVH utilize convective transport. That is, solutes simultaneously move across the filter membrane with ultrafiltered plasma water, and this is the sole modality for drug removal. This mode of transport removes larger molecules more readily than diffusion, the primary mode of drug transport during conventional hemodialysis. SCUF is primarily used to treat fluid overload states and is not used to treat renal failure *per se*. The ultrafiltrate flow rate or fluid removal rate is usually less than 5 mL/min. CAVH is predominantly used to manage patients with acute renal

Table 8-12. Effect of CAPD Peritonitis on the Pharmacokinetics of Anti-Infective Agents

Drug	Non-peritonitis evaluation					Peritonitis evaluation					References
	$t\frac{1}{2}$ (hr)	CL_{CAPD} (mL/min)	CL_T (mL/min)	V_d (L/kg)	% ABS	$t\frac{1}{2}$ (hr)	CL_{CAPD} (mL/min)	CL_T (mL/min)	V_d (L/kg)	% ABS	
vancomycin	83	2.1	8.9	1.0	59	104	1.9	6.6	1.2	81	183–185
cefamandole	91	1.7	5.0	0.6	46	184	1.4	7.0	1.2	91	186
cefazolin	8.5	2.0	25.0	0.23	71	7.6	1.4	33.0	0.26	93	187
cefotaxime	—	—	5.8	—	74	—	—	7.8	—	88	188
cefsulodin	—	—	95	—	67	—	—	250	—	90	189
ceftazidime	11.2	—	26.5	—	81	9.4	—	23.9	—	84	190
gentamicin	—	2.6	—	—	70	—	3.2	—	—	70	191
netilmicin	—	—	—	—	64	—	—	—	—	79	192
tobramycin	18.1	3.4	16.8	27.5 L	67	19.6	4.9	18.5	31.8 L	83	193
flucytosine	35.0	—	8.2	0.33	62	38.7	—	6.3	0.30	49	194
trimethoprim	—	—	—	—	81	—	—	—	—	93	195
sulfamethoxazole	23.7	5.1	66.2	2.2	90.1	—	—	—	—	93	196
	18.1	1.2	26.2	0.55	38.9	—	—	—	—	55	196

failure.[160] It employs the same basic fluid removal procedure as SCUF, but adds a substitution fluid to individualize the net fluid removal. Thus, the fluid removal and drug clearance may range from 5 to 15 mL/min.

To assess the effect of these therapies on drug disposition, a pharmacokinetic modeling approach that differs from that used for conventional hemodialysis or peritoneal dialysis must be used, since a drug's ability to pass through the filter membrane or sieving coefficient (SC) must be characterized (see Equation 8-40). Several investigators have suggested that in the clinical arena, this expression can be simplified as follows:[160,197]

$$SC = \frac{C_{UF}}{C_{ap}}$$

(Eq. 8-55)

where C_{UF} and C_{ap} are the drug concentration in ultrafiltrate and the plasma flowing into the filter, respectively. The clearance of a drug by SCUF or CAVH can be ascertained by multiplying the sieving coefficient by the ultrafiltrate flow rate (Q_F):

$$CL_{CAVH} = (SC)(Q_F)$$

(Eq. 8-56)

Several different types of filters are currently available for SCUF and CAVH therapy.[155,156] The SC of several drugs have been reported to be significantly different when filters of different membrane composition are used (see Table 8-13).[161,197,198] These differences have been hypothesized to be due to drug charge-membrane interactions which alter the transport of drug through the membrane. If the assumption is that cations are retained and anions are expelled to preserve electroneutrality, then the higher-than-predicted SC observed (based on protein

Table 8-13. *Sieving Coefficient Measured During Continuous Arteriovenous Hemofiltration*

0.75–1.0	
amikacin	metronidazole
cefotaxime	n-acetylprocainamide
ceftazidime	phenobarbital
ceftriaxone	procainamide
digoxin	sulfamethoxazole
5-fluorocytosine	theophylline
gentamicin	tobramycin
imipenem	vancomycin
0.5–0.74	
ampicillin	ganciclovir
amphotericin B	mezlocillin
cefoxitin	nafacillin
<0.5	
cefoperazone	oxacillin
clindamycin	phenytoin
clofibrate	streptomycin
erythromycin	

binding characteristics) for anionic drugs can be explained.[197] Other factors that could alter the SC and CL_{CAVH} include drug binding to the filter membrane, drug penetration into red blood cells, development of a polarized protein layer on the filter membrane surface, and altered protein binding (versus normal volunteers).

When attempting to modify the dosage regimen of a drug for the CAVH patient, literature values for SC can be utilized with the measured Q_F to calculate the CL_{CAVH}. This clearance can be added to the patient's residual total body drug clearance and the optimal dosage regimen can be designed based on the total clearance and the desired therapeutic goals.

Continuous arteriovenous hemodialysis (CAVHD) uses diffusive transport as well as convective transport to remove waste products and drugs.[157] With this therapy, dialysate is administered by gravity or by an infusion pump at an approximate rate of 15 mL/min. The dialysate and ultrafiltrate are collected and substitution fluid can be infused if the rate of ultrafiltrate generation is too great. Although there is complete equilibrium of small molecules such as urea at the low dialysate flow rates utilized with CAVHD, the diffusional clearance of drugs by this therapy has not been quantified. If similar filters are utilized with CAVHD as with SCUF and CAVH, the removal of drugs by CAVHD should exceed the clearance by these methods due to the addition of the diffusion component.

Hemoperfusion

Hemoperfusion involves the passage of blood through various adsorbent materials.[199] Activated charcoal has a large capacity for adsorbing creatinine, barbiturates, glutethimide, methaqualone, ethchlorvynol, and other drugs, but it has no affinity for urea or electrolytes, and it cannot remove water. Amberlite XAD-4, a synthetic co-polymer of styrene and divinyl benzene, has an affinity for lipophilic molecules such as barbiturates, glutethimide, digoxin, meprobamate, tricyclic antidepressants, quinidine, phenytoin, procainamide, N-acetylprocainamide, and lidocaine is also clinically available. Amberlite XAD-4, however, has no affinity for urea, creatinine, or water. Regardless of the type of adsorbent used, hemoperfusion alone is insufficient to control uremic symptoms or to remove water and electrolytes.[199] The combination of hemoperfusion with hemodialysis in a hybrid device, however, may theoretically maximize the removal of "middle" and low molecular weight compounds and may optimize patient well being.

The physical properties of drugs that restrict the effectiveness of hemodialysis (i.e., water insolubility, plasma protein binding, and molecular weight) do not appear to limit the effectiveness of hemoperfusion. With hemoperfusion, the rate-limiting factors appear to be affinity of the solute for the adsorbent, rate of movement of solute from tissues to the blood compartment, a large solute volume of distribution, and the capacity of the adsorbent for the solute. Since each molecule of adsorbed solute occupies a binding site on the column, columns of either type may become saturated and require periodic replacement if hemoperfusion is to be carried out for a prolonged period of time. The clearance of drugs by hemoperfusion can be quantitated using Equation 8-43 or by Equation 8-45 depending on the drug's distributional characteristics. The extraction ratios for acetaminophen, ethchlorvynol, glutethimide, phenobarbital, and tricyclic anti-depressants are 50% to 100% greater than those observed with conventional homodialysis when hemoperfusion with either the amberlite XAD-4 or coated or uncoated charcoal filters are used. Despite these higher extraction ratios, improvements in clinical outcome are debatable.[199]

REFERENCES

1. Kassirer JP. Clinical evaluation of kidney function-glomerular function. N Engl J Med. 1971;285:385–89.
2. Prueksaritanont T et al. Renal and non-renal clearances of iothalamate. Biopharm Drug Disp. 1986;7:347–55.
3. Reidenberg MM et al. A nonradioactive iothalamate method for measuring glomerular filtration rate and its use to study the renal handling of cibenzoline. Ther Drug Monit. 1988;10:434–37.
4. Dalmeida W, Suki WN. Measurement of GFR with non-radioisotopic radio contrast agents. Kidney Int. 1988;34:725–28.
5. Clifton GG et al. Monoexponential analysis of plasma disappearance of ^{99m}Tc-DTPA and ^{131}I-iodohippurate: a reliable method for measuring changes in renal function. J Clin Pharmacol 1989;29:466–71.
6. Farmer CD et al. Measurement of renal function with radioiodinated diatrizoate and o-iodo-hippurate. Am J Clin Pathol 1967;47:9–16.
7. Lau AH et al. Estimation of creatinine clearance in malnourished patients. Clin Pharm. 1988;7:62–65.
8. Cocchetto DM et al. Decreased rate of creatinine production in patients with hepatic disease: implications for estimation of creatinine clearance. Ther Drug Monit. 1983;5:161–68.
9. Forbes GB, Bruining GJ. Urinary creatinine excretion and lean body mass. Am J Clin Nutr 1976;29:1359–366.
10. Knoben JE, Anderson PO. Handbook of Clinical Drug Data. Hamilton, IL: Drug Intelligence Publications; 1988;11.
11. Keys A, Brozek J. Body fat in adult man. Physiol Rev. 1953;33:245–325.
12. Schwartz GJ et al. The use of plasma creatinine concentration for estimating glomerular filtration rate in infants, children, and adolescents. Pediatr Clin North Am. 1987;34:571–90.
13. Goldberg TH, Finkelstein MS. Difficulties in estimating glomerular filtration rate in the elderly. Arch Intern Med. 1987;147:1430–433.
14. Wilson R et al. Creatinine clearance in the critically ill surgical patient. Arch Surg. 1979;114:461–63.
15. Kaw DG et al. Decrease of urine creatinine *in vitro* in spinal cord injury patients. Clin Nephrol. 1988;30:216–19.
16. Hatton J et al. Estimation of creatinine clearance in patients with Cushing syndrome. Drug Intell Clin Pharm. 1989;23:974–77.
17. Dionne RE et al. Estimating creatinine clearance in morbidly obese patients. Am J Hosp Pharm. 1981;38:841–44.
18. Grossman RA et al. Nontraumatic rhabdomyolysis and acute renal failure. N Engl J Med. 1974;291:807–11.
19. Lordon RE, Burton JR. Post-traumatic renal failure in military personnel in Southeast Asia. Am J Med. 1972;53:137–38.
20. Berglund F et al. Effect of trimethoprim-sulfamethoxazole on the renal excretion of creatinine in man. J Urol. 1975;114:802–808.
21. Jacobson FL et al. Pronounced increase in serum creatinine concentration after eating cooked meat. Br Med J. 1979;21:1049–50.
22. Wesson LE. Electrolyte excretion in relation to diurnal cycles of renal function. Medicine 1964;43:547–92.
23. Bjornsson TD. Use of serum creatinine concentrations to determine renal function. In: Gibaldi M, Prescott L, eds. Handbook of Clinical Pharmacokinetics. New York: ADIS Press; 1983;277–300.

24. Walser M et al. Creatinine measurements often yield false estimates of progression in chronic renal failure. Kidney Int. 1988;34:412–18.
25. Jones JD, Burnett PC. Creatinine metabolism in humans with decreased renal function: creatinine deficit. Clin Chem. 1974;20:1204–212.
26. Dubb JW et al. Effect of cimetidine on renal function in normal man. Clin Pharmacol Ther. 1978;24:76–83.
27. Rocci ML et al. Creatinine serum concentrations and H_2-receptor antagonists. Clin Nephrol. 1984;22:214–18.
28. Mascioli SR et al. Artifactual elevation of serum creatinine level due to fasting. Arch Intern Med. 1984;144:1575–576.
29. Lott RS, Hayton WL. Estimation of creatinine clearance from serum creatinine concentration—a review. Drug Intell Clin Pharm. 1978;12:140–50.
30. Guay DRP et al. Interference of selected second- and third-generation cephalosporins with creatinine determinations. Am J Hosp Pharm. 1983;40:435–38.
31. Massoomi F et al. Positive interference with serum creatinine determination by cefpirome but no effect with cefepime and four oral cephalosporins. Pharmacother. 1991;11:281. Abstract.
32. Chow MSS, Schweizer R. Estimation of renal creatinine clearance in patients with unstable serum creatinine concentrations: comparison of multiple methods. Drug Intel Clin Pharm. 1985;19:385–90.
33. Wilson RF, Soullier G. The validity of two-hour creatinine clearance studies in critically ill patients. Crit Care Med. 1980;8:281–83.
34. Baumann TJ et al. Minimum urine collection periods for accurate determination of creatinine clearance in critically ill patients. Clin Pharm. 1987;6:393–98.
35. Smythe MA et al. Relationship between values of bioelectrical impedance and creatinine clearance. Pharmacother. 1990;10:42–46.
36. Robert S, Zarowitz BJ. Is there a reliable index of glomerular filtration rate in critically ill patients? DICP-Ann Pharmacother. 1991;25:169–78.
37. Robert S et al. Renal function assessment in the critically ill. Pharmacother. 1991;11:275.
38. Mawer GE et al. Computer-assisted prescribing of kanamycin for patients with renal insufficiency. Lancet 1972;1:12–15.
39. Jeliffe RW. Creatinine clearance: bedside estimate. Ann Intern Med. 1973;79:604–605.
40. Wagner JG. Fundamentals of clinical pharmacokinetics, Hamilton, IL: Drug Intelligence Publications; 1975;162.
41. Cockroft DW, Gault MH. Prediction of creatinine clearance from serum creatinine. Nephron 1976;16:31–41.
42. Hull JH et al. Influence of range of renal function and liver disease on predictability of creatinine clearance. Clin Pharmacol Ther. 1981;29:516–21.
43. Schwartz GJ et al. A simple estimate of glomerular filtration rate in full-term infants during the first year of life. J Pediatr. 1984;104:849–54.
44. Schwartz GJ et al. A simple estimate of glomerular filtration rate in children derived from body length and plasma creatinine. Pediatrics 1976;58:259–63.
45. Jeliffe RW, Jeliffe SM. A computer program for estimation of creatinine clearance from unstable serum creatinine concentration. Math Biosci. 1972;14:17–24.
46. Chiou WL, Hsu FH. A new simple and rapid method to monitor renal function based on pharmacokinetic considerations of endogenous creatinine. Res Com Chem Path Pharmacol. 1975;10:315.
47. Brater DC. Drug Use in Renal Disease. Balgowlah, Australia: ADIS Health Science Press; 1983;22–56.
48. Rowland M, Tozer TN. Clinical Pharmacokinetics: Concepts and Applications. Philadelphia, PA: Lea & Febiger; 1989;2:410.
49. Moller JV, Sheikh MI. Renal organic anion transport system: pharmacological, physiological, and biochemical aspects. Pharmacol Rev. 1983;34:315–58.
50. Rennick BR. Renal tubule transport of organic cations. Am J Physiol. 1981;240:F83–F89.

51. Rennick BR, Farah A. Studies of the renal tubular transport of tetraethylammonium ion in the dog. J Pharmacol Exp Ther. 1956;116:287–95.

52. Bins JW, Mattie H. The tubular excretion of benzylpenicillin in patients with cystic fibrosis. Br J Clin Pharmacol. 1989;27:291–94.

53. Bergstrom J et al. The renal extraction of para-aminohippurate in normal persons and in patients with diseased kidneys. Scand J Clin Lab Invest. 1959;11:361–75.

54. Dubb J et al. Ceftizoxime kinetics and renal handling. Clin Pharmacol Ther. 1983;31:516–21.

55. Giacomini KM et al. Renal transport of drugs: an overview of methodology with application to cimetidine. Pharm Res. 1988;5:465–71.

56. Somogyi A, Bochner F. Dose and concentration-dependent effect of ranitidine on procainamide disposition and renal clearance in man. Br J Clin Pharmacol. 1984;18:175–81.

57. Reidenberg MM et al. Aging and renal clearance of procainamide and acetylprocainamide. Clin Pharmacol Ther. 1980;28:732–35.

58. Hori R et al. Ampicillin and cephalexin in renal insufficiency. Clin Pharmacol Ther. 1983;34:792–98.

59. Regardh CG. Factors contributing to variability in drug pharmacokinetics. IV: Renal excretion. J Clin Hosp Pharm. 1985;10:337–49.

60. Shim CK et al. Prediction of renal tubular secretion of tetraethylammonium bromide by use of endogenous N^1-methylnicotinamide in the rat. J Pharmacobiodyn. 1982;5:534–37.

61. Shim CK et al. Estimation of renal secretory function of organic cations by endogenous N-1-methylnicotinamide in rats with experimental renal failure. J Pharmacokin Biopharm. 1984;12:23–42.

62. Maiza A, Daley Yates PT. Prediction of renal clearance of cimetidine using endogenous N-1-methylnicotinamide. J Pharmacokin Biopharm. 1991;19:175–88.

63. Opsahl JA, Guay DRP. Chronic renal failure and end-stage renal disease. In: DiPiro JT, Talbert RL, Hayes PE, Yee GC, Posey LM, eds. Pharmacotherapy: A Pathophysiologic Approach. New York: Elsevier; 1989;526–42.

64. Rose BD, Brenner BM. Mechanisms of progression of renal disease. In: Rose BD, ed. Pathophysiology of Renal Disease. New York: McGraw Hill; 1987;28.

65. Shah BV, Levey AS. Spontaneous changes in the rate of decline in reciprocal serum creatinine: errors in predicting the progresion of renal disease from extrapolation of the slope. J Am Soc Nephrol. 1992;2:1186–91.

66. Gambertoglio JG. Effects of renal disease; altered pharmacokinetics. In: Benet LZ, Massoud N, Gambertoglio JG, eds. Pharmacokinetic Basis for Drug Treatment. New York: Raven Press; 1984;149–72.

67. Maher JF. Pharmacologic considerations for renal failure and dialysis. In: Maher JF, ed. Replacement of renal function by dialysis. Dordrecht: Kluwer Academic Publishers; 1989;1018–76.

68. Matzke GR, Keane WF. Drug dosing in patients with impaired renal function, In: DiPiro JT, Talbert RL, Hayes PE, Yee GC, Posey LM, eds. Pharmacotherapy: A Pathophysiologic Approach. New York: Elsevier; 1989;589–98.

69. Tilstone WJ, Fine A. Furosemide kinetics in renal failure. Clin Pharmacol Ther. 1978;23:644–50.

70. Chau NP et al. Pindolol availability in hypertensive patients with normal and impaired renal function. Clin Pharmacol Ther. 1977;22:505–10.

71. Craig RM et al. Kinetic analysis of D-xylose absorption in normal subjects and in patients with chronic renal failure. J Lab Clin Med. 1983;101:496–506.

72. Guay DRP et al. Pharmacokinetics and pharmacodynamics of codeine in end stage renal disease. Clin Pharmacol Ther. 1988;43:63–71.

73. Balant LP et al. Consequences of renal insufficiency on the hepatic clearance of some drugs. Int J Clin Pharmacol Res. 1983;3:459–74.

74. Bianchetti G et al. Pharmacokinetics and effects of propranolol in terminal uraemic patients and in patients undergoing regular dialysis treatment. Clin Pharmacokinet. 1976;1:373–84.

75 Gibson TP et al. Propoxyphene and norpropoxyphene plasma concentrations in the anephric patient. Clin Pharmacol Ther. 1980;27:665–70.

76. Plaisance KI et al. Effect of renal function on the bioavailability of ciprofloxacin. Antimicrob Agents Chemother. 1990;34:1031–34.
77. Barnes JN et al. Dihydrocodeine in renal failure: further evidence for an important role of the kidney in the handling of opioid drugs. Br Med J. 1985;290:740–43.
78. Matzke GR, Flaherty FJ. Drug dosing in renal failure. In: Young LY, Koda-Kimble MA, eds. Applied Therapeutics: The Clinical Use of Drugs. Vancouver, WA: Applied Therapeutics; 1988;571–86.
79. Reidenberg MM, Drayer DE. Alteration of drug-protein binding in renal disease. Clin Pharmacokinet. 1984;9:18–26.
80. Matzke GR, Keane WF. Use of antibiotics in renal failure. In: Peterson PK, Verhoef J, eds. The Antimicrobial Agents Annual. Amsterdam: Elsevier; 1986;472–88.
81. Keller F et al. Supplementary dose after hemodialysis. Nephron 1982;30:220.
82. Gibson TP. Influence of renal disease on pharmacokinetics. In: Evans WE, Schentag JJ, Jusko WJ, eds. Applied Pharmacokinetics: Principles of Therapeutic Drug Monitoring. Vancouver, WA: Applied Therapeutics; 1986;83–115.
83. Levy RH, Moreland TA. Rationale for monitoring free drug levels. Clin Pharmacokinet. 1984;9(Suppl. 1):1–9.
84. Liponi DF et al. Renal function and therapeutic concentrations of phenytoin. Neurology 1984;34:395–97.
85. Haughey et al. Protein binding of disopyramide and elevated alpha-1-acid glycoprotein concentrations in serum obtained from dialysis patients and renal transplant recipients. Am J Nephrol. 1985;5:35–9.
86. Docci D et al. Serum alpha-1-acid glycoprotein in chronic renal failure. Nephron 1985;39:160.
87. MacKichan JJ. Pharmacokinetic consequences of drug displacement from blood and tissue proteins. Clin Pharmacokinet. 1984;9:32–40.
88. Jusko WJ et al. Pharmacokinetic design of digoxin dosage regimens in relation to renal function. J Clin Pharm. 1974;14:525.
89. Gibson TP. Renal disease and drug metabolism: an overview. Am J Kidney Dis. 1986;8:7–17.
90. Farrell GC. Drug metabolism in extrahepatic diseases. Pharmacol Ther. 1987;35:375–404.
91. Touchette MA, Slaughter RL. The effect of renal failure on hepatic drug clearance. DICP-Ann Pharmacother. 1991;25:1214–24.
92. Patterson SE, Cohn VH. Hepatic drug metabolism in rats with experimental chronic renal failure. Biochem Pharmacol. 1984;33:711–16.
93. Terner UK et al. The effects of acute and chronic uremia in rats on their hepatic microsomal enzyme activity. Clin Biochem. 1978;11:156–58.
94. Hogan EM et al. Hepatic microsomal oxidative N-demethylation in rats with renal failure. Br J Pharmacol. 1979;66:74P–5P.
95. Anders MW. Metabolism of drugs by the kidney. Kidney Int. 1980;18:636–47.
96. Bowmer CJ et al. The effect of acute renal failure on the pharmacokinetics of indocyanine green in the rat. Biochem Pharmacol. 1982;31:2531–538.
97. Leber HW et al. Enzyme induction in the uremic liver. Kidney Int. 1978;13(Suppl. 8):S43–S48.
98. Terao N, Shen DD. Reduced extraction of *l*-propranolol by perfused rat liver in the presence of uremic blood. J Pharmacol Exp Ther. 1985;233:277–84.
99. Lichter M et al. The metabolism of antipyrine in patients with chronic renal failure. J Pharmacol Exp Ther. 1973;187:612–19.
100. Maddocks JL et al. The plasma half-life of antipyrine in chronic uraemic and normal subjects. Br J Clin Pharmacol. 1975;2:339–43.
101. Harman AW et al. Salivary antipyrine kinetics in hepatic and renal disease and in patients on anticonvulsant therapy. Aust NZ J Med. 1977;7:385–90.
102. Teunissen MWE et al. Antipyrine metabolite formation and excretion in patients with chronic renal failure. Eur J Clin Pharmacol. 1985;28:589–95.
103. Awni WM et al. Hepatic blood flow (HBF) and oxidative metabolism (HOM) in hemodialysis patients (HD). Clin Pharmacol Ther. 1988;43:147. Abstract.

104. Halstenson CE et al. Comparative liver function assessment in subjects with renal impairment (RI), normal and impaired (HI) hepatic function. Pharm Res. 1989;6:S219. Abstract.

105. Gwilt PR et al. The effects of diabetes mellitus on pharmacokinetics and pharmacodynamics in humans. Clin Pharmacokin. 1991;6:477–90.

106. Narang APS et al. Impairment of drug clearance in patients with diabetes mellitus and liver cirrhosis. Indian J Med Res. 1987;85:321–25.

107. Zysset T, Wietholtz H. Differential effect of type I and type II diabetes on antipyrine disposition in man. Eur J Clin Pharmacol. 1988;34:369–75.

108. Adithan C et al. Differential effects of type I and II diabetes mellitus on antipyrine metabolism. Methods Find Exp Clin Pharmacol. 1989;11:755–6.

109. Matzke GR et al. The influence of type I and type II diabetes mellitus on antipyrine disposition. Clin Pharmacol Ther. 1992;51.

110. Ueda H et al. Disappearance rate of tolbutamide in normal subjects and in diabetes mellitus, liver cirrhosis and renal disease. Diabetes 1963;12:414–19.

111. Adithan C et al. Effect of type II diabetes mellitus on theophylline elimination. Int J Clin Pharmacol Ther Toxicol. 1989;27:258–60.

112. Adithan C et al. Effects of diabetes mellitus on salivary paracetamol elimination. Clin Exp Pharmacol Physiol. 1988;15:465.

113. Shin AF, Shrewsbury RP. Evaluations of drug interactions. St. Louis, MO: C.V. Mosby Co.; 1985;19.

114. Kosoglou T, Vlasses PH. Drug interactions involving transport mechanisms: an overview. Drug Intell Clin Pharm. 1989;23:116–22.

115. Bricker NS et al. The pathophysiology of renal insufficiency on the functional transformation in the residual nephrons with advancing disease. Pediatr Clin North Am. 1971;18:595.

116. Haberle D et al. Influence of glomerular filtration rate on the rate of para-aminohippurate secretion by the rat kidney: micropuncture and clearance studies. Kidney Int. 1975;7:385–96.

117. Lin JH, Lin TH. Renal handling of drugs in renal failure. I: Differential effects of uranyl nitrate- and glycerol-induced acute renal failure on renal excretion of TEAB and PAH in rats. J Pharmacol Exp Ther. 1988;246:896.

118. Gloff CA, Benet LZ. Differential effects of the degree of renal damage on p-aminohippuric acid and inulin clearances in rats. J Pharmacokin Biopharm. 1989;17:169.

119. Maiza A, Daley-Yates PT. The clearance of drugs in different types of renal disease. Renal Failure 1989;11:67. Abstract.

120. Westenfelder C et al. Renal tubular function in glycerol-induced acute renal failure. Kidney Int. 1980;18:432–44.

121. Chasis H et al. The use of sodium p-aminohippurate for the functional evaluation of the human kidney. J Clin Invest. 1945;24:583–88.

122. Corcoran AC et al. Functional patterns in renal disease. Ann Int Med. 1948;28:560–82.

123. Cargill WH. The measurement of glomerular and tubular plasma flow in the normal and diseased human kidney. J Clin Invest. 1949;28:533–38.

124. Bradley SE et al. Seminars on renal physiology: renal function in renal diseases. Am J Med. 1950:766–98.

125. Robertson JA et al. Renal function in diabetic nephropathy. Arch Int Med. 1951;87:570–82.

126. Bucht H et al. Renal function studies in diabetic nephropathy. Scand J Clin Lab Invest. 1956;8:309–18.

127. Nyberg G et al. Renal extraction ratios for ^{51}Cr-EDTA, PAH, and glucose in early insulin-dependent diabetic patients. Kidney Int. 1982;21:706–708.

128. Winetz JA et al. Glomerular function in advanced human diabetic nephropathy. Kidney Int. 1982;21:750–56.

129. Hori R et al. A new dosing regimen in renal insufficiency: application to cephalexin. Clin Pharmacol Ther. 1985;38:290–95.

130. von Ginneken CAM, Russel FGM. Saturable pharmacokinetics in the renal excretion of drugs. Clin Pharmacokinet. 1989;16:38–54.

131. Koren G. Clinical pharmacokinetic significance of the renal tubular secretion of digoxin. Clin Pharmacokinet. 1987;13:334–43.

132. Laskin OL et al. Effects of probenecid on the pharmacokinetics and elimination of acyclovir in humans. Antimicrob Agents Chemother. 1982;21:804–807.

133. van Crugten J et al. Selectivity of the cimetidine-induced alterations in the renal handling of organic substrates in humans. Studies with anionic, cationic and zwitterionic drugs. J Pharmacol Exp Ther. 1986;236:481.

134. Gisclon LG et al. The effect of probenecid on the renal elimination of cimetidine. Clin Pharmacol Ther. 1989;45:444–52.

135. Lam YWF. Effect of probenecid on the pharmacokinetics and pharmacodynamics of procainamide. Pharm Res. 1988;5(Suppl. 1):S181. Abstract.

136. Hedaya MA et al. Probenecid inhibits the metabolic and renal clearances of zidovudine (AZT) in human volunteers. Pharm Res. 1990;7:411–17.

137. de Miranda P et al. Alteration of zidovudine pharmacokinetics by probenecid in patients with AIDS or AIDS-related complex. Clin Pharmacol Ther. 1989;46:494–500.

138. Halstenson CE et al. Disposition of cefmetazole in healthy volunteers and patients with impaired renal function. Antimicrob Agents Chemother. 1990;34:519–23.

139. Dettli L et al. Drug dosage in patients with impaired renal function. Postgrad Med J. 1970;46(Suppl.):32–5.

140. Dettli L. Individualization of drug dosage in patients with renal disease. Med Clin North Am. 1974;58:977–85.

141. Dettli L. Drug dosage in renal failure. In: Gibaldi M, Prescrott L, eds. Handbook of Clinical Pharmacokinetics. New York: ADIS Press; 1983;261–76.

142. Tozer TN. Nomogram for modification of dosage regimens in patients with chronic renal impairment. J Pharmacokinet Biopharm. 1974;2:13–28.

143. Welling PG et al. Prediction of drug dosage in patients with renal failure using data derived from normal subjects. Clin Pharmacol Ther. 1975;18:45–52.

144. Rowland M, Tozer TN. Clinical Pharmacokinetics: Concepts and Applications. Philadelphia, PA: Lea & Febiger; 1989;2;238–54.

145. Bennett WM. Guide to drug dosage in renal failure. Clin Pharmacokinet. 1988;15:326–54.

146. Gilbert DN, Bennett WM. Use of antimicrobial agents in renal failure. Infect Dis Clin North Am. 1989;3(3):517–31.

147. Aweeka FT. Drug Reference Table. In Schrier RW, Gambertoglio JG (ed): Handbook of Drug Therapy in Liver and Kidney Disease. Boston, MA: Little, Brown and Company. 1991;285–371.

148. Sheiner LB. Methods for drug dosage individualization: past, present and future. In: Benet LZ, Levy G, Ferraiolo BL, eds. Pharmacokinetics—a modern view. New York: Plenum Press; 1984;295–314.

149. Pryka RD et al. An updated comparison of drug dosing methods. Part I: Phenytoin. Clin Pharmacokinet. 1991;20(3):209–17.

150. Erdman SM et al. An updated comparison of drug dosing methods. Part II: Theophylline. Clin Pharmacokinet. 1991;20(4):280–92.

151. Erdman SM et al. An updated comparison of drug dosing methods. Part III: Aminoglycoside antibiotics. Clin Pharmacokinet. 1991;20(5):374–88.

152. Erdman SM et al. An updated comparison of drug dosing methods. Part IV: Vancomycin. Clin Pharmacokinet. 1991;20(6):463–76.

153. Hoenich NA et al. Dialysers. In: Maher JF, ed. Replacement of renal function by dialysis. Dordrecht: Kluwer Academic Publishers; 1989;144–80.

154. Van Stone J. Hemodialysis apparatus. In: Daugirdas JT, Ing TS, eds. Handbook of Dialysis. Boston: Little Brown; 1988;21–39.

155. Daugirdas JT et al. Special procedures. In: Daugirdas JT, Ing TS, eds. Handbook of Dialysis. Boston: Little Brown; 1988;121–45.

156. Bosch JP, Ronco C. Continuous arteriovenous hemofiltration (CAVH) and the continuous replacement therapies: operational characteristics and clinical use. In: Maher JF, ed. Replacement of renal function by dialysis. Dordrecht: Kluwer Academic Publishers; 1989;347–59.

157. Geronemus R, Vlchek DL. Continuous renal replacement therapy: an overview of CAVH, CAVHD and SCUF. Nephrology News Issues 1988;24–8.

158. Gokal R. Continuous ambulatory peritoneal dialysis. In: Maher JF, ed. Replacement of renal function by dialysis. Dordrecht: Kluwer Academic Publishers; 1989;590–615.

159. Sargent JA, Gotch F. Principles and biophysics of dialysis. In: Maher JF, ed. Replacement of renal function by dialysis. Dordrecht: Kluwer Academic Publishers; 1989;87–143.

160. Bickley SK. Drug dosing during continuous arteriovenous hemofiltration. Clin Pharm. 1988;7:198–206.

161. Kronfol NO et al. Effect of CAVH membrane types on drug-sieving coefficients and clearances. Trans Am Soc Artif Inter Organs. 1986;32:85–87.

162. Sigdell JE. Technical and functional consideration in choosing a hollow-fiber dialyzer, In: Nissenson AR, Fine RN, eds. Dialysis Therapy. Philadelphia: Hanley and Belfus; 1986;51–82.

163. Sigdell JE. Parallel-plate dialyzers. In: Nissenson AR, Fine RN, eds. Dialysis Therapy. Philadelphia: Hanley and Belfus; 1986;82–85.

164. Keller F. Effect of plasma protein binding, volume of distribution and molecular weight on the fraction of drugs eliminated by hemodialysis. Clin Nephrol. 1983;19:201–205.

165. Gibson TP. Problems in designing hemodialysis drug studies. Pharmacotherapy 1985;5:23–9.

166. Lee CC, Marbury TC. Drug therapy in patients undergoing hemodialysis. Clinical pharmacokinetic considerations. Clin Pharmacokinet. 1984;9:42–66.

167. Gotch FA. Hemodialysis: technical and kinetic considerations. In: Brenner BM, Rector FC Jr, eds. The Kidney. Philadelphia: WB Saunders;1976;1672–704.

168. Barbhaiya RH et al. Pharmacokinetics of cefepime in subjects with renal insufficiency. Clin Pharmacol Ther. 1990;48:268–276.

169. Matzke GR et al. Disposition of vancomycin during hemofiltration. Clin Pharmacol Ther. 1986;40:425–30.

170. Bastani B et al. *In vivo* comparison of three different hemodialysis membranes for vancomycin clearance: cuprophan, cellulose acetate, and polyacrylonitrile. Dial Transplant. 1988;17:527–528,543.

171. Lanese DM et al. Markedly increased clearance of vancomycin during hemodialysis using polysulfone dialyzers. Kidney Int. 1989;35:1409–412.

172. Torras J et al. Pharmacokinetics of vancomycin in patients undergoing hemodialysis with polyacrylonitrile. Clin Nephrol. 1991;36:35–41.

173. Stec GP et al. N-acetylprocainamide pharmacokinetics in functionally anephric patients before and after perturbation by hemodialysis. Clin Pharmacol Ther. 1979;26:618–28.

174. Ziemniak et al. Rebound following hemodialysis of cimetidine and its metabolites. Am J Kidney Dis. 1984;6:430–35.

175. Gibson TP et al. N-acetylprocainamide levels in patients with end stage renal failure. Clin Pharmacol Ther. 1976;19:206–12.

176. Halstenson CE et al. Aminoglycoside redistribution phenomenon after hemodialysis: netilmicin and tobramycin. Intern J Clin Pharmacol Ther Toxicol. 1987;25:50–5.

177. Bauer LA. Rebound gentamicin levels after hemodialysis. Ther Drug Monit. 1982;4:99–101.

178. Ross CJ, Rutsky EA. Dialysis modality selection in the elderly patient with end-stage renal disease: advantages and disadvantages of peritoneal dialysis. Adv Perit Dial. 1990;6 (Suppl.):11–18.

179. Diaz-Buxo JA. Current status of continuous cyclic peritoneal dialysis (CCPD). Perit Dial Int. 1989;9:9–14. Editorial.

180. Paton TW. Drug therapy in patients undergoing peritoneal dialysis. Clinical pharmacokinetic considerations. Clin Pharmacokinet. 1985;10:404–26.

181. Maher JF. Influence of continuous ambulatory peritoneal dialysis on elimination of drugs. Perit Dial Bull. 1987;7(3):159–67.

182. Keane WF et al. Continuous ambulatory peritoneal dialysis (CAPD) peritonitis treatment recommendations: 1989 udpate. Perit Dial Int. 1989;9:247–56.

183. Mounier M et al. Pharmacokinetics of vancomycin following intra-abdominal administration in patients with chronic renal failure under continuous ambulatory peritoneal dialysis (CAPD). Path Biol. 1985;33:542–44.

184. Silver MR et al. Vancomycin pharmacokinetics and ototoxicity in CAPD. Kidney Int. 1987;31:255. Abstract.
185. Bastani B et al. Peritoneal absorption of vancomycin during and after resolution of peritonitis in continuous ambulatory peritoneal dialysis (CAPD) patients. Perit Dial Bull. 1988;8:135–36.
186. Walshe JJ, Morse GD. The influence of peritonitis on the pharmacokinetics of intraperitoneal vancomycin. Paper presented to 19th Annual ASN Meeting, Washington, DC: 1986 Dec 8.
187. Morse GD et al. Intraperitoneal cefamandole kinetics in continuous ambulatory peritoneal dialysis (CAPD) patients with and without peritonitis. Clin Pharmacol Ther. 1985;37:214. Abstract.
188. Paton TW et al. The disposition of cefazolin and tobramycin following intraperitoneal administration in patients on continuous ambulatory peritoneal dialysis. Perit Dial Bull. 1983;3:73 6.
189. Petersen J et al. Pharmacokinetics of intraperitoneal cefotaxime treatment of peritonitis in patients on continuous ambulatory peritoneal dialysis. Nephron 1985;40:79–82.
190. Brouard R et al. Transperitoneal movement and pharmacokinetics of cefotiam and cefsulodin in patients on continuous ambulatory peritoneal dialysis. Clin Nephrology 1988;30:197–206.
191. Ryckelynck et al. Pharmacokinetics of ceftazidime in patients on CAPD. Perit Dial Bull. 1986;6:108. Letter.
192. De Paepe M et al. Peritoneal pharmacokinetics of gentamicin in man. Clin Nephrology. 1983;19:107–9.
193. Lameire N et al. Pharmacokinetics of netilmicin after intravenous (IV) and intraperitoneal (IP) administration in CAPD. Perit Dial Bull. 1987;7:S45.
194. Halstenson CE et al. Intraperitoneal administration of tobramycin during continuous ambulatory peritoneal dialysis. Kidney Int. 1984;25:256. Abstract.
195. Krediet RT et al. Pharmacokinetics of intraperitoneally (IP) administered 5-fluorocytosine (5-FC) in CAPD patients. Perit Dial Bull. 1987;7:S43.
196. Singlas E et al. Pharmacokinetics of sulfamethoxazole-trimethoprim combination during chronic peritoneal dialysis; effect of peritonitis. Eur J Clin Pharmacol. 1982;21:409–15.
197. Golper TA, Bennett WM. Drug removal by continuous arteriovenous hemofiltration—a review of the evidence in poisoned patients. Med Toxicol. 1988;3:341–49.
198. Kronfol N et al. Clearance of drugs during continuous arteriovenous hemodialysis (CAVHD) correlates with dialysate flow rate (QDi). Clin Res. 1989;37:9A. Abstract.
199. Winchester JF. Hemoperfusion. In: Maher JF, ed. Replacement of renal function by dialysis. Netherlands: Kluwer Academic Publishers; 1989;439–59.

Chapter 9

Special Pharmacokinetic Considerations in the Elderly

Michael B. Mayersohn

It has long been an accepted principle in pharmacology and clinical medicine that aging in humans is one of many factors that may affect the response to drugs. It would seem reasonable, therefore, that we take age into consideration when designing an appropriate dosing regimen. Until just within the last several years, however, age had been ignored. Dosing regimens have been based upon information obtained in otherwise healthy young adults. There has been a growing interest in geriatric medicine, as evidenced by an expanding body of literature. It is not uncommon to see review articles in professional journals and continuing education programs designed to inform and to promote a better understanding of effective drug therapy and medical care of the aged. Although our current understanding of the aging process and its consequences is far from complete, we are now beginning to better understand the impact of age on drug therapy, and useful guidelines are emerging to improve drug use. There remains, however, a need for a great deal more information. Undoubtedly, increased research efforts during this decade will provide much of that knowledge. One such impetus to more research is the proposed guidelines of the Food and Drug Administration requiring information about elderly subjects in the clinical sections of a new drug application. Table 9-1 outlines reasons for considering the elderly as a unique group within the general population.

The purpose of this chapter is to review our current understanding of how aging influences the various processes of drug disposition (i.e., absorption, distribution, metabolism, and excretion) and what this influence implies about the design of an appropriate dosing regimen. The gerontology literature is filled with contradictions arising either from lack of controls for the many complex interacting variables or from improper experimental design and/or methods of data analysis. One cannot stress enough the need to evaluate such literature critically.

Table 9-1. *Special Considerations of the Elderly as a Unique Group within the Population*

Consideration	Characteristics
Population	The elderly (i.e., those older than age 65) currently represent about 12% of the U.S. population; this percentage is expected to increase to about 20% by year 2000.
Health	The elderly experience a greater incidence of disease, physical impairments and physiological disorders than do younger adults.
Institutionalization	The elderly occupy a greater share of hospital beds ($\approx$ 38%) and long-term care facilities than do younger adults.
Drug use	The elderly consume more drugs ($\approx$ 30% of total use) per capita than do younger adults.
Drug effects	The elderly experience a greater incidence of adverse drug effects and drug-drug interactions than do younger adults.

Perhaps in no other clinical area is there a need for more careful experimental design and adequate controls than in geriatrics research. Table 9-2 lists several of the complicating factors that need to be considered in the design and interpretation of a clinical study. One fundamental issue is the appropriate definition of age. In virtually every study which attempts to relate some parameter with chronological age, there are always marked variations among subjects even of the same age. A more fundamental and meaningful measure of age is frequently referred to as "biological age." Unfortunately there is not at present any useful means of measuring or expressing biological age, and we have little choice but to base our studies on chronological age and bear in mind the accompanying degree of variability in all its parameters.

In studies which compare some parameter with age, one of two approaches is used in age selection. First and most often, a "young" and an "elderly" group of subjects are studied. As a result, there needs to be some age demarcation between these groups. For example, an elderly person may be considered any subject older than age 55, 60, 65, or any other age that seems appropriate to that particular investigator. Indeed, there have been even further refinements applied to a description of the elderly: "young-old" (65–74 years), "middle-old" (74–84 years), and "old-old" (greater than 85 years). A young subject, on the other hand, may

Table 9-2. *Factors which Complicate the Design and Interpretation of Age-Related Studies*

Factor	Complication
Age: definition	Chronological versus biological age
Age: comparisons	Continuum over years versus arbitrary definition of elderly
Age: changes	Longitudinal design (age changes) versus cross-sectional design (age differences)
Health status	Chronic or acute illness versus good health; institutionalized versus living at home
Drug therapy	Acute or chronic drug therapy versus no drug use
Nutritional status	Good or adequate versus poor nutrition
Environment	Smoking versus not smoking; prior environmental exposure of elderly when young versus current exposure in young

represent any person in the third to fifth decades of life (i.e., 21–30, 31–40, or 41–50 years). These decisions are frequently made for convenience and represent an artificial definition of what comprises young and old ages. Most studies suggest that the majority of physiological processes associated with aging change gradually over a lifetime and not abruptly. Figure 9-1 is by now a classical representation of that argument.[1] Regardless of their exact nature and their mathematical representation, the relationships illustrated in Figure 9-1 point to a continuum of change with age. Therefore, the second of the two approaches for experimental design, to examine parameter values over as many decades of adult life as possible, would better represent the gradual nature of the aging process.

Regardless of which of the previous two approaches is taken, virtually all studies employ a cross-sectional design. That is, different people of different ages are examined to establish an age relationship. The conclusions that arise from such a design are differences in a given parameter with age. Far more desirable would be an examination of changes within an individual with age, which can only be accomplished with a longitudinal study design. In the longitudinal design the same subjects are studied over many years. There is an obvious practical limitation to that approach in terms of time and expense, although one such long-term program has been underway for many years.

There needs to be consideration of the subjects' health status in any study that examines a given parameter as a function of age. The idea that old age implies poor health is quite misleading. The elderly population is comprised of healthy individuals who are leading active lives in the community as well as those who are acutely or chronically ill and may be in a hospital or other health care facility.

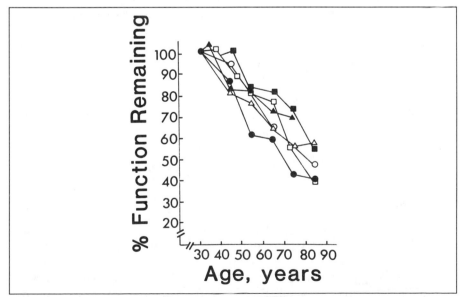

Figure 9-1. *Percentage of function remaining versus age. The values shown are relative to those at age 30 years. Key: maximal breathing capacity (●); renal plasma flow by para-amino hippurate clearance (❑); renal plasma flow by diodrast clearance (○); vital capacity (△); glomerular filtration rate by inulin clearance (■); cardiac index (▲). Adapted from reference 1.*

At the very least, the health status of the subjects needs to be determined and properly recorded in any publication. Failure to do so undoubtedly leads to many apparent discrepancies that appear in the gerontology literature.

The same principle applies to concomitant drug therapy in the subjects being studied. Drug interactions are of particular importance in elderly subjects, as they are especially likely to be receiving concomitant therapy.[2]

Nutrition is another potential complicating influence on the findings of age-related studies. The elderly, especially those living on fixed incomes, may have nutritional intake below what is considered optimal. While we have begun to recognize the influence of certain foods or food components (e.g., caffeine) on drug disposition, our current knowledge is incomplete. Therefore, there needs to be some evaluation of elderly subjects with regard to the level of nutrition, if by no other measure than history of food intake. A wide range of nutritional status among the elderly may account for some of the variability noted in certain parameters, and it therefore requires some control in experimental design.

Among confounding environmental factors, perhaps the most apparent is the difference in the disposition of certain drugs among smokers versus nonsmokers. It is important to control for this factor among subjects of all ages. Other environmental factors are likely to be important as well. An elderly person when he or she was young was exposed to a different environment than the one a young person is exposed to today (e.g., environmental pollutants and insecticides). Cross-sectional studies may suffer from the differences.

There are undoubtedly other factors, currently unrecognized, that have an impact on the results of studies that examine age relationships. Once uncovered, these factors will allow us to design better studies and to better understand our results. The importance of study design in gerontology research has been discussed by Rowe.[3] The previous discussion attempted to address some considerations in designing studies to examine, for example, the relationship between drug disposition and age. There are a host of complex interacting variables which require that such research studies be carefully designed. A similar critical attitude needs to be applied in evaluating the literature. There are a number of recent texts[4-7] and publications[8-10] that have reviewed current understanding of drug disposition and therapy as it is influenced by age and to which our readers are referred.

CLINICAL PHARMACOKINETICS

Absorption

In reviewing the gerontology literature one frequently reads general and often unqualified statements to the effect that the efficiency of drug absorption is either decreased or, alternatively, is not altered with age. Repetition of such assertions over the years appears to have given credence to their validity. Many studies of absorption (gerontologic or otherwise) are flawed by improper experimental design or incorrect methods of data analysis. For the most part, these errors reflect lack of consideration for basic pharmacokinetic principles.

There are two mistakes most frequently encountered. The first is the result of incomplete sample collections. In assessing completeness of absorption one usually relies on determination of the area under the drug plasma concentration-time curve (AUC). The ratio of AUCs within one subject resulting from different dosage forms allows assessment of the relative extent of absorption (bioavailability) or absolute absorption if an intravenous dose is given. The AUCs, however, must be complete (i.e., estimated to time infinity or about four to six elimination half-lives). Therefore, duration of sampling is not an arbitrary decision but depends upon the elimination characteristics of the drug being studied. If sample collection is arbitrarily truncated, then the estimate of absorption will be in error. This problem is easily resolved by extending blood sampling (or urine collection).

The other frequent error is the comparison of AUCs for a given drug among different subjects over a range of ages. Typically a single oral dose will be given and the AUCs determined. The problem here may be understood by examining the relationship between AUC and the extent of absorption (F, fraction of dose absorbed):

$$AUC = \frac{(F)(dose)}{CL}$$

(Eq. 9-1)

The above relationship indicates that AUC depends upon F as well as upon total or systemic body clearance (CL). In order to correctly evaluate absorption with use of Equation 9-1, one needs to assume that CL is the same in all subjects of different ages. This is a highly questionable assumption, as will be discussed below. Furthermore, Equation 9-1 is often used to assess CL after an oral dose and as a function of age. To do so requires that F be constant and unaltered by age. Again, this is a questionable assumption. If one is to rely on AUC in determining absorption there is little choice but to administer an intravenous dose of the drug as well as an oral dose. In this way, assuming that CL does not change from experiment to experiment, one will obtain a correct estimate of absolute absorption, as there is no need to assume equal values of CL for all chronological ages.

This discussion will be limited primarily to gastrointestinal (GI) absorption, as it is the most frequently used route of administration. At this time there is little if any information about the efficiency of absorption by other routes (e.g., rectal, pulmonary, intramuscular, dermal) as a function of age. Indeed, there is a need for such information, as drugs are given to the elderly by such routes. There are a number of age-related factors which may alter absorption, and these have been discussed in general terms elsewhere.[12] One point that should be borne in mind is that the GI tract is the most common site of distress in the aged,[13] possibly because of changes in eating habits and elimination.

The factors most often cited as having a potential effect on drug absorption and which may change with age include: GI fluid pH and contents; gastric emptying and intestinal transit rates; GI blood flow and surface area; nutritional intake and eating habits; age-related GI disease and drug ingestion altering gut function. In addition to these, one must also consider the physicochemical characteristics of the drug and its dosage form, as the net effect on absorption may reflect an interplay among those characteristics and the factors listed above. For example, a change in gastric emptying rate with age may have little influence on the absorption of a drug ingested as a solution, but a substantial effect may result when a solid oral dosage form is administered. There is some, albeit limited, information on how the aging process influences the factors noted previously. The impact of those changes as expressed in altered drug absorption is less clear. There is literature which indicates a substantial change in gastric fluid pH as a function of age. The incidence of achlorhydria increases dramatically in males and females from age 20 to about 79.[14] Consistent with that finding is the observation that basal and histamine-stimulated peak gastric acid secretion decline with age.[15] Atrophy of the gastric mucosa may explain this decrease in secretory function. There is less information available concerning intestinal fluid and pancreatic secretion and bile flow. Although the production and secretion of digestive enzymes may decrease with age, sufficient amounts appear to be available for digestive purposes.[13] The influence of this reduced gastric acidity on drug absorption in the aged has not been adequately addressed. It is, however, believed that the pH of GI fluid influences absorption by determining dissolution rate. Dissolution rate increases when the fluid pH results in the greatest degree of ionization (i.e., alkaline solution for acid drugs and acid solution for basic drugs). An age-related decrease in gastric fluid acidity would probably have an adverse effect on the dissolution rate of basic drugs. The less acidic gastric fluid may promote the dissolution of acidic drugs, but such drugs probably dissolve most readily in intestinal fluids which are much less acidic still.

Tetracycline affords an interesting example, as the compound is most soluble at low pH, and one report[16] indicated that exposure to acidic gastric fluids was necessary for efficient absorption. This would suggest the potential for decreased absorption in achlorhydria. In one study which addressed that issue, however, the relative absorption of tetracycline, in comparing a capsule to a solution, was unaltered in young normal subjects versus elderly achlorhydric subjects.[17] Furthermore, tetracycline absorption was not impaired in subjects who underwent surgery to remove the acid-secreting portion of the stomach.[18] These findings illustrate the interplay of dosage form and physiology, as the suggestion for the need of an acidic gastric fluid to achieve dissolution probably reflects the specific capsule dosage form examined. In the studies indicating comparable tetracycline absorption in the absence of acidic fluids, a different and probably better manufactured capsule dosage form was employed. If, for example, the solid dosage form contains diluents or disintegrants whose solubility is pH-dependent, and, in this instance, requires an acidic solution, then dissolution and absorption may be impaired. A number of studies *in vitro* have illustrated that certain dosage forms require exposure to an acidic solution in order for disintegration and dissolution to proceed.[19-21]

In addition to the previous considerations, gastric fluid pH may influence the efficiency of absorption by affecting drug stability, resulting in the production of clinically active or inactive compounds. Drugs which are unstable in acidic media (e.g., penicillin G, erythromycin) may degrade to a lesser degree in the gastric fluids of the elderly as a result of a higher pH. Also, the duration of exposure to gastric fluids, as determined by gastric emptying rate, will obviously influence the extent of chemical degradation. For example, clorazepate is a prodrug which requires acid hydrolysis for the formation of the active chemical species, N-desmethyldiazepam. The rate of hydrolysis *in vitro* is dependent upon pH with half-lives of greater than 1, 10, and 98 minutes at a pH of 3, 5, and 6, respectively.[22] Therefore, at a gastric fluid pH greater than 5 or 6, hydrolysis may be incomplete and lead to reduced bioavailability of the clinically active compound. While there is some discrepancy in the literature, it appears that elevated gastric fluid pH, achieved with coadministration of antacids, reduces the rate and the extent of absorption of N-desmethyldiazepam.[23-25] Ochs et al.[22] examined absorption in normal young and elderly subjects and in gastrectomy patients. Lower plasma concentrations and smaller areas under the 48-hour concentration-time curve were seen in the elderly and gastrectomy patients compared to the young subjects. It is difficult to judge from these data if absorption is impaired as a result of gastrectomy (and reduced acid secretion). Interestingly, these differences correlated better with age than with lack of acid secretion.

In addition to fluid pH there are components of GI fluids which may affect the absorption process. These include the quantity of enzymes and bile as well as total fluid volume. Bile salts, by virtue of their surface activity, promote particle wetting and dissolution rate of poorly water-soluble drugs.[26] Certain drugs require the presence of gut enzymes for chemical conversion to the active pharmacological form (e.g., chloramphenicol palmitate, steroid esters).[27,28] Total fluid volume may be important in permitting adequate dissolution. Unfortunately, at this time there appears to be little information about how the above factors may change with age.

By virtue of its large membrane surface area, the small intestine provides the best absorption site for all drugs, whether acids or bases. As a result, movement of drug from the stomach to the small intestine may limit the initiation of absorption. The latter is frequently expressed as gastric emptying rate or its inverse, gastric emptying time. There are a host of factors that influence gastric emptying, including specific foods, meal volume, gastric acidity, emotional status, posture, and certain drugs.[12] Although a delay in gastric emptying may in general reduce the rate or onset of absorption, only in certain circumstances is it expected to influence the extent of absorption. Emptying rate will probably exert a smaller influence on the absorption of a drug given in solution than in solid dosage form because liquids are more easily able to pass the pyloric sphincter.

GI muscle tone and motor activity are generally believed to be reduced in the elderly as a result of atrophic conditions. These differences with age may be influenced by altered eating and bowel habits and by the use of laxatives or foods high in fiber content. Other considerations may include GI disease and emotional status (e.g., anxiety, depression). Studies that have examined gastric emptying in young and elderly subjects have not clearly established a difference with age. Four recent studies examined gastric emptying half-time, and these data are summarized in Table 9-3. The results are equivocal for both liquid and solid emptying and may reflect methodological and protocol differences used for assessing emptying as well as different subject characteristics (e.g., health status, drugs taken, etc.) In all but one study, there was greater variability in emptying among the elderly. A more recent study,[32] which determined gastric residence time with use of the Heidelberg capsule, found a significantly longer residence time in a group of 12 healthy elderly subjects compared to 12 young subjects (4.5 versus 3.4 hours; mean ages, 69 versus 26 years).

If gastric emptying does change with age, the effect on absorption would be important only under certain circumstances. Emptying rate influences the absorption of compounds that are unstable in the stomach or which are best absorbed high in the small intestine. The compound L-DOPA, a prodrug for dopamine, appears to be absorbed by a specialized process in the proximal small intestine of animals.[34] The process may be inhibited by protein intake because the end products of protein digestion, amino acids, may compete with L-DOPA for absorption.[35,36] L-DOPA is metabolized in the gastric mucosa by decarboxylase enzymes;[37] hence, delay in emptying would tend to promote the metabolism of L-DOPA and thus inhibit absorption of the effective drug. On the other hand, it may improve efficiency of absorption by increasing the residence time at sites of maximal absorption. In fact, L-DOPA plasma concentrations were found to be lower in subjects with acidic gastric fluid and slower gastric emptying rates.[38] Concentrations increased when gastric fluids were made alkaline. Several reports on clinical effectiveness indicate that smaller doses of L-DOPA are required in the elderly (over 70 years old) than in younger subjects.[39,40] Another study found greater plasma concentrations in the elderly than in young subjects after oral dosing.[44] The same observation was made in a subsequent study[42] which also showed reduced gastric emptying rates in the elderly subjects compared to the young. The greater AUC in the elderly noted in those studies may reflect better absorption; however, decreased clearance could also, at least in part, explain those results, even though there was no difference in elimination half-life between the different age groups. An excellent study[43] has shown that the elderly have a lower systemic clearance and a greater oral bioavailability compared to young subjects (63% versus 41%).

Table 9-3. Comparison of Gastric Emptying Half-Times in Young and Elderly Subjects

			Gastric Emptying Half-Time in Minutes						
Age in Years			**Liquid**			**Solid**			
Mean	**(n)[a]**	**Range**	**Mean**	**(sem)[b]**	**s/ns[c]**	**Mean**	**(sem)**	**s/ns**	**References**
26	(7)	23–31	50		s				29
77	(11)	72–86	123						
31	(10)	24–51	68	(7)	ns	104	(10)	ns	30
76	(10)	71–88	94	(13)		105	(17)		
34	(22)	21–62	19	(1)	s	78	(4)	s	31
77	(13)	70–84	25	(3)		103	(8)		
24	(14)	21–28	13.7	(1.8)	ns				32
79	(14)	66–86	10.2	(1.6)					33

[a] n = Number of subjects.
[b] sem = Standard error of the mean.
[c] s = Significantly different; ns = not significantly different.

The lower oral clearance in the elderly suggests reduced decarboxylase activity in the gut. Coadministration of a decarboxylase inhibitor abolished the age difference in bioavailability (85%).

While most drugs are absorbed by a passive process, a variety of nutrients are absorbed by specialized processes. A number of these (e.g., riboflavin, ascorbic acid) are absorbed at sites high in the small intestine, and the efficiency of absorption has been shown to increase when emptying rate is reduced.[44-46] The implications of altered gastric emptying and nutrient absorption in the aged are not as yet understood, and indeed there is little information in general about nutrient absorption in the elderly. This is obviously an important consideration which requires attention.

There is little information about how intestinal transit rate may change with age. The general reduction with age in GI muscle tone and motor activity may suggest decreased intestinal motility and perhaps prolonged transit times. Slowing of motility may allow more time for drug dissolution and absorption and permit these processes to be more complete. On the other hand, the reduction of mixing motions along the tract may impede those processes. One study[32] has shown no significant difference in intestinal transit time in the elderly and the young (223 versus 208 minutes). The influence on absorption of the frequent use of laxatives and cathartics by the elderly has not been evaluated. One study examined the influence of a bran-supplemented diet on steady-state digoxin plasma concentrations in 12 elderly subjects.[47] There was no significant alteration in concentrations as a result of the diet change. As described previously for gastric emptying, the influence of dosage form must also be considered along with altered intestinal motility. For example, digoxin absorption has been studied in the presence or absence of drugs that affect gut motility.[48-50] Altered absorption in the presence of those agents (increase with propantheline; decrease with metoclopramide) will most probably be seen with poorly dissolving dosage forms, whereas there is little if any alteration of absorption for solutions or rapidly dissolving dosage forms.

The GI tract is well perfused by the blood stream, consistent with its absorption function. The splanchnic circulation, which includes portal and hepatic arterial flow, receives about 29% of cardiac output. Approximately 80% of the portal circulation perfuses the GI tract, which represents about 17% of cardiac output (approximately 850–900 mL/min in a young healthy adult).[51] Under normal circumstances blood flow to the GI tract appears to be sufficiently high to allow for rapid absorption. Blood flow may be the rate-limiting step in absorption only for those compounds that have an extremely high membrane permeability (e.g., water). The influence of altered gut blood flow on the rate of absorption and its relationship with the compounds' membrane permeability have been examined in laboratory animals.[52-55] Reduced blood flow decreases the rate of drug absorption for those compounds with high membrane permeability, and it has little effect on the rate of absorption for those compounds with low membrane permeability. Although there appear to have been no direct measurements of GI blood flow as a function of age in humans, splanchnic blood flow decreases with age.[56] Although the reduced total flow may not reflect a proportional decrease in portal and hepatic artery flow, it is likely that GI blood perfusion is diminished with age. The consequence of reduced GI blood flow with regard to absorption is not clear. It is likely that the rate of absorption will decline, but there may be little influence on the extent of absorption. A reduction in blood flow may alter the absorption of those compounds which undergo specialized transport, as a consequence of decreased delivery of oxygen and of cofactors needed to provide energy for cellular metabolism.

An additional concern, particularly pertinent to the elderly, is the presence of congestive heart failure (CHF), which may further compromise absorption by reducing GI blood flow beyond that seen as a normal consequence of aging. The majority of studies that have addressed this issue have relied upon AUC or urinary excretion measurements after a single oral dose in either different groups of subjects or in the same subjects before and after compensation of CHF. This approach is inadequate, since it is likely that CHF will also change drug clearance, thereby affecting AUC and urinary excretion and thus our conclusions about bioavailability differences. The potential influence of CHF on drug absorption has been reviewed previously,[57] and available data suggest impaired absorption of quinidine, procainamide, hydrochlorothiazide, metolazone, and possibly digoxin and furosemide.[58] Future studies need to clearly delineate the influence of disease states or physiological disorders that can influence drug disposition through their effects on absorption, especially if correlations with age are being examined.

Another consequence of age-related reduction in portal blood flow is its influence on the systemic bioavailability of those drugs that undergo substantial first-pass hepatic metabolism. Such compounds have a high hepatic clearance and a large hepatic extraction ratio. The oral clearance and systemic bioavailability of those drugs will be influenced by intrinsic hepatic metabolizing ability and, to various extents, by liver blood flow. The systemic oral bioavailability of L-DOPA,[43] chlormethiazole,[59,60] propranolol,[61] lidocaine,[62] and nalbuphine[63] is greater in the elderly than in younger subjects as a result of decreased first-pass hepatic metabolism. The same may occur with other drugs in this high clearance category; if so, greater plasma concentrations of unchanged drug could cause an increased incidence of adverse effects.

There is relatively little information in humans about how the structural integrity and barrier function of the GI tract change with age. Such alterations, if they occur, could have important implications for absorption by passive and specialized mechanisms. In one study which examined biopsy specimens from the upper jejunum of healthy young (16 to 30 years) and elderly subjects (60 to 73 years), there was a significant age-related reduction in mucosal surface area.[64] The results indicate an average reduction of about 20% in surface area, but there is substantial variability within the two age groups. It is difficult to judge the impact that this decrease in surface area might have on absorption, but assuming simple diffusion over the same length of intestine, absorption rate should decrease in direct proportion to the decrease in effective absorbing membrane surface area. This rule assumes that all other factors remain constant. It is possible, for example, that a decrease in surface area could be offset by an increase in inherent membrane permeability due to structural changes in the membranes that the drug must penetrate before reaching the blood stream. The decrease in surface area, in concert with a decrease in GI blood flow and possibly in gastric emptying rate, would argue for a decrease in absorption rate. These factors may in fact account for variability in absorption rate as a function of age. It is unlikely that these changes will decrease the extent of absorption unless the inherent absorption characteristics of the drug are so marginal as to be affected by the age-related changes discussed previously, in which case the oral route may be a questionable one to employ.

Statements to the effect that GI absorption is reduced with age are frequently based upon studies that have examined xylose absorption. This example illustrates the need to consider pharmacokinetic principles. The xylose absorption or tolerance test is often used to assess GI absorptive function when malabsorption syndromes are suspected. The same test has been used to study absorption as a function of age. While the test procedures may vary, most frequently a 5 gm or 25 gm oral dose is ingested and urine is collected for five hours. The data invariably indicate reduced xylose urinary recovery as a function of age, and this has been interpreted to indicate decreased absorption in the elderly. These studies have been reviewed, and the findings are summarized in Figure 9-2.[65] Lines B and C, which represent 5 gm and 25 gm oral xylose doses, respectively, indicate reduced urinary recovery with age. Line A, however, represents data obtained after an intravenous dose of xylose, and this line is parallel to the oral dose lines, indicating reduced urinary recovery with age. Obviously the effect of age on an intravenous dose cannot be explained by reduced absorption, but rather by decreased renal clearance, which, as is discussed below, is a natural consequence of aging. Also, the limited time period of collection may not reflect total elimination, especially after oral dosing. The interpretation of the xylose test, therefore, requires some knowledge of the subject's renal function. Line D in Figure 9-2 is the ratio of urinary recoveries after oral and intravenous dosing and suggests no

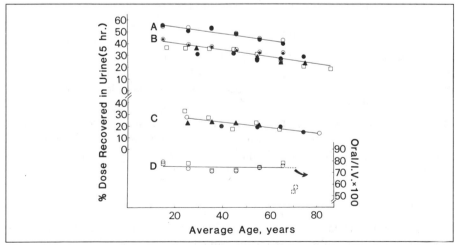

Figure 9-2. *Percentage of xylose dose recovered in a five-hour urine collection as a function of average age. Symbols reflect data obtained from different studies. Key: A) 5 gm IV dose, B) 5 gm oral dose, C) 25 gm oral dose, D) oral to IV urinary xylose recovery (y-axis on right) after a 5 gm oral and 5 gm IV dose. Reprinted by permission from reference 65.*

impairment in absorption. Xylose disposition and absorption following intravenous and oral dosing in the same group of subjects (32 to 85 years) have been reported.[66,67] Xylose absolute oral bioavailability was not related to age, indicating no apparent impairment in absorption among healthy aged subjects.

The previous discussion supports the point made in the introduction to this section, that there needs to be adequate consideration given to the disposition kinetics of the compound being studied and to basic pharmacokinetic principles. Many of the studies that have attempted to examine absorption as a function of age do not permit us to draw unequivocal conclusions. Frequently, for example, rate of absorption is determined on the basis of the time needed to achieve a maximum plasma concentration, and, based upon that value, numerous studies suggest reduced absorption rates in the elderly. That time (T_{max}), however, is influenced by the rate constants of absorption and elimination and therefore does not directly reflect rate of absorption.

A review of the literature leads to the following general conclusions: the rate of absorption is reduced or unaltered in the elderly, and the completeness of absorption is comparable to that in young adults.[68] The only exceptions to the latter rule are those drugs that undergo substantial pre-systemic elimination (i.e., first-pass metabolism), since, as noted previously, such drugs are more completely absorbed intact in the elderly.

Consideration must also be given to a variety of other factors which may alter drug absorption in the elderly. The plasma concentrations of a number of hormones that influence GI action (e.g., gastrin, motilin) are altered with age,[69] but as yet the implications of that observation are not understood. The presence of GI disorders and disease states in the elderly and the concomitant use of drugs for their treatment both have the potential for affecting absorption.[70]

Finally, as mentioned previously, absorption from routes of administration other than oral has received virtually no attention. Intramuscular absorption of diazepam,[70] lorazepam,[72] and meperidine[73] appears not to be altered with age. This may not be true of all drugs, however, because of reduced peripheral blood flow and an aqueous environment less able to maintain drugs in solution at the absorption site. Drug absorption via the transdermal route has received considerable attention during the past several years. There is little quantitative information, however, about the efficacy of transdermal absorption through aged skin, although an altered barrier function might be expected. One recent study which quantitatively examined this process for a variety of drugs indicates significantly lower penetration in aged skin (*in vivo* in humans) for hydrophilic compounds but no apparent effect of age for two lipid-soluble drugs.[74]

Distribution

There is now substantial information which indicates altered distribution for certain drugs as a function of age. Physiological and anatomical changes with age which affect distribution include blood flow and body composition, particularly with regard to water and adipose content. Relative changes in body content with age are also influenced by gender. Distribution is affected by plasma protein binding, for which there are numerous examples of its alteration with age. Less information is available about tissue binding. Altered plasma protein binding may influence elimination, clearance, and half-life and, hence, the interpretation of drug plasma concentration in the context of therapy.

Drug binding to plasma proteins as a function of age has received considerable attention in recent years. The importance of plasma protein binding rests on the generally accepted belief that only the unbound drug can distribute to extravascular sites of action and that it is therefore the unbound form which exerts a pharmacologic (or toxicologic) response. Furthermore, a change in binding can alter drug elimination in a manner that is predictable if certain disposition characteristics of the drug are known. There are a variety of factors which may affect binding which are particularly pertinent to the elderly, including protein concentration, disease states, coadministration of other drugs, and nutritional status. Another major source of variation which may to some degree explain discrepancies in the literature is in variations related to methodologic procedures. These include the technique for determining binding (usually equilibrium dialysis or ultrafiltration) and related variables (e.g., temperature, buffer, and pH), the use of "blank" (i.e., drug-free) plasma as opposed to "authentic" plasma samples, the particular concentration range examined, and the presence of other drugs and/or metabolites. In evaluating and contrasting the literature, one must keep the previous points in mind.

Although there appears to be a relatively small change with age in total serum protein concentrations,[75] albumin concentrations show a more substantial decrease.[75,76] This decrease is important because albumin is a major site of drug binding. This decrease in concentration may be more pronounced during illness; there is a shift toward lower values in the distribution of albumin concentration in the ill elderly compared to those in healthy elderly and healthy young subjects.[77] Health status, therefore, must be considered in investigating drug binding in the aged.[78] An alteration in binding with age in the absence of a change in albumin concentration implies the involvement of other factors, such as drug displacement from binding sites by drug metabolites, or endogenous compounds whose concentrations increase due to renal impairment. The possibility of displacement by metabolites illustrates the need to use authentic rather than "spiked" plasma samples. Effects of decreased renal function may in general apply to the elderly. In addition, this group's use of other drugs may also cause displacement interactions and account for altered binding. This is nicely illustrated from the results of one study which showed that the binding of several drugs (salicylate, sulfadiazine, and phenylbutazone) was decreased in elderly subjects taking other drugs compared to those not ingesting other drugs but who had equal serum albumin concentrations.[79] These data are illustrated in Figure 9-3.

Table 9-4 represents a compilation of information from studies that have examined drug plasma protein binding in young and elderly subjects. Several observations can be made from this summary, including the need to consider gender in binding studies. Other considerations, discussed previously, include health status, ingestion of other drugs, and methodologic differences in determining binding. These factors may explain why the data are contradictory for some drugs (e.g., diazepam, meperidine, phenytoin). In most instances where binding was related to age, the correlation coefficients are low (r, 0.30–0.65) and therefore age *per se* accounts for a relatively small fraction of the variation. Obviously, other explanations need to be explored (e.g., gender, illness, other drugs). In many cases decreased binding may be explained by decreased serum albumin concentration. Differences in binding in young and elderly are unlikely to be seen for those drugs which normally bind to a relatively small extent (e.g., caffeine, penicillin G, pheno-barbital, vancomycin). The general conclusion for drugs that bind to albumin is that aging is associated with either a decrease or no change in binding.

Important exceptions to the latter suggestion are those basic drugs that bind to the acute phase protein, α_1-acid glycoprotein (or orosomucoid). Since the concentration of that protein may increase in response to a variety of disorders, binding may also increase, as has been shown in elderly subjects for lidocaine[90] and propranolol.[114,122] Controversy remains, however, as to whether or not the increase in concentration of this protein is a natural consequence of aging. One recent study in 68 normal subjects (20 to 90 years of age) indicated no relationship between concentration and age.[123] These discrepancies and inconsistencies in binding and protein concentration should further impress upon investigators the need to clearly define and characterize the study population. The implications of altered plasma protein binding within an individual or of differences in binding between individuals, are not obvious. Given certain information about the drug (especially clearance and volume) one can make reasonable predictions.[124] Elimination half-life may change with altered binding, depending upon clearance and volume. This change may require an adjustment in the dosing interval, especially for a drug with a narrow therapeutic concentration range. A change in clearance due to binding will be important because clearance determines steady-state plasma concentrations.

With regard to steady-state plasma concentrations, a great deal of care needs to be exercised in the interpretation of those values, especially in conjunction with programs for therapeutic drug monitoring. For example, for restrictively cleared

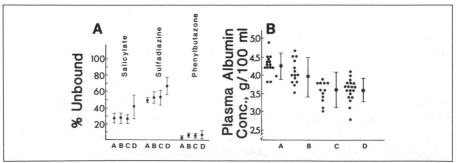

Figure 9-3. *A) Percentage unbound drug in plasma. The vertical crosshatched bars represent the standard deviation. Key: A, normal young subjects (no other drugs; n = 16; 19–40 years); B, young surgical subjects (receiving other drugs; n = 22; 14–39 years); C, elderly subjects (no other drugs; n = 16; 69–85 years); D, elderly subjects (receiving other drugs; n = 22; 74–92 years). B) Plasma albumin concentration in each of the four groups described above. The cross-hatched bars represent the standard deviation (reproduced with permission from reference 79).*

Table 9-4. *Relationship between Drug Plasma Protein Binding and Age*

Drug	Age, Years Mean	(n)[a]	Range	% Unbound drug or change in binding	Comments	References
Acetazolamide	35 79	(4) (4)	27–44 76–82	4.0 (s) 6.4		80
Amitriptyline	22 71	(7) (5)	21–23 62–81	5.2 (ns)[b] 4.4		81
Caffeine	22 71	(10) (8)	19–30 66–78	64.5 (ns) 65.0	Significantly lower serum albumin concentration in elderly.	82
Carbenoxolone		(9) (10)	< 40 > 65	% unbound drug significantly ↑ in elderly.	Significantly lower serum albumin concentration in elderly.	83
Ceftriaxone	29 71	(8) (8)	24–35 65–78	% unbound drug significantly ↑ in elderly.	Binding appears to be dependent upon drug concentration.	84
Chlordiazepoxide		(27)	16–86	No relationship between binding and age.		85
Chlormethiazole	26 76	(6) (6)	25–28 71–86	30.8 (s)[c] 40.3		59
Desalkylflurazepam		(26)	19–85	% unbound drug ↑ and correlated with age ($r = 0.56$; $p < 0.05$).		86
Desmethyldiazepam	31 68	(8) (8)	22–42 62–76	2.96 (ns; males) 2.93		87
	28 73	(7) (6)	22–31 65–85	2.67 (ns; females) 3.09		87

Table 9-4. Relationship between Drug Plasma Protein Binding and Age (cont.)

Drug	Age, Years			% Unbound drug or change in binding	Comments	References
	Mean	(n)[a]	Range			
Diazepam	28 69	(11) (11)	21–32 61–84	1.23 (s) 1.72	Significant difference in women only.	88
		(30)	15–82	No relationship between binding and age.		89
		(63)	18–88	% unbound drug ↑ and correlated with age in males (r = 0.65; p < 0.001) and females (r = 0.46; p < 0.001).	Binding related to serum albumin concentration which ↓ with age.	90
Disopyramide	30 69	(12) (7)	27–36 61–85	30 (ns) 30	Elderly subjects had a significantly higher concentration of α_1-acid glycoprotein.	91
Etodolac	27 75	(20) (20)	19–34 70–86	0.91 (ns) 0.97	Elderly subjects had osteoarthritis.	92
Fluphenazine		(19)	25–89	% unbound drug ↑ and was significantly correlated with age (r = 0.89; p <0.001).		93
Furosemide	33 83	(11) (22)	26–42 76–87	1.71 (s) 3.16	The elderly subjects had significantly lower serum albumin concentrations.	94
Ibuprofen	30 69	(17) (20)	20–44 60–88	% unbound drug not significantly different in males (1.02 vs. 1.10) or females (1.03 vs. 1.04).		95
Lidocaine		(63)	18–88	% unbound drug ↓ and correlated with age (r = 0.30; p < 0.05).	Binding related to α_1-acid glycoprotein serum concentration which ↑ with age.	90
	27 80	(6) (6)	20–34 73–87	51.9 (s) 30.5		96

Drug	%	(n)	Age (yr)	Finding	Comments	Ref.
Lorazepam	27	(15)	19–38			
	70	(15)	60–84	11.46 (s) % unbound drug ↑ 10.71 and correlated with age (r = 0.45; p < 0.01).		97
Maprotiline	23	(14)	20–32	10.5 (ns)	Elderly subjects were acutely ill and had greater serum concentrations of α_1-acid glycoprotein.	98
	82	(25)	74–95	11.0		
Meperidine		(19)	20–73	% unbound drug ↑ and correlated with age (r = 0.58; p < 0.001).		99
Midazolam	22	(12)	19–25	48 (ns)		100
	75	(11)	63–86	47		
		(40)	23–79	No relationship between binding and age.		101
Naproxen	10	(29)	22–39	% unbound drug significantly ↑ at trough concentrations (0.084 vs. 0.17) and at peak concentrations (0.23 vs. 0.51).	Binding dependent upon drug concentration.	102
	10	(71)	66–81			
Nitrazepam	35	(8)	19–44	17.8 (ns; males)		103
	67	(11)	60–80	18.9		
	27	(12)	19–44	17.9 (ns; females)		103
	69	(9)	60–80	19.0		
Oxaprozin		(42)	21–89	No relationship between binding and age.		104
Oxazepam		(13)	21–72	No relationship between binding and age.		105
		(38)	22–84	No relationship between binding and age.	% unbound drug had a tendency to ↑ with age partly due to ↓ serum albumin concentration.	106
Penicillin G		(5)	< 50	57.6 (ns)		107
		(4)	> 50	54.9		
Phenobarbital		(5)	< 50	58.2 (ns)		107
		(3)	> 50	58.1		
Phenytoin	28	(17)	20–38	Maximum binding capacity significantly ↓ with age.	Binding related to serum albumin concentration which ↓ with age.	108
	79	(19)	65–90			

Table 9-4. Relationship between Drug Plasma Protein Binding and Age (cont.)

Drug	Age, Years			% Unbound drug or change in binding	Comments	References
	Mean	(n)[a]	Range			
Phenytoin (cont.)		(6)	<50	17.6 (ns)		107
		(3)	>50	16.4		
		(40)	17–63	% unbound drug ↑ and correlated with age (p < 0.025).		109
	25	(24)	18–33	11.1 (s)	Significantly lower serum albumin concentration in elderly.	110
	75	(22)	62–87	12.5		
		(21)	65–102	No relationship between binding and age in this elderly group of subjects.		111
Piroxicam	23	(6)	20–31	0.69 (ns; males)		112
	66	(6)	62–75	0.77		
	26	(6)	20–31	0.79 (ns; females)		112
	71	(6)	62–75	0.66		
Propranolol	23	(10)	19–27	15.9 (ns)	Data shown for racemic form. There were no differences with age for either enantiomeric form. There was no difference in α_1-acid glycoprotein concentrations between groups.	113
	68	(10)	65–71	14.8		
	28	(10)	23–33	13.3 (s)	Data shown for (l)-propranolol. There was no significant difference in binding of the (d)-form. The elderly had a significantly greater concentration of α_1-acid glycoprotein.	114
	64	(10)	55–75	11.3		
Quinidine	29	(14)	23–34	24.6 (ns)		115
	66	(8)	60–69	28.2		

Drug	n[a]	Age range	Value	Comment	Ref
Temazepam	30 (14)	24–39	% unbound drug ↑ and correlated with age (r = 0.45; p < 0.01).	Binding related to serum albumin concentration which ↓ with age.	116
	70 (18)	60–84			
Tolbutamide	39 (24)	23–57	3.2 (s)		117
	72 (19)	61–87	4.0		
	(44)	23–87	% unbound drug ↑ and correlated with age (r = 0.61 - 0.72; p < 0.001).	Binding related to serum albumin concentration which ↓ with age. Binding dependent on tolbutamide concentration.	118
Triazolam	26 (16)	21–33	% unbound drug significantly greater in males only (24.7 vs. 21.3).		119
	71 (17)	61–87			
Vancomycin	24 (5)		48 (ns)		120
	69 (6)		44		
Verapamil	29 (7)	23–36	5.1 (ns)	All subjects were hypertensive males.	121
	68 (10)	61–74	6.5		
	84 (7)	75–102	5.3		

[a] Number of subjects.
[b] Not significantly different.
[c] Significantly different.

Table 9-5. *Relationship after an IV Dose between the Apparent Volume of Distribution and Age*

Drug	Age, Years Mean	(n)[a]	Range	Volume of distribution (L/kg) or relationship with age[b]	Comments	References
Acebutolol	23 79	(5) (5)	22–26 67–86	2.4 (s)[c] 1.5		131
Acetaminophen	31 70	(8) (8)	24–37 61–77	1.09 (s; male) 0.89	Volume ↓ and correlated with age (r = -0.63; p < 0.01).	132
	27 69	(8) (8)	23–33 64–78	0.94 (s; female) 0.79	Volume ↓ and correlated with age (r = -0.49; p < 0.05).	132
Alfentanil	26 65	(10) (10)		0.39 (ns) 0.34	Data shown for normal subjects. There were no significant differences between age groups for surgical patients.	133
Amitriptyline	22 71	(7) (5)	21–23 62–81	14.1 (s) 17.1		81
Ampicillin	27 81	(12) (12)	20–35 65–93	0.59 (ns) 0.59		134
Antipyrine	29 69	(14) (10)	23–43 60–76	0.66 (s; male) 0.55	Volume ↓ and correlated with age (r = -0.69; p < 0.01).	127
	28 69	(15) (12)	22–33 62–84	0.58 (s; female) 0.47	Volume ↓ and correlated with age (r = -0.73; p < 0.01).	127
Atracurium	33 75	(5) (5)	22–44 74–76	0.098(s) 0.188	The larger volume in the elderly may reflect lower plasma protein binding. Patients studied while undergoing surgery.	135
Caffeine	21 71	(8) (8)	19–24 66–78	0.613 (s) 0.524	Unbound volume significantly ↓ in elderly.	136

Drug	Age (yr)	(n)	Age range	Value	Comment	Ref
Ceftriaxone	29	(8)	24–35	0.152 (ns)[d]		84
	71	(8)	65–78	0.149		
Chlordiazepoxide		(27)	16–86	Volume ↑ and correlated with age (r = 0.60; p < 0.05).		85
Chlormethiazole	23	(6)	20–27	7.93 (s)		59, 137
	75	(8)	69–91	11.20		
Diazepam		(16)	20–70	Volume ↑ and correlated with age (r = 0.74; p < 0.001).		89
		(14)	32–78	Volume ↑ and correlated with age (r = 0.64; p < 0.05).		138
	26	(9)	21–30	1.15 (ns)		139
	79	(9)	70–88	1.71		
	28	(11)	23–37	1.11 (s; males)	Unbound volume not significantly different.	88
	69	(11)	63–76	1.83		
	28	(11)	21–32	1.73 (s; females)	Unbound volume not significantly different.	88
	69	(11)	61–84	2.64		
		(27)	20–91	Volume ↑ and correlated with age (r = 0.67; p < 0.001).	Unbound volume ↑ and correlated with age in males (r = 0.63; p < 0.001).	140
Digoxin	47	(6)	34–61	5.3 (ns)		141
	81	(7)	72–91	4.1		
Diltiazem	30	(10)		5.2 (ns)		142
	68	(10)		4.5		

Table 9-5. Relationship after an IV Dose between the Apparent Volume of Distribution and Age *(cont.)*

Drug	Age, Years		Volume of distribution (L/kg)^b or relationship with age	Comments	References
	Mean	(n)^a Range			
Diphenhydramine		(5) 20–26	4.17 (ns)		143, 144
		(12) 65–81	4.21		
L-Dopa	22	(8) 20–23	1.65 (s)		43
	71	(9) 68–75	1.01		
Ethanol		(42) 21–81	Volume ↓ and correlated with age (r = –0.40; p < 0.01).	Volume corrected for lean body mass not correlated with age. Lean body mass/surface area correlated with age (r = –0.53; p < 0.001).	129
Fentanyl	36	(5) <50	5.9 (ns)		145
	67	(4) >60	4.9		
Flunitrazepam		(20) 19–79	No relationship.		146
Lidocaine	24	(4) 22–26	0.90 (s)		147
	65	(6) 61–71	1.59		
	27	(6) 20–34	0.69 (ns)		96
	80	(6) 73–87	0.85		
Lorazepam	28	(11) 15–73	No relationship.		148
	69	(6) 22–38	1.07 (ns; male)	Unbound volume significantly ↓ in males.	72, 97
		(9) 64–76	1.02		
	27	(9) 19–32	1.14 (s; female)	Unbound volume significantly ↓ in females.	72, 97
	71	(6) 60–84	0.95		

Drug					Ref.
Meperidine	25 74	(6) (9)	18–29 67–86	5.38 (ns) 5.69	149
Metoprolol	73	(11) (10)	71–74	4.37 (ns) 3.98	150
Midazolam		(11) (11)	20–30 50–60	1.09 (s) 1.37	151
Morphine	26 67	(13) (7)	23–28 60–69	2.12 (s) 1.16	152
Pentazocine	32 76	(10) (8)	22–48 60–90	4.68 (ns) 4.31	153
Propranolol	29 78	(27) (7) (8)	21–73	No relationship. 3.0 (ns) 2.7	154 61
Propylthiouracil	33 80	(6) (9)	20–62 74–86	0.35 (ns) 0.37	155
Quinidine	29 66	(14) (8)	23–34 60–69	2.39 (ns) 2.18	115
Theophylline	56 65	(8) (13)	≤60 ≥61	0.48 (ns) 0.48	156
Thiopental	25 72	(6) (6)	20–27 65–77	0.43 (ns) 0.40	157
		(22)	25–83	Volume ↑ and correlated with age ($r = 0.64$; $p < 0.001$).	130

Subjects had chronic obstructive pulmonary disease. Data cited are for male nonsmokers. There were no differences with age for male smokers.

Table 9-5. Relationship after an IV Dose between the Apparent Volume of Distribution and Age (cont.)

Drug	Age, Years Mean	(n)[a]	Range	Volume of distribution (L/kg) or relationship with age[b]	Comments	References
Trazodone	29	(12)	18–40	0.89 (s; males)		158
	66	(7)	60–78	1.15		
	28	(13)	18–40	1.27 (s; females)		158
	69	(11)	60–78	1.50		
Valproic acid		(7)	20–35	0.13 (s)		198
		(6)	75–87	0.19		
Verapamil	29	(7)	23–36	4.3 (ns)		121
	68	(10)	61–74	4.9		
	84	(7)	75–102	6.1		
Vancomycin	23	(6)	20–26	0.64 (s)	Unbound volume significantly greater in elderly.	120
	69	(6)	61–77	0.93		

[a] Number of subjects.
[b] The volumes reported are either V_β (or V_{area}) or steady-state volume (V_{ss}).
[c] Significantly different.
[d] Not significantly different.

drugs, an increase in the unbound plasma fraction results in a decrease in total concentration but no change in the unbound concentration. Since the latter is assumed to be in equilibrium with tissue concentration and is the form responsible for eliciting a response, there is no need to change the dose rate; however, since all assays measure total concentration, and that value will decline, one may change (increase) the dose rate in error, with the resulting risk of toxicity. Therefore, for restrictively cleared drugs, if the unbound plasma fraction is noted to be greater in the elderly than in the young, there is no need to alter the regimen, provided that there is no difference in unbound intrinsic clearance (and the concentration-response relationship) between the two age groups. The same regimen will lead to different total concentrations, but, more importantly, to equal unbound concentrations. Similar concern exists for nonrestrictively cleared drugs, but different conclusions will be reached. In this instance, and assuming no difference in organ blood flow between age groups, the dose rate may need to be decreased to produce the desired unbound concentration, even though total concentration will appear to be unaltered. For certain drugs it may be necessary to determine unbound plasma concentrations in order to provide the optimum therapy or to explain an unusual response.

Tissue protein binding of drugs is more difficult to determine experimentally than is plasma protein binding. While tissue binding could theoretically change with age as a result of protein loss and decreased mass, there has been little direct evidence of its alteration. For the most part such a possibility is inferred from pharmacokinetic data analysis. The apparent volume of distribution of digoxin decreases in subjects with impaired renal function, as does the myocardium:serum concentration ratio.[125] Since digoxin is extensively bound to muscle tissue, the decreased volume may reflect reduced binding in those tissues. Furthermore, since age is associated with reduced renal function, it is likely that volume will also decrease as a function of age. Some drugs show a change in volume in the absence of a change in plasma protein binding, which may either suggest altered tissue binding or, as will be discussed, reflect a change in body composition with age.

Aging is associated with changes in body composition which may influence the distribution of certain drugs. Furthermore, the magnitude or relative change is different between males and females. There is a decline in total body and intracellular water volumes with little change in extracellular water volume.[126] In contrast, there appears to be little change with age in the various components of body water when expressed as a percentage of weight or surface area. Another study, albeit with fewer subjects, which has examined the distribution of the compound used for estimating total body water (antipyrine), indicates a decrease in that fluid volume with age (expressed as liters or as percentage of body weight).[127]

When the body is divided into lean body and fat masses as a percentage of body weight, as shown in Figure 9-4, there are substantial changes with age. Lean body mass declines with age in males and females, and fat mass increases with age. The relative changes vary with gender because males begin adult life with a greater percentage of lean body mass than do young adult females. On the other hand, females have a greater percentage of fat mass at all ages than do males. The change in body composition with age reflects the loss of muscle tissue and the increase in connective tissue and fat.

The influence this change in body composition has on drug distribution depends upon the physicochemical characteristics of the drug. Those compounds that distribute primarily into lean tissue will probably show an age-related decrease in volume of distribution, whereas compounds that distribute primarily into fatty tissue will probably show an increase in volume of distribution. For example, the volume of distribution of ethanol decreases with age because lean body mass declines with age and it is into such lean tissues that ethanol distributes.[129] In contrast, the volume of distribution of the lipid-soluble compound thiopental increases with age in women as a result of fat tissue representing a greater percentage of body weight.[130] Table 9-5 summarizes the results of studies that have examined volume of distribution with regard to age. Only those studies that used an intravenous dose have been included. It is not possible to make generalizations, as the direction of change depends upon the characteristics of the drug (e.g., oil-water partition coefficient, degree of plasma protein binding) and in some in-stances upon gender. As noted for plasma protein binding (Table 9-4), those studies that have correlated volume of distribution with age give relatively poor correlation coefficients (absolute value of r, 0.40–0.73). It seems that age *per se* explains only a small percentage of the variability.

An additional volume term which has received little attention, but which has some clinical significance, is the volume of the central compartment (V_c) or initial distribution space (V_1) in a multicompartment model. That volume finds applica-tion in the design of a loading intravenous bolus dose for certain drugs (e.g., lido-caine, rapid-acting anesthetics). The smaller dose of thiopental needed to induce

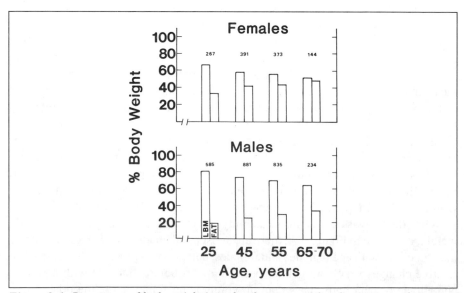

Figure 9-4. *Percentage of body weight in males (bottom) and females (top) as a function of age and expressed as lean body mass (LBM) and fat. The numbers above the bar graphs are the number of subjects. Based upon the data in reference 128.*

anesthesia in the elderly compared to that in younger adults was thought to be a result of an age-dependent decline in V_c. Recent data suggest that this is not the case but rather that there is a change in intercompartmental clearances with age.[159,160] While the central volume is not a "real" physiologic space, it is a useful concept associated with tissues and organs that are well perfused by the blood stream. A reduction in this volume with age may reflect the decline in mass of those tissues or organs and/or a reduction in blood flow. One example, is the decreased central volume of distribution of lidocaine in CHF.[161] Cardiac output and cardiac index decrease substantially with age, as reviewed by Bender[162] and as shown in Figure 9-5 under resting and exercise conditions (A and B, respectively). Also shown in Figure 9-5 are the results of a more recent study conducted in 61 subjects who had no evidence of coronary artery disease (panels C and D). Under those strict exclusion criteria one notes large variability in cardiac output among the subjects at any given age (this is also seen in A and B) and no obvious relationship with age. Therefore, aging *per se* does not appear to be associated with reduced cardiac output during resting or exercise.

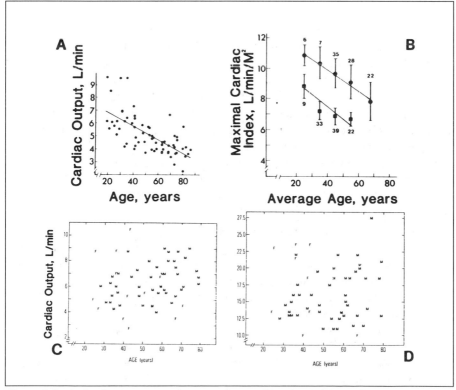

Figure 9-5. *A) Cardiac output as a function of age in 67 males. B) Maximal cardiac index after exercising as a function of average age in males (●) and females (■). The cross hatched bars represent the standard deviation and the numbers are number of subjects. C) Cardiac output as a function of age in males (M) and females (F) with no coronary artery disease. D) Cardiac output in the same subjects as in C but during exercise. Figures A, C, and D are reproduced by permission of the American Heart Association, Inc. (references 163 and 164). Figure C is based upon data in reference 162.*

Altered output is not uniform throughout the body. Cerebral blood flow decreases at a slower rate with age than does blood flow to the kidney and liver. The altered flow to the eliminating organs may have important implications in the clearance of certain drugs, as will be presented below. Blood flow to the coronary and skeletal muscles appears to be maintained throughout life in the absence of arteriosclerosis. Some care may be needed in interpreting a decrease in tissue blood flow. For example, while total flow to a tissue or organ may decrease, flow per unit weight may not be as dramatically altered, because of loss of tissue weight. In addition, there may be a differential anatomic alteration of flow within an organ which may result in a nonuniform influence on organ functions. This effect appears to apply to renal blood flow.

Further complicating the distribution process are age-related diseases or physiologic disorders which affect body composition or blood flow (e.g., CHF, hypotension).[165] Another consideration which has received little attention is the influence of bed-rest, which will in general apply to hospitalized or convalescing subjects. Bed-rest appears to influence the disposition of benzylpenicillin, for example.[166]

Metabolism

For elimination by renal excretion, certain definitive conclusions have been reached; among them is the fact that renal drug clearance is affected by a universal, age-related decline in renal function. The relationship between age and drug metabolism, on the other hand, is difficult to discuss quantitatively. There are two primary reasons for this situation. First, unlike renal excretion where one can quantitate function by creatinine clearance, hepatic function has no comparable index that can be related to drug metabolism. Second, there are a host of variables that influence hepatic drug metabolism. Even in a well-defined, normal healthy population of narrow age range, one encounters large variability in measures of drug metabolism (e.g., hepatic or metabolic clearance and half-life). Factors we are aware of which have been shown to influence hepatic drug metabolism include the following: disease states, concurrent drug use, nutritional status, environmental compounds, genetic differences, gender, liver mass, blood flow, and undoubtedly other factors that we do not currently appreciate. It is not surprising, therefore, that the influence of age on drug metabolism may be obscured by one or several of these factors. Investigators in this area need to be extremely careful in study design, especially in choice of subject population, and should attempt to control for these variables as well as possible.

The liver undergoes physiologic and anatomic changes with age which have the potential to alter drug metabolism. Liver blood flow decreases at a rate of between 0.5% and 1.5% per year after age 25. This represents a 40% to 45% decrease in flow in a 65-year-old person compared to a young adult. Indocyanine green clearance, which is a measure of hepatic blood flow (assuming an extraction ratio of about 1.0), is inversely correlated with age in males ranging in age from 22 to 73 years (r, −0.57).[167] A recent study in normal subjects indicates a significant reduction in portal blood flow with age; however, as with other age-related measurements, there is large variability (r, −0.58).[168] The clearance of those compounds that have a high hepatic extraction ratio is expected to decrease as a result of diminished flow. Hepatic blood flow per unit weight (or volume) or liver mass will probably change less with age than will the absolute value of blood flow, since liver mass also declines with age as discussed below.

Total liver mass or volume, whether as absolute values or adjusted on some basis of body size, decreases with age. The results of several studies conducted in normal subjects or at autopsy illustrate the decline in liver size with age.[169–172] The importance of these results is that the metabolic clearance of several compounds is related to liver volume. Roberts et al.[173] found a direct correlation (r, 0.69) between antipyrine clearance, which is primarily hepatic, and liver volume in young subjects (20–30 years). Antipyrine clearance also correlated with liver volume (r, 0.59) in young and elderly subjects (average ages, 29 and 84 years, respectively).[172] Antipyrine half-life was negatively correlated (r, –0.78) with liver weight in subjects ranging in age from 23 to 67 years.[169] The total and unbound clearances of phenytoin were shown to correlate with liver volume (r, 0.71 and 0.76, respectively) in young and elderly subjects.[172] Both of the above compounds have low hepatic extraction ratios and are metabolized via oxidative pathways. Other drugs in the same category may illustrate an age-dependence in clearance which is in part a result of decreased liver mass and presumably reflects decreased total enzyme activity.

Although at present there appear to be no reliable, quantitative indices of hepatic function which directly relate to the efficiency of drug metabolism, there is considerable interest in the use of exogenous marker or model compounds that might do so. Studies by different investigators using the same measurement techniques have resulted in different conclusions. Results of the aminopyrine breath test indicate no alteration in metabolism in one study[174] and a significant age-related decrease in another (r, –0.377).[175] Galactose elimination capacity has been shown to be inversely and significantly related to age in two studies (r, –0.728; –0.466).[175,176] Antipyrine has been used as a model compound for the following reasons: it is totally metabolized by oxidative pathways; it has a low hepatic extraction ratio (and therefore its clearance reflects intrinsic metabolic efficiency); it is not bound to plasma proteins; and it distributes into total body water. It has been a useful model compound for examining the influence of many variables on hepatic metabolism (for summary see reference 177). The compound has also been used rather extensively in examining the relationship between hepatic metabolism and age. Most studies indicate reduced hepatic clearance and increased half-life with age. The study of Vestal et al.[178] is particularly noteworthy, as it used a large subject population to examine the influence of smoking and caffeine ingestion, both of which alter antipyrine clearance. Antipyrine clearance was reduced with age in the three age groups examined. While cigarette smoking increased metabolic clearance in the two younger age groups, it had little influence on the oldest group. Smoking, therefore, is one factor that needs to be controlled in age-related studies of drug metabolism. This raises another interesting point for which there is no clear answer: are the elderly more or less susceptible to enzyme induction and inhibition than younger adults? The above results, along with those of Wood et al.,[167] who examined the influence of smoking on antipyrine clearance, and the findings of Salem et al.,[179] who examined the influence of another inducing agent on antipyrine and quinine metabolism, suggest that the elderly are less prone to enzyme induction than are younger adults. It appears, however, that complicating factors may make that conclusion rather equivocal. Swift et al.[171] found a longer antipyrine half-life in healthy elderly subjects than in young adults, but no prolongation of half-life in ill hospitalized elderly subjects receiving other drugs. A further complication is the finding that vitamin supplementation in nutritionally deficient elderly subjects decreased antipyrine half-life.[180] The variability of antipyrine clearance is particularly impressive, as seen in Figure 9-6.[178]

Studies that have examined the influence of age on the disposition of the benzodiazepine derivatives are particularly interesting, as these derivatives are similar chemically and they undergo either phase I or phase II metabolism. Disparities exist in the results for a given drug (e.g., diazepam). Most often there are no obvious reasons for such disparities, but given all the variables that may influence metabolism, perhaps this is not surprising. In several instances, gender influences the age relationship (e.g., desalkylflurazepam).[86] This is a relatively recent observation which suggests that age-related studies, and indeed perhaps most disposition studies, may need to be stratified according to gender. For those compounds undergoing phase I metabolism, clearance either decreases or remains unchanged with age, while half-life either increases or remains unchanged with age. It is clearance rather than half-life which serves as the better indicator of metabolic activity because the half-life is influenced by changes in plasma protein binding and volume of distribution, and because the volume of several of these compounds changes with age (see Table 9-5). Changes in plasma protein binding can also influence the value of clearance, but relatively few studies have determined unbound clearance. One study of diazepam[88] has shown a significant reduction in unbound clearance in the elderly, which suggests a decrease in

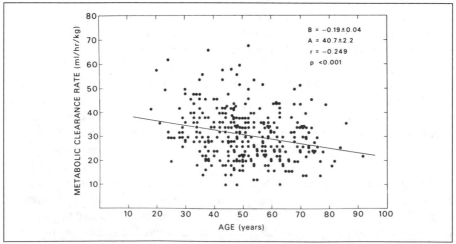

Figure 9-6. *Antipyrine clearance as a function of age in 307 healthy male subjects (18–92 years). Equation of the line is, Y = −0.19(x) + 40.7, r = −0.249 (p <0.001). Reprinted with permission from reference 178.*

intrinsic metabolic activity. An important clinical finding in the elderly is the association of the incidence of hip fractures resulting from falls and the use of benzodiazepines with a long elimination half-life.[181]

Those benzodiazepines that are metabolized via phase II (i.e., conjugation) processes generally indicate no change in clearance or half-life with age, although lorazepam may be an exception. Many investigators have the impression that there is little if any difference with age in the elimination of those compounds that are metabolized by conjugation. At present there is not enough evidence to permit a general conclusion. Benzodiazepine disposition changes and use in the elderly have been reviewed recently.[182]

Another intriguing yet complicating issue in drug metabolism is evidenced by interest in the disposition and response to enantiomeric forms of a drug. A recent study reported age-related differences in the metabolism of hexobarbital enantiomers. Elderly males had a significantly lower oral clearance for the l-form compared to younger adults, yet there were no differences in the oral clearance of d-hexobarbital.[183] Undoubtedly, other examples of differences in stereoselective metabolism with age will be uncovered. This finding also suggests the need to re-examine age-related metabolic and pharmacodynamic differences reported for racemic mixtures.

A review of studies that have examined the influence of age on the disposition of drugs eliminated primarily by metabolism indicates the same patterns noted in the previous discussion of the benzodiazepines but encompassing a wider variety of metabolic processes.[184] There are discrepancies in the results for a given drug; there are gender differences and differences in unbound clearance with age. Clearance either decreases or remains unchanged (with the exception of one study of phenytoin), and half-life either increases or remains unchanged. Once again, but not surprisingly, other than the above observations there are no general conclusions that can be drawn. Thus, dosage needs to be carefully adjusted on an individual basis in elderly patients, especially for those agents with a narrow therapeutic range.

Excretion

The two major routes of drug elimination are renal excretion and hepatic metabolism. The changes in renal function with age are by far better understood than are the changes in liver metabolism. The primary reason is that there are standard, easily employed methods for quantitating renal function, and these measures correlate with drug excretion. In contrast, there is no one test that will adequately evaluate liver function and correlate with some measure of drug metabolism. There is, in addition, a host of variables that are known to influence hepatic drug metabolism. The influence of age on renal function has been thoroughly evaluated and, for those drugs primarily excreted unchanged, there are simple, rigorous pharmacokinetic approaches available for the design of appropriate dosing regimens in the elderly.[185] Renal function declines as a natural consequence of aging, and, as a result, the elderly often require a decrease in dose and sometimes require a prolongation in dosing interval.

Creatinine clearance is perhaps the most frequently used estimate of glomerular filtration rate because creatinine is an endogenous compound that is readily measured in biological fluids and the test does not require administration of an exogenous compound (e.g., inulin). Figure 9-7 illustrates the relationship between creatinine clearance and age in 548 male subjects.[186] There is a dramatic decline with age, and, as shown in the bottom line of Figure 9-7 (which expresses the values as a percentage of the youngest age group), creatinine clearance decreases by 30% to 40% at average age 80 years. There is, however, considerable variation in clearance within any age group. The results of these cross-sectional data agree well with those found in a longitudinal study.[186]

In the majority of clinical settings, serum creatinine concentrations are deter-mined as part of a battery of blood chemistry measurements, and they are considered to reflect renal function. Creatinine clearance is less frequently meas-ured, as this involves the additional collection of urine and determination of a daily creatinine excretion. Unfortunately, serum creatinine concentrations do not corre-late with renal function across all age groups. This point is illustrated in Figure 9-8, which shows the relationship between serum creatinine concentration and daily creatinine excretion as a function of age.[186] Serum creatinine concentrations remain essentially constant, while daily creatinine excretion declines substantially. Creatinine clearance is calculated as the ratio of daily creatinine excretion to serum creatinine concentration, and, since the former decreases, creatinine clearance de-creases (see Figure 9-7). The way that serum creatinine concentration remains constant with age is analogous to the formula for steady-state drug concentrations resulting from a constant rate infusion. In the latter situation the steady-state drug concentration (C_{ss}) is equal to infusion rate (R_o) divided by systemic clearance (CL):

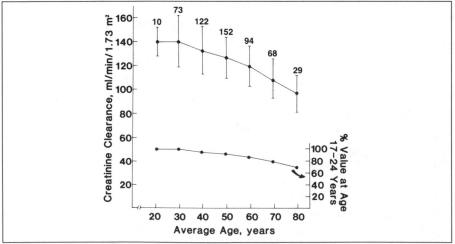

Figure 9-7. *Creatinine clearance in males as a function of average age. The cross hatched vertical bars represent the standard deviation, and the numbers above each bar are the number of subjects in each age group. The lower curve refers to the y-axis on the right, which represents the creatinine clearance as a percentage of the value of the youngest age group (17–24 years). Based upon the data in reference 186.*

$$C_{ss} = \frac{R_0}{CL}$$

(Eq. 9-2)

By analogy, steady-state serum creatinine concentration (C_{cr}) will be a function of endogenous creatinine production rate and creatinine clearance (CL_{cr}):

$$C_{cr} = \frac{\text{production rate}}{CL_{cr}}$$

(Eq. 9-3)

In order for C_{cr} to remain constant in the presence of decreasing CL_{cr}, the production rate must decrease with age at a rate comparable to the decrease in CL_{cr}. The decline in creatinine production rate with age is consistent with the fact that creatinine is an end-product of muscle metabolism and muscle mass decreases with age. Furthermore, muscle mass is also a function of body build and gender. Table 9-6 illustrates the relationship among C_{cr}, CL_{cr}, elimination half-life, and age for several drugs that are primarily excreted unchanged. It is apparent from these data that the increase in half-life seen with age is not related to C_{cr} but is inversely related to CL_{cr}. Design of a dosing regimen for a patient with renal insufficiency is usually based upon the relationship between CL_{cr} and drug elimination (most often the elimination rate constant or clearance of the drug).

The previous discussion leads to a potential dilemma: most often one has an estimate of C_{cr}, but that value is not a useful index of renal function. What is needed is a reliable relationship between C_{cr} and CL_{cr}, so that the former value may be converted into a reasonable estimate of the latter. In fact, several such relationships have been developed which take into consideration C_{cr}, age, body build (in the form of ideal body weight), and gender. One such relationship for males is:[190]

Table 9-6. *Elimination Half-Life of Kanamycin and Penicillin as a Function of Age, Serum Creatinine Concentration, and Creatinine Clearance*

Drug	Age range (years)	(n)[a]	Serum creatinine concentration (mg/dL)	Creatinine clearance (mL/min)	$t\frac{1}{2}$ (min)	References
Kanamycin	20–50	(13)	1.0		107	187
	51–70	(21)	1.1		149	
	>70	(33)	1.0		330	
	20–50	(13)	0.97	94	107	188
	50–70	(21)	0.95	75	149	
	>70	(27)	0.98	43	282	
Penicillin	<30	(7)[b]	1.03	112	21	189
	>65	(8)[b]	0.99	61	39	
	<50	(9)[c]	0.89	99	24	189
	>70	(18)[c]	1.07	44	56	

[a] Number of subjects.
[b] Male subjects. Average ages for young and elderly groups, 24 and 76 years, respectively.
[c] Female subjects. Average ages for young and elderly groups, 31 and 82 years, respectively.

$$CL_{cr} \text{ (mL/min)} = \frac{\text{(ideal body weight in kg)(140 − age in years)}}{72 \cdot C_{cr} \text{ (mg \%)}}$$

(Eq. 9-4)

For females, the above relationship is multiplied by 0.86 to reflect the smaller muscle mass.

The kidney undergoes a variety of anatomical and physiological changes with age. Kidney mass decreases by about 10% to 20% from age 40 to 80 years, along with a reduction in the size and number of nephrons.[191] Glomerular surface area and the length and volume of the proximal tubules decrease with age; however, the ratio of glomerular surface area to tubular volume remains relatively constant.[192] These changes are reflected in virtually all measures of renal function which uniformly decline with age. Figure 9-9 illustrates how various parameters of kidney function change with age.[193] Inulin clearance (see Figure 9-9, Panel A) decreases with age, as noted for creatinine clearance (see Figure 9-7) because both are measures of glomerular filtration rate. The decline in inulin clearance seen here (about 50% over the age ranges shown) is somewhat greater than that seen for creatinine clearance. The decrease in glomerular filtration rate may occur for several reasons, including decreased cortical perfusion rate, atrophy affecting the renal cortex more than the medulla, and vascular lesions of small arteries resulting in a decrease in filtration pressure in a large number of glomeruli.[191]

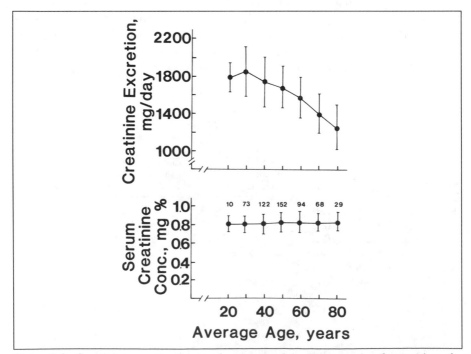

Figure 9-8. *Creatinine excretion (top) and serum creatinine concentration (bottom) in males as a function of average age. The vertical cross hatched bars represent the standard deviation, and the numbers above the bars are the number of subjects in each age group. Based upon the data in reference 205.*

Tubular function also declines with age, as measured by the excretory capacity or transport maximum (Tm) of iodopyracet (Diodrast) (see Figure 9-9, Panel B). Also affected are reabsorption mechanisms, as reflected in the decline of renal tubular glucose reabsorption. The latter decreases from a value of about 360 mg/min/1.73 m² at age 30 years to about 220 mg/min/1.73 m² at age 90 years.[194]

Renal blood flow (see Figure 9-9, Panel C) and plasma flow (see Figure 9-9, Panel D) illustrate a dramatic decrease with age. The decrease in renal blood flow appears to exceed the decrease in cardiac output and the decrease in blood flow to other tissues, as discussed in a previous section. After about the fourth decade of life, renal blood flow declines at a rate of approximately 1.5% to 1.9% per year. Thus, a 65-year-old subject will have a renal blood flow approximately 40% to 50% of that in a young adult. In a study by Hollenberg et al.,[191] in 207 normal subjects aged 17 to 76 years, renal blood flow per mass of tissue decreased with age. This suggested a limited blood perfusion rather than an effect of tissue atrophy.

A particularly interesting aspect of the data shown in Figure 9-9, which illustrates a variety of parameters of renal function, is that when all of these various measures are expressed as a percentage of the value of the youngest age group (see Figure 9-9, Panel E), the lines are virtually superimposed. This has led to a concept referred to as the "intact nephron," which in essence states that all measures of the function of the kidney decline uniformly.

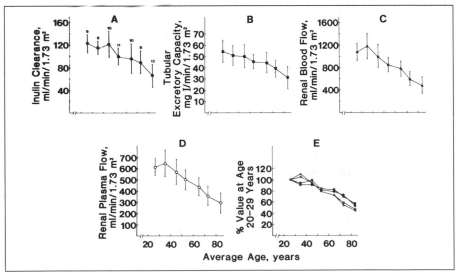

Figure 9-9. *Various parameters of renal function vs. average age in males. A) Inulin clearance (●). B) Tubular excretory capacity expressed as the transport maximum (Tm) of iodopyracet (Diodrast) (■). C) Renal blood flow (▲). D) Renal plasma flow as measured by Diodrast clearance (○). E) The values in A through D expressed as a percentage of the value of the youngest age group (20–29 years). The cross hatched vertical bars represent the standard deviation, and the numbers above the bars in A are the number of subjects in each age group. Based upon the data in reference 193.*

The previous discussion indicates that all aspects of renal function decline dramatically as a natural consequence of aging. The presence of renal disease will further compromise function and alter drug excretion. The nature of renal disease in the elderly has been reviewed elsewhere.[195] Its implications for drug therapy are quite apparent. There is a need to decrease the dose in the elderly of those drugs which are primarily excreted unchanged, especially those compounds that have a narrow therapeutic range. In the absence of a change in distribution volume, the reduction in renal drug clearance implies a prolongation in elimination half-life. The latter may require an increase in the dosing interval in conjunction with a lowered dose, depending on the method employed for adjusting the dosing regimen.[204] An additional concern of therapy is the presence of drug metabolites which are excreted by the kidney. Such compounds will accumulate in the presence of reduced renal function (and therefore in the aged). One example is the active metabolite of procainamide, N-acetylprocainamide, which is primarily excreted by the kidney and which may require careful monitoring in the aged.[196]

PROSPECTUS

The preceding discussion attempted to review our current understanding of the influence of aging on the processes of drug disposition. While our understanding of the aging process *per se* and its influence on disposition and drug therapy are far from complete, substantial progress has been made in recent years. Unquestionably our knowledge in the area of gerontology will improve during the next decade as more investigators pursue research in various basic and clinical disciplines. At the present time there is little question that age needs to be considered among the several factors that are known to alter drug disposition.

The reader will undoubtedly recognize the absence of any discussion of one of the most important considerations in therapy, that of therapeutic response. This writer believes that this area of research represents the most important challenge for the immediate future. It has received far too little attention thus far, and it has not been addressed in this chapter because of the dearth of information. For some drugs, there may well be a need to redefine the therapeutic plasma concentration range in the elderly according to response. This statement by Crooks[197] is a particularly salient and timely observation on this subject:

> Our knowledge of pharmacodynamics in the elderly is as yet grossly deficient. While there are many constraints on research into drug effects, it is difficult to escape the conclusion that the relative plethora of pharmacokinetic studies reflects the ease with which they can be done, whereas the paucity of pharmacodynamic studies is due to the methodological and logistic problems involved.

REFERENCES

1. Rowe JW, Besdine RW. Approach to the elderly patient: physiologic and clinical considerations. In: Vestal RE, ed. Drug Treatment in the Elderly. Sydney: ADIS; 1984:3–11.
2. Kurfees JF, Dotson RL. Drug interactions in the elderly. J Family Practice 1987;25:477–88.

3. Rowe JW. Clinical research on aging: Strategies and directions. N Engl J Med. 1977; 297:1332–336.
4. Vestal RE, ed. Drug Treatment in the Elderly. Sydney: ADIS; 1984.
5. Cutler NR, Narang PK, eds. Drug Studies in the Elderly—Methodological Concerns. New York: Plenum; 1986.
6. Delafuente JC, Stewart RB, eds. Therapeutics in the Elderly. Baltimore: Williams & Wilkins; 1988.
7. Schneider EL, Rowe JW, eds. Handbook of the Biology of Aging, 3rd ed. New York: Academic Press; 1990.
8. Schmucker DL. Aging and drug disposition: an update. Pharmacol Rev. 1985;37:133–48.
9. Everitt DE, Avorn J. Drug prescribing for the elderly. Arch Int Med. 1986;146:2393–396.
10. Montamat SC et al. Management of drug therapy in the elderly. N Engl J Med. 1989;321:303–309.
11. Kottke MK et al. Drug delivery systems for the elderly. Drug Devel Ind Pharm. 1989;15:1635–692.
12. Mayersohn M. Physiological factors that modify systemic drug availability and pharmacologic response in clinical practice. In: Blanchard J et al., eds. Principles and Perspectives in Drug Bioavailability. New York: S Karger; 1979:211–73.
13. Sklar M. Gastrointestinal diseases in the aged. In: Reichel W, ed. Clinical Aspects of Aging. Baltimore: Williams & Wilkins; 1978:173–81.
14. Vanzant FR et al. The normal range of gastric acidity from youth to old age. Arch Intern Med. 1932;49:345–59.
15. Baron JH. Studies of basal and peak acid output with an augmented histamine test. Gut. 1963;4:136–44.
16. Barr WH et al. Decrease of tetracycline absorption in man by sodium bicarbonate. Clin Pharmacol Ther. 1971;12:779–84.
17. Kramer PA et al. Tetracycline absorption in elderly patients with achlorhydria. Clin Pharmacol Ther. 1978;23:467–72.
18. Ochs HR et al. Absorption of oral tetracycline in patients with Billroth-II gastrectomy. J Pharmacokinet Biopharm. 1978;6:295–303.
19. O'Reilly RA et al. Physicochemical and physiologic factors affecting the absorption of warfarin in man. J Pharm Sci. 1966;55:435–37.
20. Tuttle CB et al. Biological availability and urinary excretion kinetics of oral tolbutamide formulations in man. Canad J Pharm Sci. 1973;8:31–6.
21. Bates TR et al. pH-dependent dissolution rate of nitrofurantoin from commercial suspension, tablets and capsules. J Pharm Sci. 1974;63:643–45.
22. Ochs HR et al. Effect of age and Billroth gastrectomy on absorption of desmethyldiazepam from clorazepate. Clin Pharmacol Ther. 1979;26:449–56.
23. Abruzzo CW et al. Changes in the oral absorption characteristics in man of dipotassium clorazepate at normal and elevated gastric pH. J Pharmacokinet Biopharm. 1977;5:377–90.
24. Chun AHC et al. Effect of antacids on absorption of clorazepate. Clin Pharmacol Ther. 1977;22:329–35.
25. Shader RI et al. Impaired absorption of desmethyldiazepam from clorazepate by magnesium aluminum hydroxide. Clin Pharmacol Ther. 1978;24:308–15.
26. Bates TR et al. Rate of dissolution of griseofulvin and hexoestrol in bile salt solution. Nature. 1966;210:1331–333.
27. Glazko AJ et al. Physical factors affecting the rate of absorption of chloramphenicol esters. Antibiotics Chemother. 1958;8:516–27.
28. Alibrandi A et al. Factors influencing the biological activity of orally administered steroid compounds: effect of the medium and esterification. Endocrinology. 1960;66:13–8.
29. Evans MA et al. Gastric emptying rate in the elderly: implications for drug therapy. J Am Geriatr Soc. 1981;29:201–205.
30. Moore JG et al. Effect of age on gastric emptying of liquid-solid meals in man. Digestive Dis Sci. 1983;28:340–44.
31. Horowitz M et al. Changes in gastric emptying with age. Clin Sci. 1984;67:213–18.
32. Kupfer RM et al. Gastric emptying and small-bowel transit rate in the elderly. J Amer Geriatr Soc. 1985;33:340–43.

33. Mojaverian P et al. Effects of gender, posture, and age on gastric residence time of an indigestible solid: pharmaceutical considerations. Pharmaceut Res. 1988;5:639–44.

34. Wade DN et al. Active transport of L-DOPA in the intestine. Nature. 1973;242:463–65.

35. Gillespie NG et al. Diets affecting treatment of parkinsonism with levodopa. J Am Diet Assoc. 1973;62:525–28.

36. Van Woert MH. Phenylalanine and tyrosine metabolism in Parkinson's disease treated with levodopa. Clin Pharmacol Ther. 1971;12:368–75.

37. Rivera-Calimlim L et al. Absorption and metabolism of l-dopa by the human stomach. Eur J Clin Invest. 1971;1:313–320.

38. Bianchine JR et al. Metabolism and absorption of L-3, 4-dihydroxphenylalanine in patients with parkinson's disease. Ann NY Acad Sci. 1971;179:126–40.

39. Broe GA, Caird FI. Levodopa for parkinsonism in elderly and demented patients. Med J Aust. 1973; 1:630–35.

40. Grad B et al. Effects of levodopa therapy in patients with parkinson's disease: statistical evidence for reduced tolerance to levodopa in the elderly. J Am Geriatr Soc. 1974;22:489–94.

41. Evans MA et al. Systemic availability of orally administered l-dopa in the elderly parkinsonian patient. Eur J Clin Pharmacol. 1980;17:215–21.

42. Evans JA et al. Gastric emptying rate and the systemic availability of levodopa in the elderly parkinsonian patient. Neurology. 1981;31:1288–294.

43. Robertson DRC et al. The effect of age on the pharmacokinetics of levodopa administered alone and in the presence of carbidopa. Brit J Clin Pharmacol. 1989;28:61–9.

44. Levy G, Jusko WJ. Factors affecting the absorption of riboflavin in man. J Pharm Sci. 1966;55:285–89.

45. Levy G et al. Effect of an anticholinergic agent on riboflavin absorption in man. J Pharm Sci. 1972;61:798–99.

46. Yung S et al. Ascorbic acid absorption in man: influence of divided dose and food. Life Sci. 1981;28:2505–511.

47. Woods MN, Ingelfinger JA. Lack of effect of bran on digoxin absorption. Clin Pharmacol Ther. 1979;26:21–3.

48. Manninen V et al. Altered absorption of digoxin in patients given proprantheline and metoclopramide. Lancet. 1973;1:398–99.

49. Manninen V et al. Effect of proprantheline and metoclopramide on absorption of digoxin. Lancet. 1973;1:1118–119.

50. Medin S, Nyberg L. Effect of proprantheline and metoclopramide on absorption of digoxin. Lancet. 1973;1:1393.

51. Guyton AC. Textbook of Medical Physiology, 5th ed. Philadelphia: WB Saunders; 1976:375–78.

52. Winne D. Formal kinetics of water and solute absorption with regard to intestinal blood flow. J Theoret Biol. 1970;27:1–18.

53. Winne D, Remischovsky J. Intestinal blood flow and absorption of non-dissociable substances. J Pharm Pharmacol. 1970;22:640–41.

54. Crouthamel W et al. Effects of mesenteric blood flow on intestinal drug absorption. J Pharm Sci. 1970;59:878–79.

55. Crouthamel WG et al. Drug absorption. VII. Influence of mesenteric blood flow on intestinal drug absorption in dogs. J Pharm Sci. 1975;64:664–71.

56. Sherlock S et al. Splanchnic blood flow in man by the bromsulfalein method: the relation of peripheral plasma by bromsulfalein level to the calculated flow. J Lab Clin Med. 1950; 35:923–32.

57. Benet LZ et al. Gastrointestinal absorption of drugs in patients with cardiac failure. In: Benet LZ, ed. The Effect of Disease States on Drug Pharmacokinetics. Washington, DC: American Pharmaceutical Association; 1976:33–50.

58. Greither A et al. Erratic and incomplete absorption of furosemide in congestive heart failure. Am J Cardiol. 1976;37:139.

59. Nation RL et al. The pharmacokinetics of chlormethiazole following intravenous administration in the aged. Eur J Clin Pharmacol. 1976;10:407–15.

60. Nation RL et al. Plasma levels of chlormethiazole and two metabolites after oral administration to young and aged human subjects. Eur J Clin Pharmacol. 1977;12:137–45.
61. Castleden CM, George CF. The effect of aging on the hepatic clearance of propranolol. Br J Clin Pharmacol. 1979;7:49–54.
62. Cusack B et al. Protein binding and disposition of lignocaine in the elderly. Eur J Clin Pharmacol. 1985;29:323–29.
63. Jaillon P et al. Pharmacokinetics of nalbuphine in infants, young healthy volunteers, and elderly patients. Clin Pharmacol Ther 1989;46:226–33.
64. Warren PM et al. Age changes in small-intestinal mucosa. Lancet. 1978;2:849–50.
65. Mayersohn M. The "xylose test" to assess gastrointestinal absorption in the elderly: a pharmacokinetic evaluation of the literature. J Gerontol. 1982;37:300–305.
66. Johnson SL et al. Gastrointestinal absorption as a function of age: xylose absorption in healthy adult subjects. Clin Pharmacol Ther. 1985;38:331–35.
67. Johnson SL et al. Xylose disposition in humans as a function of age. Clin Pharmacol Ther. 1986;39:687–702.
68. Mayersohn M. Special pharmacokinetic considerations in the elderly. In: Evans WE et al, eds. Applied Pharmacokinetics: Principles of Therapeutic Drug Monitoring. 2nd ed. Vancouver, WA: Applied Therapeutics, Inc.; 1986:244–46.
69. Adrian TE, Bloom SR. Gut and pancreatic hormones in the elderly. In: Hodkinson M, ed. Clinical Biochemistry of the Elderly. New York: Churchill Livingstone; 1984:237–45.
70. Shamburek RD, Farrar JT. Disorders of the digestive system in the elderly. New Engl J Med. 1990;322:438–43.
71. Divoll M et al. Absolute bioavailability of oral and intramuscular diazepam: effects of age and sex. Anesth Analg. 1983;62:1–8.
72. Greenblatt DJ et al. Lorazepam kinetics in the elderly. Clin Pharmacol Ther. 1979;26:103–13.
73. Herman RJ et al. Effects of age on meperidine disposition. Clin Pharmacol Ther. 1985;37:19–24.
74. Roskos KV et al. Effects of aging on percutaneous absorption in man. J Pharmacokin Biopharm. 1989;17:617–30.
75. Cammarata PJ et al. Serum anti-γglobulin and anti-nuclear factors in the aged. JAMA. 1967;199:445–58.
76. Greenblatt DJ. Reduced serum albumin concentration in the elderly: a report from the Boston Collaborative Drug Surveillance Program. J Am Geriatr Soc. 1979;27:20–2.
77. Hodkinson M. Test disturbances due to illness or medication. In: Hodkinson M, ed. Clinical Biochemistry of the Elderly. New York: Churchill Livingstone; 1984:24–34.
78. Woodford-Williams E et al. Serum protein patterns in 'normal' and pathological ageing. Gerontologia. 1964/65;10:86–99.
79. Wallace S et al. Factors affecting drug binding in plasma of elderly patients. Br J Clin Pharmacol. 1976;3:327–30.
80. Chapron DJ et al. Influence of advanced age on the disposition of acetazolamide. Br J Clin Pharmacol. 1985;19:363–71.
81. Schulz P et al. Amitriptyline disposition in young and elderly normal men. Clin Pharmacol Ther. 1983;33:360–66.
82. Blanchard J. Protein binding of caffeine in young and elderly males. J Pharm Sci. 1982;71:1415–418.
83. Hayes MJ et al. Changes in the plasma clearance and protein binding of carbenoxolone with age and their possible relationship with adverse effects. Gut. 1977;18:1054–1058.
84. Luderer JR et al. Age and ceftriaxone kinetics. Clin Pharmacol Ther. 1984;35:19–25.
85. Roberts RK et al. Effect of age and parenchymal liver disease on the disposition and elimination of chlordiazepoxide (librium). Gastroenterology. 1978;75:479–85.
86. Greenblatt DJ et al. Kinetics and clinical effects of flurazepam in young and elderly non-insomniacs. Clin Pharmacol Ther. 1981;30:475–86.
87. Allen MD et al. Desmethyldiazepam kinetics in the elderly after oral prazepam. Clin Pharmacol Ther. 1980;28:196–202.
88. Greenblatt DJ et al. Diazepam disposition determinants. Clin Pharmacol Ther. 1980;27:301–12.

89. Klotz U et al. The effects of age and liver disease on the disposition and elimination of diazepam in adult man. J Clin Invest. 1975;55:347–59.
90. Davis D et al. Age related changes in the plasma protein binding of lidocaine and diazepam. Clin Res. 1980;28:234A.
91. Bonde J et al. The influence of age and smoking on the elimination of disopyramide. Br J Clin Pharmacol. 1985;20:453–58.
92. Scatina J et al. Etodolac kinetics in the elderly. Clin Pharmacol Ther. 1986;39:550–53.
93. Rowell FJ et al. The effect of age and thioridazine on the *in vitro* binding of fluphenazine to normal human serum. Br J Clin Pharmacol. 1980;9:432–34.
94. Pacifici GM et al. Plasma protein binding of furosemide in the elderly. Eur J Clin Pharmacol. 1987;32:199–202.
95. Greenblatt DJ et al. Absorption and disposition of ibuprofen in the elderly. Arthritis Rheum. 1984;27:1066–1069.
96. Cusack B et al. Protein binding and disposition of lignocaine in the elderly. Eur J Clin Pharmacol. 1985;29:323–29.
97. Divoll M, Greenblatt DJ. Effect of age and sex on lorazepam protein binding. J Pharmacol. 1982;34:122–23.
98. Braithwaite RA et al. Plasma protein binding of maprotiline in geriatric patients—influence of α_1-acid glycoprotein. Br J Clin Pharmacol. 1978;6:448–49P.
99. Mather LE et al. Meperidine kinetics in man: intravenous injection in surgical patients and volunteers. Clin Pharmacol Ther. 1975;17:21–30.
100. Holmberg L et al. Pethidine binding to blood cells and plasma proteins in old and young subjects. Eur J Clin Pharmacol. 1982;23:457–61.
101. Greenblatt DJ et al. Midazolam kinetics in old age and obesity. Clin Pharmacol Ther. 1984;35:244.
102. Upton RA et al. Naproxen pharmacokinetics in the elderly. Br J Clin Pharmacol. 1984;18:207–14.
103. Greenblatt DJ et al. Age, sex, and nitrazepam kinetics: relation to antipyrine disposition. Clin Pharmacol Ther. 1985;38:697–703.
104. Greenblatt DJ et al. Oxaprozin pharmacokinetics in the elderly. Br J Clin Pharmacol. 1985;19:373–78.
105. Murray TG et al. Renal disease, age, and oxazepam kinetics. Clin Pharmacol Ther. 1981;30:805–809.
106. Greenblatt DJ et al. Oxazepam kinetics: effects of age and sex. J Pharmacol Exp Ther. 1980;215:86–91.
107. Bender AD et al. Plasma protein binding of drugs as a function of age in adult human subjects. J Pharm Sci. 1975;64:1711–713.
108. Hayes MJ et al. Changes in drug metabolism with increasing age: 2. Phenytoin clearance and protein binding. Br J Clin Pharmacol. 1975;2:73–9.
109. Hooper WD et al. Plasma protein binding of diphenylhydantoin: Effects of sex hormones, renal and hepatic disease. Clin Pharmacol Ther. 1974;15:276–82.
110. Patterson M et al. Plasma protein binding of phenytoin in the aged: *In vivo* studies. Br J Clin Pharmacol. 1982;13:423–25.
111. Gal P et al. Phenytoin and carbamazepine serum protein binding in a geriatric patient population. Clin Pharmacokinet. 1984;9(Suppl.1):92–93.
112. Richardson CJ et al. Effects of age and sex on piroxicam disposition. Clin Pharmacol Ther. 1985;37:13–8.
113. Colagelo P et al. Stereoselective binding of propranolol in the elderly. Clin Pharmacol Ther. 1989;27:519–22.
114. Lalonde RL et al. Effects of age on the protein binding and disposition of propranolol stereoisomers. Clin Pharmacol Ther. 1990;47:447–55.
115. Ochs HR et al. Reduced quinidine clearance in elderly persons. Am J Cardiol. 1978;42:481–85.
116. Divoll M et al. Effect of age and gender on disposition of temazepam. J Pharm Sci. 1981;70:1104–107.
117. Miller AK et al. Tolbutamide binding to plasma proteins of young and old human subjects. J Pharm Sci. 1978;67:1192–193.

118. Adir J et al. Effects of total plasma concentration and age on tolbutamide plasma protein binding. Clin Pharmacol Ther. 1982;31:488–93.

119. Greenblatt DJ et al. Reduced clearance in triazolam in old age: relation to antipyrine oxidizing capacity. Br J Clin Pharmacol. 1983;15:303–309.

120. Cutler NR et al. Vancomycin disposition: the importance of age. Clin Pharmacol Ther. 1984;36:803–10.

121. Abernethy DR et al. Verapamil pharmacodynamics and disposition in young and elderly hypertensive patients. Ann Int Med. 1986;105:329–36.

122. Paxton JW, Briant RH. α_1-acid glycoprotein concentrations and propranolol binding in elderly patients with acute illness. Br J Clin Pharmacol. 1984;18:806–10.

123. Veering BT et al. The effect of age on serum concentrations of albumin and alpha-acid glycoprotein. Br J Clin Pharmacol. 1990;29:201–206.

124. Mayersohn M. Special pharmacokinetic considerations in the elderly. In: Evans WE et al, eds. Applied Pharmacokinetics: Principles of Therapeutic Drug Monitoring. 2nd ed. Vancouver, WA: Applied Therapeutics, Inc.; 1986:253–54.

125. Jusko WJ, Weintraub M. Myocardial distribution of digoxin and renal function. Clin Pharmacol Ther. 1974;16:449–54.

126. Shock NW et al. Age differences in the water content of the body as related to basal oxygen consumption in males. J Gerontol. 1963;18:1–8.

127. Greenblatt DJ et al. Antipyrine kinetics in the elderly: prediction of age-related changes in benzodiazepine oxidizing capacity. J Pharmacol Exp Ther. 1982;220:120–26.

128. Forbes GB, Reina JC. Adult lean body mass declines with age: some longitudinal observations. Metabolism. 1970;19:653–63.

129. Vestal RE et al. Aging and ethanol metabolism. Clin Pharmacol Ther. 1977;21:343–54.

130. Jung D et al. Thiopental disposition as a function of age in female patients undergoing surgery. Anesthesiology. 1982;56:263–68.

131. Roux A et al. A pharmacokinetic study of acebutolol in aged subjects as compared to young subjects. Gerontology. 1983;29:202–208.

132. Divoll M et al. Acetaminophen kinetics in the elderly. Clin Pharmacol Ther. 1982;31:151–56.

133. Sitar DS et al. Aging and alfentanil disposition in healthy volunteers and surgical patients. Can J Anaesth. 1989;36:149–54.

134. Rho JP et al. Single-dose pharmacokinetics of intravenous ampicillin plus sulbactam in healthy elderly and young adult subjects. J Antimicrob Chemother. 1989;24:573–80.

135. Kitts JB et al. Pharmacokinetics and pharmacodynamics of atracurium in the elderly. Anesthesiol. 1990;72:272–75.

136. Blanchard J, Sawers SJA. Comparative pharmacokinetics of caffeine in young and elderly men. J Pharmacokinet Biopharm. 1983;11:109–26.

137. Moore RG et al. Pharmacokinetics of chlormethiazole in humans. Eur J Clin Pharmacol. 1975;8:353–57.

138. Kanto J et al. Effect of age on the pharmacokinetics of diazepam given in conjunction with spinal anesthesia. Anesthesiology. 1979;51:154–59.

139. Macleod SM et al. Age- and gender-related differences in diazepam pharmacokinetics. J Clin Pharmacol. 1979;19:15–9.

140. Ochs HR et al. Diazepam kinetics in relation to age and sex. Pharmacol Ther. 1981;23:24–30.

141. Cusack B et al. Digoxin in the elderly: pharmacokinetic consequences of old age. Clin Pharmacol Ther. 1979;25:772–76.

142. Schwartz JB, Abernethy DR. Responses to intravenous and oral diltiazem in elderly and younger patients with systemic hypertension. Am J Cardiol. 1987;59:1111–117.

143. Berlinger WG et al. Diphenhydramine: Kinetics and psychomotor effects in elderly women. Clin Pharmacol Ther. 1982;32:387–91.

144. Spector R et al. Diphenhydramine in orientals and causasians. Clin Pharmacol Ther. 1980;28:229–34.

145. Bentley JB et al. Age and fentanyl pharmacokinetics. Anesth Analg. 1982;61:968–71.

146. Kanto J et al. Effect of age on the pharmacokinetics and sedative effect of flunitrazepam. Int J Clin Pharmacol Ther Toxicol. 1981; 19:400–404.

147. Nation RL et al. Lignocaine kinetics in cardiac patients and aged subjects. Br J Clin Pharmacol. 1977;4:439–48.

148. Kraus JW et al. Effects of aging and liver disease on disposition of lorazepam. Clin Pharmacol Ther. 1978;24:411–19.

149. Holmberg L et al. Comparative disposition of pethidine and norpethidine in old and young patients. Eur J Clin Pharmacol. 1982;22:175–79.

150. Regardh CG et al. Pharmacokinetics of metoprolol and its metabolite OH-metoprolol in healthy, non-smoking, elderly individuals. Eur J Clin Pharmacol. 1983;24:221–26.

151. Avram MJ et al. Midazolam kinetics in women of two age groups. Clin Pharmacol Ther. 1983;34:505–508.

152. Owen JA et al. Age-related morphine kinetics. Clin Pharmacol Ther. 1983;34:364–68.

153. Ritschel WE et al. The effect of age on the pharmacokinetics of pentazocine. Meth Find Exptl Clin Pharmacol. 1986;8:497–503.

154. Vestal RE et al. Effects of age and cigarette smoking on propranolol disposition. Clin Pharmacol Ther. 1979;26:8–15.

155. Kampmann JP et al. Kinetics of propylthiouracil in the elderly. Acta Med Scand. 1979;624(Suppl.):93–8.

156. Au WYW et al. Theophylline kinetics in chronic obstructive airway disease in the elderly. Clin Pharmacol Ther. 1985;37:472–78.

157. Shin S-G et al. Theophylline pharmacokinetics in normal elderly subjects. Clin Pharmacol Ther. 1988;44:522–30.

158. Greenblatt DJ et al. Trazodone kinetics: effect of age, gender, and obesity. Clin Pharmacol Ther. 1987;42:193–200.

159. Avram MJ et al. The relationship of age to the pharmacokinetics of early drug distribution: the concurrent disposition of thiopental and indocyanine green. Anesthesiol. 1990;72:403–11.

160. Stanski DR, Maitre PO. Population pharmacokinetics and pharmacodynamics of thiopental: the effect of age revisited. Anesthesiol. 1990;72:412–22.

161. Thomson PD et al. Lidocaine pharmacokinetics in advanced heart failure, liver disease, and renal failure in humans. Ann Intern Med. 1973;78:499–508.

162. Bender AD. The effect of increasing age on the distribution of peripheral blood flow in man. J Am Geriatr Soc. 1965;13:192–98.

163. Brandfonbrener M et al. Changes in cardiac output with age. Circulation. 1955;12:557–66.

164. Rodeheffer RJ et al. Exercise cardiac output is maintained with advancing age in healthy human subjects: cardiac dilatation and increased stroke volume compensate for a diminished heart rate. Circulation. 1984;69:203–13.

165. Fleg JL. Alterations in cardiovascular structure and function with advancing age. Am J Cardiol. 1986;57:33C–44C.

166. Levy G. Effect of bed rest on distribution and elimination of drugs. J Pharm Sci. 1967; 56:928–29.

167. Wood AJJ et al. Effect of aging and cigarette smoking on antipyrine and indocyanine green elimination. Clin Pharmacol Ther. 1979;26:16–20.

168. Zoli M et al. Portal blood velocity and flow in aging man. Gerontology. 1989;35:61–5.

169. Pirttiaho HI et al. Liver size and indices of drug metabolism in alcoholics. Eur J Clin Pharmacol. 1978;13:61–7.

170. Thompson EN, Williams R. Effect of age on liver function with particular reference to bromsulphalein excretion. Gut. 1965;6:266–69.

171. Swift CG et al. Antipyrine disposition and liver size in the elderly. Eur J Clin Pharmacol. 1978;14:149–52.

172. Bach B et al. Disposition of antipyrine and phenytoin correlated with age and liver volume in man. Clin Pharmacokinet. 1981;6:389–96.

173. Roberts CJC et al. The relationship between liver volume, antipyrine clearance and indocyanine green clearance before and after phenobarbitone administration in man. Br J Clin Pharmacol. 1976;3:907–13.

174. Arora S et al. Effect of age on tests of intestinal and hepatic function in healthy humans. Gastroenterol. 1989;96:1560–565.

175. Schnegg M, Lauterburg BH. Quantitative liver function in the elderly assessed by galactose elimination capacity, aminopyrine demethylation and caffeine clearance. J Hepatology. 1986;3:164–71.

176. Marchesini G et al. Galactose elimination capacity and liver volume in aging man. Hepatology. 1988;8:1079–1083.

177. Mayersohn M. Drug disposition. In: Conrad KA, Bressler R, eds. Drug Therapy for the Elderly. St. Louis: C.V. Mosby; 1982:31–63.

178. Vestal RE et al. Antipyrine metabolism in man: Influence of age, alcohol, caffeine, and smoking. Clin Pharmacol Ther. 1975;18:425–32.

179. Salem SAM et al. Reduced induction of drug metabolism in the elderly. Age Ageing. 1978;7:68–73.

180. Smithard DJ, Langman MJS. The effect of vitamin supplementation upon antipyrine metabolism in the elderly. Br J Clin Pharmacol. 1978;5:181–85.

181. Ray WA et al. Benzodiazepines of long and short elimination half-life and the risk of hip fracture. J Am Med Assn. 1989;262:3303–307.

182. Greenblatt DF et al. Implications of altered drug disposition in the elderly: studies of benzodiazepines. J Clin Pharmacol. 1989;29:866–72.

183. Chandler MHH et al. Age-associated stereoselective alterations in hexobarbital metabolism. Clin Pharmacol Ther. 1988;43:436–41.

184. Mayersohn M. Special pharmacokinetic considerations in the elderly. In: Evans WE et al., eds. Applied Pharmacokinetics: Principles of Therapeutic Dug Monitoring. 2nd ed. Vancouver, WA: Applied Therapetuics, Inc.; 1986:273–77.

185. Gibson TP. Influence of renal disease on pharmacokinetics. In: Evans WE ct al., eds. Applied Pharmacokinetics, 2nd ed. Vancouver: Applied Therapeutics; 1986; 83–115

186. Rowe JW et al. The effect of age on creatinine clearance in men: A cross-sectional and longitudinal study. J Gerontol. 1976;31:155–63.

187. Lumholtz B et al. Dose regimen of kanamycin and gentamycin. Acta Med Scand. 1974; 196:521–24.

188. Kristensen M et al. Drug elimination and renal function. J Clin Pharmacol. 1974;14:307–308.

189. Hansen JM et al. Renal excretion of drugs in the elderly. Lancet. 1970;1:1170.

190. Cockcroft DW, Gault MH. Prediction of creatinine clearance from serum creatinine. Nephron. 1976;15:31–41.

191. Hollenberg NK et al. Senescence and the renal vasculature in normal man. Circul Res. 1974;34:309–16.

192. Darmady EM et al. The parameters of the aging kidney. J Pathol. 1972;109:195–207.

193. Davies DF, Shock NW. Age changes in glomerular filtration rate, effective renal plasma flow, and tubular excretory capacity in adult males. J Clin Invest. 1950;29:496–507.

194. Miller JH et al. Age changes in the maximal rate of tubular reabsorption of glucose. J Gerontol. 1952;7:196–200.

195. Samiy AH. Renal disease in the elderly. Med Clin N Am. 1983;67:463–80.

196. Galeazzi RL et al. N-acetyl-procainamide kinetics in the elderly. Clin Pharmacol Ther. 1981;29:440–46.

197. Crooks J. Aging and drug disposition-pharmacodynamics. J Chronic Dis. 1983;36:85–90.

198. Bryson SM et al. Pharmacokinetics of valproic acid in young and elderly subjects. Br J Clin Pharmacol. 1983;16:104–105.

Chapter 10

Special Pharmacokinetic Considerations in Children

Rebecca L. Milsap, Malcolm R. Hill, and Stanley J. Szefler

It was not long ago that great concern was expressed over the relative deficiency of information regarding drug therapy in children. In fact, the term "therapeutic orphan" was applied to encourage developments in this critical area of medicine.[1] The pharmacokinetic approach to drug therapy was not available to clinicians at the time of tragedies such as the chloramphenicol "gray baby syndrome," sulfisoxazole-bilirubin displacement-induced kernicterus, and the thalidomide-associated congenital anomalies. In retrospect, these unfortunate incidences exemplify the dynamic processes of growth and development and the delicate nature of drug disposition and pharmacodynamics in the pediatric patient. Application of principles of pharmacokinetics has contributed significantly to improvement in the strategy of successful treatment regimens for children.

New medications as well as new approaches to drug therapy are usually initiated in adult patients. However, dosage schedules derived in adult patients cannot be simply scaled down on a weight basis to provide an equivalent response. Children differ from adults and even from other children in regard to drug absorption, distribution, and elimination. Furthermore, advances in the measurement of drug receptors have provided insight into potential age-related differences in receptor binding characteristics.

Recent developments in sensitive and specific methods for analysis of many drugs in body tissues and fluids coupled with the advances in computer technology have facilitated the development of age-related dosage recommendations. These guidelines are increasingly substantiated by clinical studies conducted in the age and disease group for which the therapy is intended.

A significant advance in pediatric drug therapy resulted from the ability to measure serum concentrations for medications with a narrow therapeutic range or low margin of safety. New assay techniques permitted small sample volumes for serial drug analysis. The identification of elimination parameters for theophylline and digoxin provided insight into the age-related differences in drug distribution, metabolism, and renal excretion. This information provided a fundamental cornerstone for the basic principles of drug metabolism and renal function in various age groups. With the significant advance in respiratory care increasing the survival of newborn infants with birth weight as low as 500 gm, individualized dosage regimens could be derived not only for theophylline and digoxin, but also anticonvulsants, aminoglycoside antibiotics, chloramphenicol, and other medications with a low margin of safety.

This discussion will begin with a basic review of available information on age-related changes in drug absorption, distribution, elimination and drug receptor binding characteristics (see Table 10-1) including the influence of pertinent disease states. For consistency throughout this chapter, the age ranges will be defined as follows: premature infant, gestational age less than 36 weeks; full-term infant, gestational age 36 weeks to birth; neonate, first month of postnatal life; infant, one to twelve months of age; child, 1 to 12 years; adolescent, 12 to 18 years; adult, greater than 18 years. Brief summaries of age-specific information on various drug agents commonly used in pediatric patients will be included. A discussion of special considerations in clinical research investigations in pediatric patients will be presented along with a strategy for the application of pharmacokinetic principles to research design and therapeutic drug monitoring.

EFFECT OF GROWTH AND DEVELOPMENT ON DRUG ABSORPTION

Absorption

Absorption from the Gastrointestinal Tract. Absorption of drugs and nutrients is determined by multiple factors including gastric acidity, gastric and intestinal motility, enzymatic activity, permeability and maturation of the mucosal membrane, biliary function, bacterial flora, and dietary components.[2] These factors undergo considerable maturational change during the first few days, months, and years of life and influence both the rate and extent of drug absorption in pediatric patients.[3] In addition, the gastrointestinal tract represents a relatively larger portion of body weight in the neonate than in older children. The complexity of the change and interaction of these conditions hampers the ability to analyze the influence of individual components and makes prediction of bioavailability relative to adult data impossible.

The most significant changes in gastric pH occur during the neonatal period. The very high gastric pH, usually pH 6 to 8 at birth for vaginal deliveries and even more alkaline for caesarean section births, is likely related to the presence of amniotic fluid in the stomach.[4] Acid secretory capacity becomes apparent over the first 24 to 48 hours of life when the total acidity (pH 1 to 3) is equivalent to adult values.[5] Gastric acidity then decreases during the first week and remains at a low level during the first months of life.[6] Frequent feedings with milk or formula may also influence gastric pH during this period and later in childhood. A meal

Table 10-1. *Age-Dependent Physiologic Variables Influencing Drug Disposition as Compared to Adults*

Disposition parameter	Physiologic variable	Age group	Pharmacokinetic result	Example drug	References
Absorption	↑ gastric pH	neonates, infants, young children	↑ bioavailability of basic drugs; ↓ bioavailability of acidic drugs		19, 21, 31, 47
	↓ gastric and intestinal motility	neonates, infants		phenobarbital	2, 22, 31, 47
	↑ gastric and intestinal motility	older infants, children	unpredictable bioavailability	digoxin	2, 31, 47
	↓ bile acids	neonates	↓ bioavailability	vitamin E	28
Distribution	↑ total body water; ↑ extracellular water	neonates, infants	↑ volume of distribution	theophylline, aminoglycosides	47, 65, 135–138 47, 65
	↓ albumin concentration; ↓ protein binding	neonates, infants	↑ volume; ↑ free drug concentration	phenytoin	2, 31, 47, 65
Metabolism	↓ enzyme capacity	neonates, infants	↑ t½ of elimination: ↓ clearance	phenobarbital	2, 31, 47, 65
	↑ enzyme capacity	young children	↑ clearance; ↓ in t½ of elimination	theophylline	135, 142
Excretion	↓ glomerular function	neonates, infants	↑ t½ of elimination	aminoglycosides	2, 31, 47, 65
	↓ tubular function	neonates, infants	↑ t½ of elimination	penicillins; sulfonamides	31, 47, 65

containing milk significantly reduces the extent and rate of oral methotrexate absorption in children.[7] It is not until three to seven years of age that adult levels of gastric acidity are attained.[2]

Gastric emptying in the neonate and infant is considerably prolonged (up to six to eight hours) and approaches adult values at age six to eight months. Increasing feeding caloric density results in inhibition of gastric emptying in premature infants[8] and the type of feeding (breast milk or formula) influences the gastric emptying time in both premature and term infants.[9,10] Similarly, intestinal transit time may be prolonged, and peristalsis is very irregular and unpredictable.[11]

Another complexity of gastrointestinal drug absorption in this age group is the occurrence of diarrheal episodes which significantly decrease intestinal transit time. Prolonged infantile diarrhea may conversely increase the extent of drug absorption, as identified for orally administered gentamicin. The positive correlation for the duration of diarrhea and the maximum plasma gentamicin concentration suggests that the morphological and functional changes in the intestinal mucosa of infants with prolonged diarrhea may facilitate the absorption of some drugs.[12] Other examples showing that intestinal abnormalities influence transit times and thus affect drug absorption are impaired ampicillin absorption associated with gastroenteritis,[13,14] a malabsorption syndrome induced reduction in digoxin and antibiotic absorption,[15,16] and the delay in prednisone absorption associated with inflammatory bowel disease.[17] Infants with congenital heart disease exhibit a reduced capacity for gastric emptying and absorptive capacity.[18]

Consistent with the pH partition hypothesis, weak acids should be more slowly absorbed in pediatric patients than in adults due to decreased gastric acidity and weak bases would be preferentially absorbed due to the combined influence of pH and gastrointestinal motility. These theoretical conclusions have not been sufficiently examined in individual age groups. Increased bioavailabilities of penicillin G, ampicillin, and nafcillin have been observed in neonates relative to older children and adults,[19-21] whereas delayed absorption and/or reduced bioavailability of phenobarbital,[2,22] phenytoin,[23] acetaminophen,[24] and riboflavin[25] have been identified in this age group. An intensive study of enteral absorption and bioavailability in children has demonstrated increasing rates of phenobarbital absorption in relation to age.[26]

Bile salts may also influence absorption for certain medications. Premature infants and neonates have a diminished bile acid pool and biliary function develops during the first months of life.[27] The low serum levels of vitamin E in this age group may be related to the relative deficiency of bile salts and pancreatic enzymes.[28] Other factors that potentially influence drug absorption are enzymatic activity in the GI tract, specifically the increased capacity of β-glucuronidase and UDP-glucuronyl transferase of the neonatal gut.[29] Development of intestinal bacterial flora depends more upon diet than on age *per se*[30] with differences identified for bottle versus breast-fed infants. Although specific information in children is limited, the changing biochemistry of the developing GI tract highlights the potential influence these variables may have in drug absorption.

Although studies are usually directed to define the extent of absorption in both pediatric and adult subjects, only a limited effort has been extended to analyze the rate of absorption in pediatric patients. This is particularly evident in the application of sustained-release preparations in young children. The advantages for pediatric therapy were recognized because elimination in children is rapid and can be balanced by controlled-release delivery, thus diminishing the need for frequent dosage intervals.

Absorption from Extra-Intestinal Sites. Drug absorption from other sites merits a brief consideration, especially the percutaneous and intramuscular routes. Absorption through the skin is inversely related to the thickness of the stratum corneum and directly related to skin hydration.[31] The developmental biology of the skin has been reviewed.[32] Relevant factors such as thickness, vascularization, hydration, and glandular development can influence drug absorption. Systemic adverse reactions resulting from topical skin applications of hexachlorophene emulsions, boric acid powders, salicylic acid ointments, and hydrocortisone creams[31,33,34] in neonates and infants suggest increased skin permeability in this age group. Additionally, given equal applications of topical agents per area of skin, the systemic absorption in neonates and infants becomes greater than that of adults when based on surface area:body weight ratio. Therapeutic serum theophylline concentrations can be obtained in preterm infants following application of theophylline gel to the skin.[35]

Intramuscular absorption in neonates, infants, and young children may be variable and unpredictable due to blood flow and vasomotor instabilities, insufficient muscle tone and contractions, and decreased muscle oxygenation.[31] Reductions in absorption rate of intramuscularly administered digoxin[36] and gentamicin[37] have been reported in neonates.

Distribution

The specific distribution of drug in the body is impossible to determine without direct tissue analysis. Several indirect measurements are available to provide limited insight into drug distribution. The parameter most commonly used is the volume of distribution (V_d). In various forms, this parameter is a mathematical concept which relates the concentration of drug in plasma to the remaining portions of the body; the larger the volume, the greater the tissue concentrations of the drug in the body. However, this does not provide insight into the concentration of drug at the relevant receptor site. For some drugs, such as digoxin, the volume of distribution is exceedingly high and indicates extensive binding to cell membranes. Conversely, the V_d for other drugs such as theophylline and aminoglycoside antibiotics is similar to extracellular water (ECW) and total body water (TBW). Therefore, it appears that the V_d of these drugs may be related to body composition. This is an important concept in developmental pharmacology because age-related changes in the relative sizes of body water and fat compartments may result in quantitative alterations in drug distribution. Neonates have a much higher proportion of body mass in the form of water than older children and adults. Differences also exist between full-term infants (75% TBW) and small premature infants (85% TBW). The relative volume of ECW and the ratio of extracellular to intracellular water (ICW) is also higher in neonates, infants, and children. The reduction in TBW is rapid during the first year of life, and adult values (55% TBW) are gradually attained by 12 years of age (see Figure 10-1).[38,39] The percent of ICW remains stable from the first months of life through adulthood.[2] The V_d for drugs which parallel body water content are higher for infants than adults. For example, the aminoglycoside antibiotics are water soluble and distribute initially (V_c) in a volume approximating extracellular fluid volume (0.2 to 0.3 L/kg in adults as compared to 0.5 to 1.2 L/kg for neonates, infants, and children).

The effect of this increased fraction of TBW and consequent effect on the apparent V_d in infants contributes to the increasing loading dosage requirement on a body weight basis to achieve a desired serum concentration. Since V_d is a determinant of half-life and this relates to the time required to attain a desired steady-state serum concentration, this is an important consideration in designing dosage regimens, specifically the dosage interval.

Along with the age-dependent decrease in TBW content, body fat increases in normal development.[2] Approximately 16% of body weight is fat in a full-term neonate whereas the premature infant is practically devoid of body fat. Although interindividual differences occur in the amount of body fat, fat content tends to increase between five and ten years of age, followed by a decrease in boys to age 17. In girls, there is a rapid increase at puberty and from age 13 years, females have approximately twice the percentage of fat as boys.[40] The apparent volume of

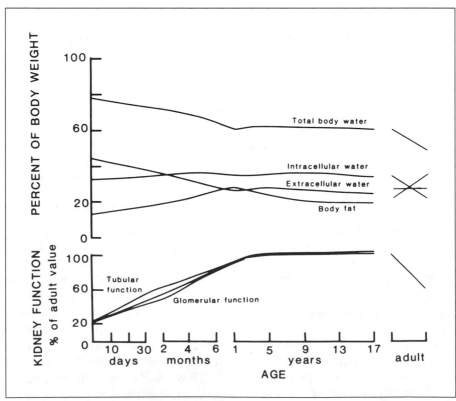

Figure 10-1. Developmental changes in total body water, intra- and extracellular water, body fat, and kidney function in infants and children expressed as percentages of body weight and adult values. Data from references 38, 39, 73, 76.

distribution of diazepam, a lipophilic drug, is smaller in neonates and infants (1.3 to 2.6 L/kg) than adults (1.6 to 3.2 L/kg), which is consistent with the high lipid solubility of the drug and with the relative lack of adipose tissue and high ECW content in young children. Additional age-dependent changes in body composition occur, specifically regarding percent of organ weights in relation to total body weight, that may influence drug distribution.[2]

Membrane permeability is frequently considered to be greater in the more immature infant, and therefore drug entry into some compartments is enhanced. Permeability of the central nervous system is thought to be increased in infancy and brain:plasma ratios of anticonvulsants vary with age.[2,41,42] Similarly, increased permeability of red blood cells has been demonstrated in infants for digoxin (erythrocyte:serum ratio of 3.6 versus 1.3 in adults)[43] and theophylline (erythrocyte:plasma ratio of 1 in neonates versus 0.5 in adults and children).[44] However, the greater toxicities of centrally acting drugs such as analgesics and anticonvulsants observed clinically in infants may not be related exclusively to their increased accumulation in the central nervous system. Increased sensitivity of specific drug receptors in the young may account for observed differences.[2]

A major factor influencing drug distribution is the extent to which the drug is protein bound. Ordinarily, in adult patients it is often assumed that the fraction of drug protein bound is relatively constant. This is inherent in the interpretation of single concentration measurements since routine therapeutic drug monitoring usually provides analysis of total drug, bound and free. For several reasons, this is not a safe assumption in the interpretation of serum drug concentrations in pediatric patients, especially the newborn infant.

Albumin is the principal binding protein, and albumin concentration increases directly in relation to gestational age. Neonatal serum contains approximately 80% as much protein as an adult. The full adult value for plasma protein binding is not reached until approximately the end of the first year of age.[2,45,46] Similarly, the affinity of albumin for many drugs (e.g., phenytoin, phenobarbital, theophylline, salicylate, and propranolol) appears less in the neonate than in the adult.[47] This lower affinity may be related to competition for binding sites by increased concentrations of endogenous substances such as bilirubin and free fatty acids, qualitatively different albumin during the fetal and neonatal period, and acid-base disturbances resulting in lower blood pH.[2,3,47] Major concern developed after the recognition of the role of sulfonamides in displacing bilirubin and, consequently, an increased risk for bilirubin encephalopathy. There are many drugs which may displace bilirubin from albumin binding sites;[3] however, the clinical significance of these *in vitro* interactions is seldom clear. Broderson has presented several guidelines for evaluating the nature of this problem.[48] α_1-acid glycoprotein binding to basic drugs such as propranolol and alprenolol has been demonstrated in neonates.[3,49] Larger free fractions of the drugs as a consequence of decreased α_1-acid glycoprotein levels have been demonstrated in this age group.

Metabolism

The capacity to metabolize drugs varies throughout development. Although drug metabolism occurs in various tissues, the liver is the major site performing the four principal pathways of oxidation, reduction, hydrolysis (all Phase I), and conjugation (Phase II). In general, studies of drug metabolism in the human neonatal period indicate that most of the enzymatic microsomal systems for biotransformation are present at birth, although their activity is reduced quantitatively in relation to adults and their capacity increases with advancing age.[2,41,50-58] Decreased hepatic uptake, low concentration of intracellular carrier proteins, and a decreased production of bile may potentiate the effect of diminished enzyme activity in neonates.[29,31,47] The insufficiency of one elimination pathway may lead to metabolism by alternate pathways, for example, the neonatal methylation of theophylline to caffeine,[59] which eventually becomes insignificant in older children and adults.

Hepatic microsomes capable of hydroxylation and major components of the mixed function oxidase system (cytochrome P450 and NADPH—cytochrome C reductase) are functional in human fetal and neonatal liver.[2,29,54,57,58] However, activity of these enzymes approximates 20% to 70% of adult values and there appears to be a positive relationship in increasing enzyme activity with fetal and postnatal age.[2] Serial antipyrine clearance studies in neonates show prolonged clearances on the first as compared to the fourth day of postnatal life.[60] Reduced hydroxylation rates have been reported for phenytoin, lidocaine, amobarbital, and diazepam in neonates.[2,31,55,56] Also, N-demethylation activity is reduced but present in neonates as indicated by urinary recovery of N-demethylated products for meperidine, theophylline, and diazepam.[29,31,55] In contrast to this general concept of reduced enzyme capacity in the newborn is the observation of full capacity for reduction[29] and increased capacity of the methylation pathway exemplified by the significantly increased proportion of methylated theophylline metabolites in neonatal studies.[59,61]

Clinical insights into developmental aspects of drug metabolism were provided by experience with bilirubin elimination in infants. Developmental aspects of glucuronidation have been reviewed by Dutton.[62] UDPG-glucuronyl transferase activity responsible for the conjugation of various endogenous substances and drugs (e.g., bilirubin, morphine, chloramphenicol) is depressed at birth and reaches adult levels in children by three years of age.[29,31,41] Agents which depend almost entirely upon this pathway for elimination are potential toxins in neonates and infants since alternate pathways of metabolism are not available for detoxification and elimination. Plasma concentration monitoring of chloramphenicol could have detected drug accumulation and saved the victims of the "gray baby syndrome." Sulfate conjugation activity is present at birth, and activity of phenosulfotransferase is more efficient in neonates than in adults.[2,29] The decreased glucuronidation of acetaminophen in neonates is compensated to some extent by their well-developed capacity for sulfate conjugation.[63] Higher rates of sulfation were found in a group of children aged seven to ten years when compared to adults.[64] In children, salicylamide and acetaminophen were excreted predominantly as sulfate conjugates whereas in adults, the major metabolite was the glucuronide conjugate. This suggests that the age-dependent interplay between these conjugation reactions may persist beyond the neonatal period. Age-related changes for drug metabolism are also apparent for other medications such as phenytoin, phenobarbital, and theophylline (see Table 10-2).

Drug metabolism studies have not been performed extensively in older children, perhaps due to the notion that children become more like adults in drug disposition after two to three years.[2] The immediate pre- and postnatal period of drug metabolism has been the subject of most drug metabolism reviews.[52,55–58] Hormonal changes occurring during puberty can affect drug disposition as can changes in tissue mass (e.g., fat and muscle) in this age group. Older children and adolescents also exhibit large interindividual differences in disposition parameters as demonstrated by theophylline, phenytoin, phenobarbital,[2,65] valproic acid,[66] and carbamazepine.[67] The mean half-life of oral quinidine for pediatric patients (ages 2 to 12 years) is shorter than reported adult values and children have significantly higher clearances than adults, perhaps reflective of faster metabolism in this age group.[68]

Another aspect important in the evaluation of drug metabolism is the phenomenon of dose-dependent or enzyme-capacity-limited drug elimination.[69–72] This is important to identify in all age groups because it will affect not only data analysis, but approaches to dosage adjustments as well. A small increment in dose could result in a more than proportionate increase in steady-state serum drug concentration. Therefore, sufficient sampling time must be provided in single-dose studies to evaluate this phenomenon, often a major technical difficulty in drug disposition studies in children. Dose-dependence for theophylline,[72] salicylate,[69] and phenytoin[70,71] has been identified in infants and children.

Renal Excretion

There are significant age-related changes in renal excretion of drugs and their metabolites. Renal function is significantly lower when normalized for surface area in infants and small children as compared to adults in relation to renal plasma flow, glomerular filtration rate, concentrating and acidifying functions, and tubular function including secretion and reabsorption. Although these values may be only 20% to 40% of the renal function of older children and adults, it is usually adequate to maintain normal homeostasis. During stressful conditions such as infection, acid-base imbalance, and dehydration, the immaturity and lack of functional reserve of the kidney may become apparent in the neonate and young infant.[73] These factors become of major concern for the excretion of drugs and are reflected in prolonged elimination which creates a risk for toxicity in the infant.

At birth, kidney blood flow is characterized by increased vascular resistance and a preferential intrarenal flow away from the outer kidney cortex.[74,75] During the postnatal period, both increases in cardiac output and decreases in intrarenal vascular resistance occur[73–75] which dramatically increase kidney perfusion. Glomerular function is more advanced than tubular function at birth, and the glomerular/tubular imbalance may persist until six months of age.[76–79] Glomerular filtration rate is

Table 10-2. *Comparative Analysis of Pharmacokinetic Parameters in Relationship to Postnatal Age*[a]

Drug	Perinatal		Newborn	Infant	Child	Adult
	Premature	Term				
Parameter: clearance (mL/hr/kg)						
Caffeine[31, 184]	(2.5–16.8)					84
Chloramphenicol[152, 161, 184]	(53–190)104	90		(25–287)152	(62–121)95	216
Mezlocillin[180, b]	52				190	150
Phenobarbital[184]		(2.7–10.7)			8.2	3.8
Phenytoin[b]						
Theophylline[31, 144–146, 184, b]	(12–25.9)			(28–161)	(31–221)	(29–124)
Parameter: Volume (L/kg)						
Caffeine[31, 184]	(0.47–1.28)0.92					0.54
Chloramphenicol[152]	(0.78–2.4)1.6			(0.25–1.99)0.76	(0.36–1.02)0.63	0.92
Mezlocillin[180]	0.38	0.38	0.49		0.24	0.16
Phenobarbital[31, 184]	0.96	0.88	(0.6–1.5)	(0.4–1.3)	0.67	(0.6–1.5)
Phenytoin[31, 152, 161, 184, 188]	1.20	1.22	(0.8–1.0)	(0.3–1.0)	0.78	0.65
Theophylline[31, 144, 145, 184]	(0.4–1.0)0.69			(0.16–0.83)	(0.2–0.68)	(0.35–0.70)0.51
Parameter: Half-life (hr)						
Caffeine[184, 186]	(36–144)	82	(2.6–26)	(2.1–5.9)3.5	(2.3–7.9)4.8	(3.5–5.2)
Chloramphenicol[187]	(2.9–21.4)10.1	(8–15)				(2–3)
Mezlocillin[180]	3.7	3.7	1.8		0.83	1.0
Phenobarbital[189, 190]	(41–380)	(102–259)	(67–99)		(53–64)	(53–118)
Phenytoin[188, 191, 192]	(12–58)	17–60			5	15(21–29)
Theophylline[65, 135, 137, 142, 180, 193]		14	4	3.4	(1.2–10.0)	(6.1–12.8)

[a] Single values represent mean data, range is presented in parentheses.
[b] Susceptible to dose-dependent kinetics.

approximately 40 mL/min/1.73 m² in the term neonate and gradually increases to adult values by three years of age,[76] although intersubject variability is great in these estimates. Premature infants have lower filtration rates than full-term infants and also develop filtration capacity more slowly postnatally.[79] Application of gentamicin dosage guidelines developed in full-term newborns resulted in extremely high serum gentamicin concentrations (see Figures 10-2A and 10-2B) when applied to premature infants.[37,80,81] Furthermore, the increase in renal function observed after the first week of life in full-term newborns, does not occur in the premature newborn. This is described in Figure 10-3.[82] Therefore, dosage must be individualized with a careful assessment for therapeutic effect. Aminoglycoside excretion may be further impaired by the effect of hypoxia and hypotension on renal function.[83–85] The practical application of serum concentration guidelines is further complicated by the apparent refractoriness for nephrotoxicity in this age group. This may be related to immature renal function altering aminoglycoside distribution in the kidney[86,87] leading to a lower renal accumulation of these antibiotics.[88]

Kidney tubular function at birth is even further reduced and is associated with decreases in glucose, phosphate, bicarbonate, and PAH clearances.[76–78] The plasma

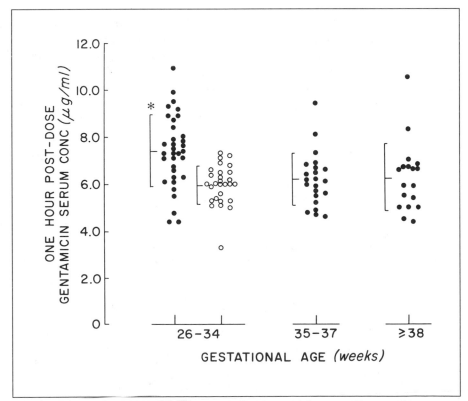

Figure 10-2A. *Relationship of one-hour post-dose gentamicin serum concentration to gestational age:* ●, *12-hour dosage interval;* ○, *18-hour dosage interval. Solid bar indicates mean ± SD. Asterisk (*) indicates significant difference (p <0.05) for comparison of the mean of that group to that of all other groups. Reproduced from reference 80 with permission of the publisher.*

half-life of intravenous PAH increases during the first month of life with adult values reached after three months of age in some children.[77] The use of PAH as a measure of renal plasma flow in neonates may be misleading since a decreased capacity to extract a PAH load (approximately 60%) has been identified.[76] Penicillins which depend mainly on tubular secretion for elimination are cleared slowly by neonates.[47] Passive tubular reabsorption may be reduced in infants and neonates,[2,31,47] and their relatively low urinary pH would also influence the rate and extent of drug absorption. Renal function in the newborn infant does not fluctuate diurnally.[89]

Differences in the renal clearance of drugs between adults and infants and children have been identified. Renal clearance of digoxin is low in neonates as compared to adults and progressively increases until adult values are reached by the first year of life[31] in parallel with the maturation of kidney function. However, digoxin renal excretion exceeds creatinine clearance in infancy, a phenomenon not observed in other age groups,[90] suggesting that both glomerular and tubular function are involved. Aminoglycoside antibiotics typify the need to carefully examine dosage guidelines for individual age groups because their urinary excretion is closely related to development of glomerular function and appears to correlate well with creatinine clearance.[91]

Cystic fibrosis, the most common genetic disorder (incidence 1/2000 live births) is a major cause of respiratory disease in childhood. Cystic fibrosis is associated with an increased volume of distribution and clearance of many

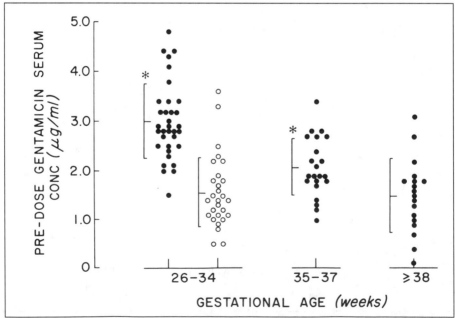

Figure 10-2B. *Relationship of pre-dosage gentamicin serum concentration to gestational age: ●, 12-hour dosage interval; ○, 18-hour dosage interval. Solid bar indicates mean ±SD. Asterisk (*) indicates significant difference (p <0.05) for comparison of the mean of that group to that of all other groups. Reproduced from reference 80 with permission of the publisher.*

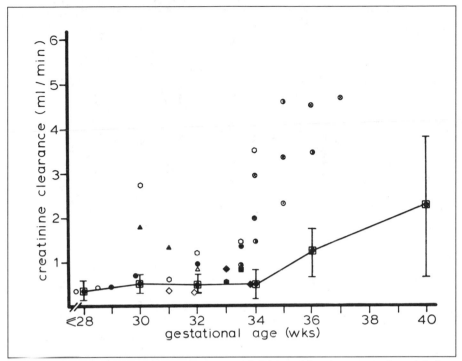

Figure 10-3. *Increase in creatinine clearance with GA (gestational + postnatal ages). Infants studied at birth were grouped for GA and are represented by mean values ± 1 SD connected by the solid line (y = 0.170 × −4.95, r = 0.51, p <0.001). Infants studied during extrauterine life are represented by a mass plot of data with GA, in which studies from one infant at different ages are indicated by the same symbol (y = 0.406 × −11.548, r = 0.68, p <0.001). Reproduced from reference 82 with permission of the publisher.*

medications used in the treatment of the pulmonary and cardiovascular complications of this disorder (see Table 10-3). It is not clear whether alterations in drug disposition are linked to the genetic defect associated with cystic fibrosis or a result of changes in body habitus due to chronic malnutrition, gastrointestinal dysfunction, increased drug metabolism, increased renal excretion, or increased renal tubular secretion.

Drug Receptors

Another concept integral to the understanding of the dose-response relationship is the evaluation of specific drug receptors. Recent developments in technology have provided insight into the nature of the cholinergic, adrenergic, steroid, opiate, and histamine receptors. *In vitro* techniques utilizing isolated tissue, such as smooth muscle from blood vessels or bronchi, are available to assess the age-related development of dose-response effects to selected stimuli. Significant advances have also taken place in the evaluation of receptor binding sites on various tissues utilizing radioligand binding techniques and autoradiography. This analysis provides the opportunity to measure the quantity of these recep-

Table 10-3. Pharmacokinetic Alterations Associated with Cystic Fibrosis as Compared to Age-Matched Volunteers. (Data are shown for a representative group of drugs used in the management of cystic fibrosis.)[c]

Drug	Clearance Total body	Clearance Renal	Non-renal	Elimination t½[a]	Volume of distribution[a]	% bound to plasma proteins[a]	Potential impact on clinically relevant alterations in dosing
Tobramycin[92]	↑ 19	↑ 10 (NS)	ND	↓ 7 (NS)	↑ 12	↓ 17.8 (NS)	+(Higher doses may be required)
Furosemide[93]	↑ 33	↑ 9 (NS)	↑ 129	↓ 10 (NS)	↑ 37 (NS)	(ND)	−(No differences in diuretic efficacy)
Ticarcillin[94]	↑ 51	↑ 42	↑ 86	↓ 18	↑ 16 (NS)	(ND)	++(Authors suggest using relatively larger daily doses)
Theophylline[95]	↑ 52	↑ 45	↑ 41	↓ 19	↑ 18	0[b]	±
Prednisolone[96]	↑ 83	↑ 60	↑ 63	↓ 5 (NS)	↑ 81	(ND)	+(Authors suggest split dosing may be necessary)

[a] Results expressed as % difference from control where % difference = (CF − control / CF) × 100. ↑ refers to a positive difference and ↓ refers to a negative difference.
[b] Mean data not reported.
[c] ND = Comparisons were not done or parameter not measured; NS = Not significantly different.

tors and their affinity for specific drugs. Information on the development of receptor function has been derived primarily from animal studies and from tissue specimens of human abortions.[2]

Some of the most detailed information on the ontogenetic modulation of pharmacologic response is related to the autonomic nervous system, specifically in regard to vascular smooth muscle, as well as to cardiac and bronchial reactivity.[97-99] One example of the differences in development of individual components is provided by an evaluation of the rat heart. Isoproterenol increases the rate and force of contraction at birth; however, stimulation of sympathetic nerves, using tyramine to release the transmitter, results in a small response which increases during the first week of life.[99] Therefore, it appears that the sympathetic control of the heart in rats less than one week of age is not fully developed. Similarly, vascular response to adrenergic nerve stimulation is not fully developed in the newborn dog. There may also be regional differences in the development of vascular response to sympathetic stimulation. One explanation may be a relatively low rate of biosynthesis of catecholamines during fetal and early postnatal life in most mammalian tissues. The concentration of adrenergic transmitters is generally low and does not approach adult levels until four to eight weeks after birth in various tissues from several different species.[100] From this information, it is apparent that there is sufficient capacity for pharmacologic response to exogenous agents, despite the immaturity of the neurotransmitter system. Detailed studies are necessary to identify the β-adrenergic receptor binding parameters in relationship to age. These studies may be useful in designing therapeutic regimens for certain pathologic conditions which occur frequently in premature newborns, such as congenital heart disease, pulmonary hypertension secondary to persistent fetal circulation, necrotizing enterocolitis, and intraventricular hemorrhages.[99]

Autonomic innervation is also important for the control of tracheal smooth muscle tone. Investigation in rabbits demonstrated that nerve fibers increase their ability to transmit nerve impulses significantly during the first four to six weeks of postnatal life.[101] Furthermore, response of rabbit tracheal smooth muscle to certain pharmacologic agents varies with age.[102] Contractile responses to nicotine, acetylcholine, histamine, and isoproterenol decrease with age suggesting the possibility that receptor function may be age-related.

With each system of analysis, caution is required in the interpretation of data. *In vivo* assessments of biologic response to a specific dose of medication may be altered by variations in pharmacokinetics between subjects or the involvement of reflex mechanisms which attenuate a physiologic action. An example of an age-related phenomenon in receptor sensitivity is that identified with digoxin receptors in neonates.[103] Traditionally, infants have been observed to "tolerate" larger doses of digoxin than adults and an *in vitro* assessment of erythrocyte digoxin binding sites revealed twice the number of binding sites on neonatal cells as on those of adults. Myocardial:plasma digoxin ratios are also reported to be considerably greater in infants and children than in adults.[104,105] However, much of these age-related differences could be subsequent to methodological error, as discussed by Wagner and co-workers.[106] Their data, evaluating specific assay techniques and using multiple regression analysis of variance, suggest that variation in digoxin concentrations and digoxin serum:tissue ratios may result primarily from variation in patient size and digoxin dose and not from age-related differences in myocardial digoxin binding or metabolism. The validity of currently accepted parameters for digoxin kinetics in infants is also being questioned since the identification of a circulating endogenous digoxin-like substance in this age group.[107] *In vitro* assessments on isolated tissue specimens could provide relevant information regarding the development of response to pharmacologic stimuli; however, isolation of the tissue removes it from vital structures which modulate response *in vivo*. Similarly, isolation and preparation of tissue will modify the interpretation of radioligand binding assays used in the analysis of receptor number and affinity. Since relatively few receptors may be necessary to produce a response, binding data must be interpreted in a relative sense with recognized limitations for evaluation of post-receptor activity. Nevertheless, the assessment of these individual investigations of pharmacologic response may be extremely useful in understanding the mechanics of age-related differences in pharmacologic response to selected agents, although methodological artifacts must be carefully eliminated before making age-related comparisons.

Despite detailed evaluation in animals, extrapolation to man, especially to an individual patient, is tenuous. Therefore, it is important to identify additional methods to measure receptor binding properties of selected drugs. One recent development in this technology is the ability to measure radioligand binding properties in peripheral blood cells. One example for the application of this technology is the measurement of β-adrenergic receptor binding parameters in peripheral leukocytes.[108] These receptors have been identified as the β_2-adrenergic receptor subtype. Leukocyte β_2-adrenergic receptors are measured in clinical studies to identify conditions which may alter receptor presentation. Conolly and Greenacre[109] suggest that observed changes reflect alterations at specific target sites, such as bronchial and vascular smooth muscle. Only limited data are available to support this hypothesis.[109]

Age-related alterations in leukocyte β-adrenergic receptor affinity have been identified. These studies suggest that β-adrenergic receptor affinity is decreased in the elderly and may explain reduced β-adrenergic sensitivity in this age group as compared to young healthy adults.[110] Similar information is not yet available for the younger age group.

Analysis of drug receptors on peripheral blood cells offers several advantages, specifically accessibility to a readily available biologic tissue and the opportunity to obtain multiple measurements in individual patients under varying conditions. With the increased availability of radioligands and identification of specific binding sites on these cells, increased applications are likely, including the evaluation of α_2-adrenergic (platelets), corticosteroids (leukocytes), and digoxin (reticulocytes) receptors. Developmental changes in receptor binding characteristics may have important implications for the identification of precise limits for serum concentrations for specific drugs in certain age groups.

SPECIFIC MEDICATIONS

The following discussion will be limited to three medications which provide examples of important considerations in pediatric drug therapy. Comprehensive summaries of the applied pharmacokinetics of these drugs are provided in separate chapters of this text.

Digoxin

Digoxin, which is excreted primarily by renal mechanisms, has been studied in detail in various pediatric age groups. As previously discussed, renal function increases with age, consequently digoxin dose is adjusted for age. For a fixed digoxin dose of 8 µg/kg/day, serum digoxin concentrations are markedly increased from 1.4 ng/mL in a 2500 gm neonate to 6.1 ng/mL in premature neonates weighing less than 1000 gm.

Considerable controversy has existed over the designated therapeutic range for serum digoxin concentrations in pediatric patients. As previously mentioned, the recent identification of a digoxin-like immunoreactive substance (DLIS) in neonatal plasma[107,111-113] complicates the interpretation of digoxin pharmacokinetic studies and the reliability of digoxin radioimmunoassays.[111] Phelps et al.[114] reported an apparent DLIS in 27% of pediatric patients ranging from less than one month to six years of age.

In adult patients the recognized limits are 1 to 2 ng/mL; however, concentrations between 2 and 3.5 ng/mL are occasionally permitted in neonates. Although toxicity has been associated with concentrations exceeding 3.5 ng/mL, other studies have noted toxicity with concentrations as low as 2 ng/mL.[111] To date a commercial assay is not available which compensates for this interference.

Although dosage must be carefully reduced in premature newborns, the dosage requirements (based on body weight) for infants and young children increase to a level that often exceeds adult requirements. Several theories are proposed to explain the increased dose in this age group and include decreased absorption or increased elimination.

In children, the oral liquid form is most commonly administered. Peak serum digoxin concentrations occur within 90 minutes, and bioavailability is approximately 72% as compared to the intravenous form.[115] Furthermore, the rate and extent of absorption is not influenced by physiologic variables, such as gastric emptying time, pH, intestinal transit time, and food.[115,116] However, the extent of absorption may be altered by severe cardiac insufficiency and intramuscular absorption is erratic and very slow.

Digoxin is distributed by infants and adults extensively to tissue sites, primarily myocardium, kidney, liver, and skeletal muscle.[104] Tissue distribution in the two age groups is similar; however, infants have a reported threefold increase in erythrocyte:plasma digoxin ratio as compared to adults[105] and a twofold higher myocardial concentration.[104] The cause of the increased erythrocyte and myocardial concentration is not known, although the variation in patient size and digoxin dose administered may partly account for the differences seen in serum:tissue digoxin ratios in children.[106] As a result of extensive tissue distribution,[117] the volume of distribution of digoxin in infants is very large and exceeds adult values during the neonatal and infant period.[118] Plasma protein binding of digoxin in neonates and adults is similar[119] and therefore does not account for the increased V_d. Measuring digoxin radioligand binding in neonatal and adult erythrocytes, Kearin et al.[103] observed an increased number and decreased affinity in neonatal erythrocytes. If erythrocytes reflect binding in cardiac tissue, this may explain the observed increase in V_d and requirement of higher serum digoxin concentrations in certain patients. Koren et al.[120] reported several cases of serum digoxin concentrations in infants and children long after cessation of therapy. Rapid development of renal failure with resulting decreases in V_d may explain the observed increases in serum digoxin concentrations. However, an increased drug concentration in the myocardium does not necessarily mean higher concentrations at receptor sites because tissue concentrations may be largely nonspecific binding.

The major routes of digoxin elimination are renal, metabolic, and biliary. The renal clearance increases with age to reach adult values at three to four months of age.[121] The total body clearance is lower and elimination half-life longer in neonates than infants and increases in parallel with development of renal excretory function.[118,122] However, the elimination half-life is shorter in infants than adults. Digoxin clearance also correlates closely with serum β_2-microglobulin clearance in neonates.[123] Information on the role of nonrenal mechanisms, such as biliary excretion, in neonates and infants is not available at this time. Drug metabolism, however, is insignificant in infants.[124]

Thus, it appears that digoxin doses in children should be carefully individualized and adjusted to maintain serum digoxin concentrations between 1 and 2 ng/mL. These limits may be exceeded with careful monitoring for adverse effects and assessment of improved clinical response. The introduction of digoxin-specific antibodies represents a major advance. Clinical experience is limited in children, but the majority of accidental digoxin ingestions are by children less than six years of age.[125]

Theophylline

Theophylline is one of the most extensively studied medications in pediatric patients. Age-related differences in pharmacokinetic parameters are of importance. Theophylline differs significantly from digoxin in its route of elimination with drug metabolism as its major route and a minor component attributed to renal excretion.

Theophylline was initially introduced into clinical medicine in 1937; however, its use became limited because of a number of adverse affects, including arrhythmias, seizures, and a significant incidence of mortality. A resurgence in use of theophylline was prompted by the identification of individual differences in theophylline elimination. Application of principles of pharmacokinetics and delineation of a therapeutic range facilitated safe and effective use of this medicine. At the present time, theophylline is used extensively in pediatric patients as a bronchodilator in the treatment of asthma and as a respiratory stimulant in neonatal apnea. For the treatment of asthma the therapeutic range is considered to be 8 to 20 µg/mL, while 2 to 15 µg/mL is recommended for neonates in preventing apnea.

Because of the narrow margin of safety, it is important to utilize theophylline preparations which provide a consistent rate and extent of absorption. Intravenous, oral liquid, and immediate-release tablet formulations and rectal solutions of theophylline are rapidly and completely absorbed. No significant food or physiologic variables affect absorption from these formulations.

Sustained-release preparations are an important addition to pediatric therapy. In young children, with theophylline half-lives frequently less than four hours, it is theoretically impossible to maintain serum theophylline concentrations between 8 to 20 µg/mL with a regimen that would assure compliance. There are considerable differences between available sustained-release preparations in their extent and rate of theophylline absorption.[126] This is summarized in detail in Chapter 13: Theophylline. Recent data suggest that theophylline absorption from certain sustained-release preparations is complete even in children two years of age.[127,128]

Theophylline absorption from sustained-release preparations may be variable between subjects and even within the same patient.[129,130] This may be related to inherent variability in gastric physiology or an effect of food.[131,132] This effect is apparent during multiple dose therapy in which diurnal patterns in serum theophylline concentrations may be observed.[133] The serum theophylline concentrations following the morning dose are higher than those following the evening dose. Our own studies indicate that this is related to decreased rate of absorption during the evening.[134] Chronopharmacokinetic studies have identified important diurnal fluctuations in C_{max} and C_{min} useful in developing guidelines for optimal sampling times for asthmatic children.[135]

Another variable which must be considered in young children is the limiting effect of intestinal transit time on the extent of absorption. Many sustained-release theophylline preparations are designed for dosage intervals of 12 and even 24 hours. Examination of absorption characteristics of these products[126,130] shows that absorption may continue beyond 12 hours. The variation within subjects may be considerable even under ideal conditions.[130]

Theophylline is distributed rapidly to peripheral sites. The average volume of distribution is 0.45 L/kg; however, the range is between 0.3 and 0.7 L/kg.[136,197] The V_d adjusted on a weight basis is larger for neonates.[137] Approximately 60% of the measured total serum concentration is bound to plasma albumin.[100] Theophylline protein binding is reduced in neonates[137] and may be altered by acidemia.[138] The higher free concentration in neonates may be related to the observation that the range of 2 to 15 µg/mL is satisfactory for the treatment of apnea in this age group.

The other significant variable which has considerable effects on theophylline dosage regimens is elimination rate. Theophylline disposition is dependent on metabolic transformation, primarily by the liver. The functional capacity of the liver may vary significantly with age, disease, and concomitant medications. In general, theophylline elimination is assumed to be a first-order process; however, the biotransformation pathways may be capacity limited in certain patients even within the therapeutic range.[139] The occurrence of both nonlinearity and possible nonstationarity in adults[140] suggests that theophylline elimination is more complex than once thought.

Recognition of conditions affecting theophylline metabolism has been related to the availability of therapeutic drug monitoring. Many observations in clinical settings led to more sophisticated investigations to confirm a hypothesis. Jenne first recognized the interpatient variability in theophylline elimination in adult patients and the individual dosage requirements necessary to attain a desired serum theophylline concentration.[141] This was followed by an array of studies which identified various conditions contributing to this interpatient variability.

Although there are no studies available which have serially examined theophylline elimination in the same patient as a function of age, individual studies suggest that this will occur. The potential for age-related change was identified by Ellis et al.[197] Further studies confirmed these observations and assisted in the development of dosage guidelines for initiating theophylline therapy.[142] There is considerable variation in elimination even within similar age groups. The relatively slow elimination of theophylline in newborn infants is attributed to continuing development of metabolic pathways.[59,143–145] The variation in metabolism and resulting plasma concentrations among pediatric patients is great (see Figure 10-4) and supports strongly the case for monitoring theophylline levels in these age groups.

Chloramphenicol

Resurgence in chloramphenicol use comes after a period of hesitancy associated with concern over potential life-threatening adverse effects, specifically aplastic anemia and the "gray baby" syndrome. With the aid of serum concentration measurements, it was determined that a certain proportion of these undesirable effects are dose-related, while others are idiosyncratic. The risk for dose-related hematopoietic suppression and the "gray baby" syndrome can be reduced by careful dose titration to avoid serum chloramphenicol concentrations that exceed 25 µg/mL. However, effective treatment of susceptible organisms often necessitates a minimum concentration of 10 µg/mL.

One aspect of chloramphenicol therapy which is important for pediatric patients is full appreciation of the limitations of available dosage forms. Chloramphenicol is very lipid-soluble and, therefore, weakly soluble in water. Aqueous solubility for liquid dosage formulations is increased by adding an ester group; and in particular, the succinate ester is added to the parenteral formulation. Chloramphenicol sodium succinate is itself inactive and requires hydrolysis, *in vivo*, to form chloramphenicol, the active agent. The hydrolysis rate is highly variable and unpredictable in infants and children.[147,148] In some patients, the ester form is detectable in serum for up to six hours after a dose.[149] The rate of hydrolysis appears to be age-related and particularly slow during the first month of life. In addition to this phenomenon, there is direct renal clearance of the succinate form by glomerular filtration and active tubular secretion. The delay in hydrolysis in young children likely affects the percent recovery in the urine. The range of recovery of chloramphenicol succinate in the urine is 6% to 80% of the administered dose.

There is also concern raised over the possibility of dose-dependent or enzyme-capacity limited hydrolysis of chloramphenicol sodium succinate. Animal studies confirm this hypothesis,[150] but it is not known whether this phenomenon occurs in humans. Therefore, the serum chloramphenicol concentration at any time during a dosage interval will be a function of the rate of hydrolysis and renal excretion of the succinate form, and of the chloramphenicol metabolism rate itself.

Bioavailability of chloramphenicol from the succinate ester appears to be age related. Increased bioavailability was observed in premature infants as compared to full-term and older infants.[151–153] This may be a function of decreased renal clearance in premature infants providing longer time periods for ester hydrolysis.

The oral form of chloramphenicol most frequently used in pediatric patients is the suspension form of the palmitate ester. It is assumed that chloramphenicol palmitate is hydrolyzed to the active form, chloramphenicol, in the gastrointestinal tract by pancreatic lipase.[154] Bioavailability is sufficient in older infants and children;[155,156] however, there is considerable variability in serum chloramphenicol concentrations when the palmitate ester is administered to premature and full-term neonatal patients.[157] It appears that only 25% to 60% of chloramphenicol is bioavailable in newborn infants, consistent with the low serum concentrations observed.[157] This may be a consequence of delays in gastric emptying or decreased hydrolysis of the palmitate ester. The crystalline form of chloramphenicol administered in capsules is rapidly absorbed and should provide satisfactory absorption for older children, adolescents, and adults.

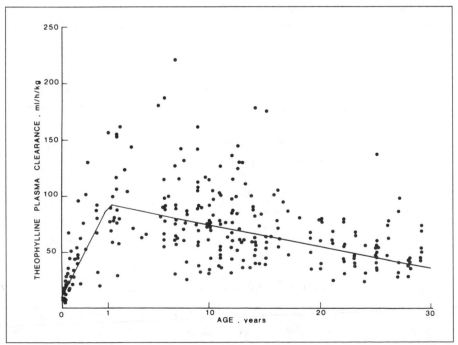

Figure 10-4. *Theophylline plasma clearance in relation to age. Data were compiled from multiple literature sources.*

Estimates of chloramphenicol volume of distribution vary considerably with an average of 0.7 L/kg from several studies with no apparent difference between adults and infants.[152,158–163] Elimination half-life for chloramphenicol also varies widely between patients with a range from one hour to indeterminate. These estimates are probably confounded significantly by variation in ester hydrolysis. Even with these limitations in interpretation, there appear to be age-related changes in chloramphenicol half-life. The average half-life in neonatal patients was reported as 27.1 hours[151] compared to 9.3 hours in older infants.[151,161]

It is generally recommended to provide dosage regimens that yield peak chloramphenicol concentrations between 10 to 25 µg/mL. Decisions regarding dosage adjustments could be influenced by impaired hydrolysis of the ester form, incomplete absorption, or delayed elimination. Increased elimination may be anticipated with advancing age or influenced by other medications, such as phenobarbital.[164]

CONSIDERATIONS IN CLINICAL PHARMACOKINETICS AND DRUG EVALUATION RESEARCH STUDIES

Determination of Dose

Absorption, distribution, metabolism, and renal excretion are primary factors contributing to the determination of correct drug dosages. Marked differences in these factors exist in the various age groups. Dosages for pediatric patients have usually been poorly derived as fractions of adult dosages and when expressed per kilogram, adult dosages are usually inadequate for pediatrics. Three parameters traditionally used for dosage calculations have been age, weight, or body surface area.[165] Many dosage rules based on age or weight are now considered outdated as our understanding of the physiologic complexities of growth, development, and drug disposition increase. Percentages of adult doses that a pediatric patient would receive based on body weight or surface area vary greatly,[2,166,167] while body surface area approximates most closely the age-dependent differences in drug disposition and is approximately proportionate to blood volume, cardiac output, renal blood flow, glomerular filtration, and caloric and fluid requirements.[168] The practicality of using surface area for dosage calculations is limited by its difficulty of calculation, the relative lack of dosages expressed this way, and the fact that not all drug requirements are linearly related to surface area.[168] Other methods for drug dosage calculation include allometric nomograms[169] and relationships of extracellular fluid water to body weight and surface area.[166,170] Table 10-4 demonstrates these relationships.

Clinical Interpretation and Application of Pharmacokinetics

Optimal application of therapeutic drug monitoring in children must consider the variables in development previously discussed in regards to absorption, distribution, and elimination. While research investigations incorporate multiple concentration determinations, clinical applications are often limited to one or two drug concentration measurements. With the limited number of samples, it is therefore important to assure that the conditions are optimal (e.g., with respect to steady-state conditions, specific sampling time, and assay specificity). Therefore, the greatest benefits of therapeutic drug monitoring are obtained when sample analysis is planned carefully to answer a specific question (e.g., adequacy of dose, risk for toxicity, suspected interactions with medications or disease states). The most frequent utilization of serum concentrations occurs with drugs having a low margin of safety, especially with life-threatening adverse effects, such as arrhythmias, seizures, or respiratory depression.

The use of simulations and curve-fitting techniques of composite pharmacokinetic profiling permits generation of parameters from single points for homogeneous patient populations, such as preterm neonates.[171] Recent applications of population kinetics[172,173] and the use of Bayesian estimators would appear to optimize the available information from a limited number of patients.[174] These techniques may be utilized more extensively in the future.

This discussion will focus on the applications of pharmacokinetics in pediatric drug therapy and special considerations in conducting pharmacokinetic research studies. Once the specific question is identified and the patient carefully assessed in regard to past history and present status, the appropriate time for blood sampling must be designated. Timing is primarily based on knowledge of the pharmacokinetics in the average patient and limitations on sample number and volume. A chronopharmacologic approach to blood sampling time would provide the optimal information, but studies on neonates and infants are lacking at the present time,[174,175] and only limited information is available for children and adolescents. There should be a clear estimate of the expected result in the individual evaluation. If the result is higher or lower than expected, a systematic assessment should be conducted before further dosage adjustments are implemented.

Serum Concentrations Lower than Expected. Conditions contributing to unexpectedly low concentrations include the dose, compliance, the time of sampling, time of drug administration, analytical error, impaired drug absorption, and accelerated elimination. The dosage regimen should be reviewed in relation to

Table 10-4. *Fraction of Adult Value for Body Weight (BW), Surface Area (BSA), and Extracellular Fluid Volume (ECF) of Children*

Age (years)	Body Weight (%)[a]	Surface Area (%)[a]	Ratio of BSA/BW	ECF (%)	Ratio of ECF child/ECF adult
0.25	8	16	2.0	178	1.8
0.50	11	20	1.8	167	1.7
1.0	15	25	1.6	148	1.5
3.0	22	34	1.5	142	1.4
7.0	37	52	1.4	122	1.2
12.0	59	69	1.2	104	1.1
Adult	100	100	1.0	100	1.0

[a] Percentages = fraction of adult dose child would receive.

dosage guidelines specific for the patient's age. One common source of low serum concentrations is the use of very low intravenous fluid flow rates for medication administration. Flow rates may be less than 10 mL/hr in neonates, requiring longer than 60 minutes for a substantial amount of medication to be delivered.[196] In this situation, alternative administration techniques such as syringe infusion pumps or "retrograde" injection may be more reliable and allow for accurate serum concentration monitoring. Occasionally serum samples are obtained later than the requested time or after a previously scheduled dose was inadvertently missed. In pediatric patients with typically rapid elimination, this may be important. It may also be necessary to review the accuracy of the laboratory analysis. A repeat analysis or the application of a second assay technique may discern analytical error or interference with the assay method from other medications or dietary constituents. An example would be the interference of a caffeine metabolite, paraxanthine, in the analysis of theophylline.[176] Impaired absorption may be a consequence of other medications, food, or disease states. Similarly, elimination could be accelerated by environmental agents, smoking, or medications causing induction of drug-metabolizing enzymes. Finally, a full pharmacokinetic evaluation may be considered and its application will be discussed.

Serum Concentrations Higher than Expected. Again, several conditions must be reviewed when concentrations are relatively high or exceed the therapeutic range. A comparison of the administered dose to the dosage guideline may indicate a dose higher than necessary. Also important to determine is whether the patient has followed medication instructions or whether the active medication is being received in more than one form. The sampling time should normally avoid the absorptive/distributive phase. Possibilities for analytical errors should be considered as above. Once these points are examined, impaired metabolism should be considered in relation to other medications and disease states (e.g., enzyme inhibitors, hepatotoxic agents, and liver or renal disease). In addition, unexpectedly high serum concentrations may be observed even after a modest increase in dose in patients who may be susceptible to dose-dependent or enzyme-capacity limited drug metabolism.

Individual Assessment of Pharmacokinetic Parameters. It may be necessary to perform detailed pharmacokinetic investigations in individual patients. Reasons for these extended evaluations may include: verification of unusually large dosage requirements; identification of the etiology of altered drug disposition, such as impaired absorption; accelerated or impaired drug elimination due to a drug interaction; or monitoring drug elimination following an overdose.

In each case, special considerations are necessary in evaluating infants and children. Careful planning must include an assessment of the study dose, sampling times, total blood volume, and methods of sample collection. The dose and sampling duration should be adequate to obtain a reliable estimate of drug elimination, preferably to include at least two half-lives. It should be designed to obtain concentrations well within the therapeutic range and also assess the potential for dose-dependent elimination. Sampling volume and methods of plasma collection (e.g., use of intravenous catheters) should provide sufficient volume for sample analysis but minimize the risk for adverse effects secondary to blood withdrawal (i.e., pain, hypotension, and infection).

Limitations to Research

A majority of drugs currently available for potential use in pediatric patients are not labeled for indications, uses, and dosages in the various developmental age groups of infants, children, and adolescents. This results from the lack of clinical research studies designed to evaluate the efficacy and disposition of these agents in pediatric subjects. The requirement that drugs be tested in infants and children before marketing raises concern over the ethics of experimentation in these age groups. Animal models have been proposed for testing, but likely are susceptible to inaccuracies when extrapolating pharmacokinetic and pharmacodynamic parameters.[177] Valuable sources of pharmacokinetic data can be obtained as a result of the direct treatment of sick infants and children when studies are carefully designed to maximize the potential investigative benefits. The development of microassay methods and the use of noninvasive procedures, such as saliva monitoring, should facilitate clinical pharmacological research in pediatrics. Pharmacokinetic studies conducted in infants and children are constrained by the number of blood samples that can be safely collected from each subject. An approach to circumvent this constraint has been to collect blood samples at different times in several children, matched for size and age, and to fit the pooled data to appropriate models.[178,179] Composite sampling from a study population of premature neonates has provided pharmacokinetic parameters and dosage recommendations for vitamin E.[179] Other approaches to maximize information from clinically obtained blood level data has been the application of population statistics, such as the use of analysis of covariance and multiple regression for factors such as age, weight, and disease.[180]

PROSPECTUS

The purpose of this discussion was to highlight the important considerations in applying pharmacokinetic principles to pediatric drug therapy and clinical investigation. Several excellent reviews are available for more detail.[2,3,31,47,65,181–185]

This summary specifically addressed conditions affecting drug disposition in children following birth. Other important topics regarding drug disposition relative to pediatric patients, such as the developing fetus and drugs in breast milk, were not discussed.

Future directions for pediatric drug therapy will continue in the present vein to apply pharmacokinetic principles in combination with a careful assessment of clinical response. Sophisticated noninvasive monitoring techniques can be utilized to carefully assess the frequency of seizures, apneic episodes, and arrhythmias. Variations in clinical response will generate questions regarding the appropriate therapeutic range for various drugs in relation to age, the reliability of drug delivery systems, and longterm effects of drug treatment in chronic disease.

REFERENCES

1. Shirkey H. Therapeutic orphans. J Pediatr. 1968;72:119–20.
2. Boreus LO. Principles of pediatric clinical pharmacology. New York, NY: Churchill Livingtone; 1982.
3. Besunder JB et al. Principles of drug biodisposition in the neonate: a critical evaluation of the pharmacokinetic-pharmacodynamic interface. Clin Pharmacokinet. 1983;189–216.
4. Avery GB et al. Gastric acidity on the first day of life. Pediatrics. 1966;37:1005–7.
5. Agunod M et al. Correlative study of hydrochloric acid, pepsin, and intrinsic factor secretion in newborns and infants. Am J Dig Dis. 1969;14:400–14.
6. Miller RA. Observations on the gastric acidity during the first month of life. Arch Dis Child. 1941;16:22–30.
7. Pinkerton CR et al. Can food influence the absorption of methotrexate in children with acute lymphoblastic leukaemia? Lancet. 1980;2:944–46.
8. Siegel M et al. Effect of caloric density on gastric emptying in premature infants. J Pediatr. 1984;118–22.
9. Cavell B. Gastric emptying in preterm infants. Acta Paediatr Scand. 1979;68:725–30.
10. Cavell B. Gastric emptying in infants fed human milk or infant formula. Acta Pediatr Scand. 1981;70:639–41.
11. Signer E, Fridrich R. Gastric emptying in newborns and young infants. Acta Paediatr Scand. 1975;64:525–30.
12. Gemer O et al. Absorption of orally administered gentamicin in infants with diarrhea. Pediatr Pharmacol. 1983;3:119–23.
13. Nelson JD et al. Absorption of ampicillin and nalidixic acid by infants and children with acute shigellosis. Clin Pharmacol Ther. 1972;13:879–86.
14. Elliot RB et al. Ampicillin in pediatrics. Arch Dis Child. 1964;39:101–5.
15. Heizer WD et al. Absorption of digoxin in patients with malabsorption syndromes. N Engl J Med. 1971;285:257–69.
16. Jussila J et al. Drug absorption during lactose-induced intestinal symptoms in patients with selective lactose malabsorption. Ann Med Exp Biol Fenn. 1970;48:33–7.
17. Milsap RL et al. Effect of inflammatory bowel disease on absorption and disposition of prednisolone. Dig Dis Sci. 1983;28:161–68.
18. Cavell B. Gastric emptying in infants with congenital heart disease. Acta Pediatr Scand. 1981;70:517–20.
19. Huang NN, High RH. Comparison of serum levels following the administration of oral and parenteral preparations of penicillin to infants and children of various age groups. J Pediatr. 1953;42:657–68.
20. O'Connor WJ et al. Serum concentrations of sodium nafcillin in infants during the perinatal period. Antimicrob Agents Chemother. 1965;5:220–22.
21. Silverio J, Poole JW. Serum concentrations of ampicillin in newborn infants after oral administration. Pediatrics. 1973;51:578–80.
22. Wallin A et al. Plasma concentrations of phenobarbitol in the neonate during prophylaxis for neonatal hyperbilirubinemia. J Pediatr. 1974;85:392–98.
23. Jalling B et al. Plasma concentrations of diphenylhydantoin in young infants. Pharmacologica Clinica. 1970;2:200–2.
24. Levy G et al. Pharmacokinetics of acetaminophen in the human neonate: formation of acetaminophen glucuronide and sulfate in relation to plasma bilirubin concentrations and d-glucaric acid excretion. Pediatrics. 1975;55:818–25.
25. Jusko WJ et al. Riboflavin absorption and excretion in the neonate. Pediatrics. 1970;45:945–49.
26. Heimann G. Enteral absorption and bioavailability in children in relation to age. Eur J Clin Pharmacol. 1980;18:43–50.
27. Murphy GM, Signer E. Progress report: bile acid metabolism in infants and children. Gut. 1974;15:151–63.
28. Dallman PR. Iron, vitamin E, and folate in the pre-term infant. J Pediatr. 1974;85:742–52.
29. Yaffe SJ, Juchau MR. Perinatal pharmacology. Ann Rev Pharmacol. 1974;14:219–38.

30. Yoshioka H et al. Development and differences of intestinal flora in the neonatal period in breast-fed and bottle-fed infants. Pediatrics. 1983;72:317–21.
31. Morselli PL et al. Clinical pharmacokinetics in newborns and infants: age-related differences and therapeutic implications. Clin Pharmacokinet. 1980;5:485–527.
32. Moynahan EJ. Developmental biology of the skin. In: Davies JA, Dobbing J, eds. Scientific foundations of pediatrics, 2nd edition. London: Heinemann Medical Books; 1981;721–41.
33. Feinblatt BI et al. Percutaneous absorption of hydrocortisone in children. Am J Dis Child. 1966;112:218–24.
34. Tyrala EE et al. Clinical pharmacology of hexachlorophene in newborn infants. J Pediatr. 1977;91:481–86.
35. Evans NJ et al. Percutaneous administration of theophylline in the preterm infant. J Pediatr. 1985;107:307–11.
36. Szefler SJ et al. Paradoxical behavior of serum digoxin concentrations in an anuric neonate. J Pediatr. 1977;91:487–89.
37. Assael BM et al. Gentamicin dosage in pre term and term neonates. Arch Dis Child. 1977;52:883–86.
38. Friis-Hansen B. Body water compartments in children: changes during growth and related changes in body composition. Pediatrics. 1961;28:169–81.
39. Friis-Hansen B. Body composition during growth. Pediatrics. 1971;47:264–74.
40. Widdowson EM. Changes in body proportions and composition during growth. In: Davies JA, Dobbing J, eds. Scientific Foundations of Paediatrics. London:Heinemann Medical Books Ltd;1974:153–63.
41. Assael BM. Pharmacokinetics and drug distribution during postnatal development. Pharmacol Ther. 1982;18:159–97.
42. Cornford EM et al. Increased blood-brain barrier transport of protein-bound anticonv-ulsant drugs in the newborn. J Cereb Blood Flow Metab. 1983;3:280–86.
43. Gorodischer R et al. Tissue and erythrocyte distribution of digoxin in infants. Clin Pharmacol Ther. 1976;19:256–63.
44. Koup JR, Hart BA. Relationship between plasma and whole blood theophylline concentrations in neonates. J Pediatr. 1979;94:320–21.
45. Darrow DC, Cary MK. The serum albumin and globulin of newborn, premature and normal infants. J Pediatr. 1933;3:573–79.
46. Metcoff J, Stare F. The physiologic and clinical significance of plasma proteins and protein metabolites. N Engl J Med. 1947;236:26–35.
47. Morselli PL. Clinical pharmacokinetics in neonates. Clin Pharmacokinet. 1976;1:81–91.
48. Broderson R et al. Drug-induced displacement of bilirubin from albumin in the newborn. Dev Pharmacol Ther. 1983;6:217–29.
49. Herngren L et al. Drug binding to plasma proteins during human pregnancy and in the perinatal period. Studies on cloxacillin and alprenolol. Dev Pharmacol. 1983;6:110–24.
50. Brown AK et al. Studies on the neonatal development of the glucuronide conjugating system. J Clin Invest. 1958;37:332–40.
51. Vest MF, Rossier R. Detoxification in the newborn: the ability of the newborn infant to form conjugates with glucuronic acid, glycine, acetate and glutathione. Ann NY Acad Sci. 1963;111:183–98.
52. Percy AK, Yaffe SJ. Sulfate metabolism during mammalian development. Pediatrics. 1964;33:965–68.
53. Vest MF, Rene S. Conjugation reactions in the newborn infant: the metabolism of para-amino-benzoic acid. Arch Dis Child. 1965;40:97–5.
54. Aranda JV et al. Hepatic microsomal drug oxidation and electron transport in newborn infants. J Pediatr. 1974;85:534–42.
55. Morselli PL. Drug metabolism during development. Paper presented to Gordon Research 4th Conference on Drug Metabolism. Plymouth, NH:1974.
56. Horning MG et al. Drug metabolism in the human neonate. Life Sci. 1975;16:651–72.
57. Juchau MR et al. Drug metabolism by the human fetus. Clin Pharmacokinet. 1980;5:320–39.
58. Rane A, Tomson G. Prenatal and neonatal drug metabolism in man. Eur J Clin Pharmacol. 1980;18:9–15.

59. Tserng KY et al. Theophylline metabolism in premature infants. Clin Pharmacol Ther. 1981;29:594–600.

60. Murdock AI et al. Serial measurements of plasma half-lives and urinary excretion of antipyrine in low-birth-weight infants. Biol Neonate. 1975;27:289–301.

61. Tserng KY et al. Developmental aspects of theophylline metabolism in premature infants. Clin Pharmacol Ther. 1983;33:522–28.

62. Dutton GJ. Developmental aspects of drug conjugation with special reference to glucuronidation. Ann Rev Pharmacol Toxicol. 1978;18:17–36.

63. Levy GL et al. Pharmacokinetics of acetaminophen in the human neonate: formation of acetaminophen glucuronide and sulfate in relation to plasma bilirubin concentration and d-glucaric acid excretion. Pediatrics. 1975;55:818–25.

64. Alam SN et al. Age-related differences in salicylamide and acetaminophen conjugation in man. J Pediatr. 1977;90:130–35.

65. Rane A, Wilson JT. Clinical pharmacokinetics in infants and children. Clin Pharmacokinet. 1976;1:2–24.

66. Hall K et al. First-dose and steady-state pharmacokinetics of valproic acid in children with seizures. Clin Pharmacokinet. 1983;8:447–55.

67. Furlanut M et al. Carbamazepine and carbamazepine-10, 11-epoxide serum concentrations in epileptic children. J Pediatr. 1985;106:491–95.

68. Szefler SJ et al. Rapid elimination of quinidine in pediatric patients. Pediatrics. 1982;70:370–75.

69. Levy G. Salicylate pharmacokinetics in the human neonate. In: Morselli PL et al., eds. Basic and Therapeutic Aspects of Perinatal Pharmacology. New York: Raven Press; 1975:319–30.

70. Richens A. Clinical pharmacokinetics of phenytoin. Clin Pharmacokinet. 1979;4:153–69.

71. Chiba K et al. Michaelis-Menten pharmacokinetics of diphenylhydantoin and application in the pediatric age patient. J Pediatr. 1980;96:479–84.

72. Weinberger MM, Ginchansky E. Dose-dependent kinetics of theophylline disposition in asthmatic children. J Pediatr. 1977;91:820–24.

73. Hook JB, Bailie MD. Perinatal renal pharmacology. Ann Rev Pharmacol Toxicol. 1979;19:491–509.

74. Jose PA et al. Intrarenal blood flow distribution in canine puppies. Pediatr Res. 1971;5:335–44.

75. Kleinmann LI, Reuter JH. Maturation of glomerular blood flow distribution in the newborn dog. J Physiol. 1973;228:91–3.

76. Barnett HL. Kidney function in young infants. Pediatrics. 1950;5:171–79.

77. Rubin MI et al. Maturation of renal function in childhood: clearance studies. J Clin Invest. 1949;2887:1144–162.

78. Guignard JP et al. Glomerular filtration rate in the first three weeks of life. J Pediatr. 1975;87:268–72.

79. Siegel SR, Oh W. Renal function as a marker of human fetal maturation. Acta Paediatr Scand. 1976;65:481–85.

80. Szefler SJ et al. Relationship of gentamicin serum concentrations to gestational age in pre-term and term neonates. J Pediatr. 1980;97:312–15.

81. Zarowitz BJM et al. High gentamicin trough concentrations in neonates of less than 28 weeks gestational age. Dev Pharmacol Ther. 1982;5:68–75.

82. Arant BS. Developmental patterns of renal functional maturation compared in the human neonate. J Pediatr. 1978;92:705–12.

83. Dauber IM et al. Renal failure following perinatal anoxia. J Pediatr. 1976;88:851–55.

84. Mirhij NJ et al. Effects of hypoxemia upon aminoglycoside serum pharmacokinetics in animals. Antimicrob Agents Chemother. 1978;14:344–47.

85. Guignard JP et al. Renal function in respiratory distress syndrome. J Pediatr. 1976;88:845–50.

86. Milner RDG et al. Tissue gentamicin concentrations in the newborn and adult rat. Pediatr Res. 1979;13:161–66.

87. Marre R et al. Age-dependent nephrotoxicity and the pharmacokinetics of gentamicin in rats. Eur J Pediatr. 1980;133:25–9.

88. Heimann G. Renal toxicity of aminoglycosides in the neonatal period. Pediatr Pharmacol. 1983;3:251–57.

89. Krauer B. The development of diurnal variation in drug kinetics in the human infant. In: Morselli PL et al., eds. Basic and Therapeutic Aspects of Perinatal Pharmacology. New York: Raven Press; 1975:347–56.

90. Gorodischer R et al. Renal clearance of digoxin in young infants. Res Commun Chem Pathol Pharmacol. 1977;16:363–74.

91. Siber GR et al. Predictability of peak serum gentamicin concentration with dosage based on body surface area. J Pediatr. 1978;94:135–38.

92. Levy J et al. Disposition of tobramycin in patients with cystic fibrosis: a prosective, controlled study. J Pediatr. 1984;105:117–24.

93. Alvan G et al. Increase renal clearance and increased diuretic efficiency of furosemide in cystic fibrosis. Clin Pharmacol Ther. 1988;44:436–41.

94. deGroot R et al. Pharmacokinetics of ticarcillin in patients with cystic fibrosis: a controlled prospective study. Clin Pharmacol Ther. 1990;47:73–8.

95. Knoppert DC et al. Cystic fibrosis: enhanced theophylline metabolism may be linked to the disease. Clin Pharmacol Ther. 1988;44:254–64.

96. Dove AM et al. Altered predisolone pharmacokinetics in patients with cystic fibrosis. Am Rev Resp Dis. 1990;141:487. Abstract.

97. Mirkin BL. Ontogenesis of the adrenergic nervous system: functional and pharmacologic implications. Fed Proc. 1973;31:65–73.

98. Pappano AJ. Ontogenic development of autonomic neuroeffector transmission and transmitter reactivity in embryonic and fetal hearts. Pharmacol Rev. 1977;29:3–33.

99. Duckles SP, Banners W. Changes in vascular smooth muscle reactivity during development. Ann Rev Pharmacol Toxicol. 1984;24:65–83.

100. Boerus LO. Drug-receptor interactions and biologic maturation. In: Mirkin BL, ed. Clinical Pharmacology and Therapeutics. Chicago: Year Book Medical Publishers Inc.; 1978:3–22.

101. Schweiler GH et al. Postnatal development of autonomic efferent innervation in the rabbit. Am J Physiol. 1970;219:391–97.

102. Hayashi S, Toda N. Age-related alterations in the response of rabbit tracheal smooth muscle to agents. J Pharmacol Exp Ther. 1980;214:675–81.

103. Kearin M et al. Digoxin "receptors" in neonates: an explanation of less sensitivity to digoxin than in adults. Clin Pharmacol Ther. 1980;28:346–49.

104. Andersson KE et al. Post-mortem distribution and tissue concentrations of digoxin in infants and adults. Acta Paediatr Scand. 1975;64:497–504.

105. Gorodischer R et al. Tissue and erythrocyte distribution of digoxin in infants. Clin Pharmacol Ther. 1976;19:256–63.

106. Wagner JG et al. Determination of myocardial and serum digoxin concentrations in children by specific and nonspecific assay methods. Clin Pharmacol Ther. 1983;33:577–84.

107. Koren G et al. Significance of the endogenous digoxin-like substance in infants and mothers. Clin Pharmacol Ther. 1984;36:759–64.

108. Williams LT et al. Identification of beta-adrenergic receptors in human lymphocytes by (–)(^{3}H)-alprenolol binding. J Clin Invest. 1976;57:149–55.

109. Conolly ME, Greenacre JK. The beta-adrenoceptor of the human lymphocyte and human lung parenchyma. Br J Pharmacol. 1977;59:17–23.

110. Feldman RD et al. Alterations in leukocyte beta-receptor affinity with aging. N Engl J Med. 1984;310:815–19.

111. Halkin H et al. Steady state serum digoxin concentration in relation to digitalis toxicity in neonates and infants. Pediatrics. 1978;61:184–88.

112. Ebara H et al. Digoxin- and digitoxin-like immunoreactive substances in amniotic fluid, cord blood, and serum of neonates. Pediatr Res. 1986;20:28–31.

113. Seccombe DW et al. Perinatal changes in a digoxin-like immunoreactive substance. Pediatr Res. 1984;18:1097–99.

114. Phelps SJ et al. Effect of age and serum creatinine on endogenous digoxin-like substances in infants and children. J Pediatr. 1987;110:136–39.

115. Wettrell G, Andersson KE. Absorption of digoxin in infants. Eur J Clin Pharmacol. 1975;9:49–55.

116. Greenblatt DJ et al. Bioavailability of digoxin tablets and elixir in the fasting and postprandial states. Clin Pharmacol Ther. 1974;16:444–48.

117. Reuning RH et al. Role of pharmacokinetics in drug dosage adjustment. I. Pharmacologic effect kineties and apparent volume of distribution of digoxin. J Clin Pharmacol. 1973;13:127–41.

118. Wettrell G, Andersson DE. Clinical pharmacokinetics of digoxin in infants. Clin Pharmacokinet. 1977;2:17–31.

119. Gorodischer R et al. Serum protein binding of digoxin in newborn infants. Res Commun Chem Pathol Pharmacol. 1974;9:387–90.

120. Koren G et al. Agonal elevation in serum digoxin concentrations in infants and children long after cessation of therapy. Crit Care Med. 1988;16:793–95.

121. Iisalo E, Ruikka I. Serum levels and renal excretion of digoxin in elderly. A comparison between three different preparations. Acta Med Scand. 1974;196:59–63.

122. Wettrell G. Distribution and elimination of digoxin in infants. Eur J Clin Pharmacol. 1977;11:329–35.

123. Ito S et al. Digoxin clearance and serum beta-2-microglobulin in neonates. J Pediatr. 1989;115:478–82.

124. Hernandez A et al. Pharmacodynamics of ^{3}H-digoxin in infants. Pediatrics. 1969;44:418–28.

125. Fazio A. Fab fragments in the treatment of digoxin overdose: pediatric considerations. South Med J. 1987;80:1553–556.

126. Hendeles L et al. A clinical and pharmacokinetic basis for the selection and use of slow release theophylline products. Clin Pharmacokinet. 1984;9:95–135.

127. Hill MR et al. The consistency of absorption from a sustained-release formulation in asthmatic children. Pharmacother. 1988;8:277–83.

128. Sallent J et al. Bioavailability of a slow release theophylline capsule given twice daily to preschool children with asthma: comparison with liquid theophylline. Pediatr. 1988;88:116–20.

129. Dederich RA et al. Intrasubject variation in sustained-release theophylline absorption. J Allergy Clin Immunol. 1981;67:465–71.

130. Pollack GM et al. Comparison of inter- and intrasubject variation in oral absorption of theophylline from sustained-release products. Int J Pharmac. 1984;21:3–16.

131. Pedersen S. Delay in the absorption rate of theophylline from a sustained-release theophylline preparation caused by food. Br J Clin Pharmacol. 1981;12:904–5.

132. Thompson PJ et al. Slow release theophylline in patients with airways obstruction with particular reference to the effects of food upon serum levels. Br J Dis Chest. 1983;77:293–98.

133. Scott PH et al. Sustained-release theophylline for childhood asthma: evidence for circadian variation of theophylline pharmacokinetics. J Pediatr. 1981;99:476–79.

134. Rogers RJ et al. Inconsistent absorption from a sustained-release theophylline preparation during continuous therapy in asthmatic children. J Pediatr. 1985;106:496–501.

135. Smolensky MH et al. Clinical relevance of theophylline chronokinetics for asthmatic children. Prog Clin Biol Res. 1987;227B:259–70.

136. Mitenko PA, Ogilvie RI. Pharmacokinetics of intravenous theophylline. Clin Pharmacol Ther. 1973;14:509–13.

137. Aranda JV et al. Pharmacokinetic aspects of theophylline in premature newborns. N Engl J Med. 1976;295:413–16.

138. Vallner JJ et al. Effect of pH on the binding of theophylline to serum proteins. Am Rev Respir Dis. 1979;120:83–6.

139. Sarrazin E et al. Dose-dependent kinetics for theophylline: observations among ambulatory asthmatic children. J Pediatr. 1980;97:825–26.

140. Efthimiou H et al. Influence of chronic dosing on theophylline clearance. Br J Clin Pharmacol. 1984;17:525–30.

141. Jenne JW et al. Pharmacokinetics of theophylline application to adjustment of the clinical dose of aminophylline. Clin Pharmacol Ther. 1972;13:349–60.

142. Hendeles L, Weinberger M. Theophylline—a "state of the art" review. Pharmacotherapy. 1983;3:2–44.

143. Grygiel JJ, Birkett DJ. Effect of age on patterns of theophylline metabolism. Clin Pharmacol Ther. 1980;28:456–62.
144. Gilman JT et al. Factors influencing theophylline disposition in 179 newborns. Ther Drug Monit. 1986;8:4–10.
145. Moore ES et al. The population pharmacokinetics of theophylline in neonates and young infants. J Pharmacokinet Biopharm. 1989;17:47–66.
146. Kolsky GB et al. The use of theophylline clearance in pediatric status asthmaticus. AJDC. 1987;141:282–87.
147. Dajani AS, Kauffman RE. The renaissance of chloramphenicol. Pediatr Clin North Am. 1981;28:195–202.
148. Smith AL, Weber A. Pharmacology of chloramphenicol. Pediatr Clin North Am. 1983;30:209–36.
149. Kauffman RE et al. Pharmacokinetics of chloramphenicol and chloramphenicol succinate in infants and children. J Pediatr. 1981;98:315–20.
150. Koup JR et al. Chloramphenicol succinate kinetics in *Macaca nemestrina:* dose dependency study. J Pharmacol Exp Ther. 1981;219:316–20.
151. Glazer JP et al. Disposition of chloramphenicol in low birth weight infants. Pediatrics. 1980;66:573–78.
152. Nahata MC, Powell DA. Comparative bioavailability and pharmacokinetics of chloramphenicol after intravenous chloramphenicol succinate in premature and older patients. Dev Pharmacol Ther. 1983;6:23–2.
153. Rajchgot P et al. Chloramphenicol pharmacokinetics in the newborn. Dev Pharmacol Ther. 1983;6:305–14.
154. Glazko AJ et al. Physical factors affecting the rate of absorption of chloramphenicol esters. Antibiot Chemother. 1958;8:516–27.
155. Kauffman RE et al. Relative bioavailability of intravenous chloramphenicol succinate and oral chloramphenicol palmitate in infants and children. J Pediatr. 1981;99:963–67.
156. Tuomanen EI et al. Oral chloramphenicol in the treatment of *Haemophilus influenza* meningitis. J Pediatr. 1981;99:968–74.
157. Shankaran S, Kauffman RE. Use of chloramphenicol palmitate in neonates. J Pediatr. 1984;105:113–16.
158. Slaughter RL et al. Chloramphenicol sodium succinate kinetics in critically ill patients. Clin Pharmacol Ther. 1980;28:69–77.
159. Sack CM et al. Chloramphenicol succinate kinetics in infants and young children. Pediatr Pharmacol. 1982;2:93–103.
160. Sack CM et al. Chloramphenicol pharmacokinetics in infants and young children. Pediatrics. 1980;66:579–84.
161. Friedman CA et al. Chloramphenicol disposition in infants and children. J Pediatr. 1979;95:1071–77.
162. Pickering LK et al. Clinical pharmacology of two chloramphenicol preparations in children: sodium succinate (iv) and palmitate (oral) esters. J Pediatr. 1980;96:757–61.
163. Yogev R et al. Pharmacokinetic comparisons of intravenous and oral chloramphenicol in patients with *Haemophilus influenzae* meningitis. Pediatrics. 1981;67:656–60.
164. Black SB et al. The necessity for monitoring chloramphenicol levels when treating neonatal meningitis. J Pediatr. 1978;92:235–36.
165. Shirkey HC. Drug dosage for infants and children. JAMA. 1965;193:105–8.
166. Bartels H. Drug therapy in childhood: what has been done and what has to be done. Pediatr Pharmacol. 1983;3:131–43.
167. Leach RH, Wood BSB. Drug dosage for children. Lancet. 1967;2:1350–351.
168. Butler AM, Richie RH. Simplification and improvement in estimating drug dosage and fluid and dietary allowances for patients of varying sizes. N Engl J Med. 1960;262:903–8.
169. Stickler GB. Drug dosage: a review of the problem in pediatrics. Clin Pediatr. 1964;3:574–77.
170. Gill MA, Ueda CT. Novel method for the determination of pediatric dosages. Am J Hosp Pharm. 1976;33:389–92.
171. Colburn WA, Gibson DM. Composite pharmacokinetic profiling. J Pharm Sci. 1984;73:1667–669.

172. Levy J, Kolski GB. The use of theophylline clearance in pediatric status astmaticus. II. The choice of appropriate dose for the intravenous theophylline infusion. AJDC. 1987;141:288–91.

173. Grasela TH, Donn SM. Neonatal population pharmacokinetics of phenobarbital derived from routine clinical data. Dev Pharmacol Ther. 1985;8:374–83.

174. Drusano GL e tal. An evaluation of optimal sampling strategy and adaptive study design. Clin Pharmacol Ther. 1988;44:232–38.

175. Reinberg A et al. Aspects of chronopharmacology and chronotherapy in pediatrics. Prog Clin Biol Res. 1987;227B:249–58.

176. Muir KT et al. Improved high-performance liquid chromatographic assay for theophylline in plasma and saliva in the presence of caffeine and its metabolites and comparisons with three other assays. J Chromatogr. 1982;231:73–82.

177. deLemos RA, Kuehl TJ. Animal models for evaluation of drugs for use in the mature and immature newborn. Pediatr. 1987;79:275–80.

178. Metzler CM, DeHaan RM. A computer study of sampling plans for blood level studies in children. Clin Pharmacol Ther. 1971;12:296A.

179. Colburn WA, Ehrenkrauz RA. Pharmacokinetics of a single intramuscular injection of vitamin E to premature neonates. Pediatr Pharmacol. 1983;3:7–14.

180. Janicke DM et al. Developmental pharmacokinetics of mezlocillin in newborn infants. J Pediatr. 1984;104:773–81.

181. Done AK et al. Pediatric clinical pharmacology and the "therapeutic orphan." Ann Rev Pharmacol Toxicol. 1977;17:561–73.

182. Cohen SN, Kauffman RE. Progress in drug therapy for children. Pediatr Clin North Am. 1981;28:1–240.

183. Berlin CM. Advances in pediatric pharmacology and toxicology. In: Barness LA, ed. Advances in Pediatrics. Chicago:Year Book Medical Publishers Inc.;1983:30:221–48.

184. Roberts RJ. Drug Therapy in Infants: Pharmacologic Principles and Clinical Experience. Philadelphia:WB Saunders; 1984.

185. MacLeod SM, Radde, eds. Textbook of Pediatric Clinical Pharmacology. Littleton:PSG Publishing Co., Inc., 1985.

186. Parsons WD et al. Elimination of transplacentally acquired caffeine in full term neonates. Pediatr Res. 1976;10:333A.

187. Sereni F, Principi N. Developmental pharmacology. Ann Rev Pharmacol. 1968;8:453–66.

188. Garrettson LK, Jusko WJ. Diphenylhydantoin elimination kinetics in overdosed children. Clin Pharmacol Ther. 1975;17:48–91.

189. Garrettson LK, Dayton PG. Disappearance of phenobarbital and diphenylhydantoin from serum of children. Clin Pharmacol Ther. 1970;116:674–79.

190. Jalling B. Plasma concentrations of phenobarbital in the treatment of seizures in newborns. Acta Paediatr Scand. 1975;64:514-524.

191. Hoppel C et al. Kinetics of phenytoin and carbamazepine in the newborn. In: Morselli PL et al., eds. Basic and Therapeutic Aspects of Perinatal Pharmacology. New York: Raven Press; 1975:341–45.

192. Reynolds JW, Mirkin DL. Urinary corticosteroid and diphenylhydantoin metabolite patterns in neonates exposed to anticonvulsant drugs *in utero*. Clin Pharmacol Ther. 1973;14:891–97.

193. Loughnan PM et al. Pharmacokinetic analysis of the disposition of intravenous theophylline in young children. J Pediatr. 1976;88:874–79.

194. Steiness E et al. Plasma digoxin after parenteral administration. Local reaction after intramuscular injection. Clin Pharmacol Ther. 1974;16:430–34.

195. Stone JA, Soldin SI. An update on digoxin. Clin Chem. 1989;35:1326–331.

196. Roberts RJ. Intravenous administration of medication in pediatric patients: problems and solutions. Pediatr Clin North Am. 1981;28:23–34.

197. Ellis EF et al. Pharmacokinetics of theophylline in children with asthma. Pediatrics. 1976;58:542–47.

198. Gal P et al. The influence of asphyxia on phenobarbitol dosing requirements in neonates. Dev Pharmacol Ther. 1984;7:145–52.

Chapter 11

Special Pharmacokinetic Considerations in the Obese

Robert A. Blouin and Mary H.H. Chandler

Before the mid-1970s, little was known about drug dosing in the obese patient population. Intuitively, the loading doses of drugs with polar characteristics were based on ideal body weight (IBW), while doses for compounds with high lipid partition coefficients (LPC) were based on actual weight in obese individuals. Since little was known about the influence of obesity on drug clearance, there were no guidelines for estimating maintenance doses. A familiar adage for that time was "when in doubt, be conservative." This empirical strategy may have been acceptable for the mildly obese patient. However, with the development of pharmacokinetic services, concerns were raised regarding the dosing of drugs with narrow therapeutic indices in the moderately to severely obese patient population. These observations stimulated several researchers to systematically evaluate the effect of obesity on the pharmacokinetics of drugs. This chapter reviews our current understanding of the effect obesity has on drug distribution and clearance and the clinical implications of these effects.

EPIDEMIOLOGY

Obesity is a serious problem for both children and adults in most industrialized countries despite recent trends toward weight-consciousness. According to the Report of the Second National Health and Nutrition Examination, approximately 26% of United States adults aged 20 to 75 years of age are overweight.[1] Others have estimated a higher prevalence of obesity in North America (United States and Canada): 45% to 50% of the adult population.[2] The percentage of people who are overweight also increases with age.[3] Morbidity and mortality increase with obesity,[4] and this poor prognosis is related to the increased incidence of hypertension, atherosclerosis, diabetes, and a variety of cancers. Consequently, the obese patient is more likely to require drug intervention much earlier in life and for a longer time than normal-weight patients. An awareness of drug disposition, particularly clearance, in the obese patient may be important to ensure appropriate drug therapy.

BODY WEIGHT PARAMETERS

Obesity is a condition characterized by an abnormally high percentage of body fat. Normally, 15% to 18% of a young male's body weight is composed of adipose tissue;[5] this percentage is slightly higher (20% to 25%) in females. Although somewhat arbitrary, obesity is frequently defined as body fat content greater than 25% and 30% of total body weight (TBW) for men and women, respectively. Accurate assessment of body fat content requires sophisticated or invasive techniques that are impractical for clinical use (e.g., whole body submersion, bioelectrical impedance, isotope or chemical dilution, measurement of the naturally occurring isotope of potassium). Numerous anthropometric approaches (e.g., the comparative measurements of the human body and its parts—usually height, weight, skinfold thickness, and wrist circumference) have been developed and correlated with body fat measurements in order to provide an indirect estimate of body fat content.[6] Although anthropometric measurements are easier to obtain, these approaches are usually restricted to research applications [e.g., Body Mass Index (BMI) = weight/height^2]. Consequently, it is difficult to obtain an accurate estimate of body fat content or obesity. Alternatively, the extent to which an individual is overweight (percent or fraction of excess body weight over "normal" for one's age, height, gender, and build) can be readily assessed using insurance actuary tables (e.g., Metropolitan Life Insurance)[7] or by arithmetic transformation of such data (e.g., method of Devine).[8] These approaches provide an assessment of an individual's ideal body weight (IBW) but not his or her fat free weight (TBW minus fat weight) or lean body mass (LBM). Although there are numerous limitations in employing this parameter, the simplicity of these methods has made them exceedingly popular in clinical practice and in the conduct of clinical pharmacokinetic studies.

To avoid confusion, we will first evaluate absolute differences between pharmacokinetic values in obese subjects and lean controls before these values have been standardized [i.e., corrected for body surface area (BSA), TBW, or IBW]. If absolute differences in these values are significant, the influence of various body measurements on the pharmacokinetic parameter can be assessed. This approach is recommended because "standardization" assumes that a linear relationship exists between total body weight or body surface area and a particular pharmacokinetic parameter. Few pharmacokinetic studies have been performed over a wide continuum of body weights, making the aforementioned assumption speculative at best. Nevertheless, the clinician must keep in mind that comparable pharmacokinetic values expressed in absolute terms will translate into marked differences in the weight-adjusted dose of medication administered to the obese patient.

ALLOMETRY AND OBESITY

The principles of allometry, the measure and study of the growth of a part in relation to the entire organism, are utilized to standardize drug dosing regimens on the basis of TBW or BSA. This practice is based upon a well defined relationship between body size (e.g., TBW, BSA), a physiologic function (e.g., cardiac output, liver or renal blood flow, glomerular filtration rate), and a pharmacokinetic parameter (e.g., clearance). Huxley[9] demonstrated a linear relationship between organ weight and body weight. Subsequently, several investigators demonstrated in mammals a linear correlation between the log of the weight[10] or function[11] of an organ and the log of body weight. The pharmacokinetic application of these principles occurred when a consistent relationship was observed between the renal clearance of urea, kidney weight, and body surface area in the rabbit.[12] Consequently, it was determined that a considerable portion of the interanimal variability in renal urea clearance could be explained by differences in BSA. These findings ultimately led to the procedure of standardizing renal clearance values to an idealized BSA of 1.73 m^2 in humans. Today, a drug's clearance (CL) and apparent volume of distribution (V_d) parameters are routinely standardized to body weight or surface area to minimize intersubject variability. The primary purpose of this chapter is to explore whether or not these fundamental allometric relationships are violated in the human obese population and to explore alternative strategies for drug dosing.

CLINICAL PHARMACOKINETICS

The evaluation and interpretation of existing pharmacokinetic data in the obese population are complicated by numerous factors. First, the etiology of obesity is rarely known in humans. It is extremely difficult to differentiate between genetic, nutritional, and hormonal factors as the sole cause of obesity in an individual. Limited work evaluating two etiologically distinct obese rodent models (genetic versus nutritional) demonstrates the importance of this issue relative to pharmacokinetic and/or toxicologic studies.[13] Second, the extent of obesity [i.e., mild, moderate, severe, or morbid (> 195% of IBW) obesity] may influence significantly the interpretation and clinical relevance of various studies. Although a systematic evaluation of physiologic differences between these obese subpopulations is lacking, it is likely that the severely obese and the morbidly obese groups (which represent a minority of the obese population) are different compared to their mildly or moderately obese counterparts. Third, obese individuals are predisposed to a number of different disease states (e.g., hypertension, diabetes, hypertriglyceridemia) which may complicate the interpretation of study results. Consequently, studies must be carefully controlled for age, disease, gender, and concomitant medications. Finally, inconsistencies in body weight measures (e.g., TBW, IBW, LBM, BMI, BSA) often make it difficult to compare and contrast studies. The reader is cautioned against making broad generalizations when interpreting such data and is encouraged to refer to several reviews on this topic.[3,14,15]

Absorption

Information about the effect of obesity on the bioavailability of drugs is scant; consequently, no generalizations can be made regarding this pharmacokinetic parameter in the overweight population. The absolute bioavailability of midazolam[16] and propranolol,[17] two relatively high-extraction compounds, was not significantly different in obese subjects compared to lean controls. The impact of body weight on cyclosporine bioavailability was evaluated in renal transplant recipients.[18] This study reported no significant effect of body weight on either the rate or extent of cyclosporine absorption.

An additional consideration in the morbidly obese population with respect to drug absorption is the potential effect gastric or jejunoileal bypass surgery may have on the rate and extent of drug absorption. As might be expected, little useful information is available on this topic. An early study evaluated antipyrine absorption in 17 obese patients 12 to 57 months following intestinal bypass surgery.[19] The investigators concluded that drug absorption and drug metabolizing capacity are unaffected by this surgical procedure.

Distribution

The rate and extent of drug distribution are determined by a number of factors including degree of tissue perfusion, tissue size, binding of drug to plasma proteins and tissue components, and permeability of tissue membranes.[20] Many of these factors will be governed by a drug's physical and chemical properties (e.g., degree of ionization, lipid solubility, polarity, molecular weight).[21] In general, the distribution of drugs can be influenced by various disease states and altered physiological conditions as a consequence of changes in vascular or tissue volume and plasma or tissue binding. Obesity is characterized by absolute increases in cardiac output,[22,23,24] blood volume,[22,23] organ mass,[25,26] LBM,[27] adipose tissue mass,[27] as well as changes in plasma binding constituents.[28,29] Thus, the distribution of many drugs may be significantly changed due to marked increases in TBW. These changes in the obese subpopulation could alter the loading dose, dosing interval, plasma half-life, and time to reach steady-state conditions.

Several studies have evaluated the impact of obesity on the volume of distribution of aqueous and lipid soluble compounds (see Table 11-1). As can be appreciated from Table 11-1, the benzodiazepines, thiopental, verapamil, and lidocaine showed the greatest difference between obese individuals and controls. Slightly to moderately higher values in obese subjects were reported for theophylline, the aminoglycosides, vancomycin, ibuprofen, prednisolone, and ifosfamide. In contrast, no significant differences were observed for digoxin, cimetidine, doxorubicin, cyclosporine, and procainamide. Propranolol's apparent volume of distribution has been shown to be increased[17] and decreased[55] as a consequence of obesity; these disparate observations are currently unexplainable.

Careful examination of the physical and chemical properties of these compounds indicates that lipid solubility plays the most important role in adipose tissue distribution.[64] Early work with the barbiturates clearly demonstrated the close relationship between lipid solubility and drug distribution. As the octanol/water

Table 11–1. Summary of Pharmacokinetic Parameters in Obesity[f]

Drug	Lean control						Obese						References
	Weight (kg) TBW	IBW	CL (mL/min)	Vd (L)	t½ (hr)	Free fraction (%)	Weight (kg) TBW	IBW	CL (mL/min)	Vd (L)	t½ (hr)	Free fraction (%)	
Acetaminophen	70.6	75.0	323.0[a]	77.0[a]	2.8	—	134.9[e]	73.0	484.0[e]	108.5[e]	2.6	—	30
	55.0	56.0	227.0[b]	51.6[b]	2.7	—	87.9[e]	57.0	312.0[e]	61.4[b]	2.3	—	
Alprazolam[d]	63.3	62.8	88.0	73.1	10.6	29.2	111.6[e]	62.0	66.4	113.5[e]	21.8[e]	30.3	31
Amikacin			—	—	—	—	166.5[c]	65.5	166.7	27.4[c]	2.1[c]	—	32
	72.4	71.9	99.2	18.6	2.2	—	147.3[c]	72.5	157.3[e]	26.8[c]	2.0	—	33
	58.5	56.7	83.2	13.4	1.8	—	132.0[e]	61.3	131.2[e]	22.1[c]	1.9	—	34
Antipyrine	62.5	64.7	47.6	39.7	10.7	—	100.3[e]	60.7	38.0	44.9	15.0[e]	—	35
Caffeine[d]	74.0	65.7	219.4	54.0	2.59	—	110.0[e]	73.0	355.4	103.3	4.37[e]	—	36
	64.0	—	112.0	43.6	5.4	—	109.0[e]	—	135.0	69.9[e]	7.2	—	37
Cefamandole	—	—	—	—	—	—	138.0[e]	59.0	275.0[e]	27.8	1.2	—	38
Cefotaxime	—	—	361.7[a]	30.0[a]	1.0[a]	—	—	—	411.7[a]	45.5[a]	1.1[a]	—	39
	—	—	264.8[b]	25.1[b]	1.1[b]	—	—	—	352.4[b]	42.9[b]	1.4[b]	—	
Cimetidine	64.0	64.6	579.0	106.0	2.1	—	113.0[e]	63.1	616.0	120.0	2.2	—	40
	62.0	—	637.0	—	1.9	—	140.0[c]	—	1147.0[c]	—	1.2	—	41
Cyclosporine	65.1	62.5	820.0	295.0	4.7	—	89.7[e]	63.2	719.0	229.0	4.4	—	18
Desmethyl-diazepam[d]	67.0	65.0	13.4	63.0	57.0	2.5	105.0[e]	62.0	13.2	159.0[e]	154.0[e]	2.4	42
Diazepam	60.4	63.3	27.3	90.7	40.0	1.3	101.1[e]	60.3	38.1[e]	291.9[e]	95.0[e]	1.5	35
	60.0	60.0	26.3	70.0	32.0	1.2	92.0[e]	62.6	32.1	228.0[e]	82.0[e]	1.4	43
	—	—	—	—	—	2.1	—	—	—	—	—	3.2	28
	78.4	—	—	—	—	1.5	108.0[e]	—	—	—	—	1.5	29
	78.4	—	—	—	—	1.5	129.0[e]	—	—	—	—	1.9[e]	
Digoxin	65.0	66.0	278.0	937.0	41.2	—	100.0[e]	61.7	328.0	981.0	35.6	—	44
Doxorubicin	66.0	—	1569.0	964.0	13.0	—	81.0[c]	—	891.0[e]	1119.0	20.4[e]	—	45

Table 11–1. Summary of Pharmacokinetic Parameters in Obesity[f] (cont.)

	Lean control						Obese						
Drug	**Weight (kg) TBW**	**IBW**	**CL (mL/min)**	**V$_d$ (L)**	**t½ (hr)**	**Free fraction (%)**	**Weight (kg) TBW**	**IBW**	**CL (mL/min)**	**V$_d$ (L)**	**t½ (hr)**	**Free fraction (%)**	**References**
Gentamicin	73.2	69.3	95.9	17.0	2.2	—	138.3[c]	68.7	135.8[e]	23.3[e]	2.2	—	33
	55.3	55.3	82.4	13.4	2.0	—	103.6[e]	59.2	128.0[c]	19.2[e]	1.8	—	46
Ibuprofen[b]	61.0	—	59.2	10.8	2.1	1.04	114.0[e]	—	83.2[e]	14.9[e]	2.0	1.07	47
Ifosfamide	64.2	64.3	72.2	33.7	5.0	—	76.8[e]	56.5	76.0	42.8[e]	6.4[e]	—	48
Lidocaine	69.0	74.2	1346.0	186.0[a]	1.6	—	124.0[e]	73.4	1427.0[a]	325.0[e]	2.7[e]	—	49
	59.0	57.8	1162.0	209.0[b]	2.1	—	96.0[e]	55.2	1089.0[b]	264.0[e]	3.0[e]	—	
Lorazepam	62.8	62.8	62.9	77.2	14.9	10.0	111.7[e]	62.5	102.0[e]	130.8[e]	16.5	10.1	50
Midazolam	65.7	69.5	530.0	114.0	2.7	3.5	116.5[e]	67.4	472.0	311.0[e]	8.4[e]	3.61	16
Nitrazepam[d]	63.0	—	66.8	137.0	23.9	17.9	107.0[e]	—	101.0[e]	290.0[e]	33.5[e]	19.7[e]	51
Oxazepam[d]	60.9	62.9	50.4	38.4	8.9	4.0	115.1[e]	63.5	156.8[e]	97.1[e]	7.7	5.1[e]	50
Phenytoin[d]	—	—	—	—	—	13.0	—	—	—	—	—	14.0	28
	78.4	—	—	—	—	11.3	108.0[e]	—	—	—	—	13.1	29
	78.4	—	—	—	—	11.3	129.0[e]	—	—	—	—	13.6	52
	67.0	72.8	39.0	40.2	12.0	14.7	124.0[e]	69.7[c]	59.0	82.2[e]	19.9[e]	13.7	53
Prednisolone	72.0	72.0	138.0	36.7	3.5	—	121.0[e]	74.0	185.0[e]	44.1	3.2	—	54
Procainamide	68.4	66.4	698.0	150.0	3.1	—	100.2[e]	63.1	862.0	158.0	2.5	—	17
Propranolol	66.8	63.8	780.0	198.0	3.0	9.9	136.5[e]	68.4	780.0	339.0[e]	5.0[e]	8.9	55
	66.7	—	1265.0	341.0	3.1	11.7	110.3[e]	—	958.0[e]	234.0[e]	3.5	9.9	28
	—	—	—	—	—	12.3	—	—	—	—	—	8.6[e]	29
	78.4	—	—	—	—	12.3	108.0[e]	—	—	—	—	12.2	
	78.4	—	—	—	—	12.3	129.0[e]	—	—	—	—	9.7[e]	

Drug													Ref.
Theophylline	—	—	—	—	—	—	114.3	61.9	65.5	—	—	—	56
	—	—	—	—	—	—	159.5	66.0	51.9	—	—	—	57
	56.7	62.9	39.5	26.9	8.4	—	91.8[c]	55.2	52.2	28.5	7.4	—	58
	61.5	—	38.7	—	6.0	—	100.5[c]	59.1	60.3	46.2	8.6[e]	20.0	59
Thiopental	57.4	73.0	198.0	111.9	6.3	20.0	137.9[c]	—	416.0[e]	1095.0[c]	27.9[e]	20.0	60
Tobramycin	71.0	69.5	101.3	18.3	2.1	—	124.5[c]	55.7	137.1	24.5[c]	2.0[c]	—	61
	58.1	58.1	108.0	17.0	1.9	—	151.1[c]	70.3	162.4[e]	29.0[e]	1.9	—	33
	—	—	—	—	—	—	85.2[e]	52.9	125.0[c]	19.2[e]	1.8	—	46
Triazolam[d]	64.2	63.9	531.2	115.5	2.6	22.2	119.7[e]	63.8	340.2[e]	116.7	4.1[e]	20.9	31
Vancomycin	74.6	72.7	80.8	33.2	4.8	—	165.7[c]	63.5	187.5[e]	50.1[c]	3.2[c]	—	62
Verapamil	—	—	1003.0	310.0	—	—	—	—	994.0	858.0[e]	—	—	63

[a] Male.
[b] Female.
[c] Statistical significance not available.
[d] Oral data.
[e] Statistically significant (obese versus control).
[f] Originally published in Clin Pharm. 1987;6:706–714, American Society of Hospital Pharmacists, Inc. All rights reserved. Reprinted and updated with permission.

lipid partition coefficient (LPC) of the various barbituric acid derivatives increased, a corresponding increase in the distribution into adipose tissue was observed.[3] Consequently, the extent to which obesity influences the volume of distribution of a drug will principally depend on its lipid solubility (octanol/water LPC). The most marked difference in drug distribution values noted to date are for thiopental and diazepam. Their volumes of distribution are 9.8 and 3.2 times higher in obese subjects (see Table 11-1) which corresponds to their very high *in vitro* octanol/water LPCs of 676[65] and 309,[66] respectively. A somewhat unexpected finding was made with the drug cyclosporine.[18] Since cyclosporine is a highly lipophilic compound exhibiting a relatively high volume of distribution in normal-weight individuals (4 L/kg), obesity would be expected to increase this drug's volume of distribution. However, two independent observations have demonstrated that cyclosporine's volume of distribution is best predicted from IBW.[18,67]

The volume of distribution values for the polar compounds, theophylline and aminoglycosides, were shown to be only slightly higher in obese subjects, consistent with their relatively low LPC values (1.0[21] and 0.1,[21] respectively). However, the clinical importance of these compounds has generated considerable interest in the development of methods to predict their volume of distribution. Numerous approaches have been proposed for theophylline.[57,59] Rizzo et al.[68] suggested the following "power" equation to predict the volume of distribution of theophylline in obese patients:

$$V_d \text{ in liters} = 1.29 \text{ TBW}^{0.74} \qquad\qquad \text{(Eq. 11-1)}$$

Their findings are in general agreement with the view of several other authors that the distribution volume for theophylline is inadequately predicted by either TBW or IBW (see Table 11-1). In contrast, the method used to predict the volume of distribution for the aminoglycoside antibiotics is generally agreed upon (see Equation 11-2 below).[46,61]

$$V_d \text{ in liters} = (0.26 \text{ L/kg}) [(IBW) + (CF \times AW)]^{32} \qquad \text{(Eq. 11-2)}$$

where, CF (correction factor) = 0.2 to 0.5; AW (adipose weight) = TBW − IBW. We have found a CF of 0.4 to work best in most of our obese patients.

Although LPC values provide some insight into the clinical consequences of obesity on volume of distribution for most drugs, there are several notable exceptions including digoxin and procainamide (see Table 11-1). The distribution of these two compounds is not significantly influenced by obesity despite their relatively high octanol/water LPC (17.8[21] and 58.9,[65] respectively). As Christoff et al.[54] pointed out, procainamide and digoxin have partition coefficients that indicate a high lipid affinity and the ability to penetrate lipophilic barriers; however, they are too low to enhance distribution into adipose tissue. Pharmacokinetic data corroborate early tissue distribution studies which suggest limited distribution of digoxin into adipose tissue.[69] Figure 11-1 demonstrates the comparable digoxin plasma concentration versus time profiles following intravenous administration to an obese and normal-weight subject.

   Ritschel and Kahl[21] recognized the limitations of using only partition coefficients to predict the impact of obesity on drug distribution. They therefore used
multiple factors (i.e., LPC, plasma protein binding, ionization, normal-weight
volume of distribution, and body weight parameters) to predict the volume of
distribution of drugs in the obese population. Based on retrospective literature data,
they developed four different equations, the application of each to be determined
by the physical and chemical properties of the drug. These equations represent a
unique approach to the prediction of apparent volumes of distribution in obese
patients. However, they have not been critically validated and should be used
cautiously. A further limitation is the poor availability of physical and chemical
characteristics for many drugs.

   Serum protein binding is an important determinant of drug disposition and a
critical factor in the correct interpretation of plasma concentration data [see
Chapter 5: Influence of Protein Binding and Use of Unbound (Free) Drug Con-
centrations]. Consequently, an appreciation of the effect obesity has on this
parameter is important for the appropriate development of therapeutic drug
monitoring strategies in this population. A variety of pathophysiologic conditions
exist in obese individuals which, theoretically, could alter the binding of drugs.
Most important, the affinity or capacity of proteins principally responsible for drug
binding [i.e., albumin, α_1-acid glycoprotein (AAG) and lipoproteins] may be
altered.

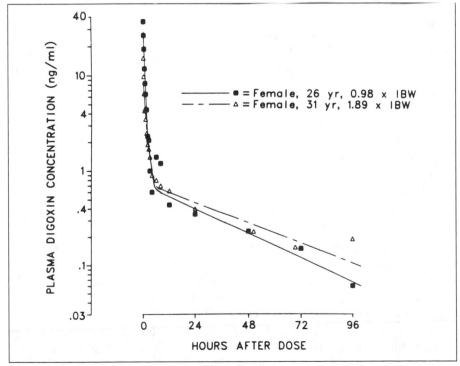

Figure 11-1. *Plasma digoxin concentration following intravenous administration to an obese
and normal-weight subject (reproduced with permission from Am Heart J. 1981;102:740–44).*

Albumin is considered the major protein to which acidic drugs are bound. Studies have shown that serum albumin and total protein were essentially unaltered in both moderately and morbidly obese subjects.[28] Consequently, the serum protein binding of drugs principally bound to albumin (e.g., phenytoin, thiopental) appears to be unchanged in the obese state. A modest, but statistically significant higher value of the percent free of diazepam[28,29] (1.9 versus 1.5), nitrazepam[15] (19.7 versus 17.9), and oxazepam[50] (5.1 versus 4.0) may be attributed to elevations in serum free fatty acids found in obese patients which subsequently could displace these drugs from their albumin binding sites.[70] Benedek et al.[28,29] suggest that an elevation in the free fraction of diazepam may be present only in extremely obese individuals.

AAG is an important binding site for basic drugs and accounts for most of the variability observed in the free fraction of these drugs. The effect of obesity on AAG and the protein binding of representative drugs is controversial. Benedek et al.[29] observed a twofold higher serum concentration of AAG in obese groups (112 and 136.4 mg/dL in intermediately and extremely obese individuals) vis-a-vis a control group (55.1 mg/dL). This corresponded to a significantly lower free fraction of propranolol in the extremely obese group (9.3 and 12.3 in obese and lean groups, respectively). In contrast, Cheymol et al.[55] observed that the AAG concentrations and the percentage of protein binding of propranolol in a group of obese subjects were similar to normal-weight controls. Unexpectedly, these authors observed a lower volume of distribution value for propranolol, a finding more consistent with increased plasma protein binding. The protein binding of verapamil, a drug known to be associated with AAG, was unaffected by obesity.[63] These discrepancies require further investigation.

Protein binding for drugs which are extensively bound to lipoproteins may also be altered in the obese population since plasma cholesterol and triglyceride levels are often elevated in this group. However, the consequence of these elevations on drugs bound to serum lipoproteins is presently unknown.

The point is frequently made that the clearance of a compound is a much more reliable parameter than is the half-life for evaluating the elimination of a drug. This is because half-life is dependent on both CL and V_d as represented by Equation 11-3.

$$t\frac{1}{2} = \frac{(V_d)(0.693)}{CL}$$

(Eq. 11-3)

The dependency of half-life on the volume of distribution of a drug is no better illustrated than with the drugs thiopental,[60] diazepam,[35,43] and desmethyldiazepam (see Table 11-1).[42] The clearance of desmethyldiazepam is unchanged as a consequence of obesity (13.2 mL/min versus 13.4 mL/min in obese versus controls); however, obese subjects exhibited prolonged plasma half-life values relative to the control group (154 hours versus 57 hours, respectively). Thus, desmethyldiazepam's extended half-life in obese subjects can be attributed to the markedly higher volume of distribution values in the obese versus the control group (159 L versus 63 L, respectively) rather than differences in the clearance values. Figure 11-2 further illustrates this point. In this example, an obese individual has the same AUC or absolute systemic clearance following a diazepam 10 mg intravenous dose compared to that of a normal-weight control. Despite similar systemic clearance values, a significant prolongation in the plasma half-life secondary to an increase in the apparent volume of distribution was observed in the obese individual. However, it will take the obese patient longer to reach steady state or reach a drug-free condition if the drug is discontinued.

Metabolism

The liver plays an important role in the metabolism of numerous xenobiotics and endogenous substances, and pathophysiologic changes associated with obesity may influence the metabolism of many of these compounds. In general, fatty infiltration characterizes the livers of most obese individuals,[71] and the degree to which this occurs appears to be proportional to the extent of obesity. Occasionally, these changes are indistinguishable from a mild alcoholic hepatitis.[71] This scenario is exaggerated greatly in the morbidly obese patient.[6]

The influence of pathophysiologic and morphologic changes associated with obesity on hepatic metabolism is not well understood. Studies correlating obesity-associated histologic changes with either hepatic drug metabolizing enzymes (e.g., hepatic cytochrome P450) or drug markers (e.g., antipyrine) are nonexistent. However, studies that provide insight into fundamental mechanisms of drug

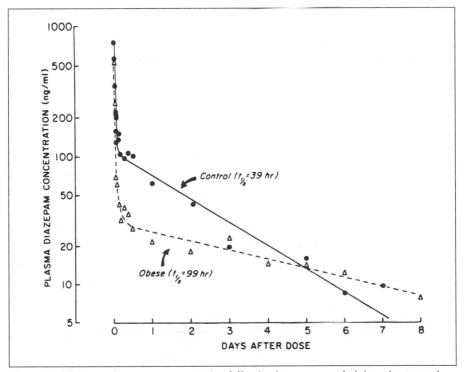

Figure 11-2. Plasma diazepam concentration following intravenous administration to an obese and normal-weight subject (reproduced with permission from J Clin Pharmacol. 1983;23:369–76).

metabolism in genetic[72-74] and nutritional[13,75-77] animal models may provide insight into the relationships between biochemical changes and pharmacokinetic parameters for compounds that are hepatically metabolized.

The influence of obesity on the pharmacokinetics of drugs which undergo either phase I or phase II metabolism has been studied extensively (see Table 11-2). The clearance for drugs undergoing phase I metabolism is increased or unchanged in the obese population. The absolute clearance for antipyrine, a drug frequently used as a marker compound to evaluate the mixed function oxidase system, was not significantly different in obese and non-obese subjects.[35] This observation is consistent with data on phenytoin,[52] caffeine,[36,37] and alprazolam.[31] In contrast, the absolute clearances of ibuprofen,[47] nitrazepam,[51] and prednisolone[53] are significantly higher in the obese population. In the case of prednisolone, the authors suggest that adipose tissue may represent a peripheral site of clearance. This is based on the presence of 11-hydroxysteroid dehydrogenase, the enzyme responsible for interconversion of prednisone and prednisolone, in adipose tissue.

Contradictory studies have been published regarding the influence of obesity on theophylline clearance.[56-59,68,78,79] Jusko et al.[78] and Gal et al.[59] recommend that theophylline maintenance dose be based on IBW since no significant change in clearance was observed between obese and lean subjects when IBW was used to standardize clearance values. In contrast, Blouin et al.[56] found a much stronger correlation between theophylline clearance and TBW than between clearance and IBW. Rohrbaugh et al.[57] also found no significant difference in theophylline clearance between obese and lean subjects when TBW was used to standardize clearance (35.9 ± 13.9 mL/kg/hr versus 42.1 ± 12.2 mL/kg/hr). Both of these studies indicate that larger absolute maintenance doses are necessary to achieve concentrations in the obese that are similar to those in lean patients. Slaughter and Lanc[58] studied theophylline clearance in obese patients in relation to smoking and congestive heart failure. They concluded that theophylline maintenance doses can be based on TBW in obese patients corroborating the findings of the latter two studies.[56,57] Rizzo et al.[68] found no improvement in predicting theophylline clearance when a power function was employed. In clinical practice, we have found an initial estimate for clearance of .035 L/kg (TBW)/hr to work best in many of our obese patients. Studies of caffeine metabolism suggest that obesity also has no significant effect on the oral clearance of this xanthine derivative.[36,37]

The effect of body weight on the elimination of cyclosporine, a low to intermediate clearance drug, was studied in 45 adult uremic candidates for renal transplantation.[18] No significant differences were observed between lean and obese

Table 11-2. *Effect of Human Obesity on Hepatic and Renal Elimination Processes[a]*

Hepatic		Renal	
Phase I	→ or ↑	Glomerular filtration	↑
Phase II	↑ glucuronidation	Tubular secretion	↑
	↑ sulfation		
	→ acetylation		

[a] ↑ = increased; → = No change.

subjects for any of the pharmacokinetic parameters evaluated (see Table 11-1). These authors recommend that cyclosporine dosage be based on IBW in the obese patient.

Drugs which are primarily biotransformed via hepatic phase II conjugation pathways (e.g., glucuronidation and sulfation) consistently demonstrate higher clearance in the obese. Abernethy et al.[50] studied the influence of obesity on glucuronidation pathways by evaluating the clearance of oxazepam and lorazepam, two benzodiazepines eliminated in the form of the glucuronide. The absolute clearance of oxazepam and lorazepam in obese subjects was, on average, 3.1 and 1.6 times greater, respectively, compared to lean controls. Consequently, clearance values for oxazepam (standardized for TBW) exceeded those of lean controls (1.39 ± 0.17 mL/min/kg versus 0.82 ± 0.08 mL/min/kg, respectively). In the case of lorazepam, standardized clearance values were similar in both groups (0.98 ± 0.12 mL/min/kg versus 1.00 ± 0.07 mL/min/kg). As a consequence of these findings, the authors concluded that maintenance doses of drugs biotransformed by glucuronidation should be increased approximately in proportion to TBW. Although no mechanism has been articulated, animal studies would suggest enhanced glucuronosyltransferase activity as a likely explanation.

Although not as dramatic, the absolute clearance for acetaminophen also was higher in obese men (484 mL/min versus 323 mL/min) and women (312 mL/min versus 227 mL/min) relative to lean controls.[30] In humans, acetaminophen is primarily eliminated as the glucuronide and sulfate conjugates.[80] Therefore, it is possible that obesity may preferentially affect some conjugation pathways over others (i.e., glucuronidation over sulfation or other minor phase II reactions). In contrast, salicylate[81] and procainamide[54] represent exceptions to this trend of enhanced conjugation pathways in the obese.[81] The oral clearance of salicylate, which is conjugated to the glycine, phenolic glucuronide and acyl glucuronide conjugates, was not significantly increased in obese subjects.[81] Additionally, Christoff et al.[54] demonstrated no difference in the acetylation of procainamide as a consequence of obesity. This further indicates that not all conjugation pathways may be enhanced in obesity.

The systemic clearance of drugs undergoing nonrestrictive drug clearance (i.e., those with high hepatic extraction values) are susceptible to changes in hepatic blood flow. Hemodynamic studies of obese patients indicate greater blood volume,[22,23] cardiac size,[22,23] cardiac output,[22,23] and splanchnic blood flow relative to lean controls.[22] However, no significant differences were observed in hepatic blood flow.[82] Pharmacokinetic studies of blood-flow dependent compounds following IV administration are consistent with this observation in that no significant differences in absolute clearances between obese and lean subjects have been noted.

Lidocaine, a highly extracted drug whose clearance closely parallels that of hepatic blood flow, was evaluated following a rapid intravenous infusion.[49] No significant differences in absolute lidocaine clearance were observed when obese men and women were compared to their lean control groups. Similar findings have been observed with verapamil.[63] These same authors[16] studied the disposition of the imidazobenzodiazepine derivative, midazolam, following oral and intravenous administration in obese and lean subjects. They reported no significant difference in absolute midazolam clearance (472 ± 38 mL/min versus 530 ± 34 mL/min) or systemic availability ($42 \pm 0.04\%$ versus $40 \pm 0.03\%$ between obese subjects and lean controls). The data for the beta blocker, propranolol, are contradictory.[17,55] Bowman et al.[17] observed no significant differences in the clearance or absolute bioavailability of propranolol in obese subjects versus lean controls. In contrast, Cheymol et al.[55] found significantly higher absolute systemic clearance values for propranolol as a consequence of obesity (1265 mL/min versus 950 mL/min in obese versus lean subjects). The basis for these discrepant results is unknown. The effect of body weight on the pharmacokinetics of doxorubicin (an intermediate to high clearance drug) was evaluated in 21 patients undergoing their initial course of chemotherapy.[45] Similar to other drugs in this category, no significant changes in absolute clearance values were observed in obese or lean subjects. Available pharmacokinetic data suggest that the absolute clearance of highly extracted compounds is not significantly affected by obesity. Consequently, obese patients should receive intravenous and oral maintenance doses of these highly extracted compounds based on IBW, not TBW.

The effect of obesity on hepatic drug clearance varies greatly from substrate to substrate, but the reasons for this are not understood. Consequently, obese animal models have been used to examine the biochemical and molecular basis of drug metabolism as a function of obesity,[13] and it appears that the overfed rat model may yield considerable insight into such mechanisms. Although these animals showed no significant difference in the concentration of total hepatic cytochrome P450 compared to lean controls, the obese animals had substantially higher absolute amounts of cytochrome P450 per liver.[13] In addition, a strong linear relationship ($r = 0.84$, $p < 0.001$) was observed between total body mass and total hepatic cytochrome P450. Increased oxidative capacity may have played an important role in the predisposition of these obese animals to liver toxicity following acetaminophen overdose[76] and exposure to halogenated anesthetics[83] since these toxicities are believed to be mediated by highly reactive metabolites formed by the cytochrome P450 mixed function oxidase system. Salazar et al.[77] recently reported that the ethanol-inducible isoenzyme of the P450 system (P4502E1), which is responsible for microsomal ethanol oxidation and the oxidative metabolism of acetaminophen and halothane, is markedly elevated in the livers of these obese, overfed rodents. The clinical implications of these toxicologic findings will require further evaluation.

Renal Excretion

The main role of the kidney is to excrete metabolic waste products and excess water. Renal clearance arises from one or more processes: glomerular filtration, tubular secretion, and tubular reabsorption. In addition, several physiologic factors influence renal function such as effective renal plasma flow, urine flow rate, and urine pH (see Chapter 8: Influence of Renal Disease on Pharmacokinetics).

Physiological changes associated with obesity may alter these processes and influence renal drug clearance (see Table 11-2). In addition, the kidney has been shown to increase in size in relation to changes in TBW and BSA.[12,25,84]

The majority of studies has focused on the effect of obesity on glomerular filtration rate (GFR). Stockholm et al.[85] reported that GFR, as determined by ^{51}Cr-EDTA plasma clearance, was significantly elevated in obese women relative to their lean counterparts (129 mL/min versus 103.5 mL/min), and this increase was positively correlated with both the plasma cortisol concentration and the urinary excretion rate of free cortisol. In a subsequent study by these same investigators,[86] a significant reduction in GFR occurred following jejunoileal bypass surgery and body weight reduction (129 mL/min versus 100 mL/min pre- and post-surgery). They concluded that obesity was responsible for the observed elevation in absolute GFR values. Similarly, Dionne et al.[87] revealed considerably higher creatinine clearance (CL_{cr}) values in 33 morbidly obese patients compared to historical controls. These higher GFR values were positively correlated with both TBW and BSA.

Several studies have evaluated the pharmacokinetics of renally excreted drugs. Absolute clearance values for drugs dependent upon glomerular filtration (e.g., vancomycin,[62] aminoglycoside antibiotics)[33,46,88,89] are consistently higher in obese subjects compared to normal-weight controls. Consequently, larger absolute total daily doses are needed to achieve similar target serum concentrations.

Renal tubular function in the obese subpopulation has not been studied extensively. No significant increase in renal blood flow has been shown to occur in the obese population,[22,88] and no studies have been performed with drugs possessing a high renal extraction in the obese.

Christoff et al.[54] studied the disposition of procainamide in obese subjects. The renal clearance (CL_R) of procainamide is dependent upon both glomerular filtration and tubular secretion. The results from this study showed that a significant increase in the CL_R of procainamide was observed beyond that which could be accounted for by the increase in GFR. In addition, the ratio between renal procainamide clearance and creatinine clearance (CL_{cr}) was significantly greater in the obese population, suggesting a disproportionate increase in tubular versus glomerular function.

Similarly, the disposition of cimetidine in obese subjects was evaluated in two separate studies.[40,41] Like procainamide, cimetidine is dependent upon both glomerular filtration and tubular secretion for its renal elimination and should serve as a useful marker in the evaluation of tubular function. Abernethy et al.[40] reported no significant differences in the pharmacokinetics of cimetidine in obese subjects. In contrast, Bauer et al.[41] observed a remarkably greater renal clearance of cimetidine in obese versus non-obese subjects (856 ± 340 mL/min versus 509 ± 176 mL/min). Bauer et al.[41] attributed differences between these studies to differences in the characteristics of the obese populations studied. Additionally, the latter study also demonstrated an increase in the ratio between renal cimetidine clearance and creatinine clearance, providing further support for a disproportionate increase in tubular versus glomerular function in the obese. Finally, the renal clearance of cefotaxime,[39] which involves both glomerular filtration and tubular function, was significantly increased in obese subjects. This higher renal clearance value may represent an increase in the acidic tubular transport mechanism in the renal tubule.

Obese animal models have also been utilized to study the effect of obesity on renal function.[90–93] As observed in humans,[86,87] the obese, overfed rodent model exhibits increased creatinine clearance values compared to those of lean controls.[92] Recently, Corcoran and Salazar[93] observed that these animals were predisposed to gentamicin-induced nephrotoxicity as evidenced by cortical necrosis, serum creatinine, and creatinine-adjusted N-acetyl hexosaminidase excretion. Nephrotoxicity occurred when gentamicin was dosed on the basis of TBW or IBW. Interestingly, in a previous report this research group also observed excessive aminoglycoside nephrotoxicity in moderately obese patients despite the fact that total aminoglycoside dosage and duration of therapy were similar to non-obese subjects.[94] This observation is particularly troublesome for the following reason. Since the clearance and volume of distribution for the aminoglycoside antibiotics are considerably larger in the obese subpopulation (see Table 11-1), higher doses must be administered at more frequent dosing intervals to achieve comparable serum concentrations in obese patients. Extreme caution must be employed with these patients and the risk/benefit ratio carefully considered.

Predicting renal clearance is an important part of clinical pharmacokinetic drug monitoring. Numerous nomograms have been developed and evaluated in the normal-weight population to develop drug dosing regimens for compounds primarily eliminated by renal mechanisms.[95,96] Dionne et al.[87] evaluated a number of these approaches in morbidly obese patients and observed that when TBW was incorporated into these relationships, erroneously high estimates of renal clearance occurred. Conversely, when IBW was utilized, renal clearance estimates were consistently underestimated. Recently, Salazar and Corcoran[92] proposed that the following formulas be utilized to predict creatinine clearance (CL_{cr}) in obese patients:

$$CL_{cr} = \frac{[137 - Age] \times [(0.285 \times Wt) + (12.1 \times Ht^2)]}{(51)(C_{cr})}$$ (Eq. 11-4)

(Males)

$$CL_{cr} = \frac{[146 - Age] \times [(0.287 \times Wt) + (9.74 \times Ht^2)]}{(60)(C_{cr})}$$ (Eq. 11-5)

(Females)

where, age is in years; weight (Wt) is in kg; height (Ht) is in meters; C_{cr} is steady-state serum creatinine in mg/dL; and, CL_{cr} is creatinine clearance in mL/min. Additional studies are needed to verify the accuracy and bias associated with this method in obese patients. It should be mentioned that the method of DuBois and DuBois[97] has been shown to accurately predict BSA in the obese when TBW is employed.[98]

PROSPECTUS

Numerous physiologic changes occur in the obese patient which could significantly alter the pharmacokinetics of various drugs. Ultimately, drugs possessing a narrow therapeutic index must be carefully monitored to ensure optimal dosing.

Higher adipose tissue mass accounts for the majority of distributional changes observed in the obese population. These effects tend to be related to the physical and chemical properties of the drug. In particular, the lipid solubility of a compound is probably the single most useful predictor of drug distribution in obesity.

The effect of obesity on the hepatic clearance of drugs primarily undergoing phase I oxidative metabolism is highly substrate dependent. A more consistent picture of enhanced elimination is observed for drugs that are glucuronidated and sulfated. Acetylation represents one example of a conjugation pathway apparently not affected by obesity. Also, the clearance of drugs possessing a high hepatic extraction ratio is not significantly affected by obesity, consistent with the physiologic finding that no significant changes in hepatic blood flow accompany this condition.

Renal elimination of drugs is increased in obese individuals due to higher glomerular filtration and tubular secretion rates relative to non-obese patients. These studies, however, involve only drugs with low to intermediate extraction properties. Furthermore, there is evidence that tubular secretion may be disproportionately increased when compared to filtration. Since obese individuals may be more susceptible to aminoglycoside nephrotoxicity despite higher clearance mechanisms, these drugs must be dosed cautiously in this patient population. The application of traditional nomograms to predict CL_{cr} values in obese patients should be avoided, and alternative methods should be employed in the absence of a measured CL_{cr} determination.

REFERENCES

1. Van Itallie TB. Health implications of overweight and obesity in the United States. Ann Intern Med. 1985;103(6pt2):983–88.
2. Chatton MJ, Ullman PM. Nutrition: nutritional and metabolic disorders. In: Krupp MA, Chatton MJ, eds. Current Medical Diagnosis and Treatment. Los Altos: Lange Medical Publications; 1983;773–96.
3. Cheymol G. Drug pharmacokinetics in the obese. Fundam Clin Pharmacol. 1988;2:239–56.
4. Lew EA. Mortality and weight: insured lives and the American Cancer Society studies. Ann Intern Med. 1985;103(6pt2):1024–29.
5. Bray GA. The obese patient. Philadelphia: WB Saunders; 1976;5–251.
6. Vaughan RW. Definitions and risks of obesity. In: Brown BR, ed. Anesthesia and the Obese Patient. Philadelphia: F.A. Davis Co.; 1982;1–8.
7. Metropolitan Life Insurance Company. New weight standard for men and women. Stat Bull Metrop Insur Co. 1959;40:3–6.
8. Devine BJ. Gentamicin therapy. Drug Intell Clin Pharm. 1974;8:650–55.
9. Huxley JS. Problems of relative growth. New York: The Dial Press; 1932;1–276.
10. Boxenbaum H. Interspecies variation in liver weight, hepatic blood flow, and antipyrine intrinsic clearance: extrapolation of data to benzodiazepines and phenytoin. J Pharmacokinet Biopharm. 1980;8:165–76.
11. Prothero J. Scaling of blood parameters in mammals. Comp Biochem Physiol. 1984;77A:133–38.

12. Taylor FB et al. The regulation of renal activity. VIII: The relation between the rate of urea excretion and the size of the kidney. Am J Physiol. 1923;65:55–61.

13. Corcoran GB et al. Pharmacokinetic characteristics of the obese overfed rat model. Int J Obes. 1989;13:69–79.

14. Blouin RA et al. Influence of obesity on drug disposition. Clin Pharm. 1987;6:706–14.

15. Abernethy DR, Greenblatt DJ. Drug disposition in obese humans: an update. Clin Pharmacokinetic. 1986;11:199–213.

16. Greenblatt DJ et al. Effect of age, gender and obesity on midazolam kinetics. Anesthesiology. 1984;61:27–35.

17. Bowman SL et al. A comparison of the pharmacokinetics of propranolol in obese and normal volunteers. Br J Clin Pharmacol. 1986;21:529–32.

18. Flechner SM et al. The impact of body weight on cyclosporine pharmacokinetics in renal transplant recipients. Transplantation. 1989;47:806–10.

19. Andreasen PB et al. Drug absorption and hepatic drug metabolism in patients with different types of intestinal shunt operation for obesity. A study with phenazone. Scand J Gastroenterol. 1977;12:531–35.

20. Rowland M, Tozer TN. Clinical Pharmacokinetics: Concepts and Applications. 2nd ed. Philadelphia: Lea and Febiger; 1989:131–47.

21. Ritchel WA, Kaul S. Prediction of apparent volume of distribution in obesity. Methods Find Exp Clin Pharmacol. 1986;8:239–47.

22. Alexander JK et al. Blood volume, cardiac output, and disposition of systemic blood flow in extreme obesity. Cardiovasc Res Cent Bull. 1962–1963;1:39–44.

23. Alexander JK. Obesity and cardiac performance. Am J Cardiol. 1964;14:860–65.

24. DeDivitiis O et al. Obesity and cardiac function. Circulation. 1981;64:477–82.

25. Naeye RL, Rode P. The sizes and numbers of cells in visceral organs in human obesity. Am J Clin Pathol. 1970;54:251–53.

26. Smith HL. The relation of the weight of the heart to the weight of the body and of the weight of the heart to age. Am Heart J. 1928;4:79–93.

27. Kjellberg J, Reizenstein P. Body composition in obesity. Acta Med Scand. 1970;188:161–69.

28. Benedek IH et al. Serum alpha₁-acid glycoprotein and the binding of drugs in obesity. Br J Clin Pharmacol. 1983;16:751–54.

29. Benedek IH et al. Serum protein binding and the role of increased alpha₁-acid glycoprotein in moderately obese male subjects. Br J Clin Pharmacol. 1984;18:941–46.

30. Abernethy DR et al. Obesity, sex and acetaminophen disposition. Clin Pharmacol Ther. 1982;31:783–90.

31. Abernethy DR et al. The influence of obesity on the pharmacokinetics of oral alprazolam and triazolam. Clin Pharmacokinet. 1984;9:177–83.

32. Bauer LA et al. Amikacin pharmacokinetics in morbidity obese patients. Am J Hosp Pharm. 1980;3:519–22.

33. Bauer LA et al. Influence of weight on aminoglycoside pharmacokinetics in normal weight and morbidly obese patients. Eur J Clin Pharmacol. 1983;24:643–47.

34. Blouin RA et al. Amikacin pharmacokinetics in morbidly obese patients undergoing gastric-bypass surgery. Clin Pharm. 1985;4:70–2.

35. Abernethy DR et al. Alterations in drug distribution and clearance due to obesity. J Pharmacol Exp Ther. 1981;217:681–85.

36. Kamimori GH et al. The effect of obesity and exercise on the pharmacokinetics of caffeine in lean and obese volunteers. Eur J Clin Pharmacol. 1987;31:595–600.

37. Abernethy DR et al. Caffeine disposition in obesity. Br J Clin Pharmacol. 1985;20:61–6.

38. Mann HJ, Buchwald H. Cefamandole distribution in serum, adipose tissue, and wound drainage in morbidly obese patients. Drug Intell Clin Pharm. 1986;20:869–73.

39. Yost RL, Derendorf H. Disposition of cefotaxime and its desacetyl metabolites in morbidly obese male and female subjects. Ther Drug Monit. 1986;8:189–94.

40. Abernethy DR et al. Cimetidine disposition in obesity. Am J Gastroenterol. 1984;79:91–4.

41. Bauer LA et al. Cimetidine clearance in the obese. Clin Pharmacol Ther. 1985;37:425–530.

42. Abernethy DR et al. Prolongation of drug half-life due to obesity: studies of desmethyldiazepam (lorazepate). J Pharm Sci. 1982;7:942–44.

43. Abernethy DR et al. Prolonged accumulation of diazepam in obesity. J Clin Pharmacol. 1983;23:369–76.

44. Abernethy DR et al. Digoxin disposition in obesity: clinical pharmacokinetic investigation. Am Heart J. 1981;102:740–44.

45. Rodvold KA et al. Doxorubicin clearance in the obese. J Clin Oncol. 1988;6:1321–327.

46. Schwartz SN et al. A controlled investigation of the pharmacokinetics of gentamicin and tobramycin in obese subjects. J Infect Dis. 1978;138:499–505.

47. Abernethy DR, Greenblatt DJ. Ibuprofen disposition in obese individuals. Arthritis Rheum. 1985;28:1117–121.

48. Lind MJ et al. Prolongation of ifosfamide elimination half-life in obese patients due to altered drug distribution. Cancer Chemother Pharmacol. 1989;25:139–42.

49. Abernethy DR, Greenblatt DJ. Lidocaine disposition in obesity. Am J Cardiol. 1984;53:1183–186.

50. Abernethy DR et al. Enhanced glucuronide conjugation of drugs in obesity: studies of lorazepam, oxazepam, and acetaminophen. J Lab Clin Med. 1983;101:873–80.

51. Abernethy DR. Obesity effects on nitrazepam disposition. Br J Clin Pharmacol. 1986;22:551–57.

52. Abernethy DR, Greenblatt DJ. Phenytoin disposition in obesity. Arch Neurol. 1985;42:468–71.

53. Milsap RL et al. Prednisolone disposition in obese men. Clin Pharmacol Ther. 1984;36:824–31.

54. Christoff PB et al. Procainamide disposition in obesity. Drug Intell Clin Pharm. 1983;23:369–76.

55. Cheymol G. Comparative pharmacokinetics of intravenous propranolol in obese and normal volunteers. J Clin Pharmacol. 1987;27:874–79.

56. Blouin RA et al. Theophylline clearance; effect of marked obesity. Clin Pharmacol Ther. 1980;28:619–23.

57. Rohrbaugh TM et al. The effect of obesity on apparent volume of distribution of theophylline. Pediatr Pharmacol. 1982;2:75–83.

58. Slaughter RL, Lanc RA. Theophylline clearance in obese patients in relation to smoking and congestive heart failure. Drug Intell Clin Pharm. 1983;17:274–76.

59. Gal P et al. Theophylline disposition in obesity. Clin Pharmacol Ther. 1978;23:438–44.

60. Jung D et al. Thiopental disposition in lean and obese patients undergoing surgery. Anesthesiology 1982;56:269–74.

61. Blouin RA et al. Tobramycin pharmacokinetics in morbidly obese patients. Clin Pharmacol Ther. 1979;26:508–12.

62. Blouin RA et al. Vancomycin pharmacokinetics in normal and morbidly obese subjects. Antimicrob Agents Chemother. 1982;21:575–80.

63. Abernethy DR et al. Verapamil dynamics and disposition in obese hypertensives. J Cardiovasc Pharmacol. 1988;11:209–15.

64. Bickel MH. The role of adipose tissue in the distribution and storage of drugs. Prog Drug Res. 1984;28:273–303.

65. Leo A et al. Partition coefficients and their use. Chem Rev. 1971;71:525–616.

66. Arendt RM et al. Predicting *in vivo* benzodiazepine distribution based on *in vitro* lipophilicity. Clin Pharmacol Ther. 1982;31:200–201.

67. Yee GC et al. Effect of obesity on CSA disposition. Transplantation. 1988;45:649–51.

68. Rizzo A et al. Effect of body weight on the volume of distribution of theophylline. Lung. 1988;166:269–76.

69. Doherty JE et al. The distribution and concentration of tritiated digoxin in human tissues. Ann Intern Med. 1967;66:116–24.

70. Bortz WM. Metabolic consequences of obesity. Ann Intern Med. 1969;71:833–43.

71. Sherlock S. Diseases of the liver biliary system. 7th ed. Boston: Blackwell Scientific Publications; 1985:384.

72. Rowse-Brouwer KL et al. Phenobarbital in the genetically obese Zucker rat. *In vivo* and *in vitro* assessments of microsomal enzyme induction. J Pharmacol Exp Ther. 1984;231:654–59.

73. Blouin RA et al. Phenobarbital induction and acetaminophen hepatotoxicity: resistance in the obese Zucker rat. Pharmacol Exp Ther. 1987;243:565–70.

74. Litterst CL. *In vitro* hepatic drug metabolism and microsomal enzyme induction in genetically obese rats. Biochem Pharmacol. 1980;29:289–96.

75. Shum L, Jusko WJ. Theophylline disposition in the obese rat. J Pharmacol Exp Ther. 1984;228:380–86.

76. Corcoran GB, Wong BK. Obesity as a risk factor in drug-induced organ injury: increased liver and kidney damage by acetaminophen in the obese overfed rat. J Pharmacol Exp Ther. 1987;241:921–27.

77. Salazar DE et al. Obesity as a risk factor for drug-induced organ injury. VI: Increased hepatic P-450 concentration and microsomal ethanol oxidizing activity in the obese overfed rat. Biochem Biophys Res Commun. 1988;157:315–20.

78. Jusko WJ et al. Factors affecting theophylline clearance: age, tobacco, marijuana, cirrhosis, congestive heart failure, obesity, oral contraceptives, benzodiazepines, barbiturates and ethanol. J Pharm Sci. 1979;68:1358–366.

79. Koup JR, Vawater TK. Theophylline pharmacokinetics in an extremely obese patient. Clin Pharm. 1983;2:181–83.

80. Cummins AJ et al. A kinetic study of drug elimination: the excretion of paracetamol and its metabolites in man. Br J Pharm Chem. 1967;29:150–57.

81. Greenblatt DJ et al. Influence of age, gender, and obesity on salicylate kinetics following doses of aspirin. Arthritis Rheum. 1986;29:971–80.

82. Messeri FH et al. Disparate cardiovascular effects of obesity and arterial hypertension. Am J Med. 1983;74:808–12.

83. Rice SA et al. Anesthetic metabolism and renal function in obese and nonobese Fisher-344 rats following enflurane or isoflurane anesthesia. Anesthesiology. 1986;65:28–34.

84. McIntosh TF et al. Studies of urea excretion III: The influence of body size on urea output. J Clin Invest. 1928;6:467–83.

85. Stockholm KH et al. Increased glomerular filtration rate and adrenocortical function in obese women. Int J Obes. 1980;4:57–63.

86. Stockholm KH et al. Glomerular filtration rate after jejunoileal bypass for obesity. Int J Obes. 1981;5:77–80.

87. Dionne RE et al. Estimating creatinine clearance in morbidly obese patients. Am J Hosp Pharm. 1981;38:841–44.

88. Korsager S. Administration of gentamicin to obese patients. Int J Clin Pharmacol Therap and Tox. 1980;18:549–53.

89. Sketris L et al. Effect of obesity on gentamicin pharmacokinetics. J Clin Pharmacol. 1981;21:228–93.

90. Shimamura T. Relationship of dietary intake to the development of glomerular sclerosis in obese Zucker rats. Exp Mol Pathol. 1982;36:423–34.

91. Fiske WD et al. Renal function in the obese Zucker rat. Int J Obes. 1986;10:175–83.

92. Salazar DE, Corcoran GB. Predicting creatinine clearance and renal drug clearance in obese patients from estimated fat-free body mass. Am J Med. 1988;84:1053–60.

93. Corcoran GB, Salazar DE. Obesity as a risk factor in drug-induced organ injury. IV: Increased gentamicin nephrotoxicity in the obese overfed rat. J Pharmacol Exp Ther. 1989;248:1–6.

94. Corcoran GB et al. Excessive aminoglycoside nephrotoxicity in obese patients. Am J Med. 1988;85:279.

95. Kampmann J et al. Rapid evaluation of creatinine clearance. Acta Med Scand. 1974;196:517–20.

96. Cockcroft DW, Gault MH. Prediction of creatinine clearance from serum creatinine. Nephron. 1976;16:31–41.

97. DuBois D, DuBois ER. The measurement of the surface area of man. Arch Intern Med. 1915;15:868–81.

98. Tucker GR, Alexander JK. Estimation of body surface area of extremely obese human subjects. J Appl Physiol. 1960;15:781–84.

Chapter 12

Dietary Influences on Drug Disposition

Mary H.H. Chandler and Robert A. Blouin

Dietary intakes and patterns vary widely among individuals. The differences may be attributed to various factors, including food preferences and availability; diet manipulations in attempts to gain or lose weight; and variations for seasonal, religious, and therapeutic reasons. Such dietary influences are likely to contribute to the observed intra- and intcrindividual variability in the pharmacokinetics of various xenobiotics (i.c., chemicals foreign to the biologic system).

Although the effects of diet and other environmental influences on drug disposition have been investigated extensively in animals, their effects in humans are less well studied.[1,2] Several factors complicate the design and interpretation of clinical studies that attempt to address the role of diet on drug disposition. These complicating factors include: age; genetic and racial influences; environmental effects (e.g., smoking); health status; concomitant drug therapy; and difficulty in controlling and standardizing diets (particularly those consumed at home). Consider, as an example, the task of documenting one's daily dietary intake. Accurate quantitation of nutrient intake is a much harder task than documenting the number of milligrams of a particular drug consumed daily. This difficulty is further complicated by the potentially varying effects that specific foods and methods of food preparation have on drug metabolism.

The purpose of this chapter is to review the effects of diet, specifically macronutrients (i.e., carbohydrate, fat, and protein), on the clinical pharmacokinetics of drugs in adults. When pertinent, findings from animal experiments are also included. Readers also are referred to several review articles that discuss the current understanding of dietary influences on drug disposition in humans.[3–8]

ABSORPTION

Food has been reported to increase, decrease, or have no effect on the bioavailability of various drugs.[3,6,9] Examples of drugs whose bioavailability is enhanced by food intake include propranolol, metoprolol, hydralazine, hydrochlorothiazide, nitrofurantoin, erythromycin (stearate), phenytoin, carbamazepine, and griseofulvin.[3,6] On the other hand, food has been shown to reduce the bioavailability of drugs, including isoniazid, rifampin, tetracycline, and penicillin. No consistent effect of food on the bioavailability of metronidazole, oxazepam, propylthiouracil, and sulfonylureas has been reported.[3,6] The type, amount, and timing of foods may influence drug dissolution and absorption. For example, high-fat meals enhance the absorption of griseofulvin, while milk and other foods containing calcium inhibit the absorption of tetracycline.[9] Mechanisms by which food may affect bioavailability of drugs include direct binding or alteration of pH, gastric emptying time, intestinal motility, mucosal absorption, and splanchnic/hepatic blood flow.[8] Additionally, food intake may increase the amount or rate of gastrointestinal absorption and delivery to the liver, thereby decreasing the bioavailability of drugs that undergo capacity-limited hepatic clearance.[6,8] A few examples of food-induced changes in drug bioavailability deserve further discussion.

Theophylline

The first example is illustrated by theophylline, specifically the Theo-24 dosage form.[10] Since dissolution of the coating on Theo-24 beads is pH dependent, the coating dissolves more rapidly after a meal. This phenomenon may lead to "dumping" of a potentially toxic amount of theophylline from Theo-24.[10]

Propranolol

Food also enhances the bioavailability of propranolol. Proposed mechanisms for this effect include a short-lasting inhibition of the presystemic conjugation of propranolol and/or a transient increase in hepatic blood flow.[11,12] Olanoff et al.[12] demonstrated that postprandially, propranolol's systemic clearance (CL) increased 38% after it was administered intravenously; its oral bioavailability, however, increased 67%.[12] These observations are consistent with a food-induced increase in liver blood flow (Q).[13,14] Propranolol has a high extraction ratio and undergoes nonrestrictive hepatic clearance. According to the "venous equilibration" perfusion model,[15]

$$CL = \frac{Q \cdot f_{up} \cdot CLu_{int}}{Q + f_{up} \cdot CLu_{int}} \qquad \text{(Eq. 12-1)}$$

where f_{up} = unbound fraction of drug in plasma and CLu_{int} = unbound intrinsic clearance of the drug.[15] Extraction ratio (E) is defined as follows:[15]

$$E = \frac{f_{up} \cdot CLu_{int}}{Q + f_{up} \cdot CLu_{int}} = \frac{CL}{Q} \qquad \text{(Eq. 12-2)}$$

The first-pass clearance of high-extraction drugs often is not flow-limited, since the relatively high concentrations presented via the portal vein (on "first pass") approach or exceed the capacity of drug metabolizing enzymes. The bioavailability (F) of a drug that is completely absorbed and eliminated solely by hepatic metabolism can be described by the equation:[13]

$$F = \frac{Q}{Q + CLu_{int}}$$

(Eq. 12-3)

According to this equation, as flow increases, F also increases substantially for a drug with high CLu_{int} (e.g., propranolol). Thus, the transient (i.e., approximately three hours in duration) increase in Q leads to decreased hepatic extraction (see Equation 12-2) and increased F (see Equation 12-3) of orally administered propranolol during the absorption phase (see Figure 12-1).[12,13] However, it is not clear that changes in flow can account completely for food-induced changes in propranolol bioavailability. For a high-extraction drug given intravenously, clearance is approximately equal to liver blood flow (i.e., $CL \approx Q$).[15] Consequently,

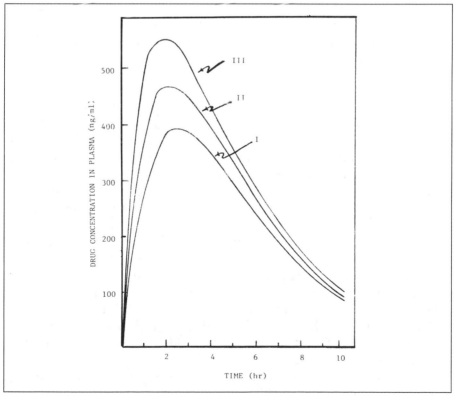

Figure 12-1. *Drug concentration in plasma after oral administration under differing conditions affecting hepatic blood flow, simulated according to the simple perfusion model. Simulation I: hepatic blood flow maintained at 1.5 L/min to mimic drug administration to fasting subjects. Simulation II: hepatic drug flow increased to 2.5 L/min after drug administration and maintained elevated for two hours then reduced to 1.5 L/min. Simulation III: hepatic blood flow increased to 4.5 L/min after drug administration and maintained elevated for 2 hr, then reduced to 1.5 L/min. Simulations II and III were intended to mimic drug administration with a meal that stimulates splanchnic blood flow (reproduced with permission from reference 13).*

food would be expected to increase the clearance of propranolol and other high-extraction drugs administered intravenously. Indeed, similar food-induced increases in clearance have been observed with intravenously administered lidocaine.[16,17]

Dietary Fiber

In general, dietary fiber decreases drug absorption to varying extents.[18-20] For example, dietary fiber increased the absorption rate of amoxicillin but significantly decreased the amount of drug absorbed.[18] Since dietary fiber increases gastric emptying and intestinal motility, it took less time for amoxicillin to reach the mucosa of the small intestine and begin its absorption. However, part of the drug may not have been available for absorption because it was trapped in the fiber matrix.[18] It is important that clinicians recognize the potential effect of fiber on drug absorption processes, particularly as our society moves toward an era of preventive medicine in which higher fiber diets are being promoted.

The above examples illustrate a number of ways food and dietary components influence drug absorption. Because food effects on drug absorption are complex, the net effect of food on drug bioavailability cannot be accurately predicted without studying the specific drug in question.

DISTRIBUTION

Dietary content also affects drug distribution. For example, high-fat meals can increase plasma free fatty acid levels. Since free fatty acid molecules bind to the same albumin binding sites occupied by drugs, they can displace various drugs from plasma albumin sites.[9] Furthermore, certain dietary factors can affect body composition (e.g., obesity) which, in turn, can influence the volume of distribution of many drugs. (See Chapter 11: Special Pharmacokinetic Considerations in the Obese: Distribution). Several clinical studies have attempted to determine whether malnutrition affects the pharmacokinetic parameters of drugs. Each described study used Body Mass Index [BMI (i.e., weight/height^2 × 100)] as an indicator of nutritional status and studied groups of well-nourished and undernourished (index values below 0.18) subjects.[21-25] Examples of drugs whose plasma protein binding is lower in undernourished or malnourished individuals include tetracycline, sulfadiazine, phenylbutazone, doxycycline, and rifampin.[21-25] In all cases, the lower plasma protein binding in the undernourished groups could be attributed to lower serum albumin levels.[21-25]

In most instances, the following relationship can be applied to explain study findings in malnourished subjects:[26]

$$V_{ss} = V_p + V_T \left(\frac{f_{up}}{f_{ut}}\right)$$

(Eq. 12-4)

where V_{ss} = volume of distribution at steady state, V_p = plasma volume, V_T = tissue volume, f_{up} = unbound fraction of drug in plasma, and f_{ut} = unbound fraction of drug in tissues. In the case of tetracycline,[21] for example, the smaller volume of distribution observed in undernourished subjects may indicate a reduction of tissue uptake and tissue binding during undernutrition.[21] An increase in f_{ut} would lead to a decrease in V_{ss}. For sulfadiazine[22] and doxycycline,[24] the larger volume of distribution values in undernourished subjects compared to well-nourished subjects were not significantly different. For phenylbutazone,[23] the significantly larger mean volume of distribution value in the undernourished group was attributed to an increase in f_{up}.[23] However, the drug was administered orally and the authors assumed that its absorption was normal.[23] Likewise, when rifampin was administered orally, differences in distribution volume between the undernourished and well-nourished groups could not be ascertained.[25]

Overall, limited data exist on the effect of diet on drug distribution. The results of several studies demonstrate differences in protein binding in undernourished versus well-nourished subjects.[21-25] Each of the clinical studies described above[21-25] was performed in India. Since genetic differences may contribute to intersubject variability in drug disposition, caution must be exercised in extrapolating these results to other populations.

METABOLISM

Most foods are complex mixtures of carbohydrate, fat, and protein. The majority of clinical investigations designed to assess the influence of diet on drug metabolism provide subjects with diets in which one macronutrient is increased, another decreased, and the third macronutrient and total caloric intake are kept constant. As noted in an earlier section (see Absorption), food can increase hepatic blood flow, a phenomenon that can increase the bioavailability of high-extraction drugs.

Carbohydrates, Protein, Fat, and Calories

Nutritional influences on oxidative metabolism also have been demonstrated in various clinical studies.[27-33] In general, high-protein diets have been associated with accelerated oxidative metabolism in humans,[27,28,30-33] while high-carbohydrate (low-protein) diets appear to have the opposite effect.[27,28,30-33] Furthermore, the substitution of fat for carbohydrate seems to have no significant effect on drug metabolism rates.[28-30] Several clinical investigators have used the low-extraction drugs, antipyrine and theophylline, as *in vivo* markers for the mixed function oxidase system.[27-33] Kappas et al.[27] found that the apparent oral clearance values of antipyrine and theophylline were higher in subjects ingesting high-protein (low-carbohydrate) diets than in those ingesting other types of diets (see Table 12-1).[27] Furthermore, protein supplementation was associated with a decrease in drug half-lives, whereas carbohydrate supplementation resulted in an increase in half-lives.[27] The findings of Kappas et al.[27] suggest that dietary protein content may have a more generalized rather than substrate-specific effect on the cytochrome P450 mixed function oxidase system, since antipyrine and theophylline clearances were affected similarly.[27]

The mechanisms by which dietary protein and carbohydrate influence oxidative metabolism in humans are not clear. In animals, increased dietary protein enhances microsomal cytochrome P450 content, whereas carbohydrate intake has an opposite effect.[34] In animals fed high-protein diets, liver weights and mitotic activity in hepatic parenchymal cells also increase.[34] Moreover, a lower level of dietary protein intake has been directly correlated *in vivo* with a lower phenobarbital clearance and prolonged anesthesia in rats.[1] The ability of carbohydrate to inhibit the synthesis of various enzymes (i.e., the "glucose effect") has been studied in bacteria and in liver.[27] For example, this "glucose effect" has been demonstrated for σ-amino-levulinate synthetase, the rate-limiting enzyme in heme biosynthesis. This effect is thought to be closely interrelated to carbohydrate's ability to lower the microsomal cytochrome P450 content, since a major portion of newly-formed heme in the liver is used to synthesize cytochrome P450.[35]

Using the same substrates (antipyrine and theophylline), Anderson et al.[28] examined the effects of increased *dietary fat content* on metabolism. The isocaloric substitution of fat for carbohydrate produced little change in the clearance of antipyrine (see Table 12-1). However, the clearance increased when subjects were changed to the high-protein diet (see Table 12-1).[28] A high-protein diet similarly increased theophylline's clearance. This study suggests that when protein is

***Table 12-1.** Effect of Diet Composition on Antipyrine Clearance*

Diets	Energy (KCal)	Protein (%)	Carbo-hydrate (%)	Fat (%)	Antipyrine CL	References
I[a]	—	—	—	—	37.0 ± 1.4 mL/min	27
II	2400–2500	44	35	21	58.0 ± 3.6 mL/min[b]	
III	2400–2500	10	70	20	38.7 ± 4.3 mL/min	
IV[a]	—	—	—	—	39.9 ± 2.6 mL/min	
I[a]	—	—	—	—	0.70 ± 0.05 mL/min/kg	28
II	2500	10	80	10	0.57 ± 0.02 mL/min/kg	
III	2500	10	20	70	0.59 ± 0.02 mL/min/kg	
IV	2500	50	20	30	0.71 ± 0.05 mL/min/kg[c]	
I	1500	10	72	18	18.8 mL/min[d]	30
II	1500	20	68	12	21.0 mL/min	
III	3000	5	63	24	19.0 mL/min	
IV	3000	10	61	21	24.9 mL/min	
V	3000	15	59	18	28.0 mL/min	
VI	1800	10	74	16	23.8 mL/min	

[a] Home diet composition values not reported; average American diet consists of 15% PRO, 50% CHO, 35% fat. See text for explanation.
[b] $p < 0.05$: I versus II; II versus III; II versus IV.
[c] $p < 0.05$: I versus II; I versus III; II versus IV; III versus IV.
[d] $p < 0.05$: I versus IV; III versus IV; III versus V.

substituted for carbohydrate or fat, hepatic drug metabolism can be accelerated. However, substitution of fat for carbohydrate has little effect on hepatic drug metabolism.[28]

The Anderson study[28] also demonstrated that the isocaloric substitution of saturated (butter) or polyunsaturated (corn oil) fat for carbohydrate produced no significant changes in antipyrine and theophylline clearance when the protein content was held constant. This was despite significant elevations in plasma levels of cholesterol and triglycerides. Thus, the degree of fatty acid saturation appears to have minimal effect on the metabolism of these two drugs.[28]

Although the clinical data suggest that fat substitution for carbohydrate has little effect on oxidative drug metabolism in humans, animal studies indicate otherwise.[6,36] In animals, dietary lipid and saturated and unsaturated fatty acids have increased the activity of the mixed function oxidase system and its inducibility by barbiturates.[36] Rats fed a diet of 3% corn oil metabolize aniline, heptachlor, and hexobarbital more quickly and have an increased cytochrome P450 content compared to those fed a fat-free diet.[6] Dietary lipid is known to affect the phospholipid composition of microsomal membranes. Phospholipid, particularly phosphatidylcholine, is an essential component of the mixed function oxidase system.[36] Consequently, the possibility exists that dietary fat intake, in amounts different from those studied by Anderson et al.,[28] may significantly affect drug oxidation in humans. This deserves further study.

Preliminary results from Mucklow et al.[29] indicate that short-term changes in the proportion of animal to vegetable fat have no influence on antipyrine clearance or debrisoquine 4-hydroxylation.[29]

Data from Krishnaswamy et al.[30] indicate that *caloric intake* also may affect drug clearances. As shown in Table 12-1 (see Reference 30), when the caloric intake was 30% to 35% below the recommended dietary intake (diet VI) drug oxidation was unaffected. However, when the energy deficit exceeded 40% (diet I), metabolism was reduced.[30] Similar findings have been observed in protein-energy malnourished animals.[37] The data from the Krishnaswamy study[30] also indicate that antipyrine clearances approach normal values at higher caloric intakes (3000 KCal) when dietary protein is adequate (i.e., 10% for diet IV or 15% for diet V). A higher protein intake (20%) combined with a low caloric intake (1500 KCal) (diet II) produced an antipyrine clearance that was greater than that associated with diet I, yet still lower than that associated with diets IV and V.[30] These data show that inadequate caloric intake appears to decrease oxidative metabolism. Increasing protein intake, however, may partially compensate for this decrease in drug clearance. Again, substituting carbohydrate or fat calories for protein did not seem to stimulate drug metabolism.[30]

Juan et al.[31] examined the effects of *low- and high-protein diets* (5% and 44% of total calories, respectively) on theophylline clearance. The mean theophylline clearance values fell 21% on the low-protein diet and rose 26% on the high-protein diet compared to the control home diet.[31] Unlike previous data on antipyrine and theophylline that suggested a generalized effect of dietary protein content on the hepatic mixed function oxidase system, the results of Juan et al.[31] suggest that caffeine N-desmethylase activity (i.e., 3-methylcholanthrene-inducible cyto-chrome P450 activity) was more responsive than aminopyrine N-desmethylase (i.e., phenobarbital-inducible cytochrome P450 activity).[31]

Fagan et al.[32] confirmed previous observations that theophylline clearance increases when protein intake rises.[27,28] This group also studied propranolol and found that increases in dietary protein had a twofold greater effect on propranolol clearance relative to theophylline. The investigators attributed this enhanced effect to the fact that propranolol is a high-clearance drug, while theophylline is a low-clearance drug.[38] They also speculated that various cytochrome P450 isoen-zymes could be differentially susceptible to dietary changes.[32] (Propranolol is metabolized by ring and side-chain oxidation reactions that, like theophylline, are cytochrome P450 mediated.)[38]

Thompson et al.[33] examined the effects of dietary components on theophylline kinetics in patients with airways obstruction as opposed to those in healthy normal subjects. The area under the plasma concentration versus time curve (AUC) for theophylline during the high-carbohydrate (low-protein) diet was 33% greater (i.e., lower clearance) than that observed during the high-protein (low-carbohy-drate) diet. These findings are in agreement with previous reports.[27,28,30-32] Each of the studies cited above[27-33] were limited by relatively small sample sizes. Further-more, in only two studies was the sequence of dietary regimens randomized.[29,32]

The principal effects of dietary factors on drug metabolism are summarized in Table 12-2. The mechanisms of these effects are, at present, unclear and warrant further study.

Vitamins and Minerals

A detailed discussion of vitamin and mineral micronutrients and their effects on drug metabolism is beyond the scope of this chapter. However, a few examples deserve mention.

The effects of vitamins and minerals on drug metabolism have been studied extensively in animals.[39] For instance, studies in laboratory animals have shown

Table 12-2. *Summary of Dietary Factors That Influence Metabolism in Humans*

Factor	Drug	Direction of effect on metabolism[a]	References
↑ protein	antipyrine theophylline propranolol	↑	27, 28, 30–33
↑ carbohydrate	antipyrine theophylline propranolol	↓	27, 28, 30–33
↑ fat	antipyrine theophylline	→	28–30
↓ calories	antipyrine	↓	30

[a] ↑ = Increase; ↓ = Decrease; → = No effect.

that the cytochrome P450 mixed function oxidase system may be affected by riboflavin, thiamine, vitamin A, vitamin C, folic acid, iron, copper, zinc, calcium, magnesium, and heavy metals.[39]

In humans, the effects of micronutrients on drug disposition have not been well studied. Although the effects of vitamin C intake or deficiency on drug metabolism have been the focus of a number of clinical studies, the findings are equivocal,[40–46] with some studies demonstrating a change in antipyrine clearance[40–42,44] and others indicating no change.[43,45] Vitamin C, in large doses, also can decrease sulfate conjugation of drugs (e.g., acetaminophen) by competing for available sulfate.[46] Other examples, in humans, include folic acid and pyridoxine.[47–52] A number of reports exist indicating that folic acid coadministration decreases both total and free plasma phenytoin concentrations.[47–49] The most likely mechanism of the interaction is the stimulation of phenytoin metabolism by folic acid.[50] However, in individuals without folate deficiency, the metabolism of phenytoin may be unaffected by folic acid coadministration.[51] Pyridoxine serves as a cofactor for dopa decarboxylase.[52] Consequently, the concomitant ingestion of pyridoxine and levodopa also can lead to an increase in the metabolism of levodopa.[52] Both of these examples (i.e., folic acid-phenytoin and pyridoxine-levodopa) may have important clinical implications in that the therapeutic effectiveness of phenytoin or levodopa may be decreased if folic acid or pyridoxine, respectively, is administered.[47 52] Overall, clinical data on the influence of micronutrient deficiencies or excesses on drug disposition are limited.

Malnutrition

Malnutrition and its effects on drug metabolism have been the focus of a number of clinical studies, many of which were performed in India.[21–25,53–55] In general, despite wide interpatient variability, adults with mild and moderate forms of undernutrition demonstrate normal or enhanced oxidative metabolism of drugs whereas those with severe malnutrition (e.g., nutritional edema) demonstrate decreased drug metabolism.[7,23–25,54]

Shastri and Krishnaswamy[21] used half-life instead of clearance as the index of metabolic capacity. Although they found the half-life of tetracycline to be significantly longer in well-nourished individuals compared to undernourished individuals, it is unclear whether this observation actually reflects altered metabolism.[21] Shastri and Krishnaswamy[22] also found the clearance of a single dose of sulfadiazine given orally or intravenously to be higher in undernourished compared to well-nourished subjects. Similar findings of increased clearance in undernourished populations have been reported for phenylbutazone,[23] doxycycline,[24] chloroquine,[54] and rifampin.[25]

In a clinical study by Bakke et al.,[53] the apparent metabolic clearance values for antipyrine varied by two- and threefold in patients with anorexia nervosa and healthy controls, respectively. However, the anorexic patients, on average, exhibited normal antipyrine metabolism. The investigators speculated that a reduced metabolic clearance of cortisol secondary to malnutrition may have been responsible for maintaining normal antipyrine metabolism in individuals with anorexia nervosa. This theory was based on reports that cortisol can shorten antipyrine's half-life and increase phenylbutazone metabolism.[53]

Tranvouez et al.[55] conducted a clinical study in patients with energy malnutrition or global protein-calorie malnutrition and in control subjects. The mean clearance of antipyrine, administered intravenously, was significantly lower in individuals who were both protein and calorie malnourished (26.5 mL/min) relative to those who were only energy malnourished or to controls (43.65 and 48.5 mL/min, respectively). The values in energy malnutrition and controls were not significantly different, suggesting that mixed function oxidase activity decreases only when protein deficiency is present but not when energy deficiency alone is present. After nutritional repletion occurred for 31 ± 4 days, antipyrine clearances approached normal values in the protein-calorie malnourished groups. There was no significant change in energy-malnourished groups following replenishment.[55]

Collectively, these findings indicate that the net effect of malnutrition on drug metabolism is determined by a number of factors such as type, degree, and duration of malnutrition as well as by other concomitant environmental and pathophysiologic influences. Generally, mild to moderately malnourished adults exhibit normal or increased drug oxidation, whereas severely malnourished individuals exhibit decreased metabolism.[7] These *in vivo* findings are supported by *in vitro* experiments which have shown that the activities of certain hepatic enzymes [benzo[a]pyrene hydroxylase and γ-glutamyl transpeptidase (GGT)] are induced in undernourished adults.[56] However, when malnutrition is severe (i.e., adaptation is inadequate and negative nitrogen balance occurs), hepatic metabolism decreases.[7]

Specific Foods, Diets and Methods of Food Preparation

Charcoal-Broiled Beef. Diets containing charcoal-broiled beef enhance the oxidative metabolism of phenacetin, antipyrine, and theophylline, but not the conjugation of acetaminophen.[57–59] Conney et al.[57] found that the average AUC_{0-7h} of phenacetin was significantly lower while subjects were on a charcoal-broiled beef diet compared to a control diet. The plasma ratios of acetaminophen (the major metabolite of phenacetin) to phenacetin also increased markedly after the charcoal-broiled beef diet. A similar study demonstrated a 30% increase in clearance for theophylline and a 38% increase for antipyrine when the subjects were fed charcoal-broiled beef.[58] While the effect of feeding charcoal-broiled beef had minimal effect on the apparent volume of distribution of the drugs, the mean half-lives for theophylline and antipyrine were both 22% lower while subjects were ingesting charcoal-broiled beef than during the control diet periods.[58] In contrast to its effects on the oxidatively-metabolized drugs, a charcoal-broiled beef diet had little or no effect on the plasma-concentration profile or urinary excretion of acetaminophen, acetaminophen glucuronide, and acetaminophen sulfate.[59] These results suggest that the human enzymes which conjugate acetaminophen are not affected significantly by charcoal-broiled beef.[59]

Charcoal-broiled beef—like cigarette smoke—contains aromatic hydrocarbons, chemicals that are potent inducers of certain metabolic enzymes.[60] The above data demonstrate that a short period of ingestion of moderate amounts of charcoal-broiled beef can significantly stimulate oxidative metabolism, but not conjugation reactions.[57-59] Rat studies have also demonstrated that charcoal-broiled beef ingestion can stimulate the *in vitro* oxidative metabolism of phenacetin and benzo[*a*]pyrene.[61]

Cruciferous Vegetables. Certain cruciferous vegetables (i.e., brussels sprouts and cabbage) contain indoles which have been shown to stimulate the oxidative metabolism of antipyrine and phenacetin and the conjugation of acetaminophen.[62,63] In healthy subjects fed a brussels sprouts and cabbage-containing diet, the mean clearance of antipyrine increased 11%, volume of distribution did not change, and the half-life decreased 13%, compared to control-diet results.[62] The AUC_{0-7h} values for phenacetin were significantly lower for the study diet compared to control diets. Additionally, the test diet increased the mean plasma ratio of conjugated acetaminophen to unconjugated acetaminophen, suggesting that the cruciferous vegetables enhanced the conjugation of acetaminophen.[62] This finding was confirmed in a later study that investigated the effects of a diet containing cabbage and brussels sprouts on the conjugation of acetaminophen and oxazepam.[63] The test diet stimulated the conjugation of acetaminophen as shown by a 16% decrease in AUC, a 17% increase in metabolic clearance, an increased plasma acetaminophen glucuronide to acetaminophen ratio, and an 8% increase in 24-hour urinary recovery of acetaminophen glucuronide. No comparable changes occurred in the metabolism of acetaminophen to acetaminophen sulfate. The dietary effects on oxazepam conjugation were less clear. The data showed a small increase in clearance of oxazepam during the study diet period which was not supported by either a decrease in half-life for oxazepam or an increase in plasma ratio of oxazepam glucuronide to oxazepam.[63]

These data suggest that cruciferous vegetables in the diet can enhance glucuronide conjugation in humans. Why there is a greater effect on acetaminophen glucuronidation relative to oxazepam conjugation is unknown. On the other hand, oxidative metabolic reactions in humans parallel those in animals.[64,65] In rats, diets containing alfalfa, brussels sprouts, cabbage, turnips, broccoli, cauliflower, or spinach have been shown to increase the intestinal activity of: benzo[*a*]pyrene hydroxylase; intestinal enzymes that O-dealkylate phenacetin and 7-ethoxycoumarin; and enzymes that hydroxylate hexobarbital.[64,65]

Vegetarian Diets. Studies of Asian vegetarians suggest that the reduced antipyrine clearance observed in this group compared to their non-vegetarian counterparts is primarily due to their low intake of dietary protein, and not to the lack of meat or any difference in fat consumption.[66] This is corroborated by the observation that the ability of Caucasian vegetarians to metabolize antipyrine, acetaminophen, and phenacetin is similar to that of their non-vegetarian counterparts. Since the daily protein consumption of the Caucasian vegetarians was similar to that of the non-vegetarians, the protein rather than meat content again appeared to be responsible for differences in drug disposition between Caucasian and Asian vegetarians.[67]

Parenteral Nutrition

The effect of intravenous nutrition on oxidative drug metabolizing capacity has been examined using antipyrine as a marker.[68-70] Findings here are similar to those of conventional oral diets.[27-33] Despite wide interpatient variability, parenteral nutrition regimens containing amino acids are associated with higher antipyrine clearances than are regimens consisting primarily of dextrose.[68,69] Existing data also suggest that parenteral refeeding of malnourished patients enhances oxidative drug metabolism.[69]

Burgess et al.[70] investigated the effect of different total parenteral nutrition (TPN) regimens on hepatic microsomal enzyme activity. Patients receiving a TPN regimen of 2000 KCal/day (TPN1: all nonprotein calories were derived from dextrose; TPN3: 25% of the nonprotein calories were given as 10% Intralipid) were compared with an unfed control patient group. Other patients received a dextrose-based TPN regimen of 1600 KCal (TPN2). All TPN regimens provided 12 to 14 gm nitrogen. Patients receiving TPN1 and TPN2 showed a 34% lower mean antipyrine clearance after seven days of TPN compared to that of controls. However, patients receiving TPN3 had a mean antipyrine clearance that was not significantly different from that of the control group. The study results demonstrate the sensitivity of hepatic microsomal oxidative function to different TPN regimens.[70] Cytochrome P450 activity and lipogenesis both depend upon NADPH. Carbohydrate-based TPN regimens lead to greater hepatic lipid synthesis than isocaloric lipid-based regimens. Consequently, increased competition for NADPH between cytochrome P450 and the lipogenesis which occurs during carbohydrate feeding may partly explain the lower antipyrine clearance following TPN1 and TPN2. However, the lipid in TPN3 regimens appeared to have a direct effect on P450 activity since the TPN2 and TPN3 regimens contained similar amounts of carbohydrate but led to different antipyrine clearances.[70]

The mechanisms by which intravenous nutrients influence oxidative drug metabolism have not been identified. Moreover, studies are needed to elucidate the mechanism by which the refeeding of nutritionally depleted patients enhances oxidative metabolism. Also unclear is the mechanism responsible for different influences of different TPN regimens.

EXCRETION

Dietary protein increases renal plasma flow and glomerular filtration rate (GFR) in humans.[71,72] A number of experiments performed in laboratory animals have demonstrated that increased dietary protein increases renal blood flow, GFR, and kidney size and weight.[71,73,74] Little information is available, however, regarding the clinical implications of these effects on the pharmacokinetics of drugs. Berlinger et al.[75] investigated the effects of a two-week high-protein (268 gm/day) and low-protein (19 gm/day) diet on the pharmacokinetics of allopurinol and its metabolite, oxypurinol. The total body clearance and renal clearance of allopurinol decreased by 31% and 28%, respectively, while the subjects were on the low-protein diet. The total body and renal clearances of oxypurinol decreased by 59% and

64%, respectively, under the same circumstances.[75] In this study, there was no control (i.e., normal protein) diet and comparisons could be made only between the high- and low-protein diets.[75] Additionally, Dickson et al.[76] found the total body clearance and urinary excretion of single doses of gentamicin to be higher after a protein meal when compared to fasting conditions.[76]

Until recently, research in the area of dietary influences on renal function focused on the possible role of dietary protein in the cause, progression, and treatment of chronic renal failure.[77] This focus has led to recent research interests in assessing the impact of dietary protein on GFR and drug disposition. It is possible that the protein-related increases in GFR are due to an amino acid-induced effect of a circulating hormone.[78] For instance, in dogs, glycine and various other amino acids have been shown to increase glucagon secretion. Glucagon secretion, in turn, can increase renal blood flow and GFR.[78] Another proposed mechanism for the protein-induced increase in GFR suggests that dietary protein intake decreases the tubuloglomerular feedback system (i.e., activation of the local or systemic renin-angiotensin system), thereby increasing GFR.[79]

Dietary protein intake appears to influence renal tubular function as well. In the Berlinger study,[75] the fractional excretion (oxypurinol renal clearance/creatinine renal clearance) was reduced by 50% during the low-protein diet. This suggests that an increase in net renal tubular reabsorption occurred in addition to a reduction in filtration for this weak acid.[75] Park et al.[80] found that the effect of protein-calorie restriction on oxypurinol was sustained for four weeks. Furthermore, renal clearance of oxypurinol was proportional to the quantity of protein in the diet.[80] Results from Kitt et al.[81] indicated that the renal clearance of oxypurinol was reduced as a result of protein restriction and not caloric restriction. Furthermore, the data showed an increase in the net tubular reabsorption of oxypurinol when dietary protein was restricted.[81] In a different study, Kitt et al.[82] determined the time of onset for changes in renal function following short-term dietary protein restriction.[82] Healthy subjects consumed a normal diet (100 gm protein, 2600 KCal) for ten days and a 400 KCal per day oral solution of glucose and electrolytes for five days. Allopurinol was administered orally on day six of the normal diet and day two of the restricted diet. Oxypurinol clearance significantly decreased on day three of the restricted diet. No further decreases occurred from day three to day five.[82]

The influence of dietary protein restriction on the renal clearance of cimetidine, a weak base, also has been studied.[83] Although the renal clearance of cimetidine did not change, protein restriction resulted in a 30% increase (as calculated by fractional excretion) in the net tubular secretion of cimetidine. This increase, coupled with a 20% decrease in filtration, could explain the lack of change in renal clearance.[83] Therefore, the studies with oxypurinol and cimetidine suggest that dietary protein restriction may result in a net increase in directional transport (i.e., secretion or reabsorption).[72] Park et al.[72] hypothesize that protein ingestion changes tubuloglomerular balance through the release of local or systemic hormones or by changing extracellular fluid volume.[72]

These preliminary findings of dietary influences on glomerular filtration and renal tubular clearance suggest that diet could alter the pharmacokinetics of drugs that are excreted renally. The clinical significance of these findings for other drugs warrants further study.

PROSPECTUS

Wide interindividual variability exists in dietary consumption. This variability reflects food preferences and availability as well as seasonal, religious, therapeutic, and weight control factors. The complex and varied components of the human diet may affect the pharmacokinetics of various drugs. We are now beginning to appreciate the significant contributions of diet on the variability in drug disposition observed within and among individuals. Nutritional factors that alter physiologic processes or pharmacokinetic parameters can have important clinical implications. Furthermore, in the design and interpretation of pharmacokinetic studies, the role of diet deserves appropriate consideration to minimize potentially confounding variables.

This chapter has provided examples of the effects of diet on drug absorption, distribution, metabolism, and excretion. In most cases, mechanistic questions still remain unanswered. Consequently, there is a need to explore the biochemical aspects of the multifaceted effects of diet on drug disposition. Other areas that warrant further study include: dietary influences on steroid hormone metabolism; the effects of diet on drug disposition in patients with various disease states; and the effects of nutrition on drug disposition in the elderly.

REFERENCES

1. Campbell TC et al. The influence of dietary factors on drug metabolism in animals. Drug Metab Rev. 1979;9:173–84.
2. Knodell RG. Effects of formula composition on hepatic and intestinal drug metabolism during enteral nutrition. JPEN. 1990;14:34–38.
3. Melander A. Influence of food on the bioavailability of drugs. Clin Pharmacokinet. 1978;3:337–51.
4. Alvares AP et al. Regulation of drug metabolism in man by environmental factors. Drug Metab Rev. 1979;9:185–205.
5. Anderson KE et al. Nutritional influences on chemical biotransformations in humans. Nutr Rev. 1982;40:161–71.
6. Welling P. Nutrient effects on drug metabolism and action in the elderly. Drug-Nutrient Interactions 1985;4:173–207.
7. Krishnaswamy K. Effects of malnutrition on drug metabolism and toxicity in humans. In: Hathcock JN, ed. Nutritional Toxicology. New York: Academic Press, Inc.; 1987;105–28.
8. Anderson KE. Influences of diet and nutrition on clinical pharmacokinetics. Clin Pharmacokinet. 1988;14:325–46.
9. Hathcock JN. Metabolic mechanisms of drug-nutrient interactions. Federation Proc. 1985;44:124–29.
10. Hendeles L et al. Food-induced dumping from a "once-a-day" theophylline product as a cause of theophylline toxicity. Chest 1985;87:758–65.
11. Liedholm H, Melander A. Concomitant food intake can increase the bioavailability of propranolol by transient inhibition of its presystemic primary conjugation. Clin Pharmacol Ther. 1986;40:29–36.

12. Olanoff LS et al. Food effects on propranolol systemic and oral clearance: support for a blood flow hypothesis. Clin Pharmacol Ther. 1986;40:408–14.

13. McLean AJ et al. Food splanchnic blood flow, and bioavailability of drugs subject to first-pass metabolism. Clin Pharmacol Ther. 1978;24:5–10.

14. Svensson CK et al. Effect of food on hepatic blood flow: implications in the food effect phenomenon. Clin Pharmacol Ther. 1983;34:316–23.

15. Wilkinson GR, Shand DG. A physiological approach to hepatic drug clearance. Clin Pharmacol Ther. 1975;18:377–90.

16. Elvin AT et al. Effect of food on lidocaine kinetics: mechanism of food-related alteration in high intrinsic clearance drug elimination. Clin Pharmacol Ther. 1981;30:455–60.

17. Daneshmend TK, Roberts CJC. The influence of food on the oral and intravenous pharmacokinetics of a high clearance drug: a study with labetalol. Br J Clin Pharmacol. 1982;14:73–78.

18. Lute M et al. Effect of structured dietary fiber on bioavailability of amoxicillin. Clin Pharmacol Ther. 1987;42:220–24.

19. Johnson BF et al. The effect of dietary fiber on the bioavailability of digoxin in capsules. J Clin Pharmacol. 1987;27:487–90.

20. Brown DD et al. Decreased bioavailability of digoxin due to hypercholesterolemic interventions. Circulation 1978;58:164–72.

21. Shastri RA, Krishnaswamy K. Undernutrition and tetracycline half-life. Clin Chim Acta. 1976;66:157–64.

22. Shastri RA, Krishnaswamy K. Metabolism of sulphadiazine in malnutrition. Br J Clin Pharmacol. 1979;7:69–73.

23. Krishnaswamy K et al. The effect of malnutrition on the pharmacokinetics of phenylbutazone. Clin Pharmacokinet. 1981;6:152–59.

24. Raghuram TC, Krishnaswamy K. Pharmacokinetics and plasma steady-state levels of doxycycline in undernutrition. Br J Clin Pharmacol. 1982;14:785–89.

25. Polasa K et al. Rifampicin kinetics in undernutrition. Br J Clin Pharmacol. 1984;17:481–84.

26. Oie S, Tozer TN. Effect of altered plasma protein binding on apparent volume of distribution. J Pharm Sci. 1979;68:1203–205.

27. Kappas A et al. Influence of dietary protein and carbohydrate on antipyrine and theophylline metabolism in man. Clin Pharmacol Ther. 1976;20:643–53.

28. Anderson KE et al. Nutrition and oxidative drug metabolism in man: relative influence of dietary lipids, carbohydrate, and protein. Clin Pharmacol Ther. 1979;26:493–501.

29. Mucklow JC et al. The influence of changes in dietary fat on the clearance of antipyrine and 4-hydroxylation of debrisoquine. Br J Clin Pharmacol. 1980;9:283.

30. Krishnaswamy K et al. Dietary influences on the kinetics of antipyrine and aminopyrine in human subjects. Br J Clin Pharmacol. 1984;17:139–46.

31. Juan D et al. Effects of dietary protein on theophylline pharmacokinetics and caffeine and aminopyrine breath tests. Clin Pharmacol Ther. 1986;40:187–94.

32. Fagan TC et al. Increased clearance of propranolol and theophylline by high-protein compared with high-carbohydrate diet. Clin Pharmacol Ther. 1987;41:402–406.

33. Thompson PJ et al. The effect of diet upon serum concentrations of theophylline. Br J Clin Pharmacol. 1983;16:267–70.

34. Argyris TS. Additive effects of phenobarbital and high protein diet on liver growth in immature male rats. Dev Biol. 1971;25:293–309.

35. Tschudy DP et al. The effect of carbohydrate feeding on the induction of σ-aminolevulinic acid synthetase. Metabolism 1964;13:396–406.

36. Wade AE et al. Lipids in drug detoxification. In: Hathcock JN, Coon J, eds. Nutrition and Drug Interrelations. New York: Academic Press, Inc.; 1978;475–503.

37. Kalamegham R et al. Metabolism of xenobiotics in undernourished rats—regulation by dietary energy and protein levels. Nutr Rep Int. 1981;24:755–68.

38. Walle UK et al. Oxidative metabolism of propranolol is catalyzed by two different P-450 activities. Pharmacologist 1986;28:218.

39. Yang CS, Yoo JH. Dietary effects on drug metabolism by the mixed-function oxidase system. Pharmacol Ther. 1988;38:53–72.
40. Beattie AD, Sherlock S. Ascorbic acid deficiency in liver disease. Gut 1976;17:571–75.
41. Smithard DJ, Langman MJS. The effect of vitamin supplementation upon antipyrine metabolism in the elderly. Br J Clin Pharmacol. 1978;5:181–85.
42. Ginter E, Vejmolova J. Vitamin C-status and pharmacokinetic profile of antipyrine in man. Br J Clin Pharmacol. 1981;12:256–58.
43. Holloway DE et al. Lack of effect of subclinical ascorbic acid deficiency upon antipyrine metabolism in man. Am J Clin Nutr. 1982;35:917–24.
44. Houston JB. Effect of vitamin C supplement on antipyrine disposition in man. Br J Clin Pharmacol. 1979;4:236–39.
45. Wilson JT et al. Failure of vitamin C to affect the pharmacokinetic profile of antipyrine in man. J Clin Pharmacol. 1976;16:265–70.
46. Houston JB, Levy G. Drug biotransformation interactions in man. VI: acetaminophen and ascorbic acid. J Pharm Sci. 1976;65:1218–221.
47. Berg MJ et al. Phenytoin and folic acid interaction: a preliminary report. Ther Drug Monit. 1983;5:389–94.
48. Berg MJ et al. Phenytoin and folic acid: individualized drug-drug interaction. Ther Drug Monit. 1983;5:395–99.
49. Furlanut M et al. Effects of folic acid on phenytoin kinetics in healthy subjects. Clin Pharmacol Ther. 1978;24:294–97.
50. Viukari NMA. Folic acid and anticonvulsants. Lancet 1968;1:980.
51. Andreasen PB et al. Folic acid and the half-life of diphenylhydantoin in man. Acta Neurol Scand. 1971;47:117–19.
52. Cotzias GC. Metabolic modification of some neurologic disorders. JAMA. 1969;210:1255–262.
53. Bakke OM et al. Antipyrine metabolism in anorexia nervosa. Br J Clin Pharmacol. 1978;5:341–43.
54. Tulpule A, Krishnaswamy K. Chloroquine kinetics in the undernourished. Eur J Clin Pharmacol. 1984;24:273–76.
55. Tranvouez JL et al. Hepatic antipyrine metabolism in malnourished patients: influence of the type of malnutrition and course after nutritional rehabilitation. Am J Clin Nutr. 1985;41:1257–264.
56. Ramesh R et al. Hepatic drug metabolizing enzymes in undernourished man. Toxicology 1985;37:259–66.
57. Conney AH et al. Enhanced phenacetin metabolism in human subjects fed charcoal-broiled beef. Clin Pharmacol Ther. 1976;20:633–42.
58. Kappas A et al. Effect of charcoal broiled beef on antipyrine and theophylline metabolism. Clin Pharmacol Ther. 1978;23:445–50.
59. Anderson KE et al. Acetaminophen metabolism in subjects fed charcoal-broiled beef. Clin Pharmacol Ther. 1983;34:369–74.
60. Conney AH. Pharmacological implications of microsomal enzyme induction. Pharmacol Rev. 1967;19:317–66.
61. Harrison YE, West WL. Stimulatory effect of charcoal-broiled ground beef on the hydroxylation of 3,4-benzpyrene by enzymes in rat liver and placenta. Biochem Pharmacol. 1971;20:2105–108.
62. Pantuck EJ et al. Stimulatory effect of brussels sprouts and cabbage on human drug metabolism. Clin Pharmacol Ther. 1979;25:88–95.
63. Pantuck EJ et al. Effect of brussels sprouts and cabbage on drug conjugation. Clin Pharmacol Ther. 1984;35:161–69.
64. Pantuck EJ et al. Stimulatory effect of vegetables on intestinal drug metabolism in the rat. J Pharmacol Exp Ther. 1976;198:278–83.
65. Wattenberg LW. Studies of polycyclic hydrocarbon hydroxylases of the intestine possibly related to cancer. Effect on diet on benzpyrene hydroxylase activity. Cancer 1971;28:99-102.
66. Mucklow JC et al. Drug oxidation in Asian vegetarians. Lancet 1980;2:151.
67. Brodie MJ et al. Drug metabolism in white vegetarians. Br J Clin Pharmacol. 1980;9:523–25.
68. Pantuck EJ et al. Effects of parenteral nutritional regimens on oxidative drug metabolism. Anesthesiology 1984;60:534–36.

69. Pantuck EJ et al. Stimulation of oxidative drug metabolism by parenteral refeeding of nutritionally depleted patients. Gastroenterology 1985;89:241–45.

70. Burgess P et al. The effect of total parenteral nutrition on hepatic drug oxidation. JPEN. 1987;11:540–43.

71. Henderson RP, Covinsky JO. Effect of protein on renal function and drug disposition. Drug Intell Clin Pharm. 1986;20:842–44.

72. Park GD et al. Effect of dietary protein on renal tubular clearance of drugs in humans. Clin Pharmacokinet. 1989;17:441–51.

73. Moise TS, Smith AH. The effect of high protein diet on the kidney: an experimental study. Arch Pathol. 1927;4:530–42.

74. Jackson H Jr, Riggs MD. The effect of high protein diets on the kidneys of rats. J Biol Chem. 1926;67:101–7.

75. Berlinger WG et al. The effect of dietary protein on the clearance of allopurinol and oxypurinol. N Engl J Med. 1985;313:771–76.

76. Dickson CJ et al. Factors affecting aminoglycoside disposition: effects of circadian rhythm and dietary protein intake on gentamicin pharmacokinetics. Clin Pharmacol Ther. 1986;39:325–28.

77. Brenner BM et al. Dietary protein intake and the progressive nature of kidney disease: the role of hemodynamically mediated glomerular injury in the pathogenesis of progressive glomerular sclerosis in aging, renal ablation, and intrinsic renal disease. N Engl J Med. 1982;307:652–59.

78. Johannesen J et al. Effect of glycine and glucagon on glomerular filtration and renal metabolic rates. Am J Physiol. 1977;233:F61–F66.

79. Seney FD Jr et al. Modification of tubuloglomerular feedback signal by dietary protein. Am J Physiol. 1987;252:F83–F90.

80. Park GD et al. Sustained reductions in oxipurinol renal clearance during a restricted diet. Clin Pharmacol Ther. 1987;41:616–21.

81. Kitt TM et al. Renal clearance of oxipurinol and insulin on an isocaloric, low protein diet. Clin Pharmacol Ther. 1988;43:681–87.

82. Kitt TM et al. Reduced renal clearance of oxypurinol during a 400 calorie protein-free diet. J Clin Pharmacol. 1989;29:65–71.

83. Gersema LM et al. The effect of dietary protein-calorie restriction on the renal elimination of cimetidine. Clin Pharmacol Ther. 1987;42:471–75.

Chapter 13

Theophylline

David J. Edwards, Barbara J. Zarowitz,
and Richard L. Slaughter

For the past two decades, parenteral theophylline has been considered the treatment of choice for the management of acute bronchospasm associated with asthma or chronic obstructive pulmonary disease (COPD). Additionally, oral theophylline therapy has been widely used as first-line therapy for chronic asthma. Recent reports, however, indicate that theophylline has limited efficacy in the early treatment of acute asthma[1,2,3] and suggest that it should not be used for the routine management of bronchospasm in the emergency room.[4,5] Theophylline therapy is of significant value in the management of chronic asthma and has been recommended for use as a first-line agent in the treatment of chronic asthma.[6] The application of pharmacokinetic and pharmacodynamic information in conjunction with readily available serum assays has allowed theophylline to be used with improved efficacy and an acceptable risk of toxicity. Therefore, understanding the pharmacodynamics and pharmacokinetics of theophylline has direct therapeutic relevance. Furthermore, because of its pharmacokinetic characteristics, theophylline has been used as a marker substance in the evaluation of factors that influence drug metabolism. Understanding the pharmacokinetics of theophylline provides a better understanding of those factors that control hepatic drug metabolism.

A MEDLINE search covering the past five years revealed almost 600 published articles dealing with the pharmacokinetics of theophylline. This chapter will not attempt to present an exhaustive review of this tremendous volume of literature. Rather, it will focus on clinical issues and recent developments that have direct relevance to practitioners using theophylline.

PHARMACODYNAMICS

Concentration-Effect Relationships for Therapeutic Effects

Theophylline produces a wide range of pharmacologic effects which have clinical relevance. It is effective in the management of asthma by relaxing bronchial smooth muscle and will prevent methacholine, histamine,[7,8] grass,[9] ragweed,[10] and exercise-induced bronchospasm;[11] it may attenuate allergen-induced hyperreactivity and the late-phase response.[12] Theophylline may be effective in the management of airflow obstruction associated with chronic obstructive airway disease,[13,14,15] and can improve diaphragmatic contractility.[16,17] While improvement is seen in respiratory mechanics and arterial blood gases,[18] the ability of theophylline to actually improve exercise tolerance in patients with irreversible airways obstruction remains controversial.[18,19] Theophylline can also be used to treat premature apnea in infants.[20] Adverse effects from theophylline are a result of its effects on the central nervous system, cardiovascular system, and renal system. Many of the therapeutic and toxic effects of theophylline have been related to serum concentrations achieved. Specific concentration-effect relationships are different for specific effects (i.e., smooth muscle bronchodilation versus seizures), and can also differ depending on the method of administration (single IV bolus versus chronic dosing). In general, the disparity between the concentration-effect relationship of beneficial effects and adverse effects provides partial justification for monitoring serum theophylline concentrations.

When administered as a single dose either intravenously[21] or orally as an elixir,[22] a lag is observed between the time theophylline serum concentrations are achieved and the time that improved pulmonary function is observed. A clearly evident counterclockwise hysteresis is present when the percent improvement in FEV_1 is plotted as a function of theophylline concentration.[21,22] This indicates a delay in the occurrence of a linear relationship between concentration and effect. The time lag ranges from 14 ± 5 minutes[23] to 70 ± 20 minutes,[22] with an average of about 60 minutes. This is an important consideration when evaluating the efficacy of theophylline in the management of acute exacerbations of asthma or COPD. Theophylline has clearly been shown not to be as effective in the management of acute bronchospasm as inhaled or injected beta adrenergic drugs when evaluated 60 minutes after drug administration.[1,2,3] It is, however, as effective when compared over a longer time frame, i.e., 24 hours.[24] The time lag is believed to be related primarily to the time required for distribution of theophylline to its target site. However, one report indicates that it may take up to 48 hours for the maximal effect of theophylline to be achieved in the management of acute bronchospasm.[25] Since this is beyond the time required to achieve steady-state concentrations, a more complex interplay may exist between serum concentration and improvement in lung function after an acute exacerbation of bronchospasm.

Current data support the concept that once theophylline is distributed to the target site, the percent improvement in pulmonary function is linearly related to the serum concentration.[23,26,27] Over the range of 5 to 20 µg/mL, pulmonary function (FEV_1 or FVC) will improve by about 2% for each µg/mL increase in drug concentration. Thus, a 20% improvement in FEV_1 can be expected when comparing patients with high theophylline concentrations (18 to 22 µg/mL) to those with low concentrations (8 to 10 µg/mL). This is quite consistent with clinical observations that have evaluated high- and low-dose theophylline therapy in patients with asthma[26] and chronic obstructive pulmonary disease.[13] Theophylline prevents both methacholine and histamine-induced bronchospasm.[7,8] The provocative methacholine dose required to increase SR_{aw}, a measure of airway resistance, by 100% ($PD_{100}SR_{aw}$) increases twofold (1.08 ± 0.72 to 2.60 ± 2.12) as concentrations increase from 3 to 6 µg/mL and again twofold (2.60 ± 2.12 to 4.98 ± 3.82) from 6 to 13 µg/mL.[7] Clearly, the degree of protection increases as a function of concentration and is evident at concentrations as low as 6 µg/mL. It should be noted that theophylline is a relatively weak bronchodilator, particularly when compared to beta agonists. Theophylline may have a more important role in preventing symptoms, despite small changes in pulmonary function. For example, theophylline is more effective than terbutaline at preventing early morning wheezing and dyspnea.[28] A relationship between concentration and appearance or disappearance of symptoms such as wheeze-free days[29] is also evident.[29,30] These beneficial effects can be seen without significant improvement in pulmonary function tests. Thus, when evaluating concentration-effect relationships for theophylline, direct measurement of symptomatology should be performed in addition to pulmonary function testing. The primary beneficial effects achieved when using theophylline to manage either asthma or chronic obstructive pulmonary disease are also concentration-related. Improvement is seen with concentrations as low as 4 to 6 µg/mL and this increases in a linear fashion up to levels of 20 µg/mL. When concentrations exceed 20 µg/mL, some improvement in pulmonary function will be realized; however, symptoms of toxicity will begin to appear. Thus, it is recommended that theophylline concentrations be maintained below 20 µg/mL in patients on chronic therapy. Conservative management dictates that concentrations should probably be maintained between 10 and 15 µg/mL. The reasons for this include: theophylline clearance is not stable; several diseases and drugs can decrease theophylline clearance (see below); and theophylline is a comparatively weak bronchodilator.

Theophylline has several effects which extend beyond the respiratory system, but the relationship of these to serum concentrations is less clear. In premature infants, concentrations of 5 to 10 µg/mL are sufficient to abolish episodes of recurring apnea.[31] Numerous other effects occur at concentrations within the therapeutic range, such as increasing diaphragmatic contractility;[16,17] metabolic effects on free fatty acids, serum glucose, and glucagon;[32] increases in gastric acid secretion;[33] and effects on neutrophil function.[34] The dependency of these effects on graded increases in concentration, however, generally are not well described.

Concentration-Effect Relationships for Toxic Effects

Adverse effects are generally associated with serum concentrations above 20 µg/mL and include: nausea, vomiting, headache, diarrhea, irritability and insomnia, supraventricular tachycardia, hypotension, ventricular arrhythmias, seizures, brain damage, and death.[35-37] The likelihood of suffering serious toxicity increases with increasing serum theophylline concentrations above 20 µg/mL.[38] For example, the probability of exhibiting an adverse reaction to theophylline is about 85% with serum concentrations over 25 µg/mL.[39] Recent studies suggest that a clear, definitive relationship between serum concentrations and the severity of toxic effects may not be as well defined as previously thought.[40,41] Occasionally, patients with theophylline concentrations well above the therapeutic range exhibit no toxicity[40] while, conversely, theophylline-induced seizures and cardiovascular toxicity can occur in patients with concentrations between 20 and 25 µg/mL.[41,42] Sustained ventricular or supraventricular tachyarrhythmias requiring antiarrhythmic therapy are uncommon.[42] Concentrations between 20 and 30 µg/mL therefore may be associated with serious adverse effects.

Seizures may occur without early warning symptoms of toxicity, particularly in patients older than 75 years who have underlying seizure disorders, hypoalbuminemia, severe pulmonary disease or liver disease; seizures frequently produce residual neurologic deficits.[43,44,280] Cardiac toxicity (most often presenting as sinus tachycardia, supraventricular and ventricular ectopic beats) is more prevalent in older adult patients with underlying cardiovascular disorders.[37,42,43,281] In patients with any of these risk factors, serum theophylline concentrations should be maintained at levels less than or equal to 10 to 15 µg/mL.[280] The circumstances surrounding the cause of toxicity can influence its symptomatology as well. For example, acute intentional intoxication will result in higher concentrations with more serious symptoms than chronic overmedication including an apparent higher incidence of fatalities.[45] In one report,[45] theophylline concentration correlated with the severity of toxicity in the patients with acute overdose, but not in those patients with chronic overdose. Aggressive management of acute theophylline overdose is essential in all cases and is independent of presenting symptoms, particularly when serum concentrations exceed 60 µg/mL (see Management of Theophylline Toxicity).

Metabolic abnormalities (including hypokalemia, hyperglycemia, leukocytosis, hypercalcemia, hypophosphatemia, hypomagnesemia, and metabolic acidosis with respiratory compensation) occur commonly when serum theophylline concentrations are greater than 40 µg/mL.[46,47] The metabolic abnormalities which are related linearly to theophylline concentration can be prevented or partially reversed by propranolol, suggesting that they are mediated by the β-adrenergic system.[47,48]

Manifestations of theophylline toxicity in neonates include failure to gain weight, sleeplessness, irritability, diuresis and dehydration, hyperflexia, and jitteriness as well as the serious cardiovascular and neurologic complications observed in adults at higher concentrations.[49]

Theophylline toxicity is relatively uncommon. The prevalence of theophylline concentrations greater than 20 µg/mL is under 10% of those samples measured in an inpatient setting.[45] However, in elderly patients undergoing chronic dosing, unintentional toxicity producing a life-threatening event occurs 16.7 times more often than in younger (less than 25 years) patients.[281] Theophylline toxicity can result in serious morbidity and mortality; thus, patients on theophylline should be monitored closely to assure they are receiving the appropriate dose.

ABSORPTION

Theophylline is well absorbed when taken as a rapid-release tablet or when administered as a liquid solution.[50,51] For both of these preparations, the extent of absorption rarely is altered to a clinically significant degree. The rate of absorption of certain formulations, however, can be influenced by food,[52] time of day,[53] and co-administration of antacids.[54] For example, antacids have a greater effect on formulations which demonstrate pH-dependent dissolution characteristics.[55] In contrast, the extent of absorption from slow-release formulations is affected by several factors as reviewed by others[56] and discussed below.

Intrapatient Variability

The absorption parameters for sustained-release theophylline products varies within subjects.[57,58] The rate of absorption can vary as much as 40% to 50% within the same subject studied on two different occasions, although the extent of theophylline absorbed fluctuates less. One group evaluated the bioavailability and fluctuations in serum theophylline concentrations in children (ages two to seven years) receiving Slo-BID. There were two study days separated by one week.[59] The absolute difference in bioavailability averaged 19.8% (range: 4% to 32%) while the percent change in serum theophylline concentration (% STC) was 59.2% (range: 26% to 94.5%). Bioavailability differed by 20% or more in five of the seven subjects and the % STC differed by more than 50% in four of the seven subjects. Patients with shorter half-lives and larger clearance values tend to exhibit greater within-subject changes in serum concentrations than those with longer half-lives and slower clearance values.

Diurnal Variation

While the clearance of theophylline is unaffected by the time of day,[53] absorption is significantly influenced.[60-62] At night, rapid-release preparations are absorbed more slowly (the time to reach peak concentrations was delayed) compared to daytime administration. The extent of absorption is unchanged.[53] With sustained-released preparations, absorption is not only slowed, it is reduced as well. This effect has been reported with Theo-Dur,[60] Uniphyl,[62] Phyllocontin,[63] and Theo-24.[63] A pronounced circadian change observed when theophylline is given at 11 a.m. and 11 p.m. is abolished when it is given at 5 a.m. and 5 p.m.[64] Thus, the time between taking the last theophylline dose and going to sleep is an important factor in this interaction. Other factors that may be involved include diurnal changes in gastric pH; the effects these changes have on formulations that show pH-dependent dissolution characteristics; and the administration of food. The diurnal effect can also be minimized by using unequal divided doses. Taking a larger percentage of the daily dose at night when absorption is decreased has been shown to be efficacious, particularly in those patients with nocturnal asthma.[62] This phenomenon can delay the absorption of the nighttime to the following morning, resulting in an increased area under the concentration-time curve (AUC) the following day.

Food

When coadministered with food, theophylline absorption is affected in various ways depending on the sustained release preparation used. For most preparations which exhibit 100% bioavailability, co-administration with food will have no effect[66] or will delay absorption.[67] There are, however, specific situations in which food can significantly alter the extent of absorption from sustained-release preparations.

Administering Theo-Dur Sprinkle with food (e.g., corn flakes cereal) reduces its bioavailability by more than 50% on average with some subjects experiencing a greater than 80% reduction in bioavailability.[68] This effect also occurs when Theo-Dur Sprinkle is administered over soft custard and then taken either ten minutes before or immediately after a meal.[69] Absorption is not affected when bead-filled capsules are taken with applesauce in an otherwise fasting condition.[70] Thus, patients using Theo-Dur Sprinkle should take it with something like applesauce which wets the sprinkles, ideally two hours before a meal. If this regimen cannot be adhered to, another theophylline formulation should be used.

When products designed for once-daily dosing are taken with food, an increase in peak concentrations and AUC as well as toxicity have been observed (see Figure 13-1).[71–75] The effect appears to be more pronounced for products that are not 100% bioavailable. Although first reported with Theo-24,[71] significant increases in theophylline serum concentrations have also been reported for Uniphyl[73–75] and Theograd.[72] The effect with Uniphyl and Theograd appears to be more delayed than that seen with Theo-24. The initial rate of absorption is slower when these two products are taken with a meal. In contrast, when Theo-24 is taken with a high fat meal, as much as 50% of the dose can be absorbed within four hours of ingestion.[71] The composition of the meal significantly influences this interaction; meals that are high in fat content cause the most pronounced changes.[76] This effect also may be more prevalent in children; their higher clearance rates necessitate the use of larger mg/kg doses.[77] These observations have resulted in labeling requirements for all once-a-day products. This subject is covered in detail in a review.[78]

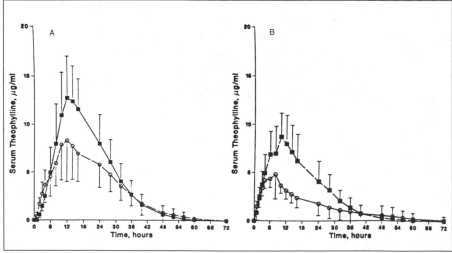

Figure 13-1. *Mean (± SD) serum theophylline concentrations in subjects given a single dose of Theo-24 900 mg (A) or Uniphyl 800 mg (B) under fasting condition (o) or following a high-fat breakfast (■).*

Once-A-Day Products

Recent innovations in the formulation of sustained-released preparations have led to the development of products recommended for once-a-day theophylline dosing. These products include Theo-24, Uniphyl, Slobid, Theo-Dur and Unidur. Both Theo-24 and Uniphyl are consistently absorbed to a lesser extent than Theo-Dur.[79,80]

The degree of fluctuation in serum theophylline concentrations during a dosing interval also tends to be large for all once-a-day products. The mean change exceeds 100% (that is, the peak concentration is more than twice that of the trough concentration within a given subject). This is particularly a problem in individuals with high clearance values who can experience fluctuations as large as 300% to 400%.[62,81] A simulation of the serum theophylline-concentration time profile for sustained-release products designed for once-daily and twice-daily dosing is shown in Figure 13-2. Note that the fluctuations in concentration that occur over a dosing interval may be acceptable for both products in patients with low theophylline clearance values. However, an unacceptable degree of fluctuation may occur for products designed for once-daily dosing in patients with high theophylline clearance values. The predicted effect of baseline theophylline clearance on fluctuations in serum concentrations is shown in Figure 13-3. This correlates well with the observation that fluctuations in theophylline concentrations depend on baseline clearance values when sustained-release products are used.[61] These data indicate how difficult it is to maintain serum concentrations within 10 to 20 μg/mL with once-a-day theophylline products.

Most products designed for twice-daily administration are 100% bioavailable and serum concentrations fluctuate 40% to 80% over a dosing interval.[56,80] Consequently, much tighter control of serum theophylline concentrations can be achieved with twice-daily formulations compared to once-daily formulations. Thus, any potential benefit that may accrue from improved compliance needs to be evaluated in light of the poorer performance of once-daily sustained-release products. Once-daily administration is recommended if the effect of food can be minimized and when alternate treatments are impractical (e.g., the use of inhaled beta agonists to treat nocturnal asthma).[61,82] These products may also be beneficial in patients who do not comply with twice-a-day regimens. In this instance one could use a product like Uni-Dur (Schering-Plough) that has a slower absorption rate than Theo-Dur and is not affected by food. However, since excessive fluctuations in theophylline concentrations still occurred in 3 out of 16 subjects,[83] this product must be used with caution as well. Using historical data, decision analysis has shown that routine use of once-a-day products is favored over twice-a-day products.[84] However, because of the problems inherent with these products, we do not recommend their routine use for the management of chronic asthma or COPD.

Substitution of Sustained-Release Theophylline Products

Significant variability in absorption patterns exist between theophylline products and thus limit the usefulness of between-brand substitution.[85] This problem was highlighted in a study that compared the serum theophylline concentrations, efficacy, and toxicity of four sustained-release preparations (Somophylline-CRT, Theo-Dur, Constant-T, and Slo-Bid).[86] Fourteen subjects were studied, and each was evaluated twice on the same product before being crossed over to the next product. Average fluctuations in theophylline concentrations were similar for all products. However, within the same subject, significant differences were apparent. For example, one subject demonstrated larger fluctuations with Theo-Dur (218% and 168%) than Constant-T (86% and 118%) even though both products were wax matrix sustained-release products. Furthermore, when products were switched,

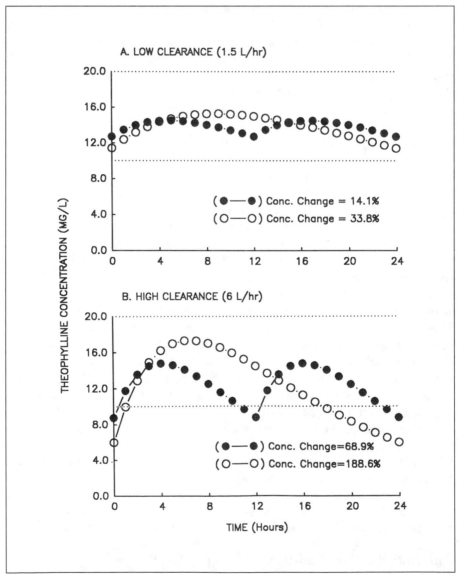

Figure 13-2. Simulated serum theophylline concentrations for products designed for once-daily ($\bigcirc$, ka = 0.10/hr) and twice-daily ($\bullet$, ka = 0.18/hr) administration. Simulations are for individuals with low (A) and high (B) theophylline clearance given the same total daily dose of each product.

pulmonary symptom scores worsened in four subjects whose concentrations dropped below 10 µg/mL. On 25 occasions, serum theophylline concentrations exceeded 20 µg/mL and symptoms of toxicity were associated with 15 of these events. This study argues strongly against routine generic substitution if a patient is responding well to a particular theophylline product. This is particularly relevant since over 30 sustained-release products are available.

Sustained-Release Suspensions

Currently, available dosage formulations designed for sustained-release administration have limited flexibility in that the patient must be able to take a solid oral dosage form. This limits their usefulness in children and patients who cannot take solid oral dosage forms (e.g., those on mechanical ventilators). Thus, a sustained-release oral suspension would have clinical utility. Theolan Suspension (Elan Pharmaceutical Corporation) is a long-acting liquid theophylline dosage form that may become commercially available. This preparation has an overall bioavailability of 89.5 ± 33% and a T_{max} of 3.4 ± 1.3 hours (compared to 1.4 ± 1 hour for theophylline liquid).[87] When dosed every 12 hours and compared to aminophylline solution dosed every eight hours, lower peak concentrations, lower max-min fluctuations, and lower variability in plasma concentrations were observed. These qualities will benefit those patients who cannot take conventional oral dosage formulations of theophylline.

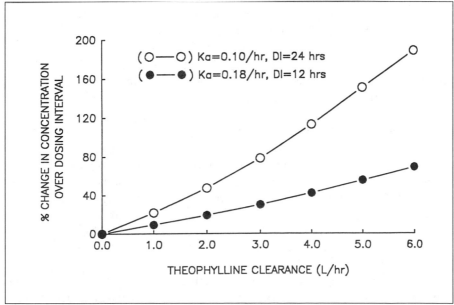

Figure 13-3. *The effect of theophylline clearance on the expected % change in theophylline concentration over a dosing interval (($(C_{max} - C_{min}/C_{min}) \times 100$) for products designed for once-daily (O) and twice-daily (●) administration.*

DISTRIBUTION

Theophylline distributes into fat-free tissues and body water and has a mean apparent volume of distribution of 0.45 L/kg (0.3 - 0.7 L/kg) in adults[88,89] and children.[90,91] The volume of distribution increases linearly with total body weight in both non-obese and obese subjects.[92-95] In obese subjects, the increase in volume of distribution is believed to be secondary to an increase in fat-free rather than fat mass. This supports the use of total body weight to estimate theophylline's volume of distribution.[96] An exception to this practice is in morbidly obese patients (i.e., those greater than 50% above their ideal body weight). Since the change in post-dose theophylline serum concentrations correlates with the degree of obesity in this group,[94] ideal body weight should be used to estimate the volume of distribution used to calculate a loading dose. This should reduce the risk of overdosing these patients.[94]

Theophylline passes freely across the placenta, into breast milk, and into the cerebrospinal fluid (CSF). Distribution into the CSF facilitates its usefulness for the treatment of apnea in premature infants and predisposes patients to central nervous system toxicity at high doses.[35,48] Saliva theophylline concentrations approximate unbound serum theophylline concentrations.[35]

Once theophylline enters the systemic circulation, distribution occurs rapidly. It is approximately 40% bound to plasma proteins, predominantly albumin. Binding decreases as the pH decreases and the temperature rises.[97] Many of the early studies did not control these conditions and this resulted in artificially high theophylline protein binding estimates of approximately 60%.[97]

Alterations in theophylline protein binding have been reported in neonates,[98] critically ill mechanically ventilated adults,[99] patients with acid/base disturbances,[100,101] hypoxemia,[102,103] cirrhosis,[104,105] protein-calorie malnutrition,[106] and in pregnant women.[107] Reduced protein binding in neonates, cirrhosis, pregnant women, and the elderly[108] is believed to be secondary to decreases in serum albumin.[35] In uncorrected acidosis, each 0.10 unit decrease in pH decreases theophylline binding by 4% and increases the apparent volume of distribution by 0.2 L/kg.[100,101] Hypoxemia and/or hypercapnea decrease theophylline volume of distribution in conscious rabbits and slightly increase the unbound fraction, suggesting a decrease in tissue distribution or an increase in the tissue unbound fraction.[103] These effects could not be isolated from the effects of acidosis alone in patients with chronic obstructive airways diseases.[102] Although the apparent volume of distribution is assumed to be approximately 0.45 L/kg, many of the above conditions can significantly alter this value; these effects are summarized in Table 13-1.

The clinical significance of protein binding alterations has received little attention because theophylline is not highly protein bound and undergoes restrictive elimination in the liver.[109] Increases in the fraction of unbound drug in the plasma do not change the unbound theophylline concentration. However, the total concentration will be lower in this situation. This could, in some patients, create an illusion of a subtherapeutic plasma concentration and lead to unnecessary and potentially dangerous dosage increases. In predisposed patients, serum albumin

Table 13-1. *Theophylline Apparent Volume of Distribution in Various Clinical Conditions*

Condition	Apparent V_d Mean ± SD (L/kg TBW)	Range	References
Normal adults	0.430 ± 0.060		108
	0.462 ± 0.087	(0.290–0.705)	88
Neonates	0.690 ± 0.950		98
Cirrhotics	0.785	(0.479–1.187)	105
	0.563 ± 0.080		104
Obese adults	0.382 ± 0.069		92
Protein-calorie malnourished children	0.725 ± 0.063		106
Elderly	0.320 ± 0.050		108
	0.550 ± 0.110		109

and arterial blood gases should be assessed to establish the likelihood of a binding aberration before the dose is increased. Patients with probable binding alterations who are maintained at serum theophylline concentrations of 15 to 20 µg/mL may be at greater risk of toxicity due to increases in unbound theophylline. Titration of the dose to serum concentrations of no more than 10 to 15 µg/mL is advised for these patients.

METABOLISM AND EXCRETION

Metabolism

Theophylline is primarily eliminated by hepatic metabolism. The primary metabolites in adults are formed by hydroxylation at the 8 position (1,3-dimethyluric acid) and by N-demethylation (3-methylxanthine and 1-methylxanthine) (see Figure 13-4). 1-methylxanthine is rapidly oxidized in the body to 1-methyluric acid which can be recovered and quantitated in the urine. Caffeine, formed by methylation of theophylline at the 7 position, is a minor metabolite but achieves serum concentrations of pharmacologic importance in neonates who eliminate caffeine more slowly than adults. In adults, approximately 35% to 40% is excreted as 1,3-dimethyluric acid, 20% to 25% as 1-methylurate and 15% to 20% as 3-methylxanthine.[110–115] Renal elimination of unchanged drug accounts for only 10% to 15% of the overall excretion of theophylline in adults but may increase up to 50% in neonates.[116]

The metabolism of theophylline is mediated via the cytochrome P450 system in the microsomal fraction of the hepatocyte.[117] It appears that CYP1A2[282] is the most important isozyme involved in theophylline metabolism. However, studies with a variety of enzyme inducers and inhibitors have suggested that the N-demethylation and 8-hydroxylation pathways are mediated by different forms, since changes in the formation of 3-methylxanthine and 1-methylurate following induction and inhibition often occur in parallel and may differ from the effect on 1,3-dimethylurate.[115,117–119,282] This is further supported by the *in vitro* observation that the V_{max} for hydroxylation is roughly fivefold higher than for the N-demethylation pathways.[120] In addition, selective inhibition of 3-methylxanthine with no effect on 1-methylurate, suggests that different isozymes may be involved in the N-demethylation of theophylline. A similar observation has been made for verapamil.[113,114] High correlations have been observed between theophylline and antipyrine metabolism; in particular, the formation of 4-hydroxyantipyrine.[121,122] This suggests the common involvement of one or more isozymes in the metabolism of both of these compounds. Certain isozymes of cytochrome P450 exhibit genetically linked differences in the rate of substrate metabolism. Studies by Miller et al.[123] suggest that genetic differences do contribute significantly to inter-individual variability in theophylline metabolism with all three metabolic pathways regulated by a common factor.

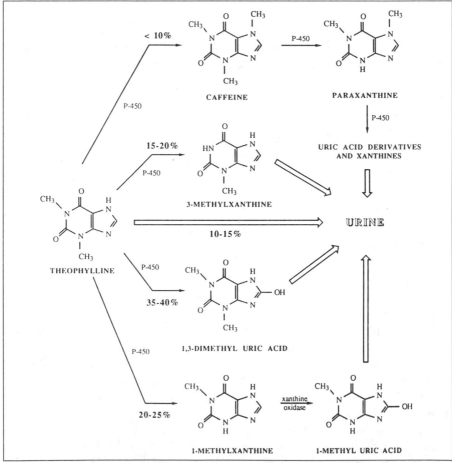

Figure 13-4. Pathways of theophylline elimination in adults and children. Solid arrows represent hepatic metabolism with enzyme involved and percentage of dose eliminated by each pathway being noted. Open arrows represent urinary excretion.

Elimination Kinetics

Theophylline elimination has traditionally been assumed to follow first-order kinetics. However, clinical reports of dose-dependency in theophylline elimination as well as studies assessing K_m and V_{max} for the individual metabolic pathways of theophylline suggest that *Michaelis-Menten kinetics* may be observed in some patients at therapeutic concentrations. The overall K_m for theophylline elimination has been estimated to be 20 to 25 mg/L with an average V_{max} of approximately 2000 mg/day.[124-126] It appears that the N-demethylation pathways exhibit lower values for V_{max} and are more susceptible to saturation than the 8-hydroxylation pathway.[110,120,124] On average, the decrease in elimination with increasing dose appears to be relatively small. Dahlqvist et al.[124] observed a 20.4% decrease in clearance over a dose range of 210 to 1260 mg/day, while Bachmann et al.[127] found that clearance was 18.8% lower following a 6 mg/kg dose compared to 2 mg/kg. Dosing simulations performed by Wagner[125] suggest that half-life will be prolonged by 17% over a dose range of 300 to 1500 mg. However, it should be noted that these are average values associated with interpatient variability and clinical studies have indicated that more significant dose-dependent kinetics may be seen in many patients.[126] At present, predicting dose-dependency in patients *a priori* is not possible.

Apparent differences in theophylline elimination following single and multiple doses have been documented.[128,129] Using stable isotope techniques, Vestal et al.[128] were able to simultaneously compare the elimination of theophylline following the oral and intravenous administration of single and multiple doses. They found that clearance appeared to be reduced with multiple-dose administration only after oral dosing. This observation was attributed to diurnal variation in absorption with slowed absorption following evening doses causing elevated morning concentrations of theophylline. Since pharmacokinetic studies with multiple dosing are frequently conducted over a single dosing interval following a morning dose, the elevated morning concentrations result in a larger area under the serum concentration-time curve being possibly misinterpreted as a lower apparent oral clearance. Although it is well documented that the absorption of theophylline is delayed at night,[60-62] there are conflicting data regarding a diurnal variation in elimination. Jonkman et al.[130] reported a 30% longer half-life during the evening, while St. Pierre et al.[131] found that despite a lower renal clearance, metabolic and total body clearance were not significantly different following morning and evening doses. Similarly, Watanabe et al.[53] found that the half-life of theophylline was not influenced by the time of day. A similar conclusion was reached in studies that found no significant differences between day and night concentrations of theophylline under steady-state conditions with a continuous intravenous infusion of theophylline.[132,133]

Physiological and Environmental Influences on Theophylline Clearance

Theophylline is primarily cleared from the body by hepatic metabolism. Since the hepatic extraction ratio is less than 0.05 in most individuals, theophylline exhibits the pharmacokinetic behavior of a poorly extracted drug. Plasma protein binding is not extensive so that metabolic and total body clearance of theophylline are primarily a function of intrinsic clearance. Therefore, any factor influencing the activity of the hepatic enzymes involved in theophylline metabolism can potentially alter theophylline clearance. Few drugs have been studied as extensively as theophylline, and numerous physiological and environmental factors, disease states, and concomitantly administered drugs have been found to affect the clearance of this drug.

Establishing a baseline value for theophylline clearance is difficult because clearance is influenced by such a wide variety of factors. However, in young adult males (20 to 30 years of age), the most commonly studied subject, the average clearance is about 0.7 mL/min/kg. If an average value for the apparent volume of distribution is assumed, the half-life of theophylline in these individuals would be seven to eight hours.

Within-Subject Variability. There are conflicting data regarding the stability of theophylline clearance within an individual subject over time. Upton et al.[134] found that the elimination rate constant of theophylline varied considerably (more than 30% in 7 of 12 subjects) when measured on five separate occasions in the same subjects. Slaughter et al.[135] reached a similar conclusion after measuring theophylline clearance on four occasions (at least three weeks apart) in six healthy volunteers. He used intravenous administration to avoid the variability associated with oral bioavailability. The within-subject coefficient of variation for clearance averaged 14.9% and clearance changes of more than 15% were observed in two of six subjects (although changes of greater than 25% occurred in five of six subjects). This wide variability in clearance has also been observed in acutely ill, hospitalized patients.[136] In contrast, Milavetz et al.[137] found that elimination rate constants determined twice in ten subjects differed by less than 10% in all cases. Studies of this type with other hepatically metabolized drugs generally support the recommendation that the clearance of theophylline should be re-evaluated frequently in acutely ill patients and periodically in those receiving long-term therapy.

Gender. Most pharmacokinetic studies with theophylline have used male subjects despite the fact that a high percentage of patients requiring the drug are female. Although few prospective studies have been published to date, current data suggest that gender differences in theophylline clearance are relatively small and unlikely to be of clinical significance.[138,139] Female smokers and nonsmokers have shorter theophylline half-life values than males.[283] Significant decrease in theophylline clearance was observed at day 20 of the menstrual cycle.[284] Significant decreases in clearance have been reported in the third trimester of pregnancy. Gender-related changes in clearance need more study.[140,141]

Age. The effect of age on the clearance of theophylline has been studied extensively (see Figure 13-5). Clearance is markedly reduced in neonates who appear to be particularly deficient in their ability to form 1,3-dimethylurate, the major metabolite of theophylline in adults. Dothey et al.[142] found that although half-life averaged 29.2 hours in nine subjects aged 12 to 191 days, it decreased significantly with postnatal age. Clearance appears to reach maximal values of roughly 1.5 mL/min/kg by one year; it remains relatively stable during the first decade of life[143,144]

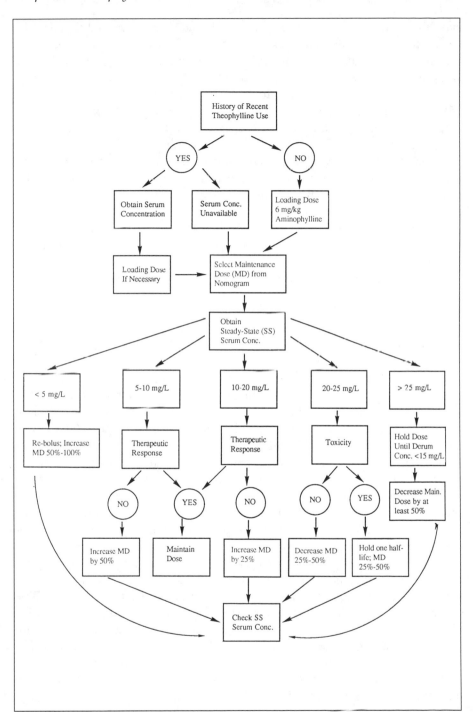

Figure 13-5. Algorithm for theophylline dosing in the adult patient with acute bronchospasm. Suggested actions for particular serum concentrations should not be misconstrued as absolute. Factors such as compliance, assay accuracy, non-attainment of steady state and the response of the individual patient can complicate interpretation and may require an alternative course of action.

and falls by approximately 50% to adult values during the second decade. The clearance in elderly adults appears to be significantly lower than in young adults. Vestal et al.[115] compared non-smoking subjects with a mean age of 27 to those with a mean age of 72 and found clearance to be 32% lower in the elderly subjects. Several other studies[112,144,145] have found similar decreases in clearance (30% to 35%) over this age range with all metabolic pathways reduced to a similar extent.[112,115] Adult age is, however, a relatively weak predictor of theophylline clearance due to the myriad of factors influencing clearance of this drug.[144]

Obesity. Since theophylline is frequently administered to obese patients, the influence of this factor on theophylline clearance is also of interest. Gal et al.[92] found that the clearance of theophylline in 14 obese subjects normalized for ideal body weight was similar to that of 57 non-obese subjects. This conclusion is supported by studies with other drugs which have found no significant alteration in oxidative drug metabolism tendencies in obese subjects.[147] In contrast, severe malnutrition reduces the oxidative metabolism of substrates like antipyrine, but well-controlled prospective studies are lacking for theophylline.[148]

Diet. A number of studies have shown dietary influences on theophylline clearance. Fagan et al.[149] confirmed earlier reports that a high-protein, low-carbohydrate diet is associated with a significantly higher theophylline clearance than a low-protein, high-carbohydrate diet. A diet high in charbroiled beef has also been shown to increase the clearance of theophylline.[150]

Cigarette Smoking. Perhaps the most significant factor influencing theophylline clearance in otherwise healthy adults is cigarette smoking. Vestal et al.[115] found that clearance was increased by 49% in young smokers and by 77% in elderly smokers compared to non-smoking subjects and that the induction was somewhat selective for the N-demethylation pathways. Other studies have confirmed that a 40% to 80% increase in theophylline clearance can be expected in smokers and that this effect is independent of patient age.[151–153] Abstinence from smoking for one week decreased the clearance of theophylline by 37.6%.[154] This observation is clinically significant since many patients stop smoking while in the hospital. Thus, the clearance determined upon admission may not be reflective of that later in the hospital stay. Matsunga et al.[155] found that passive smoking increased theophylline clearance by 47% compared to non-smokers. This suggests that classifying patients for the purpose of dosing as smokers or non-smokers may not be adequate. A further implication is that previous studies of theophylline clearance in non-smokers must be viewed with caution since it is likely that passive smokers were included in this classification. Many smokers attempt to quit with the aid of nicotine gum; Benowitz and co-workers[154,156] found that this product has no effect on theophylline clearance. Finally, patients receiving theophylline should be questioned regarding smoking of marijuana since this also has been shown to elevate theophylline clearance.[153]

Effect of Disease States on Theophylline Clearance

The clearance of theophylline is altered in a number of disease states with the largest decreases occurring in patients with cirrhosis and congestive heart failure.

Cirrhosis. Several studies[104,105,157] have found theophylline clearance to be reduced by an average of 40% to 60% in patients with cirrhosis. Mangione et al.[104] also observed a significant negative correlation between clearance and total bilirubin. However, given the experience with other drugs, all patients with active cirrhosis should be dosed with extreme caution rather than relying on the bilirubin concentration or other biochemical measures as an indicator of disease severity.

Congestive Heart Failure. Decreases in clearance of a similar magnitude have been observed in patients with congestive heart failure.[158-160] The impaired clearance is related to the degree of failure so that patients with cor pulmonale or other symptoms of severe heart failure may have much greater decreases in clearance. These patients should be treated with extreme caution. Since theophylline is a poorly extracted drug, the decreased clearance associated with heart failure is probably caused by impaired hepatocyte function rather than alterations in hepatic blood flow.[161] Renal clearance of theophylline is a small component of total body clearance (except in neonates); thus, renal disease has no significant effect on clearance.[157,162]

Infection. A matter of considerable controversy concerns the effects of acute infection on theophylline disposition. Decreased theophylline clearance has been reported in children with influenza,[163,164] and this may be related to the induction of interferon. Indeed, administration of interferon decreased theophylline clearance by about 15%.[165] In contrast, Bachmann et al.[166] found no change in theophylline clearance during and after mild upper respiratory infections in 19 adults. A decrease in antipyrine clearance of about 35% has been reported in 14 patients with pneumonia;[167] data for theophylline are limited but also suggest that its clearance is impaired as well.[160] Related to this issue is the potential effect of vaccination on clearance. Meredith et al.[168] demonstrated a transient decrease in theophylline clearance after vaccination for influenza that was accompanied by increases in interferon concentrations. However, other studies[169-172] have found no alterations in theophylline clearance following influenza vaccine. In the study by Grabowski et al.,[170] influenza vaccination did not increase concentrations of interferon, and theophylline clearance was not affected by vaccination. This provides additional support for the theory that an interferon response is needed for vaccination-induced reduction in theophylline clearance. Pneumococcal vaccine also does not affect clearance[173] although a decrease has been observed following BCG vaccination.[174]

Thyroid Disease. Alterations in thyroid function affect the disposition of several drugs. Pokrajac et al.[175] studied hyperthyroid, euthyroid, and hypothyroid patients and found the mean theophylline clearance to be 3.21, 2.33 and 1.84 L/hr, respectively. This study along with earlier work,[176] supports the conclusion that clearance is decreased in hypothyroid disease and elevated with hyperthyroidism.

Cystic Fibrosis. Theophylline clearance appears to be elevated in patients with cystic fibrosis. Total clearance normalized for weight and body surface area was 40% higher in 11 cystic fibrosis patients when compared to 15 controls matched for body size and diet.[177]

Hypoxemia. The effect of acute hypoxemia on theophylline clearance has been studied. In two studies, oxygen administration to patients with COPD had no effect on theophylline clearance suggesting that hypoxemia itself has no effect on clearance.[102,178]

Drug Interactions Altering Theophylline Clearance

The effect of other drugs on the disposition of theophylline has been widely studied because theophylline has such a narrow therapeutic range. Table 13-2 lists a number of these interactions and provides average values for expected changes in clearance.

Cimetidine. Cimetidine inhibits theophylline's metabolism. It is unlikely that any drug interaction has been studied more extensively than that between theophylline and cimetidine. A review by Powell and Donn[179] in 1984 cites more than a dozen papers on this subject. In general, these papers suggest that the inhibition occurs within one day and disappears within two to three days after cimetidine is discontinued. The decrease in theophylline clearance averages 30% with typical doses of cimetidine (1000 to 1200 mg/day). Recent studies have found a similar magnitude of inhibition and have clarified a number of clinically relevant issues concerning the interaction. Vestal et al.[115] found that cimetidine decreased theophylline clearance by 29.2% in young nonsmokers, 29.0% in young smokers, 28.8% in elderly non-smokers and 30.5% in elderly smokers. This suggests that neither age nor smoking status affects the magnitude of inhibition. Similar results have been observed by others.[180,181] Inhibition was not selective for any particular metabolic pathway for theophylline.[115] The degree of inhibition appears to be similar whether cimetidine is administered orally or intravenously (continuous

Table 13–2. *Effect of Drugs on Theophylline Clearance*[a]

Significant ↑ (>25%)	No change (<10%)	Possible ↓ (10–25%)	Significant ↓ (>25%)
Phenobarbital	Atenolol	Diltiazem	Cimetidine
Phenytoin	Famotidine	Erythromycin	Ciprofloxacin
Rifampin	Ketoconazole	Norfloxacin	Disulfiram
	Lomefloxacin	Verapamil	Enoxacin
	Methylprednisolone		Oral contraceptives
	Metoprolol		Pefloxacin
	Nifedipine		Propranolol
	Nizatidine		Troleandomycin
	Ofloxacin		
	Prednisolone		
	Ranitidine		
	Terbutaline		

[a] This list is not intended to be all inclusive and focuses on drugs which have a reasonable probability of being administered with theophylline.

infusion or intermittent bolus).[179,182,183] Other H_2-blockers have also been studied. Despite some case reports of elevated theophylline concentrations associated with ranitidine, controlled studies[184,185] have failed to show any significant alteration in clearance even at ranitidine dosages far in excess of those used clinically (up to 4200 mg/day).[184] Famotidine[186] and nizatidine[187] have not been found to alter theophylline clearance.

Quinolone Antibiotics. Several quinolone antibiotics were introduced into clinical use during the 1980s and some have been identified as potent inhibitors of theophylline disposition. Enoxacin and pipemidic acid appear to be the most significant inhibitors, typically causing dose-related[188] reductions in theophylline clearance of more than 50%.[189–191] Ciprofloxacin decreases theophylline clearance by 25% to 30% on average[189,192,193] although there have been case reports of much larger increases in theophylline concentration in elderly patients.[194–196] Pefloxacin appears to be similar to ciprofloxacin in its inhibitory potency,[189] while norfloxacin, ofloxacin and lomefloxacin reduce clearance by less than 15%.[193,197–202]

Macrolide Antibiotics. Interactions between theophylline and the macrolide antibiotics have been studied extensively as well. Troleandomycin is a potent inhibitor, decreasing theophylline clearance by 30% to 50%.[118,203] Interactions with erythromycin are of more interest, however, because it is frequently used to treat infections in COPD patients who also may be taking theophylline. More than 15 studies of this interaction have been published.[204] Erythromycin decreases theophylline clearance by approximately 20% to 25%, but this effect does not occur consistently. Many patients (perhaps the majority) exhibit little or no interaction, while others experience a greater-than-average depression in clearance. This interaction appears to be a function of erythromycin concentration and its N-demethylation metabolite and is therefore influenced by dose and bioavailability. In addition, the interaction becomes apparent only after several days of erythromycin treatment.

Beta Blockers. In several studies[119,205,206] propranolol decreased theophylline clearance by 30% to 50%. The effect is dose-dependent and more selective for the N-demethylation pathways of elimination.[119] Fortunately, propranolol is rarely used in combination with theophylline. Metoprolol[205] and atenolol[207] have not been found to affect theophylline clearance, although metoprolol appeared to have an inhibitory effect in a small number of smokers.[205] This observation, however, remains to be confirmed.

Calcium Channel Blockers. The calcium channel blockers, verapamil and diltiazem, appear to be moderate inhibitors of metabolism, decreasing theophylline clearance by 10% to 20%. The effect of nifedipine is less than 10%.[111,113,114,208,209]

Oral Contraceptives. Another interaction of clinical relevance is the potential effect of oral contraceptives on theophylline clearance. Studies of adult women have shown a 29%[137] and 34%[210] decrease in theophylline clearance. The formation of 3-methylxanthine was most extensively affected.[211] In contrast, oral contraceptives had no significant effect in adolescent females. This is possibly related to the low dose of estrogen they were taking.[212]

Other Drugs. Other drugs whose effects on theophylline disposition are of interest include *steroids*. Methylprednisolone and prednisone have not been shown to have any significant effects.[213,214] Although it has been suggested that *beta agonists* might increase theophylline clearance, studies of terbutaline suggest that it has no clinically significant effect on theophylline clearance.[206,215] *Ketoconazole* inhibits the metabolism of a number of other substrates for cytochrome P450, but appears to have no significant effect on theophylline metabolism.[118,216,217] Finally, Loi et al.[218] have observed a relatively large dose-dependent decrease in theophylline clearance secondary to *disulfiram*. The formation of 1,3-dimethylurate was affected to a greater extent than the N-demethylation pathways.

Not all drug interactions with theophylline involve inhibition of clearance. A variety of drugs that induce oxidative drug metabolism increase theophylline clearance. *Phenytoin* produces a 35% to 50% increase in theophylline clearance[219–221] on the average with all metabolic pathways being induced to a similar extent.[219] Elderly subjects appear to be induced to a similar extent as young individuals.[219] Crowley et al.[220] reported that smoking produced a 90% increase in theophylline clearance in patients receiving phenytoin compared to an 88% increase in non-induced controls (i.e., those not receiving phenytoin). Additionally, phenytoin increased theophylline clearance significantly in both smokers and non-smokers. This suggests that further induction can occur in patients already induced by either phenytoin or smoking. Studies investigating the effect of *rifampin* and *phenobarbital* on theophylline metabolism indicate that the magnitude of induction with these compounds varies widely, but is roughly similar as that for phenytoin.[222–224]

CLINICAL APPLICATION OF DATA: DOSAGE FOR ACUTE BRONCHODILATION

The therapeutic strategy used to treat acute bronchospasm is to attain maximal bronchodilation as rapidly as possible. Inhaled or injected sympathomimetic bronchodilators are the initial drugs of choice because of their rapid onset of action and high degree of efficacy.[2-4] Theophylline has been shown to have no additional benefit over inhaled beta agonists in the treatment of severe airway obstruction, but it may enhance toxicity.[2,3] Theophylline therapy should be optimized in patients presenting with severe airway obstruction who have been maintained on a theophylline product chronically. Figure 13-6 suggests a general approach to treating the adult patient with acute bronchospasm.

Theophylline loading doses should be provided by a rapidly absorbed oral formulation or, if symptoms are severe and/or the oral route is unavailable, by parenteral therapy.[35] The loading dose can be calculated to aim for a target serum concentration in the low therapeutic range by use of the following equation:

$$D_L = \frac{(C_{desired} - C_{initial})\,(V_d)}{(F)\,(S)}$$

(Eq. 13-1)

where D_L is the loading dose in mg/kg of total body weight,[92–94] $C_{desired}$ is the desired theophylline serum concentration in μg/mL, $C_{initial}$ is the measured serum concentration before the loading dose has been given, V_d is the average apparent volume of distribution (0.45 L/kg of total body weight), F is the fraction of drug absorbed (bioavailability), and S is the fraction of the salt form represented by theophylline (e.g., for aminophylline, S = 0.8). Each 1 mg/kg of theophylline yields approximately a 2 μg/mL increase in serum theophylline concentration. Individualized loading doses should target a $C_{desired}$ of 10 μg/mL because V_d varies so widely between subjects. Loading doses designed to achieved target concentrations of 10 μg/mL produced 95% confidence intervals of 4.4 to 22.5 μg/mL[160] arguing against the selection of higher initial target serum concentrations.

In general, aminophylline loading doses of 6 mg/kg (5 mg/kg theophylline) can be safely administered over 20 to 30 minutes through a peripheral line when no previous theophylline doses have been administered (assume $C_{initial}$ to be zero in this case).[26,88] When actual serum concentration data are unavailable and patients may have received theophylline within 12 to 24 hours, airway obstruction should be treated with alternate agents. Administration of partial loading doses should be guided by actual serum theophylline concentrations because patient drug histories can be unreliable and because there is poor correlation between clinical findings and serum theophylline concentrations.[225]

After administering the loading dose, a maintenance dose designed to maintain a target serum concentration of 10 μg/mL can be calculated based on a mean theophylline clearance. Estimates of clearance should take into account concomitant disease states, age, and drug therapy.[226,227] Figure 13-6 summarizes empiric theophylline maintenance doses. The addition of drugs that alter theophylline clearance (see Table 13-2) may require adjustment of the doses provided in Figure 13-6. In patients with cor pulmonale, cardiac decompensation, or endstage liver dysfunction, theophylline should be avoided if possible.[35] If this is impossible, the initial dose should not exceed 400 mg/day unless serum concentrations can be monitored at 24-hour intervals; dosage increases should be made with extreme caution.[35]

Serum theophylline concentrations should be monitored frequently until an adequate patient response at a steady state has been achieved. For adults, serum concentrations can be obtained at 12, 24, and 48 hours after initiation of a maintenance infusion. By 24 to 48 hours, most healthy adults will have reached steady state (4 $t\frac{1}{2}$s = 4 × 8 hours) and subsequent dose adjustments can be made using Equation 13-2 below. Earlier and more frequent assessment is recommended in infants, children, and patients with a known rapid theophylline clearance.

$$C_{ss} = \frac{R_o}{CL}$$

(Eq. 13-2)

where C_{ss} is the steady-state theophylline serum concentration in μg/mL, R_o is the infusion rate in mg/hour of theophylline, and CL is total body theophylline clearance in L/hour. Given a known C_{ss} and R_o, CL can be calculated and substituted back into Equation 13-2 to derive the infusion rate necessary to produce the desired C_{ss}. Usually, this is between 10 and 15 μg/mL. In general, dose increases exceeding 25% are not advised in patients with serum theophylline concentrations greater than 10 μg/mL, irrespective of the calculated adjustment. This recommendation is based on the possibility of nonlinear pharmacokinetic behavior.[110] Non-steady-state serum concentrations that are far below or above the desired range of 10 to 20 μg/mL require immediate dosage adjustment and follow-up serum concentration monitoring until the desired concentration and effect are achieved. Once steady state has been achieved, dose adjustments can be performed as suggested in Figure 13-5.

Several methods of estimating maintenance dose requirements before steady-state conditions have been attained have appeared in the literature.[160,228–238] All of the methods, except the correction factor method,[235,236] compare favorably with one another and produce actual concentrations within 22% of that predicted in the populations studied.[239–243] The method of Chiou et al.[229] relies on the measurement of two non-steady-state serum theophylline concentrations separated by at least one half-life. These concentrations are used in Equation 13-3 to estimate clearance. The estimated clearance can then be substituted into Equation 13-2 to calculate

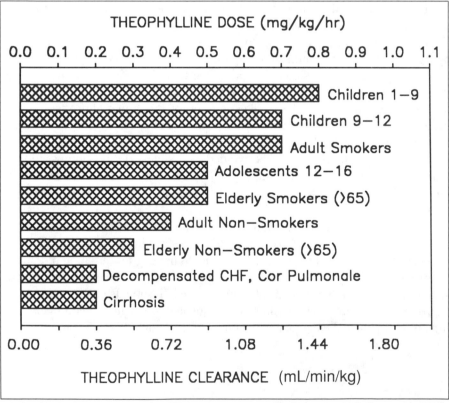

Figure 13-6. *Effect of age, disease states and smoking status on initial theophylline maintenance dose requirements and clearance. For neonates, a dose of 1 mg/kg (<24 days postnatal) or 1.5 mg/kg (>24 days) every 12 hours should be used. For infants six weeks (following the normal gestational period) to one year of age, dose should be (0.008 × Age in Weeks) + 0.21 mg/kg/hr. Maximum daily dose should not exceed 400 mg in individuals with cirrhosis or decompensated heart failure or 900 mg in others unless guided by serum concentration monitoring. Doses may need to be adjusted if theophylline is given concomitantly with drugs altering its clearance. All maintenance doses should be based on ideal body weight.*

the new infusion rate. It should be noted that if the first serum concentration is lower than the second serum concentration, the latter portion of Equation 13-3 produces a negative number and lowers the calculated clearance.

$$CL = \frac{2R_o}{C_1 + C_2} + \frac{2V_d (C_1 - C_2)}{(C_1 + C_2)(t_2 - t_1)} \qquad \text{(Eq. 13-3)}$$

where CL = total body theophylline clearance, in L/hr.
R_o = theophylline infusion rate, in L/hr.
V_d = apparent volume of distribution, 0.45 L/kg lean body weight
C_1 = the first serum theophylline concentration, in μg/mL obtained at time = t_1.
C_2 = the second serum theophylline concentration, in μg/mL obtained at time = t_2, one estimated half-life from t_1.

Use of the Chiou equation is associated with several limitations. To accurately apply this method the maintenance infusion must be constant, the serum concentrations must be separated by an interval of at least one half-life to characterize clearance, and a reliable and precise assay technique must be employed. Attempts to use this method with less than ideal conditions can result in serious errors in clearance estimates and a potential overdose.

Data consistently show that the predictive accuracy of pre-steady-state methods (such as least squares regression and Bayesian dosing) is improved as the number of serum concentration data added to the program increases.[241,242] Authors caution that while predictive methods produce comparably favorable predictions of theophylline clearance for clinical practice, steady-state assessment of theophylline clearance is still recommended.[241–243]

Clinical response to theophylline therapy should be monitored by a careful assessment of vital signs, arterial blood gases when available, one-second forced expiratory volume or peak expiratory flow rates, improvements in physical signs (i.e., wheezing) and subjective signs (i.e., decreased shortness of breath, easier breathing). Patients with distended neck veins, leg edema, S3 gallop, enlarged heart on roentgenograph are at risk for decreased theophylline clearance. They should be given lower theophylline doses and monitored aggressively.[160] Objective signs of cardiovascular, gastrointestinal, and central nervous system toxicity should be looked for as well.

When an initial response has been achieved and the patient has been stabilized on an effective intravenous regimen, oral therapy can be considered. Conversion to oral therapy is best accomplished by dividing the 24-hour intravenous theophylline requirement into two or three equal doses of a sustained-release product. Evaluation of methods used to convert patients from intravenous to oral therapy has shown that the simultaneous administration of the first oral dose when the infusion is stopped produces a minimum fluctuation of serum theophylline concentrations when Theo-Dur is used.[244,245]

DOSAGE FOR CHRONIC USE

The goal of chronic theophylline therapy is to produce the highest likelihood of successful prevention and/or management of bronchospasm with the lowest chance of intolerable side effects. In a patient for whom theophylline clearance is unknown, the initial oral dose can be estimated by converting the hourly dose rate in Figure 13-6 to a total daily dose and then dividing this dose into two or three doses of a sustained-release product depending on its rate of absorption and the patient's elimination rate. A product with proven acceptable bioavailability should be used and brand substitution is discouraged. For most patients, acceptable compliance will be achieved. If a once-a-day product is used, an F of 0.7 (Theo-24)[79,80] to 0.9 (Unidur)[83] should be assumed.

Initial oral therapy with theophylline, particularly in patients who have not received intravenous theophylline, can produce xanthine-like side effects such as nausea, headache, increased urination, agitation, and insomnia. Tolerance to these side effects will develop over time but they can be minimized by starting therapy with lower doses, for example 400 mg/day in adults, and titrating at three day intervals to the desired daily dose through 25% of the dose increments. Once the appropriate dose is achieved, serum concentrations should be obtained to assure that therapeutic and non-toxic concentrations have been attained.

Peak-trough fluctuations will be 40% to 60% in an adult patient with a low to normal clearance value who receives a twice-a-day theophylline product that is unaffected by food. Thus, at an average concentration of 12 μg/mL, peaks of 14 to 16 μg/mL and troughs of 8 to 10 μg/mL can be expected. Under these circumstances, monitoring trough concentrations will provide an acceptable guide to therapy. In patient groups with rapid clearance values, larger peak-trough fluctuations will occur. Since transient toxicity can be associated with high peak concentrations, it may be advisable in these patients to obtain a serum concentration as close to the peak as possible. When Theo-Dur is used, the peak concentration will most often occur in children at 1.5 to 3.5 hours and in adults at approximately six hours after the dose; however, considerable variability exists.[56,61] Occasionally one finds a serum concentration that is inconsistent with the clinical situation. In these circumstances, it may be useful to obtain a more complete serum-concentration-time profile to determine the actual clearance and bioavailability of the preparation being used in the individual patient.[246]

Once-a-day preparations should be monitored using peak concentrations. Even in adults, these preparations will cause large fluctuations in concentrations over a dosing interval. Most often, peak concentrations for these preparations will occur ten hours after administration.[61] If these products are administered in the evening to control nocturnal asthma, a blood sample obtained early the following morning should be suitable. If the dose is taken in the morning, then serum concentrations should be obtained late in the afternoon or in the early evening.

Once a reliable serum concentration has been obtained, dosage adjustment can be made accordingly. In most patients, serum concentrations will change in direct proportion to the change in dose. Occasional patients will exhibit nonlinearity with disproportionate increases in concentration as the dose is increased. Whenever a change in dose is made, serum concentrations should be monitored at steady state. Appropriate dosage selection coupled with monitoring of serum theophylline concentrations will allow for safe and effective use of theophylline with minimal risks of serious toxicity.

ANALYTICAL METHODS

Assays for theophylline concentration in biological fluids are conducted in a variety of settings including the research laboratory, the hospital or clinic laboratory, and the physician's office. Several different methods are available with the method of choice being largely dependent on the setting and the intended use of the result.

High performance liquid chromatography (HPLC) remains a popular technique in the research laboratory. Advantages of HPLC include excellent accuracy, specificity, precision, and sensitivity. In addition, only chromatographic methods such as HPLC are able to separate and quantitate theophylline metabolites,[247] a useful procedure for assessing alterations in the individual metabolic pathways of the drug. HPLC is, however, relatively slow. It requires sample preparation (either protein precipitation or extraction), frequent calibration, and run times of five to ten minutes per sample for most methods. In addition, equipment and maintenance costs are expensive and experienced personnel are required to operate the system. As a result of these disadvantages, HPLC is not commonly used in the clinical setting to measure theophylline concentration in the United States.

Clinically, immunoassay is the predominant method used to measure theophylline concentrations. The systems most commonly used in hospitals are the Abbott TDX system (fluorescence polarization immunoassay) and the Syva EMIT system (enzyme-multiplied immunoassay). These methods offer acceptable sensitivity, accuracy, and precision when compared to the HPLC methods,[248] although occasional problems have been noted with antibody specificity in patients with renal failure.[249] Additional advantages include little or no sample preparation, a short assay time, and a high degree of automation. The latter decreases technician costs and provides less opportunity for operator error.

There has been much interest in the past several years in developing procedures that can be used in office medical practices or in the emergency room. The cost of EMIT and TDX is prohibitive for low-volume usage such as in an office practice, and it may be difficult to justify the costs of dedicating an instrument or technician for emergency room use only. In addition, even though EMIT and TDX are relatively rapid techniques, the turn-around time is still too slow for immediate application. This is due to the delivery of samples to the laboratory and the usual practice of batching samples to be run once or twice per day.

The major products that have been developed and evaluated for this purpose are Vision (Abbott), Seralyzer (Ames), and Acculevel (Syntex).[250] All are antibody-based procedures which use blood samples obtained by finger stick. Vision is a fully automated system capable of using whole blood, plasma, or serum and is the only one which accurately quantitates concentrations below 3 µg/mL (although the clinical advantage of this is probably minimal). The Seralyzer requires initial centrifugation of whole blood. The operator must then place the serum or plasma sample onto a reagent strip, a step which can present difficulties for individuals with no laboratory experience or those who perform the assay infrequently.[251] Both Vision and Seralyzer require the purchase of equipment which must be calibrated regularly. This is in contrast to the Acculevel system which simply involves adding whole blood to a solution, placing an antibody-impregnated strip in the solution and measuring the migration of fluid up the strip. Although occasional problems with the accuracy of these methods have been reported,[252,253] the majority of studies comparing these products to conventional analytical methods such as HPLC, EMIT and TDX have found the level of accuracy to be acceptable for clinical use.[250,251,254–257] Differences of greater than 3 µg/mL from conventional techniques are relatively infrequent and the methods are clearly far superior to a clinician's judgment in estimating the theophylline concentration.[253] These products may be more susceptible to interference from competing compounds and should not be used in uremic patients.[258] All can routinely provide a result within 30 minutes (commonly, in less than 20). Vision is the fastest and Acculevel is the slowest.[250] Costs of the methods must be examined carefully. Because Vision and Seralyzer involve control and calibration costs, the cost per assay for both procedures declines with increasing volume. Clifton et al.[250] have estimated costs per assay (at a volume of 40 per month) to be $5, $15, and $14 for Seralyzer, Acculevel, and Vision, respectively. All appear to be less expensive than a standard laboratory assay.[259] The method of choice will depend upon the situation. For practices in which usage will be infrequent, the need to calibrate the instruments regularly as well as the cost of Vision in particular may make the easy-to-use Acculevel system the preferred method. However, with increased volume, Vision or Seralyzer may be more valuable, especially since the same equipment can be used for other assays (both drugs and routine biochemical tests).

MANAGEMENT OF THEOPHYLLINE TOXICITY

Ingestion of an excessive oral dose of theophylline requires immediate discontinuation of the drug and treatment with activated charcoal dissolved in water or sorbitol.[260,261] There have been several recent reports of hypernatremic dehydration associated with sorbitol administration suggesting that water may be the preferred vehicle for charcoal administration.[262–264] The oral administration of activated charcoal doubles or triples theophylline clearance depending on the population studied.[260] Patients with low theophylline clearances show the greatest improvement in clearance when charcoal is given.[260] Mathematical models suggest that the half-life of theophylline during charcoal administration will be seven hours or less even if the patient's theophylline clearance is very low.[260] Dose-response studies have suggested that the regimen which optimally increases theophylline clearance is 20 gm of high-surface-area activated charcoal orally every two hours.[261,265,266] Oral activated charcoal also effectively removes theophylline in cases of intravenous overdoses, presumably by pulling drug from the blood into the gastrointestinal tract.[267–268] Because theophylline-toxic patients may vomit, individuals with impaired pharyngeal reflexes should not receive activated charcoal unless airway protection is provided. Continuous nasogastric administration of activated charcoal with droperidol and/or metoclopramide may circumvent problems of charcoal retention in patients who are vomiting.[269,270] The prophylactic use of phenobarbital in therapeutic doses reduces the mortality of theophylline-induced seizures in mice and delays their onset.[260] Thus, phenobarbital should be considered in patients with very high theophylline serum concentrations to protect them against the onset of seizures while awaiting the effect of multi-dose charcoal.[260]

It has been emphasized that high serum theophylline concentrations are not always associated with toxicity.[40,41] As a result, previously held notions that patients exhibiting serum theophylline concentrations of greater than 40 µg/mL should undergo hemoperfusion have come into question. Since patients undergoing hemoperfusion are put at risk for bleeding, thrombocytopenia, hypotension, and hypocalcemia, this technique is now recommended only for the patients believed to be at greatest risk of adverse sequelae from theophylline toxicity.[260] This includes patients with serum theophylline concentrations of greater than 80 to 100 µg/mL after a single-dose ingestion; those who achieve concentrations greater than 60 µg/mL after multiple-dose ingestions; those who are hemodynamically unstable; those who fail to demonstrate adequate theophylline removal with oral activated charcoal or can not tolerate it; and those who exhibit seizures or severe cardiovascular manifestation of theophylline intoxication.[36,40,260,271,272]

Candidates for hemoperfusion should be admitted to an intensive care unit for aggressive monitoring and treatment.[36] Supportive care, designed to maintain normal cardiac, circulatory, respiratory, and renal function with correction of metabolic abnormalities, is indicated.[36,260] Correction of complications such as hypotension (with fluids); serious cardiac arrhythmias (with verapamil, digoxin, or a beta blocker); and seizures (with benzodiazepines and phenobarbital) is recommended, although none of these interventions is particularly effective when life-threatening ventricular arrhythmias and seizures develop.[260,273] Beta blockers must be used cautiously in patients with asthma or COPD to prevent exacerbated airway obstruction. Should difficulties arise, esmolol may offer an advantage due to its short half-life and ease of titration.[274] Serum theophylline concentrations should be monitored every six to eight hours until the concentration falls below 20 µg/mL. Additional serum concentration monitoring is recommended after the completion of hemoperfusion since rebound increases in serum theophylline concentration have been reported.[36]

Peritoneal dialysis and hemodialysis have been used to remove theophylline but are not as effective as charcoal hemoperfusion.[275-278] Peritoneal dialysis increases theophylline clearance by approximately 30% yielding little clinical utility.[275] Hemodialysis with a coil dialyzer has been estimated to increase theophylline clearance by approximately 50%.[276] With a hollow fiber dialyzer, theophylline clearance may increase to 80 to 90 mL/min, which is close to the clearance values observed with hemoperfusion.[277,278] Hemoperfusion with charcoal or resin cartridges has been estimated to increase theophylline clearance by at least two- to fourfold with an associated extraction ratio of 0.75 or higher.[260,227,279] This suggests close to complete clearance of theophylline during its passage through the hemoperfusion cartridge. If hemoperfusion is unavailable, hemodialysis may be considered when oral activated charcoal has failed to adequately decrease the theophylline concentration or the severity of the patient's clinical condition warrants aggressive intervention.

PROSPECTUS

Although the clinical use of theophylline may be declining, it remains an important drug for both acute and chronic management of bronchospasm. Pharmacokinetic studies over the past 20 years in various patient populations allow clinicians to appropriately select an initial dosage regimen. Developments in analytical techniques have allowed routine analysis of serum theophylline concentrations. Thus, the use of theophylline should be associated with minimal risks of toxicity. Furthermore, pharmacokinetic evaluation of theophylline has provided insight into the effects that various factors such as drugs, food, immune modifiers (i.e., vaccines), and the environment (i.e., passive and active smoking) have on hepatic drug metabolism. Because of this, understanding the pharmacokinetics of theophylline has much broader significance.

REFERENCES

1. Self TH et al. Is theophylline use justified in acute exacerbations of asthma? Pharmacotherapy. 1989;9:260.
2. Fanta CH et al. Treatment of acute asthma: is combination therapy with sympathomimetics and methylxanthines indicated? Am J Med. 1986;80:5.
3. Siegel et al. Aminophylline increases toxicity but not the efficacy of an inhaled beta-adrenergic agonist in the treatment of acute exacerbations of asthma. Am Rev Respir Dis. 1985;132:283.
4. Barnes PJ. A new approach to the treatment of asthma. N Engl J Med. 1989;321:1517.
5. Kelly HW, Murphy S. Should we stop using theophylline for the treatment of the hospitalized patient with status asthmaticus? DICP Ann Pharmacotherapy. 1989;23:995.
6. Weinberger M. The value of theophylline for asthma. Ann Allergy. 1989;63:1.
7. Magnussen H et al. Theophylline has a dose-related effect on the airway response to inhaled histamine and methacholine in asthmatics. Am Rev Respir Dis. 1987;136:1163.
8. McWilliams BC et al. Effects of theophylline on inhaled methacholine and histamine in asthmatic children. Am Rev Respir Dis. 1984;130:193.
9. Martin GL et al. Effects of theophylline, terbutaline and prednisone on antigen-induced bronchospasm and mediator release. J Allergy Clin Immunol. 1980;66:204.
10. Pollack J et al. Relationship of serum theophylline concentration to inhibition of exercise-induced bronchospasm and comparison with cromolyn. Pediatrics. 1977;60:840.
11. Ellis E. Inhibition of exercise-induced asthma by theophylline. J Allergy Clin Immunol. 1984;73:690.
12. Hendeles L et al. Theophylline attenuation of allergen-induced airway hyper-reactivity and late response. J Allergy Clin Immunol. 1991. Abstract in press.
13. Eaton ML et al. Efficacy of theophylline in "irreversible" airflow obstruction. Ann Intern Med. 1980;92:758.
14. Eaton ML et al. Effects of theophylline on breathlessness and exercise tolerance in patients with chronic airflow obstruction. Chest. 1982;82:538.
15. Jenne JW et al. The effect of maintenance theophylline therapy on lung work in severe chronic obstructive pulmonary disease while standing and walking. Am Rev Respir Dis. 1984;130:600.
16. Aubrier M et al. Aminophylline improves diaphragmatic contractility. N Engl J Med. 1981;305:249.

17. Aubier M. Effect of theophylline on diaphragmatic and other skeletal muscles. J Allergy Clin Immunol. 1986;78:787.
18. Vereen LE et al. Effect of aminophylline on exercise performance in patients with irreversible airway obstruction. Arch Intern Med. 1986;146:1349.
19. Sharp JT. Theophylline in chronic obstructive pulmonary disease. J Allergy Clin Immunol. 1986;78:800.
20. Dietrich J et al. Alterations in state in apneic preterm infants receiving theophylline. Clin Pharmacol Ther. 1978;24:474.
21. Levy G, Koysooko R. Pharmacokinetic analysis of the effect of theophylline on pulmonary function in asthmatic children. J Pediatr. 1975;86:789.
22. Peck CC et al. Theophylline-induced bronchodilation lags behind serum theophylline levels under non-steady-state conditions. Clin Pharmacol Ther. 1983;33:259.
23. Whiting B et al. Modelling theophylline response in individual patients with chronic bronchitis. Br J Clin Pharmacol. 1981;12:481.
24. Vozeh S et al. Theophylline serum concentration and therapeutic effect in severe acute bronchial obstruction: the optimal use of intravenous theophylline. Am Rev Respir Dis. 1982;125:181.
25. Ishizaki T. Plasma catecholamines during a 72-hour aminophylline infusion in children with acute asthma. J Allergy Clin Immunol. 1988;82:146.
26. Mitenko PA, Ogilvie RI. Rational intravenous doses of theophylline. N Engl J Med. 1973;289:600.
27. Peck CC et al. Clinical pharmacodynamics of theophylline. J Allergy Clin Immunol. 1985;76:292.
28. Heins M et al. Nocturnal asthma: slow-release terbutaline versus slow-release theophylline therapy. Eur J Respir Dis. 1988;1:306.
29. Tabachnik E et al. Sustained-release theophylline: a significant advance in the treatment of childhood asthma. J Pediatr. 1982;100:489.
30. Simons FER et al. Sustained-release theophylline for treatment of asthma in preschool children. Am J Dis Child. 1982;136:790.
31. Milsap RL et al. Oxygen consumption in apneic premature infants after low-dose theophylline. Clin Pharmacol Ther. 1980;28:536.
32. Cathcart-Rake WF et al. Metabolic response to plasma concentrations of theophylline. Clin Pharmacol Ther. 1979;26:89.
33. Foster LJ et al. Bronchodilator effects on gastric acid secretion. JAMA. 1979;241:2613.
34. Neilson CP et al. Polymorphonuclear leukocyte inhibition by therapeutic concentrations of theophylline is mediated by cyclic-3',5'-adenosine monophosphate. Am Rev Respir Dis. 1988;137:25.
35. Hendeles L, Weinberger M. Theophylline. A "state of the art" review. Pharmacotherapy. 1983;3:2.
36. Paloucek FP, Rodvold KA. Evaluation of theophylline overdoses and toxicities. Ann Emerg Med. 1988;17:135.
37. Hendeles L et al. Frequent toxicity from IV aminophylline infusions in critically ill patients. Am J Hosp Pharm. 1977;11:12.
38. Schumacher GE, Barr JT. Applying decision analysis in therapeutic drug monitoring: using decision trees to interpret serum theophylline concentrations. Clin Pharm. 1986;5:325.
39. Tschepik W et al. Therapeutic risk-assessment model for identifying patients with adverse reactions. Am J Hosp Pharm. 1990;47:330.
40. Aitken SL, Martin TR. Life-threatening theophylline toxicity is not predictable by serum levels. Chest. 1987;91:10.
41. Bertino JS, Walker JW. Reassessment of theophylline toxicity. Serum concentrations, clinical course, and treatment. Arch Intern Med. 1987;147:757.
42. Sessler CN, Cohen MD. Cardiac arrhythmias during theophylline toxicity. Chest. 1990;98:672.
43. Zwillich CW et al. Theophylline-induced seizures in adults; correlation with serum concentrations. Ann Intern Med. 1975;82:784.

44. Covelli HD et al. Predisposing factors to apparent theophylline-induced seizures. Ann Allergy. 1985;54:411.

45. Sessler CN. Theophylline toxicity: clinical features of 116 consecutive cases. Am J Med. 1990;88:567.

46. Hall KW et al. Metabolic abnormalities associated with intentional theophylline overdose. Ann Intern Med. 1984;101:457.

47. McPherson ML et al. Theophylline-induced hypercalcemia. Ann Intern Med. 1986;105:52.

48. Kearney TE et al. Theophylline toxicity and the beta-adrenergic system. Ann Intern Med. 1985;102:766.

49. Roberts RJ. Methylxanthine therapy: caffeine and theophylline. In: Roberts RJ, eds. Drug therapy in infants. Pharmacologic principles and clinical experience. Philadelphia: WB Saunders. 1984:119–37.

50. Jonkman JHG et al. Disposition and clinical pharmacokinetics of microcrystalline theophylline. Eur J Clin Pharmacol. 1980;17:379.

51. Upton RA et al. Evaluation of the absorption from 15 commercial theophylline products indicating deficiencies in currently applied bioavailability criteria. J Pharmacokinet Biopharm. 1980;8:229.

52. Welling PG et al. Influence of diet and fluid on the bioavailability of theophylline. Clin Pharmacol Ther. 1975;17:475.

53. Watanabe HK et al. Time-dependent absorption of theophylline in man. J Clin Pharmacol. 1984;24:509.

54. Reed RC, Schwartz HJ. Lack of influence of an intensive antacid regimen on theophylline bioavailability. J Pharmacokinet Biopharm. 1984;12:315.

55. Myhre KI et al. The influence of antacid on the absorption of two different sustained-release formulations of theophylline. Br J Clin Pharmacol. 1983;15:683.

56. Hendeles L et al. A clinical and pharmacokinetic basis for the selection and use of slow-release theophylline products. Clin Pharmacokinet. 1984;9:95.

57. Dederich RA et al. Intra-subject variation in sustained-release theophylline absorption. J Allergy Clin Immunol. 1981;61:465.

58. Pollarck GM et al. Comparison of inter- and intra-subject variation in oral absorption of theophylline from sustained-release products. Int J Pharmaceutics. 1984;21:3.

59. Hill M et al. The consistency of theophylline absorption from a sustained-release formulation in asthmatic children. Pharmacotherapy. 1988;8:277.

60. Martin RJ et al. Circadian variations in theophylline concentrations and treatment of nocturnal asthma. Am Rev Respir Dis. 1989;139:475.

61. Rogers RJ et al. Theophylline absorption from two sustained-release products. Am Rev Respir Dis. 1987;136:1168.

62. Smolensky MH et al. Summary and perspectus: sustained-release theophylline and nocturnal asthma, once-daily and unequal dosing schedules. Chronobiol Int. 1987;4:459.

63. Rodgers A et al. Is diurnal variation in absorption of slow-release aminophylline an age-related phenomenon? Eur J Clin Pharmacol. 1988;33:593.

64. Regazzi MB et al. A theophylline dosage regimen which reduces round-the-clock variations in plasma concentrations resulting from diurnal pharmacokinetic variation. Eur J Clin Pharmacol. 1987;33:243.

65. Sips AP et al. Food does not effect in bioavailability of theophylline from Theolin Retard. Eur J Clin Pharmacol. 1984;36:405.

66. Brazier JL et al. Influence of hyperlipidic food on the kinetics of slow-release formulations of theophylline. Eur J Clin Pharmacol. 1989;37:85.

67. Pedersen S et al. Delay in the absorption rate of theophylline from a sustained-release theophylline preparation caused by food. Br J Clin Pharmacol. 1981;12:904.

68. Pedersen S, Moller-Petersen J. Erratic absorption of a slow-release theophylline sprinkle product. Pediatrics. 1984;74:534.

69. Birkett DJ et al. Effects of time of dose in relation to food on the bioavailability of Theo-Dur sprinkle at steady state in asthmatic children. Clin Pharmacol Ther. 1989;45:305.

70. Green ER et al. Absorption characteristics of sustained-release theophylline capsules administered in applesauce. J Pediatr. 1981;98:832.
71. Hendeles L et al. Food-induced "dose-dumping" from a once-a-day theophylline product as a cause of theophylline toxicity. Chest. 1985;38:77.
72. Lagas M, Jonkman JHG. Greatly enhanced bioavailability of theophylline on postprandial administration of a sustained-release tablet. Eur J Clin Pharmacol. 1983;24:761.
73. Karim A et al. Food-induced changes in theophylline absorption from controlled-release formulations. Part 1. Substantial increased and decreased absorption with Uniphyl tablets and Theo-Dur Sprinkle. Clin Pharmacol Ther. 1985;38:77.
74. Milavetz G et al. Relationship between rate and extent of absorption of oral theophylline from Uniphyl brand of slow-release theophylline and resulting serum concentrations during multiple dosing. J Allergy Clin Immunol. 1987;80:723.
75. Arkinstall WW et al. The clinical significance of food-induced changes in the absorption of theophylline from Uniphyl tablets. J Allergy Clin Immunol. 1988;82:155-64.
76. Karim A. Effects of food on the bioavailability of theophylline from controlled-release products in adults. J Allergy Clin Immunol. 1986;78:695.
77. Steffensen G, Pedersen S. Food-induced changes in theophylline absorption from a once-a-day theophylline product. Br J Clin Pharmacol. 1986;22:571.
78. Jonkman JHG. Food interactions with sustained-release theophylline preparations. A review. Clin Pharmacokinet. 1989;16:162.
79. Hurwitz A et al. Theophylline absorption from sustained-release products: comparative steady-state bioavailability of once-daily Theo-Dur, Theo-24 and Uniphyl. J Clin Pharmacol. 1987;27:855.
80. Armstrong EP et al. Steady-state pharmacokinetics of two sustained-release theophylline products during once-daily and twice-daily dosing. Clin Pharm. 1987;6:800.
81. Purkiss R et al. A pharmacokinetic study of the recommended dosing schedules of Theo-Dur and Uniphylline. Allergy. 1984;39:634.
82. Zwillich CW et al. Nocturnal asthma therapy. Inhaled bitolterol versus sustained-release theophylline. Am Rev Respir Dis. 1989;139:470.
83. Cooper R et al. Serum theophylline concentration fluctuations with a new once-a-day product. Ann Allergy. 1991. Abstract in press.
84. Jordan TJ, Reichman LB. Once-a-day versus twice-daily dosing of theophylline. A decision analysis approach to evaluating theophylline blood levels and compliance. Am Rev Respir Dis. 1989;140:1573.
85. Kotzan JA et al. An *in vivo* single- and multiple-dose study of several marketed brands of conventional and controlled-release theophylline. DICP. 1984;18:147.
86. Baker JR et al. Clinical relevance of the substitution of different brands of sustained-release theophylline. J Allergy Clin Immunol. 1988;81:664.
87. Guill MF et al. Clinical and pharmacokinetic evaluation of a sustained-release liquid theophylline preparation. Allergy Clin Immunol. 1988;82:281.
88. Hendeles L et al. Disposition of theophylline after a single intravenous infusion of aminophylline. Am Rev Respir Dis. 1978;118:97.
89. Mitenko PA, Ogilvie RI. Pharmacokinetics of intravenous theophylline. Clin Pharmacol Ther. 1973;14:509.
90. Ellis ER et al. Pharmacokinetics of theophylline in children with asthma. Pediatrics. 1976;58:542.
91. Loughnan PM et al. Pharmacokinetic analysis of the dispostion of intravenous theophylline in young children. J Pediatr. 1976;88:874.
92. Gal P et al. Theophylline disposition in obesity. Clin Pharmacol Ther. 1978;23:438.
93. Jewesson PJ, Ensom RJ. Influence of body fat on the volume of distribution of theophylline. Ther Drug Monit. 1985;7:197.
94. Stine RJ et al. Aminophylline loading in asthmatic patients: a protocol trial. Ann Emerg Med. 1989;18:640.

95. Rizzo A et al. Effect of body weight on the volume of distribution of theophylline. Lung. 1988;166:269.
96. Shum L, Jusko WJ. Theophylline disposition in obese rats. J Pharmacol Exp Ther. 1984;228:380.
97. Shaw LM et al. Factors influencing theophylline serum protein binding. Clin Pharmacol Ther. 1982;32:490.
98. Aranda JV et al. Pharmacokinetic aspects of theophylline in premature newborns. N Engl J Med. 1976;295:413.
99. Zarowitz B et al. Alterations in theophylline protein binding in acutely ill patients with COPD. Chest. 1985;87:766.
100. Resar R et al. Kinetics of theophylline. Variability and effect of arterial pH in chronic obstructive lung disease. Chest. 1979;76:11.
101. Vallner JJ et al. Effect of pH on the binding of theophylline to serum proteins. Am Rev Respir Dis. 1979;120:83.
102. Cusack BJ et al. Theophylline clearance in patients with severe chronic obstructive pulmonary disease receiving supplemental oxygen and the effect of acute hypoxemia. Am Rev Respir Dis. 1986;133:1110.
103. Letarte L, du Souich P. Influence of hypercapnia and/or hypoxemia and metabolic acidosis on theophylline kinetics in the conscious rabbit. Am Rev Respir Dis. 1984;129:762.
104. Mangione A et al. Pharmacokinetics of theophylline in hepatic disease. Chest. 1978;73:616.
105. Piafsky KM et al. Theophylline disposition in patients with hepatic cirrhosis. N Engl J Med. 1977;296:1495.
106. Eriksson M et al. Pharmacokinetics of theophylline in Ethiopian children of differing nutritional status. Eur J Clin Pharmacol. 1983;24:89.
107. Connelly TJ et al. Characterization of theophylline binding to serum proteins in pregnant and nonpregnant women. Clin Pharmacol. 1990;47:68.
108. Fox RW et al. Theophylline kinetics in a geriatrics group. Clin Pharmacol Ther. 1983;34:60.
109. Ogilvie RI. Clinical pharmacokinetics of theophylline. Clin Pharmacokinet. 1978;3:267.
110. Tang-Liu et al. Nonlinear theophylline elimination. Clin Pharmacol Ther. 1982;31:358.
111. Robson RA et al. Selective inhibitory effects of nifedipine and verapamil on oxidative metabolism: effects on theophylline. Br J Clin Pharmacol. 1988;25:397.
112. Shin S-G et al. Theophylline pharmacokinetics in normal elderly subjects. Clin Pharmacol Ther. 1988;44:522.
113. Sirmans SM et al. Effect of calicum channel blockers on theophylline disposition. Clin Pharmacol Ther. 1988;44:29.
114. Abernethy DR et al. Substrate-selective inhibition by verapamil and diltiazem: differential disposition of antipyrine and theophylline in humans. J Pharmacol Exp Ther. 1988;244:994.
115. Vestal RE et al. Aging and drug interactions. I. Effect of cimetidine and smoking on the oxidation of theophylline and cortisol in healthy men. J Pharmacol Exp Ther. 1987;241:488.
116. Tserng K et al. Theophylline metabolism in premature infants. Clin Pharmacol Ther. 1981;29:594.
117. Robson RA et al. Characterization of theophylline metabolism by human liver microsomes. Inhibition and immunochemical studies. Biochem Pharmacol. 1988;37:1651.
118. Naline E et al. Application of theophylline metabolite assays to the exploration of liver microsome oxidative function in man. Fund Clin Pharmacol. 1988;2:341.
119. Miners JO et al. Selectivity and dose-dependency of the inhibitory effect of propranolol on theophylline metabolism in man. Br J Clin Pharmacol. 1985;20:219.
120. Robson RA et al. Characterization of theophylline metabolism in human liver microsomes. Br J Clin Pharmacol. 1987;24:293.
121. Schellens JH et al. Relationship between the metabolism of antipyrine, hexobarbitone and theophylline in man as assessed by a "cocktail" approach. Br J Clin Pharmacol. 1988;26:373.
122. Teunissen MW et al. Correlation between antipyrine metabolite formation and theophylline metabolism in humans after simultaneous single-dose administration and at steady state. J Pharmacol Exp Ther. 1985;233:770.

123. Miller CA et al. Polymorphism of theophylline metabolism in man. J Clin Invest. 1985;75:1415.
124. Dahlqvist R et al. Nonlinear metabolic disposition of theophylline. Ther Drug Monit. 1984;6:290.
125. Wagner JG. Theophylline: pooled Michaelis-Menten parameters (V_{max} and k_m) and implications. Clin Pharmacokinet. 1985;10:432.
126. Ishizaki T, Kubo M. Incidence of apparent Michaelis-Menten behavior of theophylline and its parameters (V_{max} and k_m) among asthmatic children and adults. Ther Drug Monit. 1987;9:11.
127. Bachman K et al. Theophylline kinetics: dose dependency and single sample prediction of clearance. Pharmacol. 1985;30:136.
128. Vestal RE et al. Comparison of single and multiple dose pharmacokinetics of theophylline using stable isotopes. Eur J Clin Pharmacol. 1986;30:113.
129. Efthimiou H et al. Influence of chronic dosing on theophylline clearance. Br J Clin Pharmacol. 1984;17:525.
130. Jonkman JHG et al. Chronopharmacokinetics of theophylline after sustained release and intravenous administration to adults. Eur J Clin Pharmacol. 1984;26:215.
131. St-Pierre MV et al. Temporal variation in the disposition of theophylline and its metabolites. Clin Pharmacol Ther. 1985;38:89.
132. Uematsu T et al. Circadian changes in the absorption and elimination of theophylline in patients with bronchial obstruction. Eur J Clin Pharmacol. 1986;30:309.
133. Scott PH et al. Day-night differences in steady-state theophylline pharmacokinetics in asthmatic children. Chronobiol Int. 1989;6:163.
134. Upton RA et al. Intraindividual variability in theophylline pharmacokinetics: statistical verification in 39 of 60 healthy young adults. J Pharmacokinet Biopharm. 1982;10:123.
135. Slaughter RL et al. Intraindividual variability in theophylline pharmacokinetics in subjects with mild/moderate asthma. J Allergy Clin Immunol. 1987;80:33.
136. Zarowitz BJ et al. Variability in theophylline volume of distribution and clearance in patients with acute respiratory failure requiring mechanical ventilation. Chest. 1988;93:379.
137. Milavetz G et al. Stability of theophylline elimination rate. Clin Pharmacol Ther. 1987;41:388.
138. Roberts RK et al. Oral contraceptive steroid impairs the elimination of theophylline. J Lab Med. 1983;101:821.
139. Bachmann KA et al. Use of three probes to assess the influence of sex on hepatic drug metabolism. Pharmacol. 1987;35:88.
140. Carter BL et al. Theophylline clearance during pregnancy. Obstet Gynecol. 1986;68:555.
141. Gardner MJ et al. Longitudinal effects of pregnancy on the pharmacokinetics of theophylline. Eur J Clin Pharmacol. 1987;31:289.
142. Dothey CI et al. Maturational changes of theophylline pharmacokinetics in preterm infants. Clin Pharmacol Ther. 1989;45:461.
143. Ginchansky E et al. Relationship of theophylline clearance to oral dosage in children with chronic asthma. J Pediatr. 1977;91:655.
144. Rosen JP et al. Theophylline pharmacokinetics in the young infant. Pediatrics. 1979;64:248.
145. Randolph WC et al. The effect of age on theophylline clearance in normal subjects. Br J Clin Pharmacol. 1986;22:603.
146. Jackson SH et al. The relationship between theophylline clearance and age in adult life. Eur J Clin Pharmacol. 1989;36:29.
147. Abernethy DR, Greenblatt DJ. Drug disposition in obese humans. An update. Clin Pharmacokinet. 1986;11:199.
148. Anderson KE. Influences of diet and nutrition on clinical pharmacokinetics. Clin Pharmacokinet. 1988;14:325.
149. Fagan TC et al. Increased clearance of propranolol and theophylline by high-protein compared with high-carbohydrate diet. Clin Pharmacol Ther. 1987;41:402.
150. Kappas A et al. Effect of charcoal-broiled beef on antipyrine and theophylline metabolism. Clin Pharmacol Ther. 1978;23:445.
151. Cusack BJ et al. Cigarette smoking and theophylline metabolism: effects of cimetidine. Clin Pharmacol Ther. 1985;37:330.

152. Trembath PW et al. Theophylline pharmacokinetics in patients from a geriatric hospital: influence of cigarette smoking. Human Toxicol. 1986;5:265.
153. Jusko WJ et al. Enhanced biotransformation of theophylline in marijuana and tobacco smokers. Clin Pharmacol Ther. 1978;24:405.
154. Belle LL et al. Cigarette abstinence, nicotine gum, and theophylline disposition. Ann Intern Med. 1987;106:553.
155. Matsunga SK e tal. Effects of passive smoking on theophylline clearance. Clin Pharmacol Ther. 1989;46:399.
156. Benowitz NL et al. Nicotine gum and theophylline metabolism. Biomed Pharmacother. 1989;43:1.
157. Kraan J et al. The pharmacokinetics of theophylline and enprofylline in patients with liver cirrhosis and in patients with chronic renal disease. Eur J Clin Pharmacol. 1988;35:357.
158. Jusko WJ et al. Factors affecting theophylline clearances: age, tobacco, marijuana, cirrhosis, congestive heart failure, obesity, oral contraceptives, benzodiazepines, barbiturate and ethanol. J Pharm Sci. 1979;68:1358.
159. Piafsky KM et al. Theophylline kinetics in acute pulmonary edema. Clin Pharmacol Ther. 1977;21:310.
160. Powell JR et al. Theophylline disposition in acutely ill hospitalized patients: the effect of smoking, heart failure, severe airway obstruction and pneumonia. Am Rev Respir Dis. 1978;118:229.
161. Kuntz HD et al. Theophylline elimination in congestive heart failure. Klin Wochenschr. 1983;61:1105.
162. Bauer LA et al. The effect of acute and chronic renal failure on theophylline clearance. J Clin Pharmacol. 1981;22:65.
163. Chang KC et al. Altered theophylline pharmacokinetics during acute respiratory viral illness. Lancet. 1978;1:1132.
164. Kraemer MJ et al. Altered theophylline clearance during an influenza B outbreak. Pediatrics. 1982;69:476.
165. Jonkman JH et al. Effects of alpha-interferon on theophylline pharmacokinetics and metabolism. Br J Clin Pharmacol. 1989;27:795.
166. Bachmann K et al. Theophylline clearance during and after mild upper respiratory infection. Ther Drug Monit. 1987;9:279.
167. Sonne J et al. Antipyrine clearance in pneumonia. Clin Pharmacol Ther. 1985;37:701.
168. Meredith CG et al. Effects of influenza virus vaccine on hepatic drug metabolism. Clin Pharmacol Ther. 1985;37:396.
169. Winstanley PA et al. Lack of effect of highly purified subunit influenza vaccination on theophylline metabolism. Br J Clin Pharmacol. 1985;20:47.
170. Grabowski N et al. The effect of split virus influenza vaccination on theophylline pharmacokinetics. Am Rev Respir Dis. 1985;131:934.
171. Jonkman JH et al. No effect on influenza vaccination on theophylline pharmacokinetics as studied by ultraviolet spectrophotometry, HPLC, and EMIT assay methods. Ther Drug Monit. 1988;10:345.
172. Hannan SE et al. The effect of whole virus influenza vaccination on theophylline pharmacokinetics. Am Rev Respir Dis. 1988;137:903.
173. Cupit GC et al. The effect of pneumococcal vaccine on the disposition of theophylline. Eur J Clin Pharmacol. 1988;34:505.
174. Gary JD et al. Depression of theophylline elimination following BCG vaccination. Br J Clin Pharmacol. 1983;16:735.
175. Pokrajac M et al. Pharmacokinetics of theophylline in hyperthyroid and hypothyroid patients with chronic obstructive pulmonary disease. Eur J Clin Pharmacol. 1987;33:483.
176. Vozeh S et al. Influence of thyroid function on theophylline kinetics. Clin Pharmacol Ther. 1984;36:634.
177. Knoppert DC et al. Cystic fibrosis: enhanced theophylline metabolism may be linked to the disease. Clin Pharmacol Ther. 1988;44:254.

178. du Souich P et al. Theophylline disposition in patients with COLD with and without hypoxemia. Chest. 1989;95:1028.

179. Powell JR, Donn KH. Histamine H$_2$-antagonist drug interactions in perspective: mechanistic concepts and clinical implications. Am J Med. 1984;77(Suppl.5B):57.

180. Adebayo GI, Coker HA. Cimetidine inhibition of theophylline elimination: the influence of adult age and time course. Biopharm Drug Dispos. 1987;8:149.

181. Cohen IA et al. Cimetidine-theophylline interaction: effects of age and cimetidine dose. Ther Drug Monit. 1985;7:426.

182. Cremer KF et al. The effect of route of administration on the cimetidine-theophylline drug interaction. J Clin Pharmacol. 1989;29:451.

183. Gutfeld MB et al. The influence of intravenous cimetidine dosage regimens on the disposition of theophylline. J Clin Pharmacol. 1989;29:665.

184. Kelly HW et al. Ranitidine at very large doses does not inhibit theophylline elimination. Clin Pharmacol Ther. 1986;39:577.

185. Adebayo GI. Effects of equimolar doses of cimetidine and ranitidine on theophylline elimination. Biopharm Drug Dispos. 1989;10:77.

186. Verdiani P et al. Famotidine effects on theophylline pharmacokinetics in subjects affected by COPD. Comparison with cimetidine and placebo. Chest. 1988;94:807.

187. Secor JW et al. Lack of effect of nizatidine and hepatic drug metatolism in man. Br J Clin Pharmacol. 1985;20:710.

188. Rogge MC et al. The theophylline-enoxacin interaction: I. Effect of enoxacin dose size on theophylline disposition. Clin Pharmacol Ther. 1988;44:579.

189. Wijnands WJA et al. The influence of quinolone derivatives on theophylline clearance. Br J Clin Pharmacol. 1986;22:677.

190. Beckmann J et al. Enoxacin a potent inhibitor of theophylline metabolism. Eur J Clin Pharmacol. 1987;33:227.

191. Niki Y et al. New synthetic quinolone antibacterial agents and serum concentrations of theophylline. Chest. 1987;92:663.

192. Schwartz J et al. Impact of ciprofloxacin on theophylline clearance and steady-state concentrations in serum. Antimicrob Agents Chemother. 1988;32:75.

193. Prince RA et al. Effect of quinolone antimicrobials on theophylline pharmacokinetics. J Clin Pharmacol. 1989;29:650.

194. Raoof S et al. Ciprofloxacin increases serum levels of theophylline. Am J Med. 1987;82 (Suppl.4A):115.

195. Rybak MJ et al. Effect of ciprofloxacin on theophylline serum concentrations. Drug Intell Clin Pharm. 1987;21:879.

196. Thomson AH et al. A clinically significant interaction between ciprofloxacin and theophylline. Eur J Clin Pharmacol. 1987;42:435.

197. Bowles SK et al. Effect of norfloxacin on theophylline pharmacokinetics at steady state. Antimicrob Agents Chemother. 1988;32:510.

198. Ho G et al. Evaluation of the effect of norfloxacin on the pharmacokinetics of theophylline. Clin Pharmacol Ther. 1988;44:35.

199. Sano M et al. Effects of enoxacin, oflaxacin and norfloxacin on theophylline disposition in humans. Eur J Clin Pharmacol. 1988;35:161.

200. Gregoire SL et al. Inhibition of theophylline clearance by coadministered ofloxacin without alteration of theophylline effects. Antimicrob Agents Chemother. 1987;31:375.

201. Fourtillan JB et al. Pharmacokinetics of ofloxacin and theophylline alone and in combination. Infection. 1986;14(Suppl.1):S67.

202. Nix DE et al. Effect of lomefloxacin on theophylline pharmacokinetics. Antimicrob Agents Chemother. 1989;33:1006.

203. Ludden TM. Pharmacokinetic interactions of the macrolide antibiotics. Clin Pharmacokinet. 1985;10:63.

204. Rieder MJ, Spino M. The theophylline-erythromycin interaction. J Asthma. 1988;25:195.

205. Conrad KA, Nyman DW. Effects of metoprolol and propranolol on theophylline elimination. Clin Pharmacol Ther. 1980;28:463.

206. Lombardi TP et al. The effects of a beta-2 selective adrenergic agonist and a beta-nonselective antagonist on theophylline clearance. J Clin Pharmacol. 1987;27:523.

207. Cerasa LA et al. Lack of effect of atenolol on the pharmacokinetics of theophylline. Br J Clin Pharmacol. 1988;26:800.

208. Nafziger AN et al. Inhibition of theophylline elimination by diltiazem therapy. J Clin Pharmacol. 1987;27:862.

209. Jackson SH et al. The interaction between IV theophylline and chronic oral dosing with slow release nifedipine in volunteers. Br J Clin Pharmacol. 1986;21:389.

210. Tornatore KM et al. Effect of chronic oral contraceptive steroids on theophylline disposition. Eur Clin Pharmacol. 1982;23:129.

211. Gardner MJ, Jusko WJ. Effects of oral contraceptives and tobacco use on the metabolic pathways of theophylline. Int J Pharmaceut. 1986;33:55.

212. Koren G et al. Theophylline pharmacokinetics in adolescent females following coadministration of oral contraceptives. Clin Invest Med. 1985;8:222.

213. Kuthiala C, Squire EN. Acute dosing with methylprednisolone in normal subjects does not affect theophylline clearance. Ann Allergy. 1988;61:337.

214. Fergusson RJ et al. Effect of prednisolone on theophylline pharmacokinetics in patients with chronic airflow obstruction. Thorax. 1987;42:195.

215. Jonkman JH et al. Theophylline-terbutaline, a steady-state study on possible pharmacokinetic interactions with special reference to chronopharmacokinetics aspects. Br J Clin Pharmacol. 1988;26:285.

216. Brown MW et al. Effect of ketoconazole on oxidative drug metabolism. Clin Pharmacol Ther. 1985;37:290.

217. Heusner JJ et al. Effect of chronically administered ketoconazole on the elimination of theophylline in man. Drug Intell Clin Pharm. 1987;21:514.

218. Loi C et al. Dose-dependent inhibition of theophylline metabolism by disulfiram in recovering alcoholics. Clin Pharmacol Ther. 1989;45:476.

219. Crowley JJ et al. Aging and drug interactions: II. Effect of phenytoin and smoking on the oxidation of theophylline and cortisol in healthy men. J Pharmacol Exp Ther. 1988;245:513.

220. Crowley JJ et al. Cigarette smoking and theophylline metabolism: effects of phenytoin. Clin Pharmacol Ther. 1987;42:334.

221. Miller M et al. Influence of phenytoin on theophylline clearance. Clin Pharmacol Ther. 1984;35:666.

222. Powell-Jackson PR et al. Effect of rifampicin administration on theophylline pharmacokinetics in humans. Am Rev Respir Dis. 1985;131:939.

223. Boyce EG et al. The effect of rifampin on theophylline kinetics. J Clin Pharmacol. 1986;26:969.

224. Saccar CL et al. The effect of phenobarbital on theophylline disposition in children with asthma. J Allergy Clin Immunol. 1985;75:716.

225. Emerman CL et al. Theophylline concentrations in the emergency treatment of acute bronchial asthma. Am J Emerg Med. 1983;1:12.

226. Weinberger MM et al. Intravenous aminophylline dosage. Use of serum theophylline measurement for guidance. JAMA. 1976;235:2110.

227. Mitenko PA, Ogilvie RI. Rapidly achieved plasma concentration plateau, with observations on theophylline kinetics. Clin Pharmacol Ther. 1972;13:329.

228. Koup JR et al. System for clinical pharmacokinetic monitoring of theophylline. Am J Hosp Pharm. 1976;33:949.

229. Chiou WL et al. Method for the rapid estimation of the total body drug clearance and adjustment of dosage regimens in patients during a constant-rate intravenous infusion. J Pharmacokinet Biopharm. 1978;6:135.

230. Pancorbo S et al. Use of a pharmacokinetic method for establishing dose of aminophylline to treat acute bronchospasm. Am J Hosp Pharm. 1976;38:851.

231. Slattery JT et al. Prediction of maintenance dose required to attain a desired drug concentration at steady state from a single determination after an initial dose. Clin Pharmacokinet. 1980;5:377.

232. Grambau GR et al. Reliability of theophylline clearance in determining maintenance intravenous aminophylline therapy. J Clin Pharmacol. 1985;25:381.

233. Hurley S et al. A randomized controlled clinical trial of pharmacokinetic theophylline dosing. Am Rev Respir Dis. 1986;134:1219.

234. Rizzo A et al. Early estimate of theophylline clearance during intravenous infusion. Eur J Respir Dis. 1986;68:291.

235. Haumschild MJ, Murphy JE. Prediction of theophylline clearance using condition correction factors. Clin Pharm. 1985;4:59.

236. Gotz VP et al. Evaluation of the "condition correction factor" method of estimating theophylline clearance. Ther Drug Monit. 1983;5:103.

237. McCory RW, Matzke GR. Evaluation of a single-point method for predicting theophylline dosage. Clin Pharm. 1982;1:441.

238. Coleman RW, Hedberg RL. Comparison of three methods for estimating theophylline pharmacokinetics. Clin Pharm. 1983;2:148.

239. Anderson G et al. Evaluation of two methods for estimating theophylline clearance prior to achieving steady state. Ther Drug Monit. 1981;3:325.

240. Wells TG et al. Rapid estimation of serum theophylline clearance in children with acute asthma. Ther Drug Monit. 1984;6:402.

241. Hurley SF, McNeil JJ. A comparison of the accuracy of a least squares regression, a bayesian, Chiou's and the steady-state clearance method of individualizing theophylline dosage. Clin Pharmacokinet. 1988;14:311.

242. Rodvold KA et al. Accuracy of 11 methods for predicting theophylline dose. Clin Pharm. 1986;5:403.

243. Hoon TJ et al. The relative predictive performance of two theophylline pharmacokinetics dosing programs. Pharmacotherapy. 1988;8:82.

244. Iafrate RP et al. Computer-simulated conversion from intravenous to sustained-release oral theophylline. Drug Intell Clin Pharm. 1982;16:19.

245. Hatton RC et al. Conversion from intravenous aminophylline to sustained-release theophylline: computer simulation versus *in vivo* results. Clin Pharm. 1983;2:347.

246. Kossoy AF et al. Are theophylline "levels" a reliable indicator of compliance? J Allergy Clin Immunol. 1989;84:60.

247. Muir KT et al. Simultaneous determination of theophylline and its major metabolites in urine by reverse-phase ion-pair high-performance liquid chromatography. J Chromatogr. 1980;221:85.

248. Wilson JF et al. Evaluation of chromatographic and kit immunoassay techniques for the measurement of theophylline in serum: a study based on external quality assurement measurements. Ther Drug Monit. 1988;10:438.

249. Patel JA et al. Abnormal theophylline levels in plasma by fluorescence polarization immunoassay in patients with renal disease. Ther Drug Monit. 1984;6:458.

250. Clifton GD et al. Accuracy and time requirements for use of three rapid theophylline assay methods. Clin Pharm. 1988;7:462.

251. Massoud N et al. Comparison of the Seralyzer and EMIT systems for determination of theophylline concentrations. Am J Hosp Pharm. 1986;43:1722.

252. Fling JA et al. Two rapid methods for determination of serum theophylline concentrations: a comparison. Ann Allergy. 1989;62:35.

253. Shaw KN et al. Comparison of two methods of rapid theophylline testing in clinical practice. J Pediatr. 1988;112:131.

254. Hill M, Hendeles L. Evaluation of an office method of measuring theophylline serum concentrations. J Allergy Clin Immunol. 1988;82:30.

255. Nguyen QC et al. Determination of theophylline concentration by AccuLevel. Ann Allergy. 1988;60:521.

256. Chan KM et al. The theophylline method of the Abbott "Vision" analyzer evaluated. Clin Chem. 1987;33:130.

257. Vaughan LM et al. Evaluation of the Ames Seralyzer for therapeutic monitoring of theophylline. Drug Intell Clin Pharm. 1986;20:118.

258. Jenny RW, Jackson KY. Two types of error found with the Seralyzer ARIS assay of theophylline. Clin Chem. 1986;32:2122. Letter.

259. Milavetz G et al. Comparative efficiency of a laboratory and examining room assay for therapeutic drug monitoring of theophylline in ambulatory patients. Ann Allergy. 1989;62:453.

260. Goldberg MJ et al. Treatment of theophylline intoxication. J Allergy Clin Immunol. 1986;78:811.

261. Goldberg MJ et al. The effect of sorbitol and activated charcoal on serum theophylline concentrations after slow-release theophylline. Clin Pharmacol Ther. 1987;41:108.

262. Caldwell et al. Hypernatremia associated with cathartics and overdose management. West J Med. 1987;147:593.

263. Farley TA. Severe hypernatremic dehydration after use of an activated charcoal-sorbitol suspension. J Pediatr. 1986;109:719.

264. Sullivan JB, Krenzelok EP. Repetitive doses of activated charcoal-sorbitol combination: a word of caution. Am J Emerg Med. 1988;6:201.

265. Park GD et al. Effects of size and frequency or oral doses of charcoal on theophylline clearance. Clin Pharmacol Ther. 1983;34:663.

266. Radomski L et al. Model of theophylline overdose treatment with oral activated charcoal. Clin Pharmacol Ther. 1984;35:402.

267. Berlinger WG et al. Enhancement of theophylline clearance by oral activated charcoal. Clin Pharmacol Ther. 1983;33:351.

268. Jin Ding H. Kinetics of theophylline clearance in gastrointestinal dialysis with charcoal. J Pharm Sci. 1987;76:525.

269. Ohning BL et al. Continuous nasogastric administration of activated charcoal for the treatment of theophylline intoxication. Pediatr Pharmacol (New York). 1986;5:241.

270. Amitai Y et al. Repetitive oral activated charcoal and control of emesis in severe theophylline toxicity. Ann Intern Med. 1986;105:386.

271. Olson Y et al. Theophylline overdose: acute single ingestion versus chronic repeated overmedication. Am J Emerg Med. 1985;3:386.

272. Woo OF et al. Benefit of hemoperfusion in acute theophylline intoxication. Clin Toxicol. 1984;22:411.

273. Gaudreault P et al. Theophylline poisoning: pharmacologic considerations and clinical management. Med Toxicol. 1986;1:169.

274. Seneff M et al. Acute theophylline toxicity and the use of esmolol to reverse cardiovascular instability. Ann Emerg Med. 1990;19:671.

275. Brown GS et al. Peritoneal clearance of theophylline. Am J Kidney Dis. 1981;1:24.

276. Levy G et al. Hemodialysis clearance of theophylline. JAMA. 1977;237:1466.

277. Slaughter RL et al. Hemodialysis clearance of theophylline. Ther Drug Monit. 1982;4:191.

278. Lee CS et al. Hemodialysis of theophylline in uremic patients. J Clin Pharmacol. 1979;19:219.

279. Park GD et al. The use of hemoperfusion for theophylline intoxication. Am J Med. 1983;74:961.

280. Bahls FH, et al. Theophylline-associated seizures with "therapeutic" or low toxic serum concentrations: risk factors for serious outcome in adults. Neurology. 1991;41:1309.

281. Shannon M, Lovejoy FH. The influence of age versus peak serum concentration on life-threatening events after chronic theophylline intoxication. Arch Intern Med. 1990;150:2045–2048.

282. Ratanasavanh D, et al. Methylcholanthrene but not phenobarbital enhances caffeine and theophylline metabolism in cultured adult human hepatocytes. Biochem Pharmacol. 1990;38:85.

283. Nafziger AN, Bertino JS Jr. Sex-related differences in theophylline pharmacokinetics. Eur J Clin Pharmacol. 1989;37:97.

284. Bruguerolle B, et al. Influence of the menstrual cycle on theophylline pharmacokinetics in asthmatics. Eur J Clin Pharmacol. 1990;39:59.

Chapter 14

Aminoglycosides

Darwin E. Zaske

Aminoglycoside antibiotics are among the most useful group of antimicrobial agents for gram-negative infections. This group includes streptomycin, kanamycin, neomycin, paromomycin, gentamicin, tobramycin, amikacin, and netilmicin. Some of these agents have a higher risk of toxicity or higher incidence of bacterial resistance and are not currently used. Sisomicin is marketed internationally, but not in the United States. Gentamicin, tobramycin, amikacin, and netilmicin are presently the most widely used aminoglycoside agents in the United States. These aminoglycoside antibiotics are similar in physical, chemical, pharmacologic, and toxicologic properties. They are bactericidal and rapidly induce their lethal effects. Ototoxicity and nephrotoxicity are the most frequent and troublesome side effects of these agents. The pharmacokinetic properties of these agents are influenced by a large number of physiologic changes that occur during sepsis. These changes may have a substantial effect on the pharmacologic response in patients, with some having a higher risk of treatment failure or toxicity. The following presentation describes these agents' antibacterial activity, the pharmacokinetic parameters, factors related to elimination, methods for controlling serum concentrations, and the clinical results of controlling serum concentrations of these four commonly used agents.

CLINICAL PHARMACOKINETICS

Absorption

Following oral administration, aminoglycoside antibiotics are poorly absorbed from the gastrointestinal (GI) tract, with only 0.3% to 1.5% of an administered dose appearing in the urine.[1] Nevertheless, the amount of oral absorption can lead to toxic concentrations in patients who have severe renal insufficiency. Peritoneal absorption can be substantial and can also lead to serious side effects. After two to five minutes of an intraperitoneal lavage, systemic serum concentrations of aminoglycoside can approach therapeutic values within 15 to 75 minutes.[2] The amount of aminoglycoside absorbed is additive with other systemic routes of administration.

Administration

The aminoglycoside antibiotics are administered by either intramuscular injection or intravenous infusion. These agents are generally well absorbed after intramuscular injection. In patients who have severe gram-negative sepsis, blood perfusion of the intramuscular site may be reduced because of hypotension, and the rate of drug absorption may be substantially reduced. Additionally, repeated injections at the same intramuscular site may impair absorption and result in more variation in serum concentrations.

Peak serum concentrations after intramuscular injections are generally achieved within 30 to 120 minutes after the injection. In younger patients who have normal renal function, the serum concentration peaks 30 to 60 minutes after administration. In these patients, the peak is more consistently attained, with less variability in absorption from the intramuscular site, and less variability in elimination rate. In patients 40 years of age or older, the elimination rate of aminoglycosides becomes more variable, and the absorption from the intramuscular site appears to demonstrate more interpatient variability. In patients who have compromised renal function, the peak serum concentrations are achieved later (two to five hours postadministration), depending upon the degree of renal impairment. Peak and trough serum concentrations are more difficult to maintain consistently within therapeutic guidelines after intramuscular administration. This route of administration should be used only in patients who are relatively stable or as follow-up to intravenous therapy.

Aminoglycoside antibiotics can be administered intravenously by bolus injection,[3] by 30 to 60 minute intermittent infusions,[4-6] or by continuous intravenous infusion.[6-9] Intermittent infusions of 30 to 60 minutes are thought to be safer and have additional therapeutic advantages. Theoretically, this method of administration provides an effective concentration gradient to increased interstitial concentrations. The pharmacokinetic model for aminoglycosides is simplified with 60 minute infusions as compared to shorter administration times. A 60 minute infusion may also have practical advantages for the nursing staff and may minimize the potential error in the infusion rate of the drug. Continuous infusions of aminoglycosides have been suggested to improve the efficacy of aminoglycosides, especially in neutropenic patients.[7-8] However, this method of administration is difficult in intensive care units where a patient may be receiving several intravenous medications, some of which may not be compatible with the aminoglycoside. More importantly, a higher incidence of toxicity may also occur with this method of administration.[7-8] Furthermore, the relationship of bacterial killing effect with time indicates that the aminoglycoside need only be in contact with the bacteria for a very short period of time. Hence, administration by continuous infusion would seem to lack therapeutic rationale, especially if the risk of toxicity is increased.

Bolus injections of aminoglycosides have been frequently suggested in the European literature and widely utilized.[3] This method of administration allows the drug to be rapidly injected without involving an extensive amount of nursing time or drug administration costs. These are certainly important considerations in the midst of prospective reimbursement changes. However, reports have indicated that an increased risk of ototoxicity may be associated with high transient concentrations that result from bolus injections. Most investigators from the United States have discouraged this method of administration.

Distribution

Aminoglycoside antibiotics distribute well into most body fluids including synovial, peritoneal, ascitic, and pleural fluids.[10-14] These agents distribute slowly in the bile, feces, prostate, and amniotic fluid.[15-28] Aminoglycosides distribute poorly in the central nervous system and the vitreous humor of the eye.[21-23] Binding to serum proteins is less than 10% and is not considered to be clinically important.[24-26]

Penetration of aminoglycosides in bronchial secretions varies considerably in clinical trials.[27-30] Direct administration via inhalation has been suggested[31] but not widely utilized. Aminoglycosides penetrate the eye poorly following systemic administrations.[22,23] Direct periocular injections or topical administration is necessary to treat local infections in the eye. These agents cross the placenta and achieve fetal serum concentrations which are 21% to 37% of maternal serum concentrations.[19,20]

Aminoglycoside antibiotics distribute primarily to a pharmacologic space very similar to the physiologic space of the extracellular fluid compartment. In normal volunteers, the extracellular fluid compartment approximates 20% to 25% of body weight. This physiologic space is susceptible to changes that may occur during gram-negative sepsis (e.g., dehydration, congestive heart failure). Frequently, patients in initial phases of gram-negative sepsis are febrile, nauseated, and vomiting and, consequently, are dehydrated. As a result, the extracellular fluid compartment and drug volume are decreased in the dehydrated patients. In these patients, the drug's distribution volume is markedly lower than 20% of body weight (see Figure 14-1). Additionally, several subgroups of patients have been identified who are likely to have increases in drug distribution volume. These include patients who have congestive heart failure, patients with peritonitis, patients immediately postpartum, and patients receiving intravenous hyperalimentation. In addition, newborn infants are known to have a larger extracellular fluid volume per unit of body weight. The drug's distribution volume in neonates is frequently in the range of 50% to 70% of body weight.

Initially, the distribution volume of aminoglycosides was thought to be consistent from patient to patient. However, the distribution volume demonstrates considerable variability between patients.[32-35] This interpatient variation appears to be similar for all four aminoglycosides and appears to have a substantial effect on serum concentrations and dosage requirements.

In addition to the interpatient variation, the drug's distribution volume may change during the course of antibiotic therapy. This is especially true for patients who are markedly dehydrated in the initial phases of sepsis or patients who have a large volume initially. During the course of therapy in a patient who is dehydrated, the administration of intravenous fluids replenishes the fluid deficit. As the fluid deficit is replaced, the drug's distribution volume will increase. In contrast, patients with congestive heart failure or peritonitis will eliminate their excess fluid during the course of therapy. In some patients, these changes can be substantial, and a marked change in the dosage regimen may be required to maintain therapeutic serum concentrations. This change in the distribution volume is independent of any change in renal function, but will influence the drug's half-life if total body clearance remains constant within the patient (see Figure 14-2). This change in half-life is in direct relation to the change in volume, and thus, as the volume increases, the drug's half-life will also increase. With only moderate changes in the extracellular fluid volume and drug volume, the drug's clearance remains relatively constant. In a severe state of dehydration, the drug clearance may decrease secondary to a decrease in cardiac output and shunting of blood from the kidney. In patients with large volumes, the cardiac output, renal blood flow, glomerular filtration, and drug clearance may increase, provided the cardiovascular system can tolerate the extra fluid load without failing. Thus, the patient's cardiovascular hemodynamics and the extracellular fluid compartment

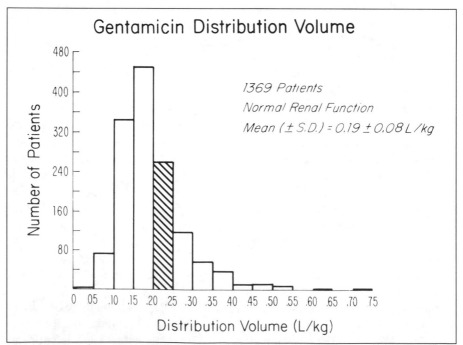

Figure 14-1. *The distribution volume for gentamicin has been reported to be consistent from patient to patient and is thought to approximate the extracellular fluid compartment of 20% to 25% of body weight. Considerably more variation was noted in the distribution volume of gentamicin in these patients.*

may change the drug's clearance and distribution volume. Clinically, monitoring of serum concentrations in patients with fluid changes is imperative to ensure therapeutic serum concentrations. Because this change in half-life via volume changes is independent of serum creatinine, measuring markers of renal function will not identify these changes in the drug's pharmacokinetic characteristics.

Pharmacokinetic Model

Aminoglycoside antibiotics are characterized by linear pharmacokinetic principles and hence would show a direct proportionality between increasing dose and increasing area under the concentration-time curve (AUC). The choice of pharmacokinetic models used to fit serum concentration-time data has received substantial discussion. Under the right set of conditions, patients may demonstrate a triphasic decay of serum concentration with time. These conditions include a rapid infusion, a slow elimination rate, or a large volume of distribution. With these conditions, a three-compartment model would fit the serum concentration-time data most precisely and would be most scientifically valid. However, the number of required serum samples (at least nine) and the difficulty in devising a useable serum sampling strategy in each patient make this approach impractical and impossible to implement clinically. Also, a question remains whether this degree of added pharmacokinetic precision will more accurately estimate dosage require-

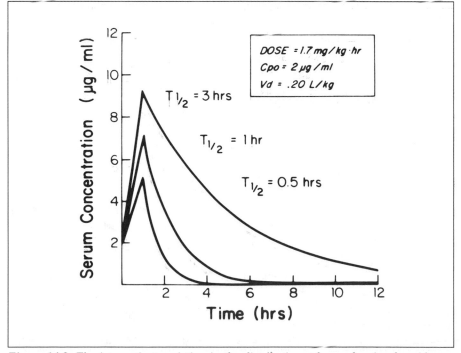

Figure 14-2. The intrapatient variation in the distribution volume of aminoglycoside can markedly affect the half-life of the drug and serum concentrations. This change is independent of a change in renal function tests. In this figure, total body clearances seem to remain constant (reproduced with permission from reference 76).

ments and better control serum concentrations than would a one-compartment model. These advantages may be doubtful when considering the large number of physiologic changes that occur in septic patients.

Generally, aminoglycosides are administered over 30 to 60 minutes as intermittent infusions. This longer infusion period, when compared to a bolus injection, decreases the infusion rate and thereby reduces or minimizes the distribution phase. In essence, the drug is allowed to distribute within the tissue compartment as rapidly as the drug is being administered. Achieving tissue equilibrium can be further altered by a slower elimination rate or by a larger distribution volume. Consequently, patients receiving high infusion rates (large doses, >1.5 mg/ kg, or short infusions, <30 minutes), having compromised renal function (CL_{cr} <50 mL/min), or having a large distribution volume (V_d >0.30 L/kg) will probably demonstrate a distribution phase in serum concentration-time data. Clinically, we have tried to avoid this phase and its potential error by increasing the infusion period (60 minutes) and thereby decreasing the infusion rate, or by altering our serum sampling strategy and simply ignoring this initial distribution phase.

A third phase or tissue compartment can also be demonstrated in many patients, especially those with compromised renal function.[36-39] This phase probably results from tissue redistribution of aminoglycoside. This phase has been proposed to explain drug accumulation in patients receiving aminoglycosides and may indicate substantial accumulation of drug within the kidney.[40,41] This accumulation phase may be associated with the risk of toxicity.[42,43] Specific patients demonstrate marked variability in the rate and extent of tissue uptake of aminoglycosides.[36] The area under the concentration-time curve represented by this terminal phase is generally a very small fraction of the total area under the concentration-time curve.[44] However, as renal function decreases, the AUC of the terminal phase becomes a larger fraction of the total area. Consequently, if this terminal phase is ignored, predicted peak and trough serum concentrations may be in error. The half-life from the terminal phase is substantially prolonged (i.e., 100 hours) and may lead to drug accumulation resulting in increased trough and peak concentrations while renal function may be stable. This terminal phase is difficult to estimate from serum concentration-time data while patients are receiving treatment for sepsis. Population estimates have been proposed for modifying dosage regimens derived from a one-compartment model.[36] These two-compartment parameters thus estimate the average tissue uptake of aminoglycoside over time. However, the predictability of these two-compartmental rate constants is extremely low, and they have limited predictive clinical utility. Tissue accumulation, however, must be an ongoing consideration in patients receiving more than seven to ten days of therapy, especially if the patients have compromised renal function.[44] Serum concentrations should be monitored during therapy in these patients to prevent excessive accumulation of drug and exposure of the patient to a higher risk of toxicity.

A one-compartment model can generally provide clinically useable estimates of drug disposition for aminoglycosides.[45,46] The infusion rate and serum sampling strategies can generally be modified to provide reliable estimates of drug elimination and distribution volume (see Figure 14-3). Also, the number of serum samples necessary to provide reliable pharmacokinetic estimates is substantially less for the one-compartment model (two to three specimens) than the number for a two- or three-compartment model (six to nine specimens). The accuracy of a one-compartment model is sufficient for determining dosage requirements of amino-glycosides and for attaining the targeted peak and trough serum concentrations.[47] It should be emphasized that the pharmacokinetic model or dosing method is only a clinical tool to assist the clinician in determining dosage requirements. During therapy, the patient's response and dosage requirement need continued monitoring and reassessment.

Excretion

Aminoglycoside antibiotics are primarily eliminated unchanged by the kidney via glomerular filtration.[48-53] Active secretion may account for a small amount of drug eliminated by the kidney. Elimination by the kidney accounts for approximately 85% to 95% of the dose administered and results in high urinary concentrations after recommended dosages. Small amounts of drug have been found in the bile and may represent an additional route of elimination.[15-17]

Wide interpatient variation in elimination of the four aminoglycosides has been recognized.[32-35] This interpatient variation occurs in patients who have a normal

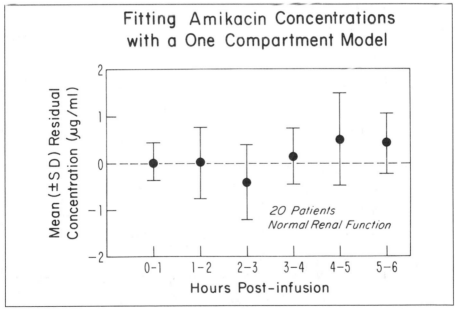

Figure 14-3. *The post-infusion serum concentration-time data were fitted by nonlinear least-squares regression analysis assuming a monoexponential decay. The difference between the measured and fitted concentrations was grouped and summed for each one-hour interval post-infusion. For each time period, the mean and standard deviation of the residual concentrations are illustrated. If the residuals were zero for all time points, the drug would display an ideal monoexponential decline. The use of the one-compartment model for amikacin demonstrated minimal bias after administering the drug as a one-hour infusion and is adequate to fit concentration-time data.*

serum creatinine or a normal creatinine clearance. The magnitude of this variation seems greater in patients being treated for gram-negative sepsis than in normal volunteers. This variation may also be greater in the initial phases of treatment, rather than later in the treatment course, when the patient's physiologic parameters have stabilized clinically. In volunteers who have normal renal function, the half-life of gentamicin was initially reported to vary between 2.5 and 4 hours,[50] and the half-life of amikacin ranged from 0.8 to 2.8 hours.[51-53] In comparison, a large group of patients were studied in the early course of sepsis. For gentamicin, the half-life ranged from 0.4 to 32.7 hours in 855 patients who had a normal serum creatinine (≤1.5 mg/dL) (see Figure 14-4) and 0.4 to 7.6 hours in 331 patients who had a normal serum creatinine clearance (≥100 mL/min/1.73 m²).[47] Thus, the half-life of gentamicin varies considerably (especially in septic patients) even if renal function tests are normal. Similar variations were also noted with tobramycin,[54] amikacin,[34] and netilmicin.[35]

The total body clearance of the aminoglycosides also demonstrated considerable patient-to-patient variability. The total body clearance for gentamicin varied from 7 to 249 mL/hr/kg in 855 patients who had a normal serum creatinine and from 8.4 to 242 mL/hr/kg in 331 patients who had a normal creatinine clearance.[47] Similar variations were also noted with tobramycin,[55] amikacin,[34] and netilmicin.[35]

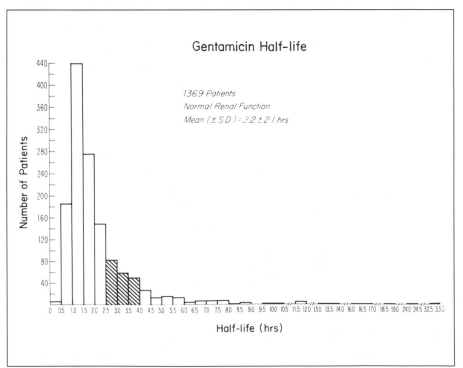

Figure 14-4. *The half-life of gentamicin demonstrates a wide interpatient variation even in patients who have a normal serum creatinine. The majority of patients have a half-life less than the previously reported range of 2.5 to 4 hours. However, a substantial number of patients have prolonged elimination rates even though they have normal renal function tests as assessed by serum creatinine.*

FACTORS RELATED TO AMINOGLYCOSIDE DISPOSITION

Several factors have been reported to alter the disposition of aminoglycoside antibiotics and thereby influence serum concentrations and dosage requirements. Additionally, specific patient conditions seem to influence the elimination of aminoglycosides and dosage requirements. Knowing these relationships, specific patients can better be selected who would benefit by more intensive serum concentration monitoring. The following variables and their relationship to aminoglycoside disposition warrant discussion.

Renal Function

Most of the early pharmacokinetic studies of aminoglycosides were conducted in volunteers with varying degrees of renal function. In volunteers, approximately 80% to 90% of the variance (r^2) in elimination of aminoglycosides was explained by changes in renal function.[50] Barza et al.[56] reported that only 52% of the variation in gentamicin elimination could be explained by changes in the serum creatinine in a group of septic patients. Kaye et al.[57] also reported that only 50% of the variation in gentamicin elimination was explained by a change in creatinine clearance in a similar group. Thus, in patients with sepsis, less variation in aminoglycoside elimi-

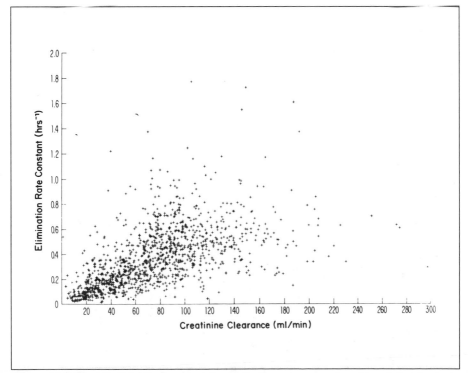

Figure 14-5. *The relationship of gentamicin elimination rate constant and creatinine clearance is illustrated for 1640 patients. At any specific creatinine clearance, the elimination rate constant demonstrated at least a tenfold variation. The amount of variance (r^2) in the elimination rate constant explained by creatinine clearance was only 34%.*

nation is explained by estimates of renal function. For amikacin, similar statistical relationships were found with serum creatinine versus amikacin half-life, elimination rate constant versus creatinine clearance, and drug clearance versus creatinine clearance (see Figure 14-5). However, only 46% of the variation in amikacin half-life was explained by a change in serum creatinine.[34] The statistical relationship between elimination rate versus creatinine clearance and total body clearance versus creatinine clearance was similar for both amikacin and netilmicin. Substantial error may thus occur in predicting drug clearance or elimination rate from estimates of glomerular filtration rate, even though renal function is the most important variable.

Age

In healthy adults, cardiac output, renal blood flow, and glomerular filtration decrease with increasing age. Pharmacologic agents which are primarily eliminated by glomerular filtration rate are influenced by these physiologic changes. The elimination and clearance of aminoglycosides decreases with increasing age.[34,47] The relationship of the elimination rate constant with age demonstrates that the rate of aminoglycoside elimination continually decreases with increasing age (see Figure 14-6). The distribution volume (L/kg) for aminoglycosides was not related to age.[47]

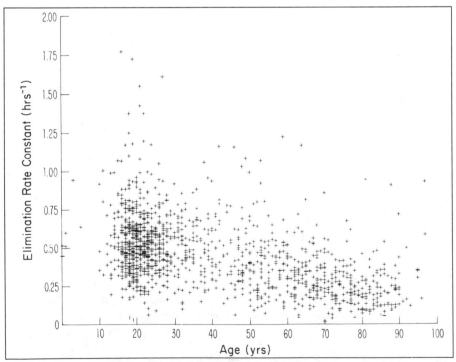

Figure 14-6. *The elimination rate constant of gentamicin continually decreased with increasing age in patients who had a normal serum creatinine (≤ 1.5 mg/dL). A substantial variation exists in this relationship.*

Distribution Volume

The relationship between half-life and distribution volume is significant with aminoglycosides.[47] The distribution volume is probably a physiologic marker for the extracellular fluid compartment; when the extracellular fluid volume decreases, the distribution volume decreases, the elimination rate increases, and the half-life decreases (see Figure 14-7). These changes are all independent of any change occurring with serum creatinine or other markers of renal function.

Fever

Fever also seems to be an important factor influencing serum concentrations and elimination of aminoglycosides.[58] In dogs pretreated with endotoxin, a 25% decrease in serum gentamicin concentrations was observed at 60 minutes post-injection when compared to corresponding values in controls. In six febrile human volunteers, serum concentrations of gentamicin were reduced by 40% at one, two, and three hours after intramuscular injection when compared to control values in each of the same subjects. Although the half-life and renal clearance of gentamicin did not appear to be affected significantly by fever, fever was the principal factor associated with the lower concentrations of gentamicin. Physiologically, fever may change the elimination of aminoglycosides by increasing heart rate and cardiac output and thereby increase renal blood flow and glomerular filtration. Thus, patients with febrile episodes may have a higher elimination rate of aminoglycosides due to underlying physiologic changes secondary to gram-negative sepsis.

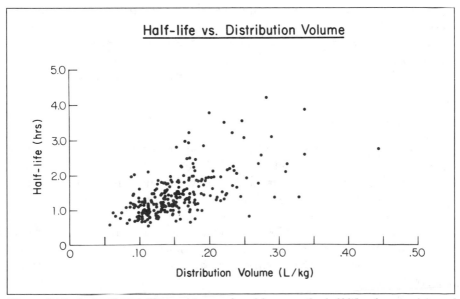

Figure 14-7. *A significant relationship was found between the half-life of gentamicin and distribution volume. The distribution volume would appear to be an indirect measurement of extracellular fluid compartment or state of hydration (reproduced with permission from reference 178.)*

Hematocrit

A nonlinear relationship was reported between the hematocrit and the half-life of gentamicin;[47,56] however, the degree of the association is low.[47] The relationship between the reciprocal of the hematocrit and drug half-life was linear and explained 42% of the variance.[56] The hematocrit is altered by changes in the patient's fluid status and thus explains the weak relationship previously observed between half-life and hematocrit.

Ideal Body Weight

Aminoglycoside antibiotics were originally thought to distribute solely into ideal body mass, and prediction of serum concentration was thought to be improved if methods used ideal body weight rather than total body weight. Later, data suggested that these agents also distributed into excess weight or adipose tissue.[56–62] Gentamicin was found to distribute into 5% to 6% of excess weight,[60] and with ideal body mass, the distribution volume was 19% of body weight. Thus the drug's distribution volume increases with increasing excess weight, presumably due to distribution into the extracellular water within the adipose tissue. However, a substantial amount of variation in the distribution volume occurred at select values of excess weight. This variation is best explained by changes in hydration and extracellular fluid volume, especially in the surgical patients.

Gender

An association between gender and the elimination rate of gentamicin was reported to be moderately significant. In a study of 1,640 patients, females eliminated gentamicin more rapidly than males.[47] The elimination rate constant, half-life, distribution volume and clearances were significantly different for males and females. Females had a lower distribution volume per unit of weight than males probably because of decreased muscle mass and decreased extracellular fluid per unit of weight.

Obstetric Patients

Several physiologic changes occur antepartum and postpartum that may influence the elimination of aminoglycosides. The extracellular fluid compartment, total body water, cardiac output, renal blood flow, and glomerular filtration are all increased during the later phases of pregnancy. The equilibrium is reestablished usually two to five days after delivery. The aminoglycosides, which distribute to the extracellular fluid and are dependent upon glomerular filtration, are markedly influenced by pregnancy. For gentamicin, the elimination is extremely rapid: 94% of 55 patients in one study had a half-life shorter than the reported range of 2.5 to 4 hours.[63]

Burn Patients

Physiologically, burn patients are "hypermetabolic," with elevated basal metabolic rates and oxygen clearance. Their caloric expenditure can be two to three times normal and can be further elevated with concurrent gram-negative sepsis and fever. Hemodynamic changes secondary to the burn appear to explain why burn patients have an extremely rapid rate of aminoglycoside elimination (see Figure 14-8).[64–67] In addition, the extracellular fluid compartment in burn patients can be extremely large immediately post-injury. Consequently, an occasional patient who develops gram-negative sepsis early in the course of burn resuscitation may have an extremely high distribution volume and a prolonged drug half-life, even though renal function tests are normal.[65] After the post-burn diuresis is completed, the volume of distribution returns to normal values (0.2 L/kg), but the clearance remains elevated until the burn injury has healed.

Pediatric Patients

The elimination rate of aminoglycosides in pediatric patients is rapid;[68–71] and the half-life of gentamicin is shortened. This rapid rate of elimination is particularly apparent in pediatric patients with cystic fibrosis, burns, and leukemia.

Internal Medicine Patients

A large number of internal medicine patients with normal serum creatinine concentrations had gentamicin half-lives of less than 2.5 hours.[72] However, a substantial number of these patients had prolonged elimination rates of the drug and required a marked dosage reduction to prevent potentially toxic serum concentra-

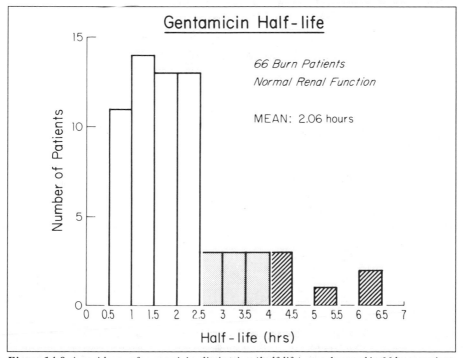

Figure 14-8. *A rapid rate of gentamicin elimination (half-life) was observed in 66 burn patients who had normal renal function (reproduced with permission from reference 65).*

tions.[72] The experience with this group of patients emphasizes the need for measuring serum concentrations and adjusting aminoglycoside dosage regimens because of substantial interpatient differences.

Ascites

The distribution volume of gentamicin is markedly increased in patients with ascites.[73,74] An expanded extracellular fluid volume attributed to the ascitic fluid explains the increase in distribution volume. Gentamicin appears to distribute rapidly into the ascitic fluid, and the large distribution volume necessitates a larger dose to achieve desired peak serum concentrations. The drug's half-life is probably prolonged in these patients due to the large extravascular distribution volume. This prolonged half-life may occur even if patients have normal renal function.

Geriatric Patients

Elderly patients have a progressive decrease in glomerular filtration rate with increasing age. Since the endogenous production of creatinine decreases with increasing age, the serum creatinine may be a misleading indicator of glomerular filtration and aminoglycoside elimination. Also, elderly patients who develop severe gram-negative sepsis may develop congestive heart failure concurrently. The resulting increase in extracellular fluid and edema results in a higher distribution volume and a longer half-life (see Figure 14-9).[75] Thus, the distribution volume and elimination rate may be difficult to accurately predict in the elderly patient from markers of renal function (i.e., serum creatinine).

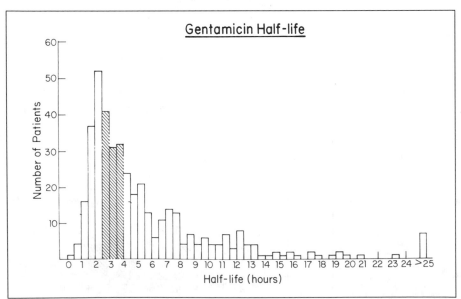

Figure 14-9. *The half-life of gentamicin demonstrated a substantial amount of variation in geriatric patients who had either normal renal function or abnormal renal function (reproduced with permission from reference 75).*

Surgery/Critically Ill Patients

A wide interpatient variation exists among surgical patients who develop gram-negative sepsis.[76] Surgical patients with infections have many underlying medical complications that may alter the elimination rate or clearance of aminoglycoside antibiotics.

Critically ill patients may be hypermetabolic or have early signs of organ failure. The hypermetabolic patients have increased oxygen consumption, cardiac output, and blood flow to vital organs, especially the kidney. The increased blood flow to the kidney explains the increased aminoglycoside clearance observed in such patients. Patients with early signs of organ failure have decreased blood flow and decreased aminoglycoside clearance. Most surgical intensive care patients have expanded distribution volumes (>0.25 L/kg) secondary to expanded extracellular fluid from undergoing surgery or to maximize oxygen delivery.

Cystic Fibrosis

Patients with cystic fibrosis often require daily doses of aminoglycosides that are much higher than those commonly recommended for gram-negative infections. From available data, creatinine clearance rates appear to be remarkably higher in these patients, as are the elimination or clearance rates of many drugs that are excreted by the kidney.[77–80] This rapid elimination may be due to the "hypermetabolic state" associated with cystic fibrosis and to the higher glomerular filtration rate associated with the younger age of these patients.

Neonates

The newborn, especially the premature patient, experiences very dynamic changes in physiologic parameters such as cardiac output, renal blood flow, renal function, and extracellular fluid. Consequently, the distribution volume, clearance, and half-life vary substantially from day to day, and therapeutic concentrations are extremely difficult to attain and maintain.[81–83] The healthy newborn infant generally has a higher extracellular fluid volume. The drug distribution volume returns to normal within the first few months of life and approaches values generally observed in normal pediatric patients. Dosing charts and nomograms have been devised to control drug concentrations in these newborn infants. Gestational age, asphyxiation, and nutritional status are additional factors associated with aminoglycoside disposition within neonates.[84,85]

Gynecologic Patients

The elimination rate of aminoglycosides in patients with gynecologic infections is generally rapid, and dosage requirements are generally increased in this group of patients.[86] The rapid elimination is probably explained by the younger age group of these patients, who may respond to fever by increasing cardiac output and renal blood flow. Increases in renal blood flow and glomerular filtration may lead to the higher clearance rate observed in these patients.

Effect of Interpatient Variation on Serum Concentrations

Wide interpatient variations in aminoglycoside elimination have marked effects on the serum concentration-time profile. Patients who have a short aminoglycoside half-life eliminate more of the drug during a one hour infusion. Consequently, the peak concentration obtained after the same dose is lower than that obtained in patients with longer half-lives. In addition, serum concentrations are below the minimum inhibitory concentrations for most gram-negative pathogens within the initial two hours of the dosing interval. Thus, with gentamicin, tobramycin, and netilmicin, serum concentrations are below inhibitory concentrations for four to six hours of the usual eight hour dosing interval. For amikacin, serum concentrations are below the minimum inhibitory concentration for *Pseudomonas aeruginosa* for nine to ten hours of the recommended 12 hour interval (see Figure 14-10). In patients with severe gram-negative sepsis, and especially in compromised hosts, the dosage interval should be decreased to prevent these excessively long periods of subinhibitory concentrations. In addition, patients who have a short

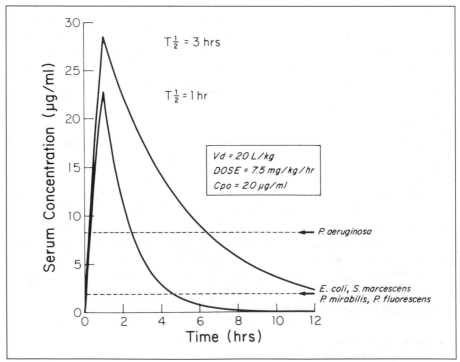

Figure 14-10. *The computer simulation illustrates a serum concentration-time profile for two hypothetical patients, one with a half-life of one hour, and one with a half-life of three hours. Each patient received the same dose, had the same distribution volume, and had the same starting concentration. The average minimum inhibitory concentrations were 8 μg/mL for* Pseudomonas aeruginosa *and 2 μg/mL for* Escherichia coli, Serratia marcescens, Proteus mirabilis, *and* Pseudomonas fluorescens. *As illustrated, the patient who had a short half-life had a lower peak serum concentration and eliminated the drug more rapidly; this tendency resulted in prolonged periods of subinhibitory concentrations (reproduced with permission from reference 179).*

half-life require a larger infusion dose over one hour to achieve therapeutic peak concentrations. In patients who have a prolonged half-life, the dosage interval should be prolonged to prevent excessively high trough concentrations.

PHARMACODYNAMICS

Clinical Response

Spectrum of Activity. The aerobic gram-negative bacilli are the primary pathogens for which aminoglycoside treatment is indicated. The spectrum of activity for the aminoglycosides includes *Escherichia coli*, *Proteus* species, *Enterobacter* species, *Klebsiella* species, *Acinetobacter* species, *Pseudomonas* species, *Serratia* species, *Providencia* species, and *Staphylococcus aureus*.[87] Other aerobic gram-negative bacilli are susceptible to aminoglycosides but are rarely indications for clinical use. These include *Neisseria gonorrhea*, *Neisseria meningitidis*, and *Hemophilus influenza*. Anaerobic bacteria are uniformly resistant to all of the aminoglycosides.

Several antibiotic groups have been demonstrated to have synergistic activity with aminoglycosides. This is especially true for the β-lactam antibiotics such as the penicillins or cephalosporins. One proposed mechanism of synergy is an increase in the porosity of the bacterial cell wall caused by the β-lactam antibiotic. This increase in cell wall porosity allows more of the aminoglycoside to penetrate the bacterial cell and hence results in higher intracellular concentrations that further increase the antibacterial effect. The combination of an aminoglycoside and a penicillin is synergistic against group-D Streptococci, *Pseudomonas aeruginosa*, and *Staphylococcus aureus*.[88,89] The aminoglycosides differ in their synergistic activity, and this effect may be specific for an individual isolate. Gentamicin generally has more synergistic activity than the other aminoglycosides.[90] Cephalosporins have shown synergistic activity with an aminoglycoside against the *Klebsiella sp*.[91] These combinations should be considered in patients with life-threatening infections such as endocarditis, pneumonia, or bacteremia. These combinations should be tested for synergy against the isolate and the most active combination of an aminoglycoside and β-lactam should be selected.

Inhibitory Concentrations. The intrinsic activity of gentamicin, tobramycin, and netilmicin is considerably higher than that reported for amikacin. The minimum inhibitory concentration (MIC) for most gram-negative pathogens is similar for gentamicin, tobramycin, and netilmicin. Most gram-negative pathogens are susceptible to 2 to 3 μg/mL or less (see Table 14-1). With amikacin, most pathogens are inhibited by concentrations of 4 to 8 μg/mL. Specific aminoglycosides have different intrinsic activity against specific bacterial strains. For example, gentamicin and netilmicin have more activity against *Serratia marcescens* than does tobramycin. Tobramycin demonstrates lower MICs with *Pseudomonas aeruginosa* than does gentamicin or netilmicin. Many institutions report susceptibility results for clinical isolates as MICs. These more quantitative values may be useful to the clinician in selecting desired peak and trough concentrations of an aminoglycoside for a specific patient.

Table 14–1. Summary of Pharmacokinetic Parameters for Gentamicin, Tobramycin, Amikacin, and Netilmicin

Parameter	Population Averages (± SD) in Patients Who Had Normal Renal Function		
	Adults	**Children**	**Neonates**
CL	Normal SCr (≤1.5 mg%): 1.33 ± 0.61 Abnormal SCr (> 1.5 mg%): 0.53 ± 0.35 CL_{cr} ≥ 100 mL/1.73 min²: 1.51 ± 0.63 (mL/min/kg)	1.31 ± 10 (mL/min/m²)	<2000 g: < 1 week: 22.1 > 1 week: 24.6 >2000 g: < 1 week: 28.4 > 1 week: 36.4 (mL/min/1.73 m²)
V_d (L/kg)	Dehydration: 0.07–0.15 Normal fluid status: 0.15–0.25 ↑ ECF: 0.35–0.70	0.07–0.7	0.20–0.70
Elimination rate constant (hr^{-1})	—[a]	—[a]	—[a]
t½ (hr)	SCr < 1.5 mg/dL: 0.5–15 CL_{cr} ≥ 100 mL/min/1.73 m²: 0.5–7.6 Age: < 30 years old: 0.5–3 hr >30 years old: 1.5–15 hr	0.5–2.5	2–9
% excreted in urine	85%–95%	85%–95%	85%–95%

[a] Varies, dependent on the following relationship: $\dfrac{CL}{V_d}$.

Mechanism of Action

Aminoglycosides are rapidly bactericidal compounds that are actively transported across the bacterial cell membrane to the site of action. Since aminoglycoside transport across the cell membrane is an oxygen-dependent process, under anaerobic conditions, aminoglycosides are not transported and thereby are not active anaerobically. Additionally, transport is enhanced in a slightly alkaline pH environment that increases the nonionized fraction of the drug. Conversely, transport and antimicrobial activity decrease in acidic environments.

Once transported across the bacterial cell membrane, the aminoglycosides attach to 30S and 50S ribosomal subunits. They cause misreading of genetic codes and defective protein synthesis. A number of other steps in protein synthesis are affected as well. The net effect of these alterations is a defective bacterial cell membrane and an increase in intracellular osmotic pressure resulting in death of the bacterial cell. Other mechanisms may also contribute to the overall antimicrobial effect of aminoglycoside antibiotics by affecting DNA and messenger RNA. These agents are effective in both the active and resting stages of the bacterial cell cycle; this characteristic may be an important difference between β-lactam and aminoglycoside antibiotics.

Adverse Effects

The two most frequently occurring toxic effects of aminoglycosides are ototoxicity and nephrotoxicity. Both toxic effects are thought to be related to serum concentrations. Ototoxicity is generally irreversible or only partially reversible and can affect cochlear and/or vestibular function. Nephrotoxicity is generally reversible upon discontinuing treatment or careful monitoring and control of serum concentrations. The results of animal studies and clinical investigations indicate significant differences do exist between aminoglycosides,[93-97] but the differences probably can be reduced clinically by carefully controlling serum concentrations. Other side-effects attributed to aminoglycosides include neuromuscular blockade;[98-101] hypersensitivity reactions; and infrequent local gastrointestinal, hematologic, and central nervous system toxicities.[102]

Substantial confusion and controversy still exist regarding the incidence of aminoglycoside-induced ototoxicity and nephrotoxicity. The incidence has varied substantially among different reports, with nephrotoxicity ranging up to 55%[103] and ototoxicity ranging up to 43%.[104] Additionally, comparative results have differed from study to study. These conflicting results have made it difficult to assess either the absolute risk of toxicity or the relative differences in risk between aminoglycosides. The importance of therapeutic monitoring to reduce the risk of toxicity has also been questioned. Several methodologic differences exist between clinical investigations which may explain these conflicting results.

Different patient populations have been utilized in several studies. Some investigators have routinely evaluated older patients or patients in a medical or surgical intensive care unit.[105,106] These patients were at a higher risk of toxicity because of their older age, concurrent medical complications (e.g., congestive heart failure), dehydration, hypotension, and concurrent drug therapy (e.g., furosemide). A higher incidence of ototoxicity and nephrotoxicity was observed in these patients[47,105] than in younger patients.[107] The higher risk populations used in these studies may partially explain the higher incidence of toxicity reported.

Different criteria have been used to study eighth cranial nerve function. Cochlear and vestibular function have been evaluated clinically for typical signs of ototoxicity (e.g., vertigo, tinnitus, hearing impairment, nausea). Audiometry and electronystagmography have been used to more objectively assess changes in eighth cranial nerve function and to determine subclinical changes which may be associated with aminoglycoside treatment.[103,108] However, several practical problems make these more objective measures difficult to perform in a clinical environment. Because of background noise or visual distractions, these tests should ideally be performed in a sound-proof room and not at the patient's bedside. Many patients receiving aminoglycosides cannot be transported because of isolation precautions or the need for supportive medical equipment. Moreover, many of these patients cannot cooperate with these tests because of altered states of consciousness secondary to sepsis or to a physical injury such as facial burns or fractures. Additionally, the results of audiometry and electronystagmography have day-to-day variations because of background changes and may lead to a false diagnosis of aminoglycoside toxicity.

Criteria used to evaluate renal function have a variable degree of precision and sensitivity[109] (see Table 14-2). Most studies have used serum creatinine concentrations to screen patients for possible nephrotoxicity. Changes greater than 0.4 mg/dL or 0.5 mg/dL from baseline have been defined as a significant change and evidence of possible nephrotoxicity. In examining our database of 1640 patients,[47] use of the criterion of 0.5 mg/dL, compared to 0.4 mg/dL, results in a three- to fourfold increase in the number of patients with possible nephrotoxicity. Also, other drugs (e.g., cephalosporins) are known to interfere with several automated techniques commonly used to measure creatinine.[124] Other criteria have also been used in some studies, including urinary enzymes, proteins, casts, and urine concentrating ability. In general, these criteria lack specificity and are imprecise in measuring changes in renal function caused by aminoglycosides.

Different methods of drug administration may also account for the variability of results. Aminoglycoside antibiotics have been administered by continuous infusion,[7,8] bolus injections,[125] and intermittent infusions. Each method of administration may have different risks of toxicity. Continuous infusions would appear to have the highest risk of toxicity.[126] Bolus injections produce high peak concentrations and a consequent risk of ototoxicity. Intermittent infusions of 30 to 60 minutes would appear to be the safest method of administration.

The method of determining dosage requirements may also be an important factor. The definition of "peak" concentrations has varied among different investigators and may have introduced additional risks of toxicity in specific patient groups. An investigator has monitored and controlled "peak" serum concentrations at one hour post-infusion.[106] For gentamicin, tobramycin, and netilmicin, the desired "peak" concentrations at the one hour time point range between 5 and 10 μg/mL, and they range between 20 and 30 μg/mL for amikacin. A large number of patients, even elderly ones, have serum half-lives approximating one hour.[75] In

Table 14-2. Relative Minimum Inhibitory Concentration to Inhibit 80% of the Isolates

	Isolates tested	Gentamicin (μg/mL)	Tobramycin (μg/mL)	Amikacin (μg/mL)	Netilmicin (μg/mL)
E.coli	284	1–1.5	1–1.5	4	1–1.5
Klebsiella pneumoniae	144	0.5–1	0.5–1	2–4	0.5–1
Proteus mirabilis	83	15.2	1.5–2	8	1.5–2
Proteus morgani	49	2–4	1–2	4–8	2
Proteus vulgaris	48	2–4	2–4	8–16	2–4
Pseudomonas aeruginosa	571	1–2	0.5–1	2–4	2
Enterobacter aerogenes	48	0.5–1	0.5–1	2–4	0.5–1
Serratia marcescens	56	1–2	2–4	4–8	2–4
Providencia stuartii	49	2–4	2–4	8	2–4

these patients with more rapid elimination, serum concentrations immediately post-infusion would range between 10 and 20 μg/mL for gentamicin, tobramycin, and netilmicin and between 40 and 60 μg/mL for amikacin. These concentrations are known to be associated with an increased risk of ototoxicity and nephrotoxicity.

In choosing which patients to include in a study, one criteria used is duration of treatment. Here is another source of variation. Many studies have used 72 hours[112] for the minimum duration of treatment, whereas other studies have used five to seven days[120] (see Table 14-2). The shorter treatment period results in a substantial increase in the number of patients enrolled for study evaluation without any appreciable increase in the number of patients at risk for toxicity. The studies with a shorter treatment duration have routinely found a lower incidence of toxicity than have similar studies with a longer treatment duration.

Ototoxicity. One problem with all aminoglycosides is the possibility of eighth cranial nerve toxicity which includes auditory and vestibular dysfunction. It can occur during treatment or up to four to six weeks after termination of treatment. The symptoms of early cochlear toxicity include a sensation of fullness and tinnitus. Aminoglycosides are thought to alter the sodium-potassium pump, thereby causing a change in the electrical potential and intracellular osmotic pressure within the endolymph. Early changes primarily affect the outer hair cells of the organ of Corti and initially affect higher frequencies such as 4000, 6000, or 8000 Hz. The early stage of toxicity generally does not affect frequencies utilized in conversational hearing. The toxic changes are generally reversible at this early stage. With more severe toxicity, the outer hair cells of the organ of Corti are destroyed, and the hair cells of the apex become damaged. Hearing impairment then occurs at lower frequencies, and conversational hearing is compromised. These auditory deficits are usually bilateral, but can be unilateral. At this later stage, the deficit is generally permanent or only partially reversible. Vestibular dysfunction generally parallels cochlear damage and is usually manifested by vertigo, nausea, dizziness, and nystagmus. The vestibular damage is usually permanent; however, the patient can generally overcome the deficit by other compensatory mechanisms (e.g., vision).

Overt ototoxicity generally occurs in 2% to 10% of patients treated with aminoglycosides.[127] Studies using audiometry or electronystagmography can more objectively measure eighth cranial nerve function and have generally reported a higher incidence of toxicity. These subclinical changes have occurred in as many as 43% of patients tested.[104] These studies frequently involved patients with an increased number of risk factors associated with ototoxicity. A wide range in the incidence of ototoxicity has been reported by various investigators (see Table 14-3). Differences in study design, patient enrollment, selected aminoglycoside, dosage control, and criterion defining toxicity may have contributed to the variability of results.

During the initial clinical trials comparing gentamicin, tobramycin, and amikacin, the incidence of ototoxicity was similar for all three aminoglycosides (see Table 14-3).[113,122] In the guinea pig model, Brummet et al.[131] demonstrated a higher safety index for netilmicin when compared to gentamicin, tobramycin, and amikacin. Recent comparative clinical investigations also have found a significantly lower

Table 14–3. Incidence of Nephrotoxicity

Patients	Dosing method[a]	Treatment duration	Criteria of toxicity			% of patients with critical change				Significance[c]	References
			In SCr	Other criteria[b]	In CL_{cr}	Gentamicin	Tobramycin	Amikacin	Netilmicin		
71	PD&I	3 days	≥ 0.5			4.9	2.7	28	38	NS	110
199	PD&I	5 days	≥ 0.5			11	11.5	8.5	2.8	NS	107
3055	—	3 days									111
68	PD&I	3 days	≥ 0.5	B_2M; NA6	33%	24	9			$p < 0.05$	108
54	PD	4 days	≥ 0.3 Doub.	SCr	—	40	28			$p < 0.01$	112
175	PD	7 days	Abnor.	Scr		20	34	15		NS	113
194	PD&I	4 days	≥ 0.5			9.8	21			NS	54
50	PD&I	—	≥ 0.5	B_2M, casts		16	7.8	20		NS	114
525	Cont	7 days		Azotemia		10				NS	7
27	PD&I	—		urinary enzymes	14%	40	58	7		NS	115
182	PD	7 days	33%			55.2	15.1			$p < 0.05$	103
279	PD&I	3 days	100%			9		8		NS	116
254	PD&I	3 days	50%				4		1	NS	117
53	PD&I	7 days	50%			15		0		NS	118
183	PD	6 days	≥ 0.5			2		6	2	NS	119
98	N	6 days	≥ 0.5			10.2	18.4			NS	120
98	I	2 days	≥ 0.5			8	16.7			NS	
229	PD&I	2 days	≥ 0.5	B_2M, casts		36	23	25		$p < 0.05$	121
201	PD&I	5 days	≥ 0.5			37	22			$p < 0.02$	105
114	PD&I	—	≥ 0.5	B_2M, casts		23	10	25		$p < 0.02$	109
74	PD&I	3 days	≥ 0.5			11		8		NS	122
167	PD&I	3 days	≥ 0.5			26	12			$p < 0.05$	106
15	PD&I	6 weeks	≥ 0.5			63	43				104
52	PD	3 days	> 100	mmol/L		27	10			NS	123

[a] PD = Dose determined by physician. PD&I = Dose determined by physician; serum concentrations used to adjust the dose. Cont = Drug infused continuously. N = Dose determined by a nomogram. I = Dosage regimen determined by measuring serum concentrations and adjusting the patient's dose.

[b] B_2M = B_2 microglobulin. NAG = N-acetyl glucosaminidase.

[c] NS = Not significant.

incidence of ototoxicity with netilmicin than with tobramycin.[117] Patients receiving repeated treatments (e.g., leukemics) or high-risk patient groups (e.g., chronic dialysis patients) may benefit from selective therapy with netilmicin.

Several factors have been associated with a higher incidence of ototoxicity (see Table 14-4). These include duration of treatment, cumulative dose, average daily dose, peak serum concentration, trough serum concentration, concurrent diuretics such as furosemide or ethacrynic acid, underlying disease states, and previous exposure to aminoglycoside therapy. Elderly patients apparently have a higher risk of toxicity than do younger patients. Patients with compromised renal function, particularly those requiring hemodialysis, may have an increased risk of toxicity. One study, however, demonstrated a similar incidence of toxicity in patients with normal and abnormal renal function when the serum concentration of aminoglycosides was maintained in the therapeutic range.[132]

Nephrotoxicity. Aminoglycoside nephrotoxicity is much more complex and difficult to separate from the complications secondary to underlying disease. Hypotension, shock, and renal failure may occur in the early phases of gram-negative sepsis and result in acute tubular necrosis. In occasional patients, these complications may occur during treatment and complicate the differential diagnosis for renal failure. Clinically and histologically, the changes in the kidney resulting from aminoglycoside toxicity, sepsis, or hypotension cannot be differentiated, and the diagnosis then is based on clinical judgment. In some instances, the changes in renal function may initially be due to underlying disease which may then decrease aminoglycoside elimination, increase serum concentrations of the aminoglycoside, and cause further damage to the nephron. Measuring serum concentrations and adjusting the dosage regimen of aminoglycoside may prevent further insult to the kidney after the septic changes have occurred.

Nephrotoxicity secondary to use of aminoglycosides classically occurs at least five days after the initiation of treatment. Typical findings generally include decreased glomerular filtration rate, increased serum creatinine, increased blood urea nitrogen, and impaired urinary concentrating ability; these factors result in non-oliguric renal failure. Additionally, proteinuria, aminoaciduria, glycosuria, and electrolyte disturbances also occur. The proximal tubule is thought to be the primary site of aminoglycoside nephrotoxicity. Markers of renal tubular function such as β_2-microglobulins, urinary casts, and urinary enzymes have been suggested as a means of detecting early renal damage and preventing severe damage to the kidney.[133,134] These markers are not specific for aminoglycoside-induced nephrotoxicity and thus have not been widely used. Patients who have a rise in serum creatinine should be evaluated for continued need of aminoglycoside therapy. In those patients requiring further therapy, serum concentrations should be monitored to prevent further accumulation and further renal damage. In most patients, the changes in renal function are reversible, provided that the infectious entity is adequately treated and further drug accumulation does not occur. During the early phases of recovery, high output failure generally occurs, and glomerular filtration generally improves slowly thereafter. The clearance of aminoglycosides may not improve in parallel with improvements in filtration, and, many times, improvement in function as estimated by aminoglycoside clearance is substan-

Table 14-4. Incidence of Ototoxicity

Patients	Critical change		% of patients with critical change				Significance[c]	References
	Cochlear[a]	Vestibular[b]	Gentamicin	Tobramycin	Amikacin	Netilmicin		
45	≥ 15 dB (1)	IWC			29	16	NS	128
114	≥ 20 dB (1)		6.2		3.4	3.4	NS	129
63	≥ 15 dB (1)	—			25	9	NS	110
1200	—	—	7.7	9.7	13.8	2.3	—	111
68	≥ 20 dB (1)	CAC	11	7			p ≤ 0.05	108
			14	7			p < 0.05	
36	≥ 15 dB (1)	—		15.7		11.7	NS	130
201	≥ 15 dB (1)		13.6		21		NS	116
33	≥ 15 dB (2)	IWC	7.7		7.4		NS	118
157	≥ 15 dB (2)	—		12		3	p < 0.05	117
90	≥ 20 dB (2)	—	6		3	3	NS	119
91	≥ 15 dB (1)	—	10	11			NS	106
81	≥ 10 dB (1)		10		6		NS	122

[a] Cochlear function was evaluated by audiograms, and a change of 10, 15, a 20 dB at one (1) or two (2) frequencies was determined to be significant.
[b] Vestibular function was evaluated by electronystagmography using either ice water calories (IWC) or cold air calories (CAC). A 33% change or 50% change from baseline was regarded as significant.
[c] NS = Not significant.

tially delayed. Dosage requirements of aminoglycosides are greatly reduced during this period of time, and serum monitoring is imperative if safe serum concentrations are to be maintained.

The incidence of nephrotoxicity has varied substantially between different studies of the same aminoglycoside and between different aminoglycosides (see Table 14-2). During comparative clinical trials, the incidence of nephrotoxicity was similar for gentamicin versus amikacin[133] and for tobramycin versus amikacin.[113] The incidence of toxicity ranged between 6% and 10%. In these studies, a change in serum creatinine of 0.5 mg/dL or greater was defined as a significant change and possible evidence of toxicity.

A recent report suggests that the incidence of nephrotoxicity may be higher ranging between 12% and 25% in patients receiving gentamicin, tobramycin, or amikacin.[106] In both studies, peak serum concentrations were obtained one hour (postinfusion) and controlled between 4 and 10 µg/mL for gentamicin and tobramycin, and between 20 and 30 µg/mL for amikacin. A substantial amount of variation will occur in the immediate postinfusion serum concentration when the one hour value is controlled within this range. The peak concentration could range from 10 to 20 µg/mL for gentamicin and tobramycin, and 40 to 60 µg/mL for amikacin, in patients who had rapid elimination rates. The variation in elimination of aminoglycosides can be relatively short, even in elderly patients.[75] Additionally, the trough concentrations were not well controlled and averaged 2.7 and 2.8 µg/mL for gentamicin and tobramycin, respectively. The elevated concentrations resulting from this dosing method may explain why the incidence of toxicity is high compared to the incidence reported previously.

The four aminoglycosides appear to have different dose-response curves when nephrotoxicity is evaluated against dose or serum concentration.[135] These differences would seemingly explain discrepancies in the data generated from animal models, as well as in the results from comparative clinical evaluations. In general, the dose-response data would indicate gentamicin to be the most toxic, followed by tobramycin and amikacin with similar degrees of toxicity, followed further by netilmicin which is the least toxic. The studies demonstrating a similar incidence of toxicity between two aminoglycosides were generally performed with doses and serum concentrations carefully controlled.[54,120] Under these conditions, the patients received doses and attained serum concentrations which placed them to the left side of the dose-response curve, where minimal differences exist between different aminoglycosides. The studies performed under less-controlled conditions exposed many patients to a higher dose and higher peak and trough serum concentrations. Thereby, many of these patients were to the right of the dose-response curve and had a higher risk of toxicity. The relative increase in risk and projected incidence of toxicity will be different for each aminoglycoside.

Several factors have been associated with a higher risk of nephrotoxicity (see Table 14-5). These include increasing age, compromised renal function, volume depletion, documented infection, total dose, duration of treatment, prior exposure to aminoglycosides, peak concentration, trough concentration, and concurrent exposure to nephrotoxic drugs (e.g., cephalosporins). Several of these risk factors may result in increased concentrations of aminoglycoside, and thereby the risk factor is more directly associated with elevated serum concentrations. For example, older patients are known to have decreased elimination of aminoglycosides. If older patients receive the standard dose, higher serum concentrations would occur and might predispose these patients to a higher risk of nephrotoxicity. Other factors may have a similar association with decreased elimination or increased serum concentrations. Controlling serum concentrations more directly may decrease the risk of toxicity associated with these specific factors.

Neuromuscular Blockade. Aminoglycoside-associated neuromuscular blockade was first thought to be rare;[98–101] however, this potentially serious side-effect may occur with a greater frequency than thought initially.[99] This reaction is more likely to occur when the aminoglycoside is administered intravenously and concurrently with other neuromuscular blocking agents or anesthetic agents such as ether, tubocurarine, succinylcholine, decamethonium, or gallamine. Additionally, patients who are hypocalcemic or who have existing neuromuscular diseases, such as myasthenia gravis or botulism, are more susceptible to neuromuscular blockade.[140] The mechanism of aminoglycoside-induced neuromuscular blockade involves interference with calcium and with the immediate release of acetylcholine presynaptically.[141] The onset is characterized by respiratory failure and/or muscle weakness. In mild cases, discontinuation of aminoglycoside usually suffices to reverse toxicity; however, in more severe cases, therapeutic intervention may be required with administration of calcium gluconate or neostigmine.

Relationship of Concentration and Toxicity

The relationship of serum concentration with toxicity has certainly been controversial. Nevertheless, a higher risk of ototoxicity and nephrotoxicity generally has been associated with elevated peak and trough serum concentrations (see Table 14-5).[135–138] For gentamicin, tobramycin, and netilmicin, risk of ototoxicity and nephrotoxicity is increased if peak concentrations are consistently maintained above 12 to 14 µg/mL. For amikacin, peak concentrations above 32 to 34 µg/mL have been associated with a higher risk of ototoxicity and nephrotoxicity.[139] For gentamicin, a higher risk of ototoxicity and nephrotoxicity has been associated with trough concentrations consistently greater than 2 µg/mL.[137,138] Tobramycin and netilmicin are thought to have a similar relationship. For amikacin, trough concentrations consistently exceeding 8 to 10 µg/mL appear to be associated with a higher risk of toxicity.[139] Recently, higher peak and trough values have been proposed for netilmicin. These peak and trough serum aminoglycoside concentrations should be used only as guidelines, and not as absolute values that are associated with toxicity. Select patients who have life-threatening infections may need serum concentrations higher than these guidelines to ensure an adequate treatment response.

Relationship of Serum Concentration and Efficacy

Improved treatment response has been demonstrated in patients who attained therapeutic serum concentrations of aminoglycosides early in their treatment course.[142,143] Measurements of serum concentrations and adjustments in a patient's dosing regimen to attain targeted concentrations have been proposed in order to improve patient response.[144] Aminoglycosides have a low therapeutic index, and concentrations necessary for optimal efficacy approximate concentrations that are associated with a risk of toxicity. Due to the large interpatient differences in pharmacokinetic parameters, serum concentrations resulting from recommended dosage regimens vary substantially. Measuring serum concentrations and adjusting an individual patient's dosage regimens are often necessary to achieve desired (therapeutic) serum concentrations.

Noone et al. studied 68 episodes of gram-negative sepsis which were treated with gentamicin.[142] They compared the treatment response in patients who had "subtherapeutic" serum concentrations to those who had "therapeutic" serum concentrations within the first 72 hours of treatment. The therapeutic concentrations were defined as peak serum concentrations greater than 5 µg/mL for patients with soft tissue infections, gram-negative septicemias, or urinary tract infections. For patients who had a gram-negative pneumonia, peak concentrations greater than 8 µg/mL were considered therapeutic. The therapeutic responses for these two groups of patients were markedly different. Eighty-four percent of the patients who achieved therapeutic serum concentrations had an optimal treatment response, while only 23% of the patients who had inadequate serum concentrations responded to treatment. Larger doses than those commonly recommended were frequently necessary to achieve desired concentrations. The authors concluded that the most direct and easiest way of ensuring adequate therapy within the first 72 hours of treatment is to measure serum concentrations and adjust the patient's dosage regimen. They further concluded that predictions of serum concentrations using estimates of renal function (i.e., serum creatinine or creatinine clearance) resulted in substantial error in individual patients.

Improved treatment response in burn patients with *Pseudomonas ecthyma gangrenosum* has been noted in patients who received individualized doses of gentamicin.[91,145] Ecthyma gangrenosum occurs infrequently in burn patients; however, it was universally fatal in these patients. This complication of Pseudomonas sepsis is characterized by the fulminant spread of Pseudomonas through the lymphatic and cardiovascular system and invasion of previously viable tissue. This

Table 14–5. *Risk Factors Associated with Toxicity*

Ototoxicity	Nephrotoxicity
Age	Age
Impaired renal function	Renal insufficiency
Dehydration	Elevated trough concentrations
Elevated trough concentrations	Elevated peak concentrations
Elevated peak concentrations	Total daily dose
Total daily dose	Cumulative dose
Cumulative dose	Concurrent nephrotoxic drugs
Concurrent ototoxic drugs	Prior aminoglycoside exposure
Prior aminoglycoside exposure	Hypovolemia
Dialysis	Gender
Duration of treatment	Duration of treatment
	Sepsis

metastatic spread of Pseudomonas occurs in visceral and cutaneous tissues. Leob and co-workers[91] successfully treated three pediatric burn patients with this complication. They attributed the favorable response to the inadvertent administration of large gentamicin doses. Additionally, four of five patients with *Pseudomonas ecthyma gangrenosum*[145] were successfully treated, but required very large aminoglycoside doses to obtain "therapeutic" serum concentrations. One patient required 30 mg/kg/day to achieve the desired therapeutic concentration. The only patient who did not survive the course of ecthyma received a maximal daily dose of 12 mg/kg/day. However, the nonsurvivor achieved a peak serum concentration of only 4.5 µg/mL. These burn patients thus required markedly increased dosages to achieve therapeutic serum concentrations, which in turn were associated with improved treatment response.

In patients with Pseudomonas bacteremias, subtherapeutic serum concentrations were identified as one of the major pharmacologic factors in explaining treatment failures with gentamicin.[144] In addition, a large group of burn patients with predominantly Pseudomonas bacteremia or burn sepsis were evaluated to determine the impact of individualized gentamicin dosage regimens.[146] Sixty-six patients received individualized dosages and were compared to a retrospective control group of 39 patients who received conventional dosage regimens of 3 to 5 mg/kg/day. The patient groups were balanced in terms of independent variables which may affect patient survival, including percent burn, age, body weight, concurrent antibiotics, topical therapy, nutritional support, gender, complications, and pre-existing disease. Those patients who were given individualized gentamicin therapy required 7.4 mg/kg/day of gentamicin to ensure therapeutic concentrations, while patients given conventional dosages received an average daily dosage of 4.5 mg/kg/day. Patient survival for the first septic episode was 51% in patients receiving conventional dosage regimens, and 86% for patients receiving individualized regimens (x^2) [1df] = 13.7; p <0.001). Improved patient response for the first septic episode contributed to an overall improvement in patient survival for the entire hospital course. Patients' survival for the entire hospital course was 33% for patients receiving conventional dosages and 64% for patients receiving individualized regimens. This difference was highly significant (x^2) [1df] = 7.8; p <0.005). A strong temporal relationship was found between increased patient survival and the implementation of individualized regimens. In addition, further statistical analysis was also performed using multivariant techniques. From these analyses, measuring serum levels for adjusting dosages was found to be the most important factor influencing patient survival.

The relationship between trough levels of antibiotics and treatment response was also evaluated.[147,148] Anderson et al.[147] demonstrated a higher failure rate in patients who had excessively long periods of antibiotic serum concentrations below the inhibitory concentration for a particular pathogen. He referred to these treatment failures as "breakthrough bacteremias," and attributed them to long periods in the dosing interval in which serum concentrations were below the inhibitory level. Many patients receiving aminoglycosides demonstrate an extremely short half-life (less than two hours) of the drug and hence would have serum concentrations below the minimum inhibitory concentration for selected pathogens early in the dosing interval. Thus, serum concentrations may be below the inhibitory level for many common gram-negative pathogens for five to six hours of the conventional eight-hour interval for gentamicin and tobramycin. For amikacin, this period of subinhibitory concentrations may be nine to ten hours of the conventional 12-hour dosing interval. Therefore, preventing excessively long periods of subinhibitory serum concentrations by adjusting the dosing interval according to the elimination rate may be an important factor in preventing treatment failures. This would appear to be more important in a severely neutropenic host with gram-negative sepsis.

Guidelines for Desired Concentrations

Serum concentrations associated with a higher treatment response rate can be used to set minimum values for peak and trough concentrations. Additionally, those concentrations associated with a higher risk of toxicity can be used to determine maximal concentrations. These data thus form the basis for designing general guidelines for peak and trough serum concentrations (see Table 14-6). Selecting concentrations within the guidelines becomes a risk-benefit judgment with each patient. Several factors should be considered in selecting a desired peak and trough concentration: the patient's clinical condition, the site of infection, and the relative sensitivity of the suspected or isolated pathogen. In patients who have infections with a higher risk of morbidity or mortality, higher peak and trough serum concentrations should be selected within the guidelines. A peak serum concentration is defined as the value attained immediately post-infusion; the trough concentration is the value attained before a dose under steady-state conditions. For gentamicin, tobramycin, and netilmicin, peak serum concentrations should range between 5 and 8 µg/mL for patients with soft tissue infections and other less severe gram-negative infections. In patients who have a life-threatening gram-negative infection, the desired peak concentrations should range between 8 and 10 µg/mL for these three aminoglycosides. The trough concentration for these three aminoglycosides should be less than 1 µg/mL for less severe gram-negative infections and 1 to 2 µg/mL for life-threatening infections. In select patients, clinicians might utilize higher peak concentrations (12 to 16 µg/mL) and trough concentrations (2 to 4 µg/mL) for netilmicin. With amikacin, the desired peak concentration for moderately severe gram-negative sepsis should range between 20 and 25 µg/mL. In patients who have life-threatening sepsis, the peak amikacin

Table 14-6. *Guideline for Desired Serum Concentration*

	Gentamicin	Tobramycin	Amikacin	Netilmicin[a]
Peaks (µg/mL)				
Serious infections	6–8	6–8	20–25	6–8
Life-threatening infections	8–10	8–10	25–30	8–10
Troughs (µg/mL)				
Serious infections	0.5–1	0.5–1	1–4	0.5–1
Life-threatening infections	1–2	1–2	4–8	1–2

[a] Higher peak and trough values have also been suggested.

concentration should range between 25 and 28 µg/mL. The desired trough amikacin concentration should range between 1 and 4 µg/mL for less severe infections and between 4 and 8 µg/mL for life-threatening infections. These suggested values for peak and trough concentrations are general guidelines which may need to be modified for select patients.

CLINICAL APPLICATION OF PHARMACOKINETIC DATA

Recommended Regimens

The recommended dosage regimen for gentamicin, tobramycin, and netilmicin in adult patients with normal renal function is 3 to 5 mg/kg/day administered in three equal doses every eight hours. The recommended dose for amikacin in adult patients with normal renal function is 15 mg/kg/day divided into two or three equal doses and administered in equally divided intervals. In patients with compromised renal function, dosage regimens should be decreased according to the degree of renal dysfunction as well as to the severity of infection. These general guidelines, however, may be substantially in error for individual patients and individualized dosing regimens are recommended.

Nomograms

Several methods have been proposed as being adequate for adjusting dosage regimens in patients with compromised renal function. These four commonly utilized methods include the "Rule of Eights,"[149] Chan method,[150] Dettli method,[151] and Hull-Sarubbi method.[152,153] These methods vary in their approach, but all use estimates of renal function to determine dosing intervals. The Hull-Sarubbi method and the Dettli method allow for a clinician to select dosage regimens according to the severity of the patient's condition.

The "Rule of Eights" suggests dosages of 1 to 1.66 mg/kg to be administered at variable intervals depending upon serum creatinine.[149] The dosing interval is determined by multiplying the serum creatinine value by eight and rounding to convenient intervals. For the Chan method,[150] a loading dose of 1.7 mg/kg is suggested, followed by a maintenance dose derived from the published nomogram. The maintenance doses are further adjusted according to calculated creatinine clearance, and a standard dosing interval of every eight hours is used. For the Dettli method,[151] the aminoglycoside elimination rate is estimated from a calculated creatinine clearance. The volume is estimated by multiplying a population average (0.25 L/kg) by the patient's ideal body weight. These two kinetic parameters are then used to calculate the dosage regimen necessary to attain selected peak and trough serum concentrations. For the Hull-Sarubbi method,[152,153] creatinine clearances are estimated for each patient. A published dosing chart is used for each aminoglycoside to determine low, medium, and high dosage regimens. The clinician must select one of these three dosage regimens according to the patient's clinical condition.

Precautions with Nomograms. Several assumptions are made in dosage nomograms, and errors inherent in these assumptions probably explain the discrepancy between predicted serum concentrations versus actual serum concentrations. In patients with gram-negative sepsis, the difference between predicted and measured creatinine clearance is much greater than that in noninfected patients. Results of comparing a measured 24-hour creatinine clearance with a calculated creatinine clearance, estimated by four commonly used methods, suggest that predicted creatinine clearances are more variable in infected patients than in normal volunteers.[154] Only 50% to 60% of the variance (r^2) in calculated creatinine clearance was explained by measured creatinine clearance for the four methods. The distribution volume of aminoglycosides varies considerably between patients and may vary during the course of a patient's treatment. With dosing nomograms, a constant volume of distribution is assumed for all patients. These factors limit the usefulness of these dosing nomograms. When the four commonly used nomograms were evaluated simultaneously in a large group of patients,[155] only a few patients attained target concentrations (see Figure 14-11). In a majority of the patients serum concentrations were subtherapeutic and in several of the patients, serum aminoglycoside concentrations were in a range that is commonly associated with a higher risk of toxicity. The method of Chan resulted in the largest number of patients who achieved potentially toxic concentrations. The methods of Dettli and Hull-Sarubbi attained targeted concentrations in the largest number of patients. Nomograms do provide the clinician with an initial dosage regimen, but further dosage adjustments based on a measured peak and trough concentration are essential for controlling serum concentrations.

INDIVIDUALIZING DOSAGE REGIMENS WITH SERUM CONCENTRATIONS

"Trial and Error" Method

Therapeutic concentrations are frequently sought by measuring serum concentrations and making necessary dosage adjustments of aminoglycoside antibiotics. Unfortunately, when serum samples are obtained clinically in an uncontrolled manner, important data such as the dose, time of sample, and time of infusion are frequently not recorded accurately.[156,157] These errors of omission may lead to incorrect interpretation of serum concentrations and incorrect dosage adjustments.[156] Many clinicians measure a peak and/or trough concentration and make empirical dosage adjustments. These empirical adjustments result in a "trial and error period" with different dosage regimens until optimal serum concentrations are achieved. This empirical, qualitative approach results in prolonged periods of suboptimal treatment, unnecessary patient cost, and incorrect dosage adjustments.[156] Under prospective reimbursement, this approach is likely to be very expensive by prolonging patient treatment and hospital stays. Serum specimens thus need to be obtained in a controlled manner and correctly interpreted to ensure optimal serum concentrations and the shortest treatment duration.

Utilizing Pharmacokinetic Principles

A method utilizing serum concentration-time data from an individual patient to calculate an optimal dosage regimen has been developed.[45,46] This method rapidly uses serum concentration-time data, preferably from the first dosing interval, to determine each patient's kinetic parameters. Dosages can be individualized within the first 12 to 24 hours of therapy. Patients quickly achieve therapeutic serum concentrations thereby improving the likelihood of therapeutic success.[142] In addition, the concentrations associated with a higher risk of toxicity are avoided.[53,56,142] Patient safety and efficacy should thus be improved.

The drug's elimination rate constant and volume of distribution are determined from the serum concentration-time data. After the clinician has determined the desired peak and trough concentrations, the kinetic parameters are used to calcu-

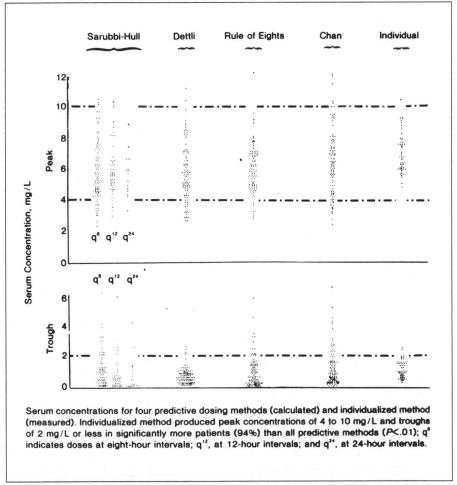

Serum concentrations for four predictive dosing methods (calculated) and individualized method (measured). Individualized method produced peak concentrations of 4 to 10 mg/L and troughs of 2 mg/L or less in significantly more patients (94%) than all predictive methods ($P<.01$); q^8 indicates doses at eight-hour intervals; q^{12}, at 12-hour intervals; and q^{24}, at 24-hour intervals.

Figure 14-11. The serum concentrations are illustrated for four predictive dosage methods and an individualized method in 96 patients consecutively treated with gentamicin. The peak or trough serum concentrations were either subtherapeutic or potentially toxic in a substantial percentage of these patients (reproduced with permission from reference 155).

late the patient's dosage interval and dose. This method allows the clinician to rapidly obtain these concentrations without the problems associated with the "trial and error" approach. The following discussion describes sampling strategy, data analysis, and dosage calculations necessary to individualize a patient's dosage regimen.

Sample Collection. Serum samples must be collected at ideal times and correctly interpreted to ensure optimal use of each serum concentration that is measured. The time and number of serum samples depend on the pharmacokinetic model, the desired accuracy of pharmacokinetic estimates, and/or the method used to make subsequent dosage recommendations. The serum concentration-time data in most patients receiving 60 minute infusions of aminoglycosides can be characterized by a one-compartment model.

When assuming a one-compartment model, there are two points on the post-infusion concentration-time curve which provide the most information describing the drug's pharmacokinetic behavior.[158] These two points are the zero-time post-infusion point, and the point at 1.5 half-lives of the drug post-infusion. The first point is necessary for estimating the drug's distribution volume. The reflection point at approximately 1.5 half-lives post-infusion is important in estimating the drug's elimination rate constant. Each patient's serum sampling strategy should be devised to obtain serum samples according to these criteria. Statistically, serum samples obtained at these time periods provide the best estimates of the patient's kinetic parameters. Additional data points will add more information describing the concentration-time curve; however, the amount of additional information diminishes markedly after three or four specimens.[159] In the individualized approach, we have chosen to obtain three post-infusion specimens, especially in critically ill patients, for whom the margin of acceptable error may be less. In select patients, two post-infusion specimens obtained under well-controlled conditions will provide adequate estimates of pharmacokinetic parameters and dosage requirements. A predose sample is required only if the patient has received a previous dose.

The serum sampling strategy must be determined for each patient to provide the most reliable information. The sampling times for each patient are influenced by factors affecting distribution and the rate of elimination. Patients receiving rapid drug infusion rates (achieved by large doses or short infusion periods), having a large distribution volume, or having a prolonged elimination rate will demonstrate an early distribution phase. This early phase can be ignored by simply delaying the first post-infusion serum sample. Patients who have impaired renal function will require prolonged serum sampling. The collection times of all serum samples should be accurately recorded, along with an accurate record of dose and infusion period.

In patients who have normal renal function and who received a 60 minute infusion, the first serum sample should be collected 15 to 30 minutes post-infusion. In patients with poor renal function, the first sample should be delayed to one to two hours post-infusion to allow for tissue distribution.

The second and third samples should be collected to characterize an estimated two to three half-lives of the drug. The timing of these samples depends primarily on the patient's renal function. For patients less than 30 years of age with normal renal function, two samples should be obtained within the initial two to three hours post-infusion. For older patients with normal renal function, the two samples should be obtained within three to four hours post-infusion. For patients with abnormal renal function, the sampling interval can be estimated by multiplying a factor of four times the serum creatinine to obtain an estimate of one half-life of the drug; the sampling times should span at least two estimated half-lives.

Data Fitting. The serum concentration-time data are fitted using least-squares regression analysis assuming a one-compartment model. This fit can be either linear or nonlinear regression analysis. Linear regression analysis fits the log of serum concentration versus time. This simplified approach requires semilog graph paper or a programmable hand-held calculator. The line of best fit using linear regression analysis is determined by the smallest vertical difference in the log of concentration. Nonlinear regression analysis fits the serum concentration versus time and requires more sophisticated computer resources. With nonlinear regression analysis, the vertical distance for 0.5 μg/mL will be greater at the lower end of the log cycle. Serum concentration-time data will then be weighted for lower values with linear fitting. In contrast, nonlinear fitting uses absolute values without inadvertently weighting the data. Generally, the estimates of kinetic parameters obtained by either method are similar as long as the data fit well. The serum concentration-time data should be plotted graphically for visual inspection of the data and the degree of fit. The visual inspection of the data may alert the clinician to transcription or analytical errors.

Calculations. The drug's elimination rate constant (k_{el}) and the serum concentration on the regression line at zero time post-infusion $(C_\infty)_{max}$ are estimated from the line of best fit. The drug's distribution volume (V_d) is calculated by the following equation, which considers the amount of drug eliminated during the infusion period:[45,46]

$$V_d = \frac{R_o}{K} \cdot \frac{1 - e^{-kt_I}}{\left[(C_\infty)_{max} - (C_\infty)_{min} \cdot e^{-kt_I}\right]} \qquad \text{(Eq. 14-1)}$$

where R_o is the infusion rate, t_I is the infusion period and $(C_\infty)_{min}$ is the predose concentration.

The patient's dosing interval (τ) is calculated from the desired peak level $(C_\infty)_{max-D}$, desired trough level $(C_\infty)_{min-D}$, and the infusion period (t_I). These values are based on the clinical status of the patient, site of infection, and pathogen isolated or suspected, as discussed above. The dosing interval is calculated from the following equation:

$$\tau = \frac{-1}{K} \ln \left[\frac{(C_\infty)_{min - D}}{(C_\infty)_{max - D}}\right] + t_I \qquad \text{(Eq. 14-2)}$$

The calculated dosage intervals are then rounded to clinically practical intervals of 4, 6, 8, 12, or 24 hours.

The infusion rate in mg/hour (R_o) required to produce desired serum concentrations is calculated by the following equation:

$$R_o = KV_d \ (C_\infty)_{max - D} \cdot \frac{(1 - e^{-K\tau})}{(1 - e^{-Kt_I})}$$

                                                                    (Eq. 14-3)

This equation considers the fraction of the dose eliminated during the infusion period and the amount of drug remaining from the previous dose under steady-state conditions. The dose in mg is determined by multiplying infusion rate by the infusion period. These calculated dosages are rounded to practical increments for the nursing staff.

With the application of this method, desired peak and trough serum concentrations have been consistently obtained with gentamicin,[32] tobramycin,[33] netilmicin,[35] and amikacin.[34] The dosage requirements for these four aminoglycosides demonstrate substantial variability from patient to patient. The variability appears similar for each aminoglycoside. In our patients who had normal renal function, the required dosage regimens ranged from 0.2 to 18.6 mg/kg/day for gentamicin (885 patients), from 0.9 to 15.3 mg/kg/day for tobramycin (46 patients), from 1.3 to 8.3 mg/kg/day for netilmicin, and from 3.7 to 53.3 mg/kg/day for amikacin (67 patients). Most patients required dosing intervals shorter than the recommended 8 or 12 hour intervals. However, a limited number of patients with normal renal function required dosing intervals beyond the recommended 8 to 12 hour interval in order to prevent excessively high trough concentrations. Thus to achieve therapeutic serum concentrations, 35% to 45% of our patients treated with aminoglycosides require dosage regimens in excess of those commonly recommended. To prevent excessively high serum concentrations, 10% to 15% of our patients require dosages less than those commonly recommended, even though they have normal renal function. The use of conventionally recommended dosages would result in a substantial number of patients who have subtherapeutic concentrations or achieve excessively high levels even though they have normal renal function.

Patient Monitoring

Patient assessment during the course of aminoglycoside therapy is imperative to ensure optimal efficacy and safety. Patients need to be evaluated clinically for overt signs of toxicity as well as for adequacy of patient response. Additional serum concentrations may be necessary to accurately calculate dosage regimens, especially in those patients who require longer treatment or have changing renal function or hydration. The application of pharmacokinetic concepts serves as a clinical tool for determining dosage requirements; the clinician must anticipate changes during the course of therapy and readjust the dosage regimens if necessary.

Many factors may change during the course of aminoglycoside therapy and affect serum concentrations and dosage requirements. Renal dysfunction may change during therapy and markedly change the elimination rate of aminoglycosides. Serum creatinine or blood urea nitrogen are clinical tests commonly used to monitor changes in elimination. Occasionally, serum concentrations may rise before a change in serum creatinine is noted. Tissue accumulation may also occur during therapy, resulting in an apparent decrease in the drug's clearance. The distribution volume of aminoglycosides may increase or decrease during therapy and can markedly effect serum aminoglycoside concentrations, half-life, and dosage regimens. Changes in physiologic parameters which affect cardiac output may be another cause of a change in the drug's clearance during therapy. The presence of fever is an example in which the heart rate and cardiac output may initially be increased and then returned to normal as the infection is successfully treated. This increase in cardiac output leads to an increase in renal blood flow and filtration. The intrinsic clearance of aminoglycosides appears to be flow-dependent, and changes in renal blood flow would be likely to cause a parallel change in aminoglycoside clearance. Thus, aminoglycoside clearance is likely to change during treatment because of changes in physiologic parameters such as cardiac output, renal blood flow, and glomerular filtration. These changes in drug clearance may not be apparent from concurrent changes in serum creatinine or blood urea nitrogen. The clinician should be aware of these possible changes to determine which patients need more intensive clinical and laboratory monitoring. Serum concentrations may need to be monitored periodically through the course of therapy, and dosage adjustments made to control serum concentrations.

Once Daily Aminoglycoside Dosing

Single daily doses of aminoglycosides have been recently recommended. A significant post-antibiotic effect for gram-negative bacilli exists.[173] Nephrotoxicity and ototoxicity in patients have been argued to be related to exposure time. Efficacy is reportedly equivalent to multiple dosing in several animal and clinical trials in patients with mild infections.[174–176]

These clinical trials, however, were limited to small patient numbers who had infections with mild-to-moderate severity.[176,177] Therefore, these clinical results are inconclusive and should not be extrapolated to routine clinical treatment. Most of the patients have had a urinary tract focus where aminoglycosides concentrate.[126,177] One study evaluated patients who had abdominal infections, but most patients had perforated appendicitis with localized infection.[176] The predominant pathogen was *E. coli*, which is extremely sensitive to the aminoglycosides (≤0.25 mg/mL).[126,176,177]

Toxicity was reportedly equivalent with once daily versus multiple dosing. However, these results are inconclusive due to small patient numbers and lack of systemic evaluation with eighth cranial nerve function.[126,176,177] Additionally, these trials frequently evaluated netilmicin, which has a different dose response curve. A paucity of information is available to compare the safety of once daily versus multiple dosing. Presently, there is inadequate experience to recommend once daily dosing routinely for life-threatening sepsis. Several centers have evaluated this new dosing approach for moderate infections.

ANALYTICAL METHODS

The analytical technology available for measuring aminoglycosides has undergone substantial advances in the last five to eight years. Fluorescence immunoassay and homogeneous enzyme immunoassay methodologies have eliminated the excessive expense and environmental concerns in handling radioactive waste resulting from radioimmunoassay techniques (see Table 14-7). Using microprocessors with the analytical instrumentation has allowed for use of a reduced number of specimens in reproducing the standard curve and has reduced the amount of technologist's time and expense. The advent of this technology has now placed most hospital laboratories, and some physician-clinic laboratories, in a position to measure serum concentrations inexpensively, accurately, and quickly.

Microbiological assays were initially used for measuring aminoglycoside concentrations, and they commonly utilized *Bacillus subtilis* as a test organism.[158,160-164] This particular methodology suffers from the major disadvantages of a delayed set-up time and long incubation time. Assay results were not generally available until 24 to 48 hours after the laboratory had received the specimens. Another major disadvantage is the several factors that influence reliability in measuring serum aminoglycoside concentrations. Temperature, pH, ion concentration in the agar, depth of agar on the plate, test strain, incubation time, and presence of other antibiotics in the serum could affect the zone diameter of inhibition and markedly affect the calculated concentration. Additionally, these microbiologic assays lacked reproducibility and sensitivity in concentrations below 2 µg/mL.

The radioimmunoassay (RIA) methods represented a major improvement over the microbiological assay. This method had a high degree of precision and sensitivity.[165,166] Also, concentrations could be measured within four to six hours after receipt in the laboratory. The disadvantages of this method were the excessive cost of the equipment and the production of radioactive waste. The radioenzymatic (REA) method offered similar advances as compared with the radioimmunoassay methods. A problem that we encountered was variation in the production of the enzyme or activity of the enzyme. These methods are presently used less frequently to assay aminoglycosides because of the cost and risk involved with the radioactive waste.

The homogeneous enzyme immunoassay (EMIT) and fluorescence immunoassay (FIA) methodologies have been substantially improved and now represent the two most common assay methods used to measure serum aminoglycosides in clinical laboratories.[167-169] These assays have similar precision and sensitivity as compared to the radioimmunoassay methods. They are substantially less expensive for the laboratory because of reduced costs in handling radioactive waste. The use of microprocessors has also facilitated the development and maintenance of a standard curve, thus further reducing the cost and the number of samples.

Gas liquid chromatography (GLC) and high performance liquid chromatography (HPLC) methods have been developed and used primarily in research settings.[170-172] These two methods have extremely high degrees of specificity for each aminoglycoside and a high degree of assay precision. However, the instrumentation can be difficult to operate consistently and may require excessive amounts of

Table 14-7. *Comparison of the Relative Advantages and Disadvantages of the Various Aminoglycoside Assay Methods*[a]

| Analytical method | Specificity for aminoglycosides | Limit of sensitivity (μg/mL) | Assayable samples | | | | Minimum sample volume required (μL) | Speed | | Analysis costs | | Specialized operatory training | Preference and rank | | | References |
			Serum	Urine	Saliva	CSF		1–10 Samples	10–100 Samples	Estimated Reagent and tech. cost per assay	Initial equipment cost		Small service	Large service	Research	
Microbiological	4	2	Y	Y	N	Y	25	3	5	2	2	4	3	5	5	158, 160–164
Radioimmunoassay (RIA)	2	0.5	Y	Y	N	Y	50	3	2	3	4	2	4	4	2	165
Radioenzymatic (REA)	2	0.5	Y	Y	N	Y	10	4	3	3	4	2	4	4	3	166
Homogeneous enzyme immunoassay (EMIT)	2	0.5	Y	Y	N	Y	50	2	2	4	3	1	2	2	3	167, 168
Fluorescent immunoassay (FIA)	2	0.5	Y	Y	N	Y	100	2	2	4	3	1	2	2	3	169
Gas liquid chromatography (GLC)	1	0.5	Y	Y	N	Y	400	3	2	4	4	4	4	4	2	170
High performance liquid chromatography (HPLC)	1	0.25	Y	Y	N	Y	500	3	2	4	4	4	4	4	2	171, 172

[a] Arbitrary ranking scale of 1 (excellent) to 5 (poor) with a score of 3 being average.

laboratory technologist's time to resolve. These methods have been useful in the research laboratories because of their extremely high specificity and precision in measuring aminoglycoside concentrations.

These assay methodologies for aminoglycosides were all originally thought to have a high degree of correlation and minimal amount of bias between different methods. However, the radioimmunoassay method now appears to have a bias when compared to the other methods.[170,171] This assay bias may result in different parameter estimates for distribution volume and elimination rate of aminoglycosides in a specific patient. The results from the radioimmunoassay generally reflect a lower distribution volume and half-life when compared to EMIT[171] or fluorescence immunoassay.[170] The microbiological assay, homogeneous enzyme immunoassay, fluorescence immunoassay, gas liquid chromatography, and high performance liquid chromatography have good interassay correlations and minimal bias.

PROSPECTUS

The aminoglycoside antibiotics have been the cornerstone in the treatment of gram-negative sepsis. Their major disadvantage is the risk of ototoxicity and nephrotoxicity. The third-generation cephalosporins have challenged the aminoglycosides. However, the rapid induction of bacterial resistance during therapy via beta-lactamases has been associated with cephalosporin treatment failures. The aminoglycosides thus remain an essential group of antibiotics in the treatment of serious gram-negative sepsis.

The changes within the health care system for reimbursement have caused major changes in the provision of services. Prospective reimbursement or similar reimbursement programs have been implemented for Medicare patients, Medicaid patients, and some patients within the private sector. Additionally, preferred provider organizations (PPOs) and health maintenance organizations (HMOs) have been organized and implemented across the county. These programs all have the intent of reducing health care costs. One of the primary goals of health care providers will be to determine the most cost-effective method of providing health care. Therefore, changes or methods which decrease institutional costs are encouraged under these reimbursement methods. These objectives might be accomplished by improving the quality of patient care or by providing systems to decrease the cost of therapy.

Greater emphasis must be placed on designing the most cost-effective therapies to reduce hospital stays and consumption of hospital resources. The application of pharmacokinetic concepts to adjust dosages and control serum concentrations has increased patient survival. The incidence of ototoxicity and nephrotoxicity would appear to be decreased with pharmacokinetic dosing, but more data from well-controlled studies are needed to confirm these observations. Clinical data suggest the severity of ototoxicity and nephrotoxicity might be reduced; however, this observation needs documentation. Individualizing a patient's dosage improves the quality of patient care by decreasing the number of treatment failures and the risk of toxicity. Both of these outcomes should have a favorable financial analysis.

The systematic methods of attaining therapeutic concentrations early in the course of aminoglycoside treatment should have a positive effect on cost benefit and cost-effectiveness. The cost of providing these services includes personnel salaries, laboratory expenditures, laboratory operating costs, and costs associated with space and physical equipment. The potential benefit derived from individualizing aminoglycoside therapy can be substantial. These savings might include shortened patient stays as a result of accelerated patient response to treatment, or shortened hospital stays through the prevention of adverse drug reactions. Additional cost savings might be realized by adding a systematic program organized to most efficiently and effectively utilize serum drug assays. This organized system might thus prevent unnecessary laboratory analysis and expense. Medical liability risks are more difficult to assess; however, medical risk analysts from insurance companies have supported individualized approaches because of the decreased potential risk of serious side-effects. Several arguments can thus be proposed to support the cost-effectiveness of individualizing aminoglycoside therapy.

The cost and benefits to society have been analyzed in septic burn patients.[110,172] The costs were balanced by the benefit realized by society by the increase in patient survival.[146] The tangible benefit to society from improved patient survival was determined, but the benefit from improved patient safety was not included in these analyses. The cost-benefit ratio was positive, indicating that society realized a favorable outcome from these services. The cost-benefit ratio was from 1:4.5 to 1:24, indicating society realized 4.5 to 24 dollars for every dollar that the service cost. Several methods are available to estimate the benefit from the improved patient survival, and each method provides a different estimate of society's benefit. This ratio of cost to benefit was similar to the cost-benefit ratio reported for the measles vaccination program. Thus, this pharmacokinetic service has a very favorable impact on patient care and a favorable cost-benefit ratio.

REFERENCES

1. Finegold SM. Kanamycin. Arch Intern Med. 1959;104:15.
2. Ericsson DC et al. Clinical pharmacology of intravenous and intraperitoneal aminoglycoside antibiotics in the prevention of wound infection. Ann Surg. 1978;188:66.
3. Mendelson J et al. Safety of the bolus administration of gentamicin. Antimicrob Agents Chemother. 1976;9:633–38.
4. Korner B. Gentamicin therapy administered by intermittent intravenous injections. Acta Pathol Microbiol Scand[B]. 1973;241(Suppl. 81):15–23.
5. Nielsen AB, Elb S. The use of gentamicin intravenously. Acta Pathol Microbiol Immunol Scand[B]. 1973;241(Suppl. 81):23–9.
6. Reiner NE et al. Nephrotoxicity of gentamicin and tobramycin given once daily or continuously in dogs. J Antimicrob Chemother. 1978;4S:85–101.
7. Keating MJ et al. Randomized comparative trial of three aminoglycosides—comparison of continuous infusions of gentamicin, amikacin and sisomicin combined with carbenicillin in the treatment of infection in neutropenic patients with malignancies. Medicine. 1979;58–9.
8. Bodie GP et al. Feasibility of administering aminoglycoside antibiotics by continuous intravenous infusion. Antimicrob Agents Chemother. 1975;8:328.
9. Issell BF et al. Continuous infusion tobramycin combined with carbenicillin for infections in cancer patients. Am J Med Sci. 1979;277:311–18.

10. Marsh DC Jr et al. Transport of gentamicin into synovial fluid. JAMA. 1974;228:607.
11. Chow A et al. Gentamicin and carbenicillin penetration into the septic joint. N Engl J Med. 1971;285:178.
12. Dee TH, Kozin F. Gentamicin and tobramycin penetration into synovial fluid. Antimicrob Agents Chemother. 1977;12:548.
13. Gerding DN et al. Antibiotic concentrations in ascitic fluid of patients with ascites and bacterial peritonitis. Ann Intern Med. 1977;86:708.
14. Chisholm GD et al. Distribution of gentamicin in body fluids. Br Med J. 1968;2:22–4.
15. Smithivas T et al. Gentamicin and ampicillin in human bile. J Infect Dis. 1971;124(Suppl.):S106.
16. Pitt HA et al. Gentamicin levels in the human biliary tract. J Infect Dis. 1973;127:299.
17. Mendelson J et al. Pharmacology of gentamicin in the biliary tract of humans. Antimicrob Agents Chemother. 1973;4:538.
18. Weinstein AJ et al. Placental transfer of clindamycin and gentamicin in term pregnancy. Am J Obstet Gynecol. 1976;124:688.
19. Yoshioka H et al. Placental transfer of gentamicin. J Pediatr. 1972;80:121.
20. Bernard B et al. Tobramycin: Maternal fetal pharmacology. Antimicrob Agents Chemother. 1977;11:688.
21. Rahal JJ Jr et al. Combined intrathecal and intramuscular gentamicin for gram-negative meningitis. Pharmacologic study of 21 patients. N Engl J Med. 1974;290:1394.
22. Barza M et al. Regional differences in ocular concentration of gentamicin after subconjuctival and retrobulbar injection in rabbit. Am J Ophthalmol. 1977;83:407.
23. Barza M. Factors affecting the intra-ocular penetration of antibiotics. The influence of route, inflammation, animal species and tissue pigmentation. Scand J Infect Dis. 1978;114(Suppl.):151.
24. Gordon RC et al. Serum protein binding of the aminoglycoside antibiotics. Antimicrob Agents Chemother. 1972;2:214–16.
25. Ramirez-Ronda CH et al. Effects of divalent cations on binding of aminoglycoside antibiotics to human serum proteins and to bacteria. Antimicrob Agents Chemother. 1975;7:239–45.
26. Myers DR et al. Gentamicin binding to serum and plasma proteins. Clin Pharmacol Ther. 1978;23:356–60.
27. Pennington JE, Reynolds HY. Pharmacokinetics of gentamicin sulfate in bronchial secretions. J Infect Dis. 1975;131:158–62.
28. Pennington JE, Reynolds HY. Concentrations of gentamicin and carbenicillin in bronchial secretions. J Infect Dis. 1973;128:63–8.
29. Wong GA et al. Penetration of antimicrobial agents into bronchial secretions. Am J Med. 1975;59:219–23.
30. Pines A et al. Gentamicin and colistin in chronic purulent bronchial infections. Br Med J. 1967;2:543–45.
31. Odio W et al. Concentrations of gentamicin in bronchial secretions after intramuscular and endotracheal administration. J Clin Pharmacol. 1975;15:518.
32. Zaske DE et al. Gentamicin pharmacokinetics in 1640 patients: Method for control of serum concentrations. Antimicrob Agents Chemother. 1982;21:407.
33. Cipolle PJ et al. Systematically individualizing tobramycin dosage regimens. J Clin Pharmacol. 1980;20:570.
34. Zaske DE et al. Amikacin pharmacokinetics: wide interpatient variation in 98 patients. In review.
35. Rotschafer JC et al. Clinical use of a one-compartment model for determining netilmicin pharmacokinetic parameters and dosage recommendations. Ther Drug Monit. 1983;5:263-67.
36. Schentag JJ et al. Gentamicin disposition and tissue aecumulation on multiple dosing. J Pharmacokinet Biopharm. 1977;5:559–77.
37. Schentag JJ et al. Comparative tissue accumulation of gentamicin and tobramycin in patients. J Antimicrob Chemother. 1978;4S:23–30.
38. Schentag JJ et al. Tissue persistence of gentamicin in man. JAMA. 1977;238:327–29.
39. Kahlmeter G et al. Multiple-compartment pharmacokinetics of tobramycin. J Antimicrob Chemother. 1978;4S:50–11.

40. Fabre J et al. Persistence of sisomicin and gentamicin in renal cortex and medulla compared with other organs and serum in rats. Kidney Int. 1976;10:444–49.
41. Schentag JJ, Jusko WJ. Renal clearance and tissue accumulation of gentamicin. Clin Pharmacol Ther. 1977;22:364–70.
42. Tulkens P, Trouet A. The uptake and intracellular accumulation of aminoglycoside antibiotics in lysosomes of cultured rat fibroblasts. Biochem Pharmacol. 1978;27:415-24.
43. Bergeron MG, Trottier S. Influence of single or multiple doses of gentamicin and netilmicin on their cortical, medullary, and papillary distribution. Antimicrob Agents Chemother. 1979;15:635–41.
44. Thiessen J. The pharmacokinetic parameters of aminoglycoside dosing. Kenilworth:Schering Corporation; 1979:7. Symposium.
45. Sawchuk RJ, Zaske DE. Pharmacokinetics of dosing regimens which utilize multiple intravenous infusions: Gentamicin in burn patients. J Pharmacokinet Biopharm. 1976;4:183–95.
46. Sawchuk RJ et al. Kinetic models for gentamicin dosing with the use of individual patient parameters. Clin Pharmacol Ther. 1977;21:360–69.
47. Zaske DE et al. Gentamicin pharmacokinetics in 1,640 patients: method for control of serum concentrations. Antimicrob Agents Chemother. 1982;21(2):407–11.
48. Clarke JT et al. Comparative pharmacokinetics of amikacin and kanamycin. Clin Pharmacol Ther. 1974;15:610-16.
49. Kirby WM et al. Clinical pharmacology of amikacin and kanamycin. J Infect Dis. 1976;134:S312–30.
50. Gyselynck AM et al. Pharmacokinetics of gentamicin: distribution of plasma and renal clearance. J Infect Dis. 1971;124:S70–6.
51. Plantier J et al. Pharmacokinetics of amikacin in patients of normal or impaired renal function: Radioenzymatic acetylation assay. J Infect Dis. 1976;134:S323–30.
52. Lode H et al. Pharmacokinetics and clinical studies of amikacin, a new aminoglycoside antibiotic. J Infect Dis. 1976;134:S316–22.
53. Clarke JT et al. Comparative pharmacokinetics of amikacin and kanamycin. Clin Pharmacol Ther. 1974;15:610-16.
54. Fong IW et al. Comparative toxicity of gentamicin versus tobramycin: a randomized prospective study. J Antimicrob Chemother. 1981;7:81–8.
55. Cipolle PJ et al. Hospital acquired gram-negative pneumonias: Response rate and dosage requirements with individualized tobramycin therapy. Ther Drug Monit. 1980;2:273–82.
56. Barza M et al. Predictability of blood levels of gentamicin in man. J Infect Dis. 1975;132:165–74.
57. Kaye D et al. The unpredictability of serum concentrations of gentamicin: pharmacokinetics of gentamicin in patients with normal and abnormal renal function. J Infect Dis. 1974;130:150–54.
58. Pennington JE et al. Gentamicin sulfate pharmacokinetics: lower levels of gentamicin in blood during fever. J Infect Dis. 1975;132:270–75.
59. Schwartz SN et al. A controlled investigation of the pharmacokinetics of gentamicin and tobramycin in obese subjects. J Infect Dis. 1978;138:499-505.
60. Sketris I et al. Effect of obesity on gentamicin pharmacokinetics. J Clin Pharmacol. 1981;21:288–94.
61. Blouin RA et al. Tobramycin pharmacokinetics in markedly obese patients. Clin Pharmacol Ther. 1979;26:508-12.
62. Bauer LA et al. Amikacin pharmacokinetics in morbidly obese patients. Am J Hosp Pharm. 1980;37:519–22.
63. Zaske DE et al. Rapid gentamicin elimination in obstetric patients. Obstet Gynecol. 1980;56:559–64.
64. Zaske DE et al. Increased dosage requirements of gentamicin in burn patients. J Trauma. 1976;16:824.
65. Zaske DE et al. Rapid individualization of gentamicin dosage regimens in 66 burn patients. Burns Incl Therm Inj. 1981;7:215.
66. Loirat P et al. Increased glomerular filtration rate in patients with major burns. N Engl J Med. 1978;299:915-19.

67. Zaske DE et al. Necessity of increased doses of amikacin in burn patients. Surgery. 1978;84:603.

68. Siber G et al. Pharmacokinetics of gentamicin in children and adults. J Infect Dis. 1975;132:637–49.

69. Evans WE et al. Use of gentamicin serum levels to individualize therapy in children. J Pediatr. 1978;93:133-37.

70. McCracken GH. Clinical pharmacology of gentamicin in infants 2 to 24 months of age. Am J Dis Child. 1972;124:884.

71. Zaske DE et al. Pharmacokinetics of gentamicin in pediatric patients. In Press.

72. Zaske DE et al. Kinetics of gentamicin in 209 internal medicine patients. In Press.

73. Gill MA, Kern JW. Altered gentamicin distribution in ascitic patients. Am J Hosp Pharm. 1979;36:1704–706.

74. Sampliner R et al. Influence of ascites on tobramycin pharmacokinetics. J Clin Pharmacol. 1984;24(1):43–6.

75. Zaske DE et al. Wide interpatient variations in gentamicin dosage requirements for geriatric patients. JAMA. 1982;248(23):3112–126.

76. Zaske DE et al. Gentamicin dosage requirements: Wide interpatient variation in 242 surgery patients with normal renal function. Surgery. 1980;87:164.

77. Bauer LA et al. Gentamicin and tobramycin pharmacokinetics in patients with cystic fibrosis. Clin Pharm. 1983;2:262–64.

78. Kearns GL et al. Dosing implications of altered gentamicin disposition in patients with cystic fibrosis. J Pediatr. 1982;100(2):312–18.

79. Kelly HB et al. Pharmacokinetics of tobramycin in cystic fibrosis. J Pediatr. 1982;100(2):318–21.

80. Michaelsen H, Bergan T. Pharmacokinetics of netilmicin in children with and without cystic fibrosis. Antimicrob Agents Chemother. 1981;19(6):1029–31.

81. Henriksson P et al. Netilmicin in moderate to severe infections in newborns and infants: A study of efficacy, tolerance and pharmacokinetics. Scand J Infect Dis. 1980;23(Suppl):155–59.

82. McCracken GH. Clinical pharmacology of gentamicin in infants 2 to 24 months of age. Am J Dis Child. 1972;124:884–87.

83. Zenk KE et al. Effect of body weight on gentamicin pharmacokinetics in neonates. Clin Pharm. 1984;3:170–73.

84. Bravo ME et al. Pharmacokinetics of gentamicin in malnourished infants. Eur J Clin Pharmacol. 1982;21:499-504.

85. Friedman CA et al. Gentamicin disposition in asphyxiated newborns: relationship to mean arterial blood pressure and urine output. Pediatr Pharmacol. 1982;2:189-97.

86. Paisley JW et al. Gentamicin in newborn infants: comparison of intramuscular and intravenous administration. Am J Dis Child. 1973;126:473–77.

87. Kagan BM. Applied pharmacology: Antimicrobial Therapy. Philadelphia:WB Saunders;1974.

88. Moellering RC Jr et al. Studies on the antibiotic synergism against enterococci. I Bacteriologic Studies. J Lab Clin Med. 1971;77:821–28.

89. Sonni M, Jawetz E. Combined action of carbenicillin and gentamicin on *Pseudomonas aeruginosa in vitro*. Appl Environ Microbiol. 1969;17:893–96.

90. Noone P et al. Experience in monitoring gentamicin therapy during treatment of serious gram-negative sepsis. Br Med J. 1974;1:477–81.

91. Loebl VC et al. Survival with ecthyma gangrenosum: a previously fatal complication of burns. J Trauma. 1974;14:370–77.

92. Brummet RE et al. Ototoxicity of tobramycin, gentamicin, amikacin and sisomicin in the guinea pig. J Antimicrob Chemother. 1978;4(Suppl.):73–83.

93. Luft FC et al. Comparative nephrotoxicities of netilmicin and gentamicin in rats. Antimicrob Agents Chemother. 1976;10:845–49.

94. Ormsby AM et al. Comparison of the nephrotoxic potential of gentamicin, tobramycin and netilmicin in the rat. Curr Ther Res. 1979;25:335–43.

95. Panwalker AP et al. Netilmicin: clinical efficacy, tolerance, and toxicity. Antimicrob Agents Chemother. 1978;13:170–76.

96. Trestman I et al. Pharmacology and efficacy of netilmicin. Antimicrob Agents Chemother. 1978;13:832–36.

97. Federspil P et al. Pharmacokinetics and ototoxicity of gentamicin, tobramycin, and amikacin. J Infect Dis. 1976;134(Suppl):200–5.

98. Warner A, Sanders E. Neuromuscular blockade associated with gentamicin therapy. JAMA. 1971;215:1153–154.

99. Pittinger CB et al. Antibiotic-induced paralysis. Anesth Analg. 1970;49:487–501.

100. McQuillen MP et al. Myasthenic syndrome associated with antibioties. Arch Neurol. 1968;18:402–15.

101. L'Hommedieu CS et al. Potentiation of magnesium sulfate-induced neuromuscular weakness by gentamicin, tobramycin, and amikacin. J Pediatr. 1983;102(4):629–31.

102. Snavely SR, Hodges GR. The neurotoxicity of antibacterial agents. Ann Int Med. 1984;1:92–104.

103. Kumin GD. Clinical nephrotoxicity of tobramycin and gentamicin: a prospective study. JAMA. 1980;244(16):1808-810.

104. Tablan OC et al. Renal and auditory toxicity of high-dose, prolonged therapy with gentamicin and tobramycin in Pseudomnas endocarditis. J Infect Dis. 1984;149(2):257-63.

105. Schentag JJ et al. Comparative nephrotoxicity of gentamicin and tobramycin: pharmacokinetic and clinical studies in 201 patients. Antimicrob Agents Chemother. 1981;19(5):859–66.

106. Smith CR et al. Double-blind comparison of the nephrotoxicity and auditory toxicity of gentamicin and tobramycin. N Engl J Med. 1980;302:1106–109.

107. Brown AE et al. Minimal nephrotoxicity with cephalosporinaminoglycoside combinations in patients with neoplastic disease. Antimicrob Agents Chemother. 1982;21:592 94.

108. Fee WE et al. Clinical evaluation of aminoglycoside toxicity: tobramycin versus gentamicin. A preliminary report. J Antimicrob Chemother. 1978;4S:31–6.

109. Schentag JJ et al. Aminoglycoside nephrotoxicity in critically ill surgical patients. J Surg Res. 1979;26:270-79.

110. Bock BV et al. Prospective comparative study of efficacy and toxicity of netilmicin and amikacin. Antimicrob Agents Chemother. 1980;17:217–25.

111. Cone LA. A survey of prospective, controlled clinical trials of gentamicin, tobramycin, amikacin, and netilmicin. Clin Ther. 1982;5:155–62.

112. Feig PU et al. Aminoglycoside nephrotoxicity: A double-blind prospective randomized study of gentamicin and tobramycin. J Antimicrob Chemother. 1982;10:217–26.

113. Feld R et al. Comparison of amikacin and tobramycin in the treatment of infection in patients with cancer. J Infect Dis. 1977;135:61–8.

114. French MA et al. Amikacin and gentamicin accumulation pharmacokinetics and nephrotoxicity in critically ill patients. Antimicrob Agents Chemother. 1981;19:147–52.

115. Keys TF et al. Renal toxicity during therapy with gentamicin or tobramycin. Mayo Clin Proc. 1981;56:556–59.

116. Lau MY et al. Comparative efficacy and toxicity of amikacin/carbenicillin versus gentamicin/carbenicillin in leukopenic patients. A randomized prospective trial. Am J Med. 1977;62:959–66.

117. Lerner AM et al. Randomized controlled trial of the comparative efficacy, auditory toxicity, and nephrotoxicity of tobramycin and netilmicin. Lancet. 1983;1123–126.

118. Lerner SA et al. Comparative clinical studies of ototoxicity and nephrotoxicity of amikacin and gentamicin. Am J Med. 1977;62:919–23.

119. Love LJ et al. Randomized trial of empiric antibiotic therapy with ticarcillin in combination with gentamicin, amikacin or netilmicin in febrile patients with granulocytopenia and cancer. Am J Med. 1979;66:603–10.

120. Matzke GR et al. Controlled comparison of gentamicin and tobramycin nephrotoxicity. Am J Nephrol. 1983;3:11–8.

121. Plaut ME et al. Aminoglycoside nephrotoxicity: comparative assessment in critically ill patients. J Med. 1979;10:257–66.

122. Smith CR et al. Controlled comparison of amikacin and gentamicin. N Engl J Med. 1977;296:349–51.

123. Weintraub RG et al. Comparative nephrotoxicity of two aminoglycosides: gentamicin and tobramycin. Med J. 1982;2:129–32.

124. Swain RR, Briggs SL. Positive interference with the Jaffe reaction by cephalosporin antibiotics. Clin Chem. 1977;23:1340–342.
125. Meondelan J et al. Safety of bolus administration of gentamicin. Antimicrob Agents Chemother. 1976;9:633–38.
126. Powell SH et al. Once daily vs. continuous aminoglycoside dosing: efficacy and toxicity in animal and clinical studies of gentamicin, netilmicin, and tobramycin. J Infect Dis. 1983;147:918–32.
127. Jackson GG, Arcieri G. Ototoxicity of gentamicin in man: a survey and controlled analysis of clinical experience in the United States. J Infect Dis. 1971;124(Suppl.):S130.
128. Barza M et al. Prospective randomized trial of netilmicin and amikacin, with emphasis on eighth-nerve toxicity. Antimicrob Agents Chemother. 1980;17:707–14.
129. Bender JF et al. Comparative auditory toxicity of aminoglycoside antibiotics in leukopenic patients. Am J Hosp Pharm. 1979;36:1083–87.
130. Gatell JM et al. Comparison of the nephrotoxicity and auditory toxicity of tobramycin and amikacin. Antimicrob Agents Chemother. 1983;23:897–901.
131. Huang MY, Schacht J. Drug induced ototoxicity, pathogenesis and prevention. Med Toxicol Adverse Drug Exp. 1989;4:452–67.
132. Smith CR et al. Relationship between aminoglycoside induced nephrotoxicity and auditory toxicity. Antimicrob Agents Chemother. 1979;15:780.
133. Davey PG et al. Study of alanine aminopeptidase excretion as a test of gentamicin nephrotoxicity. J Antimicrob Chemother. 1983;11:455–65.
134. Schentag JJ, Plaut ME. Patterns of urinary β_2-microglobulin excretion by patients treated with aminoglycosides. Kidney Int. 1980;17:654–61.
135. Herting RL et al. Netilmicin: chemical development and overview of clinical research. Scand J Infect Dis. 1980;23(Suppl):20–9.
136. Falco FG et al. Nephrotoxicity of aminoglycosides and gentamicin. J Infect Dis. 1969;119:406–9.
137. Dahlgren JG et al. Gentamicin blood levels: a guide to nephrotoxicity. Antimicrob Agents Chemother. 1975;8:58-62.
138. Mawer GE et al. Prescribing aids for gentamicin. Br J Clin Pharmacol. 1974;1:45–50.
139. Gooding PV et al. A review of results of clinical trials with amikacin. J Infect Dis. 1976;134:S441–45.
140. Albiero L et al. Comparison of neuromuscular effects and acute toxicity of some aminoglycoside antibiotics. Arch Int Pharmacodyn Ther. 1978;233:343–50.
141. Finegold SM. Toxicity of kanamycin in adults. Ann NY Acad Sci. 1966;132:942–56.
142. Noone P et al. Experience in monitoring gentamicin therapy during treatment of serious gram-negative sepsis. Br Med J. 1974;1:477–81.
143. Moore RD et al. The association of aminoglycoside plasma levels with mortality in patients with gram-negative bacteremia. J Infect Dis. 1984;149(3):443–48.
144. Jackson GG, Riff LJ. Pseudomonas bacteremia. Pharmacologic and other bases for failure of treatment with gentamicin. J Infect Dis. 1971;124(Suppl.):S185–91.
145. Solem LD et al. Ecthyma gangrenosum, survival with individualized antibiotic therapy. Arch Surg. 1979;114:580–83.
146. Zaske DE et al. Increased burn patient survival with individualized dosages of gentamicin. Surgery. 1982;91(2):142–49.
147. Anderson ET et al. Simultaneous antibiotic levels in "breakthrough" gram-negative rod bacteremia. Am J Med. 1976;61:493–97.
148. Weinstein MP, Reller LB. Clinical importance of "breakthrough" bacteremia. Am J Med. 1984;76:175–80.
149. McHenry MC et al. Gentamicin dosage for renal insufficiency: adjustments based on endogenous creatinine clearance, and serum creatinine concentrations. Ann Int Med. 1971;74:192–97.
150. Chan RA et al. Gentamicin therapy in renal failure: a nomogram for dosage. Ann Intern Med. 1978;76:775.
151. Dettli LC. Drug dosage in patients with renal disease. Clin Pharmacol Ther. 1974;16:274.

152. Sarubbi FA, Hull JH. Amikacin serum concentrations: predictions of levels and dosage guidelines. Ann Intern Med. 1978;89:612–18.

153. Hull JH, Sarubbi FA. Gentamicin serum concentrations: pharmacokinetic predictions. Ann Intern Med. 1976;85:183-89.

154. Lott RS et al. Correlation of predicted versus measured creatinine clearance values in burn patients. Am J Hosp Pharm. 1978;35:717.

155. Lesar TS et al. Gentamicin dosage errors with four commonly used nomograms. JAMA. 1982;248:1190–193.

156. Anderson AC et al. Determination of serum gentamicin sulfate levels. Arch Intern Med. 1976;136:785.

157. Greenlaw CW et al. Aminoglycoside serum assays restricted through a pharmacy program. Am J Hosp Pharm. 1979;36:1080-83.

158. Waterworth PM. An enzyme preparation inactivating all penicillins and cephalosporins. J Clin Pathol. 1973;26:596–98.

159. Rodman JH et al. Effect of analytical error in sampling schemes on precision of parameters and model prediction. Paper presented at Academy of Pharmaceutical Sciences. Hollywood, FL:1978.

160. Winters RE et al. Relation between dose and levels of gentamicin in blood. J Infect Dis. 1971;124(Suppl.):S90-5.

161. Alcid DV, Seligman SJ. Simplified assay for gentamicin in the presence of other antibiotics. Antimicrob Agents Chemother. 1973;3:559–61.

162. Lund ME et al. Rapid gentamicin bioassay using a multiresistant strain of *Klebsiella pneumoniae*. Antimicrob Agents Chemother. 1973;4:569–73.

163. Stevens P et al. Radioimmunoassay, radioenzymatic assay, and microbioassay of gentamicin. J Lab Clin Med. 1975;86:349–59.

164. Giamarellou H et al. Assay of aminoglycoside antibiotics in clinical specimens. J Infect Dis. 1975;132:399–406.

165. Smith DH et al. A rapid chemical assay for gentamicin. N Engl J Med. 1972;286:583–86.

166. Casc RV, Mezei LM. An enzymatic radioassay for gentamicin. Clin Chem. 1978;24:2145–150.

167. Standefer JC, Saunders GC. Enzyme immunoassay for gentamicin. Clin Chem. 1978;24:1903–907.

168. Rubenstein KE et al. Homogenous enzyme immunoassay a new immunochemical technique. Biochem Biophys Res Commun. 1972;42:846–51.

169. Burd JF et al. Homogenous reactant labeled fluorescent immunoassay for therapeutic drugs exemplified by gentamicin determination in human serum. Clin Chem. 1977;23:1402–408.

170. Anhalt JP, Brown SD. High performance liquid chromatographic assay of aminoglycoside antibiotics. Clin Chem. 1978;24:1940–947.

171. Mayhew JW, Gorbach SL. Assay for gentamicin and tobramycin by Gas-Liquid Chromatography. Antimicrob Agents Chemother. 1978;14:851–55.

172. Maitra SK et al. Gentamicin assay by high performance liquid chromatography. Clin Chem. 1977;23:2275–278.

173. Craig WA, Vogelman B. The postantibiotic effect. Ann Intern Med. 1987;106:900–2.

174. Wood CA et al. The influence of tobramycin dosage regimens on nephrotoxicity, ototoxicity and antibacterial efficacy in rat model of subcutaneous abcess. J Infect Dis. 1988;158:13–22.

175. Kapusnik JF et al. Single large daily dosing versus intermittent dosing of tobramycin for treating experimental Pseudomonas pneumonia. J Infect Dis. 1988;158:7–12.

176. Hollender LF et al. A multicenter study of netilmicin once daily versus thrice daily in patients with appendicitis and other intra-abdominal infections. J Antimicrob Chemother. 1989;23:773–83.

177. Strum AW. Netilmicin in the treatment of gram-negative bacteremia: single daily versus multiple daily dosage. J Infect Dis. 1989;159:931–7.

178. Zaske DE et al. Increased gentamicin dosage requirements: rapid elimination in 249 gynecology patients. Obstetrics and Gynecology. 1981;139:896–900.

179. Zaske DE, Crossley K. Amikacin: a new aminoglycoside antibiotic. Minnesota Med. 1978;61:123–26.

Chapter 15

Vancomycin

Gary R. Matzke

Vancomycin (from the word "vanquish") was originally obtained from the fermentation broth of *Streptomyces orientalis*, an organism that was first isolated in 1956 by picric acid precipitation applied to a soil sample from Borneo.[1 5] The pharmaceutical products presently available for clinical use include a chromatographically purified form (claimed purity greater than 90%) which was introduced by Lilly in 1986 and products of slightly lower purity (80% to 90%) produced by several other manufacturers.[6]

Despite improvement of the vancomycin formulation, development of the anti-staphylococcal penicillins and cephalosporins in the 1960s resulted in a marked decrease in the clinical use of this agent. However, new indications, treatment of endocarditis in patients allergic to penicillins and treatment of antibiotic-associated colitis, have stimulated renewed interest in this compound.[4,7–10]

The pharmacokinetics of vancomycin have been more extensively characterized during the last decade than any other time period in the drug's developmental history. These new findings are reviewed here in the light of earlier observations. Areas of controversy are discussed, and a rational pharmacokinetic approach to the use of vancomycin in various patient populations and settings is proposed.

CLINICAL PHARMACOKINETICS

Geraci et al.,[11] as well as Kirby and Divelbiss,[12] first described vancomycin disposition in the 1950s. Dosage schedules derived from these early assessments were still in use well into the 1980s.

During the 1960s and 1970s, only modest advances in our knowledge of vancomycin pharmacokinetics were reported.[13] The disposition of vancomycin in many patient populations, including those with renal insufficiency, was well characterized for the first time in the 1980s.[14–18] Although several investigators reported serum concentration-time data after vancomycin administration to hemodialysis patients,[19–23] it was not until the 1980s that the pharmacokinetic characteristics of vancomycin in patients with end-stage renal disease were reported.[15,18,23-26] These recent investigations have provided therapeutic dosing guidelines that are applicable to most patients.

Absorption

Although early reports suggested that the oral absorption of vancomycin was minimal,[27,28] substantial serum concentrations have been observed in subjects with antibiotic-associated colitis.[29-32] Serum vancomycin concentrations of 10 to 20 mg/L and 13 to 34 mg/L were observed in two subjects with pseudomembranous colitis after the oral administration of 500 mg and 250 mg of drug every six hours, respectively.[29,30] These findings suggest that, under some conditions, orally administered vancomycin may be absorbed in quantities sufficient to produce serum concentrations within the therapeutic range. Oral absorption of vancomycin was recently evaluated in five patients with end-stage renal disease and culture-positive *Clostridium difficile* pseudomembranous colitis.[33] Serum concentrations were detectable in four of these patients (range 3 to 12 mg/L). A significant relationship was observed between the administered dose of vancomycin and the measured serum concentration [concentration (in mg/L) = [dose (in mg) · 0.027] – 2.8; $r = 0.86$; $p < 0.01$.]

Although the risk of ototoxicity or nephrotoxicity due to vancomycin therapy appears low, periodic monitoring of serum vancomycin concentrations is recommended for colitis patients with severe renal failure, especially those receiving greater than 2 gm/day for ten days or more.

Intramuscular administration of vancomycin causes severe local pain; hence, the intravenous route is almost always chosen. Although vancomycin can be administered as a slow intravenous bolus, the recommended parenteral administration method is as a slow intravenous infusion at a rate no greater than 7.5 to 15 mg/min.[15,34]

Distribution

The serum concentration-time profile of vancomycin has been described with one-, two-, and three-compartmental models in subjects with normal renal function.[15-18,35-37] The half-life of the first distributive phase is approximately 0.4 hours, while the half-life of the second distributive phase has ranged from 1.6 to 3.6 hours in adults with normal renal function and end-stage renal disease, respectively[25,26,35] (see Table 15-1). The terminal elimination half-life has ranged from 2.6 to 9.1 hours in subjects with normal renal function.[15-18] Because of the relationship between terminal elimination half-life and renal function, an understanding of this terminal elimination phase may be useful in designing dosage regimens and therapeutic monitoring strategies.

The central compartment volume of distribution derived from two- and three-compartment analyses approximates 0.2 to 0.6 L/kg and 0.13 L/kg, respectively.[16,17,35,37] The apparent steady-state volume of distribution is also highly variable and mean values have ranged from 0.5 to 0.9 L/kg. Although early evidence suggested that vancomycin was minimally bound (less than 10%) to

Table 15-1. Vancomycin Pharmacokinetics in Adults

Investigator	Patient type	n	Age (years)[b]	CL$_{cr}$ (mL/min)[b]	t½ α	t½ β	t½ λ	V$_c$ (L/kg)[b]	V$_{SS}$ (L/kg)[b]	CL$_S$ (mL/min)[b]	CL$_R$ (mL/min)[b]
Brater[63]	Burn	10	41 (4)	105 (19)	—	—	—	—	—	93.9 (56.4)	—
Garrelts[62]	Burn	9	27.8 (13.2)	131 (25)	—	—	3.8 (1.0)	—	0.51 (0.09)[c]	97.0 (27.8)	—
	Control	8	28.1 (9.2)	117 (24)	—	—	5.2 (1.3)	—	0.50 (0.05)[c]	72.7 (22.3)	—
Rybak[38]	Burn	10	36.4 (14.9)	111 (28.3)	—	—	—	—	0.59 (0.17)	142.8 (34.5)	124 (40.7)
	IVDA	14	36.0 (6.2)	85.5 (23)	—	—	—	—	0.56 (0.12)	98 (29.7)	77.4 (24.1)
	VDRF	10	38.0 (11.9)	68.3 (30.4)	—	—	—	—	0.52 (0.15)	67.7 (21.2)	58.4 (15.9)
Rodvold[17]	VDRF	10	46.3 (11.6)	93.4 (28.3)	0.4 (0.30)	—	5.2 (2.6)	0.21 (0.11)	0.50 (0.20)	98.4 (24.3)	88.0 (33.6)
		14	49.5 (14.3)	51.0 (8.3)	0.49 (0.32)	—	10.5 (3.6)	0.21 (0.14)	0.59 (0.27)	52.6 (17.7)	48.2 (10.8)
		13	61.6 (18.4)	23.9 (8.2)	0.51 (0.21)	—	19.9 (10.2)	0.24 (0.12)	0.64 (0.18)	31.3 (14.9)	19.8 (7.9)
Comstock[25]	ESRD	10	37.7 (13.1)	3.6 (1.4)	0.15 (0.12)	3.6 (2.8)	156 (45)	0.12 (0.09)	0.71 (0.16)	3.2 (1.2)	—
Tan[26]	ESRD	6	59.3 (4.6)	3.9 (1.0)	0.42 (0.09)	2.9 (0.45)	142.6 (11.1)	0.38 (0.09)	1.07 (0.11)	5.4 (0.11)	—
Healy[34]	NV	11	24.7 (2.1)	110 (19)	0.23 (0.23)	1.6 (0.88)	8.1 (2.2)	0.14 (0.06)	0.92 (0.24)	84.8 (11.5)	—
Golper[36]	NV	9	21–34	110 (30)	0.62 (0.30)	—	5.7 (1.8)	0.58 (0.19)	0.89 (0.19)	138 (29)	88 (14)

a Burn = Thermal injury; Control = Non burn acutely ill; IVDA = Intravenous drug abuser; VDRF = Various degrees of renal function; ESRD = End stage renal disease; NV = Normal volunteer.

b Mean (SD).

c V$_{area}$.

plasma proteins,[20] recent observations in healthy volunteers and patients with normal renal function suggest that approximately 30% to 55% of circulating vancomycin is bound.[17,38,39] The degree of binding in patients with end-stage renal disease is somewhat lower (mean 18.5 %, range 0% to 30.6%).[26]

Therapeutic concentrations of vancomycin have been measured in pleural, pericardial, ascitic, and synovial fluids and in lung, lymph, feces, and bile.[11,28,40] Vancomycin concentrations in bone and heart valves after an intravenous dose of 15 mg/kg have also been observed to exceed the minimum inhibitory concentration (MIC) of susceptible *staphylococci* for six to nine hours.[41,42] The majority of the distribution data have been generated from single-dose studies, and it is notable that concentrations at all sites have been higher in the few multiple-dose studies that have been conducted.[11]

Although vancomycin penetration across the uninflamed meninges is minimal, therapeutic cerebrospinal fluid (CSF) concentrations have been reported in some adults and children.[43-48] However, since adequate concentrations are not achieved in all patients, intrathecal administration of the drug in a dose of 10 to 20 mg every 24 hours has been recommended.[49-52] Intraventricular vancomycin has also been proposed to treat CSF shunt infections.[53-56,189] Although Swayne et al.[53] reported that 100% of their patients responded without experiencing adverse events when 20 mg (adults) and 10 mg (children) were administered by this route once a day, others have suggested that this dosage regimen may produce excessive CSF concentrations[54,56,57] which may be related to alterations in consciousness.[54] The utilization of 10 mg or less once a day in adults has led to unacceptable failure rates.[55,58] Thus, although peak CSF concentrations of 30 to 50 mg/L may be attained with this dosage regimen, this may not represent the optimal therapeutic range for the treatment of CSF shunt infections. Thus, prospective monitoring of CSF concentrations and dosage adjustment will be required to obtain the desired clinical response.

Metabolism

Kirby and Divelbiss[12] reported that 80% to 100% of 1 gm and 2 gm intravenous doses were recovered in the urine in the first 24 hours after drug administration. Lee et al.[59] more extensively evaluated the distribution, excretion, and renal clearance of vancomycin in animal studies. From results indicating "no vancomycin or only a low concentration" in the liver and a very small amount excreted in the bile, they concluded that the drug was not metabolized to any great extent.

Brown and associates[60] evaluated the effects of liver function on vancomycin disposition. Although distribution half-lives did not differ significantly, the terminal elimination half-life was 2.6 ± 1.3 hours in six patients with normal hepatic function and 37.0 ± 74.3 hours in nine patients with impaired hepatic function (bilirubin 7.1 ± 5.3 mg/dL). These studies were conducted after patients had received 500 mg of vancomycin intravenously over 30 minutes every six hours for up to seven days. The short observation period during the dosing interval may have affected the accuracy with which the elimination half-life could be determined. Furthermore, it is not known whether these patients had concomitant renal impairment.

Narang et al.[61] and Rodvold et al.[17] observed no significant relationship between the presence of clinical hepatic disease or liver function tests and vancomycin pharmacokinetic parameters among acutely ill adult patients with various degrees of renal function (n = 47). Thus, although some nonrenal clearance of vancomycin occurs, it does not appear to warrant any alterations of vancomycin dosage in patients with hepatic impairment.

Excretion

The extent of vancomycin renal excretion has now been evaluated in multiple studies of healthy volunteers and acutely ill patients.[12,17,35,36,38] Eighty to ninety percent of the intravenous administered dose has been recovered intact in the urine of adults with normal to moderately impaired renal function.

The ratio of renal clearance to creatinine clearance for vancomycin was first assessed in dogs and found to be 0.69 ± 0.05 (mean ± SD).[59] Almost 20 years later, Nielson et al.[13] reported that in humans the ratios of vancomycin renal clearance to iothalamate and creatinine clearances were 0.79 ± 0.11 and 0.53 ± 0.11, respectively. The relationship between vancomycin renal clearance and inulin clearance has been reported recently to be 0.89 ± 0.06.[36] These observations that vancomycin renal clearance is consistently less than creatinine clearance suggest that vancomycin may either undergo renal tubular reabsorption or may be significantly bound to proteins. Although the differences in renal vancomycin and creatinine clearances may be related to the binding of this drug to plasma proteins, the observations of Rodvold et al.,[17] Goper et al.,[36] and Rybak et al.[38] suggest that tubular secretion may be a significant component of vancomycin's net renal excretion.

Effects of Disease and Aging

In the last five years, the disposition of vancomycin has been characterized in patients with various acute and chronic disease states. The serum concentration-time profiles of vancomycin in these studies have been described in terms of one-, two-, and three-compartment pharmacokinetic models.

Regardless of the pharmacokinetic model used to assess the serum concentration-time profiles, the terminal elimination half-life of vancomycin is prolonged (see Figure 15-1) and the total body clearance is reduced in subjects with impaired renal function (see Table 15-1).[14–18,25,26,38] The degree of decline in vancomycin total body clearance and elimination rate constant associated with particular degrees of renal impairment have been characterized by numerous investigators. Although there is marked variability in the kinetic parameters of vancomycin within a defined range of renal function, the relationship between vancomycin total body clearance and creatinine clearance has generally been found to be highly significant.

Macias et al.[62] observed that early in the course of oliguric acute renal failure, there was substantial preservation of the nonrenal clearance of vancomycin. The nonrenal clearance which approximated 16 mL/min (range 3.8 to 23.3 mL/min), however, appeared to decrease as the duration of renal failure increased and eventually approached the total clearance previously observed in patients with chronic renal failure (i.e., 4 to 6 mL/min). These data suggest that patients with acute renal failure handle vancomycin and perhaps other drugs differently from patients with stable chronic renal insufficiency.

Patients with thermal injury require higher vancomycin doses than non-burn patients to achieve similar target serum concentrations.[63,64] Brater et al.[64] reported that the CL_s of vancomycin in burn patients was significantly correlated with renal function and that this relationship ($CL_s = 12.5 + 0.69\ CL_{cr}$) was similar to that observed in other patient populations.[13-15] Rybak et al.[38] have recently confirmed that vancomycin CL_s is increased in burn patients. Their data indicate that the protein binding of vancomycin is not altered in these patients; furthermore, the increase in vancomycin CL_s and renal excretion was predominantly due to enhanced tubular secretion.

The disposition of vancomycin has also been evaluated in intravenous drug abusers and critically ill patients.[38,61,65] These investigations indicated that the CL_s was considerably increased in these patient populations. Although CL_s was significantly correlated with renal function by two of the three investigators,[38,61] the utility of CL_{cr} to guide dosage regimen design has not been rigorously assessed.

The effects of aging on vancomycin pharmacokinetics have been evaluated in infants and pediatric patients.[44] Schaad et al.[44] evaluated the disposition of vancomycin in 55 pediatric patients after single and/or multiple intravenous infusions. In 21 premature infants (gestational age range, 32 to 40 weeks) an increase in total

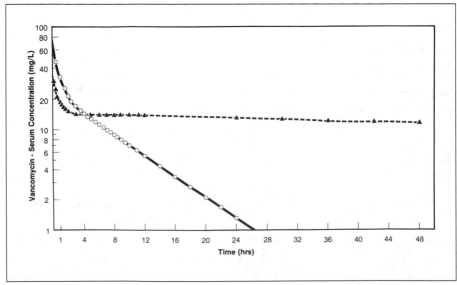

Figure 15-1. *Vancomycin serum concentration-time curve for a patient with normal renal function (○) and end-stage renal disease (▲), after one-hour IV infusion of 1 gm.*

body clearance from 15 to 30 mL/min/1.73 m^2 was observed in association with an increase in gestational age. The increase in clearance was associated with a decrease in the terminal elimination half-life and no significant change in the volume of distribution.

More recently, several investigators have evaluated the disposition of vancomycin in 116 infants between 25 and 56 weeks of age (post conceptional) (see Table 15-2).[66-73] The observed mean steady-state volume of distribution, although lower than reported by Schaad et al., is quite similar among these studies (mean 0.55 L/kg; range 0.38 to 0.97). Significant correlations between CL_s and post-conceptional age have been reported by several investigators (see Figure 15-2).[68-72] Although multiple dosage guidelines based on postconceptional age have been proposed, additional studies will be needed to ascertain if any one of the guidelines is superior to the others.

The disposition of vancomycin has also been evaluated in older infants and in children up to 7.8 years of age.[38] A progressive increase in vancomycin clearance was observed with increasing age, reaching a peak in the 3.9 year age group. No further increase in vancomycin clearance was observed in children whose ages ranged from four to eight years. Terminal elimination half-lives range from 2.2 to 3 hours. Similarly, no significant increase or decrease in vancomycin distribution volume was noted with age. Hence, the clearance of vancomycin in pediatric patients appears to be related primarily to the degree of renal maturation, with no age-specific difference associated with the elimination of vancomycin when adjusted for renal function.

The pharmacokinetic characteristics of vancomycin in geriatric patients were evaluated by Cutler et al.[37] who reported that elderly males with normal renal function have a significantly longer elimination half-life (12.1 hours) than do young males with normal renal function (7.2 hours). They also reported significant changes in volume of distribution (0.93 L/kg old versus 0.64 L/kg young) and total body clearance (4.7 L/hr young versus 3.6 L/hr old), neither of which was correlated with creatinine clearance. Furthermore, no significant difference in protein binding of vancomycin was observed between the two patient groups. These investigators hypothesized that the difference in the pharmacokinetic parameters of vancomycin in the geriatric population may be a result of altered tissue binding and/or tissue distribution volume.

The investigations of Healy et al.[35] and Golper et al.[36] revealed a mean V_{ss} of 0.92 L/kg and 0.89 L/kg in patients in their 20s and 30s, respectively. These large V_{ss} values differ from the lower values observed in young patients by Culter et al.[37] and subsequently replicated by Rodvold et al.[17] and Rybak et al.[38] The marked variability in V_{ss} among these studies, which utilized similar study designs, suggests that age may not be the predominant factor which affects V_{ss}.

Effect of Dialysis on Vancomycin Pharmacokinetics

Numerous factors affect the removal of a drug by dialysis,[74] including physical-chemical properties of the drug, mechanical properties of the dialysis system, the blood flow and/or dialysate flow during the dialysis procedure, and the

Table 15-2. *Pharmacokinetics of Vancomycin in Acutely Ill Infants*

Population size	Age (weeks)[b]	t½ (hr)		V_{ss} (L/kg)	CL_s (mL/min/kg)	References
		α	β			
7	32	0.15	9.8	0.74	0.85	44
7	34	0.05	5.9	0.71	2.41	
7	40	0.25	6.7	0.69	2.05	
3	30	—	9.9	0.97	1.1	66
6	33	—	5.3	0.45	1.0	
5	32	—	7.0	0.48	0.90	67
6[c]	29	—	24.6	0.71	0.38	
14	32–41	—	4.9	0.48	1.33	68
6	40–62	—	3.0	0.38	1.70	
15	25–34	—	6.0	0.50	0.96	70
20	25–41	—	3.5–24	0.69	0.4–1.8	71
7	29–35	—	7.0	0.48	0.87	72
6	39–56	—	2.9	0.47	2.11	
17	30.5	—	5.5	0.48	1.12	73

[a] All values indicated are mean values.
[b] Postconceptional.
[c] These six infants had patent ductus arteriosus and received indomethacin therapy.

pharmacokinetic characteristics of the drug. The primary impact of dialysis procedures is to enhance clearance by providing an additional route for vancomycin elimination.

Lindholm et al.[20] reported in 1966 that vancomycin was dialyzable, but so slowly that the dosage schedule need not be modified for persons undergoing hemodialysis. These conclusions were drawn from studies *in vitro* based on a two-pool dialysis experimental technique. This method of assessment did not simulate the blood flow rate or the dialysate flows that are used during clinical dialysis procedures. Although several reports of vancomycin utilization in patients receiving chronic hemodialysis therapy were reported in the 1970s, none of these studies was designed to evaluate the impact of the dialysis procedure on vancomycin.[19,21,22]

In 1984, Salem et al.[75] evaluated the dialysis clearance of vancomycin in six subjects with end-stage renal disease. The dialysis clearance, calculated by quantitating the amount of vancomycin removed in the dialysate, exceeded the patient's total body clearance of vancomycin fivefold. However, only 7.6% (approximately 45 mg) of the vancomycin dose was removed during the dialysis procedure. These observations suggest that no vancomycin dosage supplementation would be required after a dialysis procedure in which a cuprophane filter membrane is used.

The development of new hemodialysis filter membranes and the clinical introduction of rapid high-efficiency and high-flux dialysis, as well as hemofiltration, during the late 1980s has necessitated a re-evaluation of the impact of dialysis on the disposition of many drugs.[76] Nine studies have evaluated the impact of dialysis filter selection on vancomycin clearance and disposition during hemodialysis[77-82] and hemofiltration (see Table 15-3).[83-86] Conventional cuprophane filters remove vancomycin to a minimal degree (clearance 9 to 10 mL/min, and less than 7% of a dose is removed during dialysis).[77,79] Cellulose acetate filters are slightly more efficient in clearing vancomycin from blood.[77,78,81] The high-flux filter membranes (polysulfone, polyamide, and polyacrylonitrile) when used in hemo-

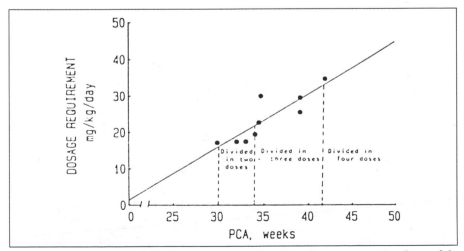

Figure 15-2. Vancomycin daily dosage nomogram based on the post conceptional age of the infant. Reproduced with permission from reference 191.

Table 15-3. Effect of Hemodialysis and Hemofiltration on Vancomycin Disposition

Investigator	Extra-corporeal perfusion method[a]	Number studied	Filter composition/SA[b]	Clearance (mL/min)	t½ (hr)
Bastani[77]	HD	5	Cellulose acetate/1.4 m²	21.1 (3.3)	19.0 (1.1)
			Polyacrylonitrile/1.0 m²	31.3 (2.2)	12.0 (1.5)
			Cuprophane/1.1 m²	8.9 (3.0)	38.5 (9.4)
Lanese[79]	HD	6	Cuprophane/0.8 m²	9.6 (2.9)	35.1 (11.2)
			Polysulfone F-40/0.65 m²	44.7 (6.7)	11.8 (5.6)
			Polysulfone F-60/1.2 m²	73.0 (5.0)	6.7 (1.0)
			Polysulfone F-80/1.9 m²	85.2 (7.0)	4.5 (−0.1)
Schoumcher[78]	HD	1	Cellulose acetate/0.9 m²	13.8	6.0
Pollard[80]	HD	6	Polysulfone F-80/1.9 m²	146 (23)	NR
Minakata[81]	HD	23	Cellulose diacetate/C-D 4000	53	NR
			Cellulose triacetate/FB-1504	21	NR
			Polymethylmethacrylate	72–116	NR
Matzke[83]	HF	5	Gambro polyamide	152.6 (21.5)	4.1 (1.2)
Rawer[86]	HF	4	Gambro HF88	61-157	NR
Lau[85]	CAVH	1	Polysulfone D-10	0.67–0.83	NR
Dupuis[84]	CAVH	1	Polysulfone D-10	62-6.6	45

[a] HD = Hemodialysis; HF = Hemofiltration; CAVH = Continuous arteriovenous hemofiltration; HD clearances are blood flow rate dependent; HF and CAVH clearances are ultrafiltrate flow rate dependent.
[b] SA = Surface area.

dialysis or hemofiltration delivery systems are far more efficient in clearing vancomycin from blood than cuprophan or cellulose acetate filters. Lanese et al.[79] demonstrated that the clearance of vancomycin increases and the half-life decreases as the surface area of the polysulfone filter increases (see Table 15-3). Utilization of the largest surface area filter produced clearances of 95.2 ± 7 mL/min, and the observed half-life during dialysis was 4.5 ± 0.1 hour. Pollard et al.[80] reported a vancomycin clearance of 146 ± 23 mL/min with the same filter evaluated by Lanese et al. Minakata et al.[81] reported that the clearances with a polymethylmethacrylate filter ranged from 72 to 116 mL/min. These observations suggest that vancomycin dosage regimens will need to be individualized for patients who are dialyzed with these new filters.

The use of continuous renal replacement therapies such as continuous arteriovenous hemofiltration (CAVH) and continuous arteriovenous hemodialysis (CAVHD) have increased dramatically in the 1980s.[87] Drug clearance by these modalities of therapy differs from that of hemodialysis in that the filter membranes are almost always of the high-flux type and the blood flow rates to the filter are markedly reduced. Thus, the clearances on a mL/min basis are less. However, since this therapy is continuous, the impact on vancomycin disposition can be significant. Individualization of therapy will be necessary due to the dependence of clearance on filter type,[88] ultrafiltrate flow rate, and duration of therapy.[87]

The disposition of vancomycin during intermittent and continuous ambulatory peritoneal dialysis procedures has been evaluated by several investigators.[89-98] The total body clearance of vancomycin is generally only minimally increased (1 to 2 mL/min) during intermittent peritoneal dialysis.[89-92] The peritoneal clearance values observed in continuous ambulatory peritoneal dialysis patients are also reasonably consistent and approximate 1 to 3 mL/min.[93-98] In the presence of active peritonitis, the peritoneal clearance may be moderately increased to 2 to 5 mL/min.[96-98] Due to the high degree of variability in peritoneal clearance, especially in patients with peritonitis, individualization of therapy is recommended. Current dosage guidelines for vancomycin in this patient population are 30 mg/kg administered intraperitoneally in one six-hour exchange every seven days.[99] Alternatively, vancomycin may be administered continuously utilizing a regimen of 15 to 25 mg/L in each dialysate exchange.

Vancomycin serum concentrations have been monitored in 38 patients who underwent open-heart surgery.[100-103] The primary objective of two of these studies was to ascertain whether vancomycin (15 mg/kg) maintained adequate anti-staphylococcal activity in the blood for the duration of the bypass procedure. The peak concentrations of vancomycin reported in these studies were consistent with previous reports.[11] Although multiple serum concentrations were determined by all three groups of investigators, only two groups reported the precise times at which these samples were obtained and performed an analysis of the pharmacokinetic data.[102,103] A marked redistribution phenomenon was observed by Klamerus et al.[102] at the time of reperfusion and rewarming; however, further studies are needed to confirm this observation. These data suggest cardiac bypass has no significant deleterious effect on the pharmacokinetics of vancomycin and that a 15 mg/kg dose administered intravenously one hour before bypass to adult and pediatric patients provides therapeutic serum concentrations for up to six hours.

PHARMACODYNAMICS

Clinical Response

Vancomycin inhibits cell wall synthesis by a mechanism that differs from those of the penicillins and cephalosporins.[104,105] It binds very tightly to peptides that contain D-alanyl-D-alanine at the free carboxyl end. It is postulated that the resultant steric hindrance prevents substrate binding to the enzyme peptidoglycan synthetase, thus blocking the synthesis of peptidoglycan. In addition to this effect on peptidoglycan synthetase, vancomycin also alters the permeability of the cell membrane. At clinically achievable concentrations, vancomycin is active against essentially all gram-positive organisms.[1,104,106,107,109]

The minimal bactericidal concentration (MBC) is not usually significantly different from the MIC. However, a significant discrepancy between MIC and MBC has been reported for some organisms, notably enterococci.[106,108,109] This characteristic of enterococci and streptococcal isolates is an important consideration in the use of vancomycin for treating endocarditis.[109] Synergy between vancomycin and aminoglycosides, rifampin or cephalosporins is variable.[106,107] Synergy testing *in vitro* should be done to document the efficacy of any proposed vancomycin combination.

Since MIC or MBC determinations indicate the relative degree of an organism's susceptibility to an antibiotic, they are useful in selecting the most effective and least toxic drug. However, MIC and MBC are of little value unless the clinician also knows what drug concentrations can be achieved in various body fluids. The inhibitory quotients (i.e., the ratio of the expected peak antibiotic serum concentration to the MIC of the organism) may aid the clinician in choosing the most appropriate antibiotic.[110] A further consideration in the selection of an antibiotic is the length of time following the administration of the dose that the serum concentration will exceed the MIC. By these criteria, vancomycin has exceptional peak activity against most gram-positive organisms and should show prolonged activity.

As early as 1961, a relationship between bactericidal levels of vancomycin and therapeutic efficacy was apparent. Louria et al.[111] observed a relationship between dose, serum concentration, and serum bactericidal (but not bacteriostatic) concentrations and clinical outcome. Only two of the eight patients they treated had serum bactericidal titers of less than 1:8, and neither subject showed evidence of significant reduction of staphylococci at the infected site. Sorrell et al.,[108] some 20 years later, reported similar observations. All eight patients whose staphylococcal isolates had an MBC of less than 32 mg/L were cured, contrasted with only three of the six patients with MBCs greater than 32. The MBC:MIC ratio appeared to be predictive of successful vancomycin therapy. All ten patients with MBC:MIC ratios of less than 32 were cured; whereas only one of four with higher ratios was cured. The authors concluded that there is not a simple relationship between *in vitro* tests and clinical response to vancomycin therapy,[108] but that tolerance (MBC:MIC >32) was associated with poor therapeutic response.

The relationship between antistaphylococcal activity and vancomycin serum concentrations has also been evaluated by Schaad et al.[44] and Lisby-Sutch and Nahata.[72] A bactericidal titer of 1:8 or greater was observed when the vancomycin serum concentration (peak or trough was not specified) exceeded 12 mg/L. The attainment of a bactericidal titer of 1:8 in these patients was associated with cure of the staphylococcal disease.[44] Lisby-Sutch and Nahata[72] reported that peak concentrations of 25 to 35 mg/L and troughs of 5 to 10 mg/L resulted in bactericidal titers of ≥1:8 and 1:2 to 1:8, respectively. Although these investigations in approximately 30 patients and two earlier reports represent a small database,[112,113] the attainment of peak titers of ≥1:8 and trough titers of 1:2 appear to correspond with a favorable clinical outcome. These reports suggest that individualization of vancomycin dosage may be required to provide optimum therapy.

Adverse Effects

Although the toxicity of vancomycin has been well publicized, the actual number of patients who have experienced adverse effects from the drug is quite small. Review of the literature from 1956 to 1992 revealed two major and six minor or rare adverse effects. Until the late 1980s, ototoxicity and nephrotoxicity had been reported in less than 30 and 60 patients, respectively, who were receiving or had recently received vancomycin at the time the adverse event was identified.[7,114] The incidence of both of these adverse effects does not appear to have changed significantly during the years in which vancomycin has been in clinical use. A clear picture of the potential toxicity of vancomycin is difficult to draw from early reports because many of these patients were receiving concomitant aminoglycoside therapy (frequently streptomycin or neomycin), had pre-existing renal disease, and/or had life-threatening staphylococcal infections with accompanying failure of a major organ (e.g., congestive heart failure). Furthermore, assessment of ototoxicity was not sensitive or specific, since most patients did not receive audiometric testing during the course of antibiotic therapy. Thus, these early studies would not have revealed a hearing loss unless it was a substantial one at lower frequencies (i.e., 2000 Hz to 3000 Hz).

Relating ototoxicity and/or nephrotoxicity to vancomycin serum concentrations is difficult because most reports do not specify how long after a dose the serum samples were taken. Despite this lack of precision, there was growing appreciation as early as 1960 that the ototoxicity of vancomycin was associated with serum concentrations in the range of 80 to 100 mg/L.[115]

Attempts to clarify the relationship between vancomycin serum concentration and ototoxicity have been less than conclusive. In seven of nine subjects in whom "ototoxicity" was reported, the maximum observed vancomycin concentrations ranged from 25 to 50 mg/L, and trough concentrations obtained just before the next scheduled dose ranged from 13 to 32 mg/L.[11,115-119] In these nine subjects, there was no clinical deficit in auditory acuity, and in five subjects tinnitus was reversible and high-frequency hearing loss (greater than 4000 Hz) either stabilized or improved with reduction in vancomycin dose. These data suggest a causal relationship between vancomycin administration, vancomycin serum concentration, and auditory toxicity. Furthermore, they suggest that ototoxicity may be reversed, if not prevented, by close monitoring of vancomycin serum concentrations. Unfortunately, it is not clear whether excessive peak or trough vancomycin serum concentrations are primarily related to the development of ototoxicity. In fact, some experts have concluded that vancomycin may only be "ototoxic" when it is administered with other ototoxic agents.[120,121]

Over 50% of the reported cases of vancomycin nephrotoxicity appeared in the medical literature within the first six years of the drug's discovery.[11,12,111,115,122–130] These early assessments of toxicity were generally not part of the prospective evaluation of the compound, but were observations that were made after completion of drug therapy. Despite this fact, concern about nephrotoxicity was one of the factors limiting the clinical use of vancomycin. It was not until the 1980s that systematic assessments were carried out to ascertain its nephrotoxic potential.

Several investigations of the nephrotoxic potential of vancomycin when it is administered alone or in combination with an aminoglycoside were reported between 1981 and 1992.[131–140] These data suggest that vancomycin has some potential for causing nephrotoxicity (range 5% to 15%). In contrast, when vancomycin was administered concomitantly with an aminoglycoside to adults, the incidence of nephrotoxicity increased in some, but not all, studies (range 22% to 35%).[131,136–138] Those patients who developed nephrotoxicity more commonly had trough vancomycin concentrations which exceeded 10 mg/L before the rise in serum creatinine levels. Furthermore, these elevated serum creatinine levels generally returned to baseline following dosage adjustment. Thus, vancomycin trough concentrations greater than 10 mg/L should be avoided whenever possible. Furthermore, patients with neutropenia, peritonitis, increased age, liver disease, concurrent amphotericin B therapy and those of the male gender appear to have an increased risk of developing nephrotoxicity.[138]

Although Dean et al.[132] reported an increased incidence of nephrotoxicity in pediatric patients who received vancomycin in combination with an aminoglycoside, the serum concentrations of the aminoglycoside were not reported. Swinney et al.[140] and Nahata,[141] however, have suggested that combination therapy, at least in pediatric patients, may not result in a change in the incidence of nephrotoxicity if the serum concentrations of the aminoglycoside are maintained within the therapeutic range.

The early formulations of vancomycin were associated with a high incidence of chemical thrombophlebitis, chills, and fever.[7] With elimination of the impurities, solutions of the drug became clear and colorless, and side effects were less frequent. The incidence of phlebitis decreased from a rate of 50% during the 1950s to approximately 10% during the 1980s.[7] Intravenous administration of vancomycin may result in a histamine-like reaction characterized by flushing, tingling, pruritus, tachycardia, and an erythematous macular rash involving the face, neck, upper trunk, back, and arms with sparing of the rest of the body. Systemic arterial hypotension or shock has also been noted. This "red neck syndrome" which appears to be associated with bolus or rapid intravenous infusion, was initially described in the 1950s.[142]

The adverse reaction is mediated in part by histamine release and a correlation between the area under the histamine concentration-time curve and severity of the reaction has been observed in some,[34,143,144] but not all, investigations.[145] The incidence of this syndrome in healthy volunteers who received 1 gm of vancomycin as a one hour intravenous infusion was 80% to 95%.[34,143-147] The incidence of this reaction in patients has been reported to be 24% and 47% in those who were and were not receiving concomitant antihistamines.[148] Reduction in the administration rate of vancomycin to 15 mg/min in patients[7,149] and from approximately 15 mg/min to 7.5 mg/min in volunteers reduces the frequency and the severity of this syndrome.[34]

Maculopapular erythematous skin rashes have been observed in 2% to 6.5% of patients treated with vancomycin.[7] The incidence of rash was highest during the 1950s and appears to have stabilized during the 1970s and 1980s to a rate of approximately 2% to 3%. Transient neutropenia and drug-induced fever have also been reported as complications of vancomycin therapy. That 13 of the 17 reported cases of vancomycin drug fever occurred during the 1950s suggests that it may have been related to impurities present in the early formulations. By contrast, the number of reported cases of neutropenia increased dramatically during the 1970s and 1980s. The development of neutropenia has been reported to be both dose- and time-dependent. Neftel et al. reported an incidence of 17% in patients treated for 14 or more days.[150] Furthermore, significantly higher daily doses were utilized in those patients who developed neutropenia.

Vancomycin appears to be a relatively safe antistaphylococcal antibiotic with a low incidence of allergic reactions. The most common side effect currently associated with vancomycin use is the histamine-like reaction following rapid administration, which can be minimized by slow infusion of the drug. Although ototoxicity and nephrotoxicity have been associated with vancomycin therapy, the incidence is generally less than 2% and 5%, respectively. Further evaluation will be required to identify the mechanism responsible for the apparent increased incidence of nephrotoxicity in patients who receive concomitant aminoglycoside and vancomycin therapy.

CLINICAL APPLICATION OF PHARMACOKINETIC DATA

The unpredictability with which peak and trough serum vancomycin concentrations are attained may be related to inherent interpatient variability in drug disposition as well as the use of different infusion times,[34,35,149] altered distribution of the drug,[37] altered renal function,[14-18] and other variables such as age[37,44,66-73] and concomitant disease states.[61-65] In view of the complex nature of these variables and the potential for multiple interactions within a given patient, it seems impractical to rely on nomograms based on renal function alone.

In addition to these pharmacokinetic factors, the specific infectious and clinical status of the patient must be considered when one is designing the initial dosing regimen. Variables to be considered include the site of infection, the severity of the infection, and the suspected pathogen. Since median minimal inhibitory concentrations for vancomycin-susceptible gram-positive organisms vary by more than fivefold,[7] and the vancomycin body fluid-to-serum concentration ratio varies from 4 to 4000,[7] individualization of vancomycin dosing may be required.

Dosing Considerations

Several dosage initiation methods were proposed in the 1980s.[14,15,17,151,152] The Moellering et al.[14] dosing nomogram and the Brown and Mauro[151] dosing chart are designed to yield average serum concentrations of 15 mg/L. The nomogram of Matzke et al.[15] is designed to attain concentrations one hour after the end of the infusion of 30 mg/L (range 25 to 35 mg/L) and 7.5 mg/L (range 5 to 10 mg/L) at the end of the dosing interval. The Lake and Peterson dosing method is designed to attain concentrations 15 minutes after the end of the infusion of 20 to 30 mg/L and 5 to 10 mg/L at the end of the dosing interval.[152] The accuracy with which the desired serum concentrations are attained by four of these methods has been prospectively evaluated.[153–155]

Rybak and Boike[153] evaluated the predictive accuracy of the Moellering et al., Matzke et al., and an individualized method of vancomycin dosage adjustment in 50 patients. Peak and trough concentrations were significantly underpredicted by the Moellering method. The Matzke et al. method also significantly under-predicted peak concentrations (22.7 ± 6.5 versus 30.3 ± 5.7 mg/L). However, no significant difference in trough concentrations were observed.

Zokufa et al.[154] evaluated three of these methods in 37 patients with various degrees of renal function. The frequency with which the desired peak or trough concentrations were attained varied from 3% to 40%. However, less than 20% of patients would have achieved the peak and trough concentrations recommended by the individual dosing method. They concluded that no method performed satisfactorily and that the use of these methods to derive the initial dosage regimen is only reasonable if serum concentrations are prospectively monitored to adjust the dosage regimen further.

Dosing recommendations for the initiation of vancomycin therapy in pediatric patients were not well defined in the early 1980s.[149] Schaad et al.[44,47] reported excellent agreement between desired and actual serum concentrations when they used their age-specific guidelines. Alpert et al.,[156] however, using the same dosing guidelines, found that 30% to 70% of peak vancomycin concentrations and 25% to 53% of trough concentrations exceeded the desired maximum values of 30 mg/L and 12 mg/L, respectively. Subsequent investigations have confirmed the exces-siveness of these dosing guidelines.[70–72] Currently, initial dosage recommendations for infants can be derived from the relationship between postconception age and vancomycin clearance (see Figure 15-2).[71,72] Dosage in older children should be guided by the child's renal function.

Initial assessment of the patient's renal function, the type and site of infection, and other risk factors should result in an improved approach to initial dosing of vancomycin. Adults with impaired renal function, elderly patients, morbidly obese patients and pediatric patients, may derive additional benefit from an individualized dosing approach based on serum concentrations.

Although the pharmacokinetic profile of vancomycin is best described by a two- or three-compartment model, the collection of a sufficient number of serum concentrations to perform these characterizations has not been practical or cost-justified in routine clinical practice. Therefore, an approach similar to that used for the aminoglycoside antibiotics was proposed in the 1970s and utilized during most of the 1980s (see Figure 15-3).

This approach for individualization of vancomycin therapy begins with the calculation of a loading dose on the basis of: 1) the patient's total body weight (kg); 2) the appropriate volume of distribution estimate from population data (L/kg); 3) the desired peak serum concentration (mg/L); and 4) an estimate of the patient's terminal elimination rate constant.

The desired peak and trough serum concentrations for the individual patient will depend on the infection site and organism. Peak concentrations should be about eight times the MIC. Trough concentrations of one to two times the MIC should also be adequate. The elimination rate constant of vancomycin in adults can be estimated from the relationship between creatinine clearance and the terminal elimination rate constant appropriate for the patient population.[15,17,63,157] In some subjects with serum creatinine levels of less than 1 mg/dL, the calculated creatinine clearance may be exceedingly high. In these subjects, use of 120 mL/min as a conservative estimate of creatinine clearance is recommended as the basis for initial dosing until vancomycin clearance can be measured. The terminal elimination rate constant can be approximated for infants as described previously.[72]

Blood samples for measuring vancomycin serum concentrations after an intravenous infusion should be designed to encompass one elimination half-life, whenever possible. To determine the blood sampling times, one may use an estimate of the patient's creatinine clearance or use population-average kinetic parameters to obtain a projection of the patient's elimination half-life.

The question of what constitutes a "peak" vancomycin concentration, and its relationship to efficacy and toxicity remains controversial. The true peak concentration would be expected to occur immediately at the end of the intravenous infusion. Data on toxicity and efficacy of vancomycin, however, have been based primarily on concentrations determined from immediately after, to one hour after, bolus administration, or 15 minutes to two hours after an intravenous infusion. This variability in the times at which "peak" concentrations have been obtained and the expected alteration in peak concentrations when the dose is administered over a different time interval, make interpretation of the relationship between toxicity and/or efficacy and serum concentration extremely difficult. (See Figures 15-4a and 15-4b.)

In the clinical setting, vancomycin is usually monitored in a manner similar to that used for the aminoglycosides. Peak vancomycin concentrations, for the purpose of clinical pharmacokinetic monitoring and for the establishment of toxicity and efficacy correlations, should be determined 15 minutes to one hour

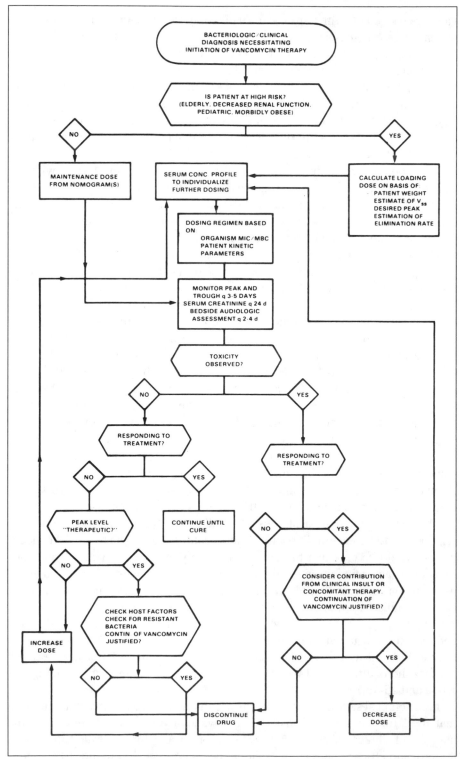

Figure 15-3. *Algorithm for the application of pharmacokinetics to vancomycin therapy.*

after the end of the intravenous infusion, depending on the desired therapeutic goal.[14,15,17,151,152] Trough concentrations should be obtained just before or within one hour of the next scheduled dose.

The serum concentration-time data can be analyzed by linear or nonlinear regression analysis to calculate the patient's vancomycin terminal elimination rate

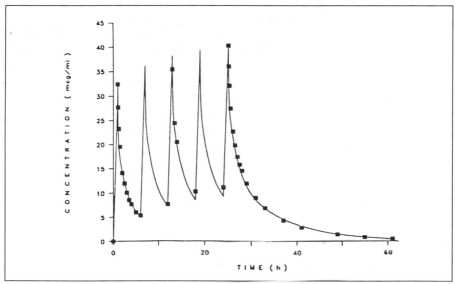

Figure 15-4a. *Mean observed (■) and three-compartmental computer predicted (-) concentrations of vancomycin in serum at a dosage of 500 mg every 6 hours. Reproduced with permission from reference 35.*

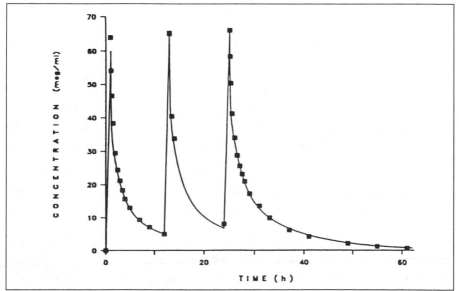

Figure 15-4b. *Mean observed (■) and three-compartmental computer predicted (-) concentrations of vancomycin in serum at a dosage of 1000 mg every 12 hours. Reproduced with permission from reference 35.*

constant. The steady-state volume of distribution can then be estimated either by model-independent techniques[158] or by standard one-compartment first-order equations.[159] Once the patient's pharmacokinetic parameters for vancomycin have been calculated, the most appropriate dose and dosage interval to achieve the desired serum concentrations can be determined using the method advocated by Sawchuk and Zaske[159] for aminoglycosides. The limitations and potential errors assumed with this approach have been discussed by Ackerman et al.[160]

Alternatively, a monoexponential Bayesian method could be utilized to guide the initiation of therapy and to evaluate vancomycin serum concentration time data. Several studies have shown that this method yields less biased and at least as precise serum concentration predictions as the individualized approach proposed by Sawchuk and Zaske while requiring less serum concentration-time data.[161–163] Several commercially available kinetic computer programs now utilize this method of data analysis as their primary or sole technique of data analysis.

Recently, biexponential Bayesian methods have been developed and evaluated.[164–166] A two-compartment Bayesian program was superior to the one-compartment program when population parameters and non-steady-state feedback concentrations were analyzed.[165] However, no difference in the two programs was evident when steady-state concentrations were used to predict future steady-state concentrations. The availability of the biexponential Bayesian method allows the kineticist the first opportunity to utilize this more complex pharmacokinetic model that better describes the drugs' disposition in the clinical setting.[166] A Bayesian method of data analysis and preferably a biexponential model would thus appear to be optimal for use in most clinical settings, particularly early in the course of therapy.

For patients with stable renal function, peak and trough vancomycin serum concentrations should be determined when the patient has reached steady state on the new dosing schedule. If the serum concentrations are inconsistent with the desired values, a new dosing regimen should be designed. This dosage regimen should then be re-evaluated when the patient has reached steady state.

For patients with fluctuating renal function, a pre-dose serum concentration and a series of post-dose serum concentrations should be obtained early during the course of therapy. These values should be used to re-estimate the patient's pharmacokinetic parameters. Appropriate modifications of the patient's dosage regimen may then be made to maintain peak and trough serum concentrations within the desired ranges.

Intermittent peritoneal dialysis[89–92] and hemodialysis[75,77,79] with a cuprophane filter minimally alters the pharmacokinetics of vancomycin. Although the total body clearance of vancomycin is enhanced during the time of the dialysis procedure, the amount of vancomycin removed is minimal. However, the effect of continuous ambulatory peritoneal dialysis[93–98] and rapid high efficiency and high flux dialysis[77–81] or hemofiltration[82–85] on the pharmacokinetics of vancomycin may be significant. Guidelines for the initiation of vancomycin therapy in CAPD patients have been proposed and may be used for initial dosing recommendations.[99] However, since significant variability has been reported in the dialysis clearance, the elimination half-life, and steady-state volume of distribution of vancomycin, doses that are individualized on the basis of serum concentration measurements are recommended for all dialysis patients.

Monitoring for Adverse Effects

Nephrotoxicity and ototoxicity are serious complications of vancomycin administration in a small number of patients. These few sensitive patients appear to be clinically indistinguishable from the majority who tolerate vancomycin without toxic reactions. Present monitoring techniques (i.e., serial serum concentration measurements, serum creatinine measurements, and hearing evaluations) can only confirm that damage has already occurred. The goal in monitoring vancomycin therapy is to develop sensitive methods to detect early renal or auditory damage. Methods for monitoring aminoglycoside antibiotics may prove useful in the assessment of vancomycin therapy. A more complete discussion of the tools used to monitor the pharmacologic effects is presented in the Chapter 14: Aminoglycosides.

ANALYTICAL METHODS

Six assay methods are available for determining vancomycin concentrations in biologic fluids. They include the microbial assay,[167–169] radioimmunoassay (RIA),[170,171] fluorescence polarization immunoassay (FPI),[172–177,179,180] fluorescence immunoassay (FIA),[177] enzyme multiplied immunoassay technique (EMIT),[178–180] and high-performance liquid chromatography (HPLC).[180–186] HPLC is the only chemical method available for determining vancomycin concentrations. The relative advantages and disadvantages of the available methods are summarized in Table 15-4. Although the microbiologic plate assays require minimal capital investment and can be completed at a low cost, they are subject to interferences from other antimicrobials and require an extended period of time to perform. Radioimmunoassay can be performed in high volume and is rapid, sensitive, and accurate. It may not, however, be economical for small laboratories because of the substantial initial investment required for equipment and reagents. An extension of fluorescence polarization immunoassay technology for the measurement of vancomycin concentrations has been reported.[174] This method can be performed in high volume, and it is rapid, sensitive, and extremely accurate. Like radioimmunoassay, it may not be economical for small laboratories, although the instrument is capable of running many other drug assays.

Good agreement between bioassay, radioimmunoassay, and fluorescence polarization immunoassay has been demonstrated by several independent investigators.[172,173,175–177] During the 1980s fluorescence polarization immunoassay became the technique most commonly used in clinical laboratories. As a fully automated assay, it eliminates much of the variability in test results associated with manual pipetting of samples and the reading and calculation of results. Furthermore, sample turnaround time is less than five minutes. The stability of the standard curve, which exceeds one month, eliminates the need for standardization before

Table 15-4. *Comparison of the Relative Advantages and Disadvantages of the Various Vancomycin Assay Methods*

Analytical method	Specificity[a]	Limit of sensitivity (mg/L)	Assayable samples				Minimum sample volume required in microliters	Coefficient of variation		Speed[a]		Cost[a]		Preference[a]		References
			Serum	Plasma	Urine	Tissue		Within run	Between run	1–10 Samples	10–100 Samples	Reagent and tech	Equipment	Clinical services	Research	
Microbiological																
A. *Bacillus subtilis*	4	0.8	Yes	—[b]	—	—	80	<10	<10	3	3	1	1	3	4	167–169
B. Multiresistant str.	3	0.8	Yes	—	—	—	50–80	<10	≤25	4	4	1	1	3	4	
Radioimmunoassay																
A. I^{125}	2	1.0[c]	Yes	Yes	Yes	Yes	100	9.5	12.2	2	1	3	3	2	2	170–171
B. H^{3}	2	0.04–0.1	Yes	Yes	Yes	Yes	50–100	—	—	2						
High performance liquid chromatography	1	2–5	Yes	ND[d]	ND	ND	100–500	2.8–3.4	3.1–5.9	2	3	2	2	4	1	181–186
Fluorescence polarization immunoassay	2	0.6	Yes	Yes	Yes	Yes	50	1.5–2.5	2.3–4.6	1	2	4	4	1	3	172–177, 179, 180
Fluorescence immunoassay	2	ND	Yes	ND	ND	ND	100	8.9–14.5	12.2–16.2	2	1	3	2	4	4	177
Enzyme multiplied immunoassay	1	0.5	Yes	Yes	Yes	Yes	50–100	4.1–6.9	4.1–6.9	1	2	3	2	1	1	178–180

[a] Arbitrary performance ranking scale of 1 (best, fastest, least costly) to 4 (worst, slowest, most expensive).
[b] Requires standard curve in fluid to be assayed.
[c] Enhanced sensitivity may be possible in some situations; however, this value reflects usual clinical environment.
[d] No data regarding use available.

each run and, thereby, considerably reduces the cost associated with emergency and routine analyses. The primary disadvantage of this technique is its nonspecificity, which results in an overestimation of true vancomycin concentrations when vancomycin degradation products are present.[179,180] The degree of overestimation in clinical specimens from patients with renal insufficiency has ranged from 13% to 53%.[180,187] *In vitro* evaluations have indicated that the degree of overestimation increases over time from less than 10% at two days to greater than 200% at 15 days.[187,188] Thus, vancomycin concentrations measured by this technique in patients with renal insufficiency should be interpreted with caution.

Results of fluorescence immunoassay and bioassay in the analysis of reference samples have correlated well.[177] However, the precision of the former method is inferior to that of other established methods, and the within-run coefficient of variation exceeds 10%. Thus, in its present state, the fluorescence immunoassay cannot be recommended for clinical use.

Several HPLC methods that quantify vancomycin concentrations in serum have been described.[180–186] Although HPLC methods are more specific, they are not nearly as sensitive as the fluorescence polarization immunoassay. In addition, the HPLC assays require relatively large sample volumes and have not been evaluated for several common biologic fluids. Despite these shortcomings, comparative studies have indicated excellent correlations between vancomycin serum concentrations determined by HPLC and the biologic techniques.[175,177,180,182] HPLC techniques provide a relatively inexpensive, timely, and accurate means of assessing vancomycin therapy, and can be primarily recommended for research use. Routine use in clinical service laboratories is also an option, although one of the immunoassays may be preferable.

Either the enzyme multiplied immunoassay technique or the fluorescence polarization immunoassay is recommended for established and high-volume clinical services. Both techniques have high-volume capacities, rapid turnaround times, and are extremely specific. The EMIT, however, may be preferred because of its superior specificity, particularly in patients with renal insufficiency.[179,180,187,188] Regardless of which analytical technique is used, the clinical pharmacokineticist should have a thorough understanding of the analytical technique and employ rigid quality control to ensure that accurate results are obtained.

PROSPECTUS

The clinical application of vancomycin has markedly increased in recent years and, barring unforeseen developments, it will probably continue. The evolving use of serum concentrations to guide therapy has been enhanced by the recent availability of simple, yet rapid and specific analytical techniques.

The kinetic profile of vancomycin has been rigorously characterized in infants and adults with normal renal function and various degrees of renal insufficiency during the last decade. However, expansion of clinical pharmacokinetic monitoring services will probably not occur until some critical issues are resolved. For example, the kinetics of vancomycin in pediatric and geriatric patients is not well characterized. In addition to a more complete characterization of the pharmacokinetics of vancomycin in patients with altered physiologic and disease states, a clearer picture is needed of the correlation between dose, serum concentration, and serum bactericidal activity and efficacy or toxicity. These assessments are crucial to the development of more rational approaches to the use of vancomycin.

REFERENCES

1. McCormick MH et al. Vancomycin, a new antibiotic. I. Chemical and biologic properties. Antibiotic Ann. 1955;606–11.
2. Ziegler DW et al. Vancomycin, a new antibiotic. II. *In vitro* antibacterial studies. Antibiot Ann. 1955–1956. 1956;612–18.
3. Griffith RS, Peck FB. Vancomycin, a new antibiotic. III. Preliminary clinical and laboratory studies. Antibiot Ann. 1956;619–22.
4. Griffith RS. Introduction to vancomycin. Rev Infect Dis. 1981;3:S200–204.
5. McHenry MC, Gavan TL. Vancomycin. Pediatr Clin North Am. 1983;30:31–47.
6. Anon. New preparations of vancomycin. The Med Letter. 1986;28:121–2.
7. Matzke GR. Vancomycin. In: Evans WE et al., eds. Applied Pharmacokinetics: Principles of Therapeutic Drug Monitoring. 2nd ed. Vancouver. Applied Therapeutics; 1986:399.
8. Cook FV, Farrar WE. Vancomycin revisited. Ann Intern Med. 1978;88:813–18.
9. Bartlett JG. Treatment of antibiotic-associated pseudomembranous colitis. Rev Infect Dis. 1984;6:S235–41.
10. Esposito AL, Gleckman RA. Vancomycin: a second look. JAMA. 1977;238:1756–757.
11. Geraci JE et al. Some laboratory and clinical experiences with a new antibiotic, vancomycin. Antibiotic Ann. 1957;90–106.
12. Kirby WMM, Divelbiss CL. Vancomycin: clinical and laboratory studies. Antibiot Ann. 1956–1957. 1957:107–17.
13. Nielsen HE et al. Renal excretion of vancomycin in kidney disease. Acta Med Scand. 1975;197:261–64.
14. Moellering RC et al. Vancomycin therapy in patients with impaired renal function: a nomogram for dosage. Ann Intern Med. 1981;94:343–46.
15. Matzke GR et al. Pharmacokinetics of vancomycin in patients with various degrees of renal function. Antimicrob Agents Chemother. 1984;25:433–37.
16. Rotschafer JC et al. Pharmacokinetics of vancomycin: observations in 28 patients and dosage recommendations. Antimicrob Agents Chemother. 1982;22:391–94.
17. Rodvold KA et al. Vancomycin pharmacokinetics in patients with various degrees of renal function. Antimicrobial Agents Chemother. 1988;32:848.
18. Dunn G et al. Vancomycin pharmacokinetics in end stage renal disease patients on hemodialysis. Paper presented to the 19th Annual ASHP Midyear Clinical Meeting. Dallas, TX: 1984 December.
19. Morris AJ, Bilinskey RT. Prevention of staphylococcal infections by continuous vancomycin prophylaxis. Am J Med Sci. 1971;262:87–92.
20. Lindholm DD, Murray JS. Persistence of vancomycin in the blood during renal failure and its treatment by hemodialysis. N Engl J Med. 1966;274:1047–51.
21. Eykyn S et al. Vancomycin for staphylococcal shunt site infections in patients on regular haemodialysis. Br Med J. 1970;3:80–2.
22. Barcenas CG et al. Staphylococcal sepsis in patients on chronic hemodialysis regimens. Intravenous treatment with vancomycin given once weekly. Arch Inter Med. 1976;136:1131–134.
23. Bierman MH et al. Vancomycin therapy for serious staphylococcal infections in chronic hemodialysis patients. J Dialysis. 1980;4:179–84.
24. Lam FY et al. Pharmacokinetics of vancomycin in chronic renal failure. Kidney Int. 1981;19:152. Abstract.
25. Comstock TJ et al. Multicompartment vancomycin (V) kinetics in patients with end-stage renal disease (ESRD). Clin Pharmacol Ther. 1988;43:172. Abstract.

26. Tan CC et al. Pharmacokinetics of intravenous vancomycin in patients with end-stage renal failure. Ther Drug Monit. 1990;12:29.

27. Griffith RS. Vancomycin: continued clinical studies. Antibiot Ann. 1956–1957. 1957;118–22.

28. Bryan CS, White WL. Safety of oral vancomycin in functionally anephric patients. Antimicrob Agents Chemother. 1978;14:634–35.

29. Thompson CM et al. Absorption of oral vancomycin—possible associated toxicity. Int J Pediatr Nephrol. 1983;4:1–4.

30. Spitzer PG, Eliopoulos GM. Systemic absorption of enteral vancomycin in a patient with pseudomembranous colitis. Ann Intern Med. 1984;100:533–34.

31. Dudley MN et al. Absorption of vancomycin. Ann Intern Med. 1984;101:144.

32. Tedesco F et al. Oral vancomycin for antibiotic-associated pseudomembranous colitis. Lancet. 1978;2:226–28.

33. Matzke GR et al. Systemic absorption of oral vancomycin in patients with renal insufficiency and antibiotic-associated colitis. Am J Kid Dis. 1987;9:422.

34. Healy DP et al. Vancomycin-induced histamine release and "red man syndrome": comparison of 1- and 2-hour infusions. Antimicrob Agents Chemother. 1990;34:550.

35. Healy DP et al. Comparison of steady-state pharmacokinetics of two dosage regimens of vancomyin in normal volunteers. Antimicrob Agents Chemother. 1987;31:393.

36. Golper TA et al. Vancomycin pharmacokinetics, renal handling, and nonrenal clearance in normal human subjects. Clin Pharmacol Ther. 1988;43:565.

37. Culter NR et al. Vancomycin disposition: the importance of age. Clin Pharmacol Ther. 1984;36:803–10.

38. Rybak MJ et al. Vancomycin pharmacokinetics in burn patients and intravenous drug abusers Antimicrobial Agents Chemother. 1990;34:792.

39. Ackerman RP et al. Vancomycin serum protein binding determination by ultrafiltration. Drug Intell Clin Pharm. 1988;22:300.

40. May DG et al. Vancomycin entry into lung lymph in sheep. Antimicrob Agents Chemother. 1987;31:1689.

41. Graziani AL et al. Vancomycin concentrations in infected and noninfected human bone. Antimicrob Agents Chemother. 1988;32:1320.

42. Daschner FD et al. Pharmacokinetics of vancomycin in serum and tissue of patients undergoing open-heart surgery. J Antimicrob Chemother. 1987;19:359.

43. Moellering RC et al. Pharmacokinetics of vancomycin in normal subjects and in patients with reduced renal function. Rev Infect Dis. 1981;3:S230–235.

44. Schaad UB et al. Clinical pharmacology and efficacy of vancomycin in pediatric patients. J Pediatr. 1980;96:119–126.

45. Sutherland GE et al. Sterilization of ommaya reservoir by instillation of vancomycin. Am J Med. 1981;71:1068–70.

46. Congeni BL et al. Kinetics of vancomycin (V) after intraventricular and intravenous administration. Pediatr Res. 1979;13:459. Abstract.

47. Schaad UB et al. Pharmacology and efficacy of vancomycin for staphylococcal infections in children. Rev Infect Dis. 1981;3:S282–288.

48. Fan-Harvard et al. Pharmacokinetics and cerebrospinal fluid (CSF) concentrations of vancomycin in pediatric patients undergoing CSF shunt placement. Chemotherapy. 1990;36:103–8.

49. Chan GLC, Joy ME. Vancomycin in the treatment of central nervous system infections. Drug Intell Clin Pharm. 1988;22:486–88.

50. Kay EA et al. Disposition of intrathecal vancomycin. Drug Intell Clin Pharm. 1988;22:267–68. Letter.

51. Arroyo JC, Quindlen EA. Accumulation of vancomycin after intraventricular infusions. South Med J. 1983;76:1554–555.

52. Young EJ et al. Staphylococcal ventriculitis treated with vancomycin. South Med J. 1981;74:1041–42.

53. Swayne et al. Intraventricular vancomycin for treatment of shunt-associated ventriculitis. J Antimicrob Chem. 1987;19:249–53.

54. Golledge CL, Mckenzie T. Monitoring vancomycin for treatment concentrations in CSF after intraventricular administration. J Antimicrob Chem. 1988;20:283–92.
55. Bayston R. Intraventricular vancomycin for treatment of shunt-associated ventriculitis. J Antimicrob Chem. 1987;20:283–92.
56. Reesor C et al. Kinetics of intraventricular vancomycin in infections of cerebrospinal fluid shunts. J Infect Dis. 1988;158:1142–143.
57. Pau AK et al. Intraventricular vancomycin: observations of tolerance and pharmacokinetics in two infants with ventricular shunt infections. Ped Infect Dis. 1986;5:93–6.
58. Younger JJ et al. Failure of single-dose intraventricular vancomycin for cerebrospinal fluid shunt surgery prophylaxis. Ped Infect Dis. 1987;6:212–13.
59. Lee CC et al. Vancomycin, a new antibiotic. V. Distribution, excretion and renal clearance. Antibiot Ann. 1956–1957. 1957;82–8.
60. Brown N et al. Effects of hepatic function on vancomycin clinical pharmacology. Antimicrob Agents Chemother. 1983;23:603–9.
61. Narang PK et al. Vancomycin multiple-dose kinetics in critically ill patients. Clin Pharmacol Ther. 1985;37:216. Abstract.
62. Marcias WL et al. Vancomycin pharmacokinetics in acute renal failure: preservation of nonrenal clearance. Clin Pharmacol Ther. 1991;50:688.
63. Garrelts JC, Peterie JD. Altered vancomycin dose vs. serum concentration relationship in burn patients. Clin Pharmacol Ther. 1988;44:9.
64. Brater DC et al. Vancomycin elimination in patients with burn injury. Clin Pharmacol Ther. 1986;39:631.
65. Garaud JJ et al. Vancomycin pharmacokinetics in critically ill patients. J Antimicrob Chemother. 1984;14(Suppl.):53.
66. Gross JR et al. Vancomycin pharmacokinetics in premature infants. Pediatr Pharmacol. 1985;5:17.
67. Spivey JM, Gal P. Vancomycin pharmacokinetics in neonates. Am J Dis Child. 1986;140:859.
68. Naqvi SH et al. Vancomycin pharmacokinetics in small, seriously ill infants. Am J Dis Child. 1986;140:107.
69. Schaible DH et al. Vancomycin pharmacokinetics in infants: relationships to indices of maturation. Ped Infect Dis. 1986;5:304–8.
70. Reed MD et al. The clinical pharmacology of vancomycin in seriously ill preterm infants. Pediatr Res. 1987;22:360–3.
71. James A et al. Vancomycin pharmacokinetics and dose recommendations for preterm infants. Antimicrobial Agents Chemother. 1987;31:52.
72. Lisby-Sutch SM, Nahata MC. Dosage guidelines for the use of vancomycin based on its pharmacokinetics in infants. Eur J Clin Pharmacol. 1988;35:637.
73. Kildoo C et al. Vancomycin kinetics in infants: relationship to gestational age (GA), chronological age (CA) and renal function. Clinical Research. 1988;36:202a. Abstract.
74. Lee CC, Marbury TC. Drug therapy in patients undergoing haemodialysis clinical pharmacokinetic considerations. Clin Pharmacokinet. 1984;9:42–66.
75. Salem NG et al. Clearance of vancomycin by hemodialysis. 30th Annual Meeting, American Society for Artificial Internal Organs. Washington, DC: 1984.
76. Vlchek DL. Staying tuned into the high-tech world. Dial Transplant. 1989;18:306.
77. Bastani B et al. In vivo comparison of three different hemodialysis membranes for vancomycin clearance; cuprophan, cellulose acetate, and polyacrylonitrile. Dial Transplant. 1988;17:527.
78. Schoumacher R et al. Enhanced clearance of vancomycin by hemodialysis in a child. Pediatr Nephrol. 1989;3:83.
79. Lanese DM et al. Markedly increased clearance of vancomycin during hemodialysis using polysulfone dialyzers. Kidney Int. 1989;35:1409.
80. Pollard TA et al. Impact of vancomycin (Vanc) redistribution on dosing recommendations following high flux hemodialysis. J Am Soc Nephrology. 1991;2:345. Abstract.
81. Minakata T et al. Comparison of vancomycin (VCM) clearance during HD between high flux and conventional membranes. J Am Soc Nephrology. 1991;2:339. Abstract.

82. Quale JM et al. Effects of high flux dialyzers on vancomycin pharmacokinetics. Presented at the 31st Interscience Conference on Antimicrobial Agents and Chemotherapy. Chicago, IL. 1991. Abstract 1299.

83. Matzke GR et al. Vancomycin disposition during continuous arteriovenous hemofiltration. Clin Pharmacol Ther. 1986;40:425.

84. Dupuis RE et al. Vancomycin disposition during continuous arteriovenous hemofiltration. Clin Pharm. 1989;8:371.

85. Lau AH, John E. Vancomycin removal by continuous arteriovenous hemofiltration (CAVH). Clin Pharmacol Ther. 1988;43:154. Abstract.

86. Rawer P, Seim KE. Elimination of vancomycin during hemofiltration. Eur J Clin Microbial Infection Dis. 1989;8:529.

87. Bickley SK. Drug dosing during continuous arteriovenous hemofiltration. Clin Pharm. 1988;7:198.

88. Kronfol NO et al. Effect of CAVH membrane types on drug-sieving coefficients and clearances. Trans Am Soc Artif Intern Organs. 1986;32:85.

89. Nielsen HE et al. Peritoneal transport of vancomycin during peritoneal dialysis. Nephron. 1979;24:274–77.

90. Ayus JC et al. Peritoneal clearance and total body elimination of vancomycin during chronic intermittent peritoneal dialysis. Clin Nephrol. 1979;11:129–32.

91. Glew RH et al. Vancomycin pharmacokinetics in patients undergoing chronic intermittent peritoneal dialysis. Int J Clin Pharmacol Ther Toxicol. 1982;20:559–63.

92. Magera BE et al. Vancomycin pharmacokinetics in patients with peritonitis on peritoneal dialysis. Antimicrob Agents Chemother. 1983;23:710–14.

93. Pancorbo S, Comty C. Peritoneal transport of vancomycin in 4 patients undergoing continuous ambulatory peritoneal dialysis. Nephron. 1982;31:37–9.

94. Bunke CM et al. Vancomycin kinetics during continuous ambulatory peritoneal dialysis. Clin Pharmacol Ther. 1983;34:631–37.

95. Blevins RD et al. Pharmacokinetics of vancomycin in patients undergoing continuous ambulatory peritoneal dialysis. Antimicrob Agents Chemother. 1984;25:603–6.

96. Morse GD et al. Comparative study of intraperitoneal and intravenous vancomycin pharmacokinetics during continuous ambulatory peritoneal dialysis. Antimicrob Agents Chemother. 1987;31:173.

97. Harford AM et al. Vancomycin pharmacokinetics in continuous ambulatory peritoneal dialysis patients with peritonitis. Nephron. 1986;43:217.

98. Whitby M et al. Pharmacokinetics of single dose intravenous vancomycin in CAPD peritonitis. J Antimicrob Chemother. 1987;19:351.

99. Keane WF et al. Continuous ambulatory peritoneal dialysis (CAPD) peritonitis treatment recommendations: 1989 update. Peritoneal Dial Inter. 1989;9:247.

100. Austin TW et al. Vancomycin blood levels during cardiac bypass surgery. Can J Surg. 1981;24:423–25.

101. Farber BF et al. Vancomycin prophylaxis in cardiac operations: determination of an optional dosage regimen. J Thorac Cardiovasc Surg. 1983;85:933–40.

102. Klamerus KJ et al. Effect of cardiopulmonary bypass on vancomycin and netilmicin disposition. Antimicrob Agents Chemo. 1988;32:631–35.

103. Hatzopoulos F et al. Vancomycin (V) dosage for prophylaxis in pediatric cardiac pulmonary bypass (CPB) surgery. Clin Pharmacol Ther. 1990;47:186. Abstract.

104. Watanakunakorn C. The antibacterial action of vancomycin. Rev Infect Dis. 1981;3:S210–15.

105. Pfeiffer RR. Structural features of vancomycin. Rev Infect Dis. 1981;3:S205–9.

106. Tuazon CU, Miller H. Comparative *in vitro* activities of teichomycin and vancomycin alone and in combination with rifampin and aminoglycosides against staphylococci and enterococci. Antimicrob Agents Chemother. 1984;25:411–12.

107. Watanakunakorn C, Tisone JC. Synergism between vancomycin and gentamicin or tobramycin for methicillin-susceptible and methicillin-resistant staphylococcus aureus strains. Antimicrob Agents Chemother. 1982;22:903–5.

108. Sorrell TC et al. Vancomycin therapy for methicillin-resistant staphylococcus aureus. Ann Intern Med. 1982;97:344–50.

109. Geraci JE, Hermans PE. Vancomycin. Mayo Clin Proc. 1983;58:88–91.

110. Ellner PA, Neu HC. The inhibitory quotient. A method for interpreting minimum inhibitory concentration data. JAMA. 1981;246:1575–578.

111. Louria DB et al. Vancomycin in severe staphylococcal infections. Arch Intern Med. 1961;107:225–40.

112. Klasterky J et al. Significance of antimicrobial synergism for the outcome of gram negative sepsis. Am J Med Sci. 1977;273:57.

113. Prober CG, Yeager AS. Use of the serum bactericidal titer to assess the adequacy of oral antibiotic therapy in the treatment of acute hematogenous osteomyelitis. J Pediatr. 1979;95:131.

114. Bailie GR, Neal D. Vancomycin ototoxicity and nephrotoxicity a review. Med Tox. 1988;3:376.

115. Kirby WMM et al. Treatment of staphylococcal septicemia with vancomycin. N Engl J Med. 1960;262:49–55.

116. Hook EW, Johnson WD. Vancomycin therapy of bacterial endocarditis. Am J Med. 1978;65:411–15.

117. Traber PG, Levine DP. Vancomycin ototoxity in a patient with normal renal function. Ann Intern Med. 1981;95:458–60.

118. Mellor JA et al. Vancomycin ototoxity in patients with normal renal function. Br J Audiology. 1984;18:179.

119. Ahmad R et al. Vancomycin: a reappraisal. Br Med J. 1982;284:1953–954.

120. Brummett RE. Effects of antibiotic-diuretic interactions in the guinea pig model of otoxicity. Rev Infect Dis. 1981;3:S216–223.

121. Brummett RE, Fox KE. Vancomycin- and erythromycin-induced hearing loss in humans. Antimicrob Agents Chemother. 1989;33:791.

122. Spears RL, Koch R. The use of vancomycin in pediatrics. Antibiot Ann. 1959–1960. 1960;798–803.

123. Geraci JE et al. Antibiotic therapy of bacterial endocarditis. VII. Vancomycin for acute micrococcal endocarditis. Mayo Clin Proc. 1958;33:172–81.

124. Waisbren BA et al. The comparison toxicity and clinical effectiveness of vancomycin, ristocetin, and kanamycin. Antibiot Ann. 1959–1960. 1960;497–515.

125. Riley HD, Ryan NJ. Treatment of severe staphylococcal infections in infancy and childhood with vancomycin. Antibiot Ann. 1959–1960. 1960;908–16.

126. Ehrenkranz NJ. The clinical evaluation of vancomycin in treatment of multi-antibiotic refractory staphylococcal infections. Antibiot Ann. 1958-1959. 1959;587–94.

127. Dangerfield HG et al. Clinical use of vancomycin. Antimicrob Agents Ann. 1960;428–38.

128. Geraci J, Heilman FR. Vancomycin in the treatment of staphylococcal endocarditis. Mayo Clin Proc. 1960;35:316–27.

129. Woodley DW, Hall WH. The treatment of severe staphylococcal infections with vancomycin. Ann Intern Med. 1961;55:235–49.

130. Geraci JE et al. Vancomycin in serious staphylococcal infections. Arch Intern Med. 1962;109:53–61.

131. Farber BF, Moellering RC. Retrospective study of the toxicity of preparations of vancomycin from 1974 to 1981. Antimicrob Agents Chemother. 1983;23:138–41.

132. Dean RP et al. Vancomycin/aminoglycoside toxicity. J Pediatr. 1985;106:861.

133. Mellor JA et al. Vancomycin toxicity: a prospective study. J of Antimicrob Chemother. 1985;15:773.

134. Sorrell T, Collignon PJ. A prospective study of adverse reactions associated with vancomycin therapy. J Antimicrob Chemother. 1985;16:235.

135. Cimino MA et al. Relationship of serum antibiotic concentrations to nephrotoxicity in cancer patients receiving concurrent aminoglycoside and vancomycin therapy. Am J of Med. 1987;83:1091.

136. Rybak MJ et al. Nephrotoxicity of vancomycin, alone and with an aminoglycoside. J Antimicrob Chemother. 1990;25:679.

137. Downs NJ et al. Mild nephrotoxicity associated with vancomycin use. Arch Intern Med. 1989;149:1777–781.
138. Pauly DJ et al. Risk of nephrotoxicity with combination vancomycin-aminoglycoside antibiotic therapy. Pharmacotherapy. 1990;10:378.
139. Odio C et al. Nephrotoxicity associated with vancomycin-aminoglycoside therapy in four children. J Ped. 1984;105:491–93.
140. Swinney VR et al. Nephrotoxicity of vancomycin-gentamicin therapy in pediatric patients. J Ped. 1987;110:497–98.
141. Nahata MC. Lack of nephrotoxicity in pediatric patients receiving concurrent vancomycin and aminoglycoside therapy. Chemotherapy. 1987;33:302–4.
142. Rothenberg HJ. Anaphylactoid reaction to vancomycin. JAMA. 1959;171:1101–102.
143. Polk RE et al. Vancomycin and the red-man syndrome: pharmacodynamics of histamine release. J Infect Dis. 1988;156:502.
144. Sahai J et al. Influence of antihistamine pretreatment on vancomycin-induced red man syndrome. J Infect Dis. 1989;160:876.
145. Sahai J et al. Comparison of vancomycin- and teicoplanin-induced histamine release and "red man syndrome." Antimicrob Agents Chemother. 1990,34:765.
146. Boeckh M et al. Pharmacokinetics and serum bactericidal activity of vancomycin alone and in combination with ceftazidime in healthy volunteers. Antimicrob Agents Chemother. 1988;32:92.
147. Lagast HP et al. Comparison of pharmacokinetic and bactericidal activity of teicoplanin and vancomycin. J Antimicrob Chemother. 1986;18:513.
148. Wallace MR et al. Incidence of vancomycin induced red man syndrome in hospitalized patients. Paper presented at 29th Interscience Conference on Antimicrobial Agents and Chemotherapy Meeting. Houston, TX: 1989 September 19.
149. Banner W, Ray CG. Vancomycin in perspective. Am J Dis Child. 1984;138:14–6.
150. Neftel K et al. Vancomycin induced neutropenia impact of duration of therapy and blood level monitoring. Paper presented at 28th Interscience Conference on Antimicrobial Agents and Chemotherapy Meeting. Los Angeles, CA: 1988 October 24.
151. Brown DL, Mauro LS. Vancomycin dosing chart for use in patients with renal impairment. Am J Kid Dis. 1988;11:15–9.
152. Lake KD, Peterson CD. A simplified dosing method for initiating vancomycin therapy. Pharmacother. 1985;5:340–4.
153. Rybak MJ, Boike SC. Individualized adjustment of vancomycin dosage: comparison with two dosage nomograms. Drug Intell Clin Pharm. 1986;20:64.
154. Zokufa HZ et al. Simulation of vancomycin peak and trough concentrations using five dosing methods in 37 patients. Pharmacotherapy. 1989;9(1):10.
155. Lake KD, Peterson CD. Evaluation of a method for initiating vancomycin therapy: experience in 205 patients. Pharmacother. 1988;8:284–86.
156. Alpert G et al. Vancomycin dosage in pediatrics reconsidered. Am J Dis Child. 1984;138:20–2.
157. Birt JK, Chandler MH. Using clinical data to determine vancomycin dosing parameters. Ther Drug Monit. 1990;12:206.
158. Gibaldi M, Perrier D. Pharmacokinetics. New York, NY: Marcell Dekker; 1982.
159. Sawchuk RJ, Zaske DE. Pharmacokinetics of dosing regimens which utilize multiple intravenous infusions: gentamicin in burn patients. J Pharmacokinetic Biopharm. 1976;4:183–95.
160. Ackerman BH et al. Errors in assuming a one-compartment model for vancomycin. Ther Drug Monit. 1990;12:304–5. Letter.
161. Uaamnuichai M et al. Bayesian and least-squares methods for vancomycin dosing. Am J Med Sci. 1987;294(2):100.
162. Garrelts JC et al. Accuracy of bayesian, sawchuk-zaske, and nomogram dosing methods for vancomycin. Clin Pharm. 1987;6:795.
163. Burton ME et al. Evaluation of a bayesian method for predicting vancomycin dosing. DICP—Annal Pharmacother. 1989;23:294.

164. Rodvold KA et al. Evaluation of a two-compartment bayesian forecasting program for predicting vancomycin concentrations. Ther Drug Monit. 1989;11:269.
165. Pryka RD et al. Individualizing vancomycin dosage regimens; one- versus two-compartment bayesian models. Ther Drug Monit. 1989;11:450.
166. Hurst AK. Application of a bayesian method to monitor and adjust vancomycin dose regimens. Antimicrob Agents and Chemother. 1990;34:1165.
167. Sabath LD et al. Rapid microassay of gentamicin, kanamycin, neomycin, streptomycin, and vancomycin in serum or plasma. J Lab Clin Med. 1971;78:457–63.
168. Walker CA, Kopp B. Sensitive bioassay for vancomycin. Antimicrob Agents Chemother. 1978;13:30–3.
169. Walker CN. Bioassay for determination of vancomycin in the presence of rifampin or aminoglycosides. Antimicrob Agents Chemother. 1980;17:730–31.
170. Crossley KB et al. Comparison of a radioimmunoassay and a microbiological assay for measurement of serum vancomycin concentrations. Antimicrob Agents Chemother. 1980;17:654–57.
171. Fong KL et al. Sensitive radioimmunoassay for vancomycin. Antimicrob Agents Chemother. 1981;19:139–43.
172. Ackerman BH et al. Comparison of radioimmunoassay and fluorescent polarization immunoassay for quantitative determination of vancomycin concentrations in serum. J Clin Microbiol. 1983;18:994–95.
173. Filburn BH et al. Evaluation of an automated fluorescence polarization immunoassay for vancomycin. Antimicrob Agents Chemother. 1983;24:216–20.
174. Schwenzer KS et al. Automated fluorescence polarization immunoassay for monitoring vancomycin. Ther Drug Monitor. 1983;5:341–45.
175. Ristuccia PA et al. Comparison of bioassay, high-performance liquid chromatography, and fluorescence polarization immunoassay for quantitative determination of vancomycin in serum. Ther Drug Monitor. 1984;6:238–42.
176. Pohlad DJ et al. Comparison of fluorescence polarization immunoassay and bioassay of vancomycin. J Clin Microbiol. 1984;20;159–61.
177. Pfaller MA et al. Laboratory evaluation of five assay methods for vancomycin: bioassay, high-pressure liquid chromatography, fluorescence polarization immunoassay, radioimmunoassay, and fluorescence immunoassay. J Clin Microbiol. 1984;20:311–16.
178. Yeo KT et al. Clinical performance of the EMIT vancomycin assay. Clin Chem. 1989;95:1504–507.
179. Anne L et al. Potential problems with fluorescence polarization immunoassay cross-reactivity to vancomycin degradation product CDP-1: its detection in sera of renally impaired patients. Ther Drug Monit. 1989;11:585.
180. Hu MW et al. Measurement of vancomycin in renally impaired patient samples using a new high-performance liquid chromatography method with vitamin B_{12} internal standard: comparison of high-performance liquid chromatography, EMIT, and fluorescence polarization immunoassay methods. Ther Drug Monit. 1990;12:562
181. Kirchmeier L, Upton RP. Simultaneous determination of vancomycin, anisomycin and trimethoprim lactate by high pressure liquid chromatography. Anal Chem. 1978;50;349–51.
182. Uhl JR, Anhalt JP. High performance liquid chromatographic assay of vancomycin in serum. Ther Drug Monit. 1979;1:75–83.
183. McClaim JB et al. Vancomycin quantitation by high performance liquid chromatography in human serum. J Chromatogr. 1982;231:463–66.
184. Hoagland RJ et al. Vancomycin: a rapid HPLC assay for a potent antibiotic. J Anal Toxicol. 1984;8:75–7.
185. Rosenthal AR et al. Simplified liquid-chromatographic determination of vancomycin. Clin Chem. 1986;32:1016.
186. Jehl F et al. Determination of vancomycin in human serum by high-pressure liquid chromatography. Antimicrob Agents Chemother. 1985;27:503.

187. Morse GD et al. Overestimation of vancomycin concentrations utilizing fluorescence polarization immunoassay in patients on peritoneal dialysis. Ther Drug Monit. 1987;9:212.

188. White LO et al. The *in vitro* degradation at 37 °C of vancomycin in serum, CAPD fluid and phosphate-buffered saline. J Antimicrob Chemother. 1988;22:739.

189. Hirsch et al. Instillation of vancomycin into a CSF reservoir to clear infection: pharmacokinetic considerations. J Infect Dis. 1991;163:197–200.

190. Shenep J et al. Vancomycin, ticarcillin, and amikacin compared with ticarcillin-clavulamate and amikacin in the emperical treatment of febrile, neutropenic children with cancer. New Engl J Med. 1988;319:1053–58.

Chapter 16

Chloramphenicol

Milap C. Nahata

Chloramphenicol was first isolated from the bacterium *Streptomyces venezuela*, in 1947. This antibiotic quickly gained wide popularity because of its broad spectrum of antimicrobial activity *in vitro* and its excellent clinical efficacy for the treatment of a variety of serious infections. The initial enthusiasm was dampened when serious idiosyncratic and dose-related toxicities developed in association with chloramphenicol's use. Despite its adverse effects, this drug is currently considered useful for the treatment of central nervous system infections, typhoid fever, rickettsial diseases, anaerobic infections, and certain infections of the eye.[1]

The use of chloramphenicol increased markedly because of the emergence of ampicillin-resistant *Haemophilus influenzae* type b.[2] Since this microorganism is the most common cause of meningitis in infants and children, pediatric patients with severe infections due to *H. influenzae* are initially treated with chloramphenicol or certain third-generation cephalosporins, pending the results of bacterial culture and evidence of sensitivity.

Both efficacy and dose-related toxicity of chloramphenicol correlate with its serum concentrations. Because this drug has a narrow therapeutic index (10 to 20 µg/mL therapeutic and greater than 25 µg/mL toxic) and there is substantial variability in its pharmacokinetics, chloramphenicol serum concentrations are routinely monitored to optimize therapy. Recent studies using sensitive and specific analytical methods have generated extensive data on the bioavailability and pharmacokinetics of chloramphenicol. The major objective of this chapter is to provide a proper perspective on the importance of factors to be considered for therapeutic monitoring of chloramphenicol.

OVERVIEW OF CLINICAL PHARMACOKINETICS

For systemic use, chloramphenicol is available in three pharmaceutical preparations: chloramphenicol base, a bitter-tasting powder marketed in capsules for oral administration; chloramphenicol palmitate, an inactive prodrug in tasteless oral suspension which is hydrolyzed in the intestine to active chloramphenicol;[3] and chloramphenicol sodium succinate, another inactive prodrug for parenteral administration, which is hydrolyzed to chloramphenicol primarily in the liver.[5]

Absorption

Chloramphenicol palmitate is the most commonly used oral preparation in pediatric patients. This prodrug is thought to be hydrolyzed by pancreatic lipase in the duodenum to microbiologically active chloramphenicol. Glazko et al.[3] have shown that 96% of the chloramphenicol palmitate is hydrolyzed to chloramphenicol in the rat duodenum in two hours at 38° C. However, clinical data demonstrating these findings in humans are not available.

In pediatric patients beyond the neonatal age group receiving chloramphenicol palmitate, the highest measured steady-state serum concentrations of chloramphenicol have averaged 19.3[6] and 18.5[7] μg/mL after 25 mg/kg doses; 21 to 25 μg/mL after 19 mg/kg and 22 to 27 μg/mL after 25 mg/kg doses;[7] and 27.5 μg/mL after 15 to 27 mg/kg doses;[9] these values were determined at 1.5 to 3.0 hours after the dose was administered. In newborn infants, the highest measured chloramphenicol serum concentration ranged from 5.5 to 23 μg/mL at ≥4 hours after 12.5 mg/kg doses.[10] In preterm infants, the dose of chloramphenicol palmitate had to be increased from 25 mg/kg/day to 50 mg/kg/day to achieve a therapeutic serum concentration.[10] These data suggest that the absorption of chloramphenicol from chloramphenicol palmitate may be incomplete, delayed, and variable in neonates, possibly because of delayed gastric emptying or decreased intraluminal hydrolysis of chloramphenicol palmitate.[10]

Two studies have shown that the area under the serum concentration-time curve (AUC) of chloramphenicol after the same oral dose was higher with chloramphenicol capsules than with chloramphenicol palmitate suspension.[3,11] In adults receiving an equivalent chloramphenicol dose of 1.5 gm, the AUC was 143 and 126 μg × hr/mL after administration of capsules and the suspension, respectively;[3] a similar difference was reported in children.[11]

In patients (mean age, 22 years) with cystic fibrosis (CF), the highest peak serum concentration and AUC were obtained after a single-dose administration of chloramphenicol (base) capsule, followed by IV chloramphenicol succinate and oral chloramphenicol palmitate suspension. The peak serum concentrations of chloramphenicol were within the therapeutic range in CF patients receiving chloramphenicol capsules and IV chloramphenicol succinate. However, subtherapeutic peak concentrations were associated with chloramphenicol palmitate, and these were attributed to decreased amounts of pancreatic lipase, which is necessary for the conversion of palmitate ester to chloramphenicol. Mean peak serum concentrations of chloramphenicol were 5.4 μg/mL and 3.2 μg/mL in patients receiving chloramphenicol palmitate (mean dose, 19.5 mg/kg), with and without pancreatic enzyme replacement, respectively. Thus, patients with CF are likely to achieve lower-than-expected serum concentrations of chloramphenicol from its palmitate suspension.[127]

Intramuscular administration of chloramphenicol succinate results in slow absorption of chloramphenicol, and peak concentrations have been shown to be only 5% to 66% of those obtained by intravenous or oral drug administration.[12] Intramuscular administration of chloramphenicol also has been associated with a delayed therapeutic response and increased relapse rate in adults with typhoid fever.[13] It should be noted, however, that comparable peak serum concentrations and AUC of chloramphenicol have been reported in infants and children (age one month to six years) after intravenous and intramuscular doses of chloramphenicol succinate, 25 mg/kg.[128] Because of these conflicting results, the intramuscular route is not widely used.

Although bioavailability is generally considered only for drugs administered orally, it should also be determined for drugs derived *in vivo* from the prodrugs administered parenterally. The bioavailability of chloramphenicol from the intravenously administered prodrug, chloramphenicol succinate, is determined by the extent of hydrolysis of chloramphenicol succinate to chloramphenicol and the efficiency of renal elimination of unchanged chloramphenicol succinate. In our studies,[14,15] the bioavailability of chloramphenicol averaged 0.93 in premature infants (mean gestational age, 32 weeks; postnatal age, 8.4 weeks); 0.72 in full-term infants (mean age, 0.64 year); and 0.64 in children (mean age, 10.7 years) (see Figure 16-1). These data showed that chloramphenicol was incompletely bioavailable, partly because a considerable amount of the prodrug, chloramphenicol succinate, was eliminated by the kidney before it was hydrolyzed to chloramphenicol. This finding conflicts with an earlier study which reported complete hydrolysis of chloramphenicol succinate to chloramphenicol;[15] however, it is consistent with the substantial loss of chloramphenicol succinate in the urine

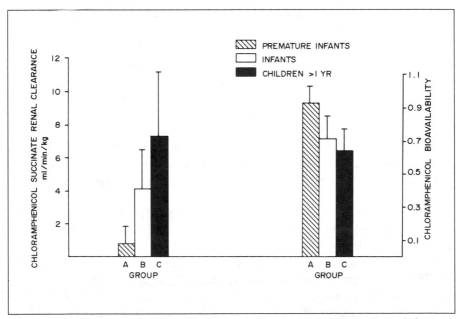

Figure 16-1. Chloramphenicol bioavailability and chloramphenicol succinate renal clearance in three groups of patients (reproduced with permission from reference 15).

observed in another study.[17] The increased bioavailability of parenteral chloramphenicol succinate in premature infants appeared to be a result of decreased renal clearance of chloramphenicol succinate, causing a greater fraction of the chloramphenicol succinate dose to be hydrolyzed to chloramphenicol.[15]

Comparative studies of oral palmitate and intravenous succinate esters in pediatric patients receiving equivalent doses have reported a higher AUC of chloramphenicol after oral chloramphenicol palmitate than after chloramphenicol succinate,[6-9] except in the premature infants or those with cystic fibrosis.[10] Thus, oral administration of chloramphenicol palmitate can be considered for patients beyond the neonatal age group or in patients with suspected pancreatic disease.

Since there is no intravenous preparation of chloramphenicol base or chloramphenicol palmitate, the bioavailability of chloramphenicol from these oral chlormphenicol formulations has been determined by urinary recovery of total nitro compounds.[4] With this method, the bioavailability of chloramphenicol was 0.76 to 0.93 from capsules containing chloramphenicol base[47,48] and 0.8 from a suspension containing chloramphenicol palmitate.[3] In patients with CF receiving pancreatic enzyme supplementation, the mean relative bioavailability of chloramphenicol was 0.69 after IV chloramphenicol succinate and 0.64 after oral chloramphenicol palmitate suspension compared with chloramphenicol base capsule; the bioavailability was substantially lower (0.42) after chloramphenicol palmitate in patients not receiving pancreatic enzymes.[127]

Distribution

Chloramphenicol has excellent distribution characteristics. The highest tissue concentration occurs in the liver and kidney; the lowest concentrations are found in the brain and cerebrospinal fluid (CSF).[18-20] It should be noted that penetration of chloramphenicol into the brain and CSF is independent of meningeal inflammation.[19-20] Average cerebrospinal fluid concentrations of chloramphenicol have ranged from 4.2 to 13 µg/mL or 23% to 84% of the concomitant serum concentration after administration of the recommended doses.[6-8,18,21] The penetration of chloramphenicol into the ventricular CSF was found to be variable in two infants; the ventricular CSF concentration was 57.5% and 22.5% of the simultaneous serum concentration of chloramphenicol.[22]

Despite a significant correlation between serum and saliva chloramphenicol concentrations, the saliva:serum concentration ratio was too variable (0 to 0.45) to permit the use of saliva concentrations for monitoring chloramphenicol therapy.[23]

Chloramphenicol distributes well into various body fluids. It diffuses into the aqueous and vitreous humor of the eye.[24] In the gravid female, chloramphenicol crosses the placenta, resulting in fetal concentrations between 30% to 80% of the maternal serum concentration,[25,26] although no evidence of teratogenicity is available. It also has been shown that chloramphenicol is present in breast milk.[26] It has been estimated that infants may receive about 7% of the maternal dose by breast milk.[137] Thus, large doses should be avoided in mothers breast feeding infants of any age; even normal doses should not be used in mothers feeding infants less than

34 weeks postconceptional age.[137] Therapeutic concentrations of chloramphenicol have also been reported in pleural and ascitic fluid.[27,28] Bile primarily contains the inactive glucuronide conjugate.

The average plasma protein binding of chloramphenicol was 53% in normal adults, 42% in adult cirrhotic patients, and 32% in premature infants.[29] The average apparent volume of distribution of chloramphenicol succinate was 0.42 to 2.1 L/kg in pediatric patients[14,30,31] and 0.30 L/kg in adult patients.[30] As summarized in Table 16-1, the mean apparent volume of distribution of chloramphenicol has ranged from 0.63 to 1.55 L/kg in pediatric patients[14,15,31,32] and 0.55 to 0.98 L/kg in adult patients.[29,30]

Metabolism

As shown in Figure 16-2, both microbiologically inactive prodrugs, chloramphenicol succinate and chloramphenicol palmitate, undergo hydrolysis to yield active chloramphenicol. The enzyme systems and sites of hydrolysis of these prodrugs are discussed above (see Absorption).

Chloramphenicol is metabolized in the liver, primarily to a monoglucuronide (75% to 90%).[35,36] In microsomal systems, chloramphenicol glucuronyl transferase has been shown to differ from the bilirubin glucuronyl transferase.[36] This major glucuronide metabolite of chloramphenicol has no antimicrobial activity. Chloramphenicol also undergoes reduction at the nitro position to an amine.[35] This reduction primarily occurs in the gastrointestinal tract after excretion of glucuronide and chloramphenicol into the bile. Many enterobacteriaceae possess an aromatic nitro reductase that can reduce chloramphenicol to the corresponding amine.[35] No antibacterial activity has been reported for this reduced metabolite.

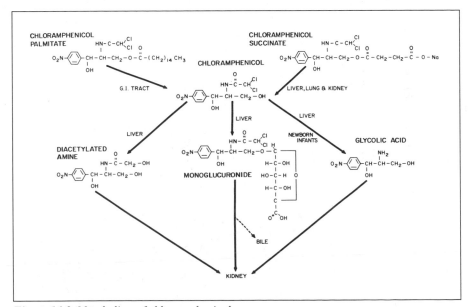

Figure 16-2. Metabolism of chloramphenicol.

Table 16-1. Pharmacokinetic Data of Chloramphenicol After IV Administration of Chloramphenicol Succinate

Number of patients	Age	Dose (mg/kg/day)	Bioavailability	Total clearance (mL/min/kg)	Renal clearance (mL/min/kg)	Nonrenal clearance (mL/min/kg)	Distribution volume (L/kg)	Elimination t½ (hr)	References
5	31.8±3.42 wk[a] / 8.4±3.4 wk[b]	36–75	0.93±0.10	1.73±1.00	0.36±0.32	1.37±0.72	1.55±0.67	10.1±6.9	15
8	0.64±0.28 yr	100	0.71±0.14	2.54±1.79	0.43±0.20	2.05±1.71	0.76±0.65	3.48±1.52	14
4	10.7±7.50 yr	100	0.64±0.13	1.59±0.44	0.44±0.38	1.15±0.46	0.63±0.29	4.84±2.41	
17	4–72 mo	75	ND[d]	4.68±1.95	ND	ND	1.39±0.34	3.93±1.75	32[c]
24	0.4–84 mo	100	ND	1.50	ND	ND	0.64	4.60	31
10	3–18 mo	100	ND	2.11	ND	ND	ND	ND	33[c]
9	31.2±1.9 wk[a] / 10.4±3.3 days[b]	50–80	ND	1.10±0.20	ND	ND	ND	1.61±2.90	34[c]
8	43–72 yr	32–114	ND	1.29	0.14	1.16	0.55	5.10	30
8	19–64 yr	30–80	ND	3.21	0.33	2.88	0.81	3.20	139
4	Adults	NR[e]	ND	3.57±1.72	ND	ND	0.92	2.25	29[c]
8[f]	Adults	NR	ND	1.99±1.49	ND	ND	0.98	3.91	

[a] Gestational age.
[b] Postnatal age.
[c] Because these studies assumed a complete hydrolysis of chloramphenicol succinate to chloramphenicol, clearance and distribution volumes are likely to be overestimated.
[d] Not determined.
[e] Not reported.
[f] Cirrhosis patients.

In the newborn infant, a glycolic acid metabolite of chloramphenicol has also been found; this metabolite has 2% to 4% of the antimicrobial activity of chloramphenicol against *Shigella sonnei*.[37] Initial attempts to implicate this metabolite as a cause of gray baby syndrome were unsuccessful.[27]

The mean nonrenal clearance of chloramphenicol succinate is about 83% of its mean total clearance in adult patients.[30] A substantial variation has been observed in nonrenal clearance of chloramphenicol succinate in pediatric patients; the mean nonrenal clearance is about 93%, 77%, and 40% of the mean total clearance in newborn infants, full-term infants greater than two months of age, and children, respectively.[14,15] In another study involving infants and children (age 0.4 months to seven years), the nonrenal clearance was found to be 59% of total clearance.[31] The difference in these values may partly be due to difference in age of patients.

The mean nonrenal clearance of chloramphenicol is about 90% of its mean total clearance in adult patients.[32] In pediatric patients, the mean nonrenal clearance has ranged from 72% to 81% of the mean total clearance of chloramphenicol in premature and full-term infants and in children.[14,15]

Chloramphenicol has been shown to interact with a number of drugs, usually as a consequence of competition for hepatic microsomal enzymes. It has been suggested that chloramphenicol inhibits the metabolism of tolbutamide, chlorpropamide, phenytoin, and warfarin.[38–40] On the other hand, chloramphenicol metabolism can be influenced by other drugs. Simultaneous administration of phenobarbital, phenytoin, or rifampin (known inducers of glucuronyl transferase), may lead to increased metabolism of chloramphenicol.[41–43,129] There was one report[43] of a decrease in chloramphenicol metabolism by phenytoin, which is difficult to explain. Acetaminophen was reported to prolong the elimination half-life of chloramphenicol in one patient,[44] but this was not confirmed in subsequent studies.[8,15,130]

Liver disease has been shown to affect the serum concentration of chloramphenicol.[29,45,46] Apparent total clearance of chloramphenicol was about 40% lower in patients with cirrhosis of the liver than in normal adults.[29] Four seriously ill infants and children with underlying liver dysfunction developed acidosis during chloramphenicol succinate therapy. The peak serum concentration of chloramphenicol ranged from 62 to 84 µg/mL in three patients receiving chloramphenicol succinate, 100 mg/kg/day; the peak concentration was 30 µg/mL in one receiving 75 mg/kg/day.[131] It should be understood, however, that due to the lack of a clear relationship between chloramphenicol clearance and routinely measured biochemical indices of hepatic function, no specific guidelines are available for dosage modification in patients with liver disease.

Excretion

About 30% of intravenous chloramphenicol succinate is eliminated unchanged in the urine of pediatric and adult patients.[14,17,30] However, newborn infants may not excrete as much chloramphenicol succinate in the urine.[15] The mean renal clearance of chloramphenicol succinate is about 19% of its total clearance in adult patients.[30] A marked variation has been reported in the renal clearance of chloramphenicol succinate in pediatric patients: the mean renal clearance is about 7%, 29%, and 61% of the total clearance in newborn infants, full-term infants greater than two months of age, and children, respectively.[14,15] In another study with infants and children (age 0–4 months to seven years), the renal clearance of chloramphenicol succinate was found to be 41% of its total clearance.[31]

Urinary recovery of chloramphenicol has ranged from about 5% to 29% of the administered dose.[14,15,35,47] The mean renal clearance of chloramphenicol is about 12% of its total clearance in adult patients.[30] In pediatric patients, the mean renal clearance has ranged from 19% to 28% of the mean total clearance of chloramphenicol in premature and full-term infants and children.[14,15] About 85% of the chloramphenicol dose is excreted in the urine as its inactive glucuronide metabolite.[48,50]

Renal clearance of chloramphenicol succinate was found to be 4.0 times and 1.4 times creatinine clearance in pediatric and adult patients, respectively;[30] this finding suggests active secretion by the renal tubule. Because the ratio of chloramphenicol succinate clearance to creatinine clearance may be variable in critically ill patients, the relative importance of glomerular filtration and tubular secretion cannot be resolved.[30] Chloramphenicol is filtered and partially reabsorbed

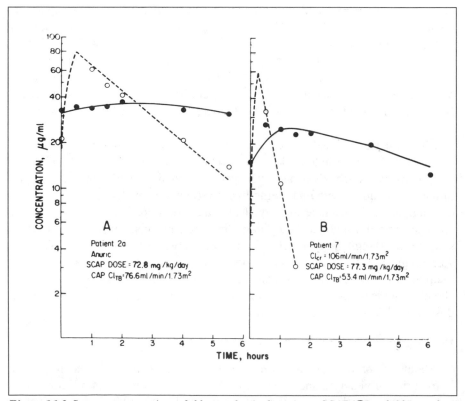

Figure 16-3. *Serum concentrations of chloramphenicol succinate, SCAP (○) and chloramphenicol, CAP (●) in an anuric patient (A) and in a patient with normal renal function (B). Solid line is a computer-generated best fit for chloramphenicol and dashed line is best fit for a chloramphenicol succinate (reproduced with permission from reference 30).*

by the renal tubule; a linear correlation has been observed between chloramphenicol renal clearance and inulin clearance.[47] Increasing the tubular perfusion rate, as with osmotic diuresis, increases the renal clearance of chloramphenicol.[52]

The renal clearance of chloramphenicol succinate and chloramphenicol decreases in patients with underdeveloped or compromised renal function. The decrease in chloramphenicol succinate clearance can be clinically significant because a greater fraction of chloramphenicol succinate is available for hydrolysis, yielding higher serum concentrations of active chloramphenicol.[15,30] Serum concentrations of chloramphenicol have been reported to be higher in patients with severe renal disease than in those with normal renal function (Figure 16-3).[30] Cardiovascular collapse has been reported in an anephric patient (age 19 years), who received normal doses of chloramphenicol succinate (0.8 gm and then 0.5 gm every six hours). The serum concentration of chloramphenicol and chloramphenicol succinate was 161 and 75 µg/mL, respectively, at one hour after the dose.[132] Because no specific guidelines are available for dosage modification in decreased renal function, serum concentrations of chloramphenicol should be monitored in these patients when they receive intravenous chloramphenicol succinate.

It has been estimated that about 3% of chloramphenicol and 5% of its glucuronide metabolite may be excreted in the bile.[48,50,52]

PHARMACODYNAMICS

Clinical Response

Chloramphenicol possesses a broad spectrum of antibacterial activity. The antimicrobial action depends on the binding of chloramphenicol to the 50-S subunit of bacterial ribosomes. This binding appears to prevent attachment of a complete aminoacetyl transfer RNA to the ribosome,[53] thereby inhibiting formation of peptide bonds.[54]

Chloramphenicol inhibits growth *in vitro* of large numbers of both gram-positive and gram-negative bacteria.[55] Although early studies suggested that the drug was strictly bacteriostatic, more recent data have demonstrated its bactericidal activity against important human pathogens such as *Haemophilus influenzae* and *Streptococcus pneumoniae*. Rahal and Simberkoff[56] showed that 100% of 11 strains of *H. influenzae* were killed with a concentration of 0.78 µg/mL; while 100% of 10 strains of *Neisseria meningiditis*, another important human pathogen, were killed at concentrations up to 50 µg/mL,[56] but such concentrations are not achievable for prolonged periods *in vivo* without the risk of hematologic side effects.

Because of the bacteriostatic activity of chloramphenicol, the issue of antagonism of bactericidal antibiotics has been raised. When *H. influenzae* and *S. pneumoniae* have been tested *in vitro* with combinations of a penicillin and chloramphenicol, antagonism has not been demonstrated.[55,60] On the contrary, some studies have shown additive or synergistic effects.[59,61] Although controlled clinical trials have not been conducted comparing the therapeutic efficacy of combined ampicillin and chloramphenicol versus single-drug therapy in bacterial meningitis,[61,62] these *in vitro* data support the current recommendations to initiate therapy with both drugs in patients with suspected *H. influenzae* meningitis.[2]

Until recently, complete antibacterial resistance to chloramphenicol has been limited to *Pseudomonas aeruginosa*, indole-positive proteus, acinetobacter, and a few strains of *Serratia marcescens*. Of much greater clinical importance has been the recent emergence of chloramphenicol resistance among strains of *H. influenzae*, type b. In 1972, a type b strain with a minimum inhibitory concentration (MIC) of 50 µg/mL was reported from Texas.[62] Subsequent isolates with similarly high MICs have been reported from Philadelphia,[63] Washington,[64] and England.[65] The reports of *H. influenzae* type b resistant to both chloramphenicol and ampicillin are of concern.[66–68] Such organisms have accounted for the death of at least three children from an orphanage in Bangkok, Thailand, where 47% of *H. influenzae* type b strains isolated from the nasopharynx of 38 children were found to be resistant to both drugs.[69] These findings raise great concern for the future first-line antibiotic coverage of childhood bacterial meningitis. Fortunately, several third-generation cephalosporins have proven effective for the treatment of meningitis.

The only other clinically significant form of bacterial resistance has been the emergence of salmonella strains resistant to chloramphenicol.[70] While a frequency of chloramphenicol-resistant strains may be no more than one per 1,000 isolates of salmonella, such resistance has been shown to emerge during chloramphenicol treatment in several cases.[71] Strains of *Salmonella typhae* and *Shigella dysenteriae* resistant to chloramphenicol accounted for epidemic disease in Mexico and Central America in the early 1970s.[71]

Chloramphenicol resistance is usually plasmid-mediated and occurs from the production of chloramphenicol acetyltransferase.[64] Conjugative transmission has been demonstrated between strains of haemophilus and from haemophilus to other gram-negative bacteria.[72] Resistance among certain strains of pseudomonas and serratia may depend on alterations in membrane permeability[73] and may be transmitted chromosomally.[74]

Adverse Effects

Major impediments to the widespread use of chloramphenicol have been the associated hematologic adverse effects and the gray baby syndrome.

Hematologic Toxicity. Hematologic toxicity manifests as either common and reversible serum-concentration-related bone marrow suppression or rare and irreversible idiosyncratic aplastic anemia.

The onset of reversible bone marrow suppression is characterized uniformly by a decrease in red cell iron uptake, an increase in circulating serum iron with saturation of iron-binding uptake and of iron-binding globulin, and a depression of erythropoiesis, manifested as reticulocytopenia.[75] Continuation of therapy may lead to a progressive decline in the circulating hemoglobin concentration in five to ten days.[76] Accompanying the early reticulocytopenia is an increase in erythroid:myeloid ratio in the bone marrow and vacuolization of bone marrow precursors.[77,78] With prolonged chloramphenicol use (generally longer than ten days), mild thrombocytopenia and neutropenia may also occur, particularly in children.[76]

These adverse effects are dose-related and most common when peak serum concentrations exceed 25 µg/mL.[79] While these changes are usually reversed soon after discontinuation of the drug, one recent case report[80] demonstrated possible progression to irreversible marrow suppression and suggests the need to discontinue therapy if leukopenia becomes severe.

The reversible form of bone marrow suppression is believed to result from chloramphenicol binding to 70-S ribosomes resulting in mitochondrial ultrastructural changes and a decrease in mitochondrial protein synthesis. With impaired production of mitochondrial membrane-binding proteins and enzymes such as ferrochelatase, mitochondrial heme synthesis is blocked.[79]

Aplastic anemia, the more dreaded form of bone marrow suppression, was recognized shortly after commercial distribution of chloramphenicol.[81] Several epidemiologic surveys in the 1960s led to the conclusion that this complication occurs with a frequency of one in 24,000 to one in 200,000 individuals treated with chloramphenicol.[82,83] An average incidence is approximately one in 40,000, with the highest occurrence in children[84] and females.[85] This complication is not related to dose or duration of therapy and has been described after single doses of chloramphenicol[83] and after the administration of chloramphenicol eye drops.[86] The onset of anemia may occur weeks or months after the termination of therapy.[83] Although the mechanism underlying this irreversible suppression of heme synthesis has not been determined, it is postulated that previous exposure to chloramphenicol is necessary, suggesting the possibility of some form of hypersensitivity reaction. The occurrence of aplastic anemia in identical twins[87] has led to the speculation of possible genetic predisposition involving pathways of DNA synthesis. Yunis[79] has postulated that p-nitrosulfathiazole groups on the chloramphenicol molecule may inhibit DNA synthesis in marrow stem cells of certain predisposed individuals.

There continues to be debate whether aplastic anemia occurs exclusively following oral administration of the drug or is a complication of parenteral chloramphenicol as well. Holt[88] postulated that the fatal marrow suppression was the result of a toxic metabolite resulting from colonic bacterial degradation of oral chloramphenicol. Despite several articles[82,89,91,138] reporting cases of aplastic anemia following parenteral drug administration, there is still concern that many of these patients had other reasons for their aplastic anemia, including exposure to oral drug, severe infections, concomitant cimetidine, or old age.[92,138] This debate is important in light of the recent literature suggesting higher bioavailability and more predictable peak serum concentrations following the administration of oral chloramphenicol palmitate than of intravenous chloramphenicol succinate.[6–9] Certainly, the parenteral form of chloramphenicol should not be withheld from individuals with serious and potentially life-threatening illnesses. The impression that aplastic anemia is associated with oral chloramphenicol may reflect the pattern of drug utilization during the decade when most cases were reported.[10] Definitive studies on the epidemiology and pathophysiology of aplastic anemia are needed.

Gray Baby Syndrome. The other major fatal form of chloramphenicol toxicity is the gray baby syndrome.[93] This problem was first observed in 1958 when neonates born following premature rupture of the membranes were given prophylactic chloramphenicol. The mortality rates in these infants were significantly higher than in untreated infants.[94,95] Typically, these babies received the drug within the first several days of life in doses of 100 to 300 mg/kg/day. Serum concentrations of chloramphenicol in two of the infants studied immediately before their death were recorded as 180 and 75 μg/mL.[94] The classic picture of the gray baby syndrome begins three to four days after initiation of chloramphenicol therapy, with vomiting, abdominal distension, anorexia, and respiratory distress. Soon thereafter, infants develop hypotension, a characteristic gray color, greenish diarrhea, and progressive shock. Within two to three days, 40% of affected infants die; the remainder recover completely upon cessation of chloramphenicol.[93] This syndrome has occasionally been reported in older infants and adults,[96,98] without obvious preceding liver or renal damage. While the underlying mechanism of action is unknown, studies in rats have shown that chloramphenicol, at high serum concentrations, blocks mitochondrial electron transport at the site of NADH dehydrogenase, and results in reduced oxygen consumption with disruption of energy metabolism.[99,100] Because of the high risk of the gray baby syndrome developing in infants with chloramphenicol serum concentrations in excess of 50 μg/mL, infants who receive a chloramphenicol overdose should be treated with either charcoal column hemoperfusion[101] or multiple whole blood exchange transfusions.[102]

As with any antibiotic, a host of worrisome, nonfatal complications have also been described. These include diarrhea and glossitis,[103] bacterial superinfection, allergic maculovesicular rash,[104] hemorrhagic allergic skin rash,[105] central nervous system (CNS) disturbance in young patients with cystic fibrosis,[106,107] alterations in humoral immune responsiveness,[108,109] acute hemolysis in G-6PD deficiency,[110] and acute left ventricular cardiac dysfunction.[111] There does not appear to be a definitive relationship between these toxicities and chloramphenicol serum concentrations.

CLINICAL APPLICATION OF PHARMACOKINETIC DATA

Serum concentrations of chloramphenicol are routinely monitored to assure efficacy and minimize toxicity. It is important to consider the factors discussed above, which may affect the serum concentration of chloramphenicol, including age, liver and renal function, and concomitant drugs. Two additional variables, infusion method and repeated therapy, should also be taken into account when monitoring chloramphenicol serum concentrations.

Effect of Infusion Method

Our *in vitro* studies show that the times required to deliver a dose of chloramphenicol succinate by IV infusion may exceed the predicted delivery time by threefold (based upon the infusion rate).[112] We delivered chloramphenicol succinate through various sites on the IV setup (an injection port in the IV tubing—Flash-ball, a y-site, and Buretrol) at three flow rates. The actual time required to deliver 95% of the dose was compared to the predicted times. For the Buretrol site, the actual delivery time exceeded the predicted time by 2.5-fold at flow rates of 15 and 29 mL/hr. At a slow rate (5 mL/hr), only 85% of the dose had been delivered at six hours. The clinical relevance of these data was demonstrated by significantly lower peak serum concentrations of chloramphenicol succinate and chloramphen-icol, as well as delayed peak concentrations when chloramphenicol succinate was injected into the Buretrol instead of the Flashball site.[112]

These data point to several potential problems in clinical care. Alterations in IV flow rates and injection site of an IV system may be made under the false assumption that the total amount of antibiotic has been delivered.[113] For example, in children receiving IV fluids for the sole purpose of drug delivery, chloramphen-icol succinate is often injected into the Buretrol; the IV rate is increased to 25 to 30 mL/hr for 30 to 60 minutes, and thereafter it is decreased to a keep-open rate of ≤5 mL/hr. Even at the end of 60 minutes at the fastest rate, as much as 25% of the chloramphenicol succinate may not have been infused. Further, since IV sets are routinely replaced every 24 hours to minimize the risk of bacterial contamina-tion,[112] as much as a total dose of chloramphenicol succinate may be discarded, depending on the rate and site of drug infusion and the timing of replacement.

Finally, in clinical monitoring of serum concentrations, samples are frequently drawn at an arbitrary time after the start of drug infusions. Without consideration of the rate and infusion site, anticipated peak serum concentrations may be very inaccurate, leading to unjustified and potentially harmful alterations in the dose of chloramphenicol succinate to be administered.[112]

Effect of Repeated Therapy

To evaluate the effect of repeated therapy, chloramphenicol succinate and chloramphenicol kinetics were examined on two occasions within the same course of therapy at steady state, separated by 2 to 17 days, in ten pediatric patients on the same intravenous dose of chloramphenicol succinate. The steady-state peak serum concentration of chloramphenicol succinate fell from an average of 77.1 µg/mL during the first study to 42.2 µg/mL during the second. The steady-state peak serum concentration of chloramphenicol also decreased from an average of 27.8 µg/mL to 24.9 µg/mL. There was a marked decrease in the steady-state trough serum concentration of chloramphenicol, which averaged 8.4 µg/mL in the first study and 5.3 µg/mL in the second study. The concurrent decrease in the serum concentrations and AUCs of chloramphenicol succinate and chloramphenicol is shown in Figure 16-4.[114]

The decrease in the AUCs of both chloramphenicol succinate and chloramphen-icol may be due to either a decrease in bioavailability or an increase in body clearance. Our studies[112] have shown that the method used for intravenous chlor-amphenicol succinate delivery may affect steady-state serum concentrations and AUCs of chloramphenicol succinate and chloramphenicol. These data were con-sidered in conducting our study, and the same intravenous dose of chloramphenicol succinate was given to each patient by the same research nurse. Thus, the decrease in the serum concentrations and AUCs of chloramphenicol succinate and chloramphenicol may have been caused by an increase in clearance. This may have been due to an unknown alternate pathway of chloramphenicol succinate metabolism, concurrent stimulation of chloramphenicol succinate and chloramphenicol metabolism, or an increase in renal clearance of chloramphenicol succinate.[114] Thus, it seems appropriate to repeat the measurement of chloramphenicol serum concentration, especially in patients responding poorly to a given dose of chloramphenicol succinate.

Monitoring Serum Concentration

Inter- and intrasubject variation in chloramphenicol pharmacokinetics and a narrow therapeutic index support the need for individualizing chloramphenicol therapy. Chloramphenicol peak serum concentrations should be measured in all patients with serious infections. In general, the goal is to achieve a minimum peak serum concentration of 10 µg/mL and a maximum peak serum concentration of 25 µg/mL. Although it has been suggested that the trough serum concentrations of chloramphenicol should fall between 5 and 10 µg/mL,[133] no studies have found a correlation between trough serum concentration and efficacy or adverse effects. The recommendations for achieving a peak serum concentration between 10 and 25 µg/mL is based on the premise that it should exceed the MIC of common susceptible pathogens by severalfold to achieve therapeutic efficacy. Limited data exist about direct relationships between serum concentrations, AUC or duration for which the serum concentration must exceed the MIC, and efficacy or adverse effects in patients receiving usual doses. Close monitoring is required for certain

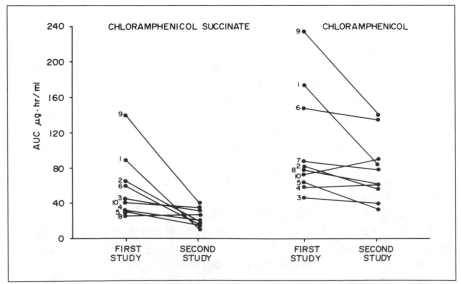

Figure 16-4. *AUC of chloramphenicol and chloramphenicol succinate on two occasions in patients during repeated doses within one course of therapy. The subjects are identified by patient numbers (reproduced with permission from reference 114).*

patients, including those with liver or pancreatic disease; those who are unresponsive or showing symptoms of toxicity to a prescribed dose; those with underdeveloped or compromised renal function receiving chloramphenicol succinate; those receiving repeated doses of interacting drugs, such as phenobarbital, phenytoin, and rifampin; and those with serious illnesses. A general approach for monitoring chloramphenicol therapy is presented in the algorithm (Figure 16-5). Since the antimicrobial efficacy and certain adverse effects have been related to the peak serum concentration, blood samples should be obtained at appropriate peak times after drug administration. As discussed previously, the chloramphenicol peak serum concentration after administration of oral chloramphenicol palmitate may occur 1.5 to 3.0 hours after the dose, whereas peaks after intravenous chloramphenicol succinate may be more variable because of variable rates of hydrolysis, rates of administration, and sites of drug infusion. The peak serum concentration of chloramphenicol generally occurs 0.5 to 1.5 hours after the completion of 0.5-hour chloramphenicol succinate intravenous infusion. Similar general guidelines can be used to determine the time to obtain a blood sample in premature infants receiving chloramphenicol succinate; however, in these patients the infusion period is usually longer than that of older patients. In premature infants, it is not possible to recommend a precise time to draw a blood sample after administration of chloramphenicol palmitate.[10] Based on an average elimination half-life of two to five hours in various patient populations (Table 16-1), about 12 to 24 hours of therapy may be required to achieve steady-state conditions. In newborn infants with a mean elimination half-life of 10 to 16 hours, a minimum of two to three days of therapy may be required to attain steady-state conditions. Serum concentration monitoring during initial therapy, however, may decrease the possibility of gray baby syndrome.

After chloramphenicol therapy has been initiated, a peak serum concentration should be measured at steady state so that subsequent doses can be modified to attain a therapeutic and a safe peak serum concentration. Certain patients, as identified earlier, may need repeated measurement of chloramphenicol serum concentrations. The measurement of chloramphenicol succinate serum concentration is generally not necessary, but it may explain uninterpretable chloramphenicol serum concentrations. For example, an unusually low chloramphenicol serum concentration and a high chloramphenicol succinate serum concentration may suggest limited capacity for the hydrolysis of chloramphenicol succinate to chloramphenicol. In unresponsive or toxic patients, multiple measurements may be required during a dosing interval.

It should be noted that the "dose-related" hematologic adverse effects may not be predicted by monitoring chloramphenicol serum concentration. No relationship was seen between chloramphenicol peak serum concentration and the occurrence of neutropenia, leukopenia, eosinophilia, anemia, and thrombocytopenia in infants and children.[134] Two other studies in pediatric patients also reported a lack of association between chloramphenicol peak concentration and development of hematologic toxicity.[128,135] There was a trend for a higher cumulative dose of chloramphenicol succinate in patients who developed toxicity (1.2 to 1.8 gm/kg versus 0.9 to 1.1 gm/kg), but the relationship was not statistically significant.[134]

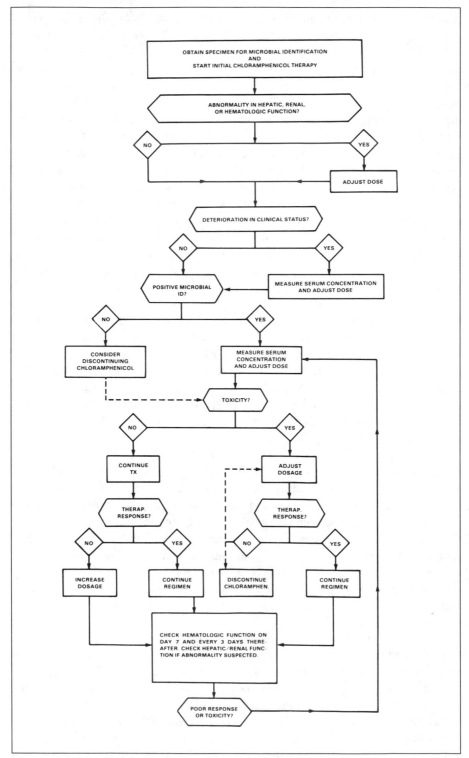

Figure 16-5. *Algorithm for monitoring chloramphenicol therapy.*

These data suggest that factors other than serum concentration may be important in predicting hematologic toxicity due to chloramphenicol. For example, genetic factors or concentration of chloramphenicol in the marrow may be important, but no data are available to support these possibilities.

Because of substantial variation in the bioavailability and pharmacokinetics of chloramphenicol after the administration of its prodrug, and because of the multitude of factors affecting the serum concentration of chloramphenicol, it is difficult to predict serum concentrations in an individual patient. Koup et al.[115] reported good agreement between predicted and observed chloramphenicol clearance in infants and children from a single serum sample obtained at six hours after the initial chloramphenicol succinate dose. This approach has not been tested by others and requires exclusion of patients with low or changing chloramphenicol clearance (a reported change in serum concentration is discussed above)[114] and those in shock or receiving vasoactive or interacting drugs.

Monitoring Hematologic Function

Specific recommendations are available to detect and minimize the hematologic adverse effects of chloramphenicol. It has been suggested that complete blood cell count including differential, reticulocyte count, platelet count, and hemoglobin should be measured at the start of chloramphenicol therapy. It has been recommended that these laboratory studies be repeated after one week of chloramphenicol therapy and every three days thereafter during continued therapy.[76]

Initial Dosage Recommendations

Recent pharmacokinetic studies have led to new pediatric dosage recommendations for chloramphenicol. Although 100 mg/kg/day was routinely prescribed for the treatment of serious infections, this dose has been shown to result in chloramphenicol peak serum concentrations exceeding 25 µg/mL in many.[8,9,14] Thus, the current initial dosage recommendation is 75 mg/kg/day (divided in four equal doses) for most patients beyond the newborn period.[8,9,116] Initial doses of 25 to 50 mg/kg/day are recommended for newborns, 25 mg/kg/day for patients 1 week of age or younger, and 25 mg/kg/12 hours (50 mg/kg/day) for infants one to four weeks of age.[17,116] Initial adult doses are 12.5 to 25 mg/kg/6 hours, with a maximum dose of 1 gm/4 hours.[116] It is important to note that these are only initial dosage guidelines which may require modification after the assessment of chloramphenicol serum concentrations.

Analytical Methods

Routine monitoring of chloramphenicol serum concentrations requires the availability of an accurate, precise, and specific analytical method. A comparison of five analytical techniques is provided in Table 16-2.

Colorimetric methods measure the amine formed after the reduction of aromatic nitro groups of chloramphenicol.[117] Thus, the inactive prodrug and the glucuron-

Table 16-2. Comparison of Chloramphenicol Assay Methods

Method	Specificity[a]	Limit of sensitivity (μg/mL)	Assayable samples			Minimum sample volume (μL)	Speed[a]	Cost[a]		Application[a]			References
			Prodrug/ metabolite	Serum and urine	CSF			Estimated reagent and technical	Initial equipment	Small service	Large service	Research	
Colorimetric	5	NA	No	Yes	Yes	NA	3	2	2	5	5	5	117,118
Microbiologic	4	2.0	No	Yes	Yes	25	4	2	2	3	3	4	119
Radioenzymatic	2	0.2–0.5	No	Yes	Yes	25	2	3	5	4	4	3	118,120,121
EMIT	2	2.5	No	Yes	Yes	50	1	1	3	2	1	3	136
HPLC	1	0.5–1.0	Yes	Yes	Yes	50	4	2	4	3	2	1	122–124
GLC	1	0.1–0.5	Yes	Yes	Yes	50–100	4	2	4	4	3	2	118, 125, 126

[a] Arbitrary ranking scale of 1 (excellent) to 5 (poor); NA, not available.

ide-metabolite-containing nitro groups interfere with chloramphenicol measurement.[118] Although this method is inexpensive, it suffers from poor specificity. This method is not recommended for the measurement of chloramphenicol concentration.

Microbiologic methods are relatively inexpensive and easy to use, but their limitations include poor sensitivity and specificity, and delay in obtaining results.[119,120] This method also suffers from variations in precision and accuracy of interpreting the zone of inhibition. This method may be useful in an established microbiology laboratory for measuring chloramphenicol in patients not receiving other antibiotics, when the serum concentration of the prodrug is not desired.

The radioenzymatic assay is rapid, precise, sensitive, and specific, but its disadvantages include high cost, the need to dispose of radioactive materials, and the assay's inability to measure the prodrug or chloramphenicol metabolites.[121,122]

An enzyme-mediated immunoassay technique (EMIT) became available in 1986 for the measurement of chloramphenicol. It is rapid, precise, specific, and easy-to-use for the quantitation of chloramphenicol, but the prodrug and metabolites cannot be measured.[136]

High-performance liquid chromatography (HPLC) methods are accurate, precise, sensitive, and specific for the measurement of chloramphenicol as well as its prodrug and major metabolite.[123-125] Gas liquid chromatographic (GLC) methods are also accurate, precise, sensitive, and specific but generally require several extraction steps and thus are more cumbersome than HPLC.[126] Further, the reported GLC methods have not been utilized to measure the prodrug of chloramphenicol.

Based on the above criteria, as presented in Table 16-2, HPLC is currently a preferred method for the measurement of chloramphenicol in research or large service laboratories. EMIT is useful for routine monitoring of chloramphenicol concentrations in biological fluids.

PROSPECTUS

Because of chloramphenicol's serious adverse effects, its substantial variation in bioavailability and pharmacokinetics, and the severity of clinical illnesses for which it is generally prescribed, few would question the need for monitoring serum concentrations. Additional information, however, is needed in the following areas: dosage guidelines in patients with liver or renal disease; cost-benefit analysis of chloramphenicol serum concentration monitoring; confirmation of pharmacodynamic (efficacy and adverse effect) relationships using specific analytical techniques; assessment of metabolism during chronic therapy; studies of the effect of disease states on chloramphenicol; and studies of the epidemiology and pathogenesis of aplastic anemia.

Based on present knowledge, chloramphenicol serum concentrations should be monitored to maximize therapeutic benefits and minimize potential toxicity.

REFERENCES

1. Feigin RD, Cherry JD. Textbook of Pediatric Infectious Diseases. Philadelphia: WB Saunders; 1981.
2. Report of Committee on Infectious Diseases. *Hemophilus influenzae* infections. Redbook, 18th ed. In: Steigman AJ, ed. Evanston:American Academy of Pediatrics; 1977.
3. Glazko AJ et al. Physical factors affecting the rate of absorption of chloramphenicol esters. Antibiot Chemother. 1958;8:516–27.
4. Ambrose PI. Clinical pharmacokinetics of chloramphenicol and chloramphenicol succinate. Clin Pharmacokinet. 1984;9:222–38.
5. Schmidt FH, Vomel W. Uber die Spaltung von Chloramphenicol-Succinate durch tierische unk menschliche Gewebe. Iuin Wochenschr. 1965;43:535.
6. Pickering LK et al. Clinical pharmacology of two chloramphenicol preparations in children: sodium succinate (iv) and palmitate (oral) esters. J Pediatr. 1980;96:757–61.
7. Yogev R et al. Pharmacokinetic comparison of intravenous and oral chloramphenicol in patients with *Haemophilus influenzae* meningitis. Pediatrics. 1981;67:656–60.
8. Tuomanen EI et al. Oral chloramphenicol in the treatment of *Haemophilus influenzae* meningitis. J Pediatr. 1981;99:968–74.
9. Kauffman RE et al. Relative bioavailability of intravenous chloramphenicol succinate and oral chloramphenicol palmitate in infants and children. J Pediatr. 1981;99:963–67.
10. Shankaran S, Kauffman RE. Use of chloramphenicol palmitate in neonates. J Pediatr. 1984;105:113–16.
11. Ross S et al. The use of chloromycetin palmitate in infants and children: A preliminary report. Antibiot Chemother. 1952;2:199.
12. Glazko AJ et al. Absorption and excretion of parenteral doses of chloramphenicol sodium succinate (CMS) in comparison with peroral doses of chloramphenicol (CM). Clin Pharmacol Ther. 1977;21:104. Abstract.
13. Roy TE et al. Studies on the absorption of chloramphenicol in normal children in relation to the treatment of meningitis. Antibiot Chemother. 1952;11:505-16.
14. Nahata MC, Powell DA. Bioavailability and clearance of chloramphenicol after intravenous chloramphenicol succinate. Clin Pharmacol Ther. 1981;30:368–72.
15. Nahata MC, Powell DA. Comparative bioavailability and pharmacokinetics of chloramphenicol after intravenous chloramphenicol succinate in premature infants and older patients. Dev Pharmacol Ther. 1983;6:23–32.
16. McCrumb FR et al. The use of chloramphenicol acid succinate in the treatment of acute infection. In: Antibiotics Annual. New York: Medical Encyclopedia, Inc.; 1957–1958;837–41.
17. Kauffman RE et al. Pharmacokinetics of chloramphenicol and chloramphenicol succinate in infants and children. J Pediatr. 1981;98:315–20.
18. Kelly RS et al. Studies on absorption and distribution of chloramphenicol. Pediatrics. 1951;8:362.
19. Schoenbach EB et al. Treatment of *Hemophilus influenzae* meningitis with aureomycin and chloramphenicol. Am J Med. 1952;12:263.
20. Roy TE. Studies on absorption of chloramphenicol in normal children in relation to treatment of meningitis. Antibiot Chemother. 1952;2:505.
21. Glazer JP et al. Disposition of chloramphenicol in low birth weight infants. Pediatrics. 1980;66:573–78.
22. Yodev R, Williams T. Ventricular fluid levels of chloramphenicol in infants. Antimicrob Agents Chemother. 1979;16:7–8.
23. Koup JR et al. Relationship between serum and saliva chloramphenicol concentrations. Antimicrob Agents Chemother. 1979;15:658–61.
24. George FJ, Hanna C. Ocular penetration of chloramphenicol. Effects of route of administration. Arch Ophthalmol (Copenh). 1977;95:879–82.
25. Ross S et al. Placental transmission of chloramphenicol (chloromycetin). JAMA. 1950;142:1361.

26. Scott WC, Warner RF. Placental transfer of chloramphenicol (chloromycetin). JAMA. 1950;142:1331.
27. Meissner HC, Smith AL. Current status of chloramphenicol. Pediatrics. 1979;64:348–56.
28. Williams B, Dart RM. Chloramphenicol concentration in cerebrospinal, ascitic and pleural fluid. Boston Med. 1950;1:7.
29. Koup JR et al. Chloramphenicol pharmacokinetics in hospitalized patients. Antimicrob Agents Chemother. 1979;15:651–57.
30. Slaughter RL et al. Chloramphenicol succinate kinetics in critically ill patients. Clin Pharmacol Ther. 1980;28:69–77.
31. Sack CM et al. Chloramphenicol succinate kinetics in infants and young children. Pediatr Pharmacol. 1982;2:93.
32. Sack CM, Koup JR, Smith AL. Chloramphenicol pharmacokinetics in infants and young children. Pediatrics. 1980;66:579–84.
33. Burckart GJ et al. Chloramphenicol clearance in infants. J Clin Pharmacol. 1982;22:49–52.
34. Rajchgot P et al. Chloramphenicol pharmacokinetics in the newborn. Dev Pharmacol Ther. 1983;6:305–14.
35. Kunin CM et al. Persistence of antibiotics in blood of patients with acute renal failure. II. Chloramphenicol and its metabolic products in the blood of patients with severe renal disease or hepatic cirrhosis. J Clin Invest. 1959;38:1498.
36. Young WS III, Lietman PS. Chloramphenicol glucuronyl transferase: assay, ontogeny, and inducibility. J Pharmacol Exp Ther. 1978;204:203–11.
37. Dill WA et al. A new metabolite of chloramphenicol (chloromycetin). J Biol Chem. 1950;183:679.
38. Christensen KK, Skousted L. Inhibition of drug metabolism by chloramphenicol. Lancet. 1969;2:1397–399.
39. Petitpierre B, Fabre J. Chlorpropamide and chloramphenicol. Lancet. 1970;1:789.
40. Rose JQ et al. Intoxication caused by chloramphenicol. Lancet. 1969;2:1397–399.
41. Powell DA et al. Interactions among chloramphenicol, phenytoin, and phenobarbital in a pediatric patient. J Pediatr. 1981;98:1001–3.
42. Bloxham RA et al. Chloramphenicol and phenobarbitone: A drug interaction. Arch Dis Child. 1979;54:76.
43. Krasinski K et al. Pharmacological interactions among chloramphenicol, phenytoin and phenobarbital. Pediatr Infect Dis. 1982;1:232–35.
44. Buchanan N, Moodley GP. Interaction between chloramphenicol and paracetamol. Br Med J. 1979;2:307.
45. Azzollini F et al. Elimination of chloramphenicol and thiamphenicol in subjects with cirrhosis of the liver. Int J Clin Pharmacol Ther Toxicol. 1972;6:130–43.
46. Narang APS et al. Pharmacokinetic study of chloramphenicol in patients with liver disease. Eur J Clin Pharmacol. 1979;15:651.
47. Schuck O et al. Excretion of chloramphenicol and its metabolites by the chronically diseased kidney. Int J Clin Pharmacol Res. 1974;10:33.
48. Glazko AJ et al. Biochemical studies on chloramphenicol (chloromycetin). J Pharmacol Exp Ther. 1949;96:445–49.
49. Glazko AJ et al. An evaluation of the absorption characteristics of different chloramphenicol preparations in normal human subjects. Clin Pharmacol Ther. 1968;9:472-83.
50. Glazko AJ et al. Biochemical studies on chloramphenicol (chloromycetin). J Biol Chem. 1950;1983:679.
51. Schuck O et al. Consequences of osmotic diuresis in residual nephrons for urinary drug excretion. Int J Clin Pharmacol Res. 1977;15:201–4.
52. Glazko AJ et al. Observations on the metabolic disposition of chloramphenicol in the rat. J Pharmacol Exp Ther. 1952;104:452.
53. Pratt WB. Chemotherapy of Infection. New York, NY:Oxford University Press;1977:132–34.
54. Pongs O et al. Identification of chloramphenicol-binding protein in *Escherichia coli* ribosomes by affinity labeling. Proc Natl Acad Sci USA. 1973;70:2229–233.

55. Barry AL, Thornsberry C. Susceptibility testing, appendix 2. In: Leneetee EH et al., eds. Manual of clinical microbiology, 3rd ed. Washington, DC: American Society for Microbiology; 1980.

56. Rahal JJ, Simberkoff JS. Bactericidal and bacteriostatic action of chloramphenicol against meningeal pathogens. Antimicrob Agents Chemother. 1979;16:13–8.

57. Turk DC. A comparison of chloramphenicol and ampicillin as bactericidal agents for *Haemophilus influenzae* type b. J Med Microbiol. 1977;10:127–31.

58. Klastersky J, Husson M. Bactericidal activity of the combination of gentamicin with clindamycin or chloramphenicol against species of *Escherichia coli* and *Bacteroides fragilis*. Antimicrob Agents Chemother. 1977;12:135–38.

59. Feldman WE, Zweighaft T. Effect of ampicillin and chloramphenicol against *Streptococcus pneumoniae* and *Neisseria meningitidis*. Antimicrob Agents Chemother. 1979;15:240–42.

60. Cole FS et al. Effect of ampicillin and chloramphenicol alone and in combination on ampicillin-susceptible and -resistant *Haemophilus influenzae* type b. Antimicrob Agents Chemother. 1979;15:415–19.

61. Feldman WE. Effect of ampicillin and chloramphenicol against *Haemophilus influenzae*. Pediatrics. 1978;61:406-9.

62. Barrett FF et al. A 12-year review of the antibiotic management of *Hemophilus influenzae* meningitis. Comparison of ampicillin and conventional therapy including chloramphenicol. J Pediatr. 1972;81:370–77.

63. Long SS, Phillips SE. Chloramphenicol-resistant *Hemophilus influenzae*. J Pediatr. 1977;90:1030–31.

64. Roberts MC et al. Characterization of chloramphenicol resistant *Hemophilus influenzae*. Antimicrob Agents Chemother. 1980;18:610–15.

65. Kinmonth A et al. Meningitis due to chloramphenicol resistant *Haemophilus influenzae* type b. Br Med J. 1978;1:694.

66. Uchiyama N et al. Meningitis due to *Haemophilus influenzae* type b resistant to ampicillin and chloramphenicol. J Pediatr. 1980;97:421–24.

67. Kennedy JF et al. Meningitis due to *Haemophilus influenzae* type b resistant to both ampicillin and chloramphenicol. Pediatrics. 1980;66:14–6.

68. Ampicillin and chloramphenicol resistant in systemic *Haemophilus influenzae* disease. 1984;33:35–7.

69. Simasathien S et al. *Haemophilus influenzae* type b resistant to ampicillin and chloramphenicol in an orphanage in Thailand. Lancet. 1980,2:1214–217.

70. Chau PY et al. Resistant to chloramphenicol and ampicillin *Salmonella johannesburg* in Hong Kong: observations over a five-year period 1973–977. J Hyg(London). 1978;81:353–51.

71. Cherubin CE et al. Emergence of resistance to chloramphenicol in *Salmonella*. J Infect Dis. 1977;135:807-12.

72. Van luingeren B et al. Plasmid-mediated chloramphenicol resistance in *Haemophilus influenzae*. Antimicrob Agents Chemother. 1977;11:383–87.

73. Irvin JE, Ingram JM. Chloramphenicol-resistant variants of *Pseudomonas aeruginosa* defective in amino acid transport. Can J Biochem. 1980;58:1165–171.

74. Traub WH, Fukushima PI. Nonspecific resistance of *Serratia marcescens* against antimicrobial drugs. Resistance or decreased susceptibility of phenotypic variants against chloramphenicol, nalidixic acid, nitrofurantoin, sulfonamides, and trimethoprim. Chemotherapy. 1979;25:196-203.

75. Scott JL et al. A controlled double-blind study of the hematologic toxicity of chloramphenicol. N Engl J Med. 1965;272:1137–142.

76. Oski FA. Hematologic consequences of chloramphenicol therapy. J Pediatr. 1979;94:515–16.

77. Rosenbach L et al. Chloramphenicol toxicity: reversible vacuolization of erythroid cells. N Engl J Med. 1960;263:724–28.

78. Saidi P et al. Effect of chloramphenicol on erythropoiesis. J Lab Clin Med. 1961;57:247–56.

79. Yunis AA. Chloramphenicol-induced bone marrow suppression. Semin Hematol. 1973;10:225–34.

80. Daum RS et al. Fatal aplastic anemia following apparent "dose related" chloramphenicol therapy. J Pediatr. 1979;94:403–6.

81. Rich ML et al. A fatal case of aplastic anemia following chloramphenicol therapy. Ann Intern Med. 1950;33:1459-461.
82. Wallerstein RO et al. Statewide study of chloramphenicol treatment and fatal aplastic anemia. JAMA. 1969;208:2045–50.
83. Best WR. Chloramphenicol-associated blood dyscrasias. JAMA. 1967;201:181–88.
84. Hugeley CM Jr et al. Drug related blood dyscrasias. JAMA. 1961;177:23–6.
85. Welch H et al. Blood dyscrasias: a nationwide survey. Antibiot Chemother. 1954;4:607–23.
86. Rosenthal RL, Blackman A. Bone-marrow hypoplasia following use of chloramphenicol eyedrops. JAMA. 1965;191:136–37.
87. Nagao T, Mauer AM. Concordance for drug-induced aplastic anemia in identical twins. N Engl J Med. 1969;281:7–11.
88. Holt R. The bacterial degradation of chloramphenicol. Lancet. 1967;1:1259–260.
89. Domart A et al. Fatal bone marrow aplasia after intramuscular chloramphenicol administration in two adults. Sem Hop Paris. 1961;37:2256–258.
90. Grilliat JP et al. Fatal cytopenia after chloramphenicol hemisuccinate therapy. Ann Med. 1966.5:754–62.
91. Restrepo MA, Zambrano F. II. Late-onset aplastic anemia secondary to chloramphenicol. Report of ten cases. Antioquia Medica. 1968;18:593–606.
92. Klein JO. Antimicrobial agents for infants and children. In: Feigin RD, Cherry JD, eds. Textbook of pediatric infectious diseases. Philadelphia: WB Saunders; 1981:1695-712.
93. Lietman PS. Chloramphenicol and the neonate-1979 view. Clin Pharmacol. 1979;6:151–62.
94. Burns LE et al. Fatal circulatory collapse in premature infants receiving chloramphenicol. N Engl J Med. 1959;261:1318–321.
95. Lambdin MA. On the "gray syndrome" and chloramphenicol toxicity. Pediatrics. 1960;25:935–40.
96. Craft AW et al. The "gray toddler": Chloramphenicol toxicity. Arch Dis Child. 1974;49:235–37.
97. Morton K. Chloramphenicol overdosage in a 6-week-old infant. Am J Dis Child. 1961;102:430.
98. Thompson WL et al. Overdoses of chloramphenicol. JAMA. 1975;234:149–50.
99. Freeman KB, Haldar D. The inhibition of mammalian NADH oxidation by chloramphenicol and its isomers and analogues. Can J Biochem. 1968;46:1003–8.
100. Hallman M. Oxygen uptake in neonatal rats: A developmental study with particular reference to the effects of chloramphenicol. Pediatr Res. 1973;7:923–30.
101. Mauer SM et al. Treatment of an infant with severe chloramphenicol intoxication using charcoal-column hemoperfusion. J Pediatr. 1980;96:136–39.
102. Kessler DL et al. Chloramphenicol toxicity in a neonate treated with exchange transfusion. J Pediatr. 1980;96:140–41.
103. Krakoff IH et al. Effect of large doses of chloramphenicol on human subjects. N Engl J Med. 1955;253:7–10.
104. Woodward TE, Weissman CL. Chloromycetin (chloramphenicol). Antibiotics monograph No.8. New York: Medical Encyclopedia; 1958.
105. Felix NS. Chloramphenicol: Applied pharmacology. Pediatr Clin North Am. 1966;3:317–27.
106. Cocke JG et al. Optic neuritis with prolonged use of chloramphenicol on human subjects. N Engl J Med. 1955;253:7–10.
107. Keith CG et al. Side effects to antibiotics in cystic fibrosis. Arch Dis Child. 1966;41:262–66.
108. Ambrose CT, Coons AH. Studies on antibody production: VII. Inhibitory effect of chloramphenicol on synthesis of antibody in tissue culture. J Exp Med. 1963;117:1075–88.
109. Weisberger AS, Daniel TM. Suppression of antibody synthesis by chloramphenicol analogs. Proc Soc Exp Biol Med. 1969;131:570–75.
110. Beutler E. Drug-induced hemolytic anemia. Pharmacol Rev. 1969;21:73–103.
111. Biancaniello T et al. Chloramphenicol and cardiotoxicity. J Pediatr. 1981;98:828-30.
112. Nahata MC et al. Effect of intravenous flow rate and injection site on *in vitro* delivery of chloramphenicol succinate and *in vivo* kinetics. J Pediatr. 1981;99:463-66.
113. Gould T, Roberts RJ. Therapeutic problems arising from the use of the intravenous route for drug administration. J Pediatr. 1979;95:465–71.

114. Nahata MC, Powell DA. Chloramphenicol serum concentration falls during chloramphenicol succinate dosing. Clin Pharmacol Ther. 1983;33:308–13.

115. Koup JR et al. Rapid estimation of chloramphenicol clearance in infants and children. Clin Pharmacokinet. 1981;6:83–8.

116. Nelson JD, ed. Pocketbook of Pediatric Antimicrobial Therapy. Dallas:Jodone Publishing;1981.

117. Glazko AJ, Wolf LM, Dill WA. Biochemical studies on chloramphenicol (Chloromycetin). Arch Biochem. 1949;23:411.

118. Mason EO Jr et al. Modification of the colorimetric assay for chloramphenicol in the presence of bilirubin. Antimicrob Agents Chemother. 1979;15:544–46.

119. Schuck O et al. Excretion of chloramphenicol and its metabolites by the chronically diseased kidney (with respect to the theory of adaptive nephrons). Int J Clin Pharmacol Res. 1974;10:33–43.

120. Bannatyne RM, Cheung R. Chloramphenicol bioassay. Antimicrob Agents Chemother. 1979;16:43–5.

121. Smith AL, Smith DH. Improved enzymatic assay of chloramphenicol. Clin Chem. 1978;24:1452–457.

122. Robison LR et al. Simplified radioenzymatic assay for chloramphenicol. Antimicrob Agents Chemother. 1970;13:25-9.

123. Aravind MK et al. Simultaneous measurement of chloramphenicol and chloramphenicol succinate by high performance liquid chromatography. J Chromatogr. 1980;221:176–81.

124. Nahata MC, Powell DA. Simultaneous determination of chloramphenicol and its succinate ester by high-performance liquid chromatography. J Chromatogr. 1981;223:247–51.

125. Aravind MK et al. Determinations of chloramphenicol glucuronide in urine by high performance liquid chromatography. J Chromatogr. 1982;232:461–64.

126. Least CJ et al. Quantitative gas-chromatographic flame ionization methods for chloramphenicol in human serum. Clin Chem. 1977;23:220–22.

127. Dickinson CJ et al. The effect of exocrine pancreatic function on chloramphenicol pharmaco-kinetics in patients with cystic fibrosis. Pediatr Res. 1988;23:388–92.

128. Shann F et al. Absorption of chloramphenicol sodium succinate after intramuscular administration in children. N Engl J Med. 1985;313:410–414.

129. Kelly HW et al. Interaction of chloramphenicol and rifampin. J Pediatr. 1988;112:817–20.

130. Kearns GL et al. Absence of pharmacokinetic interaction between chloramphenicol and acet-aminophen in children. J Pediatr. 1985;107:134–39.

131. Evans LS, Kleiman MB. Acidosis as a presenting feature of chloramphenicol toxicity. J Pediatr. 1986;108:475–77.

132. Phelps SJ et al. Chloramphenicol-induced cardiovascular collapse in an anephric patient. Pediatr Infect Dis J. 1987;6:285–88.

133. Ristuccia AM. Chloramphenicol: clinical pharmacology in pediatrics. Ther Drug Monit. 1985;7(2):159–67.

134. Nahata MC. Lack of predictability of chloramphenicol toxicity in pediatric patients. J Clin Pharm Ther. 1989;14:297–303.

135. Sherry B et al. Anemia during *Haemophilus influenzae* type b meningitis: lack of an effect of chloramphenicol. Dev Pharmacol Ther. 1989;12(4):188–89.

136. EMIT Chloramphenicol Assay. 1986. Syva Co. Palo Alto, CA.

137. Atkinson HC et al. Drugs in human milk: clinical pharmacokinetic considerations. Clin Pharmacokin. 1988;14:217–40.

138. West BC et al. Aplastic anemia associated with parenteral chloramphenicol: review of 10 cases, including the second case of possible increased risk with cimetidine. Rev Infect Dis. 1988;10:1048–51.

139. Burke JT et al. Pharmacokinetics of intravenous chloramphenicol sodium succinate in adult patients with normal renal and hepatic functions. J Pharmacokin Biopharm. 1982;10:601–14.

Chapter 17

Dual Individualization with Antibiotics: Integrated Antibiotic Management Strategies for Use in Hospitals

Jerome J. Schentag, Charles H. Ballow,
Joseph A. Paladino, and David E. Nix

The common goal of clinical pharmacokinetics practice is to individualize drug regimens and thus optimize the treatment of disease. Antibiotics provide frequent examples of improved clinical response as a consequence of individualized therapy.[1-5] In current practice, pharmacokinetic principles are used to maintain serum concentrations within a rather narrow therapeutic range for drugs such as aminoglycosides.[6-10] However, there are a growing number of reasons why "individualization" of antibiotic therapy means *more* than attaining a target range of serum concentrations, particularly in an outcome oriented health care system. Incorporation of both pharmacokinetics and bacterial pharmacodynamics into the mathematical process of dosage adjustment can cure patients more rapidly, and often lower the cost of antibiotic therapy. In contrast to the variable rate of response associated with a standard, average dose, the outcome of therapy can be controlled by using a dosing regimen designed with consideration of the pharmacologic response of the bacteria. Since few antibiotics are currently individualized on the basis of both pharmacokinetic and pharmacodynamic characteristics, this chapter will review and update an evolving methodology for antibiotic selection and proper dosing regimen design applicable to virtually all hospitalized patients.

Aminoglycosides are often underdosed in hospitalized patients. Although outcome of therapy can be greatly improved by making dosage adjustments based on blood levels, this process alone oversimplifies the interactions between patient and bacteria shown in Figure 17-1. The current target blood level strategy assumes that fixed concentrations kill susceptible bacteria at equal rates. Under this assumption, dosage individualization considers only pharmacokinetics and toxicity. The remaining four interactions in the relationship between bacteria, host, and antibiotic are generally neglected.

The situation with all the other antibiotics is worse, since the aminoglycosides and vancomycin are often the only antibiotics where any attempt at dosage adjustment is made. For other antibiotics (such as β-lactams), there is the general belief that it makes little difference what dose or regimen is chosen since nearly all regimens produce concentrations greater than required.[11] Some studies have tested this hypothesis by using very small doses to treat urinary tract infection (UTI),[12] but if the β-lactams were consistently given in excessive dosages, there should be no treatment failures. Furthermore, we should be able to reduce dosages in most patients and save enormous amounts of money. Neither of these goals has been realized, but only now are there early efforts underway to individualize dosages of β-lactam and quinolone antibiotics in an attempt to avoid treatment failures and reduce antibiotic costs. With the rising costs of antibiotics and the emphasis on favorable outcomes at the lowest necessary cost, it becomes advantageous to consider the previously neglected portions of the dynamic system portrayed in Figure 17-1. Since there are four remaining variables relevant to drug treatment of infection (pharmacodynamics, resistance, toxicity, and pharmacokinetics), there have been attempts to integrate the pharmacodynamic relationship between drug and bacteria into the individualized approach to treatment regimens.

Methods that incorporate pharmacodynamics (i.e., concentration-dependent effect of the antibiotic on bacteria) into antibiotic use are logical and can alter the

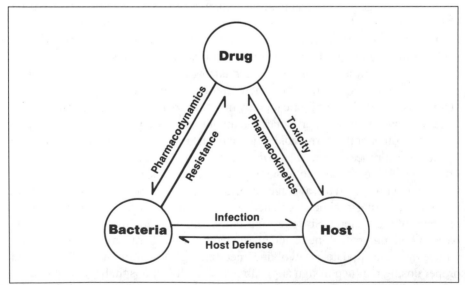

Figure 17-1. *Schematic representation of the interactions between bacteria, patient, and antibiotic. Each of the six possible interactions is characterized and defined by the arrows between categories. A major purpose of this chapter is to identify areas where these interactions can be optimized to the benefit of clinical pharmacy practitioners and their patients.*

clinical outcome if appropriate changes in the antibiotic dose or dosing intervals are made. When these methods are computer assisted, they also represent an increasingly practical cost-containment strategy. An integrated pharmacokinetic-pharmacodynamic dosing methodology can be used prospectively to change doses, thereby altering clinical outcome and directly benefiting the patient. Adoption of this strategy produces an immediate change in the focus of day-to-day activities of clinical antibiotic use. Its use in the clinic places the selection of antibiotics, dosages, and dosing intervals into a system designed to take important pharmacokinetic and pharmacodynamic variables into account in both product selection and monitoring. The proposed expansion of the narrow antibiotic kinetics perspective into an outcome-oriented mode can be readily distinguished from the common practice of dosage based on target blood levels. Antibiotic strategies which consider both kinetics and dynamics will be distinguished by use of the term "dual individualization."[13]

DUAL INDIVIDUALIZATION: BACKGROUND AND HISTORICAL PERSPECTIVE

The theories which foster the development of dual individualization are not new, and there is a large body of literature over the course of its development. It has long been assumed that there is a mathematical relationship between the antimicrobial serum concentration and bacterial killing. The general acceptance of *in vitro* susceptibility testing as a rationale for antibiotic selection is also a major founding principle. The assumption that antibiotic activity was related to concentration led to the notion of bacterial susceptibility, defined as minimal inhibitory concentration (MIC). The MIC was then integrated with blood levels with the object of achieving antibiotic concentrations above the MIC. This tendency to combine *in vitro* susceptibility with *in vivo* pharmacokinetic perspectives eventually led investigators to propose inhibitory indices. Examples include the Inhibitory Quotient,[14] Intensity Index,[15] bactericidal titers,[16,17] bactericidal rate,[18] bactericidal AUC,[19] and area of free concentration above MIC.[20]

Parameters like AUC above MIC, Inhibitory Quotients, and Intensity Index are promising techniques. Their disadvantage is that they assume that antibiotic blood levels are predictable when patients are given standard doses.[21] Thus, they do not account for the marked pharmacokinetic variance in serum antibiotic concentrations which may occur as a consequence of disease. All are based on a single factor: relative susceptibility. Aminoglycosides, above all, teach us that the assumption of predictable antibiotic serum concentrations is clearly not valid, particularly in diseased populations.

General success with *in vitro* susceptibility testing and the incorporation of *in vitro* susceptibility indices into dosing strategy design comprised half of the process of dual individualization. An appreciation for disease-dependent antibiotic kinetics comprised the other half. What remained was a method to conveniently integrate both factors into the design of dosage regimens so that *in vivo* bacterial exposure to antibiotics could be further optimized. The only possible means of accomplishing dual individualization on a hospital-wide scale was to incorporate population kinetic data, patient-specific demographic and organ function factors, measured serum concentrations, and a known MIC into a computerized monitoring program.

In the course of developing and computerizing this model, it became apparent that the post-antibiotic effect (PAE) could seriously complicate the application of dual individualization to patients. This was because direct extrapolation of the equations would require measurement of the PAE in each patient. Although we developed a way to rapidly measure PAE so that we could calculate the dose accurately,[22] we have postulated that the PAE is only of potential importance for aminoglycosides[23] and probably of little importance for the quinolones,[24] vancomycin,[25] or β-lactams.[26] In order to maintain our focus on gram-negative infections while avoiding the PAE, we decided to use the antibiotics other than the aminoglycosides to test dual individualization initially. Both the aminoglycosides and quinolones exhibit *in vitro* PAE of variable duration against gram-negative organisms.[27–30] There were other reasons which made aminoglycosides poor candidates for the initial development of dual individualization principles: they were seldom used alone, making it impossible to isolate their *in vivo* antibacterial effects, and they had a rigidly defined concentration range. Thus, if we considered variable susceptibilities in making dosage adjustment, serum levels could drop well below the generally accepted range when treating very susceptible bacteria or, in contrast, exceed the usually accepted values when treating more resistant bacteria.[23] In view of this, we decided to use drugs that did not carry the liability of a rigidly defined therapeutic window. Conversely, β-lactam and quinolone antibiotics do not normally exhibit an *in vivo* PAE on gram-negative organisms,[27,30] although β-lactams do with gram-positive bacteria.[31]

As this antibiotic management strategy was evolving, Craig and associates were rigorously testing the underlying concepts using β-lactam antibiotics against Pseudomonas in animal models such as the neutropenic mouse.[27,28,32] These animal model studies yielded virtually the same relationships between β-lactam antibiotic kinetics and dynamics as did our human studies using dual individualization. Not all animal models yielded useful data, however. Of the available animal models, only the studies of Gerber[28] and Roosendaal[33] validate dual individualization because most experimental models gave doses to achieve peak concentrations similar to those in patients, but employed dosing intervals that were too long to match the trough values typical of patients.[34–39]

RATIONALE FOR DUAL INDIVIDUALIZATION STRATEGY APPLIED TO GRAM-NEGATIVE PNEUMONIA

Initial testing of dual individualization in patients required the selection of a single infection site in order to minimize the potential for variance introduced by host factors. Neutropenic patients would be a rigorous test of the dosing strategy, but in most cases, there is no bacterial isolate on which to determine dosing regimens or evaluate response. Furthermore, all of these patients are treated with combinations of two to four drugs.

Abdominal sepsis is a condition we have extensively studied.[40] However, this was also considered a poor initial site for testing dual individualization because cure primarily depends on surgical correction of the underlying problem, and resolution is minimally dependent on the antibiotic. In surgical sepsis, no antibiotic combination or single agent succeeds in cases where the underlying problem is not surgically repaired, and virtually all broad spectrum single agents or antibiotic combinations are effective when the surgical problem is corrected.

Urinary tract infections are also cured by virtually all regimens, and the difficulty of distinguishing between upper and lower urinary tract disease complicates the diagnosis of this disease. There is a relationship between urine concentration and MIC and bacterial killing rate with aminoglycosides[41] and cephalosporins,[42] but thus far, it has not been rigorously evaluated in infected patients.

Gram-negative nosocomial pneumonia was the infection site most adaptable to our initial dual individualization protocol. Nosocomial gram-negative pneumonia is the leading cause of death from nosocomial infection.[43] The disease is common in the elderly patient who has been hospitalized for prolonged periods of time, and who often resides in the intensive care unit due to other clinical conditions. Nosocomial pneumonia is considered a major factor in as many as 6% of deaths in hospitals[44] and is a source of significant financial loss to hospitals.[45] The disease is relatively simple to identify and stage,[46] and its course is easy to monitor. It is not self-limiting and often becomes a therapeutic failure, even when the causative bacteria are susceptible *in vitro*.[47–49] Patients we encounter are elderly and often nutritionally compromised, but they are not neutropenic.[50,51] Pathogens are readily extracted from tracheal aspirates, and tracheal secretions can be serially cultured in order to assess the day of bacterial eradication. Finally, there is a spectrum of different bacteria which cause this disease, and they exhibit a wide range of *in vitro* susceptibilities to antibiotics. The varied susceptibility of causative organisms plus the wide interpatient variation in antibiotic excretion caused by different degrees of renal function justifies the development of better individualization strategies.

ASSUMPTIONS IN THE DEVELOPMENT OF DUAL INDIVIDUALIZATION

Assumptions must be made to develop a dosing strategy, and dual individualization is no exception. We assumed that serum concentrations of aminoglycosides, cephalosporins, and quinolones were either equal to or proportional to concentrations at a well-perfused infection site.[54] For reasons more extensively described elsewhere by us[52–54] and others,[55–58] this premise appears reasonable for infection sites other than closed spaces or abscesses. At well-perfused sites, bacteria and antibiotics, such as β-lactams, quinolones, and aminoglycosides are confined to the extracellular space, and interstitial fluids are similar to those in serum after the initial rapid distributive phase.[54] The distribution of cephalosporins into true interstitial fluids is only minimally influenced by serum protein binding. Penetration through capillaries is rapid, and interstitial fluid contains similar fluid and protein, as does serum.[53–58] Our findings of a good correlation between serum concentrations and bacterial killing[51] and between ciprofloxacin and bacterial killing[24] strongly support this premise. Animal models support this premise for β-lactams and aminoglycosides.[28,29,33] Quinolones have not yet been rigorously studied.

Our second assumption was that there is a relationship between bacterial killing *in vitro* and *in vivo* at controlled exposure to drug. This does not necessarily assume that the rate of killing is identical *in vitro* and *in vivo*—only that the two rates are proportional. It is doubtful that the rates are equal, since bacteria are generally eradicated more slowly *in vivo* than *in vitro*.[59] There are a number of hypotheses advanced to account for slower *in vivo* killing of bacteria.[60]

The pharmacodynamic relationships between antibiotic concentration and rate of *in vivo* killing needed to be evaluated by conducting a concentration-controlled clinical trial. It was one of the purposes of our studies to evaluate these relationships. We standardized the patient population by age and disease and focused our attention on gram-negative pneumonia in elderly ICU patients who were intubated. Patients had gram-negative pneumonia in Stage III.[46] We carefully stratified patients by disease and then assumed that variances in underlying disease or host demographics would not play a major role in the rate of bacterial eradication. Accordingly, this study standardized the host and tested the remaining two sources of variance (drug concentration versus bacteria).

PHARMACODYNAMIC AND PHARMACOKINETIC INTEGRATION IN PATIENTS WITH PNEUMONIA

Two major reasons for the slow evolution of practical methods to apply dual individualization have been the time lag required to determine quantitative susceptibility and the need for computer systems capable of merging both patient and bacterial kinetics into the prospective design of dosing regimens. The first of these two problems has been partially solved by the development of automated microbiology equipment. The second problem required computer hardware capable of handling a large database and considerable software development.

The major source of variance for patients in the ICU is disease and the associated alterations in antibiotic clearance. The aminoglycosides have been extensively studied in relation to disease in critical care patients, and the wide variance which can be encountered is well documented.[3,7,8] Serum concentration monitoring is a normal practice in ICU patients. For β-lactam antibiotics like cefmenoxime and for quinolones like ciprofloxacin, there have been only a few studies conducted.[24,51] Not surprisingly, when these studies were performed there was at least as much pharmacokinetic variance in peak, clearance, and volume of distribution in critical care patients as that found previously for the aminoglycosides.[7] A standard dose of cefmenoxime or ciprofloxacin is no more likely to produce uniform peak concentrations than is a standard dose of an aminoglycoside. Cefmenoxime peaks produced by the same dose vary from 40 to 400 µg/mL, and clearance may range fivefold.[51]

Both sources of variance must be controlled to accomplish dual individualization in ICU patients with pneumonia. Pharmacokinetic factors which alter the serum profile in the patient often require measurement of serum concentrations, even when the bacteria are susceptible. A simulation was performed to illustrate the effect that the interaction of these two sources of variance would have on dosing in the same patient. We used the clinically tested target AUC above MIC of 140 µg × hr/mL for the simulations in Table 17-1. Using population kinetic averages and the range in MIC of susceptible bacteria, we simulated cefmenoxime doses (see Table 17-1) that would be required for patients with varied renal function and a varied, but susceptible, MIC. These dosing regimens make it clear that about half of the variance in dose requirements is a result of the pharmacokinetic effects of renal function changes; the other half is a consequence of the differences in bacteria susceptibility. The data in Table 17-1 clearly establish that cefmenoxime dosage requirements can easily vary fivefold between some combinations of the MIC and creatinine clearance when the target AUC is predetermined. These data further demonstrate why dual individualization must successfully integrate both sources of variance into dosage calculations. If random dosages are given without attention to bacterial susceptibility, then various combinations of patient factors, bacteria, and drug can easily produce variances that are ten- or twentyfold from the optimal range. Similar principles, problems, and variations hold for the aminoglycosides and quinolones.

Since the combinations of kinetics and susceptibility can be complex, this process is best accomplished by interfacing a microcomputer with the antimicrobial susceptibility testing system. If population parameters are used for the antibiotic, then the dual individualization process only requires a bacterial isolate and its MIC value. This value is then integrated into the computer program which calculates dosage based on measured or predicted blood levels of the antibiotic. The entire process of dosage calculation using this method can be performed as soon as the bacterial MIC is determined. In this manner, the same computer that performs the calculation of MIC for the bacteria can be used to calculate serum concentrations, AUC, and AUC above MIC thereby completing the process of dual individualization.

Table 17-1. *Simulated Cefmenoxime Dosage (gm every 6 hours) Needed to Produce AUC of 140 µg × hr/mL Above MIC at Various Degrees of Creatinine Clearance[a,b]*

Creatinine clearance	MIC 0.2	MIC 2.0	MIC 25.0
10 mL/min	0.5	0.5	1.0
50 mL/min	1.0	1.0	2.0
100 mL/min	1.5	1.5	2.5

[a] Values are rounded to the nearest 50 mg unit.
[b] Reproduced with permission from reference 51.

Dual Individualization Applied to Treatment of Pneumonia

Development and validation of the dual individualization methodology has now been completed using cefmenoxime[51] and ciprofloxacin.[24] All studies have been conducted in gram-negative nosocomial pneumonia patients. For each patient, daily cultures of endotracheal tube aspirates were also taken in order to identify the day of bacterial eradication. Response (both clinical and bacteriologic) was assessed in each study patient, as eradication and cure in relation to kinetic/dynamic parameters. Essentially, these studies show that higher exposure in relation to the MIC produces more rapid bacterial eradication. Secondly, they show that dosage adjustment to optimize the AUC and the time above MIC can speed the rate of bacterial eradication in the individual patient. Finally, the study data reveal that high MIC organisms like Pseudomonas are often underexposed (low AUC in relation to high MIC) with conventional dosages and often develop resistance to the antibiotic. Higher dosages prevented this development. Also, patients with abnormal renal function are often given higher dosages than needed to rapidly eradicate the pathogens. In these patients, dosages can be lowered to produce rapid bacterial eradication at a lower cost.

Our optimal treatment results may have occurred because of careful standardization of host factors during the development of dual individualization. However, a sufficient proportion of the relationship could be explained by considering only the interactions between drug versus bacteria. This correlation also documents that the rate of bacterial killing *in vitro* is related to the rate of bacterial killing *in vivo*, a finding also observed in animal models.[29] Although the rates of killing *in vitro* and *in vivo* are related, this does not imply that both rates are the same. The *in vivo* killing rate appears to be slower than that *in vitro*.[59] One complicating factor in other studies has been the post-antibiotic effect. However, an *in vivo* PAE could not be demonstrated for ciprofloxacin in our patients.[24] Additional study revealed an even better marker of the relationship between antibiotic pharmacokinetics and dynamics, as shown by the correlation ($r = 0.89$) between the time above MIC and days to bacterial eradication.[24,51]

In precise agreement with the animal models of Craig,[29] time above MIC was the most accurate explanation of the eradication of gram-negative bacteria by cephalosporins in nosocomial pneumonia patients. It made little difference what the species of bacteria were, as all were eradicated in relationship to time over their individually measured MICs.[51] Clinical parameters such as nutrition, fever, baseline disease, and specific bacteria did not influence the results.[50] Protein binding and consideration of free cefmenoxime did not further improve either the relationship between time or AUC above MIC, indicating little effect of serum protein binding on bacterial eradication. The correlations further support the assumption that cefmenoxime concentrations at the infection site are either equal to or proportional to serum concentrations.[53,54]

In the patients with rapid bacterial eradication, fever, WBC, and both the quantity and purulence of bronchial secretions declined rapidly. In contrast, these signs and symptoms resolved more slowly in those patients with slow bacterial eradication. In most cases, it was possible to stop cefmenoxime or ciprofloxacin after the patient was afebrile for five days. Radiological improvement occurred more slowly and often lagged behind improvement in the other clinical parameters. However, even those patients in whom we stopped antibiotics before pulmonary infiltrates had resolved had subsequent radiological improvement. Thus, while dosage adjustments were performed with an endpoint of bacterial eradication, there appears to be parallelism between bacterial eradication and the time antibiotics can be stopped (because of resolution of symptoms). An interesting goal would be to accelerate bacterial eradication and then determine if antibiotics could be stopped even earlier. This hypothesis was prospectively tested by a second study of cefmenoxime in nosocomial pneumonia. The second study was therefore organized to test the concept of a therapeutic window for the cephalosporin, cefmenoxime.

PROSPECTIVE CLINICAL STUDIES OF DUAL INDIVIDUALIZATION: A TEST OF THE SYSTEM FOR DOSAGE ADJUSTMENT

The relationships presented thus far were derived from analysis of clinical, bacteriologic, and pharmacokinetic data collected during and after treatment. These data provided evidence of a therapeutic target AUC above MIC in patients. A prospective study was initiated in April 1984 to test the clinical effectiveness of a prospective dosage regimen design to achieve the target AUC above MIC. This study was therefore designed to prospectively test dual individualization. The clinical purpose of the prospective study was to eradicate bacteria causing pneumonia within four days by adjusting the cefmenoxime dose to produce an AUC above MIC of 140 µg × hr/mL. From Table 17-1 and Figure 17-2, one can appreciate that combinations of high MIC values and/or low serum AUC values are associated with a much slower eradication time, and that a very low MIC or very high serum AUC are associated with a very fast eradication time. We sought to control these relationships within a narrow range along the regression by prospectively altering the cefmenoxime dose to maintain an AUC above MIC of 140 µg × hr/mL. It was the hypothesis for testing that this practice should produce four-day eradication and remove all the variance in the clinical relationship between dosage and bacterial eradication. Dosage regimens designed to produce an AUC above MIC of 140 µg × hr/mL, like those in Table 17-1, are able to cluster eradication time tightly around treatment day four as shown in Figure 17-2.

As before, all study patients had Stage III pneumonia,[46] and all patients were managed in the same manner by the same physicians. Only the dosage adjustment process was different. Each patient who entered into the prospective study had measurements of serum cefmenoxime concentration profiles on the first dose, and measurements of MIC on the bacteria isolated from tracheal aspirates. From the computerized integration of these two variables, a dose was chosen to produce an AUC above MIC of 140 µg × hr/mL as well as 100% of time above MIC. We then administered this regimen to the patients with gram-negative pneumonia and cultured their tracheal aspirates daily to determine day of eradication. The data from the first 18 treated patients are shown in Figure 17-2. The bacteria of the earlier study are shown as triangles, and solid circles denote the individual points for each bacteria prospectively treated using dual individualization.

The results with the prospective application of dual individualization were striking in that essentially all bacteria were eradicated within the narrow time window. There were no bacteria that persisted for long periods of time, in direct contrast to results in patients on the fixed dose of 1 gm every six hours. In the concentration-controlled trial, there were a number of patients who had pretreatment isolation of several gram-negative bacteria with a range of MIC values. When these situations were encountered, the dosage chosen was directed to eradicate the most resistant isolate. This was an effective process, but the data in Figure 17-2 shows variance in achieved AUC above MIC because of the presence of several

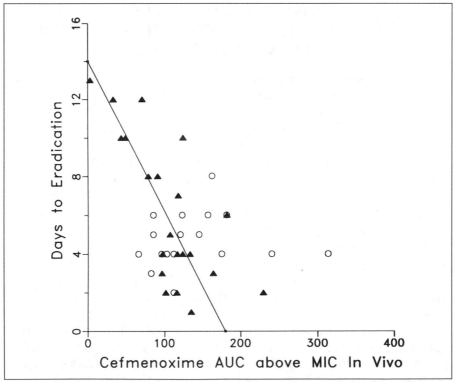

Figure 17-2. *Relationship between the cefmenoxime serum concentrations (i.e., AUC) above the MIC for retrospectively assessed (○) and prospectively treated (▲) patients, and the days to bacterial eradication in vivo. Each data point represents one bacteria. The regression line describing the retrospective data took the form of the equation:*

$$\text{Days to Eradication} = 13.96 - 0.07 \, \frac{\text{AUC}}{\text{MIC}} \, ; \; r = 0.71, \; p < 0.001$$

The dual individualized dosage method clustered the eradication day tightly around days four to six. It should be noted that patients had more than one bacteria. Since all data are plotted on this graph, treatment of a mixed culture would produce some very high AUC above MIC values for the susceptible strains. This accounts for most, but not all, of the deviant prospective data points in this figure (adapted with permission from reference 51).

bacteria. Thus, the greatest source of x-axis variation in Figure 17-2 is the presence of more than one bacterial isolate in the baseline culture. Of interest, the dosage actually given ranged from 1.5 to 12 gm/day in contrast to the fixed dosage of 4 gm/day given to virtually all patients in the first study.[50] Even though there was a wider range of dosage in the second study, the average dose between the two studies did not differ significantly. Prospectively treated patients who received an average dosage of 5 gm/day did not differ from the 4 gm/day average dose of the patients in the first study.[51]

Our conclusions from this prospective dual individualization study were that bacteria can be eradicated on a desired schedule, but it requires more careful attention to dosage to achieve the target range of concentrations above MIC. Treatment duration was significantly shorter (p <0.05) in cases of bacterial eradication. The data indicate that five days is the minimum treatment duration for the patients with ICU pneumonia. Thus, it appears from the cefmenoxime studies that dosage determination using dual individualization can shorten the duration of treatment by producing more rapid bacterial eradication.

RESULTS OF DUAL INDIVIDUALIZATION STUDIES WITH INTRAVENOUS CIPROFLOXACIN

Studies were conducted in 50 patients given intravenous doses of ciprofloxacin.[24] It was found that ciprofloxacin also demonstrated a relationship between the serum concentration, MIC, and day of bacterial eradication. Intravenous doses of 200 to 300 mg every 12 hours rapidly eradicated bacteria with MIC values below 0.25 µg/mL, while bacteria with higher MIC values often failed to respond at these doses.[24] These findings led to a prospective study using an intravenous dosage of 400 mg every eight hours. At these higher dosages, the bacterial isolates with MIC values up to 0.8 to 1 µg/mL were eradicated, while organisms with MIC values of 1 to 2 µg/mL failed to respond and often became resistant.[61] These two studies illustrate the value of dual individualization in that failures become more predictable, and successes can be achieved by selectively raising dosages in patients with high-MIC organisms or rapid clearances. The cure rate of Pseudomonas pneumonia with intravenous ciprofloxacin was increased from 30% to 75% by increasing the dose from 300 mg every 12 hours to 400 mg every eight hours, illustrating the potential of this approach in clinical practice. Moreover, the dosage increase we made could be predicted from population pharmacokinetics of ciprofloxacin and the MIC of the patient's organism. It required only 11 patients studied prospectively to identify that the initial 300 mg every 12 hours dosage was too low for organisms with MIC values above 0.25 µg/mL.[62]

DUAL INDIVIDUALIZATION AND ITS ROLE IN THE ERA OF ANTIBIOTIC CONTROL AND COST EFFECTIVENESS: AN OPPORTUNITY FOR PRACTITIONERS OF APPLIED PHARMACOKINETICS

There have been sweeping changes in the methods used to reimburse hospitals in the past few years, forcing them to deliver optimal care in the fastest possible manner using the lowest expenditure for drugs, supplies, and personnel. Complications of disease (or its treatment) such as nosocomial pneumonia prolong hospital stays,[63] add to the costs of delivering health care, and narrow or reverse the margin between the fixed reimbursement provided and the actual costs of providing care. Intensive care is at least four times more costly than management on the floor.[64] Since any patient managed in the ICU is already in a position to cause a loss of revenues to the hospital, a series of additional complications in this type of patient has the potential for financial disaster. Nosocomial pneumonia is precisely that disastrous complication, and it is not often a primary diagnosis under the DRG system. Rather, it is nearly always a nonreimbursable complication which prolongs ICU stay and further weakens the patient.[64,65] New complications often follow even if the patient survives the episode of pneumonia. Gram-negative pneumonia is the leading infectious cause of death in critical care patients.[43] Costs quickly accumulate in an arena in which the price of each day's delay to cure and the continuing need for ICU management is very high. The goal is to cure it as rapidly as possible. Dual individualization can potentially cure these patients more rapidly through the use of higher doses, particularly when bacteria are less susceptible or when the patient's drug clearance is more rapid due to a hyperdynamic septic state. The problems which limit dose are toxicity and cost. In some cases, dosage adjustments may increase the time to cure if new, more resistant organisms are selected more rapidly. There are also limited data which suggest that problems also occur above the optimal dosage. Because of the link between dosage and the development of resistance, very high doses of these agents not only can be unnecessarily expensive, but also may hasten the development of resistance.[66]

Besides providing a role for clinical pharmacists in making dosing adjustments for newer antibiotics, the cost effectiveness implication of the dual individualization strategy is that it can shorten the duration of treatment for gram-negative pneumonia. In a review of nosocomial pneumonia, the average stay was 12 ± 7 days in ICU with a 20% mortality.[65] These values are in close agreement with our initial study of cefmenoxime at a standard dosage of 1 gm every six hours; there was a 78% cure rate and a 13-day average duration of treatment.[50] Compared with the 13-day average duration of treatment with cefmenoxime at 1 gm every six hours, those patients given cefmenoxime by dual individualization were treated with similar average doses for nine days ($p < 0.05$). Since there were no baseline clinical differences between the two study populations, and because treatment cessation remained fixed at approximately four to five days after bacterial eradication, it appears that the earlier eradication of bacteria by the use of dual individualization produced more rapid resolution of the pneumonia and allowed earlier cessation of antibiotic treatment.[51]

A method which allows precise dosage individualization by making antibiotic treatment more specific to the requirements of patient and pathogen can potentially improve the quality of life and the quality of care and lower the hospital costs of managing serious infections. This is particularly relevant to the problems associated with ICU treatment where the price of failure is very high in relation to the price of drugs. Average drug costs in a population of patients given regimens by dual individualization may change only slightly, depending on how resistant the bacteria are and how fast patients excrete the antibiotic. Using these data, the care of individuals can be greatly improved.[51]

In some cases, dual individualization results in the administration of doses that are higher or lower than the standard recommended doses. However, even if drug costs are higher, real cost savings accrue from more rapid resolution of disease and earlier transfer to less intensive care units. Each day in a high technology ICU may cost $2000 to $5000; drugs comprise less than 10% of this cost.[67] The principle of more rapidly resolving disease is particularly applicable to complications like nosocomial pneumonia which are not reimbursed under the DRG system because they are not considered a primary diagnosis. The improper use of antibiotics can lead to progression, slow resolution of infection, and excessive costs. This has been documented for outpatient pneumonia[73] as well as nosocomial pneumonia.

The costs of initiating a dual individualization service is approximately $60,000 (a full-time clinical pharmacist paid $45,000 plus the hardware and software costs). If 100 patients are treated for pneumonia at a savings of $1000 each (less than one day in ICU), the dual individualization service could show a profit in the first year. As hospital administrators begin to appreciate *where* the costs of health care accumulate,[45] they will become quite receptive to cost-saving measures that focus on rapid cure of complications such as nosocomial pneumonia in ICU patients. A growing focus on "outcomes" will also support this type of approach to care.

ANTIBIOTIC INTERVENTIONS BASED ON DOSING AND MONITORING STRATEGIES: THE ROLE OF COMPUTERIZED MONITORING OF ANTIBIOTICS USING DUAL INDIVIDUALIZATION PRINCIPLES

A number of strategies have been advanced to contain antibiotic costs in hospitals.[68–70] Many of these retrospectively enforce formulary guidelines, but the more successful strategies focus on intervention.[69] To determine the value of these new antibiotic management strategies to an institution, we began a series of outcome-oriented evaluations to document safety, efficacy, and cost benefit. It was our hypothesis that well-planned and appropriately executed antibiotic interventions would improve patient outcome at less cost to the institution. Furthermore, it was agreed in advance that the institution would use documented cost savings to fund the salary of a clinical pharmacist whose full-time responsibility would become antibiotic management and documentation of clinical outcome. In the initial study we monitored 266 interventions in 240 patients managed over six months.[71] All patients were identified through formal consultation or culture reports of bacterial isolates during routine surveillance of patients in critical care units and selected units. In addition to focusing on dual individualization, we continued to monitor aminoglycosides and vancomycin. Culture data were used to propose changes in antibiotic regimens, route, or dosage, regardless of the antibiotic prescribed. Creatinine clearance was calculated and the appropriate dose requirements were reviewed for all antimicrobials; β-lactam dosages were changed on the basis of renal function and/or MIC.

The types of interventions performed and their associated cost savings are listed in Table 17-2. The greatest cost savings were associated with interventions made on β-lactams; regimens were streamlined, patients were switched to oral therapy from single agents or combinations administered intravenously. Aminoglycosides were important only because they were used in such high volume. Table 17-2 shows the types of interventions and drugs involved, as well as the outcomes of these activities. Clinical outcomes were favorable in 91% of the interventions, particularly those which involved antibiotic changes, streamlining, and the "oral switch" protocol. As a result of aggressive shortening of the aminoglycoside course, only 8% of the patients developed nephrotoxicity. Other safety-related issues were favorable.

The major benefit to the hospital was cost savings in antibiotic expenditures. These data readily justified a clinical pharmacist's salary. Although the pharmacy budget increased from $3 to $3.4 million between 1988 and 1989, antibiotic costs fell from 30% to 22% of the total budget during this period. About half of the total dollar savings could be directly or indirectly traced to antibiotic intervention by a clinical pharmacist. This represented the first real decline in the real dollar outlay for antibiotics recorded at Millard Fillmore Hospital since 1979.

These results further reinforce the contention of others that all patients receiving antibiotics should be reviewed by a clinical pharmacist on a daily basis.[74,75] We

Table 17-2. *Categories of Interventions Performed on Antibiotic Therapy*

	Frequency	Drug cost	Cost savings/ intervention
Dosing adjustment	40%	$ 13,540	$ 127
Discontinue antibiotic[a]	18%	$ 5,677	$ 116
Change regimen[b]	14%	$ 4,828	$ 134
Change IV to oral[c]	17%	$ 5,038	$ 117
Enroll in clinical trial	11%	$ 8,791	$ 326
Totals	**100%**	**$ 37,764**	

[a] Reasons for discontinuation: negative cultures (45%), redundant antibiotics (33%), end of treatment (10%), miscellaneous (12%).
[b] Reasons for change: culture results (78%), risk of toxicity (14%), poor choice for the patient (8%).
[c] Types of oral antibiotics used: quinolone (43%), cephalosporin (11%), penicillin (13%), trimethoprim-sulfamethoxazole (20%), other (13%).

estimate that one specialist can cover about 250 beds if all reports and orders are personally reviewed. Based on pilot projects elsewhere,[76,77] we believed that if the raw data could be assembled in a computer and then prescreened according to an algorithm, then the antibiotic specialist could spend less time searching for intervention candidates and more time consulting with physicians. We therefore electronically interfaced the pharmacy computer and the microbiology computer, and wrote software to prescreen patients for the situations of interest. The computer surveyed all data and then printed names, room numbers, and the type of intervention suggested by the antibiotic management algorithm. The clinical specialist saw each targeted patient and intervened as appropriate. The computer linkages and algorithm enhanced our ability to monitor every hospitalized patient receiving antibiotics. Properly designed software should make it possible to accurately document outcomes in a large hospital with one full-time, dedicated specialist. The cost savings demonstrated here create a role for these specialists which is highly responsible and highly interactive. Clinical specialist interventions contribute in an important way to patient care, fulfill the JCAHO requirements, and save hospitals money.

Only small per patient cost savings are associated with monitoring the aminoglycosides and vancomycin. These latter drugs have great toxic potential and should be monitored hospital wide, but the cost of monitoring is high in relation to the potential for cost savings. One approach to offset these costs is to incorporate the financial burden of aminoglycoside monitoring with β-lactam and quinolone monitoring and intervention services. The large cost savings that accrue from monitoring β-lactams offset the otherwise high and unrecoverable personnel costs associated with aminoglycoside monitoring.

The key to this successful strategy is collecting and organizing culture reports and antibiotic orders in a timely manner. Dual individualization enables the clinician to use this type of information optimally, but it must be done prospectively, not retrospectively. Rapid screening of MICs and population kinetics justifies the dosing changes with β-lactams and quinolones; this approach can be readily incorporated into software to screen every dose against every bacterial isolate. Some patients benefit because it raises their dosage to improve efficacy; for others, the dose may be reduced or the drugs may be stopped. The software calculates the costs of each possible regimen automatically and allows the clinician to rapidly review the options.

DESIGNING NEW APPROACHES TO THE TREATMENT OF HOSPITALIZED PATIENTS WITH SERIOUS INFECTIONS: THE ROLE OF ORAL ANTIBIOTICS

Even with an active dual individualization strategy in place, the costs of parenteral antibiotics are high. This is particularly true for the newest parenteral agents such as imipenem and the third-generation cephalosporins (e.g., ceftazidime and ceftriaxone). Costs of new oral drugs like ciprofloxacin are also higher than earlier agents, but they are considerably lower than the intravenous dosage forms and provide equivalent coverage.

In our hospital, we have many seriously ill patients, and like most hospitals, we treat them empirically when they become infected—often with combinations of two or three intravenous antibiotics. The cost of these regimens frequently exceeds $100 per day. We hypothesized that oral ciprofloxacin might be as efficacious as some of these intravenous regimens and could save the institution significant costs. Because there was resistance to the empirical use of oral antibiotics in seriously or critically ill patients, we elected to evaluate the possibility of replacing intravenous drugs with oral agents after three days of therapy. At this point, the patient often has improved and can tolerate oral antibiotics; furthermore, culture and sensitivity data are generally available as an aid to switching.

To be eligible for this study, the patient had to be hospitalized with a serious infection, and the identified organisms had to exhibit *in vitro* sensitivity to the antibiotics initially chosen. Each patient was randomized (1:1) at day three after informed consent. Patients were either continued on an intravenous regimen, or were switched to oral ciprofloxacin at usual doses of 750 mg every 12 hours. No concomitant antibiotics were allowed except for oral metronidazole to cover the documented or suspected presence of anaerobes (e.g., patients with diabetic foot ulcers).

Costs assessed for each patient were: 1) acquisition cost of antibiotics; 2) costs of preparation and administration (a conservative estimate of $3 per intravenous dose); and 3) costs of monitoring aminoglycosides and vancomycin (serum concentrations and renal function tests).

Ninety-nine patients were enrolled in this study over one year. The infections treated were similar to those represented in many of our previous studies of hospitalized patients.[24,33,51] The study population was well balanced between the sites of infection, with the majority of infections in the respiratory tract, skin, and/or bone. The organisms causing initial infection were typically staphylococci, Pseudomonas, or other enterobacteriaceae. All were susceptible to both the intravenous regimen selected initially (usually aminoglycosides and/or cephalosporins) and to oral ciprofloxacin. Approximately one-half of the patients were started on more than one parenteral antibiotic. Three or more antibiotics were given to 5% of the patients.

Both the patients given intravenous antibiotics for their entire treatment and those given intravenous antibiotics followed by oral ciprofloxacin responded well to treatment. There were no statistically significant differences in efficacy or overall prevalence of adverse effects. No unexpected adverse effects were encountered.

The comparative cost analysis of the two regimens revealed that patients given oral ciprofloxacin after three days of intravenous antibiotics had significant cost savings. Savings averaged $293 per patient if decreased length of stay was not considered. Savings increased to $1291 per patient if decreases in length of stay were taken into account.

When used as continuation therapy, oral ciprofloxacin can be at least as safe and effective as intravenous antibiotics in selected serious infections, and it is certainly more convenient. Potential intravenous access complications (e.g., phlebitis) are likely to be avoided, and some patients may benefit from a decreased length of hospital stay. Finally, the cost of oral ciprofloxacin is markedly less than that of intravenous antibiotics, whether the patient is hospitalized or is receiving home intravenous services.[72] These findings lead us to regularly identify patients for which this type of intervention is appropriate. Switching intravenous combination antibiotics to oral agents like ciprofloxacin routinely accounts for up to one-third of our monthly cost savings. The dosage of ciprofloxacin is tailored to the MIC of the bacteria isolated and this yields even greater cost reductions with this agent.

PROSPECTUS

In 1985, we could not advocate the routine application of dual individualization to all patients who are given antibiotics. At that time, the technology was too new to make the assumptions that it would work with population kinetic parameters or estimates of the MIC. We confined these methods to the critically ill population who we believed had the greatest potential to benefit, but we seriously doubted that this technology should be considered for greater than 10% of all patients given antibiotics in hospitals. Since that time, we and others have confirmed the value of dual individualization in the ICU and are now convinced that this method has broader application. This is because computer software-assisted surveillance and intervention technology makes it possible to apply dual individualization to all patients on antibiotics with potentially enormous cost savings in the present economic environment. In most hospitals, there are large numbers of patients who would benefit from dose optimization even if it were done on a population kinetic basis. Nearly all can potentially be switched to oral antibiotics earlier than thought possible even five years ago.

We have outlined the potential of dual individualization for the practice of applied pharmacokinetics. Now that it can be computerized and operated on a large scale hospital-wide, there will be great demand for this technology, and other disciplines will begin to apply it. The potential for prospectively testing dual individualization as a rational method for establishing optimal dosages for new and existing antibiotics is enormous. New infections, resistant bacteria, and new, highly active drugs present a broad scope of potential research endeavors.

REFERENCES

1. Bootman JL et al. Individualizing gentamicin dosage regimens in burn patients with gram-negative septicemia: a cost-benefit analysis. J Pharm Sci. 1979;68:267–72.
2. Schentag JJ et al. Antibiotic tissue penetration in liver infection: a case of tobramycin failure responsive to moxalactam. Am J Gastroenterol. 1983;78:641–44.
3. Noone P et al. Experience in monitoring gentamicin therapy during treatment of serious gram-negative sepsis. Br Med J. 1974;1:477–81.

4. Dahlgren JG et al. Gentamicin blood levels: a guide to nephrotoxicity. Antimicrob Agents Chemother. 1975;8:58–62.

5. Jackson GG, Riff LJ. Pseudomonas bacteremia: pharmacologic and other bases for failure of treatment with gentamicin. J Infect Dis. 1971;124(Suppl.):S185–S191.

6. Schentag JJ, Adelman MH. A microcomputer program for tobramycin consult services, based on the two compartment pharmacokinetic model. Drug Intell Clin Pharm. 1983;17:528–31.

7. Schentag JJ et al. Clinical and pharmacokinetic characteristics of aminoglycoside nephrotoxicity in 201 critically ill patients. Antimicrob Agents Chemother. 1982;21:721–26.

8. Cipolle RJ et al. Hospital acquired gram-negative pneumonias: response rate and dosage requirements with individualized therapy. Ther Drug Monit. 1980;2:358–63.

9. Dettli L. Individualization of drug dosage in patients with renal disease. Med Clin North Am. 1974;58:977-985.

10. Bootman JL et al. Cost of individualizing aminoglycoside dosage regimens. Am J Hosp Pharm. 1979;36:368–70.

11. Kunin CM. Dosage schedules of antimicrobial agents: an historical review. Rev Infect Dis. 1981;3:4–11.

12. Redjeb SB et al. Effects of ten milligrams of ampicillin per day on urinary tract infections. Antimicrob Agents Chemother. 1982;22:1084–86.

13. Schentag JJ et al. Dual individualization—antibiotic dosage calculation from the integration of *in vitro* pharmacodynamics and *in vivo* pharmacokinetics. J Antimicrob Chemother. 1985;15(Suppl.A):47–57.

14. Ellner PD, Neu HC. The inhibitory quotient: a method for interpreting minimum inhibitory concentration data. JAMA. 1981;246:1575–578.

15. Schumacher GE. Pharmacokinetic and microbiologic evaluation of dosage regimens for newer cephalosporins and penicillins. Clin Pharmacokinet. 1983;2:448–57.

16. Wolfson JS, Swartz MN. Serum bactericidal activity as a monitor of antibiotic therapy. N Engl J Med. 1985;312:968–75.

17. Klastersky J et al. Antibacterial activity in serum and urine as a therapeutic guide in bacterial infections. J Infect Dis. 1974;129:187–93.

18. Drake TR et al. Value of serum tests in combined drug therapy of endocarditis. Antimicrob Agents Chemother. 1983;24:653–57.

19. Barriere SL et al. Analysis of a new method for assessing activity of combinations of antimicrobials: area under the bactericidal activity curve. J Antimicrob Chemother. 1985;16:49–59.

20. Drusano GL et al. Integration of selected pharmacologic and microbiologic properties of three new beta-lactam antibiotics: a hypothesis for comparison. Rev Infect Dis. 1984;6:357–63.

21. Schentag JJ et al. Dual individualization with antibiotics. In: Evans WE et al., eds. Applied Pharmacokinetics. Vancouver, WA: Applied Therapeutics, Inc.; 1985:463–92.

22. Rescott DL et al. Comparison of two methods for determining *in vitro* postantibiotic effect of three antibiotics on *Escherichia coli*. Antimicrob Agents Chemother. 1988;32:450–53.

23. McCormack JP, Schentag JJ. The potential impact of quantitative susceptibility tests on the design of aminoglycoside regimens. Drug Intell Clin Pharm. 1987;21:187–91.

24. Peloquin CA et al. Intravenous ciprofloxacin in patients with nosocomial lower respiratory tract infections: impact of plasma concentrations, organism MIC, and clinical condition on bacterial eradication. Arch Intern Med. 1989;149:2269–273.

25. Blaser J et al. Impact of dosing regimens on antibacterial activity of vancomycin in an *in vitro* pharmacokinetic model. Proceedings of the Third European Congress of Clinical Microbiology. The Hague, Netherlands. 1987 May 11–14. Abstract #512.

26. Leggett JE et al. Comparative antibiotic dose-effect relations at several dosing intervals in murine pneumonitis and thigh infection models. J Infect Dis. 1989;159:281–92.

27. Gerber AU et al. Impact of dosing intervals on activity of gentamicin and ticarcillin against *pseudomonas aeruginosa* in granulocytopenic mice. J Infect Dis. 1983;147:910–17.

28. Gerber AU et al. Antibiotic therapy of infections due to *pseudomonas aeruginosa* in normal and granulocytopenic mice: comparison of murine and human pharmacokinetics. J Infect Dis. 1986;153:90–97.

29. Vogelman B et al. Correlation of antimicrobial pharmacokinetic parameters with therapeutic efficacy in an animal model. J Infect Dis. 1988;158:831–47.
30. Gudmundsson S et al. Postantibiotic effect (PAE) for newer antimicrobials. 24th ICAAC. 1984;1120:289. Abstract.
31. McDonald PJ et al. Persistent effect of antibiotics on *Staphylococcus aureus* after exposure for limited periods of time. J Infect Dis. 1977;135:217–23.
32. Vogelman B et al. Correlation of pharmacokinetic parameters of beta-lactam and aminoglycoside antibiotics with efficacy against gram-negative bacilli in an animal model. 24th ICAAC. 1984;24:93. Abstract.
33. Roosendaal R et al. Therapeutic efficacy of continuous versus intermittent administration of ceftazidime in experimental klebsiella pneumonia in rats. J Infect Dis. 1985;152:373–78.
34. Schaad UB et al. Pharmacokinetics and bacteriologic efficacy of moxalactam, cefotaxime, cefoperazone, and ceftriaxone in experimental bacterial meningitis. J Infect Dis. 1981;143:156–63.
35. Hook EW III et al. Antimicrobial therapy of experimental enterococcal endocarditis. Antimicrob Agents Chemother. 1975;8:564–70.
36. Carizosa J et al. Effectiveness of nafcillin, methicillin, and cephalothin in experimental *Staphylococcal aureus* endocarditis. Antimicrob Agents Chemother. 179;15:735–37.
37. Peterson LR et al. Comparison of azlocillin, ceftizoxime, cefoxitan, and amikacin alone and in combination against *Pseudomonas aeruginosa* in a neutropenic-site rabbit model. Antimicrob Agents Chemother. 1984;25:545–52.
38. Tauber MG et al. The postantibiotic effect in the treatment of experimental meningitis caused by *Streptococcus pneumoniae* in rabbits. J Infect Dis. 1984;149:575–83.
39. Schiff JB, Pennington JE. Comparative efficacies of piperacillin, azlocillin, ticarcillin aztreonam, and tobramycin against experimental *pseudomonas aeruginosa* pneumonia. Antimicrob Agents Chemother. 1984;25:49–52.
40. Schentag JJ et al. A randomized clinical trial of moxalactam alone versus tobramycin plus clindamycin in abdominal sepsis. Ann Surg. 1983;198:35–41.
41. Peloquin CA et al. Kinetics and dynamics of tobramycin action in patients with bacteriuria given single doses. Antimicrob Agents Chemther. 1991;35:1191–195.
42. Helm EB et al. Kinetics of bacterial elimination in urine during antimicrobial treatment. J Antimicrob Chemother. 1979;5(Suppl B):191–99.
43. Gross PA et al. Deaths from nosocomial infections: experience in a university hospital and a community hospital. Am J Med. 1980;68:219–23.
44. Daschner F et al. Surveillance, prevention and control of hospital-acquired infections. III: Nosocomial infections as a cause of death: retrospective analysis of 1,000 autopsy reports. Infection 1978;6:261–65.
45. Spengler RF, Greenough WB III. Hospital costs and mortality attributed to nosocomial bacteremias. JAMA. 1978;240:2455–458.
46. Schentag JJ et al. Treatment with aztreonam or tobramycin in critical care patients with gram-negative pneumonia. Am J Med. 1985;78(Suppl.2A):34–41.
47. Bradsher RW Jr. Overwhelming pneumonia. Med Clin North Am. 1983;67:1233–250.
48. Stevens RM et al. Pneumonia in an intensive care unit. Arch Intern Med. 1974;134:106–11.
49. Johanson WG Jr et al. Nosocomial respiratory infections with gram-negative bacilli: the significance of colonization of the respiratory tract. Ann Intern Med. 1972;77:701–706.
50. Reitberg DP et al. Cefmenoxime in the treatment of nosocomial pneumonia in critical care patients. J Antimicrob Chemother. 1984;14:81–91.
51. Schentag JJ et al. Role for dual individualization with cefmenoxime. Am J Med. 1984;77(Suppl.6A):43–50.
52. Schentag JJ, Gengo FM. Principles of antibiotic tissue penetration and guidelines for pharmacokinetic analysis. Med Clin North Am. 1982;66:39–49.
53. Schentag JJ. Antimicrobial kinetics and tissue distribution: concepts and applications. In: Cunha BA, Ristuccia AM, eds. Antimicrobial Therapy. New York: Raven Press; 1984:81–94.
54. Schentag JJ. Clinical significance of antibiotic tissue penetration. Clin Pharmacokinet. 1989;16(Suppl.1):25–31.

55. Whelton A, Stout RL. An overview of antibiotic tissue penetration. In: Cunha BA, Ristuccia AM, eds. Antimicrobial Therapy. New York: Raven Press; 1984:365–78.

56. Ryan DM, Cars O. Antibiotic assays in muscle: are conventional tissue levels misleading as indicators of antibacterial activity? Scand J Infect Dis. 1980;12:307–309.

57. Ryan DM et al. Simultaneous comparison of three methods for assessing ceftazidime penetration into extravascular fluid. Antimicrob Agents Chemother. 1982;22:995–98.

58. Ryan DM. Implanted tissue-cages: a critical evaluation of their relevance in measuring tissue concentrations of antibiotics. Scand J Infect Dis. 1978;13(Suppl.):58–62.

59. Klaus U et al. Bacterial elimination and therapeutic effectiveness under different schedules of amoxicillin administration. Chemotherapy 1981;27:200–208.

60. Costerton JW. The etiology and persistence of cryptic bacterial infections: a hypothesis. Rev Infect Dis. 1984;6(Suppl.3):S608–S616.

61. Schentag JJ et al. Safety of high dose intravenous ciprofloxacin in the treatment of *pseudomonas aeruginosa* and staphylococcal infections. Proceedings of the 3rd International Symposium on New Quinolones. Vancouver, B.C.: 1990 July 12–14. Abstract #12.

62. Nix DE et al. Dual individualization of intravenous ciprofloxacin in patients with nosocomial lower respiratory tract infections. Am J Med 82. 1987;(Suppl.4A):352–56.

63. McGowan JE Jr. Antimicrobial resistance in hospital organisms and its relation to antibiotic use. Rev Infect Dis. 1983;5:1033–48.

64. Wagner DP et al. The hidden costs of treating severely ill patients: charges and resource consumption in an intensive care unit. Health Care Financ Rev. 1983;5:81–86.

65. Craig CP, Connelly S. Effect of intensive care unit nosocomial pneumonia on duration of stay and mortality. Am J Infect Control. 1984;12:233–38.

66. Freeman J, McGowan JE Jr. Methodologic issues in hospital epidemiology. III. Investigating the modifying effects of time and severity of underlying illness on estimates of cost of nosocomial infection. Rev Infect Dis. 1984;6:285–300.

67. Kolar R et al. Identification of drug costs within diagnosis related groups. Hosp Pharm. 1984;19:731–34.

68. Catania HF, Catania PN. Using clinical pharmacy interventions to cost-justify additional pharmacy staff. Hosp Pharm. 1988;23:544–48.

69. Briceland LL et al. Streamlining antimicrobial therapy through review of order sheets. Am J Hosp Pharm. 1989;46:1376–380.

70. Hirschman SZ et al. Use of antimicrobial agents in a university teaching hospital. Arch Intern Med. 1988;148:2001–2007.

71. Ballow CH et al. Development of an outcome oriented antimicrobial interventions program at a 460-bed teaching hospital. Proceedings of the 11th American College of Clinical Pharmacy. San Francisco: 1990 August 5–8. Abstract #132.

72. Paladino JA et al. Clinical and economic evaluation of oral ciprofloxacin following an abbreviated course of standard intravenous antibiotics. Am J Med. 1991;91:462–70.

73. Dans PE et al. Management of pneumonia in the prospective payment era. Arch Intern Med. 1984;144:1392–397.

74. Job ML et al. Seven years' experience with a pharmacokinetic service. Hosp Pharm. 1989;24:512–19.

75. Von Seggern RL. Culture and antibiotic monitoring service in a community hospital. Am J Hosp Pharm. 1987;44:1358–362.

76. Scarafile PD et al. Computer assisted concurrent antibiotic review in a community hospital. Am J Hosp Pharm. 1985;42:313–15.

77. Evans RS et al. Computer surveillance of hospital acquired infections and antibiotic use. JAMA. 1986;256:1007–11.

Chapter 18

Commentary on Dual Individualization with Antibiotics

Michael N. Dudley

The integration of pharmacokinetic and, more recently, pharmacodynamic properties into the design of dosage regimens for anti-infectives has gained increasing emphasis in the evaluation of anti-infectives and dosage design.[1-4] This is due in part to the availability of new classes of drugs to treat certain infections (e.g., antiretroviral drugs and AIDS), drug resistance, cost of therapy, and the desire to distinguish between a multitude of agents that often exhibit only subtle differences in pharmacology.

In deriving linked pharmacokinetic/pharmacodynamic relations for "dual-individualization," it is important to acknowledge the components, assumptions, and limitations of the parameters that are used to develop current models for antimicrobial effects *in vivo*. This commentary will review some key aspects and assumptions used in the development and application of linked pharmacokinetic/pharmacodynamic parameters for antibacterial agents (i.e., dual individualization) and suggest strategies for future study.

ASSESSING THE PHARMACODYNAMIC PROPERTIES OF ANTI-INFECTIVES

Minimum Inhibitory Concentration (MIC)

The MIC is the benchmark used to assess the *in vitro* antibacterial activity of drugs in the screening phase and in the clinical setting. In view of the use of this measurement in both research and clinical settings, it is not surprising that MIC testing has been incorporated into the development of pharmacokinetic/pharmacodynamic models which have been proposed to more effectively predict the antibacterial effects of antibiotics in patients. Although standardization has been instrumental in achieving sufficient reproducibility for clinical and research applications, MIC testing remains an incomplete measure of antibiotic pharmacodynamics. This is because the endpoint of growth/no growth (as assessed by turbidity) measured after an 18 to 24 hour incubation period (MIC) represents the net effect of several events. These events may include any or all of the following: bacterial killing, stasis, and growth. The net results, as read by growth (turbidity) or no growth (clarity) in each tube (or well) during MIC determinations, reflect differential effects of a given drug concentration on several bacterial subpopulations in the test inoculum.

The possible influence of bacterial subpopulations on the MIC determination is depicted in Figure 18-1. Curves A through D show the change in bacterial counts over time for four hypothetical bacterial strains exposed to a drug during MIC testing. Curve A depicts data for a strain that represents what might be considered "classical" bacterial resistance; bacterial growth is steady and continues seemingly unimpaired by drug, with turbidity easily readable after several hours of incubation. Curve B also depicts an organism resistant to the drug concentration tested; however, early killing of a significant portion of the initial inoculum occurs, followed by regrowth of a resistant bacterial subpopulation present in the initial inoculum. This subpopulation ultimately increases to produce a visually turbid (resistant) result. Although there was significant killing of an initial (susceptible) bacterial inoculum during the early stages of incubation, this strain is considered resistant to the drug concentration tested.

Curves C and D depict results for antibiotic "susceptible" organisms. Curve D depicts the simplistic example of an organism rapidly and completely inhibited/killed by a drug. In contrast, Curve C has a similar killing/regrowth pattern similar to Curve B, where an initial period of bacterial killing is followed by regrowth of a resistant bacterial subpopulation. Although the result read at the end of the incubation period indicates that the organism is "susceptible," a resistant bacterial subpopulation clearly was selected during incubation; however, in contrast to Curve B, the number of resistant bacteria did not increase enough to exceed the

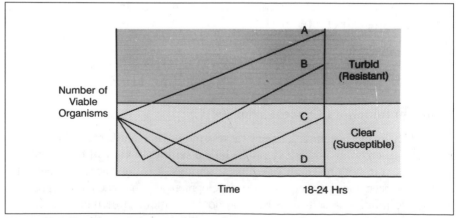

Figure 18-1. Hypothetical change in bacterial counts during MIC testing. The ordinate is a log scale. See text for description.

threshold for turbidity by the end of the incubation period. This latter example is compatible with recommendations for the use of prolonged incubation periods to detect "true resistance" in certain bacterial strains.[1,49]

Curves B and C suggest that a sufficiently large bacterial inoculum should be considered a "swarm" and not a clone. Depending on the shape of the population distribution curve and drug concentration tested, different parts of the distribution curve may be obliterated, with persisting bacteria reflecting those requiring higher concentrations of drug to be eliminated (see Figure 18-2). The situation is analogous to heterogeneity in receptor site affinity for an agonist, where the observed pharmacological response is determined by the "mix" of receptors. In the face of low drug concentrations, a bacterial strain with heterogeneous subpopulations may have resistant subpopulations selected during therapy.

The importance of the development of resistance on treatment outcome has been illustrated for several classes of drugs. Milotovic and Braveny concluded that the development of resistance during therapy was linked to treatment failure in approximately 50% of cases for third-generation cephalosporins, imipenem, and ciprofloxacin and 85% of cases for aminoglycosides.[5] Antibiotic-resistant bacterial subpopulations exist for a number of human pathogens (see Table 18-1). The selection of aminoglycoside-resistant subpopulations and the adaptive resistance of *Pseudomonas aeruginosa* after exposure to aminoglycosides at doses and concentrations used to treat human infection have been demonstrated *in vitro*[6-8] and in hospitalized patients.[9] Bacterial resistance and clinical unresponsiveness to third-generation cephalosporins have occurred in patients with infections caused by certain gram-negative bacilli. This resistance has been associated with the selection of stably derepressed mutant bacteria which produce large amounts of the Richmond-Sykes Type I β-lactamase.[10] Fluoroquinolone resistance in *P.*

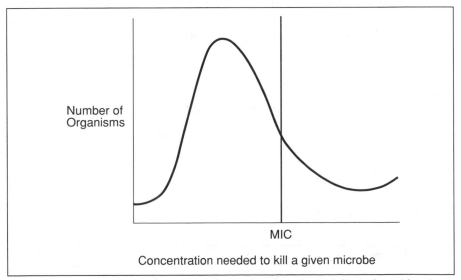

Figure 18-2. *Skewed population distribution curve for a large bacterial inoculum with resistant bacterial subpopulations showing that the MIC does not correspond to concentration at which all bacteria in the inoculum tested are inhibited.*

aeruginosa due to spontaneously occurring *gyr-A* mutants has been described; the selection of these resistant bacteria has been linked to treatment failure of certain infections.[11]

Postantibiotic Effect (PAE)

The persistent inhibition of bacterial growth following exposure to an antibiotic is known as the postantibiotic effect.[12,13] Although this phenomenon has been demonstrated *in vitro* and *in vivo* for several bacteria and drug classes, much remains to be understood regarding the mechanisms and factors modulating this effect.

Although the PAE has become an accepted parameter to consider in determining dosage frequency *in vivo*, a few caveats are in order. First, most experiments examining the importance of an *in vivo* postantibiotic effect in animal or in *in vitro* models of infection have studied relatively short courses of therapy; the presence of a PAE following several cycles of drug exposure has not been fully evaluated. Recent laboratory experiments demonstrated loss of an *in vitro* PAE in a strain of *Pseudomonas aeruginosa* following three tobramycin exposure-regrowth cycles (as occurs during therapy of an infection *in vivo*). In contrast, there was no change when this experiment was performed with imipenem.[50] Secondly, as noted by Schentag and colleagues (see Chapter 17: Dual Individualization with Antibiotics), the reproducibility of a PAE across different strains of the same bacterial species or members of a similar drug class has not been established.[14-16] We have noted significant variation in the presence and duration of a PAE induced by amikacin among strains of *P. aeruginosa* (unpublished data). Indeed, studies using electron microscopy have demonstrated significant variability among cells examined during the PAE-phase with fluoroquinolones; this may indicate drug effects on only certain bacterial populations.[17] Despite these questions concerning the mechanism and reproducibility of the PAE, data in animals, *in vitro* models of infection,[8,18-23] and patients[24-29] support the use of dosage regimens that exploit the PAE by the use of longer dosage intervals.

Table 18-1. *Frequency of Resistant Bacterial Subpopulations for Selected Drug Classes and Bacterial Species*

Drug	Frequency of resistant mutants
Fluoroquinolones	
gyr-A mutants: *E. coli*	10^{-11}
P. aeruginosa	10^{-7} to 10^{-9}
Beta-lactams	
Stably-derepressed β-lactamase producers	10^{-5} to 10^{-8}
(e.g., *E. cloacae*, *P. aeruginosa*)	
Aminoglycosides	
Small colony variants	$>10^{-5}$

INTEGRATION OF PHARMACOKINETICS AND PHARMACODYNAMICS

Theoretical Considerations

The study of antimicrobial pharmacokinetics and pharmacodynamics has facilitated the development of a more rational basis for regimens to treat infection. In Figure 18-3 several pharmacokinetic parameters are correlated with the MIC, the most frequently employed parameter reflecting the pharmacodynamic activity of antibiotics. The ratio of the peak concentration to the MIC is perhaps the most familiar parameter; this parameter can be calculated or derived directly through measurement of the serum inhibitory or bactericidal titer (SIT or SBT).[1] The duration of expected "inhibitory effect" can be expressed by the time serum drug concentrations exceed the MIC. To further integrate peak and duration effects, the AUC exceeding the MIC can be calculated by subtracting the "sub-MIC" trapezoid from the total AUC for a given dose of drug or by dividing the total AUC by the MIC. A similar relation has been developed by calculating the area under the serum bactericidal titer-versus-time curve.[30]

While these parameters provide useful comparisons and are particularly easy to derive, there are some conceptual and statistical pitfalls associated with their use. As described previously, the MIC as a pharmacodynamic parameter often fails to consider several other important drug effects, including the PAE and concentration-dependent effects on bacterial subpopulations; the latter includes the effects of sub-MIC concentrations on bacterial adherence.[1] Further, the relation between drug concentration and MIC is too simplistic in that it forces an "on/off" effect model as drug concentrations fall below the MIC. This is not the case for certain beta-lactams where antimicrobial effects persist during exposure to sub-inhibitory drug concentrations following brief exposure to a high peak. Perhaps one of the greatest pitfalls is failure to recognize the twofold error assumption implicit in MIC determinations when serial twofold dilutions are used; unless

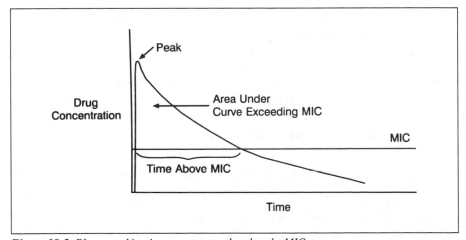

Figure 18-3. Pharmacokinetic parameters related to the MIC.

geometric dilutions are used when determining MIC or SIT/SBT values, the parameters depicted in Figure 18-2 (especially area measurements) will have significant errors in estimation, particularly when MIC values are large.

When comparing peak and duration effects with serum drug concentration, one must also recognize the covariance between peak, duration of time, and AUC values related to the MIC. For example, a larger dose increases all of these parameters. Therefore, careful studies with varying doses as well as dose frequencies (and if possible, adjustment of drug half-life) are needed to fully distinguish the importance of changes in each specific pharmacokinetic-pharmacodynamic parameter on outcome. This is particularly important when small animal models of infection are used since the elimination of many drugs is markedly more rapid than that which occurs in humans.[31]

Studies in Animal and *In Vitro* Models

Despite theoretical shortcomings, studies in carefully designed animal and *in vitro* models of infection have established relations between certain pharmacokinetic parameters and the MIC.

Aminoglycosides. For aminoglycosides, the total dose (expressed as an AUC) appears to be linked to increased bacterial killing of a small homogeneous bacterial inoculum in some animal models; the dosing interval is relatively unimportant unless very long dosing intervals (e.g., greater than 8 to 12 hours) are used.[18] Other *in vitro* models as well as animal models have demonstrated the importance of peak concentrations in avoiding the selection of resistant bacterial subpopulations.[7,8,21,32] The discrepancy in results between studies may be due to use of larger bacterial inocula that included spontaneously occurring resistant bacterial subpopulations which were suppressed by high peak concentrations.

β-lactams. Studies of gram-negative bacilli and beta-lactams in animal and *in vitro* models support the use of regimens that provide prolonged exposure to drug concentrations at or just above threshold levels (e.g., the MIC).[33–35] However, these conclusions are based largely on studies that used "susceptible" (based on MIC breakpoint values) bacterial strains. Thus, the conclusions may not apply in cases where spontaneously occurring mutants (such as stably derepressed bacteria producing the Richmond-Sykes Class I beta-lactamase) are frequent; peak drug concentrations may be important in some strains to avoid selection of these drug-resistant subpopulations.

Fluoroquinolones. Few studies have examined the pharmacokinetic/pharmacodynamic relationships for the fluoroquinolones. *In vitro* and animal studies have demonstrated the importance of peak drug concentration for rapid bacterial killing and minimizing the selection of resistant bacteria.[21,36,37,57]

HUMAN STUDIES

A major obstacle to the clinical application of results from experimental models is determining whether the findings of pharmacokinetic/pharmacodynamic studies carried out *in vitro* and in animal models are of clinical significance in patients.

For example, the endpoints used (extent of bacterial killing in a tissue or eradication of bacteria) may not have direct application in human infection. Furthermore, pharmacokinetic/pharmacodynamic models derived from animal studies are often based on experiments using bacterial inocula too small to include resistant bacterial subpopulations. Unfortunately, the use of a larger inoculum often overwhelms the animal and thus does not allow investigators to assess drug effects because of rapid death. However, if resistant bacterial subpopulations were included and selected during drug exposure, the observed extent of bacterial killing and ultimately the model used to describe antibiotic effects would be altered. Finally, the clinical relevance of statistically significant, but perhaps minor differences in the extent bacterial killing, must be considered.

In view of the above, it is possible that one set of pharmacokinetic/pharmacodynamic relations for a given drug class and bacteria may apply in some models, while others apply in other infections with a different inoculum size or other local factors. For example, the rate and extent of bacterial killing of a relatively small inoculum of *Pseudomonas aeruginosa* by an aminoglycoside can be linked with the AUC,[18] whereas the peak concentration seems to be important in models where the test bacterial inoculum is larger and the selection of resistance leads to "failure" in the experimental model or clinical setting.

Controlled studies relating pharmacokinetic and pharmacodynamic parameters to outcome in the treatment of gram-negative bacillary infections are scant. The confounding effects of adjunct therapy, underlying disease, and a good clinical prognosis in many types of infections may obscure the importance of pharmacokinetics and pharmacodynamics. A critical test of the effectiveness of antimicrobial therapy occurs in gram-negative bacteremia, particularly in profound, persistently neutropenic patients. Large, randomized prospective studies have been capable of detecting important differences between regimens evaluating drugs with similar *in vitro* profiles.[38,39] Several studies have demonstrated the efficacy and safety of once-daily aminoglycoside doses. A randomized, prospective trial comparing single- versus multiple-daily doses of amikacin was recently concluded by the European Organization for Research and Treatment of Cancer (EORTC) Antimicrobial Therapy Project Group. The preliminary results indicate that a single-daily dose of amikacin is as effective as traditional dosage regimens, but further analysis is required of these data.[56]

The detailed, intensive, "data rich" studies of critically ill patients described by Schentag and colleagues (see Chapter 17: Dual Individual with Antibiotics), are without peer and have provided some of the most extensive data on pharmacokinetic factors associated with antibacterial effects in patients.[40,41] As described, they chose to examine the effect of drug regimens on the eradication of bacterial pathogens from the tracheal secretions of intubated patients in an intensive care unit. Although respiratory secretions appear to be a logical and convenient site for study of bacterial eradication, the clinical significance of the recovery of bacteria in tracheal specimens is difficult to evaluate as it is an *expected* finding in many patients in ICU settings.[42] For example, in a study of patients with nosocomial pneumonia whose deaths were associated with adult respiratory distress syndrome, bacterial pneumonia was misdiagnosed from these secretions in up to 30%

of patients.[43] Furthermore, the significance and standard of practice of using systemic antimicrobials to treat tracheobronchitis in intubated patients based on bacteria recovered in secretions "colonized" with bacteria has been challenged.[44] Indeed, the presence of several different "pathogens" in baseline cultures from patients studied by Schentag et al. brings into question the clinical significance of bacterial presence and the relationship between their eradication from secretions and clinical response. Investigators studying other patient populations (e.g.; those with cystic fibrosis) have similarly challenged the clinical significance of eradication versus a simple reduction in bacterial counts on clinical illness. Several clinical factors besides antimicrobial therapy (e.g., prior respiratory disease, quantity of secretions, infection control procedures, and duration of intubation) are likely to affect the recovery of bacteria from tracheal secretions.[42]

Although the clinical significance of the eradication of bacteria from respiratory secretions in this patient population may be questioned, these studies do serve as a useful *in vivo* "model" for studying bacterial killing with different dosing regimens which vary the type of exposure to drug. Studies using cefmenoxime showed a statistically significant relationship between both the AUC and time above the dynamic response concentration (DRC, an apparent correlate of the MIC based on the Abbott MS-2 Automated Susceptibility Testing system) and eradication of a specific pathogen from respiratory secretions.[40] The effect of peak drug concentration on eradication was not reported. However, close inspection of the figures provided in the original paper suggests that the relation was made possible by the few strains of *P. aeruginosa* and *Acinetobacter sp.* studied; these pathogens often persisted in sputum and became resistant during therapy. Although the prospective phase of the study targeted a specific AUC above DRC (MIC) value, there was significant imprecision in attaining target levels. Further, a poor correlation between the actual observed values and the time to bacterial eradication can be noted.

A second study was conducted using intravenous ciprofloxacin in the same type of patient population.[41] In this study, both length of time that serum concentrations exceeded the MIC and the ratio of the peak serum concentration to the MIC were associated with bacterial eradication; overall, the number of days required for bacterial eradication from sputum was markedly shorter than that for cefmenoxime.[40] Because ciprofloxacin is excreted both renally and by hepatic metabolism, drug half-life was similar among patients; thus, the covariance between peak and duration effects could not be controlled. Further, the authors collected the first plasma level at one hour and extrapolated back using a one-compartment pharmacokinetic model to calculate a peak; this technique would seriously underestimate the "true" peak since the pharmacokinetics of intravenous ciprofloxacin are best described using a two-or-three-compartment pharmacokinetic model.[50] Although the authors conclude that time above MIC was the "best" predictor (based on a slightly lower p value), inspection of raw data suggest that a peak:MIC ratio greater than eight was highly predictive of eradication; this is consistent with previous studies in *in vitro* models.[21,36,37,57]

COMBINATION THERAPY

The pharmacokinetic determinants associated with enhanced antimicrobial effects of drug combinations are not known. Several studies have examined the importance of dose timing when using aminoglycoside/beta-lactam combinations to treat gram-negative bacillary infections. Bacterial killing with gentamicin and piperacillin in *in vitro* timed-kill curve experiments was greatest when the concentrations of each drug corresponded to those that occurred following the simultaneous administration of both drugs.[45] In contrast, studies in *in vitro* kinetic models of infection demonstrated greater killing of drug-susceptible *P. aeruginosa* when the first dose of an aminoglycoside was followed two to four hours later by the first dose of an antipseudomonal penicillin;[46,47] however, when azlocillin preceded the first dose of sisomicin by two hours, less killing was observed.[46]

An *in vitro* model was used to study the combined effects of amikacin and ceftriaxone against ceftriaxone-susceptible or -resistant strains of *P. aeruginosa*. Bacterial regrowth and resistance occurred when either drug was used alone (single- or multiple-daily doses). No significant differences in bacterial killing were observed when single-daily doses of amikacin-ceftriaxone were used in combination (dosed simultaneously or staggered by six hours).[32] In contrast, simultaneous administration of ticarcillin and gentamicin (by continuous infusion) compared to bolus administration of one or both drugs in an animal model of infection resulted in greater bacterial killing and lower mortality in rats infected with a strain of *P. aeruginosa* resistant to both drugs but synergistically inhibited.[48]

Resistance to ciprofloxacin has occurred during therapy in patients with *P. aeruginosa* infections in some settings. Using an *in vitro* model, we evaluated simulated doses of ciprofloxacin 200 mg alone or combined with azlocillin. The dosing interval for both drugs was 12 hours. The drugs were given simultaneously or staggered (by six hours, with either azlocillin or ciprofloxacin given first). All combination regimens prevented the selection of ciprofloxacin-resistant bacterial subpopulations; simultaneous administration gave the most reliable results for all strains, including a strain initially resistant to both drugs. These data suggest that adequate contact time between drugs, particularly at high concentrations, is needed to kill drug-resistant bacteria.[37]

The data derived in experimental models and human studies are concordant with each other when bacterial cell population dynamics are considered in interpreting results. Approved product labeling (i.e., "package inserts") for antibacterials has often defined dose schedules in terms of "mild," "moderate," or "severe" infections. While vague, these categories imply the need to individualize antimicrobial dosage regimens. An alternative approach would emphasize the need for more aggressive dosage regimens based on the size of the bacterial inoculum, the susceptibility of expected bacterial subpopulations, and drug's pharmacological properties. For example, larger doses or regimens yielding higher peaks would be preferred for infections involving large bacterial inocula in which development of resistance during therapy is often associated with clinical failure. Table 18-2 integrates of these considerations with pharmacological properties such that one might forecast optimal dosage regimens for antibacterial agents with similar properties.

Table 18-2. *Important Pharmacokinetic Parameters for Antibacterial Agents According to In Vitro Pharmacodynamic Properties and Characteristics of Bacterial Inoculum*

Parameter	PAE	Conc. dependent bacterial killing	Inoculum size/ resistant subpopulations[a]	Examples/comments
		Characteristics of drug pharmacodynamics and infectious inocula that dictate importance of parameter in treatment of bacterial infection		
Time serum drug concentration exceed MIC[b]	Short or absent	Absent, or saturated at low concentrations	Small/none	Beta-lactams vs. aerobic gram-negative bacilli
Drug AUC[c]	Present	Present over therapeutic range	Small/none	Aminoglycosides vs. small inocula of *E. coli*
Peak drug concentration[d]	Present	Present over therapeutic range	Large/yes	Fluoroquinolones, aminoglyosides versus *Pseudomonas aeruginosa*

[a] Bacterial subpopulations in the initial inoculum resistant to the drug.

[b] The duration of time serum concentrations exceed some index of activity, usually the MIC or MBC. However, other measures of activity may be applicable as well.

[c] Sometimes this parameter is related to the MIC or MBC by either a ratio (e.g., AUC/MIC) or a difference (e.g., area exceeding the MIC).

[d] Sometimes related to the MIC or MBC by either a ratio (e.g., PK:MIC) or difference (e.g., PK–MIC).

PROSPECTUS

Perhaps the best application of linked pharmacokinetic and pharmacodynamic models for antimicrobials is yet to come. The availability of effective antiviral and immunomodulating agents, many of which have narrow therapeutic indices and exhibit significant interpatient variability in pharmacokinetic properties, provide a challenge for the application of existing models as well as the development of new ones. The need for chronic, lifelong therapy with antiretroviral and immune-enhancing agents in patients with the acquired immunodeficiency syndrome (AIDS) introduces the concept of chronic management into infectious disease pharmacotherapy. The identification of effective dosage regimens through use of linked pharmacokinetic/pharmacodynamic models assists in the determination of effective and nontoxic dosage regimens using several surrogate pharmacodynamic endpoints instead of death or progression of HIV infection.[52] The impact of development of linked pharmacodynamic-pharmacokinetic models on individualization of dosage on drug development and clinical management of patients will be enormous.[53]

REFERENCES

1. Dudley MN. Use of the laboratory in infectious diseases. In: DiPiro J et al., eds. Pharmacotherapy: A Pathophysiologic Approach. 2nd ed. New York: Elsevier; 1992.
2. Drusano GL. Role of pharmacokinetics on the outcome of infections. Antimicrob Agents Chemother. 1988;32:289–97.
3. LeBel M, Spino M. Pulse dosing versus continuous infusion of antibiotics. Pharmacokinetic-pharmacodynamic considerations. Clin Pharmacokinet. 1988;14:71–95.
4. Ebert SC, Craig WA. Pharmacodynamic properties of antibiotics: application to drug monitoring and dosage regimen design. Infect Control Hosp Epidemiol. 1990;11:319–26.
5. Milatovic D, Braveny I. Development of resistance during antibiotic therapy. Eur J Clin Microbiol. 1987;6:234–44.
6. Daikos GL et al. Adaptive resistance to aminoglycoside antibiotics from first-exposure down-regulation. J Infect Dis. 1990;162:414–20.
7. Daikos GL et al. First-exposure adaptive resistance to aminoglycoside antibiotics *in vivo* with meaning for optimal clinical use. Antimicrob Agents Chemother. 1991;35:117–23.
8. Blaser J et al. Efficacy of intermittent versus continuous administration of netilmicin in a two-compartment *in vitro* model. Antimicrob Agents Chemother. 1985;27:343–49.
9. Olson B et al. Occult aminoglycoside resistance in *Pseudomonas aeruginosa*: epidemiology and implications for therapy and control. J Infect Dis. 1985;152:769–74.
10. Livermore DM. Clinical significance of beta-lactamase induction and stable derepression in gram-negative rods. Eur J Clin Microbiol. 1987;6:439.
11. Wolfson JS, Hooper DC. Bacterial resistance to quinolones: mechanisms and clinical importance. Rev Infect Dis. 1989;11(5):S960–S968.
12. Craig WA, Vogelman B. The postantibiotic effect. Ann Intern Med. 1987;106:900–902.
13. Vogelman B et al. *In vivo* postantibiotic effect in a thigh infection in neutropenic mice. J Infect Dis. 1988;157:287–98.
14. Potel G et al. Impact of dosage schedule on the efficacy of gentamicin, tobramycin, or amikacin in an experimental model of *Serratia marcescens* endocarditis: *in vitro-in vivo* correlation. Antimicrob Agents Chemother. 1991;35:111–16.
15. Ingerman MJ et al. The importance of pharmacodynamics in determining dosing interval in therapy for experimental *Pseudomonas endocarditis* in the rat. J Infect Dis. 1986;153:707–14.
16. Bustamante CI et al. Postantibiotic effect of imipenem on *Pseudomonas aeruginosa*. Antimicrob Agents Chemother. 1984;26:678–82.

17. Gottfredsson M et al. Metabolic and ultrastructural effects induced by ciprofloxacin in *S. aureus* during the postantibiotic phase. Scand J Infect Dis. 1991;74(Suppl.):124–28.

18. Leggett JE et al. Comparative antibiotic dose-effect relationships at several dosing intervals in murine pneumonitis and thigh-infection models. J Infect Dis. 1989;159:281–92.

19. Powell SH et al. Once-daily vs continuous aminoglycoside dosing: efficacy and toxicity in animal and clinical studies of gentamicin, netilmicin and tobramycin. J Infect Dis. 1983;147:918–32.

20. Kapusnik JE et al. Single, large daily dosing vs. intermittent dosing of tobramycin for treating experimental *Pseudomonas* pneumonia. J Infect Dis. 1988;158:7–12.

21. Blaser J et al. Comparative study with enoxacin and netilmicin in a pharmacodynamic model to determine importance of ratio of antibiotic peak concentration to MIC for bactericidal activity and emergence of resistance. Antimicrob Agents Chemother. 1987;31:1054–60.

22. Wood CA et al. The influence of tobramycin dosage regimens on nephrotoxicity, ototoxicity, and antibacterial efficacy in a rat model of subcutaneous abscess. J Infect Dis. 1988;158:13–22.

23. Kovarik JM et al. Once-daily aminoglycoside administration: new strategies for an old drug. Eur J Clin Microbiol Infect Dis. 1989;8:761–69.

24. DeVries PJ et al. Toxicity of once daily netilmicin in patients with intra-abdominal infections. 27th Interscience Conference for Antimicrobial Agents and Chemotherapy, American Society for Microbiology. New York: 1987. Abstract 608, Program and Abstracts.

25. Fan ST et al. Once daily administration of netilmicin compared with thrice daily, both in combination with metronidazole, in gangrenous and perforated appendicitis. J Antimicrob Chemother. 1988;22:69–74.

26. Maller R et al. A study of amikacin given once versus twice daily in serious infections. J Antimicrob Chemother. 1988;22:75–79.

27. Hollender LF et al. A multicenter study of netilmicin once daily versus thrice daily in patients with appendicitis and other intra-abdominal infections. J Antimicrob Chemother. 1989;23:773–83.

28. Sturm AW. Netilmicin in the treatment of gram-negative bacteremia: single daily versus multiple daily dosage. J Infect Dis. 1989;159:931–37.

29. Tulkens PM et al.. Safety and efficacy of aminoglycosides once-a-day: experimental data and randomized, controlled evaluation in patients suffering from pelvic inflammatory disease. J Drug Develop. 1988;1(Suppl.3):71–82.

30. Barriere SL et al. Analysis of a new method for assessing activity of combinations of antimicrobials: area under the bactericidal activity curve. J Antimicrob Chemother. 1985;16:49–59.

31. Gerber AU et al. Antibiotic therapy of infections due to *Pseudomonas aeruginosa* in normal and granulocytopenic mice: Comparison of murine and human pharmacokinetics. J Infect Dis. 1986;153:90–97.

32. Dudley MN et al. Pharmacodynamics and subpopulation analysis of single and combination therapy of *Pseudomonas aeruginosa* with single or divided daily dosing of amikacin with simultaneous or staggered ceftriaxone. Pharmacotherapy 1990;10:234.

33. Zinner SH et al. Effect of dose and schedule on cefoperazone pharmacodynamics in an *in vitro* model of infection in a neutropenic host. Am J Med. 1988;85(Suppl.1A):56–58.

34. Vogelman B et al. Correlation of antimicrobial pharmacokinetic parameters with therapeutic efficacy in an animal model.

35. Daenen S, De Vries-Hosper H. Cure of *Pseudomonas aeruginosa* infection in neutropenic patients by continuous infusion of ceftazidime. Lancet 1988;1:937.

36. Dudley MN et al. Pharmacokinetics and pharmacodynamics of intravenous ciprofloxacin. Am J Med. 1987;82(Suppl.4A):363–68.

37. Dudley MN et al. Combination therapy with ciprofloxacin plus azlocillin against *Pseudomonas aeruginosa*: effect of simultaneous vs. staggered administration in an in vitro model of infection. J Infect Dis. 1991;164:499-506.

38. Klastersky J et al. Prospective randomized comparison of 3 antibiotic regimens for empirical therapy of suspected bacteremic infection in febrile granulocytopenic patients. Antimicrob Agents Chemother. 1986;29:263–70.

39. EORTC International Antimicrobial Therapy Cooperative Group. Ceftazidime combined with a short or long course of amikacin for empirical therapy of gram-negative bacteremia in cancer patients with granulocytopenia. N Engl J Med. 1987;317:1692–698.

40. Schentag JJ et al. Role of dual individualization with cefmenoxime. Am J Med. 1984;77(Suppl.6A):43–50.

41. Peloquin CA et al. Evaluation of intravenous ciprofloxacin in patients with nosocomial lower respiratory tract infections: impact of plasma concentrations, organism, minimum inhibitory concentration, and clinical condition on bacterial eradication. Arch Intern Med. 1989;149:2269–273.

42. Pennington JE. Nosocomial respiratory infection. In: Mandell GL et al., eds. Principles and Practice of Infectious Diseases. 3rd ed. New York: Churchill Livingstone; 1990:2199–205.

43. Andrews CP et al. Diagnosis of nosocomial bacterial pneumonia in acute, diffuse lung injury. Chest 1981;80:254–8.

44. DiNubile MJ. Antibiotics: the antipyretics of choice? Am J Med. 1990;89:787–88.

45. Tisdale JE et al. Antipseudomonal activity of simulated infusions of gentamicin alone or with piperacillin assessed by serum bactericidal rate and area under the killing curve. Antimicrob Agents Chemother. 1989;33:1500–505.

46. Guggenbichler JP et al. Spaced administration of antibiotic combinations to eliminate *Pseudomonas* from sputum in cystic fibrosis. Lancet 1988;II:749–50.

47. Haller I. Combined action of decreasing concentrations of azlocillin and sisomicin on *Pseudomonas aeruginosa* as assessed in a dynamic in vitro model. Infection 1982;10 (Suppl.3):229–33.

48. Mordenti JJ et al. Combination antibiotic therapy: comparison of constant infusion and intermittent bolus dosing in an experimental animal model. J Antimicrob Chemother. 1985;15(Suppl.A):313–21.

49. Greenwood D. *In vitro veritas?* Antimicrobial susceptibility tests and their clinical relevance. J Infect Dis. 1981;144:380–85.

50. McGrath B et al. Effect of repeated antibiotic exposure on the *in vitro* postantibiotic effect. 31st Interscience Conference on Antimicrobial Agents and Chemotherapy. Chicago, IL: 1991 September 29–October 2. Abstract 416.

51. Dudley MN et al. Effect of dose on serum pharmacokinetics of intravenous ciprofloxacin with identification and characterization of extravascular compartments using noncompartmental and compartmental pharmacokinetic models. Antimicrob Agents Chemother. 1987;31:1782–786.

52. Dudley MN et al. Study of antiretroviral pharmacodynamics using an *in vitro* model. 31st Interscience Conference on Antimicrobial Agents and Chemotherapy. Chicago, IL: 1991 September 29–October 2. Abstract 363.

53. Dudley MN, Horton C. Pharmacokinetics and pharmacodynamics in antiviral therapy. Clin Pharmacokinet. 1992. [In press.]

54. Gilbert DN. Once-daily aminoglycoside therapy. Amtimicrob Agents Chemother. 1991;35:399–405.

55. Odenholt-Tongvist I et al. Pharmacodynamic effects of subinhibitory concentrations of antibiotics. Scand J Infect Dis. 1991;74(Suppl.):94–101.

56. EORTC. Single vs. multiple daily doses of amikacin combined with ceftriaxone or ceftazidime for empirical therapy of fever in the granulocytopenic cancer patient. 31st Interscience Conference on Antimicrobial Agents and Chemotherapy. Chicago, IL: 1991 September 29–October 2. Abstract 292.

57. Radandt JM et al. Single or divided dosing of high-dose ciprofloxacin against *Pseudomonas aeruginosa*: pharmacodynamics and effect on selection of *gyr-A* mutants. 31st Interscience Conference on Antimicrobial Agents and Chemotherapy. Chicago;IL:1991 September 29–October 2. Abstract 813.

Chapter 19

Zidovudine

Gene D. Morse

$\mathbf{S}$ ince the recognition of the acquired immunodeficiency syndrome (AIDS) in 1981[1] and the subsequent discovery of the etiologic agent, human immunodeficiency virus (HIV) in 1985,[2-4] there has been an ongoing, intensive search for effective treatment modalities. The *in vitro* observation of anti-retroviral activity of zidovudine [ZDV—formerly azidothymidine (AZT)] was rapidly followed by a randomized, double-blinded, placebo-controlled, multicenter clinical trial to assess ZDV efficacy in HIV-infected patients with AIDS or advanced AIDS-related complex (ARC).[5] The decreased mortality noted in this study,[5] as well as the beneficial experience with ZDV in subsequent studies,[6,7] led to the widespread use of this agent in both comparative Phase II studies and a compassionate-use, investigational new drug (IND) protocol.[8,9] More recently, clinical efficacy in asymptomatic HIV-infected individuals and early ARC patients has been demonstrated.[10] In addition, the results of phase I studies with other nucleoside analogs, dideoxyinosine (ddI), and dideoxycytidine (ddC) appear promising (see Figure 19-1).[11-14]

GENERAL CONSIDERATIONS

The urgent need for a drug with activity against HIV necessitated a rapid transition from preclinical testing through Phase I and II investigations for ZDV. Since dosage form development and alternative administration techniques have evolved concurrently with clinical studies, pharmacokinetic data obtained for different formulations have been reported in the literature. Initial pharmacokinetic data were derived from the oral administration of the intravenous preparation and a capsule as well as one hour intravenous (IV) infusion studies.[15] Since many infants and children are now infected with HIV, continuous IV infusions and, more recently, an oral suspension have been studied in this population.[16-18] In addition to formulation differences, the dosage administered, the subpopulation of HIV-infected patients studied, and the duration of study have all varied. Lastly, the degree of HIV disease progression has varied between studies. Therefore, even within a specific subpopulation, important interindividual differences may have influenced study results.

CLINICAL PHARMACOKINETICS

Absorption

ZDV is a thymidine analog which is well absorbed and subjected to first-pass hepatic glucuronidation; peak serum concentrations occur 30 minutes to 1 hour after administration in the fasted state (see Figure 19-2).[15,19] While the time to reach maximum concentrations (T_{max}) is fairly consistent among patients, peak serum concentrations can vary.[20] A high-fat meal taken before ZDV administration will delay the T_{max} and decrease the AUC following a single dose.[21,71] First-pass hepatic glucuronidation contributes to interpatient variability in ZDV exposure. The bioavailability (F) of an oral solution (5 mg/kg) of ZDV has been reported to be 0.63 ± 0.10 in AIDS and ARC patients,[19] and a capsule dosage form has yielded an F = 0.64 ± 0.10 (see Figure 19-2).[15,19] Data obtained in pediatric patients (data reported as solution and capsules) and in asymptomatic hemophiliac patients (capsules) are similar but more variable (F = 0.68 ± 0.25).16,20 In addition, intrapatient bioavailability may increase or decrease up to twofold during chronic dosing.[22]

Distribution

Following IV administration (one hour infusion), ZDV serum concentrations decay in a biexponential pattern with a rapid alpha phase and a beta phase half-life of 0.9 to 1.4 hours.[15,19] The rapid decline of serum concentration presumably reflects intracellular accumulation of ZDV; this conclusion is based on ZDV's mechanism of action (see below) as well as its known metabolism to GZDV. Because the beta half-life is so short, ZDV is administered every four hours around

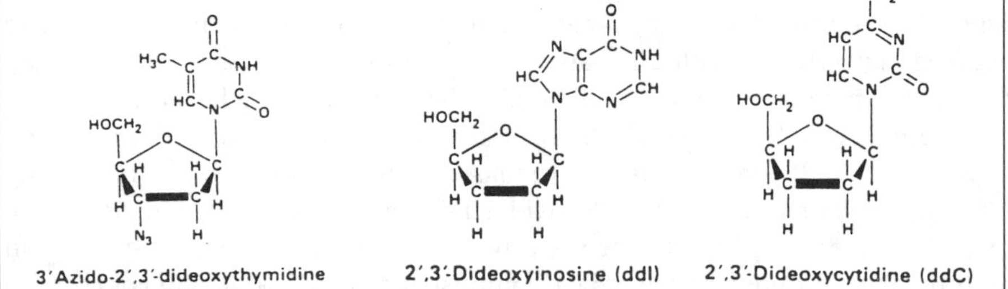

3′Azido-2′,3′-dideoxythymidine   2′,3′-Dideoxyinosine (ddI)   2′,3′-Dideoxycytidine (ddC)
(AZT, zidovudine)

Figure 19-1. Chemical structure of zidovudine (ZDV), dideoxyinosine (ddI), and dideoxycytidine (ddC).

the clock in an attempt to maintain serum concentrations above a target *in vitro* virustatic concentration of 1 μmol.[23] In a study of HIV-infected, asymptomatic hemophilia patients receiving a 300 mg oral dose of ZDV, a gamma phase of ZDV was identified.[22] However, the intensive blood sampling protocol required to clearly define each exponential phase was prohibitive in this population. Thus, the resultant serum profiles did not fit well into two- or three-compartment models when analyzed with nonlinear least squares regression analysis. More studies are needed to confirm the existence of a slower (or gamma) phase of ZDV elimination and to delineate its significance.

ZDV distributes throughout body water and tissues with a distribution volume (V_{ss}) of 1.6 ± 0.6 L/kg.[15,19] One report utilizing a population pharmacokinetic analysis of ZDV found a volume of distribution of 3 ± 0.6 L/kg in ARC patients.[24] The penetration of ZDV into the central nervous system is of special importance because of the known ability of HIV to infect the brain directly or via macrophages.[25] Most evidence of ZDV diffusion across the blood-brain barrier is derived from analysis of ZDV in the cerebrospinal fluid (CSF) following a continuous intravenous infusion (children)[17] or intermittent intravenous or oral administration (adults).[15] Although these studies are not directly comparable because of the differing methods of administration, the data from pediatric patients indicate a CSF/serum ratio of 0.28; in adults, the ratio ranges from 0.15 to 1.35. The mean CSF concentrations of ZDV in children ranged from 0.31 ± 0.1 to 0.87 ± 0.3 μmol/L over a dose range of 0.5 to 1.8 mg/kg/hr given as a continuous intravenous infusion.[17] In adults, the CSF concentration ranged from 0.14 to 2.3 μmol/L over a dosage range of 2 to 15 mg/kg given either intravenously or orally.[15] The association between CSF and CNS concentrations of the active metabolite, ZDV-TP is unknown; however, the beneficial neurologic outcome attained in some HIV-infected patients[8] and reports of ZDV-associated neurotoxicity[26,27] suggest that a significant degree of CNS distribution occurs. The distribution of ZDV into the CSF is partly due to low plasma protein binding (20%).[28]

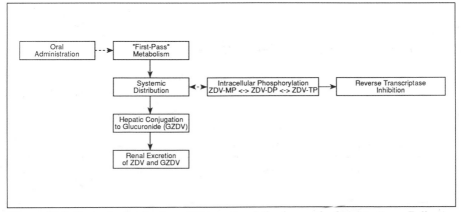

Figure 19-2. Systemic distribution of Zidovudine following oral administration. Following diffusion into cells, ZDV is sequentially phosphorylated to Zidovudine-monophosphate (ZDV-MP), Zidovudine-diphosphate (ZDV-DP) and ZDV-triphosphate (ZDV-TP). ZDV-TP is the active moiety incorporated into the growing DNA molecule, resulting in chain termination.

Because an increasing number of pregnant women are HIV-infected, concern over ZDV penetration into breast milk and transplacental diffusion has arisen. Data obtained in monkeys and mice indicate that ZDV is present in breast milk and crosses the placental membrane.[29,30] Reports in humans have confirmed these data with umbilical cord serum concentrations ranging from 113% to 127% of maternal serum concentrations[72] and evidence that fetal glucuronidation of ZDV is impaired.[31] The potential for sexual transmission of HIV also makes ZDV concentrations in semen a relevant question. The semen:serum ratio ranges from 1.3 to 20, but the reason for such accumulation of drug remains unclear.[32] Stimulated saliva concentrations of ZDV are approximately 70% of concurrent serum concentrations, consistent with reported values for protein binding.[73]

ZDV diffuses into host cells and is phosphorylated by thymidine kinase to ZDV-monophosphate (ZDV-MP). Subsequently, ZDV-MP is converted to ZDV-diphosphate (ZDV-DP) and then to ZDV-triphosphate (ZDV-TP).[33] ZDV-TP, a competitive inhibitor of the HIV reverse transcriptase, may also be incorporated into the growing strand of DNA and act as a chain terminator.[33] The intracellular phosphorylated ZDV derivatives are in a dynamic equilibrium with intracellular and extracellular ZDV (see Figure 19-2) and are currently under investigation as a potential method for monitoring intracellular ZDV.[74,75]

Metabolism

The metabolic fate of ZDV is summarized in Figure 19-2. While intracellular conversion of ZDV to ZDV-TP is essential for the antiviral effect, there is a delicate balance between attaining successful inhibition of reverse transcriptase activity and inhibition of host kinase activity.[35] Figure 19-3 illustrates that k_m value for each step in the phosphorylation of ZDV to ZDV-TP. It is noteworthy to

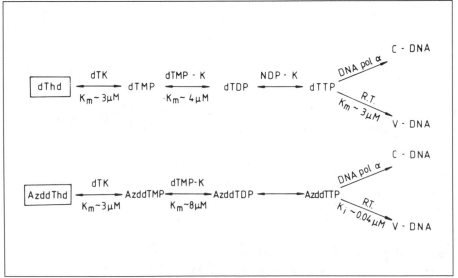

Figure 19-3. *Schematic of deoxythymidine (aThd) and Zidovudine (AZddThd) intracellular phosphorylation (reproduced with permission from reference 36).*

examine the k_m values for ZDV and deoxythymidine phosphorylation since the conversion of ZDV-MP to ZDV-DP ($k_m \approx 8$ µmol) appears to be the rate-limiting step in the ultimate formation of ZDV-TP.[36] Excessive accumulation of ZDV-MP may decrease the conversion of the host cell thymidine-MP to thymidine-DP ($k_m \approx 4$ µmol) and thus lead to cellular toxicity.

Figure 19-2 also provides insight into the potential for interpatient variation in hepatic glucuronidation rates that could affect intracellular concentrations of ZDV-TP. About 80% of an IV dose of ZDV is recovered as a renally excreted metabolite, 5'-0-glucuronide (3'-azido-3'-deoxy-5-B-D-glucopyranuronosylthymidine— formerly GAZT, now GZDV).[19] Interestingly, studies of UDP-glucuronyltransferase (UDGPT) obtained from rat and human liver indicate that large differences in their substrate efficiencies for ZDV exists; this may explain the discrepancy between the preclinical and Phase I results.[37]

Since the extracellular pool of unbound ZDV serves as the driving force in the diffusion of ZDV into cells, individual pharmacokinetic parameters will have an important impact on the extent of ZDV-TP formation. While gastrointestinal absorption and the extent of first-pass metabolism will determine the peak serum concentration of unbound ZDV, total clearance (hepatic and renal) and volume of distribution of ZDV will influence the serum concentration decay profile, and therefore, the intracellular diffusion gradient. The total clearance of ZDV (following intravenous administration of 1 to 5 mg/kg) ranges from 1.7 to 2.1 L/min/kg in adults, indicating a pattern of high clearance.[15,16,19] Similar values (641 ± 161 mL/min/m²) have been noted in children (see Table 19-1).[17] Since many studies are conducted in ambulatory HIV-infected patients, the oral ZDV clearance (CL_{oral}) is more commonly reported. However, CL_{oral} of ZDV does not distinguish changes in bioavailability from hepatic clearance. Bioavailability can vary between and among patients;[22] thus, oral clearance alone may be an unreliable indicator of alterations in ZDV metabolism.

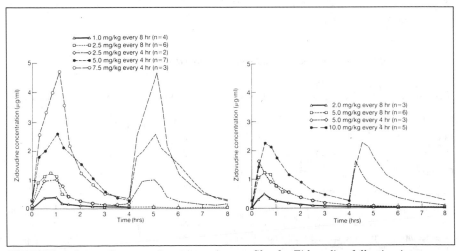

Figure 19-4. *Serum concentration versus time profiles for Zidovudine following intravenous and oral administration (reproduced with permission from reference 19).*

Excretion

ZDV is eliminated from plasma by at least three routes: uptake into human cells with conversion to ZDV-TP; hepatic glucuronidation to GZDV; and renal excretion of the parent compound. Both GZDV and ZDV are eliminated via renal excretion. In AIDS and ARC patients, 18% ± 5% of an intravenous ZDV dose is excreted unchanged, while 60% ± 10% is eliminated as GZDV. After oral dosing, recovery in the urine comprises 14% ± 3% ZDV and 75% ± 15% GZDV. The mean urinary recovery GZDV:ZDV ratio after oral dosing has been reported to be 5.7 and 6.9 in two separate studies in patients with AIDS.[19,38] In contrast, the GZDV:ZDV urinary recovery ratio in patients with hemophilia may be higher (up to 20) and may vary within a patient during multiple dosing.[39]

Renal clearances in AIDS patients with good renal function (estimated creatinine clearance 102 ± 29 mL/min) are reported to be 188 ± 65 mL/min for ZDV and 293 ± 46 mL/min for GZDV).[38] Tubular secretion is a component of the renal excretion for both ZDV and GZDV.

Determination of the renal excretion of GZDV and ZDV during probenecid administration indicates that a decreased tubular excretion of GZDV contributes to a higher GZDV AUC, while the ZDV AUC is increased as a result of decreased hepatic glucuronidation caused by the probenecid.[38]

The apparent renal clearance of ZDV decreases to 17 ± 2 mL/min in seronegative (non-HIV-infected) uremic patients (mean creatinine clearance 18 ± 2 mL/min).[40] In anuric, seronegative patients, hemodialysis clearance does not contribute appreciably to the removal of ZDV; however, GZDV is efficiently removed, with interdialytic half-life and dialysis half-life values of 52 ± 11 hours and 1.7 ± 0.1 hours, respectively. Studies of ZDV disposition in peritoneal dialysis patients are lacking. Despite the apparent lack of change in ZDV half-life, many dialysis patients do not tolerate the recommended daily dose of ZDV and require dosage reduction and/or dosing interval prolongation (i.e., 100 mg every 8 to 12 hours). Further studies are needed to clarify the optimal dosing schedule for ZDV in renal failure patients.

Table 19–1. Summary of Zidovudine Pharmacokinetic Parameters[a]

Parameters	Normal Volunteer	AIDS	Adult Hemophilia	Renal	Pediatric
CL_S (mL/min/kg)[b]	36.7 ± 2.0	22 ± 5	28.3 ± 14.9	17.3 ± 2.0[b]	641 ± 161[d]
CL_R (mL/min/kg)	3.2 ± 0.8	5.0	3.8	0.2 ± 0.03	—
V_β (L/kg)	3.2 ± 0.5[c]	1.6 ± 0.6	1.4	2.2 ± 0.2	45 ± 28
F (oral)	—	0.63 ± 0.1	0.15–0.99	—	0.68 ± 0.25
$t\frac{1}{2}\,\alpha$ (min)	—	—	—	—	0.25 ± 0.05
$t\frac{1}{2}\,\beta$ (hr)	1.0 ± 0.2	1.1 ± 0.2	3.5 ± 2.8	1.4 ± 0.1	1.5 ± 0.2

[a] Data compiled from references 15–20, and 39.
[b] Cl_S/F
[c] V_{area}/F
[d] $CL = mL/min/m^2$; $V_\beta = L/m^2$.

PHARMACOLOGIC EFFECT

Anti-HIV Effect

In contrast to bacterial infections in which the effects of antibiotics on bacterial growth can be assessed, the effect of an antiviral agent is less easily evaluated. A cell culture line which is not killed by HIV is required to culture the virus or to directly assess its antiviral effect. Common cell lines that are employed to preliminarily screen compounds for anti-retroviral activity and human cellular toxicity are H9 and TM3.[23] Antiviral effects are detected indirectly by measuring reverse transcriptase activity or directly, by detection of HIV antigen in the culture supernatant (an indicator of HIV replication), viral culture, or DNA probes.[41]

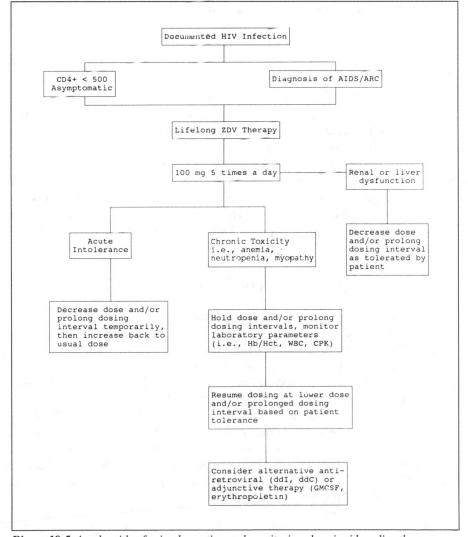

Figure 19-5. An algorithm for implementing and monitoring chronic zidovudine therapy.

Although an "inhibitory" concentration of ZDV is often quoted to be 0.1 μmol, it should be pointed out that *in vitro* ED_{50} values may differ according to the cell line used, and that the relationship between an ED_{50} value and the plasma or intracellular concentration necessary for a desirable *in vivo* effect remain to be determined.

Clinical assessment of anti-HIV effect is also difficult to directly assess. Since the initial beneficial effect of ZDV in AIDS patients was based on decreased mortality, subsequent studies have searched for more practical endpoints. The term "surrogate marker" is now used to describe the *in vivo* assessment of anti-HIV effects.[42,43] As the retroviral body burden is lowered during ZDV treatment, the ability to culture HIV from peripheral blood mononuclear cells decreases, and the detection of HIV antigen in serum decreases, while the absolute CD4+ count, the CD4+:CD8+ ratio, and the absolute CD8+ count may vary. Clinical findings are also used as indirect evidence of an anti-HIV effect. These include regression of lymphadenopathy or Kaposi's sarcoma, decreased occurrence of opportunistic infections, weight gain, increased Karnofsky rating, and increased responsiveness to skin antigen testing.

Adverse Effects

The adverse effect profile of ZDV has primarily been delineated in patients receiving 1200 to 1500 mg/day.[26] Symptoms of acute intolerance, including fever, nausea, and headache are observed most frequently; the more severe hematologic adverse effects (i.e., anemia, neutropenia) tend to be dose related and dose limiting. Other less common, although severe, complications include neurotoxicity,[24] hepatitis,[44] and myopathy.[45] It is difficult to incriminate ZDV as the sole offender in many of these toxicity reports since HIV disease and its complications can produce similar effects (see Progression of HIV Disease). With the recent recommendation to decrease the daily dose of ZDV from 1200 mg to 500 mg, hematologic toxicity has decreased.[10]

PROGRESSION OF HIV DISEASE

HIV infection can alter the function of the immune system, central nervous system, hematopoietic system, gastrointestinal tract, kidneys, and endocrine system.[46-49] The frequent occurrence of Kaposi's sarcoma[50] requiring chemotherapy and opportunistic infection[51] may also alter hepatic and kidney function, which can, in turn, influence drug disposition. Therefore, the clinical status of the patient at the time of evaluation (i.e., asymptomatic, ARC, AIDS) may lead to differences in the observed pharmacokinetics and/or pharmacologic effects of ZDV. An important recent observation is that asymptomatic, HIV-infected patients may have an enteropathy that can cause malabsorption.[46] In this report, patients with no clinical manifestations of opportunistic gastrointestinal infection were shown to have HIV antigen present in duodenal brush border cells, and decreased intestinal enzyme activity was noted.

DRUG INTERACTIONS

In vitro Data

Since patients with HIV disease often require chronic therapy with multiple drugs, it is important to consider the combined effects of antiviral drugs and immunomodulators on HIV growth. Isoprinosine does not appear to enhance viral replication and neither increases nor diminishes the antiviral effect of ZDV.[52] Castanospermine, an inhibitor of HIV envelope protein glycosylation, does result in synergistic anti-retroviral activity when combined with ZDV.[53] Acyclovir has been shown to have synergistic activity with ZDV,[54] while ribavirin antagonizes the activity of ZDV.[55] Synergistic inhibition of HIV has also been reported with recombinant soluble CD4 (a soluble retroviral receptor),[56] interferon-alpha,[57] and phosphonoformate (Foscarnet).[58]

Granulocyte-macrophage colony stimulating factor (GMCSF) is one of a number of cytokines with myelostimulative properties currently under investigation. With the recognition of neutropenia as a dose-limiting adverse effect of zidovudine, GMCSF has been under Phase I evaluation as adjunctive therapy in ZDV-induced neutropenic AIDS patients. The data of Perno et al. indicate that combined GMCSF/ZDV therapy may be a double-edged sword. While retroviral replication in monocytes was increased and the dose of virus needed to induce a productive infection was decreased during GMCSF exposure, the net anti-HIV effect of ZDV was increased as a result of enhanced ZDV cell entry and subsequent phosphorylation.[59] Preliminary clinical experience with GMCSF and ZDV to date indicates that GMCSF does elevate neutrophil counts in some neutropenic AIDS patients.[60]

In vivo Data

Hepatic glucuronidation is the predominant clearance mechanism for ZDV; both the parent compound (10% to 30%) and the metabolite (GZDV, 70% to 90%) are excreted renally. Probenecid, which inhibits organic acid secretion in the proximal tubule (e.g., penicillin), also competes with ZDV for hepatic glucuronidation.[38] The combined use of ZDV and probenecid is currently under investigation as a method of prolonging the ZDV dosing interval. Other glucuronidated drugs that are commonly prescribed for HIV-infected individuals, (e.g., sulfamethoxazole, sulfadiazine) were initially theorized to impair ZDV metabolism; however, in-depth evaluations have not identified an interaction.[61,62] For example, an initial observation from the multicenter ZDV efficacy study suggested that acetaminophen may have potentiated ZDV hematologic toxicity by impairing hepatic glucuronidation. Subsequent pharmacokinetic studies have not documented any influence of acetaminophen on ZDV disposition.[63,64,76]

CLINICAL APPLICATION OF PHARMACOKINETIC DATA

Methods to maximize the efficacy and minimize the toxicity of zidovudine have continued to evolve through ongoing multicenter studies. For example, a recently completed AIDS Clinical Trials Group (ACTG) study found that a lower daily dose of ZDV (100 mg five times daily) was as effective as, and perhaps less toxic than, the originally prescribed dose of 1200 mg/day. Another ACTG study[10,65] has reported that disease progression is slowed in asymptomatic, HIV-infected patients by ZDV therapy if the CD4+ count is less than 500/mm³. Other studies are currently investigating ZDV efficacy in hemophilia patients, pediatric patients, and neonates.

Few studies have attempted to examine the *in vivo* relationship between plasma ZDV concentrations and its anti-HIV effect. Balis et al. have reported the first human concentration:effect relationship data in pediatric AIDS patients receiving a continuous infusion of zidovudine.[17] In this study, 21 patients received 0.5 to 1.8 mg/kg/hr over one year. There was a significant difference in the nadir of the absolute neutrophil count between those patients who maintained a mean steady-state ZDV concentration (C_{ss}) of ≤ 2.5 μmol versus those with a $C_{ss} \geq 3.0$ μmol. It seems likely that a lower C_{ss} would decrease the intracellular exposure to ZDV and the accumulation of ZDV-MP.

Kornhauser et al. attempted to utilize a target ZDV AUC while administering probenecid with lower doses of ZDV, with the goal of decreasing the frequency of ZDV administration.[66] Although hypersensitivity reactions may limit the clinical application of this combination, the concept of a target AUC is an innovative approach to chronic ZDV therapy. In addition, Stretcher et al. have developed and conducted preliminary investigations of intracellular ZDV phosphorylated metabolites.[74,75] More studies are needed to correlate a target serum AUC with concurrent intracellular concentrations of ZDV phosphorylated derivatives.

Larder et al. reported that HIV isolates obtained during chronic ZDV therapy demonstrated decreased *in vitro* sensitivity.[67,68] The clinical significance of the impact of HIV resistance during long-term ZDV administration is currently under investigation; however, this finding is intriguing with regard to the potential future role for therapeutic monitoring of ZDV to ensure that plasma ZDV levels exceed the *in vitro* inhibitory concentration for an individual patient's isolate.

ANALYTICAL METHODS

Initial pharmacokinetic studies of ZDV were conducted using two different HPLC methods.[13,69] While both methods have similar variability (8% to 12%) and sensitivity (30 to 50 ng/mL), the method by Good et al.[69] has the advantage of measuring the glucuronide metabolite concurrently. More recently, a radio-immunoassay and a fluorescence polarization immunoassay have been reported.[34,70] These methods offer greater sensitivity (approximately 5 ng/mL), a quality which has taken on added significance since the recommended daily dose of ZDV has decreased. The RIA method can also determine GZDV; however, additional samples, to which glucuronidase is added, are required.

OTHER NUCLEOSIDE ANALOGS FOR HIV

Because the therapeutic range for ZDV is so narrow, a massive effort has been underway to develop alternative anti-retroviral agents. Two additional reverse transcriptase inhibitors have reached comparative Phase II evaluation against ZDV: dideoxyinosine (ddI) and dideoxycytidine (ddC). While ddC is also phosphorylated to an active triphosphorylated nucleotide analog (ddC-TP), ddI is ultimately converted to ddATP. Both agents are partially renally excreted; ddI is also metabolized to uric acid. Phase I studies indicate that both compounds have an anti-HIV effect.[11-14] Preliminary pharmacokinetic data indicate that although ddI has a short plasma half-life, the intracellular half-life of ddATP ranges from 12 to 24 hours. As a result, once or twice daily administration regimens for ddI are currently under investigation.

PROSPECTUS

While ZDV has clearly become the established agent for HIV, certain limitations to successful, long-term therapy exist. The delicate balance between suppression of HIV replication and host cell toxicity underscores the need for clinical research efforts to identify new dosing methods that will broaden the therapeutic window for this agent. The cumulative nature of ZDV toxicity and the recent observations of resistant HIV strains indicate that the use of alternating nucleoside analog regimens in combination with drugs that have different mechanisms of action may provide the safest, most effective treatment protocols. Ongoing basic and clinical research of other anti-HIV agents, including CD4 receptor analogs, protease inhibitors, glycosylation inhibitors, and others, offers hope that patients with HIV infection eventually can be managed on a chronic basis with decreased morbidity and mortality.

REFERENCES

1. Pneumocystis pneumonia. Los Angeles. MMWR. 1981;30:250–52.
2. Barre-Smoussi F et al. Isolation of a T-lymphotropic retrovirus from a patient at risk for acquired immune deficiency syndrome (AIDS). Science. 1983;22:868–71.
3. Gallo RC et al. Frequent detection and isolation of cytopathic retroviruses (HTLV-III) from patients with AIDS and at risk for AIDS. Science. 1984;224:500–3.
4. Levy JA et al. Isolation of lymphocytopathic retroviruses from San Francisco patients with AIDS. Science. 1984;225:840–42.
5. Fischl MA et al. The efficacy of azidothymidine (AZT) in the treatment of patients with AIDS and AIDS-related complex. A double-blind, placebo-controlled trial. New Engl J Med. 1987;317:185–91.
6. Dournan E et al. Effects of zidovudine in 365 consecutive patients with AIDS or AIDS-Related complex. Lancet. 1988;(1):1297–302.
7. Lane HC et al. Zidovudine in patients with human immunodeficiency virus (HIV) infection and Kaposi's sarcoma. Ann Intern Med. 1989;111(1):41–50.
8. Schmitt F et al. Neuropsychological outcome of zidovudine (AZT) treatment of patients with AIDS and AIDS-related complex. New Engl J Med. 1988;319(24):1573-78.
9. Creagh-Kirk T et al. Survival experience among patients with AIDS receiving zidovudine: Follow-up of patients in a compassionate plea program. JAMA. 1988;260(20):3009–15.
10. Volberding PA et al. Zidovudine in asymptomatic human immunodeficiency virus infection. New Engl J Med. 1990;322:941–49.
11. Yarchoan R et al. *In vivo* activity against HIV and favorable toxicity profile of 2',3'-Dideoxyinosine. Science. 1989;245:412–15.

12. Lambert JS et al. Administration 2',3'-dideoxyinosine (ddI) to patients with AIDS and ARC. New Engl J Med. 1990;322:1333–40.

13. Cooley TP et al. Once daily administration of 2'3'-dideoxyinosine (ddI) in patients with AIDS or ARC. New Engl J Med. 1990;322:1340–45.

14. Yarchoan R et al. Phase I studies of 2',3'-dideoxytidine in severe human immunodeficiency virus infection as a single agent and alternating with zidovudine (AZT). Lancet. 1988;1:76–80.

15. Klecker RW et al. Plasma and cerebrospinal fluid pharmacokinetics of 3'-azido-3'-deoxythymidine: A novel pyrimidine analog with potential application for the treatment of patients with AIDS and related diseases. Clin Pharmacol Ther. 1987;41:407–12.

16. Balis FM et al. Pharmacokinetics of zidovudine administered intravenously and orally in children with human immunodeficiency virus infection. J Pediatr. 1989;114(5):880–14.

17. Balis FM et al. The pharmacokinetics of zidovudine administered by continuous infusion in children. Ann Intern Med. 1989;110(4):279–85.

18. Drew RH et al. Bioequivalence assessment of zidovudine (Retrovir) syrup, solution, and capsule formulations in patients infected with human immunodeficiency virus. Antimicrob Agents Chemother. 1989;33:1801–3.

19. Blum MR et al. Pharmacokinetics and bioavailability of zidovudine in humans. Am J Med. 1988;84(Suppl. 2A):189—94.

20. Morse GD et al. Pharmacokinetics of orally administered zidovudine among patients with hemophilia and asymptomatic human immunodeficiency virus infection. Antivirual Res. 1989;11:57–66.

21. Unadkat JD et al. Pharmacokinetics of oral zidovudine (azidothymidine) in patients with AIDS when administered with and without a high fat meal. J Acq Imm Def Syn. 1990;4:229–32.

22. Morse GD et al. Multiple-dose pharmacokinetics of oral zidovudine in hemophilia patients with human immunodeficiency virus infection. Antimicrob Agents Chemother. 1990;34:394–97.

23. Mitsuya H et al. 3'-Azido-3'-deoxythymidine (BW A509U): an antiviral agent that inhibits the infectivity and cytopathic effect of human T-lymphotrophic virus type III/lymphadenopathy-associated virus *in vitro*. Proc Natl Acad Sci. USA. 1985;82:7096–100.

24. Gitterman SR et al. Population pharmacokinetics of zidovudine. Clin Pharmacol Ther. 1990;48:161–67.

25. Koenig S et al. Detection of AIDS virus in macrophages in brain tissue from AIDS patients with encephalopathy. Science. 1986;233:1089–93.

26. Richman DD et al. The toxicity of azidothymidine (AZT) in the treatment of patients with AIDS and AIDS-related complex. A double-blind, placebo-controlled trial. New Engl J Med. 1987;317:192–97.

27. Hagler DN, Frame PT. Azidothymidine neurotoxicity. Lancet. 1986;II:1392–93.

28. Collins JM et al. Pyrimidine dideoxyribonucleosides: selectivity of penetration into cerebrospinal fluid. J Pharmacol Exp Ther. 1988;245:466–70.

29. Ruprecht RM et al. Therapy against neurotropic retroviruses: a rapid murine model involving transplacental or neonatal infection. In: Bolognesi D ed. Human retroviruses, cancer and AIDS. AR Liss, New York; 1988:461–477.

30. Unadkat JD et al. Transplacental transfer and the pharmacokinetics of zidovudine (ZDV) in the near term pregnant macaque. Proceedings of the 28th Interscience Conference on Antimicrobial Agents and Chemotherapy. Los Angeles, CA: 1988:372.

31. Gillet JY et al. Fetoplacental passage of zidovudine. Lancet I; 1989:269–70.

32. Henry K et al. Concurrent zidovudine levels in semen and serum determination by radioimmunoassay in patients with AIDS or AIDS-related complex. JAMA. 1988;259:3023–26.

33. Furman PA et al. Phosphorylation of 3'-azido-3'-deoxythymidine and selective interaction of the 5'-triphosphate with human immunodeficiency virus reverse transcriptase. Proc Natl Acad Sci. 1986;83:8333–37.

34. Product Information. ZDV-Track[R] RIA Incstar Corp. Stillwater, MN.

35. Frick LW et al. Effects of 3'-azido-3'-deoxythymidine on the deoxynucleotide triphosphate pools of cultured human cells. Biochem Biophys Res Comm. 1988;154:124–29.

36. Balzarini J, Broder S. Principles of antiretroviral therapy for AIDS and related diseases. In: DeClerq E ed. Clinical Use of Antiviral Drugs. Martinus-Nijhoff Publ (Boston); 1988.

37. Resetar A, Spector T. Glucuronidation of 3-azido-3'-deoxythymidine: human and rat enzyme specificity. Biochem Pharmacol. 1989;38:1389–93.

38. deMiranda P et al. Alteration of zidovudine pharmacokinetics by probenecid in patients with AIDS-related complex. Clin Pharmacol Ther. 1989;46:494–500.

39. Morse GD et al. Renal excretion of zidovudine and zidovudine-glucuronide during multiple dosing. Clin Pharmacol Ther. 1990;47:177. Abstract.

40. Singlas E et al. Zidovudine disposition in patients with severe renal impairment: influence of hemodialysis. Clin Pharmacol Ther. 1989;46:190–97.

41. Schleupner CJ. Detection of HIV-1 infection. In: Mandell GL et al, ed. Principles and Practice of Infectious Disease. New York: Churchill Livingstone; 1990:1092–102.

42. Lange JMA et al. Markers for progression to acquired immune deficiency syndrome and zidovudine treatment of asymptomatic patients. J Infect. 1989;18(Suppl. I):85–91.

43. Jackson GG et al. Human immunodeficiency virus (HIV) antigenemia (p24) in the acquired immunodeficiency syndrome (AIDS) and the effect of treatment with zidovudine (AZT). Ann Intern Med. 1988;108:175–80.

44. Dubin G, Braffman MN. Zidovudine-induced hepatotoxicity. Ann Intern Med. 1989;110:85–6.

45. Simpson DM, Bender AN. Human immunodeficiency virus-associated myopathy: analysis of 11 patients. Ann Neurol. 1988;24:79–84.

46. Ullrich R et al. Small intestine structure and function in patients infected with human immunodeficiency virus (HIV): Evidence for HIV-induced enteropathy. Ann Intern Med. 1989;11:15–21.

47. Lopez AP et al. Diarrhea in AIDS. Infect Dis Clin Nor Amer. 1988;2:705–18.

48. Sreepada TK et al. The types of renal disease in the acquired immunodeficiency syndrome. New Engl J Med. 1987;316:1062–68.

49. Glassock RJ et al. Human immunodeficiency virus (HIV) infection and the kidney. Ann Intern Med. 1990;112:35–49.

50. Kovacs JA et al. Combined zidovudine and interferon-alpha therapy in patients with Kaposi's sarcoma and the acquired immunodeficiency syndrome (AIDS). Ann Intern Med. 1989;111(4):280–7.

51. Lerner CW, Tapper ML. Opportunistic infection complicating acquired immune deficiency syndrome. Medicine. 1984;63:155–64.

52. Schinazi RF et al. Combinations of isoprinosine and 3'-azido-3'-deoxythymidine in lymphocytes infected with human immunodeficiency virus type 1. Antimicrob Agents Chemother. 1988;32:1784–87.

53. Johnson VA et al. Synergistic inhibition of human immunodeficiency virus type 1 and type 2 replication *in vitro* by castanospermine and 3'-azido-3'-deoxythymidine. Antimicrob Agents Chemother. 1989;33:53–7.

54. Mitsuya H, Broder S. Strategies for antiviral therapy in AIDS. Nature. 1987;325:773–78.

55. Vogt MW et al. Ribavirin antagonizes the effect of azidothymidine on HIV replication. Science. 1987;235:1376-79.

56. Johnson VA et al. Synergistic inhibition of human immunodeficiency virus type 1 (HIV-1) replication *in vitro* by recombinant soluble CD4 and 3'-azido-3'-deoxythymidine. J Infect Dis. 1989;159:837–44.

57. Hartshorn KL et al. Synergistic inhibition of human immunodeficiency virus in vitro by azidothymidine and recombinant alpha A interferon. Antimicrob Agents Chemother. 1987;31:168–72.

58. Ericksson BFH, Schinazi RF. Combinations of 3'-azido-3'-deoxythymidine (Zidovudine) and phosphonoformate (Forscarnet) against human immunodeficiency virus type 1 and cytomegalovirus replication *in vitro*. Antimcrob Agents Chemother. 1989;33:663–69.

59. Perno CF et al. Replication of human immunodeficiency virus in monocytes: granulocyte/macrophage colony-stimulating factor (GMCSF) potentiates viral production yet enhances the antiviral effect mediated by 3'-azido-2'3'-dideoxythymidine (AZT) and other dideoxynucleotide congeners of thymidine. J Exp Med. 1989;169:933–51.

60. Hewitt R et al. Concurrent administration of granulocyte-macrophage colony stimulating factor and zidovudine in patients with AIDS/ARC. Sixth International Conference on AIDS. San Francisco, CA: 1990.

61. Hardy WD et al. Clinical and pharmacokinetic interactions of combined zidovudine and sulfadozine-pyrimethamine prophylaxis in post-PCP AIDS patients. Fifth International Conference on AIDS 1989: Abstract. T.B. P.46. Montreal, Canada.

62. Ptachcinski RJ et al. Influence of trimethoprim-sulfamethoxazole on zidovudine pharmacokinetics (Abstract): J Clin Pharmacol. 1991 (In Press).

63. Koda RT et al. Effect of acetaminophen on the pharmacokinetics of zidovudine. Fifth International Conference on AIDS 1989: Abstract. W.B.O.5., Montreal, Canada.

64. Pazin GJ et al. Interactive pharmacokinetics of zidovudine and acetaminophen. Fifth International Conference on AIDS 1989: Abstract. M.B.P. 338, Montreal, Canada.

65. Fischl MA et al. The safety and efficacy of zidovudine in the treatment of subjects with mildly symptomatic human immunodeficiency virus type I (HIV) infection. Ann Int Med. 1990;112:727–37.

66. Kornhauser DM et al. Effects of quinine sulfate and probenecid alone and in combination on the pharmacokinetics of zidovudine. Program and abstracts of the twenty-eight Interscience Conference on Antimicrobial Agents and Chemotherapy. Los Angeles, CA: 1988 October. Abstract 1467:371.

67. Marx JL. Drug-resistant strains of AIDS virus found. Science. 1989;243:1551–52.

68. Larder BA et al. HIV with reduced sensitivity to zidovudine (AZT) isolated during prolonged therapy. Science. 1989;243:1731–734.

69. Good SS et al. Simultaneous quantification of zidovudine and its glucuronide in serum by high-performance liquid chromatography. J Chromatog. 1988;431:123–33.

70. Granich GG et al. Fluorescence polarization immunoassay for zidovudine. Antimicrob Agents Chemother. 1989;33:1275-279.

71. Lotterer E et al. Decreased and variable systemic availability of zidovudine in patients with AIDS if administered with a meal. Eur J Clin Pharmacol. 1991;40:305–308.

72. Watts DH et al. Pharmacokinetic disposition of zidovudine during pregnancy. J Infect Dis. 1991; 163:226–232.

73. Rolinski B et al. Evaluation of saliva as a specimen for monitoring zidovudine therapy in HIV-infected patients. J Acq Imm Def Syn 1991;5:885–88.

74. Stretcher BN et al. *In vitro* measurement of phosphorylated zidovudine in peripheral blood leucocytes. Ther Drug Monit. 1990;

75. Stretcher BN et al. Concentrations of phosphorylated zidovudine (ZDV) in patient leukocytes do not correlate with ZDV dose or plasma concentrations. Ther Drug Monitor. 1991;13:325–31.

76. Sattler et al. Acetaminophen does not impair clearance of zidovudine. Ann Intern Med. 1991;114;937–40.

Chapter 20

Digoxin

Richard H. Reuning, Douglas R. Geraets,
Mario L. Rocci, Jr., and Peter H. Vlasses

The indications for digoxin therapy in current clinical practice are limited to congestive heart failure (CHF) and control of supraventricular tachyarrhythmias.[1] Progressive revision of the role of digoxin therapy in these pathologies has intensified in the past few years, mainly due to the availability of alternative or complementary drugs. As a result, the outcome of therapy has improved.

In **chronic CHF** the usual combination of a diuretic to reduce filling pressure and congestion, as well as digoxin for positive inotropy, has been complemented by vasodilators capable of reducing preload and afterload.[2] Angiotensin-converting enzyme (ACE) inhibitors balance arteriolar dilation and venodilation and have improved both symptoms and survival.[3] There is debate regarding the question of whether ACE inhibitors or digoxin should be the first addition to CHF therapy after diuretics.[4,5,6] Concurrently, there is increasing evidence of the effectiveness of digoxin for patients in sinus rhythm with substantially impaired left ventricular systolic function [New York Heart Association (NYHA) classes III and IV, usually having a dilated left ventricle[7] and a third heart sound], whether digoxin is added to diuretic therapy or to both diuretic and vasodilator therapy.[5-9] In mild heart failure (NYHA class II), digoxin is usually unnecessary in asymptomatic patients with good exercise tolerance and in patients with symptoms of heart failure but with preserved left ventricular systolic function.[5] Although digoxin improves left ventricular performance and hemodynamic status, several authors have pointed out that this does not lead to improved symptomatology or exercise capacity in those with mild to moderate heart failure[6,10,11] like it does in patients with more severe failure.[8,12] However, some argue that the negative exercise results are due to flawed methodology for measuring exercise capacity.[13,14] When digoxin is withdrawn in mild heart failure, a varying fraction of patients deteriorate clinically,[5,10] and this deterioration is accompanied by changes in receptor binding and receptor function in erythrocytes.[10] Thus, identification of the subsets of patients with chronic CHF that have a favorable risk:benefit ratio for digoxin therapy requires further clarification.[5]

In **atrial fibrillation of acute onset**, the traditional approach of administering intravenous digoxin is being challenged. Spontaneous reversion to sinus rhythm is common and digoxin has not been shown to be more effective than placebo in aiding the reversion.[15,16] In contrast, intravenous verapamil has been shown in numerous studies to consistently reduce the ventricular response rate in a rapid manner,[16] as has amiodarone in one study.[17] If atrial fibrillation is accompanied by CHF, however, intravenous digoxin is the preferred initial therapy because of its positive inotropic effect and the negative inotropic effect of verapamil.[18]

In **chronic atrial fibrillation**, oral digoxin has limited ability to decrease resting heart rate and does not control exercise heart rate.[16] However, the substantial effect of oral verapamil on both resting and exercise heart rate via a direct depressant action on conduction through the atrioventricular node is enhanced by digoxin's augmentation of vagal tone.[16,19] Diltiazem, another calcium channel-blocking agent, has effects similar to verapamil with only a small negative inotropic effect and with no pharmacokinetic interaction with digoxin.[20,21] If atrial fibrillation is accompanied by reduced ventricular function, the use of digoxin and diltiazem together is superior to either drug alone.[21] The combination of digoxin and a beta-adrenergic blocking agent has also shown considerable promise for reducing both resting and exercise heart rates in atrial fibrillation.[22]

Some miscellaneous observations in the recent literature regarding digoxin therapy are also worthy of note. It has been hypothesized that after acute myocardial infarction digoxin may adversely affect survival.[23] However, even suggesting this as an hypothesis has been vigorously criticized[24,25] in light of the lack of evidence for such an effect.[24,26] As with heart failure of other origins, it is recommended by several authors that digoxin use after acute myocardial infarction be restricted to chronic CHF patients with left ventricular systolic dysfunction and a dilated left ventricle.[1,13,25,26] In another vein, two recent publications have provided data relative to improved left ventricular performance after digoxin in patients with aortic regurgitation[27] and cardiac failure due to severe sepsis.[28]

CLINICAL PHARMACOKINETICS

Absorption

The intestinal absorption of digoxin from solution exhibits the properties of a passive, nonsaturable transport process in animal studies.[29] Although digoxin can be absorbed from solution in the stomach or colon in humans, the predominant site for absorption after oral administration is the upper part of the small intestine.[30–32] The portal vein transports absorbed drug to the liver, with little digoxin being transported by thoracic-duct lymph[33] and no significant first-pass effect.

The dosage forms of digoxin include conventional tablets, pediatric elixir and injection solution as well as the newer Lanoxicaps. Various studies have reported mean systemic availability of 70% to 85% for the elixir and 50% to 85% for conventional tablets.[34–36] Values in the upper part of these ranges appear to be more accurate because of improved methods of bioavailability assessment in more recent studies. Use of area under the concentration-time curve (AUC) values extrapolated to time infinity or cumulative urinary excretion data for several days results in higher and apparently more accurate bioavailability estimates than does use of AUC zero to six hours.[36–38] Thus, the current literature would indicate that one can expect the **systemic availability** of conventional digoxin **tablets** and **elixir** to average 70% to 80% and 75% to 85%, respectively (see Figure 20-1). Both ranges have been shown to apply to patients with severe, chronic renal failure.[39] In addition, severe right or left heart failure does not appear to influence bioavailability of digoxin from tablets.[40,41] Bioavailability from digoxin tablets has been shown to be independent of dose over an eightfold range.[42]

Lanoxicaps are soft gelatin capsules containing a solution of digoxin. The aqueous solvent contains polyethylene glycol, ethyl alcohol, and propylene glycol. As illustrated in Figure 20-1, this new dosage form has **improved bioavailability** (although at greater cost per dose), with reported values in the 90% to 100% range for both single-dose and steady-state conditions.[38,43,44] The digoxin content of Lanoxicaps is 80% of that in conventional tablets, so that the bioavailable dose

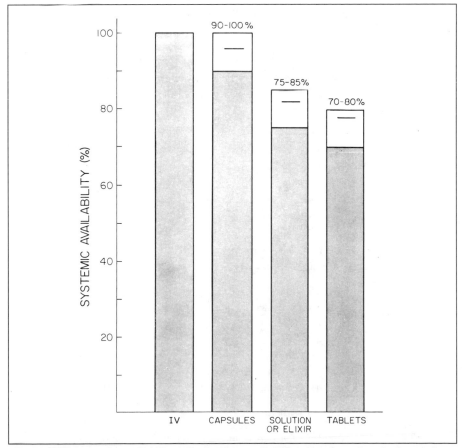

Figure 20-1. *Systemic availability (absolute bioavailability) of various digoxin dosage forms in humans. The lighter area indicates the range of mean values from several studies judged to be more accurate (see text). The horizontal lines within the lighter area indicate mean values from a recent multicenter study.[38]*

will be approximately equivalent for the two dosage forms. The bioavailability advantage of liquid-filled capsules containing digoxin also appears to extend to patients with heart disease.[45]

Considerable **metabolism** of digoxin **within the gastrointestinal tract** may occur either by hydrolysis of digitoxose glycosidic moieties in the acidic environment of the stomach or by reduction of the lactone double bond by intestinal bacteria (see Clinical Pharmacokinetics: Metabolism and Figure 20-2). Although the mechanism of enhanced digoxin bioavailability from liquid-filled soft gelatin capsules is not known, one attractive hypothesis is that this dosage form avoids metabolic breakdown at both ends of the gastrointestinal (GI) tract. Perhaps the soft gelatin capsule shields the contents long enough to avoid stomach acid-catalyzed hydrolysis of the digitoxose moieties, yet releases the digoxin in a rapidly absorbable form in the upper intestine. Support for this hypothesis is available from the substantially reduced urinary excretion of digoxin reduction products in "dihydro-formers" after administration of liquid-filled capsules as compared to conventional tablets.[46] The expected reduction in intra- and interpatient variability in bioavailability when liquid-filled capsules are substituted for conventional

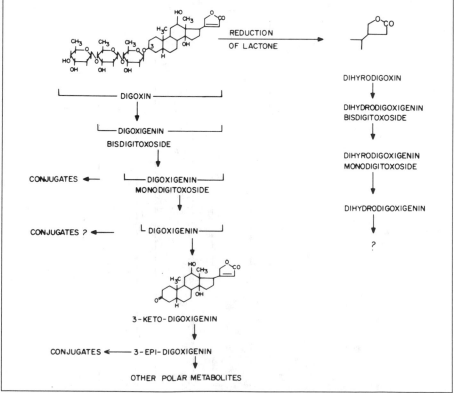

Figure 20-2. *Metabolic pathways for digoxin in humans. The first three steps in the pathway on the left represent sequential hydrolysis of digitoxose sugar moieties and result in active metabolites. This occurs in the stomach and perhaps other sites as well. The pathway on the right, involving hydrogenation of the lactone double bond, results in metabolites that are nearly inactive. This hydrogenation is carried out by intestinal bacteria (see text).*

tablets was not realized in a recent study in 28 patients with CHF and/or atrial fibrillation.[47] However, these authors observed a reduction in intrapatient variability in urinary excretion of reduced digoxin metabolites for liquid-filled capsules in a subgroup of six patients who formed the largest amounts of reduced metabolites. The bioavailability data for digoxin are summarized in Figure 20-1 and Table 20-1.

In newborn infants, the bioavailability of digoxin from a solution administered orally averaged 72% in four subjects, which is within the range observed for adults.[48] In elderly patients, there may be a reduction in bioavailability from tablets,[49] but further study is needed. Although administration of digoxin tablets with a meal may delay absorption, a normal breakfast does not appear to influence bioavailability.[50] Administration with a meal high in fiber content decreased digoxin absorption from tablets an average of 21%[51] and from capsules an average of 7%.[52] Volume of coadministered water had no effect on amount of digoxin absorbed from either dosage form.[53]

The effects of various gastrointestinal conditions on digoxin absorption have been studied. Surgical removal of two-thirds of the stomach (ten patients with Billroth II gastric resection) and most of the small intestine (seven patients with jejuno-ileal bypass leaving 12 inches of jejunum anastomosed to 6 inches of distal ileum) yielded no evidence of substantial reduction in absorption of digoxin tablets.[54–56] In 16 patients with surgical removal of part of the intestinal tract (12

Table 20-1. *Summary of Pharmacokinetic Parameters*[a, b]

	Population Averages (± SD) (Normal renal & hepatic function)		
	Adults	**Children**	**Neonates**
CL_S (mL/min/kg)	2.7	c	c
CL_R (mL/min/kg)	1.86 (0.32)	—	—
CL_{NR} (mL/min/kg)	0.82 (0.23)	—	—
V_1 (L/kg)	0.54 (0.11)	—	—
V_{ss} (L/kg)	6.7 (1.4)	16	7.5–10
F (oral) Tablets	0.75 (0.14)	—	—
Elixir	0.80 (0.16)	—	0.72 (0.13)
Liquid-filled capsules	0.95 (0.13)	—	—
% excreted in urine as			
parent drug (IV)	72 (8)	—	—
parent drug (PO)	54	—	—
$t^{1/2}\ \lambda_N$ (hr)	36 (8)	18–37	37

a Values obtained using radioimmunoassayed serum and urine concentrations of apparent digoxin. Values from the several studies cited in the text were averaged where possible. All values in neonates are open to serious question because of likely assay interference from endogenous digoxin-like immunoreactivity.

b These parameters were obtained from data in references 34–38, 43, 44, 48, 111, 121, 131, 155, 162, 174, 175, and 177–183.

c Clearance in premature infants is highly variable.[180,182] A recent study in 166 patients receiving intravenous digoxin at steady state yielded the following mean values for clearance (mL/min/kg): <3 months, <1500 gm—0.75; <3 months, 1500–2500 gm—1.33; <3 months, >2500 gm—1.70; 3–12 mo—3.10; 1–5 yr—3.70; 6–10 yr—3.17; 11–20 yr—2.70.[183]

of whom had the terminal ileum removed), the absorption of digoxin at steady state from tablets and liquid-filled capsules was comparable to that in normal volunteers.[57] In contrast, patients with various malabsorption syndromes, including untreated subtotal villus atrophy, hypermotility and diarrhea, and abdominal radiation have reduced absorption from digoxin tablets.[56,58] Prior chemotherapy, and total body irradiation reduced the bioavailability of digoxin tablets to 54% of the value before chemotherapy whereas the reduction for liquid-filled capsules was to 85%.[59] Use of the elixir improved digoxin bioavailability compared to tablets in one patient with radiation-induced malabsorption.[60] The lack of an effect of removing of a substantial portion of the gastrointestinal tract on bioavailability of digoxin tablets would seem to be inconsistent with the incomplete bioavailability of the drug from this dosage form and its potential for absorption throughout the GI tract. Further studies are needed to test the hypothesis that absorption occurs predominantly within a relatively short portion of the upper intestine and other hypotheses related to digoxin metabolism within the GI tract. The effects of physiological and pathological variables on digoxin absorption are summarized in Table 20-2.

The extent of absorption of digoxin from tablets can be reduced by a number of coadministered agents. Kaolin-pectin is the most significant of these. Coadministration of 90 mL decreased the extent of absorption of digoxin by 62%.[61] Administration of the antidiarrheal two hours after digoxin avoided the interaction.[61] Certain **antacids** (i.e., aluminum hydroxide 4%, magnesium hydroxide 8%, and magnesium trisilicate), given in large doses (60 mL), appear to reduce digoxin absorption by about 25% to 35%, whereas **cholestyramine** reduces digoxin bioavailability by 20% to 35%.[51,62,63,64] Decreasing intestinal motility by coadministration of **propantheline** increases digoxin bioavailability, whereas bioavailability is decreased when intestinal motility is increased by coadministration of **metoclopramide**.[64,65] The interactions of digoxin with these coadministered agents are minimized with liquid-filled capsules as compared to tablets (see Table 20-3 on page 20-9).[64-66] **Sulfasalazine**, **neomycin**, and **para-aminosalicylic** acid have also been shown to decrease digoxin absorption from tablets by an unknown mechanism.[51,62,67] These interactions are summarized in Table 20-3 on page 20-9.

Distribution

Distribution of digoxin has been studied in animals and humans through the use of nonspecific radioactivity measurements or the partially specific extraction-RIA (see Assay). Thus, the results reviewed herein represent a mixture of digoxin and metabolites ("apparent" digoxin), with the predominant compound being digoxin, as judged from studies of urinary excretion rates and serum concentration kinetics using more specific analytical methodology (see Pharmacokinetics: Metabolism). The distribution studies have been carried out in animals and human autopsy specimens.

After intravenous administration of tritiated digoxin to dogs, most tissues achieve a constant ratio of tissue radioactivity to serum radioactivity within eight hours,[68] which corresponds to the onset of the terminal pharmacokinetic exponen-

Table 20-2. *Influence of Physiological and Pathological Factors on Digoxin Absorption, Disposition, and Response*

Factor	Description	Clinical implications	References
Age: newborn	Evidence indicates no unusual bioavailability of solution dosage form. ↓ CL_s and V_{ss}.	↓ mg/kg loading and maintenance doses recommended.	48
Age: infants and young children	CL_s and V_{ss} ↑ with age up to about 5 years, then ↓ gradually until puberty.	↑ mg/kg dosage requirements; poor predictability of clearance necessitates selective apparent SDC[a] monitoring.	162, 163, 183, 240, 241
Obesity	Little distribution to body fat.	Dosage based on lean body weight.	96
Enterohepatic cycling	Conflicting evidence for the extent of cycling.	Efficacy of adsorbants for digoxin intoxication requires further evaluation. Activated charcoal is promising.	141, 172, 173, 184
Physical exercise	↓ serum and ↑ skeletal muscle concentrations of digoxin.	A standardized rest period before blood sampling may be needed.	99–103, 243
Administration with a meal	Evidence indicates no influence on bioavailability of tablets.	Relative timing of drug administration and meals is not important.	50
Administration with a high fiber meal	↓ bioavailability of tablets.	Effect minimized by administration of digoxin in liquid-filled capsules.	51, 52
Surgical removal of part of GI tract	Unchanged bioavailability of tablets or capsules for certain surgical categories.	Evidence suggests that dosage adjustment is unnecessary for surgical categories studied.	54–57
Malabsorption (disease-related or chemotherapy/ radiation induced)	↓ bioavailability of tablets.	Elixir or liquid-filled capsules may ↑ absorption; monitor SDCs[a], and adjust dosage appropriately.	56, 58–60
Hypoalbuminemia	↓ plasma protein binding.	Changes in free drug concentration in plasma appear to be clinically insignificant.	107
Hypokalemia	Enhanced cardiac effects and toxicity.	Usual therapeutic range does not apply. Replace potassium.	222, 223
Hypomagnesemia	Enhanced toxicity, perhaps due to ↓ intracellular potassium.	Usual therapeutic range does not apply. Replace magnesium.	223–225

Table 20-2. Influence of Physiological and Pathological Factors on Digoxin Absorption, Disposition, and Response (cont.)

Factor	Description	Clinical implications	References
Coronary artery disease or old myocardial infarction	Enhanced toxicity, even when SDCs[a] in usual therapeutic range.	↓ dosage, monitor both SDCs[a] and toxic responses.	216, 217, 229
Atrial fibrillation	Possible ↓ sensitivity to digoxin, conflicting data in literature.	Usual therapeutic range may be too low in some patients.	210, 231
Chronic pulmonary heart disease (*cor pulmonale*)	Possible enhanced toxicity.	Monitor for toxic effects.	216, 232, 233
Hyperthyroidism	↓ sensitivity to digoxin.	Usual therapeutic range does not apply; toxicity may be difficult to avoid.	56, 62
Hypothyroidism	↑ sensitivity to digoxin.	↓ dosage and use a lower therapeutic serum level range; monitor for toxicities.	56, 62
Chronic renal failure	↓ renal excretion and potential distribution changes.	↓ loading and maintenance doses, using CL$_{cr}$ as a guide. Monitor SDCs[a] and for toxicities.	69, 104, 106, 108–110, 121, 131, 152, 161, 235–239

[a] SDC = Serum digoxin concentration.

Table 20-3. Drug Interactions with Digoxin

Factor	Interaction description	Clinical implications	References
Antacids, oral	Concurrent administration of large doses ↓ digoxin absorption about 25%–35%.	Space doses apart (e.g., administer digoxin 1 hr before or 2–3 hr after antacid dose).	62, 63
Antibiotics, oral	Concurrent therapy may enhance absorption by ↓ the population of colonic bacteria which metabolize digoxin to inactive DRPs.[a] Only tetracycline and erythromycin have been tested thus far, yielding enhanced SDCs[b] in "DRP formers" (thought to comprise about 10% of the population).	↑ SDCs[b] may lead to toxic symptoms; avoid if possible. If not, monitor SDCs[b] with a method that is not characterized by interference from DRPs.[a]	140
Cholestyramine or Colestipol	Binds digoxin in gut ↓ bioavailability by 20%–35%.	Space doses apart (e.g., administer digoxin 1 hr before or 2–3 hr after resin dose).	62, 63
Kaolin-pectin	Concurrent administration of large doses ↓ absorption by about 60%.	Space doses apart (e.g., anti-diarrheal 2 hr after digoxin).	62, 63
Metoclopramide	Coadministration with slow-dissolving digoxin tablets ↓ bioavailability by about 25% due to ↑ intestinal motility.	Effect minimized by administration of digoxin in capsules.	65
Neomycin	Coadministration results in ↓ digoxin absorption by unknown mechanism.	Space doses apart or avoid concurrent use.	62
Propantheline	Coadministration with slow-dissolving digoxin tablets ↑ GI absorption.	Effect minimized by administration of digoxin in capsules.	64
Sulfasalazine	Same as neomycin.	Same as neomycin.	67
Amiodarone	Up to 70% ↑ in apparent SDCs[b] occurring over 5–7 days of concurrent therapy; mechanism involves ↓ renal/nonrenal digoxin elimination.	Digoxin toxic symptoms may develop; monitor SDCs[b] and anticipate dosage reduction.	167, 246, 247

Table 20–3. Drug Interactions with Digoxin (cont.)

Factor	Interaction description	Clinical implications	References
Cyclosporine	Marked elevations in SDC[b] after initiation of cyclosporine in several cardiac transplant patients. ↓ apparent volume of distribution and plasma clearance. Patients also had renal compromise which contributed to rise in SDC.[b]	Monitor SDCs[b] and renal function carefully when cyclosporine therapy is initiated or stopped.	256
Propafenone	Approximately 30% ↓ in total and renal clearance of digoxin in cardiac patients.	Monitor SDCs[b] carefully when propafenone therapy is initiated.	257
Quinidine	Two- to threefold ↑ in SDC[b] in about 90% of patients receiving both agents. Mechanism: ↓ volume of distribution, renal and nonrenal elimination and possible ↑ rate and extent of absorption.	Elevated SDC[b] may produce toxic symptoms. Monitor SDCs[b] and anticipate dosage reduction.	252, 253
Spironolactone	↑ in SDC,[b] possibly by ↓ renal and nonrenal clearance and ↓ apparent volume of distribution.	Monitor SDCs[b] frequently and anticipate reduction of digoxin dose. Check assay for interference from spironolactone and/or its metabolites.	248–251
Verapamil	Coadministration results in up to 70% ↑ in SDC[b] in majority of patients secondary to ↓ renal and nonrenal elimination.	Elevated SDC[b] may produce toxicity; reduce dosage, with frequent monitoring of SDC.[b] Diltiazem may avoid this interaction.	20, 21, 167, 254, 255

[a] DRP = Digoxin reduction product.
[b] SDC = Serum digoxin concentration.

tial phase in humans.[69] In human post-mortem samples, kidney, heart, liver, choroid plexus, adrenals, diaphragm, and intestinal tract have the highest concentrations on a mg/gm basis.[70-72] The overall distribution of apparent digoxin to various organs and tissues appears to be largely related to the body distribution and activity of the enzyme Na^+,K^+-ATPase to which digoxin binds.[73,74] Thus, **skeletal muscle** appears to account for about 50% of apparent digoxin in the body. The binding capacity of the skeletal muscle pool was 52-fold higher than that of the heart ventricular muscle pool.[75] Thus, small variations in the occupancy of digitalis binding sites in skeletal muscle can influence the serum concentrations available for binding to the heart. The concentration of digitalis binding sites in skeletal muscle (Na^+,K^+-ATPase) was not dependent on age (one-day to 80-year-old humans) but was increased in hyperthyroidism and decreased in hypothyroidism.[75,76] Significant correlations have been observed between concentrations of apparent digoxin in **heart tissue** and in serum or blood in patients on maintenance digoxin therapy undergoing surgical procedures[77] (sampling carried out at least six hours after dosing) or autopsy.[71] Ratios of heart tissue digoxin concentration (ng/gm) to serum concentration (ng/mL) average about 70 in surgery patients on chronic digoxin therapy.[77,78] Digoxin does not distribute appreciably into body fat,[79] a characteristic that has dosage implications. Digoxin readily distributes across the **placental barrier** and has recently been administered to pregnant mothers to resolve several cases of fetal supraventricular tachycardia.[80,81]

Digoxin distributes from blood to other body fluids to varying extents. The concentration measured by RIA in **saliva** 20 to 24 hours after a single dose was correlated with serum digoxin concentration, with the average saliva:serum ratio being 1.1:1.[82] Although the authors suggest monitoring digoxin concentrations in saliva, sufficient predictability for application has not been demonstrated. Collection of stimulated saliva results in a digoxin concentration in saliva that most closely approximates the unbound digoxin concentration in serum.[83] In contrast to salivary concentrations, **cerebrospinal fluid** (CSF) concentrations of apparent digoxin averaged only 14% of the steady-state serum digoxin concentration.[84] Presence of digoxin in CSF may be related to the effects of this drug on the central nervous system. Likewise, presence of apparent digoxin in the eye (localized in the iris and inner retinal layers in the rat)[85] may be related to visual side effects.

The **binding** of digoxin to **plasma proteins** is independent of concentration over a very wide range and averages 20% to 30% in normal humans.[86-88] The important binding protein is albumin.[89] Digoxin in plasma water also partitions into erythrocytes by passive diffusion, with a mean transit time for equilibration of less than 0.5 minute at 37 °C.[88] The concentration ratio (cells:plasma) is approximately 0.9.[90]

The distribution of tritiated digoxin is influenced by several physiologic variables. Body **electrolytes** are intimately connected with digoxin distribution, particularly potassium. Acute **hyperkalemia** is associated with decreased distribution of ^{3}H-digoxin to several tissues in the dog, including the heart and skeletal muscle.[91] Conversely, acute **hypokalemia** is associated with increased ^{3}H-digoxin distribution to the heart and skeletal muscle in dogs.[92,93] **Age** also influences digoxin distribution. There is a higher degree of distribution to the heart and red blood cells in very young humans[94] and to these tissues as well as the kidney, liver and skeletal muscle in young animals.[95] **Obesity** does not alter digoxin distribution appreciably in humans, since digoxin distributes to body fat to a very small degree.[96] **Physical exercise** affects digoxin distribution, possibly by altering Na^+,K^+-ATPase to a high-affinity conformation in skeletal and heart muscle.[97–99] Joretag and Jogestrand have studied healthy men taking digoxin chronically and have shown that physical exercise increases biopsied skeletal muscle digoxin concentration with a concurrent decrease in serum digoxin concentration, as measured by radioimmunoassay (preceded by extraction for muscle).[99] The degree of change in concentration was related primarily to frequency of neuromuscular activation and to a lesser extent to work load, with a mean increase in skeletal muscle digoxin of 29% and a mean decrease in serum digoxin of 39% at the high pedalling rate (80 rpm) in a one-hour bicycle exercise test.[100] Even routine physical activity can result in substantial lowering of digoxin serum levels and this causes problems of interpretation in serum concentration monitoring of digoxin.[101,102] A standardized rest before blood sampling has been recommended.[101,103]

The apparent **volume of distribution** (V_d) for digoxin decreases in **chronic renal failure**, as originally pointed out by Reuning et al.[69] and confirmed by others.[104] The clinical significance of the decreased V_d depends on the mechanisms responsible for the observation and these are controversial.

Analytical limitations are important to consider. A substance in serum from patients with renal failure has digoxin-like immunoactivity[105] that contributes to the "blank level" (less than 0.2 ng/mL for the majority of patients); however, this amount is insufficient to explain the decreased V_d. Furthermore, some studies indicating a decreased V_d in renal failure were done using tritiated digoxin and liquid scintillation quantitation,[106] methods which are not influenced by endogenous digoxin-like immunoactivity. Another analytical limitation to consider is the lack of specificity for digoxin metabolites by both the radioactivity and RIA procedures (see Analytical Methods). This is important because serum concentrations of the metabolites may be higher in renal failure thus contributing to the higher measured serum digoxin concentrations measured by the radioactivity or RIA methods. These "higher" levels cause the V_d for digoxin to appear low.

Another possible mechanism for a decreased V_d is an alteration in the distribution of digoxin in renal failure. Plasma protein binding of digoxin does not change appreciably in renal failure except during hemodialysis. When heparin is administered the latter releases fatty acids which displace digoxin from protein binding sites.[107] Renal dysfunction may also cause decreased binding of digoxin to tissues. Decreased distribution of digoxin from serum (direct RIA) to left ventricular tissue (extraction-RIA) occurred in patients with renal failure, and the myocardium:serum concentration ratio was dependent on creatinine clearance.[108] However, Jogestrand and Ericsson,[109] using similar methodology, found that the ratio of biopsied skeletal muscle digoxin concentration to serum concentration was not significantly different in patients with renal failure than in subjects with normal renal function. A reduced tissue mass (e.g., skeletal muscle) because of chronic renal failure also does not seem to be an important factor.[69,110] Differences between patients with respect to electrolyte balance may play a role in whether differences in distribution are detected in renal failure.[109,110]

The ultimate clinical significance of the reduced digoxin V_d in renal failure depends on the quantitative relationship between concentration of digoxin (and possibly its metabolites) in serum and the intensity of therapeutic and toxic responses to digoxin. Aronson and Grahame-Smith presented evidence in three patients that the usual therapeutic serum concentration (0.5 to 2 ng/mL) was applicable in the presence of renal dysfunction, and that toxicities occurred above 2 ng/mL.[110] However, these authors pointed out that differences in these patients' electrolyte balance may have influenced the relationship between serum digoxin concentration and response. Further direct evidence is needed to define the relationship of serum digoxin concentrations to therapeutic and toxic responses when the V_d is diminished in renal failure. The effects of various physiological and pathological factors on the distribution of apparent digoxin are summarized in Table 20-2.

Digoxin disposition can be described by a **three-compartment pharmacokinetic model** that is consistent with a triexponential serum concentration-time curve.[111] An essentially constant ratio between concentration of apparent digoxin in serum and in tissues occurs about eight hours after an intravenous dose in humans and animals; thereafter, there is a parallel exponential decline of serum and tissue levels.[68,69,112]

Only a small fraction of digoxin in the body is present in blood. This finding, together with the rather **slow rate of distribution** between blood and tissues, is consistent with observations that little digoxin is removed from the body by hemodialysis (despite effective dialyzer clearance)[113] or by exchange transfusion[114,115] in humans. However, continuous arteriovenous hemofiltration over 20 hours was long enough to allow redistribution and this removed a substantial amount of body digoxin and resolved a case of digoxin intoxication in one patient.[116] After intravenous infusion, digoxin-specific Fab-antibody fragments also appear to persistently bind digoxin for a sufficient time to allow for redistribution, elimination, and resolution of digoxin intoxication in an adult,[117] child,[118] and functionally anephric patient.[119] This slow distribution is also undoubtedly responsible for the observation of somewhat higher tissue:serum ratios for apparent digoxin after chronic intravenous administration than in samples obtained at the same time (24 hours) after a single dose in dogs; there was also a two- to fourfold increase in the tissue:serum concentration ratio for the central nervous system after chronic digoxin administration.[120] A similar accumulation pattern for erythrocytes has been observed in human infants when chronic therapy is compared to a single loading dose.[94]

The V_d for digoxin averages 6 to 7 L/kg (total body weight) in patients with normal renal function and 4 to 5 L/kg in patients with renal failure (see Table 20-1). However, the V_d varies widely in individual patients, with a range of 4 to 9 L/kg in normal subjects and 1.5 to 8.5 L/kg in those with renal failure.[121] Patients with severe renal failure treated with hemodialysis have a V_d that is about midway between that for normal subjects and that for patients with severe renal failure who are off dialysis.[113]

Metabolism

The known pathways of digoxin metabolism in man are illustrated in Figure 20-2. One pathway consists of sequential hydrolysis of the digitoxose sugar moieties attached to the 3-position of the steroid nucleus to form digoxigenin bis-digitoxoside, digoxigenin mono-digitoxoside and digoxigenin. The latter two compounds may be further metabolized by conjugation.[122,123] However, further metabolism of digoxigenin is mainly by oxidation to 3-keto-digoxigenin, which can subsequently be reduced to 3-alpha-digoxigenin (3-epi-digoxigenin). Subsequent conjugation of 3-epi-digoxigenin and conversion to other polar metabolites ensues. The bis- and mono-digitoxosides are considered to be approximately as cardioactive as digoxin,[124,125] whereas digoxigenin and subsequent, more polar metabolites are considered to be much less active (see Pharmacodynamics).[125,126] The second pathway is the reduction of the double bond in the lactone ring of digoxin to form dihydrodigoxin, which is only slightly cardioactive.[127,128] Dihydrodigoxin may be further metabolized to hydrolyzed reduction products.[129,130]

The **hydrolysis pathway** of digoxin metabolism was once thought to be minor, with less than 15% of the total urinary excretion of glycoside due to the sum of digoxigenin, digoxigenin mono-digitoxoside and digoxigenin bis-digitoxoside and their enzyme-hydrolyzable conjugates.[123,131] However, the work of Gault et al.[125,132,133] extended our understanding of this pathway to include the subsequent, more polar metabolites shown in Figure 20-2. Unidentified polar metabolites account for about one-third of the radioactivity in plasma six hours after an oral dose of tritiated digoxin for patients with or without renal failure.[125] Because these metabolites are so polar, they are considered to be inactive, but they do interfere substantially with apparent digoxin concentration measured by the I-RIA assay.[125] The same holds for the glucuronide metabolites.[134]

The hydrolysis pathway of digoxin metabolism involves sequential hydrolysis of the digitoxose sugars and originates within the stomach.[132,133,135] This hydrolysis is minimized by an enteric coat on the tablet.[136] Another potential site of hydrolysis is the liver.[137,138] Anaerobic incubation with feces does not hydrolyze digoxin.[138] Under normal conditions of stomach acidity, the bis-and mono-digitoxosides combined with digoxigenin accounted for ≤10% of the total radioactivity in urine, whereas the unidentified polar metabolites were ≤14%. When pentagastrin was infused for 30 minutes before and 60 minutes after oral digoxin administration, the sum of the percentage of hydrolyzed metabolites in urine approximately doubled, and the unidentified polar metabolites increased to 32% to 54%.[133] These results suggest that hydrolysis of digoxin by stomach acid is an important determinant of further metabolism by this pathway. Therefore, disease conditions that promote gastric acidity may increase the formation of inactive polar metabolites.

The importance of the formation of **dihydro (reduced) metabolites** as a major metabolic pathway for digoxin, at least in certain subjects, has been documented in several studies.[129,139,140] There is convincing evidence that formation of these metabolites is accomplished by intestinal bacteria in humans.[139,140] About 10% of normal volunteers are substantial dihydro metabolite formers (greater than 40% of the urinary excretion of digoxin plus metabolites attributed to dihydro metabolites. In three "substantial reduced-metabolite formers" that took a constant daily dose of digoxin,the coadministration of an antibiotic (tetracycline or erythromycin), which presumably killed most of the intestinal bacteria, nearly doubled the steady-state serum digoxin concentration.[140] A threefold increase has been reported in another patient.[141] The RIA method, which is not influenced by reduced metabolites, was used to measure digoxin concentrations. The absence of reduced metabolites after antibiotic treatment suggests that other metabolizing organs are not involved in this particular reaction. If the absorption of orally administered digoxin is delayed (e.g., ingestion of a capsule containing slowly dissolving, enteric-coated granules) the extent of dihydro metabolite formation can increase in dihydro formers.[136] The single microorganism found capable of carrying out this reduction is *Eubacterium lentum*.[142] Serum concentrations of dihydrodigoxin are substantial in certain subjects that are "reduced-metabolite formers,"[136,143,144] but the appearance of dihydrodigoxin in serum is delayed for several hours after a single dose.[136] Recent evidence suggests that the capability to reduce digoxin develops over a protracted period after age eight months.[145] The environment during intestinal bacterial colonization in early life seems to influence the adult pattern of reduction, with urban residence during childhood correlating positively with dihydro-metabolite formation.[146,147] Dietary differences do not appear to influence digoxin reduction.[146]

Although the **GI tract** plays a key role in both major metabolic pathways for digoxin, the **liver** and other organs also contribute. The oxidation of digoxigenin to the 3-keto product, subsequent reduction to 3-epi-digoxigenin, and conjugation probably occur predominately in the liver.[137,148,149] In addition, conjugation of digoxigenin mono-digitoxoside appears to occur in the human liver.[138] Very polar metabolites or conjugates of the hydrolyzed metabolites are present in serum at substantial concentrations in some normal volunteers and patients.[136,144,150]

Although many studies of digoxin metabolism and pharmacokinetics in various disease states have been carried out using the nonspecific radioimmunoassay and radioisotopic analytical methods, their results do not clarify influence of disease on digoxin metabolism. Chromatography combined with RIA or radioisotope detection has led to most of our current understanding of digoxin metabolism. Thus far, **renal failure** is the only disease that has been studied using these specific analytical methods. In one study of patients with chronic renal failure,[125] the relative percentage of digoxin and its metabolites in 0- to 24-hour urine samples and 6-hour plasma samples did not change appreciably. In another investigation the percentage of unchanged digoxin in serum ranged from 33% to 100% in dialysis-dependent renal failure patients and 52% to 100% in subjects with normal renal function.[151] Overall, in patients with renal failure, urinary excretion of digoxin plus its metabolites decreases substantially and fecal excretion increases.[131,152] Marked elevations in serum digoxin concentrations were observed in a patient with combined renal and hepatic impairment after the drug had been discontinued. This was due to accumulation and immunoassay cross-reactivity of digoxigenin mono-digitoxoside conjugates.[153]

Because most analytical methods for digoxin lack specificity for its metabolites (see Analytical Methods), the literature concerning digoxin "metabolism" is ambiguous and the implications for therapeutic drug monitoring are unclear. The foregoing summary represents research with the more specific chromatographic methodology which yields less ambiguous results.

Excretion

Investigations of total body clearance as well as the renal clearance of digoxin have usually been carried out using nonspecific radioimmunoassay (RIA) procedures. Thus, there is the possibility that the clearances represent the sum of unchanged digoxin and assayable metabolites. With the foregoing in mind, we have summarized several determinations of the renal clearance and total body clearance of "apparent" digoxin (by RIA). The total body clearance for apparent digoxin in adults with normal renal and hepatic function averages about 180 mL/min/1.73 m^2, with a range of 100 to 300 mL/min/1.73 m^2.[154,155] **Renal clearance** accounts for most of this, (averaging 140 mL/min/1.73 m^2 in one study)[154] and exceeds creatinine and inulin clearances (thus indicating a tubular secretion component).[154,156] When a specific assay was used, renal digoxin clearance in three normal volunteers was 20% to 25% higher than that measured by RIA.[144] The clearance ratio of unbound digoxin to inulin was found to be 1.9 for radioimmunoassayable material.[156] The correlation between the renal clearance of "apparent" digoxin and the blood flow-limited renal clearance of para-amino-hippurate[157] suggests a dependence of digoxin renal clearance on blood flow.[157] This is also consistent with a tubular secretion component for digoxin, since para-aminohippurate is a marker for blood flow-limited tubular secretion. An acute increase in renal blood flow induced by vasodilators in CHF patients is associated with a 50% increase in renal digoxin clearance.[158] Some dependence of "apparent" digoxin renal excretion on diuresis suggests a tubular reabsorption component also, although the magnitude of this does not appear to be clinically significant.[156,159,160] In renally impaired patients, the clearance of "apparent" digoxin is linearly correlated with creatinine clearance; however, the renal clearance of "apparent" digoxin is consistently higher than that of creatinine.[161] This is illustrated schematically in Figure 20-3.

The renal clearance of "apparent" digoxin may change in infants and young children as a function of age. In one study[162] renal clearance increased with age up to five months. Another has reported decreasing clearance and a high digoxin:creatinine clearance ratio (1.5 to 2.0) up to the age of puberty, at which time the clearance ratio has decreased to the adult level of about 1.0.[163] This enhanced renal excretory function for "apparent" digoxin in the young appears to be due to an enhanced tubular secretory component and is one factor responsible for the higher dosage requirements in children.[162,163] It has also been observed[163] that the apparent digoxin:creatinine clearance ratio in adult volunteers (about 1.4) is greater than the clearance ratio for digitalized adult patients (about 1.0). The clinical significance of this finding is not clear. However, Pederson et al.[164] have demonstrated a difference between normal physical activity and complete immobilization with respect to the renal clearance of apparent digoxin. The clearance ratio, digoxin:creatinine, was 1.23 during physical activity and 1.03 during immobilization. This may at least partly explain the difference observed in clearance ratio between adult volunteers and adult patients. Physical activity also results in increased binding of digoxin to skeletal muscle (see Distribution). Chronic congestive heart failure appears to reduce renal digoxin clearance with a digoxin:creatinine clearance ratio of 0.73 compared to a ratio of 1.09 in controls without heart failure.[165]

Since the renal clearance of "apparent" digoxin has a significant secretory component, the efficiency of renal excretion may be influenced by interacting factors. Thus tubular secretion has been shown to be inhibited by hypokalemia,[166] spironolactone,[156] quinidine,[167] verapamil,[168] and amiodarone.[168]

Nonrenal excretion of digoxin and/or digoxin metabolites includes biliary excretion, possible intestinal secretion, and subsequent fecal elimination of digoxin

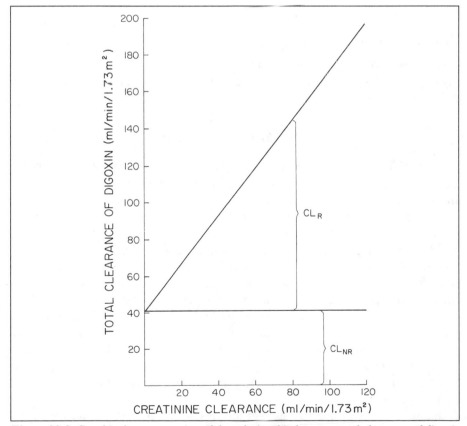

Figure 20-3. *Graphical representation of the relationship between total clearance of digoxin and creatinine clearance. The mathematical relationship is from reference 104 and includes the nonrenal and renal components of total digoxin clearance (CL_{NR} and CL_R, respectively). Patients with severe heart failure may have a smaller CL_{NR} component.*

and/or metabolites that are not absorbed. The five-day cumulative fecal excretion of radioactivity after an oral dose of tritiated digoxin ranged from 4% to 45% of the dose, with an average of 20%.[169] After an intravenous dose, the total fecal excretion of radioactivity averaged 11%.[170] Some of the radioactivity excreted in feces after oral administration may originate from unabsorbed digoxin or from unabsorbed gastrointestinal metabolites of digoxin. However, excretion of radioactivity in feces after intravenous administration indicates excretion into the intestine via the bile or by alternative pathways. Evidence for secretion of digoxin and/or metabolites by the intestinal mucosa has been obtained in rats,[171] but has not been studied in humans. However, **biliary excretion** after administration of digoxin has been studied in humans. Using an intestinal perfusion technique which minimally interrupted enterohepatic circulation, Caldwell et al.[172] studied biliary excretion of digoxin in five subjects. Over 24 hours, these investigators recovered an average of 30% of an intravenous dose of tritiated digoxin from a 15-cm segment of intestine into which the bile drains. There is substantial evidence for enterohepatic cycling of "apparent" digoxin[141] and one method of treating digoxin intoxication is to interrupt the cycling by oral administration of activated charcoal.[173]

Pharmacokinetics Summary

The pharmacokinetics of digoxin are considered to be linear within the therapeutic dosage range.[161,174–176] Pharmacokinetic parameters for radioimmunoassayed digoxin are summarized in Table 20-1.

PHARMACODYNAMICS

Digoxin has a direct positive inotropic and electrophysiologic action on the heart which has been well-documented in laboratory animals[185] and humans.[186,187] In one review, Smith[188] made the following conclusion: "the only unifying concept regarding cardiac glycoside action is that, at pharmacologically relevant doses, these drugs act by binding with high affinity and specificity to a site on the **Na+, K+- AT Pase** complex that faces the outer surface of virtually all eukaryotic cells. Alternative receptors, if they exist, have eluded recognition." This binding to an inhibitory site decreases outward transport of Na^+, leading to increased intracellular sodium concentration. It is currently thought that, in the myocardial cell, by means of a Na^+-Ca^{++} exchange mechanism, intracellular calcium increases and is stored in the sarcoplasmic reticulum for subsequent release to the contractile elements, thus leading to a positive inotropic effect.[188,189] Alternatives to this sequence of events have also been considered.[188] Those metabolites of digoxin that exhibit cardioactive properties may contribute to the overall pharmacologic and toxicologic response.

Potency ratios of the various **metabolites**, determined experimentally from several models of glycoside activity,[190] are presented in Table 20-4. Because animal and *in vitro* systems were used to measure the effects of metabolites, one should be cautious in extending these results to humans. Despite these limitations, the data presented in Table 20-4 consistently suggest that the bis- and mono-digitoxosides have cardioactivity at least comparable to that of digoxin, that digoxigenin is considerably less active, and that the 3-keto digoxigenin and the dihydro metabolites are nearly inactive.[62,127,191]

The **toxic effects** encountered with digoxin remain a significant complication of cardiac therapy. Adverse effects are most commonly associated with the heart (70% to 95% of toxic patients have cardiac toxicities), the GI tract (50% to 75% of toxic patients), and the CNS (infrequent and less worrisome).[192-194] The most serious adverse effects are premature ventricular contractions and varying degrees of atrioventricular block. However, cardiac toxicity may present as virtually any of the other types of cardiac dysrhythmias. Anorexia, nausea, vomiting, and diarrhea, often accompanied by abdominal discomfort and pain, are the common adverse effects of digoxin associated with the gastrointestinal tract. CNS toxicity includes headache, fatigue, malaise, neurologic pain, confusion, frank delirium, acute psychoses, and seizures. Visual symptoms and disturbed color vision are also frequent complaints in patients with digitalis toxicity[192] and the degree of color vision impairment is related to serum digoxin concentration.[195]

Inotropic Response

Evidence for a relationship between digoxin concentrations and pharmacologic response has been obtained from isolated *in vitro* preparations and laboratory animals.[196-198] In humans, inotropic response can be estimated noninvasively using systolic time intervals (STIs). Shortening of electromechanical systole, QS_2I, best reflects the positive inotropic effect of digoxin.[199] The use of STIs has been criticized because they can be affected by changes in preload or afterload which limits their reproducibility. However, QS_2I is minimally affected by changes in loading conditions and, when sources of variation are minimized, STIs are highly reproducible.[200] An inotropic response estimate for digoxin is plotted as a function of time in Figure 20-4, along with the time profile of "apparent" digoxin concentration in serum. The plots were obtained by computer simulations of mean pharmacokinetic and pharmacodynamic parameters obtained from a single dose of digoxin in 12 healthy volunteers.[177]

Table 20–4. *Comparative Potency Ratios of Digoxin and Metabolites*[a]

	(Digoxin = 1.0)		
Digoxin Metabolite	**Lethality[127]**	***In Vitro* Inotropy[191]**	**RBC Cation Flux[62]**
Digoxigenin bisdigitoxoside	0.75	—	1.60
Digoxigenin monodigitoxoside	0.68	—	2.31
Digoxigenin	0.21	0.1	0.17
3–epidigoxigenin	—	—	—
3–ketodigoxigenin	<0.02	0.02	—
Dihydrodigoxin	<0.024	—	0.02
Dihydrodigoxigenin	<0.005	—	—

[a] Ratio of metabolite potency to digoxin potency.

Over the **first six to eight hours** after a dose there is **no relationship between apparent digoxin serum concentration, and inotropic response intensity,** the former increases and then decreases rapidly, and the latter increases gradually (see Figure 20-4). However, the slow declines of both serum concentration and response are approximately parallel from 12 to 24 hours. Because the ratio of response to serum concentration remains reasonably constant during this period, it is the most appropriate time interval to sample blood for therapeutic drug monitoring. Samples obtained within eight hours of administration can be very misleading as an indicator of digoxin response (see Figure 20-4).

Whether the inotropic response is linearly or nonlinearly related to digoxin serum concentrations in the therapeutic range is unclear. Some investigations suggest that the inotropic response increases with "apparent" digoxin serum concentration in a stepwise fashion[201,202] while others suggest increases in the inotropic response are less-than-proportional to changes in serum digoxin concentration.[177,203] Using computer simulations, Kolibash and colleagues[203] have provided a picture of the nonlinear relationship between steady-state, post-distributive serum digoxin concentrations and response (QS_2I). (See Figure 20-5.) This suggests that increasing the dose of digoxin in patients with higher serum concentrations could result in toxic serum concentrations with only a small increase in the inotropic response. There are limitations to this study which warrant caution relative to clinical situations. First, computer simulations were based on data from single intravenous and oral doses. Second, the study was conducted in healthy volunteers whose response may differ from patients with cardiac failure. Finally,

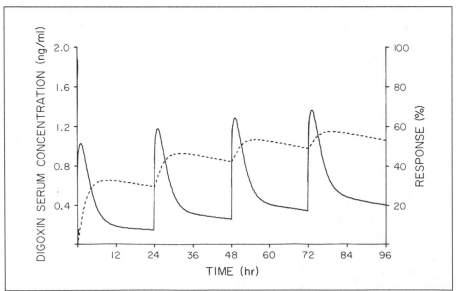

Figure 20-4. *Simulated time profile of digoxin serum levels (solid line) and response (dashed line) over a four-day time period. The response is the change in QS_2 index (ΔQS_2I), which is an estimate of inotropy, and is plotted as a percent of the maximum response. Pharmacokinetic and pharmacodynamic constants for the simulation were obtained from single dose studies of digoxin serum levels and ΔQS_2I in 12 normal subjects.[177] The dosage regimen for the simulation was 0.375 mg digoxin tablets per day with a bioavailability of 0.8.*

other therapeutic and toxic responses to digoxin are ignored. Additional studies are needed to examine the serum concentration-response relationship of digoxin in patients with CHF.

Clinical studies in which digoxin serum concentrations were measured in **toxic and nontoxic patients** have reported statistically significant differences between the two groups.[204] In a study of 116 patients,[205] "apparent" digoxin serum concentrations varied from nontoxic, subtherapeutic levels to toxic levels. These patients were divided into four groups based on clinical considerations: Group I, no toxicity, patients with CHF; Group II, no toxicity, subjects without CHF; Group III, possible toxicity; Group IV, definite toxicity. A rank-order correlation was found between the apparent serum digoxin concentration and the clinical cardiac status of the patient (see Figure 20-6). In addition, the mean digoxin concentration of each group was significantly different from those of the other three groups, and the "apparent" digoxin concentration was a better predictor of clinical response of the patient than were diagnostic classifications of cardiac and renal function.

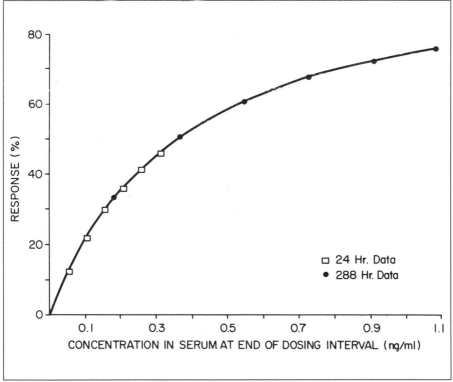

Figure 20-5. *Nonlinear relationship between response (percent of maximum) at 24 hours after a digoxin dose and the concentration of the digoxin in serum at the same time. Data were obtained from reference 203 and are based on mean pharmacokinetic/pharmacodynamic parameters in 12 healthy adult subjects. The relationship applies only to the post-absorptive, post-distributive phase of the serum level-time curve (about 12 to 24 hours after each dose) and does not depend on the number of doses administered. Simulated data at 24 hours and 12 days were selected for presentation (reprinted with permission from reference 203).*

Chronotropic Response

In producing a negative chronotropic response, digoxin acts by a direct effect, a vagally mediated indirect mechanism, and via sympathetic withdrawal to prolong the effective refractory period and slow conduction through the atrioventricular (AV) node.[202,206,207] This slows and blocks atrial impulse conduction to the ventricles, **thereby reducing the ventricular rate** in the presence of such arrhythmias as atrial fibrillation or flutter. The pharmacodynamics of this chronotropic effect have been studied to a limited degree; most investigators have examined the relationship between serum concentration and ventricular rate.[208–210] One group[208] also examined subjective symptoms and physical working capacity relative to apparent digoxin serum concentration. Although comparison between these studies is difficult, it appears that the chronotropic effect of digoxin is not consistently related to serum digoxin concentration in any graded fashion in individual patients.[208–212] A rank-order relationship between mean heart rate and mean serum digoxin concentration was observed only when patients with atrial fibrillation were

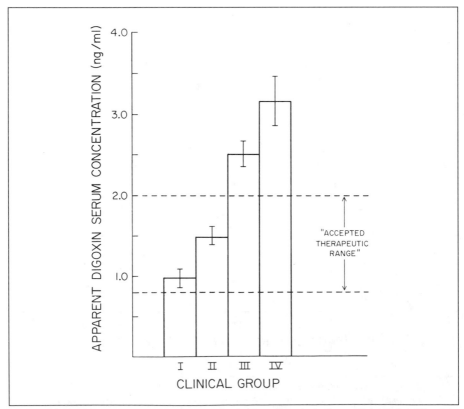

Figure 20-6. Mean serum concentration of apparent digoxin in four clinical classifications related to therapeutic responses in humans taking digoxin tablets chronically (plotted from data in reference 205). Group I, not toxic, in congestive heart failure; Group II, not toxic, not in congestive heart failure; Group III, possibly toxic; Group IV, definitely toxic. Vertical bars represent the standard deviation. The sampling time for blood withdrawal was six to eight hours subsequent to the previous dose.

grouped by serum digoxin concentration: nil (less than 0.5 ng/mL), low (mean 0.8 ng/mL), and high (mean 1.8 ng/mL).[213] One must conclude, therefore, that **ventricular rate is not a good measure for assessing the chronotropic effect of digoxin in an individual patient**. This is not surprising, considering that conduction via the AV node is affected by a number of interplaying factors including intrinsic AV blockade, endogenous catecholamines, and the underlying parasympathetic tone.[210,214] A variety of disease conditions can alter these factors and affect conduction through the AV node (e.g., hyperthyroidism, sepsis, post-thoracotomy, hypoxemia). Attempts to "push" digoxin until the desired decrease in rate is obtained may result in dangerous and potentially toxic serum concentrations.[212]

Adverse Effects

The concept of a **therapeutic range** for digoxin has been evolving over the past 20 years, subsequent to the development of radioimmunoassays capable of measuring low concentrations of the glycoside in serum. Most studies report a statistically significant, two to threefold difference in the mean "apparent" digoxin serum concentration between patients with and without electrocardiographic evidence of toxicity.[215] However, significant overlap exists between effective and toxic ranges of digoxin serum concentrations. The results of four of the most representative of these studies[216-219] are presented in Figure 20-7, together with the therapeutic range for serum digoxin concentration. For example, an early study reported that 90% of patients without toxicity had serum digoxin concentrations of 2 ng/mL or less, 87% of the toxic group had levels above 2 ng/mL; the range of overlap between the two groups extended from 1.6 to 3 ng/mL.[216] Others observing this overlap have questioned the usefulness of the serum digoxin concentration in differentiating between therapeutic and toxic levels.[220] In one study, 44% (54/123) of patients with serum digoxin concentrations greater than 3 ng/mL had no signs or symptoms of toxicity at the time blood was sampled for serum digoxin determination.[221]

The variability of digoxin serum concentrations associated with effective and toxic responses is due to the multiple factors which influence individual response. Of these, the one most frequently encountered clinically is alteration of serum electrolyte concentrations. Serum potassium, magnesium, and calcium are known to influence the response to digoxin.

Hypokalemia increases the cardiac effects of digitalis glycosides and enhances the potential for digoxin toxicity.[222] Depletion of intracellular potassium, which may be associated with digoxin-induced arrhythmias, is potentially even more important than low serum potassium. A group of 28 patients with depleted intracellular potassium (as reflected by metabolic alkalosis) exhibited digoxin-induced dysrhythmias at "therapeutic" concentrations.[223] Twenty-six of these twenty-eight patients were receiving potassium-depleting diuretics. This study points out the inadequacy of serum potassium concentration as an estimate of intracellular potassium and suggests that clinicians look for other potential sequelae of intracellular potassium depletion as markers of this condition. These include hypo-natremia, hypochloremia, and hypochloremic alkalosis, especially if the alkalosis is associated with aciduria.

Hypomagnesemia has also been implicated in the potentiation of digoxin toxicity.[224] However, this may be due to decreased intracellular potassium induced by low magnesium.[223] Evidence from patients with atrial fibrillation indicates that hypomagnesemia necessitates larger intravenous doses of digoxin to control heart rate, despite the increased risk of toxicity. The authors recommend replacement of magnesium to improve response and avoid toxicity.[225] Specific recommendations for magnesium replacement have been published.[226]

Hypercalcemia may enhance digoxin toxicity, but this is only associated with extremely high levels.[227] In another study, digoxin-induced abnormal automaticity in 19 patients was accompanied by higher than normal calcium:potassium ratios and higher pH values in the serum, even through apparent serum digoxin concentrations were in the therapeutic range.[228]

The toxic response to digoxin is also influenced by the nature and severity of the **underlying heart disease**. In one report, a group of ten patients was identified who exhibited definite digitalis toxicity accompanied by relatively low (less than

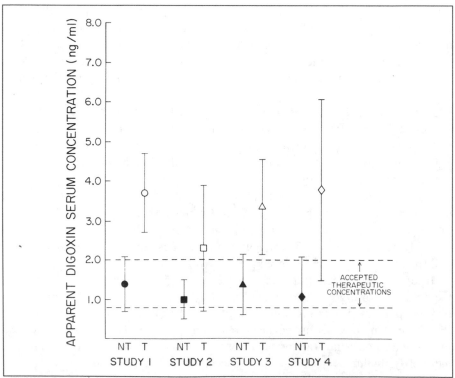

Figure 20-7. *Mean serum concentration of apparent digoxin in four representative studies in which toxic (T) and nontoxic (NT) patients taking digoxin tablets chronically were differentiated. Study 1, reference 216; study 2, reference 217; study 3, reference 218; study 4, reference 219. Vertical bars indicate standard deviation. The sampling time for blood withdrawal was at least five hours subsequent to the previous dose.*

1.7 ng/mL) serum digoxin concentrations. Nine of these patients had coronary atherosclerotic heart disease and that five had evidence of old myocardial infarction.[217] This increased sensitivity to digoxin due to underlying cardiac disease has been noted by others[216,229] and documented by studies in laboratory animals.[230]

Several investigators have reported decreased sensitivity and increased tolerance to high serum concentrations of digoxin in patients with atrial fibrillation. Goldman et al.[210] noted that high serum concentrations (2.5 to 5 ng/mL) failed to elicit gastrointestinal or cardiovascular signs or symptoms of digoxin toxicity in most instances. However, according to others such high concentrations are not needed to achieve a therapeutic response in patients with atrial fibrillation and are associated with toxicity.[231]

A higher incidence of digitalis toxicity has been reported in patients with **chronic pulmonary heart disease** (cor pulmonale), and this is probably related to the arterial hypoxia associated with this disease.[216] The use of digitalis in these patients has been controversial, but is increasingly recommended with careful dose selection and close monitoring for the development of adverse effects.[232] There is some evidence that the pulmonary heart disease patients most likely to respond to digoxin can be identified and selectively treated (i.e., those with left heart failure in combination with right heart failure resulting from pulmonary heart disease).[233]

Thyroid disease is known to alter the normal response to digoxin. Hyperthyroid patients appear to be more resistant to digoxin, while hypothyroid patients require a decreased dose relative to that required by euthyroid patients.[56] The mechanisms for these alterations are not completely understood, but evidence is available to implicate altered distribution to tissue, altered absorption, altered renal excretion, and an altered sensitivity of digitalis receptors in patients with thyroid disease.[56,62] Aronson[62] has pointed out that hyperthyroid patients with atrial fibrillation may not respond to the usual therapeutic serum concentrations of digoxin and that increasing the dose above the usual therapeutic range may result in frank digitalis toxicity. Thus, the interpretation of serum digoxin concentrations in patients with thyroid disease is fraught with uncertainty.

CLINICAL APPLICATION OF PHARMACOKINETIC DATA

Population-Based Approach

In the late 1960s and 1970s a number of methods were published for dosing digoxin using population-based estimates of pharmacokinetic parameters.[104,234-237] The equations associated with this approach were summarized in the previous edition of this text.

Hyneck et al.[238] compared five population-based methods for determining digoxin dosing regimens and found severe limitations of the formulas for predicting concentrations in serum. Furthermore, Koup et al.[104] evaluated several methods which were dependent on population-based estimates of a patient's pharmacokinetic parameters, as well as a method that used digoxin renal clearance measured in patients. Koup noted that predictions within ± 30% of the measured serum digoxin concentrations were achieved with 6 of 16 patients using the Jelliffe method,[234] 9 of 16 using the estimated digoxin body clearance, and 12 of 16 using the measured digoxin renal clearance. The limitations of the first two approaches are obvious. Though the latter approach can be technically difficult, the use of patient-specific information in the selection of digoxin dosage appears advantageous. Even this approach, however, resulted in digoxin serum concentrations falling outside of a rather wide predictive range in 25% of patients.

Individualized Approach

Because of the limitations of population-based methods, a more individualized pharmacokinetic approach seems warranted when monitoring patients on digoxin. Such an approach **relies heavily on actual measurements of serum digoxin concentration**, with the interpretation of these values based on a thorough understanding of the factors affecting digoxin pharmacokinetics and pharmacodynamics. The individualized method employs selection of the initial dose empirically followed by adjustments based on the interpretation of serum digoxin concentration measurements. The remainder of this section will review the components of this individualized approach.

Loading Dose. The need for a loading dose of digoxin requires careful consideration. Jelliffe[239] has argued that patients being initiated on digoxin should receive a loading dose of digoxin to evaluate its effect and toxicity under controlled circumstances. However, there is little therapeutic rationale for a loading dose in most situations. Heart failure usually does not require immediate resolution of symptoms. In acute pulmonary edema due to CHF, administration of digoxin is no longer deemed essential for reversing the emergent situation. Loading doses of digoxin were commonly used in the past to slow down ventricular response in patients with symptomatic supraventricular tachyarrhythmias. Intravenous verapamil, however, has superseded digoxin as the drug of first choice in many of these patients. However, intravenous loading doses of digoxin are justified for the treatment of symptomatic supraventricular tachyarrhythmias accompanied by CHF because of the negative inotropic effect of verapamil.

For cases in which a loading dose of digoxin is desired, the literature is replete with recommended regimens. In adult patients with creatinine clearances greater than 20 mL/min, one recommended loading dose procedure is to administer two 0.5 mg oral tablet doses (or two 0.375 mg intravenous doses) of digoxin separated by six hours. In patients with renal insufficiency, the volume of distribution of digoxin is reduced.[69,104] For this reason, the administration of two 0.25 mg oral tablet doses (or two 0.1875 mg intravenous doses) separated by six hours is recommended for patients with creatinine clearances less than 20 mL/min. Patients with a low body weight (less than 40 kg) should also receive the latter loading dose.

Loading doses of digoxin for CHF in **premature infants** (20 µg/kg), full-term **neonates** (less than two months of age: 30 µg/kg), **infants** (less than two years of age: 40 to 50 µg/kg), and **children** (greater than two years of age: 30 to 40 µg/kg) tend to be higher, on a µg/kg basis, than those recommended in adults. This is due to the higher, weight-normalized volume of distribution observed in these patient populations.[240,241]

Maintenance Therapy. If loading doses of digoxin are well tolerated, or if a loading dose is deemed unnecessary, maintenance therapy can be initiated empirically at a dose of 0.25 mg/day in adult patients with creatinine clearances greater than 20 mL/min. In patients with creatinine clearances less than 20 mL/min or body weight less than 40 kg, maintenance doses of 0.125 mg/day of digoxin are recommended. In each of these situations, measurement of the serum digoxin concentration is advocated after three days of therapy. Although not a steady-state measurement, evaluation of this digoxin serum concentration can prove valuable for proper dose adjustment. The individualized dosing algorithm presented in Figure 20-8 outlines suggested dosage adjustment schemes based on the results of the serum digoxin concentration measurement taken at this time. Actual dosing decisions must be based on a careful evaluation of the patient's overall clinical condition.

Higher maintenance doses, when expressed on a µg/kg basis, may be required for **neonates, infants**, and **children** due to their potentially higher renal and nonrenal clearances of digoxin. Suggested daily maintenance doses for premature infants, full term neonates (less than two months of age), infants (less than two years of age), and children (greater than two years of age) are 5, 8 to 10, 10 to 12, and 8 to 10 µg/kg, respectively.[240] **Lower maintenance doses**, compared to the usual doses, may be appropriate for the **elderly**.[242]

Indications for Serum Concentration Monitoring. Digoxin serum concentrations should be monitored in the following circumstances: 1) to assess patient compliance; 2) to investigate clinical deterioration following an initial good response; 3) in patients with marked alterations in renal function; 4) when digoxin toxicity is suspected; 5) to evaluate the need for continued digoxin therapy; 6) when conditions known to alter the therapeutic response to digoxin (e.g., thyroid disease), develop; and 7) when there is a suspected drug interaction.

When to Obtain Blood Samples. The selection of the optimal time to collect blood for determination of a patient's serum digoxin concentration requires an understanding of the relationship between pharmacodynamic response and the serum concentration-time profile (see Pharmacodynamics). The relationship between response intensity and serum concentration most closely approximates a constant ratio 12 to 24 hours following dose administration. In addition, assessments of the "therapeutic range" for digoxin were carried out using blood samples drawn at least six hours after dosing. To avoid the segment of the serum concentration-time curve that shows no relationship to either response or the defined therapeutic range (see below), **blood samples** should optimally be drawn **at least 12 and preferably 24 hours following the administration of a dose.**[231] The potential influence of exercise on digoxin serum concentration (see Distribution and Excretion) suggests that a **period of rest** may be needed before blood sampling to avoid an exercise-induced decrease in serum digoxin concentration. In one study of 56 outpatients taking chronic digoxin, a two-hour rest increased the mean serum digoxin concentration by about 25%; also, the fraction of patients in the therapeutic range increased from 32% to 58%.

Maximal response from any maintenance dose regimen of digoxin will occur when steady state has been achieved. Any adjustment of digoxin dose or alteration in digoxin pharmacokinetics necessitates a waiting period of four to five times the half-life before a new steady state is achieved.

Response Monitoring. The electrocardiogram (ECG) is of limited value in monitoring digoxin response. There are numerous possible ECG changes which can occur during normal therapy; however, there is no defined parallel between the degree of these changes and the effect of digoxin.[244] Before serum concentrations were monitored, it was common practice to permit the development of toxicity to signify an adequate therapeutic dose. The risk of this method lies in the development of potentially life-threatening cardiac arrhythmias which frequently are the first and only signs of toxic concentrations. Inotropic response is assessed by improvement in the symptoms (dyspnea, fatigue, weakness, peripheral edema) and signs (improvement in chest x-ray, decreased blood urea nitrogen concentration, weight gain) of CHF. The use of systolic time intervals has been advocated as a noninvasive assessment of inotropic response. They have not, however, proven useful for monitoring digoxin response in the clinical setting.[245]

The chronotropic response to digoxin has been assessed traditionally by the change in ventricular response rate to atrial fibrillation. A variety of clinical conditions disrupt the relationship between ventricular response and digoxin concentration, resulting in a weak correlation.[212] If adequate ventricular slowing is not obtained at digoxin serum concentrations of 1 to 2 ng/mL in a patient who is not exhibiting signs or symptoms of toxicity, then increasing concentrations to 2 to 3 ng/mL may be cautiously attempted. The practice of increasing the dose until a desired ventricular rate is achieved should be discouraged, since some patients may respond minimally while others may exhibit toxicity before achieving the desired response. Addition of a second agent (a beta blocker or verapamil) should be considered when therapeutic serum concentrations of digoxin fail to elicit a response or when dose-related adverse effects occur.

Dose Adjustment Based on Serum Concentrations. Assuming that digoxin bioavailability (F) and clearance (CL) remain stable in a patient, then a linear relationship exists between digoxin dose (D) and the average serum digoxin concentration at steady state (C_{ss}). This is illustrated in Equation 20-1, where τ is the dosing interval.

$$C_{ss} = \frac{FD}{CL \cdot \tau}$$

(Eq. 20-1)

The C_{ss} which is achieved at a particular steady-state dosage regimen can be used with Equation 20-1 to predict the C_{ss} that will be achieved at another digoxin dose rate, assuming F and CL remain constant.

Drug Interactions. Numerous studies have been undertaken to identify, quantitate, and evaluate the mechanisms of drug interactions involving digoxin. Clinicians need to be aware of clinically significant drug interactions in order to appropriately dose and monitor patients. Because digoxin continues to be widely prescribed and has a narrow therapeutic index, the Food and Drug Administration (FDA) recommends the evaluation of potential interactions between new agents and digoxin before they are marketed.

A complete review of the interaction studies with digoxin is beyond the scope of this chapter and the reader is referred to the many excellent drug interaction texts available. Table 20-3 summarizes a number of potentially important interactions with digoxin.[246–257] The criteria for inclusion in this table was a consensus in the literature for a greater than 20% change in mean clearance, AUC, or response; such interactive potential may have clinical relevance in a given patient.

It is important to assess the potential for significant drug interactions with digoxin and take corrective steps which will minimize adverse patient outcomes. Although some authors advocate dose adjustments for certain interactions (e.g., reduce the digoxin dosage by 50% when quinidine or amiodarone therapy is initiated), such recommendations do not take into account interpatient variability in the magnitude and significance of the interaction. In fact, some authors argue that the rise in digoxin serum concentration after the addition of quinidine may be associated with a displacement of digoxin from cardiac binding sites, making a reduction in digoxin dosage ill-advised.[258] An individualized approach attempts to weigh the potential for an interaction in relation to the patient's clinical status. Careful monitoring of serum concentrations and patient response in light of the potential interaction is the most appropriate course of action.

Therapeutic Range. Figure 20-7 illustrates an important point. The literature is replete with references on the therapeutic range for digoxin. In some investigations there was no overlap between the range for nontoxic and toxic patients, while in others, the ranges were virtually the same. Thus, one is struck with the limitations of interpreting the therapeutic or toxic potential of a serum digoxin concentration in a particular patient. Factors affecting digoxin sensitivity have not been considered in many of these studies. Thus, serum digoxin concentration ranges are useful only as guides and the patient's values must be interpreted in the context of other patient variables.

Nonetheless, inspection of Figure 20-7 suggests that the arbitrary steady-state serum digoxin concentration range of 0.8 to 2 ng/mL is a useful initial goal in all patients, if efficacy and toxicity are evaluated carefully. This is based on the fact that serum concentrations greater than 2 ng/mL have been frequently associated with toxicity in almost all studies. The same therapeutic range has been recommended for infants and children with CHF.[240] Higher digoxin concentrations may be required in and tolerated by certain patients, such as those with atrial fibrillation. Thus, each time digoxin is prescribed for a patient, a **therapeutic experiment is begun** in which an individual's response to, and tolerance for digoxin should be prospectively evaluated; digoxin serum concentrations serve as only one of the measures of evaluation. Eraker and Sasse[259] analyzed the value of serum digoxin concentrations in decision making relative to toxicity using a Bayesian approach and suggested that the test had an important impact on therapeutic decisions.

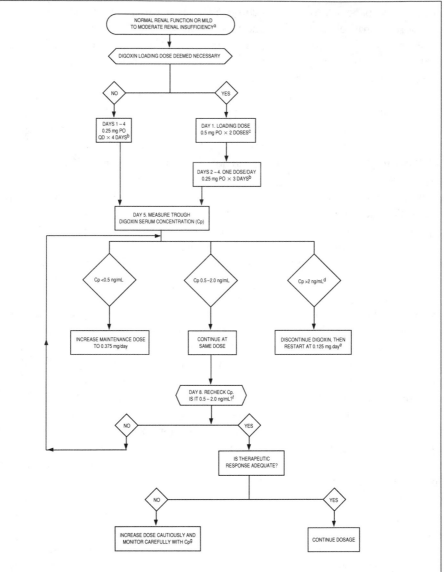

[a] Adult with Cl$_{cr}$>20 mL/min.

[b] Initial maintenance dose or schedule may need to be modified in some patients(e.g., emaciated, obese, pregnant, hypo- or hyperthyroid).

[c] The two doses should be separated by at least 6 hours. a more aggressive loading dose schedule can be initiated if necessary.

[d] If signs or symptoms of toxicity are present (even if Cp <2.0 ng/mL), discontinue digoxin and monitor Cp (about 6 hours after last dose). Consider factors that can decrease digoxin clearance (e.g., decrease in renal function or drugs such as quindine) or decrease digoxin sensitivity (e.g., hypokalemia, hypomagnesemia).

[e] When signs or symptoms of toxicity clear and/or Cp approachs 1ng/mL.

[f] In patients with normal renal function (creatinine clearance >60 mL/min.). This level may be used to approximate the ultimate steady-state level. Adjustments in therapy to achieve a different dsc may be made by adjusting the dose proportionately to the change in Cp desired in patients with CL$_{cr}$ between 20 to 50 mL/min. further assessment of Cp is recommended to evaluate the ultimate steady-state level achieved.

[g] Consider that patient may be a digoxin non-responder.

Figure 20-8a. *Individualized approach to initiating and adjusting digoxin therapy in adults with normal renal function or mild-to-moderate renal insufficiency (CL$_{CR}$ >20 mL/min).*

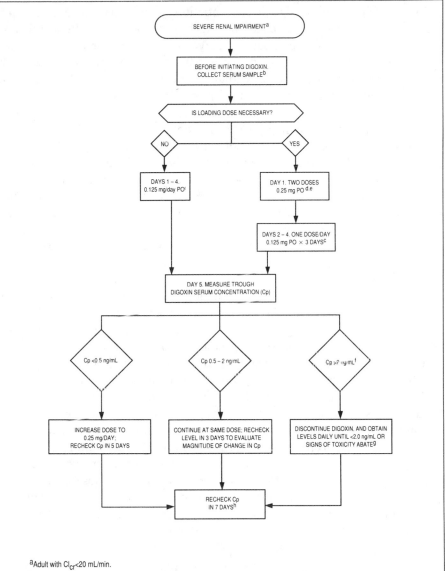

aAdult with Cl_{cr}<20 mL/min.

bThe presence of digoxin immunoreactive substances may need to be determined later.

cInitial maintenance dose or schedule may need to be modified in some patients (e.g. emaciated, obese, pregnant, hypo- or hyperthyroid).

dThe two doses should be separated by at least 6 hours. a more aggressive loading dose schedule can be initiated if necessary.

eThe need to modify loading dose in renal failure is controversial.

fIf signs or symptoms of toxicity are present (even if Cp <2.0 ng/mL), discontinue digoxin and monitor Cp (about 6 hours after last dose). consider factors that can decrease digoxin sensitivity (e.g., hypokalemia, hypomagnesemia) ordecrease digoxin clearance (e.g., decrease in renal function or drugs such as quinidine).

gRestart at maintenance dose at O.625 mg/day.

hIn severe renal failue, steady state may not be achieved for weeks. Therefore, Cp monitoring may be indicated. Consider that a patient may be a digoxin non-responder.

Figure 20-8b. *Individualized approach to initiating and adjusting digoxin therapy in adults with severe renal impairment (CL_{CR} <20 mL/min).*

Interpretation of serum digoxin concentration measurements in relationship to the established "therapeutic range" for digoxin can be complicated further by assay-related variables. In particular, the digoxin-like immunoreactive substance or digoxin metabolites that accumulate in patients with renal insufficiency can increase "apparent" digoxin concentrations measured by the RIA technique. Likewise, when Fab fragments of digoxin-specific antibodies are used to treat digoxin intoxication, the Fab fragment can interfere with the measurement of digoxin serum concentrations by some (but not all) immunoassays.[260-262] For a complete discussion of these confounding factors, see Analytical Methods.

Algorithm. An individualized approach to the use of digoxin is presented in Figure 20-8. This algorithm is intended for use in adult patients treated with oral digoxin tablets which possess consistent intra- and inter-lot bioavailability (e.g., Lanoxin). Use of intravenous or other oral dosage forms requires appropriate adjustment of the proposed doses.

The approach employs **digoxin serum concentration monitoring early in the treatment course** to identify how each patient is handling the drug and to prevent the achievement of concentrations greater than 2 ng/mL. Once steady state has been achieved, the method utilizes Equation 20-1 to make dose adjustments as necessary. If serum concentrations increase on the same dosage, or if the predicted increase in serum concentration resulting from a dosage change is exceeded, factors which may alter digoxin disposition should be evaluated. Evidence of toxicity at concentrations less than 2 ng/mL requires careful assessment of other variables that may be affecting the patient's sensitivity to digoxin.

The use of a minimum of two serum digoxin measurements is an important feature of this method. In a recent study, a population-based method for digoxin dosing based on serum urea and body weight was supplemented with a serum digoxin concentration on day three.[263] The fraction of patients within the therapeutic range at ten days improved from 68% of 41 control patients without the day three dosage adjustment to 80% of 30 patients with the single dosage adjustment. However, five of the latter group were in the potentially toxic range as compared to one in the control group. Thus, the second serum digoxin measurement in Figure 20-8 is designed to further individualize the dosage regimen.

ANALYTICAL METHODS

Radioimmunoassay

The basic principles of the radioimmunoassay (RIA) for digoxin are as follows. Digoxin in the serum sample competes with a radiolabeled (^{125}I) digoxin derivative for binding sites on the antibody to digoxin. The unbound digoxin (both labeled and unlabeled) is then separated from the bound form. One of these is quantitated by radioactivity counting, and the concentration of unlabeled digoxin in the serum sample is calculated by comparison to digoxin standards. RIA has become the most popular method of digoxin analysis for both clinical therapeutic drug monitoring and scientific purposes because it is sensitive, precise, and easy to perform. The sensitivity of most current RIA kits is 0.2 to 0.4 ng/mL of serum (below the therapeutic range), and one author has reported a modified procedure sensitive to 0.05 ng/mL.[264] For several different RIA kits, the coefficient of variation for repetitive determinations is in the range of 5% to 15% at therapeutic concentrations.[264-266]

The main problem with digoxin immunoassays is **low specificity**. Interference by endogenous digoxin-like immunoreactive substances (DLIS) occurs in patients with renal failure, hepatic failure, combined renal and hepatic failure, in pregnant women during the third trimester, and in neonates.[267] This interference is clinically significant and varies among different RIA methods and antibody lots.[150,267] Various methods have been used to decrease this interference with the most effective being a solid phase extraction pretreatment.[267-269]

Despite the high precision of the digoxin RIA, potential problems in the interpatient reproducibility of RIA results have been reported. Hypoalbuminemic serum samples yield falsely low serum digoxin concentrations.[270] In addition, tracer binding to the antibody is increased when the usual ^{125}I-digoxin derivative (3-O-succinyl-digoxigenin-^{125}I-tyrosine) is used with sera having a low thyroxine concentration.[271] This results in a falsely lowered apparent digoxin concentration. Quantitation of the gamma-emitting ^{125}I-digoxin derivative in serum is influenced by the presence of gamma-emitting radioisotopes from various diagnostic tests.[272]

Drug-related substances also have the potential to interfere with the RIA for digoxin, but this appears to be manageable. Interference by concurrent therapy with spironolactone depends on the individual patient and on the source of the RIA procedure.[251] When Fab fragments of digoxin-specific antibodies are used to treat digoxin intoxication, the unbound digoxin can be determined by pretreating serum with ultrafiltration before immunoassay[260] or by the use of certain RIA procedures shown to estimate free digoxin in the presence of Fab fragments.[261,262] Other cardiac glycosides may also react with the antibody used in the digoxin RIA, usually to a relatively small extent. However, cross-reactivity with digitoxin can be clinically significant.[266,273]

Lack of specificity of the digoxin RIA with respect to both active and inactive metabolites has been reported for certain RIA kits. The pharmacologically active, sugar-hydrolyzed metabolites, digoxigenin bis-digitoxoside and digoxigenin mono-digitoxoside, were comparable to digoxin in RIA cross-reactivity. The less potent digoxigenin was also highly cross-reactive in the RIA.[273] Most authors have viewed this similarity in pharmacologic potency and RIA cross-reactivity as a fortunate coincidence that permits clinical use of the RIA to measure a serum concentration that is a reflection of total digitalis-like activity. However, this ignores the digoxigenin mismatch and one should be aware that the degree of cross-reactivity of these metabolites varied widely in a comparative study of six commercial RIA procedures.[274] In another survey of six different commercial ^{125}I-RIA kits, the greatest cross-reactivity for dihydrodigoxin was about 11%, a value judged to be clinically insignificant.[275] This low cross-reactivity has been confirmed by others.[273] However, the polar metabolites have high cross-reactivity and can be an important contributor to the assayed serum digoxin concentration.[150]

An experimental antibody has also been prepared that minimizes interference from hydrolyzed metabolites, but interference by dihydrodigoxin may still be substantial.[276]

The preceding summary of literature pertaining to the digoxin RIA yields a confusing and sometimes contradictory picture of the important factors that influence RIA results. The major reason for this is that the procedures, and especially the antibodies, are not the same for kits from different manufacturers. Despite these limitations, RIA has proven to be very helpful in the management of patients requiring digoxin. For the ^{125}I-RIA kits, one must be alert for spironolactone administration, diagnostic radioisotopes, hypoalbuminemia, and hypothyroidism, any of which may influence assay results. Information regarding the degree to which these potential problems are important for a particular antibody should be demanded from the manufacturer. In addition, information from individual manufacturers regarding cross-reactivity with endogenous substances in serum and with known digoxin metabolites (and preferably lot-to-lot variability in cross-reactivity) must be available for intelligent interpretation of RIA results, particularly in patients with renal failure and in infants.

Enzyme Immunoassay

Enzyme immunoassays are a more recent development than RIAs and are closely related. In this technique, digoxin-enzyme (digoxin chemically bonded to an enzyme) competes with serum digoxin for digoxin-antibody binding sites. Depending on the particular procedure, either free or antibody-bound digoxin-enzyme is then reacted with excess substrate for the enzyme along with cofactors. The enzyme reaction produces a chromophore which is measured spectrophotometrically or fluorometrically. The precision and sensitivity of the enzyme immunoassay are similar to those of the RIAs[277] (see Table 20-5). Several variants of this basic scheme have been developed by certain manufacturers.

Because enzyme immunoassays depend on competition for an antibody binding site, they suffer from most of the same disadvantages as the RIAs. Interference from DLIS occurs unless there is solid phase extraction pretreatment[267,278] and interference from spironolactone administration is suspected.[267,277] Essentially complete cross-reactivity with the active, hydrolyzed metabolites of digoxin has been demonstrated, whereas the inactive dihydrodigoxin did not cross-react.[273,279]

Enzyme immunoassays do not suffer from disadvantages related to radioactivity measurement. One distinct advantage of many of these procedures is the quantitation of a UV chromophore which is technically easier and requires less investment in equipment.

Fluorescence Polarization Immunoassay

Another addition to the array of immunoassays for digoxin is the fluorescence polarization immunoassay (TD$_x$, see Table 20-5). The method is based on the ability of a fluorescein-labeled digoxin tracer to compete with unlabeled serum digoxin for antibody binding sites. Upon excitation by single-wavelength, polarized light, the unbound label and antibody-bound fluorescent label exhibit widely different degrees of polarization of emission fluorescence, upon which quantitation is based. This method has excellent reproducibility with a coefficient of variation of less than 6% for inter-day replicates.[280] Data provided by the manufacturer indicate a high degree of cross-reactivity for all of the hydrolyzed metabolites, including the less-active digoxigenin. Little cross-reactivity was found for dihydrodigoxin and digitoxin. The DLIS found in neonates and infants and in patients with hepatic and renal failure interferes with the fluorescence polarization immunoassay.[281–283] Ultrafiltration appears to be effective in removing this interference.[284] Total serum protein can also influence the fluorescence polarization immunoassay of digoxin.[285]

Chromatographic Methods

Chromatographic analytical methods offer potentially greater specificity with respect to interferences from metabolites and endogenous plasma constituents than do immunologic methods. However, the usual means of detection in chromatography (e.g., UV absorbance, fluorescence) do not permit analysis of serum concentrations because of the general lack of detectable functional groups on the digoxin molecule. Thus, the only chromatographic methods that have been applied to analysis of serum samples have utilized tritiated digoxin administration coupled with liquid scintillation counting of separated fractions[144] or have coupled chromatographic separation with RIA.[150,286,287] Such methods are labor intensive and are not feasible for routine clinical use, but offer the advantage of assaying metabolites as well as unchanged digoxin; they can also be used to analyze these substances in urine and tissues.[286]

Another approach that potentially offers both specificity and adequate sensitivity is the combined use of chemical derivatization of digoxin and its metabolites with chromatographic separation. The preparation of UV-absorbing or fluorescent derivatives for subsequent chromatographic separation (pre-column derivatization) is a method that has been used to analyze digoxin, its three hydrolyzed metabolites, and dihydrodigoxin in urine.[288,289] Fluorescent derivatives[289] or the use of microbore HPLC technology with UV-absorbing derivatives[290] offer the potential for sub-nanogram sensitivity, which is necessary for analysis of serum concentrations of digoxin and its metabolites. The preparation of chemical derivatives following chromatographic separation (post-column derivatization) has attracted recent attention and has potential for the analysis of digoxin and its hydrolyzed and reduced metabolites at therapeutic serum concentrations; it also has the potential for automation.[291,292] Although chromatographic analysis is not currently feasible for routine therapeutic drug monitoring due to its limited sensitivity, difficulty of performance, and long turn-around time (see Table 20-5), it is an important evolving technique for investigations of digoxin metabolism and pharmacokinetics. A summary of all of the analytical methods is provided in Table 20-5.

Table 20-5. Comparison of the Relative Advantages and Disadvantages of the Various Digoxin Assay Methods

Analytical method[a]	Specificity for digoxin[b]	Limit of sensitivity (ng/mL)	Metabolite analysis	Assayable samples				Minimum sample volume required (mL)	Speed		Analysis cost[c]		Specialized operatory training[d]	Preference rank[e]			Comments
				Plasma/serum	Urine	Saliva	CSF		1–10 Samples	10–100 Samples	Estimated reagent and tech. cost per assay	Initial equipment cost		Small service	Large service	Research	
RIA	4	0.2–0.4	No	Yes	Yes	Yes	Yes	0.1	0.25–0.5 hr	0.5–3 hr	2	5	2	3	2	4	Metabolite & endogenous interference
Enzyme immunoassay	4	0.3–0.5	No	Yes	Yes	?	?	01.–0.2	0.1–0.3 hr	0.3–3 hr	3	3	3	3	3	4	Metabolite & endogenous interference
Fluorescence polarization immunoassay	4	0.2	No	Yes	?	?	?	0.2	0.1–0.2 hr	0.2–2 hr	3	3	3	2	3	4	Metabolite & endogenous interference
Derivatization HPLC	1	≥10	Yes	No	Yes	?	?	1–10	0.5–1 day	1–3 days	5	4	5	5	5	1	Sensitivity inadequate for serum
HPLC-RIA	1	≈0.1	Some	Yes	Yes	?	?	1	0.5–1 day	1–3 days	5	5	5	5	5	1	Some metabolites not immunologically active

[a] HPLC = High performance liquid chromatography; RIA = radioimmunoassay.
[b] Arbitrary ranking scale of 1 (excellent) to 5 (poor).
[c] 1 = Least expense.
[d] 1 = Least training.
[e] 1 = Preferred method.

PROSPECTUS

One striking theme in the digoxin pharmacokinetics and pharmacodynamics literature is the **unavailability of specific procedures** to measure concentrations of unchanged digoxin and its active metabolites in serum or to evaluate the inotropic and chronotropic effect in humans. One must question the value of the extensive research that has been carried out using the currently available, but limited techniques. Future investment in more basic research that addresses methodology development would indeed be well placed. Analytical procedures that differentiate between active and inactive metabolites and that are not influenced by endogenous substances must be developed. Although the potential approaches for solving the analytical problems are limited, they have not been systematically and thoroughly explored. Likewise, methodology must be developed to quantitate the therapeutic responses to digoxin, independent of interference by common physiologic perturbations. It seems likely that such development will depend upon an improved understanding of the basic pharmacologic mechanisms that mediate the response to digoxin.

The **gastrointestinal tract** has a unique role in mediating the primary pathways of digoxin metabolism. This offers novel research challenges that must be met to further improve our understanding of the disposition of this drug in diseased patients. Obviously, the influence of GI diseases that affect stomach acid output, intestinal bacterial populations, GI transit, and intestinal permeability should be investigated with respect to their influence on digoxin metabolism and the patient's response to this drug. The importance of potential interactions with various anti-infectives that alter intestinal bacterial populations should be better defined.

Finally, **endogenous digitalis-like immunoreactive substance(s)** (DLIS) are being intensively investigated and have been associated with pathologies connected with increased intravascular volume in the central circulation.[293,294] The finding that digoxin-free patients with renal failure, hepatic failure, low renin hypertension, pregnant women during the third trimester, neonates, and infants all exhibit assayable levels of DLIS (often in the "therapeutic range") has raised serious doubts about the validity of pharmacokinetic studies and therapeutic drug monitoring using the immunoassay technique in these groups of patients. There is evidence that in these conditions there is redistribution of tightly plasma-protein-bound DLIS to weakly bound and unbound DLIS.[295] Recently, increased DLIS concentrations in serum have also been associated with acromegaly,[296] insulin-induced hypoglycemia,[297] essential hypertension,[298] and the hypertension associated with multiple alkylating agents used in autologous bone marrow transplantation.[299] DLISs that interfere with immunoassays include fatty acids, phospholipids, steroids and bile acids; however, these are not the natriuretic hormone that has been hypothesized and that interacts with Na^+,K^+-ATPase.[267] The structures of the natriuretic DLISs have not yet been identified, but peptide and glycosteroid structures have been hypothesized.[267] It has been postulated that DLIS is formed in the hypothalamus and/or adrenal gland,[294] and there is considerable excitement about its potential role in Na^+ homeostasis, hypertension, and the transitional period of volume contraction in the newborn.[294]

REFERENCES

1. Smith TW. Digitalis—mechanisms of action and clinical use. New Engl J Med. 1988;318:358–65.
2. Erdmann E. The value of positive inotropy in acute and chronic heart failure. J Cardiovasc Pharmacol. 1989;14(Suppl. 3):S36–S41.
3. Parmley WW. Treatment of congestive heart failure—state of the art and future trends. Br J Clin Pharmacol. 1989;28:31S–39S.
4. Parmley WW. Should digoxin be the drug of first choice after diuretics in chronic congestive heart failure? I. Introduction. J Am Coll Cardiol. 1988;12:265–67.
5. Smith TW. Should digoxin be the drug of first choice after diuretics in chronic congestive heart failure? II. Protagonist's viewpoint. J Am Coll Cardiol. 1988;12:267–71.
6. Pitt B. Should digoxin be the drug of first choice after diuretics in chronic congestive heart failure? III. Antagonist's viewpoint. J Am Coll Cardiol. 1988;12:271–73.
7. Lee DC et al. Heart failure in out-patients. A randomized trial of digoxin vs. placebo. N Engl J Med. 1982;306:699–705.
8. Guyatt GH et al. A controlled trial of digoxin in congestive heart failure. Am J Cardiol. 1988;61:371–75.
9. Gheorghiade M et al. Comparative hemodynamic and neurohormonal effects of intravenous captopril and digoxin and their combinations in patients with severe heart failure. J Am Coll Cardiol. 1989;13:134–42.
10. Pugh SE et al. Clinical, haemodynamic, and pharmacological effects of withdrawal and reintroduction of digoxin in patients with heart failure in sinus rhythm after long term treatment. Br Heart J. 1989;61:529–39.
11. The captopril-digoxin multicenter research group. Comparative effects of therapy with captopril and digoxin in patients with mild to moderate heart failure. JAMA. 1988;259:539–44.
12. Beaune J. Comparison of enalapril versus digoxin for congestive heart failure. Am J Cardiol. 1989;63:22D–5D.
13. Kimmelstiel C, Benotti JR. How effective is digitalis in the treatment of congestive heart failure? Am Heart J. 1988;116:1063–70.
14. Sullivan M et al. Increased exercise capacity after digoxin administration in patients with heart failure. J Am Coll Cardiol. 1989;13:1138–143.
15. Falk RH et al. Digoxin for converting recent-onset atrial fibrillation to sinus rhythm. Ann Intern Med. 1987;106:503–6.
16. Klein HO, Kaplinsky E. Digitalis and verapamil in atrial fibrillation and flutter—is verapamil now the preferred agent? Drugs. 1986;31:185–97.
17. Cowan JC et al. A comparison of amiodarone and digoxin in the treatment of atrial fibrillation complicating suspected acute myocardial infarction. J Cardiovasc Pharmacol. 1986;8:252–56.
18. Lewis RP. Digitalis: a drug that refuses to die. Crit Care Med. 1990;18:S5–S13.
19. Pomfret SM et al. Relative efficacy of oral verapamil and digoxin alone and in combination for the treatment of patients with chronic atrial fibrillation. Clin Sci. 1988;74:351–57.
20. Roth A et al. Efficacy and safety of medium- and high-dose diltiazem alone and in combination with digoxin for control of heart rate at rest and during exercise in patients with chronic atrial fibrillation. Circulation. 1986;73:316–24.
21. Maragno I et al. Low- and medium-dose diltiazem in chronic atrial fibrillation: comparison with digoxin and correlation with drug plasma levels. Am Heart J. 1988;116:385–92.
22. Zoble RG et al. Comparative effects of nadolol-digoxin combination therapy and digoxin monotherapy for chronic atrial fibrillation. Am J Cardiol. 1987;60:39D–45D.
23. Bigger JT et al. Effect of digitalis treatment on survival after acute myodardial infarction. Am J Cardiol. 1985;55:623–30.
24. Yusuf S et al. Digitalis—a new controversy regarding an old drug. Circulation. 1986;73:14–8.
25. Johnston GD. Digoxin after myocardial infarction—does it have a role? Drugs. 1989;37:577–82.
26. Muller JE et al. Digoxin therapy and mortality after myocardial infarction—experience in the MILIS study. New Engl J Med. 1986;314:265-70.
27. Crawford MH et al. Effect of digoxin and vasodilators on left ventricular function in aortic regurgitation. Int J Cardiol. 1989;23:385–93.

28. Nasraway SA et al. Inotropic response to digoxin and dopamine in patients with severe sepsis, cardiac failure, and systemic hypoperfusion. Chest. 1989;95:612–15.

29. Caldwell JH et al. Intestinal absorption of digoxin-3H in the rat. Am J Physiol. 1969;217:1747–751.

30. Hall WH, Doherty JE. Tritiated digoxin XVI. Gastric absorption. Am J Digest Dis. 1971;16:903–8.

31. Ochs H et al. Absorption of digoxin from the distal parts of the intestine in man. Eur J Clin Pharmacol. 1975;9:95–7.

32. Andersson KE et al. Absorption of digoxin in man after oral and intrasigmoid administration studied by portal vein catheterization. Eur J Clin Pharmacol. 1975;9:39–47.

33. Beermann B et al. Elimination of orally administered digoxin and digitoxin by thoracic duct drainage in man. Eur J Clin Pharmacol. 1972;5:19–21.

34. Marcus FI. Current status of therapy with digoxin. Curr Probl Cardiol. 1978;3:1.

35. Huffman DH. Clinical use of digitalis glycosides. Am J Hosp Pharm. 1976;33:179–85.

36. Kramer WG, Reuning RH. Use of area under the curve to estimate absolute bioavailability of digoxin. J Pharm Sci. 1978;67:141–42.

37. Beveridge T et al. Absolute bioavailability of digoxin tablets. Arzneimittelforsch. 1978;28:701–3.

38. Doherty JE et al. A multicenter evaluation of the absolute bioavailability of digoxin dosage forms. Curr Ther Res. 1984,35:301–6.

39. Ohnhaus EE et al. Absolute bioavailability of digoxin in chronic renal failure. Clin Nephrol. 1979;11:302–6.

40. Ohnhaus EE et al. Untersuchungen zur resorption von digoxin bei patientin mit dekompensierter rechtsherzinsuffizienz. Schweiz Med Wochenschr. 1975;105:1782–783.

41. Meister W et al. Unchanged absorption of digoxin tablets in patients with cardiac failure. Pharmacology. 1984;28:90–4.

42. Ochs HR et al. Effect of dose on bioavailability of oral digoxin. Eur J Clin Pharmacol. 1981;19:53–5.

43. Johnson BF et al. A completely absorbed oral preparation of digoxin. Clin Pharmacol Ther. 1976;19:746–51.

44. Johnson BF et al. The comparability of dosage regimens of Lanoxin tablets and Lanoxicaps. Br J Clin Pharmacol. 1977;4:209–11.

45. Astorri E et al. Bioavailability and related heart function index of digoxin capsules and tablets in cardiac patients. J Pharm Sci. 1979;68:104–6.

46. Rund DG et al. Decreased digoxin cardioinactive reduced metabolites after administration as an encapsulated liquid concentrate. Clin Pharmacol Ther. 1983;34:738–43.

47. Johnson BF et al. Variability of steady-state digoxin kinetics during administration of tablets or capsules. Clin Pharmacol Ther. 1986;39:306–12.

48. Wettrell G, Andersson KE. Absorption of digoxin in infants. Eur J Clin Pharmacol. 1975;9:49–55.

49. Grimm R et al. Estimated versus measured serum digoxin levels. Am J Hosp Pharm. 1978;35:1346.

50. White RJ et al. Plasma concentrations of digoxin after oral administration in the fasting and postprandial state. Br Med J. 1971;1:380–81.

51. Brown DD et al. Decreased bioavailability of digoxin due to hypercholesterolemic interventions. Circulation 1978;58:164–72.

52. Johnson BF et al. The effect of dietary fiber on the bioavailability of digoxin in capsules. J Clin Pharmacol. 1987;27:487–90.

53. Bustrack JA et al. Bioavailability of digoxin capsules and tablets: effect of coadministered fluid volume. J Pharm Sci. 1984;73:1397–400.

54. Ochs H et al. Biologische verfugbarkeit von digoxin bei patienten mit und ohne Magenresektion nach Billroth II. Deut Med Woch. 1975;47:2430–434.

55. Marcus RI et al. The effect of jejunoileal bypass on the pharmacokinetics of digoxin in man. Circulation. 1977;55:537–41.

56. Ochs HR et al. Disease-related alterations in cardiac glycoside disposition. Clin Pharmacokinet. 1982;7:434–51.

57. Heizer WD et al. Absorption of digoxin from tablets and capsules in subjects with malabsorption syndromes. DICP, The Ann Pharmacother. 1989;23:764–69.

58. Kolibash AJ et al. Marked decline in serum digoxin concentrations during an episode of severe diarrhea. Am Heart J. 1977;94:806–7.

59. Bjornsson TD et al. Effects of high-dose cancer chemotherapy on the absorption of digoxin in two different formulations. Clin Pharmacol Ther. 1986;39:25–8.

60. Jusko WJ et al. Digoxin absorption from tablets and elixir. The effect of radiation-induced malabsorption. JAMA. 1974;230:1554–555.

61. Albert KS et al. Influence of kaolin-pectin suspension on digoxin bioavailability. J Pharm Sci. 1978;67:1582–586.

62. Aronson JK. Clinical pharmacokinetics of digoxin 1980. Clin Pharmacokinet. 1980;5:137–49.

63. Binnion PF. Absorption of different commercial preparations of digoxin in the normal human subject, and the influence of antacid, antidiarrheal and ion-exchange agents. In: Storstein O, ed. *Symposium on digitalis.* Oslo: Glydendal Norsk Forlag;1973:216–23.

64. Brown DD et al. A steady-state evaluation of the effects of propantheline bromide and cholestyramine on the bioavailability of digoxin when administered as tablets or capsules. J Clin Pharmacol. 1985;25:360–64.

65. Johnson BF et al. Effect of metoclopramide on digoxin absorption from tablets and capsules. Clin Pharmacol Ther. 1984;36:724–30.

66. Allen MD et al. Effect of magnesium-aluminum hydroxide and kaolin-pectin on absorption of digoxin from tablets and capsules. J Clin Pharmacol. 1981;21:26–30.

67. Juhl RP et al. Effect of sulfasalazine on digoxin bioavailability. Clin Pharmacol Ther. 1976;20:387–94.

68. Doherty JE, Perkins WH. Tissue concentration and turnover of tritiated digoxin in dogs. Am J Cardiol. 1966;17:47–52.

69. Reuning RH et al. Role of pharmacokinetics in drug dosage adjustment. I. Pharmacologic effect kinetics and apparent volume of distribution of digoxin. J Clin Pharmacol. 1973;13:127–41.

70. Doherty JE et al. The distribution and concentration of tritiated digoxin in human tissues. Ann Intern Med. 1967;66:116–24.

71. Karjalainen J et al. Tissue concentrations of digoxin in an autopsy material. Acta Pharmacol Toxicol. 1974;34:385–90.

72. Andersson KE et al. Post-mortem distribution and tissue concentration of digoxin in infants and adults. Acta Paediatr Scand. 1975;64:497–504.

73. Dutta S et al. Effect of metabolic inhibitors on the accumulation of digitaloids by the isolated guinea-pig heart. J Pharmacol Exp Ther. 1972;180:351–58.

74. Aronson JK, Grahame-Smith DG. Monitoring digoxin therapy II. Determinants of the apparent volume of distribution. Br J Clin Pharmacol. 1977;4:223–27.

75. Kjeldsen K. Regulation of the concentration of 3H-ouabain binding sites in mammalian skeletal muscle - Effects of age, K-depletion, thyroid status and hypertension. Dan Med Bull. 1987;34:15–46.

76. Kjeldsen K, Gron P. Skeletal muscle Na,K-pump concentration in children and its relationship to cardiac glycoside distribution. J Pharmacol Exp Ther. 1989;250:721–25.

77. Hartel G et al. Human serum and myocardium digoxin. Clin Pharmacol Ther. 1976;19:153–57.

78. Coltart J et al. Myocardial and skeletal muscle concentration of digoxin in patients on long-term therapy. Br Med J. 1972;2:318–19.

79. Harrison CE Jr et al. The distribution and excretion of tritiated substances in experimental animals following the administration of digoxin-3H. J Lab Clin Med. 1966;67:764–77.

80. King CR et al. Successful treatment of fetal supraventricular tachycardia with maternal digoxin therapy. Chest. 1984;85:573–75.

81. Wiggins JW et al. Echocardiographic diagnosis and intravenous digoxin management of fetal tachyarrhythmias and congestive heart failure. Am J Dis Children. 1986;140:202–4.

82. Jusko WJ et al. Digoxin concentrations in serum and saliva. Res Commun Chem Pathol Pharmacol. 1975;10;189–92.

83. Haeckel R, Muhlenfeld HM. Reasons for intraindividual inconstancy of the digoxin saliva to serum concentration ratio. J Clin Chem Clin Biochem. 1989;27:653–58.
84. Gayes JM et al. Cerebrospinal fluid digoxin concentrations in humans. J Clin Pharmacol. 1978;18:116–20.
85. Lissner W et al. Localization of tritiated digoxin in the rat eye. Am J Ophthalmol. 1971;72:608–14.
86. Storstein L. Studies on digitalis V. The influence of impaired renal function, hemodialysis, and drug interaction on serum protein binding of digitoxin and digoxin. Clin Pharmacol Ther. 1976;20:6–14.
87. Ohnhaus EE et al. Protein binding of digoxin human serum. Eur J Clin Pharmacol. 1972;5:34–6.
88. Hinderling PH. Kinetics of partitioning and binding of digoxin and its analogues in the subcompartments of blood. J Pharm Sci. 1984;73:1042–53.
89. Evered DC. The binding of digoxin by the serum proteins. Eur J Pharmacol. 1972;18:236–44.
90. Abshagen U et al. Distribution of digoxin, digitoxin and ouabain between plasma and erythrocytes in various species. Nauyn-Schmiedebergs Arch Pharmacol. 1971;270:105–16.
91. Morgan LM, Binnion PF. The distribution of 3H-digoxin in normal and acutely hyperkalemic dogs. Cardiovasc Res. 1970;4:235–41.
92. Marcus FI et al. The effect of acute hypokalemia on the myocardial concentration and body distribution of tritiated digoxin in the dog. J Pharmacol Exp Ther. 1971;178:271–81.
93. Francis DJ et al. The effect of insulin and glucose on the myocardial and skeletal muscle uptake of tritiated digoxin in acutely hypokalemic and normokalemic dogs. J Pharmacol Exp Ther. 1974;188:564–74.
94. Gorodischer R et al. Tissue and erythrocyte distribution of digoxin in infants. Clin Pharmacol Ther. 1976;19:256–63.
95. Kroening BH, Weintraub M. Age-associated changes in tissue distribution and uptake of 3H-digoxin in mice and guinea pigs. Pharmacology. 1980;20:21–6.
96. Ewy GA et al. Digoxin metabolism in obesity. Circulation. 1971;44:810–14.
97. Lullmann H, Peters T. Action of cardiac glycosides on the excitation-contraction coupling in heart muscle. Prog Pharmacol. 1979;2:3–57.
98. Lullmann H et al. Kinetic events determining the effects of cardiac glycosides. Trends Pharmacol Sci. 1979;1:102–6.
99. Joreteg T, Jogestrand T. Physical exercise and digoxin binding to skeletal muscle:relation to exercise intensity. Eur J Clin Pharmacol. 1983;25:585–88.
100. Joreteg T, Jogestrand T. Physical exercise and binding of digoxin to skeletal muscle—effect of muscle activation frequency. Eur J Clin Pharmacol. 1984;27:567–70.
101. Jogestrand T. Influence of everyday physical activity on the serum digoxin concentration in digoxin-treated patients. Clin Physiol. 1981;1:209–14.
102. Hall PD et al. The effect of everyday exercise on steady state digoxin concentrations. J Clin Pharmacol. 1989;29:1083–88.
103. Jogestrand T, Nordlander R. Serum digoxin determination in out-patients; need for standardization. Br J Clin Pharmacol. 1983;15:55–8.
104. Koup JR et al. Digoxin pharmacokinetics: role of renal failure in dosage regimen design. Clin Pharmacol Ther. 1975;18:9–21.
105. Graves SW et al. An endogenous digoxin-like substance in patients with renal impairment. Ann Intern Med. 1983;99:604–8.
106. Doherty JE et al. Studies with tritiated digoxin in renal failure. Am J Med. 1964;37:536–44.
107. Storstein L. Protein binding of cardiac glycosides in disease states. Clin Pharmacokinet. 1977;2:220–33.
108. Jusko WJ. Weintraub M. Myocardial distribution of digoxin and renal function. Clin Pharmacol Ther. 1974;16:449–54.
109. Jogestrand T, Ericsson F. Skeletal muscle digoxin binding in patients with renal failure. Br J Clin Pharmacol. 1983;16:109–11.
110. Aronson JK, Grahame-Smith DG. Altered distribution of digoxin in renal failure— a cause of digoxin toxicity? Br J Clin Pharmacol. 1976;3:1045-51.

111. Kramer WG et al. Pharmacokinetics of digoxin. Comparison of a two- and a three-compartment model in man. J Pharmacokinet Biopharm. 1974;2:299–312.

112. Okita GT. Species difference in duration of action of cardiac glycosides. Fed Proc. 1967;26:1125–130.

113. van der Vijgh WJF, Oe PL. Pharmacokinetic aspects of digoxin in patients with terminal renal failure. Int J Clin Pharmacol. 1977;15:249–59.

114. Wettrell G et al. Effect of exchange transfusion on the elimination of digoxin in neonates. Eur J Clin Pharmacol. 1976;10:25–9.

115. Rosegger H et al. Digoxin elimination by exchange transfusion. Eur J Pediatr 1977;124:217–22.

116. Lai KN et al. Hemofiltration in digoxin overdose. Arch Intern Med. 1986;146:1219–220.

117. Sinclair AJ et al. Kinetics of digoxin and anti-digoxin antibody fragments during treatment of digoxin toxicity. Br J Clin Pharmacol. 1989;28:352–56.

118. Rossi R et al. Severe digoxin intoxication in a child treated by infusion of digoxin-specific Fab-antibody-fragments. Eur J Pediatr. 1984;142:138–40.

119. Nuwayhid NF, Johnson GF. Digoxin elimination in a functionally anephric patient after digoxin-specific Fab fragment therapy. Ther Drug Monit. 1989;11:680–85.

120. Cook LS et al. Comparison of the canine tissue distribution of digoxin after acute and chronic administration: implications for digitalis therapy. Am J Cardiol. 1984;53:1703–706.

121. Aronson JK. Clinical pharmacokinetics of cardiac glycosides in patients with renal dysfunction. Clin Pharmacokinet. 1983;8:155–78.

122. Kuhlmann J et al. Pharmacokinetics and metabolism of digoxigenin- mono-digitoxoside in man. Eur J Clin Pharmacol. 1974;7:87–94.

123. Magnusson JO et al. Excretion of digoxin and its metabolites in urine after a single oral dose in healthy subjects. Biopharm Drug Dispos. 1982;3:211–18.

124. Marcus FI et al. The reactivity of digoxin as measured by the Na-K-ATPase displacement assay and radioimmunoassay. J Lab Clin Med. 1975;85:610–20.

125. Gault MH et al. Digoxin biotransformation. Clin Pharmacol Ther. 1984;35:74–82.

126. Gierke KD et al. Metabolism and rate of elimination of digoxigenin bisdigitoside in dogs before and during chronic azotemia. J Pharmacol Exp Ther. 1980;212:448–51.

127. Lage GL, Spratt JL. Structure-activity correlation of the lethality and central effects of selected cardiac glycosides. J Pharmacol Exp Ther. 1966;152:501–8.

128. Bach EJ, Reiter M. The difference in velocity between the lethal and inotropic action of dihydrodigoxin. Naunyn-Schmiedeberg's Arch Exp Pathol Pharmacol. 1964;248:437–49.

129. Peters U et al. Digoxin metabolism in patients. Arch Intern Med. 1978;138:1074–76.

130. Clark DR, Kalman SM. Dihydrodigoxin: a common metabolite of digoxin in man. Drug Metab Dispos. 1974;2:148–50.

131. Gault MH et al. Biotransformation and elimination of digoxin with normal and minimal renal function. Clin Pharmacol Ther. 1979;25:499–13.

132. Gault H et al. Influence of gastric pH on digoxin biotransformation. I. Intragastric hydrolysis. Clin Pharmacol Ther. 1980;27:16–21.

133. Gault H et al. Influence of gastric pH on digoxin biotransformation. II. Extractable urinary metabolites. Clin Pharmacol Ther. 1981;29:181–90.

134. Flasch VH et al. Affinitat von polaren digoxin-und digitoxin-metaboliten zu digoxin-und digitoxin-antikorpern. Arzneimittelforschung. 1977;27:269–653.

135. Magnusson JO. Metabolism of digoxin after oral and intrajejunal administration. Br J Clin Pharmacol. 1983;16:741–42.

136. Magnusson JO et al. Increased metabolism to dihydrodigoxin after intake of a microencapsulated formulation of digoxin. Eur J Clin Pharmacol. 1984;27:197–202.

137. Schmoldt A, Ahsendorf B. Cleavage of digoxigenin digitoxosides by rat liver microsomes. Eur J Drug Metab Pharmacokinet. 1980;5:225–32.

138. Abshagen U et al. Formation and disposition of bis- and monoglycosides after administration of 3H-4-methyldigoxin to man. Eur J Clin Pharmacol. 1974;7:177–81.

139. Lindenbaum J et al. Urinary excretion of reduced metabolites of digoxin. Am J Med. 1981;71:67–74.

140. Lindenbaum J et al. Inactivation of digoxin by the gut flora: reversal by antibiotic therapy. N Engl J Med. 1981;305:789–94.

141. Norregaard-Hansen K et al. The significance of the enterohepatic circulation on the metabolism of digoxin in patients with the ability of intestinal conversion of the drug. Acta Med Scand. 1986;220:89–92.

142. Dobkin JF et al. Digoxin-inactivating bacteria: identification in human gut flora. Science. 1983;220:325–27.

143. Watson E et al. Identification by gas chromatography-mass spectrometry of dihydrodigoxin—a metabolite of digoxin in man. J Pharmacol Exp Ther. 1973;184:424–31.

144. Hinderling PH et al. Comparative *in vivo* evaluation of a radioimmunoassay and a chromatographic assay for the measurement of digoxin in biological fluids. J Pharm Sci. 1986;75:517–21.

145. Linday L et al. Digoxin inactivation by the gut flora in infancy and childhood. Pediatrics. 1987;79:544–48.

146. Alam AN et al. Interethnic variation in the metabolic inactivation of digoxin by the gut flora. Gastroenterol. 1988;95:117–23.

147. Mathan VI et al. Geographic differences in digoxin inactivation, a metabolic activity of the human anaerobic gut flora. Gut. 1989;30:971–77.

148. Talcott RE et al. Metabolites and some characteristics of the metabolism of 3H-digoxigenin by rat liver homogenates. Biochem Pharmacol. 1972;21:2001–6.

149. Schmoldt A, Promies J. On the substrate specificity of the digitoxigenin monodigitoxoside conjugating UDP-glucuronyltransferase in rat liver. Biochem Pharmacol. 1982;31:2285–289.

150. Gault MH et al. Combined liquid chromatography/radioimmunoassay with improved specificity for serum digoxin. Clin Chem. 1985;31:1272–277.

151. Gault H et al. Interpretation of serum digoxin values in renal failure. Clin Pharmacol Ther. 1986;39:530–36.

152. Marcus FI et al. The metabolism of tritiated digoxin in renal insufficiency in dogs and man. J Pharmacol Exp Ther. 1966;152:373–82.

153. Vlasses PH et al. False-positive digoxin measurements due to conjugated metabolite accumulation in combined renal and hepatic dysfunction. Am J Nephrol. 1987;7:355–59.

154. Koup JR et al. Pharmacokinetics of digoxin in normal subjects after intravenous bolus and infusion doses. J Pharmacokinet Biopharm. 1975;3:181–92.

155. Ochs HR et al. Single- and multiple-dose kinetics of intravenous digoxin. Clin Pharmacol Ther. 1980;28:340–45.

156. Steiness E. Renal tubular secretion of digoxin. Circulation. 1974;50:103–7.

157. Gibson TP et al. Effect of acute changes in serum digoxin concentration on renal digoxin clearance. Clin Pharmacol Ther. 1984;36:478–84.

158. Cogan JJ et al. Acute vasodilator therapy increases renal clearance of digoxin in patients with congestive heart failure. Circulation. 1981;64:973–76.

159. Steiness E et al. Renal digoxin clearance: dependence on plasma digoxin and diuresis. Eur J Clin Pharmacol. 1982;23:151–54.

160. Halkin H et al. Determinants of the renal clearance of digoxin. Clin Pharmacol Ther. 1975;17:385–94.

161. Okada RD et al. Relationship between plasma concentration and dose of digoxin in patients with and without renal impairment. Circulation. 1978;58:1196–203.

162. Gorodischer R et al. Renal clearance of digoxin in young infants. Res Commun Chem Pathol Pharmacol. 1977;16:363–74.

163. Linday LA. Maturation and renal digoxin clearance. Clin Pharmacol Ther. 1981;30:735–38.

164. Pedersen KE et al. Effects of physical activity and immobilization on plasma digoxin concentration and renal digoxin clearance. Clin Pharmacol Ther. 1983;34:303–8.

165. Naafs MAB et al. Decreased renal clearance of digoxin in chronic congestive heart failure. Eur J Clin Pharmacol. 1985;29:249–52.

166. Steiness E. Suppression of renal excretion of digoxin in hypokalemic patients. Clin Pharmacol Ther. 1978;23:511–14.

167. Hager WD et al. Digoxin-quinidine interaction: pharmacokinetic evaluation. N Engl J Med. 1979;300:1238–241.
168. Koren G. Clinical pharmacokinetic significance of the renal tubular secretion of digoxin. Clin Pharmacokinet. 1987;13:334–43.
169. Doherty JE et al. Tritiated digoxin studies in human subjects. Arch Intern Med. 1961;108:531–39.
170. Doherty JE. The clinical pharmacology of digitalis glycosides: a review. Am J Med Sci. 1968;255:382–414.
171. Caldwell JH et al. Intestinal secretion of digoxin in the rat. Naunyn-Schmiedeberg's Arch Pharmacol. 1980;312:271–75.
172. Caldwell JH, Cline CT. Biliary excretion of digoxin in man. Clin Pharmacol Ther. 1976;19:410–15.
173. Lalonde RL et al. Acceleration of digoxin clearance by activated charcoal. Clin Pharmacol Ther. 1985;37:367–71.
174. Koup JR et al. Pharmacokinetics of digoxin in normal subjects after intravenous bolus and infusion doses. J Pharmacokinet Biopharm. 1975;3:181–92.
175. Ochs HR et al. Dose-independent pharmacokinetics of digoxin in humans. Am Heart J. 1978;96:507–11.
176. Schenck-Gustafsson K et al. Skeletal muscle binding and renal excretion of digoxin in man. Eur J Clin Pharmacol. 1987;31:601–3.
177. Kramer WG et al. Pharmacokinetics of digoxin. Relationship between response intensity and predicted compartmental drug levels in man. J Pharmacokinet Biopharm. 1979;7:47–61.
178. Dungan WT et al. Tritiated digoxin XVIII. Studies in infants and children. Circulation. 1972;46:983–88.
179. Nyberg L. Andersson KE, Bertler A. Bioavailability of digoxin from tablets. II. Radioimmunoassay and disposition pharmacokinetics of digoxin after intravenous administration. Acta Pharma Suec. 1974;11:459–70.
180. Collins-Nakai RL et al. Total body digoxin clearance and steady-state concentrations in low birth weight infants. Dev Pharmacol Ther. 1982;4:61–70.
181. Sumner DJ et al. Digoxin pharmacokinetics: multicompartmental analysis and its clinical implications. Br J Clin Pharmacol. 1976;3:221–29.
182. Gortner, Hellenbrecht D. Estimation of digoxin dosage in VLBW infants using serum creatinine concentrations. Acta Paediatr Scand. 1986;75:433–38.
183. Hastreiter AR et al. Maintenance digoxin dosage and steady-state plasma concentration in infants and children. J Pediatr. 1985;107:140–46.
184. Klotz U, Antonin KH. Biliary excretion studies with digoxin in man. Int J Clin Pharmacol. 1977;15:332–34.
185. Walton RP et al. Comparative increase in ventricular contractile force produced by several cardiac glycosides. J Pharmacol. 1950;98:346–57.
186. Arnold SB et al. Long-term digitalis therapy improves left ventricular function in heart failure. N Engl J Med. 1980;303:1443–448.
187. Ferrer MI et al. Some effects of digoxin upon the heart and circulation in man. Digoxin in combined left and right ventricular failure. Circulation. 1960;21:372–85.
188. Smith TW. Basic mechanisms of cardiac glycoside action. In: Smith TW, ed. Digitalis glycosides. New York: Grune & Stratton; 1986:5.
189. Akera T. The function of Na+,K+-ATPase and its importance for drug action. In: Erdmann E, Greef K, Skou JC, eds. Cardiac glycosides 1785–1985. Darmstadt, West Germany: Steinkopff Verlag; 1986:19.
190. Reuning RH, Geraets DR. Digoxin. In: Evans WE et al., eds. Applied pharmacokinetics: principles of therapeutic drug monitoring. Vancouver: Applied Therapeutics; 1986:570–623.
191. Brown BT et al. Chemical structure and pharmacologic activity of some derivatives of digitoxigenin and digoxigenin. Br J Pharmacol. 1962;18:311–24.
192. Smith TW et al. Digitalis glycosides: mechanisms and manifestations of toxicity. Prog Cardiovasc Dis. 1984;27:21–56.
193. Fowler NO. Digitalis intoxication and electrolyte imbalances. In: Cardiac diagnosis and treatment. Hagerstown, MD: Harper and Row; 1980;1129–152.

194. Mahon WA. Cardiac glycosides and drugs used in dysrhythmias. In: Dukes MN, ed. Meyler's side effects of drugs. Amsterdam: Excerpta Medica; 1980:280–305.
195. Chuman MA, LeSage J. Color vision deficiences in two cases of digoxin toxicity. Am J Ophthalmol. 1985;100:682–85.
196. Mason DT et al. The digitalis inotropic-dose-response curve: demonstration of linearity and attenuation by potassium. Circulation. 1972;46(Suppl. II):30.
197. Klein M et al. Correlation of the electrical and mechanical changes in the dog heart during progressive digitalization. Circ Res. 1971;29:635–45.
198. Lee G et al. Similarity of the inotropic time course of differing digitalis preparations in isolated cardiac muscle. Circulation. 1972;46(Suppl. II):31.
199. Lewis RP et al. Systolic time intervals. In: Weissler AM, ed. Noninvasive cardiology. New York: Grune and Stratton; 1974:301–68.
200. Kupari M. Reproducibility of the systolic time intervals: effect of the temporal range of measurements. Cardiovasc Res. 1983;17:339–43.
201. Hoeschen RJ, Cuddy TE. Dose-response relation between therapeutic levels of serum digoxin and systolic time intervals. Am J Cardiol. 1975;35:469–72.
202. Partanen J et al. Effect of digoxin on the heart in normal subjects: influence of isometric exercise and autonomic blockade: a noninvasive study. Br J Clin Pharmacol. 1988;25:331–40.
203. Kolibash AJ et al. Extension of the serum digoxin concentration-response relationship to patient management. J Clin Pharmacol. 1989;29:300–6.
204. Smith TW. Digitalis toxicity: epidemiology and clinical use of serum concentration measurements. Am J Med. 1975;470:470–76.
205. Huffman DH et al. Association between clinical cardiac status, laboratory parameters, and digoxin usage. Am Heart J. 1976;91:28–34.
206. Hoffman BF, Bigger JT Jr. Digitalis and allied cardiac glycosides. In: Gilman AG et al., eds. The pharmacological basis of therapeutics. New York: Macmillian Publishing Co; 1980:729–60.
207. Partanen J. Effect of intravenous digoxin on the heart at rest and during isometric exercise: a noninvasive study in normal and autonomically blocked volunteers. J Cardiovasc Pharmacol. 1988;11:158–66.
208. Redfors A. The effect of different digoxin doses on subjective symptoms and physical working capacity in patients with atrial fibrillation. Acta Med Scand. 1971;190:307–20.
209. Redfors A. Plasma digoxin concentration—its relation to digoxin dosage and clincal effects in patients with atrial fibrillation. Br Heart J. 1972;34:383–91.
210. Goldman S et al. Inefficacy of "therapeutic" serum levels of digoxin in controlling the ventricular rate in atrial fibrillation. Am J Cardiol. 1975;35:651–55.
211. Halkin H et al. Value of serum digoxin concentration measurement in the control of digoxin therapy in atrial fibrillation. Isr J Med Sci. 1979;15:490–93.
212. Masuhara JE, Lalonde RL. Serum digoxin concentrations in atrial fibrillation. A review. Drug Intell Clin Pharm. 1982;16:543–46.
213. Beasley R et al. Exercise heart rates at different serum digoxin concentrations in patients with atrial fibrillation. Br Med J. 1985;290:9–11.
214. Ogden PC et al. The relationship between inotropic and dromotropic effects of digitalis. the modulation of these effects by autonomic influences. Am Heart J. 1969;77:628–35.
215. Lee TH, Smith TW. Serum digoxin concentration and diagnosis of digitalis toxicity-current concepts. Clin Pharmacokinet. 1983;8:279–85.
216. Smith TW, Haber E. Digoxin intoxication: the relationship of clinical presentation to serum digoxin concentration. J Clin Invest. 1970;49:2377–386.
217. Beller GA et al. Digitalis intoxication. A prospective clinical study with serum level correlations. N Engl J Med. 1971;284:989–97.
218. Evered DC, Chapman C. Plasma digoxin concentrations and digoxin toxicity in hospitalized patients. Br Heart J. 1971;33:540 45.
219. Park HM et al. Clinical evaluation of radioimmunassay of digoxin. J Nucl Med. 1973;14:531–33.
220. Ingelfinger JA, Goldman P. The serum digitalis concentration—does it diagnose digitalis toxicity? N Engl J Med. 1976;294:867–70.

221. Park GD et al. Digoxin toxicity in patients with high serum digoxin concentrations. Am J Med Sci. 1987;29:423–28.
222. Sampson JJ et al. The effect on man of potassium administration in relation to digitalis glycoside, with special reference to blood serum potassium, the electrocardiogram, and ectopic beats. Am Heart J. 1943;26:164–79.
223. Brader DC, Morrelli HF. Digoxin toxicity in patients with normokalemic potassium depletion. Clin Pharmacol Ther. 1977;22:21–33.
224. Sellar RH et al. Digitalis toxicity and hypomagnesemia. Am Heart J. 1970;79:57-68.
225. DeCarli C et al. Serum magnesium levels in symptomatic atrial fibrillation and their relation to rhythm control by intravenous digoxin. Am J Cardiol. 1986;57:956–59.
226. Landauer JA et al. Magnesium deficiency and digitalis toxicity. JAMA. 1984;251:730.
227. Nola GT et al. Assessment of the synergistic relationship between serum calcium and digitalis. Am Heart J. 1970;79:499–507.
228. Sonnenblick M et al. Correlation between manifestations of digoxin toxicity and serum digoxin, calcium, potassium, and magnesium concentrations and arterial pH. Br Med J. 1983;286:1089–91.
229. Mason DT, Foerster JM. Side effects and intoxication of cardiac glycosides: manifestations and treatment. In: Greef K, ed. Cardiac glycosides, part II pharmacokinetics and clinical pharmacology. New York: Springer-Verlag; 1981:275–97.
230. Morris JJ et al. Digitalis and experimental myocardial infarction. Am Heart J. 1969;77:342–55.
231. Miyashita H et al. The problems of digitalis therapy from the viewpoint of serum concentration with special reference to the sampling time, to the overlapping range of serum concentraion where intoxicated and non-intoxicated patients are located, and to atrial fibrillation. Jap Circulation J. 1986;50:628–35.
232. Ferrer MI. Management of patients with cor pulmonale. Med Clin North Am. 1979;63(1):251–65.
233. Mather PN et al. Effects of digoxin on right ventricular function in severe chronic outflow obstruction: a controlled clinical trial. Ann Int Med. 1981;95:283–88.
234. Jelliffe RW. An improved method of digoxin therapy. Ann Intern Med. 1968;69:703–17.
235. Jusko WJ et al. Pharmacokinetic design of digoxin dosage regimens in relation to renal function. J Clin Pharmacol. 1974;14:525–35.
236. Gault MH et al. Studies of digoxin dosage, kinetics, and serum concentrations in renal failure and review of the literature. Nephron. 1976;17:161–87.
237. Keller F et al. Digoxin in renal insufficiency: impracticality of basing it on the creatinine clearance, body weight, and volume of distribution. Eur J Clin Pharmacol. 1980;18:433–41.
238. Hyneck ML et al. Comparison of methods for estimating digoxin dosing regimens. Am J Hosp Pharm. 1981;38:69–73.
239. Jelliffe RW. Factors to consider in planning digoxin therapy. J Chronic Dis. 1971;24:407–16.
240. Park MK. Use of digoxin in infants and children, with specific emphasis on dosage. J Pediatr. 1986;108:871–77.
241. Wettrell G, Andersson KE. Clinical pharmacokinetics of digoxin in infants. Clin. Pharmacokinet. 1977;2:17–31
242. Impivaara O, Iisalo E. Serum digoxin concentrations in a representative digoxin-consuming adult population. Eur J Clin Pharmacol. 1985;27:627–32.
243. Jogestrand T et al. Clinical value of serum digoxin assays in outpatients: improvement by the standardization of blood sampling. Am Heart J. 1989;117:1076–83.
244. Grosse-Brockhoff F, Peters U. Clinical indications and choice of cardiac glycoside, clinical conditions influencing glycoside effects. In: Greef K, ed. Cardiac Glycosides, part II, pharmacokinetics and clinical pharmacology. New York: Springer-Verlag; 1981:239–74.
245. Aronson JK. Indications for the measurement of plasma digoxin concentration. Drugs. 1983;26:230–42.
246. Oetgen WJ et al. Amiodarone-digoxin interaction: clinical and experimental observations. Chest. 1984;86:75–9.
247. Nademanee K et al. Amiodarone-digoxin interaction: clinical significance, time course of development, potential pharmacokinetic mechanisms, and therapeutic implications. J Am Coll Cardiol. 1984;4:111–16.

248. Waldorff S et al. Spironolactone-induced changes in digoxin pharmacokinetics. Clin Pharmacol Ther. 1978;24:162–67.
249. Waldorff S et al. Interactions between digoxin and potassium-sparing diuretics. Clin Pharmacol Ther. 1983;33:418–23.
250. Fenster PE et al. Digoxin-quinidine-spironolactone interaction. Clin Pharmacol Ther. 1984;36:70–3.
251. Morris RG et al. Spironolactone as a source of interference in commercial digoxin immunoassays. Ther Drug Monit. 1987;9:208–11.
252. Pedersson KE et al. Effect of quinidine on digoxin bioavailability. Eur J Clin Pharmacol. 1983;24:41–7.
253. Bigger JT Jr. The quinidine-digoxin interaction. Int J Cardiol. 1981;1:109–16.
254. Pederson KE et al. Digoxin-verapamil interaction. Clin Pharmacol Ther. 1981;30:311–16.
255. Elkayam U et al. Effect of diltiazem on renal clearance and serum concentration of digoxin in patients with cardiac disease. Am J Cardiol. 1985;55:1393–395.
256. Dorian P et al. Cyclosporine nephrotoxicity and cyclosporine-digoxin interaction prior to heart transplantation. Transplant Proceed. 1987;19:1825–827.
257. Calvo MV et al. Interaction between digoxin and propafenone. Ther Drug Monit. 1989;11:10–5.
258. Moses HW, Mikell FL Jr. Antiarrhythmic drugs. In: Wang RIH, ed. Practical drug therapy. Milwaukee: Medstream Press, Inc.; 1987:44.
259. Eraker SA, Sassc L. The digoxin test and digoxin toxicity: a bayesian approach to decision making. Circulation. 1981;64:409–20.
260. Hursting MJ et al. Determination of free digoxin concentrations in serum for monitoring Fab treatment of digoxin overdose. Clin Chem. 1987;33:1652–655.
261. Hansell JR. Effect of therapeutic digoxin antibodies on digoxin assays. Arch Pathol Lab Med. 1989;113:1259–262.
262. Ujhelyi MR et al. Effect of digoxin Fab antibodies on five digoxin immunoassays. Ther Drug Monit. (In press).
263. Taggart AJ ct al. A simple aid to digoxin prescribing. Eur J Clin Pharmacol. 1987;33:441–45.
264. Wagner JG et al. Sensitive radioimmunassay for digoxin in plasma and urine. Steroids. 1977;29:787–807.
265. MacKinney AA Jr et al. Comparison of five radioimmunoassays and enzyme bioassay for measurement of digoxin in blood. Clin Chem. 1975;21:857–59.
266. Kubasik NP et al. Problems in measurement of serum digoxin by commercially available radioimmunassay kits. Am J Cardiol. 1975;36:975–77.
267. Stone JA, Soldin SJ. An update on digoxin. Clin Chem. 1989;35:1326–331.
268. Longerich L et al. Disposable-column radioimmunoassay for serum digoxin with less interference from metabolites and endogenous digitalis-like factors. Clin Chem. 1988;34:2211–216.
269. Skogen WF et al. Endogenous digoxin-like immunoreactive factors eliminated from serum samples by hydrophobic silica-gel extraction and enzyme immunoassay. Clin Chem. 1987;33:401–4.
270. Voshall DL et al. Effect of albumin on serum digoxin radioimmunoassays. Clin Chem. 1975;21:402–6.
271. Kroening BH, Weintraub M. Reduced variation of tracer binding in digoxin radioimmunoassay by use of (125I)-labeled tyrosine-methyl-ester derivative: relation of thyroxine concentration to binding. Clin Chem. 1976;22:1732–734.
272. Cerceo E, Elloso CA. Factors affecting the radioimmunoassay of digoxin. Clin Chem. 1972;18:539–43.
273. Valdes R et al. Variable cross-reactivity of digoxin metabolites in digoxin immunoassays. Am J Clin Pathol. 1984;82:210–13.
274. Belpaire FM et al. Radioimmunassay of digoxin in renal failure: a comparison of different commercial kits. Clin Chim Acta. 1975;62:255–61.
275. Malini PL et al. Cross reactivity of digoxin radioimmunoassay kits to dihydrodigoxin. Clin Chem. 1982;28:2445–446.

276. Thong B et al. Lack of specificity of current anti-digoxin antibodies, and preparation of a new, specific polyclonal antibody that recognizes the carbohydrate moiety of digoxin. Clin Chem. 1985;31:1625–631.

277. Sadee W, Beelen GCM. Drug level monitoring-analytical techniques, metabolism and pharmacokinetics. New York: John Wiley and Sons, Inc.; 1980.

278. Kulaots IA et al. Endogenous digoxin-like immunoreactive substances eliminated from serum samples from patients with liver disease by the EMIT column digoxin assay. Clin Chem. 1987;33:1490–491.

279. Linday L, Drayer DE. Cross reactivity of EMIT digoxin assay with digoxin metabolites, and validation of the method for measurement of urinary digoxin. Clin Chem. 1983;29:175–77.

280. Al-Fares AM et al. Evaluation of the fluorescence polarization immunoassay for quantitation of digoxin in serum. Ther Drug Monit. 1984;6:454–57.

281. Hicks JM, Bret EM. Falsely increased digoxin concentrations in samples from neonates and infants. Ther Drug Monit. 1984;6:461–64.

282. Bianchi P. Interferences in TDx digoxin assay in dialysis patients. Clin Chem. 1986;32:2099.

283. Frye R, Mathews SE. Effect of digoxin-like immunoreactive factor on the TDx digoxin II assay. Clin Chem. 1987;33:629–30.

284. Christenson RH et al. Digoxin-like immunoreactivity eliminated from serum by centrifugal ultrafiltration before fluorescence polarization immunoassay of digoxin. Clin Chem. 1987;33:606–8.

285. Porter WH et al. Effect of protein concentration on the determination of digoxin in serum by fluorescence polarization immunoassay. Clin Chem. 1984;30:1826–829.

286. Morais JA et al. Specific and sensitive assays for digoxin in plasma, urine and heart tissue. Res Commun Chem Pathol Pharmacol. 1981;31:285–98.

287. Loo JCK et al. The estimation of serum digoxin by combined HPLC separation and radio-immunological assay. J Liquid Chromatogr. 1981;4:879–86.

288. Bockbrader HN, Reuning RH. Digoxin and metabolites in urine: a derivatization-HPLC method capable of quantitating individual epimers of dihydrodigoxin. J Chromatogr. 1984;310:85–95.

289. Shepard TA et al. Digoxin and metabolites in urine and feces: a fluorescence derivatization-high-performance liquid chromatographic technique. J Chromatogr. 1986;380:89–98.

290. Fujii Y et al. Micro HPLC separation of 3,5-dinitrobenzoyl derivatives of cardiac glycosides and their metabolites. J Chromatogr Sci. 1983;21:495–99.

291. Reh E. Determination of digoxin in serum by on-line immunoadsorptive clean-up high-performance liquid chromatographic separation and fluorescence-reaction detection. J Chromatogr. 1988;433:119–30.

292. Kwong E, McErlane KM. Analysis of digoxin at therapeutic concentrations using high-performance liquid chromatography with post-column derivatization. J Chromatogr. 1986;381:357–63.

293. Wilkins MR. Endogenous digitalis: a review of the evidence. Trends Pharmacol Sci. 1985;6:286–88.

294. Hastreiter AR et al. Digitalis, digitalis antibodies, digitalis-like immunoreactive substances, and sodium homeostasis: a review. Clinics in Perinatol. 1988;15:491–522.

295. Valdes R. Endogenous digoxin-like immunoreactive factors: impact on digoxin measurements and potential physiological implications. Clin Chem. 1985;31:1525–532.

296. Deray G et al. Evidence of an endogenous digitalis-like factor in the plasma of patients with acromegaly. N Engl J Med. 1987;316:575–80.

297. Graves SW et al. Increases in plasma digitalis-like factor activity during insulin-induced hypoglycemia. Neuroendocrinol. 1989;49:586–91.

298. Clerico A et al. Endogenous cardiac glycoside-like substances in newborns, adults, pregnant women and patients with hypertension or renal insufficiency. Drugs Exp Clin Res. 1988;14:603–7.

299. Graves SW et al. Endogenous digoxin-like immunoreactive factor and digitalis-like factor associated with the hypertension of patients receiving multiple alkylating agents as part of autologous bone marrow transplantation. Clin Sci. 1989;77:501–7.

Chapter 21

Lidocaine

John A. Pieper and Kenneth E. Johnson

L idocaine is considered the parenteral drug of choice for the acute treatment or prevention of ventricular arrhythmias associated with acute myocardial infarction or cardiovascular surgery and ventricular tachycardia.[1-5] Lidocaine was introduced as a local anesthetic in 1948 and as an antiarrhythmic agent in the 1960s. This drug is widely used because it is effective against ventricular arrhythmias of diverse etiology, because effective serum concentrations can be attained and controlled with intravenous dosage with a low incidence of adverse hemodynamic complications, and because drug clearance is relatively rapid compared to that of other antiarrhythmic agents.

Clinical application of pharmacokinetic principles requires a reliable relationship between clinical measure(s) of response and measured drug concentrations. The use of pharmacokinetic principles and monitoring of drug concentrations are indicated for drugs with significant interpatient variability in pharmacokinetic and pharmacodynamic characteristics, for drugs with a narrow therapeutic index, and when clinical endpoints of therapy are absent or obscure. There is sufficient evidence to suggest that the pharmacologic effects of lidocaine are correlated with blood (serum or plasma) concentrations. Concentration monitoring is warranted by lidocaine's extensive interpatient variability in disposition and by its narrow therapeutic index.[6-9]

The need for individualizing lidocaine therapy is evidenced by past experience with standard dosage regimens in normal volunteers.[10,11] These standard regimens consisted of an intravenous loading dose of 50 to 150 mg, followed by a continuous intravenous infusion of 1 to 4 mg/min.[12-14] Empiric dosage reductions were advised in patients with congestive heart failure (CHF) or liver disease.[15] When this dosing approach was used, serum concentrations outside the therapeutic range were observed in 38% of patients and evidence of toxicity was reported in approximately 15% of patients.[17] It has been further reported that 19% of lidocaine serum concentration determinations in 32 patients administered the standard regimen were subtherapeutic and 30% were above the usual therapeutic range.[18] The reasons for these observations include intersubject variability in lidocaine volume of distribution,[19-22] plasma protein binding[23-25] and systemic clearance,[5,9,22,26] and the potential for differences in effective concentrations required for prevention versus treatment of ventricular arrhythmias.

When lidocaine is used for the treatment of ventricular tachycardia or persistent, high-grade ventricular ectopy, titration of the dose to suppression of the arrhythmia can guide the clinician. However, application of pharmacokinetic principles will provide a more precise determination of the dose necessary for the desired therapeutic effect with an acceptable risk of toxicity. When lidocaine is administered for the prophylaxis of primary ventricular fibrillation after acute myocardial infarction, or for suppression of transient ventricular arrhythmias, a precise clinical endpoint for therapy is not available to the clinician. Thus, the dosage regimen must be individualized to attain appropriate therapeutic concentrations. There is now considerable evidence that the individualization of lidocaine therapy should improve the effective use of the drug in the treatment of potentially life-threatening arrhythmias.[15,16,44,67,83,108]

CLINICAL PHARMACOKINETICS

Absorption

Following oral administration, lidocaine is extensively and rapidly absorbed.[19,27,28] It has been reported that 84% of an administered oral dose was recovered as parent compound and metabolites in the urine from two volunteers receiving 250 mg of lidocaine.[27] After 250 and 500 mg oral doses, peak blood concentrations ranged from 0.3 to 0.8 and 0.6 to 1.1 µg/mL, respectively, at 30 to 60 minutes.[27,28] Despite rapid absorption, presystemic hepatic metabolism (first-pass effect) causes low and variable systemic availability. Following a 250 mg oral dose in five normal volunteers, mean bioavailability was 35.6% ± 12.8%, and 33.8% ± 9.8% after a single 500 mg dose.[27] The bioavailability of lidocaine following single lidocaine doses of 100, 300, and 500 mg averaged 30% in three volunteers, although intersubject variability was large (range 18% to 46%). A linear relationship between dose and area under the concentration-time curve (AUC), and superposition of dose-normalized concentration-time data, were observed.[28] Hepatic presystemic elimination is further documented by Huet and colleagues,[29] who reported a bioavailability of 38.7% ± 4.9% in nine normal volunteers and 90.6% ± 5.5% in 12 cirrhotic patients who underwent end-to-end portocaval shunt surgery.[29] Significant increases in lidocaine bioavailability have also been reported in ten cirrhotic patients before and two to three weeks after portocaval shunt surgery.[152] Absolute lidocaine bioavailability, determined after single 100 mg oral and intravenous doses, increased from a mean of 0.77 ± 0.05 to 0.98 ± 0.03 after surgery. These data demonstrate that lidocaine is extensively metabolized before reaching the systemic circulation. Due to the variability in the rate and extent of absorption[19] and the nausea, vomiting, and abdominal discomfort observed after oral administration, this route is not recommended.

Rectal administration of lidocaine has been evaluated in six normal volunteers[43] and compared to intravenous and oral administration. Following a rectal dose of

300 mg, lidocaine bioavailability ranged from 45% to 107% (mean 71%) using whole blood concentrations as compared to 31% after a 300 mg oral dose. The mean peak blood concentration was approximately 1.5 µg/mL and occurred at 20 minutes after the rectal dose.

Intramuscular administration avoids the first-pass effect of the oral route and has been extensively evaluated in patients and normal volunteers. Antiarrhythmic effects of lidocaine have been observed with doses of 200 to 400 mg.[30–36] Lidocaine concentrations measured in all studies usually exceeded 1.0 µg/mL at 10 minutes and persisted above 1.0 µg/mL for 90 to 120 minutes.[30–36] Peak concentrations after intramuscular doses of 200 to 400 mg were 1.5 to 6.5 µg/mL[8,30,31,34,36]

The site of intramuscular administration is an important factor in determining peak lidocaine concentrations.[34–36] Peak lidocaine concentrations were achieved earlier and were significantly higher with deltoid administration than with vastus lateralis administration or with gluteus administration. In one study,[37] absorption half-life was approximately 12 minutes after injection into the deltoid muscle and 26 minutes after injection into the vastus lateralis or gluteus.

Lidocaine is absorbed systemically when administered as a local anesthetic.[40,41] In general, studies have found that peak lidocaine concentrations achieved by local anesthesia are linearly related to the administered dose and that the rate of absorption depends upon the vascularity of the site of administration.[13] Coadministration of epinephrine appears to decrease peak lidocaine concentrations from all sites of administration.[13] A table of peak concentrations and their times of occurrence with different routes of administration is presented in a recent review.[13] Lidocaine and its two major metabolites, monoethylglycinexylidide (MEGX) and glycinexylidide (GX), have been measured in subjects given nebulized 4% lidocaine before fiberoptic bronchoscopy.[42] The mean administered dose was 287 mg, and the mean peak lidocaine plasma concentration was 1.54 µg/mL (range 0.6 to 3.3 µg/mL). Measurable but clinically insignificant metabolite concentrations were found in 11 of 19 patients.

Significant concentrations of lidocaine have also been reported in patients receiving 1% lidocaine solution for local anesthesia before electrophysiologic study.[154] Following subcutaneous administration, at anesthetic doses of 1 to 5 mg/kg in 17 patients, Nattel et al. reported that peak lidocaine concentrations occurred at 60 minutes and ranged from 0.3 to 1.5 µg/mL. Other investigators have observed therapeutic concentrations following similar anesthetic doses.[155,156] At anesthetic doses less than 2.5 mg/kg, therapeutic concentrations are unlikely. To minimize the influence of lidocaine on the interpretation of electrophysiologic studies, the lowest dose of lidocaine (i.e., 1% solution) should be utilized. Since therapeutic and occasionally toxic concentrations of lidocaine are achieved from anesthetic doses of lidocaine, it seems prudent to monitor lidocaine concentrations in patients with conditions known to reduce lidocaine clearance or when high doses are required.

Distribution

Appropriate use of lidocaine requires a knowledge of its extravascular distribution. Blood concentrations fall rapidly after intravenous bolus administration[10,11,19] due to lidocaine's large volume of distribution. In addition, distributional changes have been reported in patients with CHF or acute myocardial infarction receiving lidocaine for treatment or prophylaxis of arrhythmias.[15,44] Lidocaine partitions extensively into body tissues in man and animals.[46-48] There is no direct information about lidocaine tissue-to-plasma partition coefficients in man. However, using information on extraction ratios and blood flows in normal volunteers, together with partition values measured in monkeys, Benowitz and colleagues suggest that lidocaine initially distributes to the lungs, then to the heart and kidneys, followed by redistribution of drug into muscle and adipose tissue. They report steady-state tissue-to-plasma partition coefficients in normal rhesus monkeys of 3.46 for the spleen, 3.08 for the lungs, 2.80 for the kidneys, 2.43 for the stomach, and 2.00 for adipose tissue. Lower values are reported for the heart (0.96), brain (1.21), and muscle (0.65).[46,47] Partition coefficients in patients with cardiovascular disease, in aged patients, or in patients receiving lidocaine continuous infusions have not been investigated. This information would greatly increase knowledge of lidocaine behavior in the clinical setting.

Extensive tissue distribution of lidocaine is supported by values found for central and steady-state volumes of distribution. Representative volumes of distribution in young, healthy, normal volunteers following single-bolus doses are 0.48 ± 0.12 L/kg for volume of central compartment (V_1), 1.08 ± 0.12 L/kg for steady-state volume of distribution (V_{ss}), and 1.58 ± 0.30 for volume of distribution by the area method (V_{area}).[10] These values are similar to those reported by other investigators.[11,15,19,49,50] Steady-state volume of distribution does not appear to change during long-term (24-hour) infusions.[50] The volume of distribution, as calculated by the area method, has been reported to be similar in young (mean age 29 years) and elderly (mean age 70 years) males. Volume of distribution (V_{area}), is also similar in young (mean age 28 years) and elderly (mean age 72 years) females.[52] Volume of distribution (V_{area}) uncorrected for total body weight is greater in young obese subjects as compared to young normal subjects and is correlated with percent ideal body weight.[51] When corrected for total body weight, there were no significant differences between obese and nonobese populations. Lidocaine volume of distribution also appears to be approximately 33% greater for young healthy women than for men.[51,52]

Patients with CHF appear to have a smaller mean V_1 (0.31 L/kg) than do normal subjects,[15,44] although V_1 may be increased in patients with acute myocardial infarction but no heart failure.[44] V_{ss} may be slightly reduced in CHF.[15] V_1 and V_{ss} are increased in patients with acute viral hepatitis to 1.0 ± 0.6 L/kg and 3.1 ± 1.8 L/kg, respectively.[53] Renal disease has not been shown to influence distribution.[15] A two-compartment open pharmacokinetic model can adequately describe lidocaine's blood concentration-time profile[10,11,15,49] and has been used in planning dosage regimens.[67] Table 21-1 lists the median and mean two-compartment parameters determined in 20 patients receiving lidocaine for ventricular arrhythmias.[67] Of particular note is the higher value for V_{ss} than that reported for normals and the variable, non-normal distribution of parameters.

The binding of drug to tissue and blood proteins is a major determinant of the volume of distribution.[54,55] The apparent volume of distribution (V_d) can be conceptualized as the sum of the volume of circulating blood plus the product of the volume of body tissues and the ratio of unbound drug in blood and tissues.[54,55] Differences in plasma protein binding in different patients and disease-induced alterations in plasma binding are important determinants of lidocaine pharmacokinetics.[45,62,63]

The extent of lidocaine protein binding appears to be variable in plasma of normal volunteers[23,25] and is dependent upon the method of sample collection,[23,56] lidocaine concentrations,[23,57,58] pH of sample,[23,59] and binding technique utilized.[57] Investigations that have avoided Vacutainer collection tubes, studied concentrations of 2 to 3 µg/mL, controlled pH at 7.4 and utilized equilibrium dialysis techniques have reported the percentage of *unbound* lidocaine in serum and plasma to range from 21% to 39% (mean 28% to 30%).[23,25] Part of this variability can be explained by the tobacco smoking habits of the volunteers since tobacco smokers have a lower percentage of free lidocaine (26 ± 4) than do nonsmokers (31 ± 3).[60] The major binding site for lidocaine in plasma is α_1-acid glycoprotein (AAG).[25,61-63] Plasma AAG concentrations are known to vary widely in normal volunteers[25,64] and to correlate with the binding ratio of lidocaine.[24,25] The percentage of unbound lidocaine decreases with age from 48% ± 5% in neonates (30 to 36 weeks); 32% ± 7% in infants (1 to 12 months); 26% ± 7% in children (1 to 5 years) and 26% ± 6% in adolescents (12 to 18 years).[153] The percentage of lidocaine binding to isolated human serum albumin (4.0 to 4.5 gm/dL) has been reported as 20% to 22%.[23,25] These studies documented that AAG binds 60% to 70% of lidocaine that is bound in serum and that albumin binds approximately 30% of lidocaine bound at therapeutic concentrations. Therefore, if 70% of lidocaine is bound in serum, approximately 20% of the total is bound to albumin and approximately 50% to AAG (30% and 70% of the bound fraction, respectively).

The effects of lidocaine metabolites, drugs, and disease states on lidocaine binding have been evaluated. The lidocaine metabolites, 3-OH lidocaine, 4-OH lidocaine, MEGX and GX, at concentrations of 1 µg/mL, do not significantly alter

Table 21-1. Two-Compartment Parameters for Lidocaine

Parameter	Median	Mean (± SEM)
k_{10}	0.0133 min^{-1}	0.316 min^{-1} (± 0.015)
k_{12}	0.0471 min^{-1}	0.0865 min^{-1} (± 0.024)
k_{21}	0.0194 min^{-1}	0.0315 min^{-1} (± 0.009)
V_1[a]	0.49 L/kg	0.49 min^{-1} (± 0.25)
V_β[a]	2.52 L/kg	2.97 L/kg (± 1.69)
V_{ss}[a]	2.10 L/kg	2.72 L/kg (± 1.26)

[a] Based on actual (total) body weight.

serum binding of lidocaine. However, therapeutic concentrations of quinidine and disopyramide significantly increased the percentage of free lidocaine, by 34% and 21%, respectively.[23] Plasma concentrations of AAG have been reported to be higher (103 mg/dL) in epileptic patients receiving phenytoin, carbamazepine, primidone, and phenytoin plus phenobarbital than in age and gender-matched controls (65 mg/dL).[63] The mean percentage of free lidocaine in the plasma of epileptic patients (28%) was lower than in control subjects (34%). The percentage of unbound lidocaine in the plasma of females taking estrogen-progestogen oral contraceptives (37% ± 3.8%) was significantly greater than in the control females (34% ± 5%). The females receiving the oral contraceptives showed significantly lower AAG concentrations (52 ± 10 mg/dL versus 62% ± 12 mg/dL).[65] Percent free lidocaine was the same in males (32% ± 4%) and contraceptive-free females. Various drugs can alter lidocaine protein binding by either displacing lidocaine from binding sites and/or altering AAG concentrations. The clinical significance of these findings has not been thoroughly investigated. However, these changes could potentially have important effects on both the pharmacokinetics of unbound lidocaine and on the interpretation of total concentrations.

AAG concentrations, along with other acute phase reactant proteins, are known to increase after acute myocardial infarction[66] and have been shown to cause significant changes in the binding of lidocaine.[62] It has been reported that a significant increase in AAG concentrations occurs in acute myocardial infarction patients 36 hours after admission to a coronary care unit (140 mg/dL, as compared to 117 mg/dL at the time of admission). The percentage of free lidocaine was significantly reduced, from 30.2% to 25.6%, over this 36-hour period. These changes in AAG concentrations and lidocaine binding may explain in part the accumulation of lidocaine that has been observed in myocardial infarction patients given long-term lidocaine infusions.[26,62,82] Following nonurgent cardiac surgery in 13 males, AAG concentrations increased from a mean preoperative value of 63 ± 23 mg/dL to 72 ± 18 at 12 hours postoperation, 112 ± 34 at 24 hours, 150 ± 72 hours and 157 ± 39 at 120 hours.[158] Percent lidocaine unbound actually increased above preoperative values (31%) immediately postoperation (58%) but decreased at 72 hours (23%) and 150 hours (22%). This biphasic alteration in lidocaine binding should be considered when interpreting total lidocaine concentrations.

Metabolism

The metabolic fate of lidocaine has been extensively presented in previous reports.[13,27,70,71] The proposed pathways for the metabolism of lidocaine are summarized in Figure 21-1. Lidocaine is metabolized primarily by the liver.[27,28,68-71] Sequential oxidative N-dealkylation of lidocaine by the cytochrome P450 system in hepatic microsomes produces MEGX and GX. It has been suggested that cytochrome P450IIIA4 is responsible for microsomal MEGX formation.[159] The hepatic extraction ratio for lidocaine has been reported between 62% and 81%[27-29,68] in man and as 99% in a perfused rat liver preparation.[72] Approximately 2% of an administered oral dose of lidocaine is excreted as intact drug in the urine over 24 hours.[27] The primary metabolite found in the urine was 4-hydroxy 2,6-xylidine, which comprised 73% of the dose. MEGX and GX are found in small quantities: 4.0% and 2.5%, respectively.[27,70,71] Other metabolic products recovered in the urine in amounts of less than 1.0% of an administered dose included 3-hydroxy lidocaine, 3-hydroxy MEGX and 2,6-xylidine.[27] Approximately 10% to 20% of a dose is excreted as N-hydroxy derivatives of lidocaine and MEGX.[71] In a perfused rat liver preparation, data suggest that lidocaine disposition is best predicted where a low-affinity, high-capacity N-de-ethylation system is anterior to a high-affinity, low-capacity hydroxylation system.[160]

In animal models of arrhythmia, MEGX has been shown to have 80% to 90% and GX, 10% to 26%, of the antiarrhythmic potency of lidocaine[69,81] based on total drug concentrations. In isolated guinea pig ventricular myocytes, GX appears to competitively displace lidocaine from sodium channel receptors. The clinical significance of this observation is unknown.[161]

In the study by Thompson et al. lidocaine (104 mg), MEGX (102 mg) and lidocaine plus MEGX, were administered intravenously to eight male volunteers.[157] Transient side effects were experienced by all subjects, with side effects most pronounced with the combination, somewhat less with lidocaine and mild

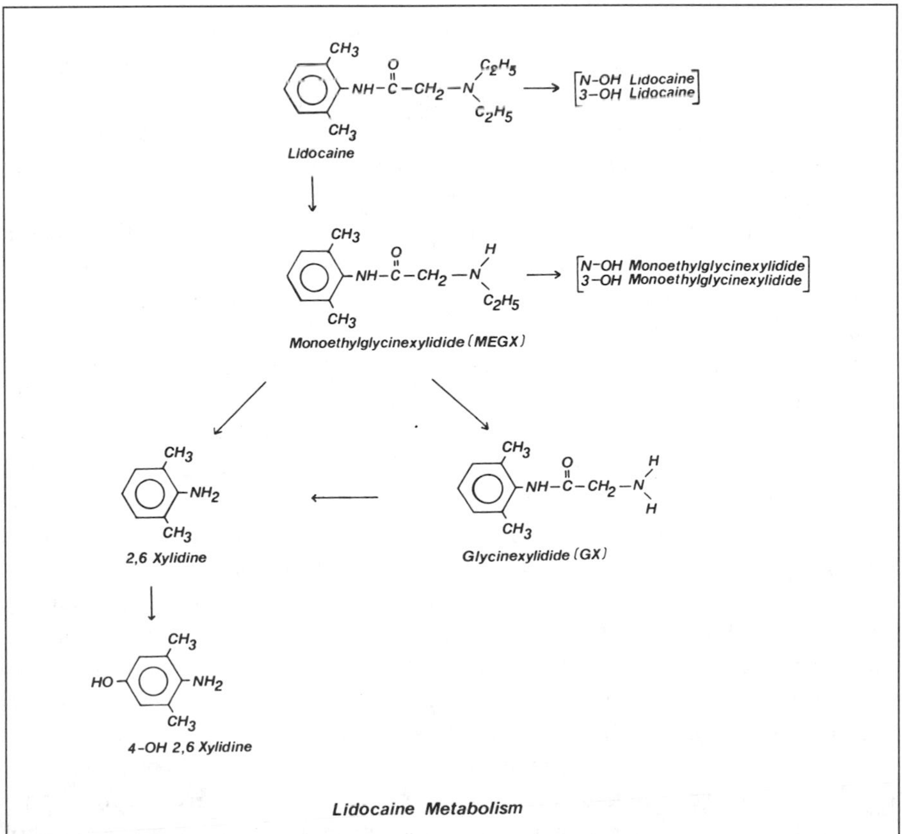

Figure 21-1. *The predominant metabolic routes for lidocaine are summarized above. See text for further discussion.*

with MEGX.[157] The most common side effects tinnitus, dizziness, light light-headedness, and other CNS effects were transient, lasting less than 15 minutes in all cases. The toxicity of GX was evaluated by Strong et al. who demonstrated that GX (276 and 697 mg doses) produced high clinically-achievable concentrations (1.5 to 6.0 µg/mL).[69] No CNS or cardiovascular adverse effects were observed; however, headache and impaired ability to concentrate were reported.

There is no convincing evidence that MEGX and GX independently contribute to the spectrum of toxicities observed after lidocaine administration. The contribution of MEGX and GX to the side effect profile observed during prolonged lidocaine infusions has not been rigorously investigated.

MEGX and GX have been identified in the blood of patients receiving lidocaine infusions.[74,76–79] The mean ratio of serum concentrations of MEGX to lidocaine after a 10- to 24-hour lidocaine infusion is reported to be 0.11 to 0.36 in cardiac patients without cardiac failure[4,76,79] and 0.28 in patients with cardiac failure.[76] The mean ratio of GX to lidocaine in cardiac patients is between 0.05 and 0.11.[74,79]

In four patients with renal failure given 12-hour lidocaine infusions, MEGX concentrations ranged from 20% to 66% of the lidocaine values.[77] The protein binding of lidocaine, MEGX, and GX in serum from five normal volunteers, at 20 °C, averaged 50% ± 9%, 15% ± 3%, and 5% ± 4%, respectively.[79] In seven patients, two days after acute myocardial infarction, mean lidocaine binding was 55% ± 6% and that of MEGX was 14% ± 3%. Therefore, the mean free fraction in patient serum was 45% for lidocaine and 86% for MEGX. Since the intensity of drug effect is thought to be better related to unbound drug concentrations, total MEGX:lidocaine concentration ratios should be corrected for differences in protein binding before one can assess the activity of MEGX relative to lidocaine. The estimated free MEGX:lidocaine ratio averaged 0.68 ± 0.49 in these seven patients with myocardial infarction. Since MEGX is 0.8 to 0.9 times as potent as lidocaine, MEGX may contribute to the pharmacologic effects of lidocaine in a substantial number of patients.

The serum concentration of MEGX following intravenous bolus doses of lidocaine (1 mg/kg) to liver donors has been used to predict liver graft survival in recipients.[162–164] In addition, the magnitude of MEGX concentrations in liver transplant recipients may be useful for post-transplant follow-up.[165] The survival rate for transplant recipients was higher, for up to 100 days post-transplant, if recipients received livers from donors with MEGX concentrations greater than 90 ng/mL at 15 minutes as compared to recipients receiving livers from donors with MEGX concentrations less than 90 ng/mL.[162] Use of this approach is clinically applicable with the recent introduction of a fluorescence polarization immunoassay technique (Abbott Laboratories, Chicago Illinois, USA) for MEGX. The limit of sensitivity of the assay is 10 ng/mL with coefficients of variation of less than 4% and an analysis time of 20 minutes or less.[166]

Lidocaine is more lipophilic than its two metabolites and has an octanol:buffer (pH 7.4) partition coefficient of 65.0. The coefficients for MEGX and GX are 5.7 and 1.3. Differences in these partition coefficients mirror differences in extent of protein binding. There was no effect of age on steady-state MEGX plasma concentrations normalized for lidocaine infusion rate; however, GX concentrations, normalized for lidocaine infusion rate, decreased with age.[79] This is to be expected, since 50% of GX is eliminated unchanged in the urine.[69]

The mean elimination half-life of MEGX was 2.33 ± 0.35 hours after an intravenous bolus dose of 100 mg MEGX base in eight healthy male volunteers.[167] Mean volume of distribution was 154 ± 47 L and mean systemic clearance was 50.3 ± 12.3 L/hr. The formation and elimination kinetics of MEGX are independent of dose or time following single intravenous and oral doses of lidocaine.[28] The concentrations of MEGX are much less than those of lidocaine after intravenous doses, but similar to those of lidocaine after oral administration. Although concentrations differ, the dose-normalized area under the MEGX concentration-time curve is similar for oral and intravenous administration.[28]

Following intravenous administration of 4 mg/kg of GX to two normal volunteers, the mean elimination half-life was 9.8 hours and the mean clearance 168 mL/min. The mean renal clearance of GX was 82 mL/min, and renal elimination of GX accounted for 49% of the dose.[69] Metabolism of GX to xylidine accounted for 4.5% of the dose. The fate of the remaining 40% to 50% of the dose is unknown.

Clearance and Half-Life

The systemic clearance and elimination half-life of lidocaine have been determined in healthy young volunteers, children, elderly, and obese volunteers (see Table 21-2), and in patients with various disease states (see Table 21-3). The mean systemic clearance and half-life of lidocaine following single intravenous bolus doses of 25 to 200 mg in young, healthy male volunteers is 15.6 ± 4.6 mL/min/kg and 1.6 ± 0.18 hours, respectively. The mean metabolic (hepatic) clearance in normal male subjects is 15.3 ± 4.6 mL/min/kg. Greater than 98% of an administered lidocaine dose can be recovered in the urine as metabolites and parent compound. These values and all subsequent values were calculated from the individual studies referenced. Because of potential differences in subject definition, drug administration, data analysis, etc., these values represent approximate estimates for mean half-life and clearance. Young female volunteers appear to have an increased clearance and half-life and a larger volume of distribution than do young, healthy male volunteers.[51,52] The systemic clearance and half-life of lidocaine in children, ages six months to three years, is not significantly different than normal adult volunteers.[168] Elderly men and women demonstrate a reduced clearance and a prolonged half-live as compared to young controls. This would suggest that for comparable lidocaine concentrations, elderly subjects should have lidocaine infusion rates reduced 20% to 30%. Lidocaine clearance, adjusted to ideal body weight in young, obese volunteers, was similar to that in normal controls.[51] However, half-life is significantly prolonged and volume of distribution increased. Lidocaine loading doses should be based then, on total body weight and maintenance infusions adjusted using ideal body weight.

As lidocaine is eliminated primarily by the liver, systemic clearance is controlled by the three factors responsible for hepatic clearance: rate of drug delivery

Table 21-2. Lidocaine Half-Life and Clearance Values (Population Means ± Estimated SD)

Population	Number of subjects	Dose	Age (years)	Terminal t½ (hr)	Clearance (mL/min/kg)
Normal males[10, 11, 15, 19, 28, 49–52]	75	25–200 mg IV bolus	25–54	1.6 ± 0.18	15.6 ± 4.6
Normal females[28, 51, 52]	22	25–100 mg IV bolus	22–38	2.11 ± 0.18	20.2 ± 1.0
Children[168]	10	1 mg/kg IV bolus	0.5–3	0.97 ± 0.32	11.1 ± 1.8
Normal elderly males[49, 52]	12	25–50 mg IV bolus	61–88	2.51 ± 0.75	10.5 ± 2.8
Normal elderly females[52]	7	25 mg IV bolus	64–88	2.27 ± 0.21	18.3 ± 2.0
Young obese male[51]	14	25 mg IV bolus	29–40	2.69 ± 0.20	19.5 ± 1.6[a]
Young obese female[51]	11	25 mg IV bolus	26–38	2.88 ± 0.31	19.7 ± 1.5[a]

[a] Clearance normalized for ideal body weight.

Table 21-3. *Lidocaine Half-Life and Clearance Values (Population Means ± Estimated SD)*

Population	Number of subjects	Duration of infusion	Age (years)	Terminal t½ (hr)	Clearance (mL/min/kg)
Congestive heart failure (CHF)[15,16,22,49]	30	24 hr	44–73	3.66 ± 2.46	5.5 ± 1.7
Acute myocardial infarction (AMI)[22,26,82,85]	58	16 hr	41–70	4.22 ± 1.79	9.1 ± 2.0
CHF + AMI[22,82,84]	29	24 hr	36–83	7.81 ± 2.48	6.3 ± 1.4
Chronic liver disease[15,86]	29	(PO, n = 21) (IV bolus, n = 8)[a]	45–68	6.13 ± 4.15	6.0 ± 3.2[a]
Renal disease[15,77]	10	(IV bolus, n = 6) (12-hr, n = 4)	24–38	1.76 ± 0.64	13.2 ± 3.2[a]
Orthostatic hypotension[87]	5	(IV bolus)	53–75	2.23 ± 0.17	8.6 ± 1.4

[a] Only IV data were used to determine clearance.

to the liver (Q_H, hepatic blood flow); ability of the liver to irreversibly remove drug from the blood (CLu_{int}, intrinsic free clearance) and the fraction of drug unbound in the blood (f_{ub}, free fraction).[55] Effective hepatic blood flow (Q_H) is influenced directly by cardiac output and indirectly by shunts bypassing the metabolic site(s) in the liver. The venous equilibrium or "well-stirred" model incorporates these factors as follows:

$$CL_s \approx CL_H = Q_H E = \frac{Q_H \cdot f_{ub} \cdot CLu_{int}}{Q_H + f_{ub} \cdot CLu_{int}}$$

(Eq. 21-1)

where CL_H is hepatic (metabolic) clearance; Q_H is hepatic blood flow; E is extraction ratio; f_{ub} is fraction unbound in blood; and CLu_{int} is free intrinsic clearance.

Using mean values from normal volunteers for f_{ub} (0.3), Q_H (21.5 mL/min/kg) and CL_H (15.3 mL/min/kg), the estimated value of CLu_{int} for lidocaine is 170 mL/min/kg.

Since estimated free intrinsic clearance is several fold larger than hepatic blood flow, hepatic clearance seems to be primarily determined by hepatic blood flow,[88] and will be altered in disease states characterized by changes in effective hepatic blood flow (e.g., CHF, liver disease, hypotension).

Elimination half-life ($t\frac{1}{2}$) is dependent on CL_s and distribution:

$$t\frac{1}{2} = \frac{0.693 \, V_d}{CL_S}$$

(Eq. 21-2)

Thus, changes in hepatic blood flow and drug binding are major determinants of lidocaine half-life.

Decreased hepatic blood flow associated with reduction in cardiac output from CHF,[15,16,49] age,[49,52] or acute myocardial infarction[22,26,82–85] reduces lidocaine clearance. Mean systemic clearance of lidocaine in patients with CHF is 35% of normal values, and mean half-life is prolonged by more than twofold.[15,16,22,29] Although most heart failure patients are elderly, the reductions in clearance with heart failure are greater than can be explained by age. In patients suffering with acute myocardial infarction, mean systemic clearance of lidocaine is reduced by about 40%, to 9.1 ± 2.0 mL/min/kg (see Table 21-3). These changes are not great enough to explain the changes in half-life; apparently distribution is also altered. Serum protein binding of lidocaine is increased following myocardial infarction (see Clinical Pharmacokinetics: Distribution) and, along with reduced hepatic clearance, this increase explains the prolonged elimination observed in patients.[26,49,67,68] In patients with CHF and myocardial infarction, mean half-life may be prolonged to over seven hours (see Table 21-3). Maintenance lidocaine infusion rates must be reduced in proportion to reduction in systemic clearance in order to maintain therapeutic concentrations (see Clinical Pharmacokinetics).

The systemic clearance of lidocaine is reduced to variable degrees in patients with chronic liver disease.[15] Whether this reduction is due to a decrease in effective hepatic blood flow[89] or to impaired metabolism, infusion regimens must be reduced to prevent lidocaine accumulation. Lidocaine clearance has been reported to be normal or decreased in patients with active hepatitis[53] and reduced in chronic cirrhosis.[15,86] Although the presence of abnormal serum albumin and prothrombin time has been reported to be associated with a prolonged lidocaine half-life in patients with chronic liver disease, these indices are not sufficiently sensitive to be useful guides for adjusting dosage regimens.

Hepatic blood flow and intrinsic free clearance can be altered by other drugs, including propranolol,[90,91] cimetidine,[75,92] and anticonvulsants[33,63] (see Table 21-4). Lidocaine may alter hepatic blood flow[94] during constant-rate infusions of 2 to 4 mg/min, and this change would alter its clearance; but other data suggest lidocaine has little effect on cardiovascular hemodynamics.[95,96]

Propranolol, in moderate beta-blocking doses, reduces lidocaine systemic clearance by 40% to 50%.[90,91] Metoprolol reduces systemic clearance by approximately 30%. These changes are attributed largely to a beta-blocker-induced reduction in cardiac output and hepatic blood flow, although the changes in clearance are greater than would be predicted from the observed reductions in cardiac index induced by propranolol.[97,98] Since propranolol has been shown to reduce antipyrine clearance (a marker of intrinsic clearance),[99,100] propranolol may, in addition, reduce the hepatic oxidative metabolism of lidocaine. A 15% to 45% reduction in lidocaine clearance has been observed after coadministration of cimetidine.[75,92,169–172] Cimetidine significantly reduces lidocaine intrinsic clearance. Cimetidine appears to have no significant effect on lidocaine free fraction. Powell and colleagues[182] have reported that lidocaine systemic clearance is reduced by 15% and mean half-life increased from 1.5 to 2.02 hours by an oral cimetidine regimen of 300 mg every six hours for two days. One hour pretreatment with a 300 mg intravenous cimetidine dose has no significant effects on lidocaine disposition. No interaction was observed between lidocaine and ranitidine.[93] To date, there are no reports in the literature regarding an interaction between lidocaine and other H_2-antagonists.

Excretion

The renal clearance of lidocaine contributes less than 5% to the total systemic clearance.[27,70,71,73,79] Renal elimination accounts for 40% to 60% of the overall elimination of GX.[75] Acidification of the urine to pH less than 5.5 has been reported to increase renal elimination of unchanged lidocaine to 3% to 7%,[71,73] but this fact is not likely to be clinically significant. The results of two studies of patients with chronic renal failure suggest that volume of distribution, elimination half-life, and clearance[15,77] are similar to those found in normal subjects (see Tables 21-3 and 21-4). MEGX concentrations appear to plateau and decline in parallel with lidocaine concentrations in patients with renal failure. GX concentrations appear to persist relatively unchanged for 12 hours after lidocaine is discontinued.[77] Renal failure does not appear to cause accumulation of MEGX. GX concentrations may accumulate, but are unlikely to cause significant toxicity.

Table 21-4. Drug-Induced Alteration in Lidocaine Clearance and Half-Life

Drugs	Population	Number of subjects	Dose lidocaine	Drug	Age (years)	Terminal t½ (hr)		Clearance (mL/min/kg)[b]		References
						Pre-drug	Post-drug	Pre-drug	Post-drug	
Propranolol	Healthy males	6	3 mg/kg	40 mg Q 6 hr × 4	22–31	1.5 ± 0.3	2.0 ± 0.3	14.6 ± 4.7	7.8 ± 2.8	90
Metoprolol	Healthy males	6	3 mg/kg	50 mg Q 6 hr × 4	22–31	1.6 ± 0.3	1.9 ± 0.5	14.6 ± 4.7	10.1 ± 3.3	90
Propranolol	Healthy males (4)	7	150–300 mg	80 mg Q 8 hr × 9	18–25	1.08 ± 0.37	1.68 ± 0.6	18.0 ± 7.6	10.7 ± 3.1	91
Cimetidine	Healthy males (15)	24	1 mg/kg (76 mg)	1000–1200 (mg/day)	20–43	1.8 ± 0.2	2.5 ± 0.4	12.04 ± 5.4	9.34 ± 3.7	75, 92
	Healthy males	7	2 mg/kg	1200 mg/day	21–28	1.2 ± 0.2	1.8 ± 0.2	16.6 ± 4.4	11.6 ± 3.4	169
	Healthy males	6	100 mg	1200 mg/day	21–33	1.5 ± 0.4	2.02 ± 0.6	12.1 ± 4.8	10.3 ± 5.0	172
Ranitidine	Healthy males (4) Healthy females (2)	6	1 mg/kg (65 mg)	150 mg Q 12 hr × 2	21–35	1.2 ± 0.5	1.3 ± 0.5	12.9 ± 5.4	12.8 ± 5.4	93

a Half-life reported as mean values ± SD.
b Clearance is reported as mean values ± SD.

PHARMACODYNAMICS

Relationship Between Concentration and Therapeutic Effect

The earliest and most widely quoted work on the concentration-therapeutic response relationship of lidocaine was reported by Gianelly and colleagues in 1967.[6] They studied 21 post-myocardial infarction patients who received lidocaine infusions of 7 to 128 µg/kg/min for 2 to 65 hours. Lidocaine blood samples were collected on at least four occasions and analyzed by a gas liquid chromatographic method. A beneficial effect was defined as a 50% or greater reduction in the number of premature ventricular contractions (PVCS). Although a quantitative relationship between arrhythmia control and lidocaine concentrations was not reported, blood concentrations of 2 to 5 µg/mL were recommended for treatment of ventricular arrhythmias.

Three studies have reported relationships between concentrations of lidocaine administered intramuscularly and antiarrhythmic effect.[31,32,34] Eleven patients with greater than five PVCs per minute were administered 4.5 mg/kg lidocaine hydrochloride 10% into the deltoid muscle.[34] Seventy-five percent PVC suppression was achieved at five minutes at a mean whole blood lidocaine concentration of 1.8 µg/mL. At 60 minutes, PVC suppression remained at 75% at a mean concentration of 2.2 µg/mL. In a similar group of 15 patients given 250 mg of intramuscular lidocaine, greater than 75% suppression of PVCs occurred in 7 of 15 patients at 30 minutes at a mean concentration of 2.9 ± 1.7 µg/mL (range 0.7 to 5.9 µg/mL).[32] Mean reduction of greater than 75% of baseline ectopic frequency was also observed at 60 minutes at a mean concentration of 2.4 µg/mL. In ten patients with various cardiovascular diseases, greater than 75% reduction in PVCs was observed in all patients for up to 45 minutes following a 300 mg intramuscular dose.[31] Whole-blood concentrations measured at 15, 30, and 45 minutes averaged 2.6, 2.7, and 2.4 µg/mL, respectively. Plasma or serum concentrations may be as much as 20% lower than whole blood concentrations because of observed concentration-dependent erythrocyte uptake over the therapeutic range.[58,60]

In nine patients with acute myocardial infarction, greater than 75% reduction in ectopic beats was observed at a mean concentration of 2.5 µg/mL following a 100 mg intravenous bolus and a simultaneous 300 mg intramuscular dose. When concentrations fell below 1.5 µg/mL, PVC frequency was similar to that observed before treatment.[101] Although it appears that a majority of patients demonstrate greater than 75% suppression of arrhythmia frequency at mean blood lidocaine concentrations of 2 to 2.5 µg/mL, higher concentrations are often required for arrhythmia control. Furthermore, adverse effects to the central nervous system may be observed before an antiarrhythmic effect is achieved.[7,102]

Lidocaine concentrations of greater than 1.5 µg/mL are required for effective prophylaxis against primary ventricular fibrillation (PVF) following acute myocardial infarction.[17] A multiple-bolus-plus-infusion regimen that is reported to be highly successful in preventing PVF attains mean plasma lidocaine concentrations greater than 2.0 µg/mL ten minutes after initiation.[44] The lidocaine concentration required to minimize the risk of PVF with an acceptable risk of toxicity is 1.5 to 2.0 µg/mL.

Further research is required to define a therapeutic range for lidocaine. Questions that remain unanswered include the effects of intersubject variability in the protein binding of lidocaine, the effects of metabolites, and the effects of concomitant disease and drug therapy on the concentrations required for the treatment and prevention of ventricular arrhythmias.

Relationship Between Concentration and Toxicity

The relationship between lidocaine blood concentrations and CNS toxicity was first reported in 1960.[103] Lidocaine, 0.5 mg/kg/min, was infused intravenously to ten healthy male volunteers until symptoms of central nervous system toxicity (e.g., twitching, convulsions, muscular fasciculations, disorientation) developed. The mean time to onset of symptoms was 12.8 ± 1.1 minutes (6.4 mg/kg), at which time mean blood concentrations were 5.3 ± 0.6 µg/mL. Signs of cortical irritability (fasciculations or twitching) were observed in all subjects. These data have been used since the 1960s to define the upper end of the lidocaine therapeutic range. Limitations of this study include: 1) the use of a colorimetric assay with limited information available regarding its reproducibility, specificity, and precision; 2) the difficulty of extrapolating results from a small number of young, healthy male volunteers to patients; and 3) the differences in response to acute, high-dose administration and to conventional lidocaine dosing.

Several studies have measured lidocaine concentrations in cardiac patients with lidocaine-associated toxicity.[6,7,17,18,22,24,104] These studies suggest that subjective CNS effects such as drowsiness, dizziness, paresthesias, and euphoria can occur at concentrations of 3 to 6 µg/mL. Objective signs of toxicity, such as fasciculations, visual disturbances, and tinnitus, usually occur at concentrations from 6 to 8 µg/mL. Serious signs of toxicity (seizures, obtundation) are most frequently seen at concentrations greater than 8 µg/mL.

Total and free lidocaine serum concentrations have been measured in 22 patients with clinically assessed lidocaine toxicity during long-term (>12 hours) intravenous infusions.[24] Toxicity was classified as 1+ (slurred speech, numbness, dizziness, trembling, dry mouth); 2+ (loss of coordination, confusion, visual disturbances, agitation, somnolence); and 3+ (muscular fasciculation, hallucinations, unresponsiveness and seizures).[151] Mean (± 1 SD) total lidocaine concentrations in the three groups were 4.3 ± 1.4 µg/mL (n = 8); 5.9 ± 2.7 µg/mL (n = 11); and 6.6 ± 2.5 µg/mL (n = 5). Corresponding mean (± 1 SD) free lidocaine concentrations were 1.9 ± 0.8, 2.3 ± 0.9, and 3.4 ± 2.0 µg/mL. There were no statistical differences among these mean concentrations. However, the expected trend of increased concentrations of both free and total drug with increased severity of toxicity was observed. The patients in group 3+ had the highest percentage of free lidocaine (51%) and the lowest mean AAG concentrations (102 mg/dL). The inability to statistically differentiate severity of toxicity by total or free concentrations, or to confirm that free concentrations are a better indicator of toxicity was probably due to the small number of patients and the large variability in concentrations and protein binding in each group. Variable sensitivity of central nervous system receptors may also be a factor, as may interpatient variability in penetration of lidocaine into the central nervous system.

Several factors have been associated with lidocaine toxicity in cardiac patients.[105] Four percent of 750 lidocaine recipients were reported to have adverse CNS effects associated with lidocaine. Adverse effects were more frequent in patients experiencing acute myocardial infarction and/or CHF, in patients weighing less than 70 kg, and in patients greater than 70 years of age. Since lidocaine clearance is known to be reduced in the presence of these factors and doses may not have been appropriately adjusted, these findings are expected. The incidence of toxicity has been reported to be 15% to 20% in smaller studies where side-effects were closely monitored.[17,106] Although the majority of adverse effects of lidocaine involved the CNS, 17% to 20% of adverse effects were cardiovascular, representing a 1% incidence in all patients who received lidocaine.[105] The most common cardiovascular adverse effects are conduction disturbances, bradyarrhythmias, and hypotension. Hypotension or decreased cardiac output is probably uncommon unless sustained concentrations are greater than 9 µg/mL,[107] but the data on the relationship between lidocaine concentrations and cardiovascular adverse effects are limited.

Contribution of the lidocaine metabolites MEGX and GX to lidocaine toxicity has not been firmly established. There have been reports of lidocaine toxicity in patients with total lidocaine concentrations of less that 5 µg/mL,[69,75] GX concentrations above 2 µg/mL and MEGX concentrations greater than 4 µg/mL.[76] However, these observations could be explained by altered lidocaine protein binding and/or receptor sensitivity in these patients. There have been no reports to date that elevated metabolite concentrations can be definitively associated with toxic effects.

Definition of the Therapeutic Range

Based on the preceding discussion, total lidocaine blood (or serum or plasma) concentrations of 2 to 6 µg/mL constitute a rational therapeutic range. Suppression of ventricular arrhythmias at concentrations greater than 2 µg/mL are likely. At concentrations exceeding 6 µg/mL, the frequency of objective signs of CNS toxicity increases. There are, however, a significant number of patients who may require concentrations of 6 to 9 µg/mL for arrhythmia control.[7] The benefits and risks of lidocaine concentrations above 6 µg/mL must be determined carefully for patients who do not respond to usual therapeutic concentrations.

When lidocaine is administered for suppression of ventricular tachycardia, the electrocardiogram (ECG) can be used to monitor and individualize therapy. When lidocaine is administered for the prevention of PVF and for treatment of ventricular arrhythmias, no acceptable clinical endpoints of therapy exist. Lidocaine therapy in these patients should be tailored to ensure lidocaine concentrations of greater than 2 µg/mL. This population may also benefit from monitoring of free lidocaine concentrations, since protein binding is altered in patients with acute myocardial infarction (see Clinical Pharmacokinetics: Distribution). A therapeutic range for free lidocaine concentrations of 0.5 to 2.0 µg/mL can be suggested based on the concentration-dependent binding of lidocaine and the toxicity data discussed above. A better understanding of the factors that influence lidocaine concentration-response relationships and a better definition of intersubject variability would improve the utility of measured lidocaine concentrations.

CLINICAL APPLICATION OF PHARMACOKINETIC DATA

When intravenous lidocaine is administered as an initial loading dose followed by a constant-rate infusion, plasma concentrations fall after the loading dose because of distribution, then gradually rise to steady-state concentrations in 12 to 48 hours. Further, a two- to fourfold variability in concentrations is observed throughout a dosage regimen because of interpatient pharmacokinetic variability. Therefore, when a fixed-dosage scheme is used some patients have subtherapeutic concentrations, some have therapeutic concentrations, and some experience toxicity. In designing individualized dose regimens, there are three important principles that govern the clinical use of lidocaine: 1) lidocaine rapidly distributes from the blood following intravenous loading doses (multicompartmental pharmacokinetics); 2) during constant-rate intravenous infusion, lidocaine accumulates to a degree greater than predicted from single intravenous loading-dose data (time-dependent pharmacokinetics); and 3) lidocaine clearance is largely determined by hepatic blood flow and, therefore, indirectly, by cardiac output. The individualization schemes discussed below require that initial loading and infusion regimens be selected for specific clinical endpoints and adjusted based on a sound pharmacokinetic rationale.

Dosage Regimen Design

Loading Dose Regimens. The usual lidocaine regimen consists of a loading dose of 50 to 100 mg and a constant-rate maintenance infusion of 1 to 4 mg/min. However, because of rapid distribution, lidocaine concentrations often fall below the therapeutic range even when a constant-rate infusion is initiated at the time of the loading dose. This "dip" in concentrations below the usual therapeutic range is referred to as the "therapeutic gap"[4] and persists for 90 to 120 minutes after initiation of bolus and infusion therapy, when acute myocardial infarction patients are most susceptible to either ventricular arrhythmias or PVF.[20,83] Increasing the size of the loading dose to 200 to 300 mg to ensure that concentrations remain above 2 µg/mL increases the probability of toxicity.[109,110] Increasing the maintenance rate would cause toxic concentrations to accumulate at steady state.

To rapidly attain and maintain therapeutic lidocaine concentrations throughout the duration of lidocaine therapy, several loading-dose approaches have been proposed.[44,67,83,110,111,113] These proposed regimens involve either 1) the use of multiple bolus injections over 15 to 30 minutes along with a constant-rate infusion,[44,114,151] 2) an exponentially declining infusion,[110,113] or 3) stepwise-tapering infusions.[67,83,111]

The multiple-loading-dose technique consists of an initial 75 mg injection, followed by up to six 50 mg bolus injections every five minutes if necessary for arrhythmia control.[44,151] The reduction of ectopic ventricular beats to fewer than five per minute *and* complete suppression of complex ventricular arrhythmias during each four minute observation period between bolus doses is used as a measure of effectiveness. Three hundred acute myocardial infarction patients required between two and four bolus injections. PVF occurred in only 0.6% of patients. In a subset of patients without CHF who received five 50 mg injections, mean plasma lidocaine concentrations were approximately 1.1 µg/mL immediately after the initial 75 mg bolus (one minute), 1.7 µg/mL after the first 50 mg bolus (six minutes), 2.4 µg/mL after the second 50 mg bolus (11 minutes), 3.0 µg/mL after the third bolus (16 minutes), 3.5 µg/mL after the fourth bolus, and 4.3 µg/mL after the fifth and sixth bolus doses.[151] This regimen appeared to be clinically effective in either the presence or absence of CHF.

This multiple-bolus regimen has been compared to a rapid-infusion method.[112] All patients received a 75 mg loading dose over two minutes, and 150 mg during the loading period. Twelve patients received 150 mg as an 8.33 mg/min infusion over 18 minutes and six patients received three 50 mg injections every five minutes. There were no significant differences in plasma concentrations achieved by the two regimens over the first hour of therapy. However, the number of patients demonstrating mild CNS side effects was greater with the multiple-bolus technique (6 in 6) than with the infusion technique (1 in 12). Further, it has been reported that a similar regimen [1.5 mg/kg loading dose, 120 µg/kg/min for 25 minutes (8 mg/min/70 kg), and 30 µg/kg/min maintenance infusion] produced concentrations between 2 and 4 µg/mL in 70% of all measurements in 17 cardiac patients. Only 8% were higher than 4 µg/mL. However, 48% were lower than 2.5 µg/mL during the initial six hours of therapy.

Using an exponentially declining infusion rate method (87 mg loading dose and 8.3 mg/min, exponentially declining to 2.0 mg/min over 35 to 40 minutes; half-life of 40 minutes), the mean maximum lidocaine plasma concentration was 3.5 ± 1.2 µg/mL, and the mean six hour concentration was 2.5 ± 1.1 µg/mL, in eight normal male volunteers.[110] During the six hour infusion, all concentrations were in the range of 1.9 to 4.6 µg/mL (mean 2.9 ± 0.6 µg/mL).

These loading regimens appear to be capable of maintaining lidocaine concentrations in the therapeutic range for the majority of patients evaluated. The multiple-bolus technique has significant merit in that it can be easily implemented and it permits the clinician to administer the minimum amount of drug required to suppress ventricular tachycardia, as opposed to administering predetermined high-rate infusions. This regimen has also been demonstrated to be effective in 19 of 21 patients with ischemic heart disease who were considered refractory to 225 mg of lidocaine administered as multiple doses over 16 minutes.[151] Effectiveness was judged as reduction of PVCs to less than five per minute and complete suppression of complex ventricular arrhythmias. When lidocaine is administered prophylactically in patients with acute myocardial infarction but with no ectopic ventricular beats, a fixed loading regimen of 75 mg followed by 50 mg in five minutes, and an appropriate infusion, has proven highly effective in the prevention of PVF.[44]

The feasibility of more sophisticated approaches is rapidly developing. The optimal general dosage strategy of a loading regimen declining exponentially to a maintenance rate[46,67,109] for drugs exhibiting bi-exponential decline in concentrations has now been shown to be feasible[67,113 111] for routine clinical use.

A prospective, comparative evaluation of alternative dosage strategies has not been, and perhaps cannot be, done. The number of patients required would be extremely large and the cost prohibitive, if an objective clinical endpoint such as prevention of ventricular fibrillation or mortality was to be used for comparison. A retrospective clinical comparison has been done which demonstrates improved efficacy of the tapering-infusion regimen when compared to conventional therapy.[67] However, the conventional-therapy regimen evaluated was not completely consistent with the more aggressive multiple-bolus regimen that has been advocated.[114,151] Several studies have documented the ability of pharmacokinetically designed tapering-dosage regimens to provide acceptable precision in controlling lidocaine concentrations in patients.[67,111–113] Advanced computer systems and in fusion devices are currently available to provide optimal lidocaine therapy in a clinical setting.[67]

Loading-dose schemes for obese patients have not been proposed or evaluated, and the initial volume of distribution of lidocaine (V_1) in obese subjects is not known. It has been reported that V_{area} is correlated with percent ideal body weight, although no differences in V_{area} are observed between control and obese groups when corrected for total body weight.[51] These data suggest that loading doses may best be based on total body weight, but unfortunately, V_1 data were not reported in this study.

The initial volume of lidocaine is reduced in patients with CHF by 40% to 50%.[15,44,151] However, these patients also exhibited an increased rate of decline of initial plasma concentrations, so that distribution clearance was similar in CHF and non-CHF groups.[44] Reduced loading doses for patients with heart failure are commonly recommended, but supporting data is limited.

Maintenance Dose Regimens. The maintenance infusion rate of lidocaine is dependent upon the systemic clearance of lidocaine (CL_s) and the desired steady-state concentrations (C_{ss}). Since lidocaine is metabolized primarily by the liver, systemic clearance is approximated by hepatic clearance (CL_H). For a high-extraction drug like lidocaine, hepatic blood flow (Q_H) is the primary determinant of CL_s. CL_s and C_{ss} can be used to calculate maintenance infusion rates (k_o) for patients with and without various diseases as follows:

$$k_O = C_{ss} \cdot CL_s \qquad \text{(Eq. 21-3)}$$

Appropriate maintenance infusion rates can be calculated for patients with varying degrees of hepatic blood flow (cardiac output) using several approaches.[13,15,16,44,67,114–116] Proposed guidelines for maintenance dose selection include 1) use of a linear, two-compartment model where k_{10} is adjusted for age and estimated cardiac index[67] (see Appendix); 2) use of population averages for systemic clearance to calculate maintenance infusion rates (see Table 21-5); and 3) use of population estimates of clearance and volumes of distribution for selection of initial infusion rates coupled with serum concentrations for feedback information.[115–117,150,173–177]

A significant problem in designing dosage regimens is the observation that lidocaine half-life and clearance appear to change during constant-rate infusions in acute myocardial infarction and CHF patients.[22,26,50,82,84,91,119,120] This phenomenon was first reported in 1976 in a group of post-acute myocardial infarction patients with and without CHF.[82] Lidocaine half-life values of 4.3 ± 2.0 hours were reported in six acute myocardial infarction patients without clinical signs of CHF, and 10.2 ± 5.3 hours in the infarction group with CHF. It was also reported that mean lidocaine concentrations did not reach steady state during infusions of up to 46 hours in patients with or without CHF. Mean half-life values in normal volunteers are reported to be one to two hours. Therefore, steady state should be achieved within 7 to 12 hours. Mean lidocaine half-life values of three to five hours have consistently been reported in uncomplicated acute myocardial infarction patients following 15- to 65-hour infusions.[22,26,84,118] Systematic clearance values are reduced to 8.5 to 10 mL/min/kg in uncomplicated acute myocardial infarction patients.[22,84,119]

Several mechanisms have been proposed to explain nonlinear lidocaine clearance and include product inhibition,[80,178–180] alterations in lidocaine protein binding secondary to increases in AAG concentrations,[62,66,120] alterations in hepatic blood flow,[68,179] saturation of metabolism,[121,122] and lidocaine tissue binding.[180] Data suggest that the observed time-dependent pharmacokinetics of lidocaine are not

Table 21-5. *Mean Systemic Clearance and Recommended Infusion Rates for Selected Patient Populations*

Population	Mean (± SD) systemic clearance (mL/min/kg)	Infusion rate (mg/kg/min) to achieve 3 μg/mL	Infusion rate (mg/min/70 kg)
		Mean (Range)	Mean (Range)
Normal	15.6 ± 4.6	47 (33–61)	3.3 (2.3–4.3)
Congestive heart failure	5.5 ± 1.7	17 (11–22)	1.2 (0.8–1.5)
Acute myocardial infarction	9.1 ± 2.0	27 (21–33)	1.9 (1.5–2.3)
Congestive heart failure plus acute myocardial infarction	6.3 ± 1.4	19 (15–23)	1.3 (1.1–1.6)
Chronic liver disease	6.0 ± 3.2	18 (8–27)	1.3 (0.6–1.9)
Renal disease	13.2 ± 3.2	40 (30–49)	2.8 (2.1–3.4)
Propranolol coadministration	9.4 ± 3.1	28 (19–38)	2.0 (1.3–2.7)

due to changes in hepatic blood flow or plasma protein binding because nonlinear pharmacokinetics are observed *in vitro* at fixed perfusion rates with protein-free perfusate.[50,91,178] Isolated perfused rat liver studies indicate that saturation of metabolism is not a significant factor in reduction of lidocaine clearance during infusions.[178,179] Tam and colleagues[178] suggested that the deethylation of lidocaine to MEGX is dose independent. These workers and Suzuki et al. have demonstrated that MEGX and lidocaine compete for hydroxylation systems.[178,180] Inhibition of lidocaine hydroxylation by MEGX is unlikely since saturation of hydroxylation by MEGX occurs while lidocaine extraction ratio is greater than 0.9. Evidence that product inhibition is not a significant factor is provided by *in vitro* data, in that lidocaine extraction ratio is unaltered in the perfused rat liver model over a wide range of MEGX steady-state concentrations.[178] However, MEGX appears to have a modest effect on lidocaine clearance after single intravenous doses of concomitant lidocaine and MEGX in man.[157] Lidocaine systemic clearance was reduced from 58 ± 18 to 48 ± 13 L/hr (p <0.02). This 17% mean reduction in clearance does not explain the reductions in clearance observed during sustained infusions, suggesting product inhibition is not the primary factor. Irreversible lidocaine tissue binding and enzyme inactivation have been proposed as contributory factors to the observed time-dependent pharmacokinetics.[178,179] Our most current understanding is that no one mechanism can account for the nonlinear accumulation of lidocaine. Product inhibition, tissue binding and enzyme inactivation probably all play a role. These studies illustrate the potential shortcomings of time-invariant models for designing lidocaine dosing regimens.

It has been proposed[13,15] that lidocaine maintenance can be individualized using infusion rates calculated from population averages of clearance. The infusion rate required to produce steady-state concentrations (C_{ss}) of 3 µg/mL can be determined with Equation 21-5 and the mean population values for systemic clearance listed in Tables 21-2 and 21-3. Table 21-5 shows the mean values for systemic clearance and the infusion rates calculated to achieve "steady-state" concentrations of 3 µg/mL. The mean infusion rate, based on population averages of clearance is 47 µg/kg/min for normals, 17 µg/kg/min for CHF patients, 27 µg/kg/min for acute myocardial infarction patients, and 19 µg/kg/min for CHF + acute myocardial infarction patients. It has been suggested[51] that infusion rates for obese patients (actual weight 50% greater than ideal weight) be calculated from ideal body weight adjusted values, since clearance appears to be similar for obese and nonobese healthy subjects when normalized for ideal body weight.

The limitations to the use of population averages are that steady state is assumed to be reached at 16 to 24 hours and that this approach has not been compared to others. Effective use of this population-average method requires close clinical monitoring for CNS side effects and awareness that some patients will be inadequately treated with these initial infusion rates.

Several investigators have reported that lidocaine dosages can be successfully individualized using a Bayesian forecasting technique and a single lidocaine serum concentration.[115-117,181-183] This method has been used to individualize doses in patients with acute myocardial infarction, CHF, and acute ventricular arrhythmias.

Approaches that utilize a one-compartment model have been found to consistently underestimate lidocaine concentrations beyond 12 hours[116] while a two-compartment model produced unbiased predictions for up to 24 hours.[181,183,184]

Access to computer support and to facilities for rapid turnaround time of lidocaine assays is required for patient-specific design of lidocaine dosage regimens. If such facilities are not available, the use of mean population clearance values for initial selection of maintenance infusion rates is recommended. Clinical observation and a knowledge of the time course of drug accumulation are required for adjustment in infusion rate during therapy.

Principles of Monitoring Lidocaine Concentration

The precise role of measured lidocaine concentrations for monitoring and individualizing maintenance infusions is not fully defined. Because of the relatively long turnaround time required in many institutions for analysis of samples and the short duration of lidocaine therapy (usually <24 hours), routine monitoring of lidocaine concentrations is not usually performed. The guidelines provided here reflect an analysis of benefits in light of practical limitations.

A second evolving area is the role that measuring free lidocaine concentrations plays in monitoring lidocaine therapy in acute myocardial infarction patients. Since plasma protein binding of lidocaine is concentration-dependent over the therapeutic range, and because binding can change markedly during lidocaine infusions after acute myocardial infarction, total concentrations are less useful than free concentrations. Measurement of total concentrations and AAG concentrations allow one to predict free concentrations using published equations.[115] However, AAG concentrations do not explain all of the intersubject variability in lidocaine plasma protein binding.

Clinical indications for measuring lidocaine concentrations include, but are not limited to, the following:

- **Patients at high risk for toxicity.** This group includes those patients with cardiogenic shock, liver disease, moderate-to-severe heart failure, arrhythmias likely to require lidocaine for more than 24 hours, or rapidly changing clinical status (e.g., trauma, surgery, sepsis).

- **Patients whose arrhythmias fail to respond to maximum recommended doses.** Failure to control arrhythmias with usual doses of lidocaine occurs in 8% to 19% of patients treated,[7,114] depending on the definition used. Lack of response in these patients could be due to a higher systemic clearance than predicted, and these patients may respond to doses above the usual maximum. Measured concentrations can be used to distinguish between patients with low concentrations and those who have arrhythmias that do not respond to maximum safe concentrations, thus assisting in the decision to change the antiarrhythmic agent or increase the dose. These concentrations would also be useful retrospectively to determine the incidence of lidocaine-resistant arrhythmias.

- **Patients in whom prophylactic efficacy of lidocaine must be assured.** Patients with suspected acute myocardial infarction are at high risk for PVF, and achieving a safe, effective lidocaine concentration is a necessary, effective prophylaxis.

It would seem rational to obtain samples at one to two hours and 12 to 24 hours after the start of an infusion to ensure both efficacy during the "therapeutic gap" and to prevent unexpected accumulation and toxicity at infusion times greater than 24 hours.

Summary and Recommendations for Application of Pharmacokinetic Data

The individualization of a dosing scheme should start with consideration of the indication for lidocaine therapy. In post-acute myocardial infarction patients administered lidocaine for prevention of PVF, a loading regimen (75 mg bolus followed in five minutes by a 50 mg bolus) or the exponentially declining infusion-rate method should be used. If the drug is administered for treatment of ventricular arrhythmias, either the multiple-bolus loading regimen described previously or the exponentially declining infusion-rate method is recommended. When a sustained arrhythmia is present, the dose can be titrated to control the arrhythmia, and the maintenance dosage can then be adjusted to maintain the estimated or measured effective lidocaine concentration. At the very least, individualization of maintenance infusions should include weight-corrected infusion rates based on mean population values for systemic clearance. Computer-assisted methods using Bayesian parameter estimation are currently available and hold much potential for improvement of lidocaine therapy (see Figure 21-2).

ANALYTICAL METHODS

Lidocaine has been measured by a wide variety of analytical methods (see Table 21-6) over the past 40 years. The first to be developed was a methyl orange colorimetric procedure.[127–129] This procedure was time-consuming and lacked sensitivity, specificity, and precision. This procedure is important from a historical perspective, since it was used in the original studies of the toxicity of lidocaine.[103] This spectrophotometric procedure was replaced by gas liquid chromatographic (GLC) methods[130–137] which provided increased sensitivity (<0.5 µg/mL). Early procedures[130–133] were not specific for lidocaine, as known metabolites could co-elute with it, thus preventing both the specific quantitation of lidocaine and a description of metabolite disposition. In 1971, the first method for separating MEGX and GX was described[134] Later methods allowed for quantitation of GX and MEGX in blood and plasma.[135–137] GC-MS procedures were developed; in spite of enhanced specificity and sensitivity,[74,138] these procedures are time-consuming and technically difficult. A GLC procedure, with a reported sensitivity of 5 ng/mL, is particularly well suited for single-dose studies, but requires attention to detail that limits its clinical utility.[139] The GLC techniques currently in use are sensitive and reproducible and can quantitate lidocaine metabolites in clinical samples. The disadvantages of all the GLC procedures are the technical training required for proficient operation and the limited number of other pharmaceutical compounds that can be analyzed by GLC in the clinical chemistry laboratory setting.

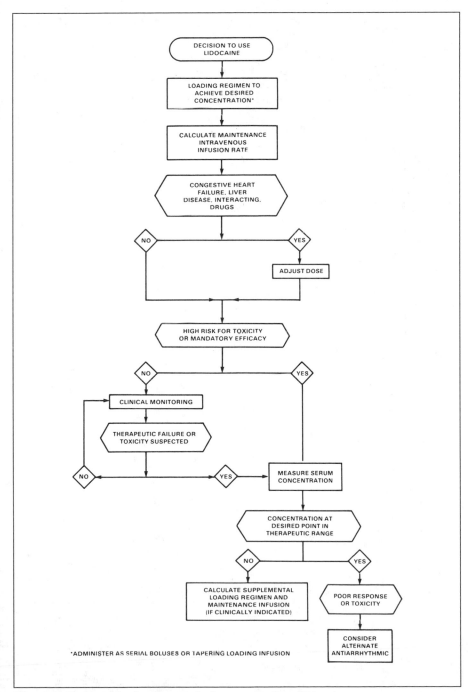

Figure 21-2. *Algorithm for therapeutic drug monitoring of lidocaine.*

Table 21-6. *Comparison of Relative Advantages and Disadvantages of Lidocaine Analytical Methods[a]*

Analytical method[b]	Specificity for lidocaine	Sensitivity	Metabolite analysis	Assayable samples					Minimum sample volume	Speed per sample		Cost		Specialized operator training	Preference		Comments
				Blood	Plasma/serum	Urine	CSF	Saliva		1–10 Samples	10–100 Samples	Reagent/technician	Initial equipment		Clinical	Research	
Colorimetric	4	1 µg/mL	no	yes	yes	?	?	?	2 mL	0.5 hr	0.5 hr	2	2	3	5	5	Poor specificity
GLC-NPD	2	5 ng/mL	yes	yes	yes	yes	yes	yes	1 mL	0.5 hr	0.5 hr	4	4	4	5	2	
GLC-MS	1	2 ng/mL	yes	yes	yes	yes	yes	yes	1 mL	2 hr	2 hr	5	5	5	5	1	Impractical
HPLC	2	20 ng/mL	yes	yes	yes	yes	yes	yes	1 mL	0.5 hr	0.5 hr	4	4	4	3	1	UV detection
EMIT	3	100 ng/mL	no	?	yes	?	?	?	100 µL	10 min	20 min	4	4	2	2	3	Syva Co.
TDx	3	100 ng/mL	no	?	yes	?	?	?	100 µL	5 min	5 min	4	4	1	1	3	Abbott Diag.

[a] Arbitrary ranking scale of 1 (excellent) to 5 (poor).
[b] GLC-NPD = Gas liquid chromatography with nitrogen phosphorous detection; GLC-MS = Gas liquid chromatography with mass spectroscopy; HPLC = High-performance liquid chromatography; EMIT = Enzyme immunoassay; TDx = Fluorescence polarization assay.

Several high-performance liquid chromatographic (HPLC) techniques have been reported.[140-144] The methods are generally capable of quantitating lidocaine, MEGX, and GX at concentrations of 10 to 20 ng/mL using ultraviolet detection (200 to 210 nm). These procedures are highly reproducible, with coefficients of variations reported to range from 5% to 8% for lidocaine, MEGX, and GX at 0.5 µg/mL. The HPLC methods are characterized by low sample volume requirements, simple one-step extraction procedures, and wide applicability in the general analytical laboratory. For these reasons, the HPLC methods are now preferred in the research laboratory and in the clinical setting where metabolite concentration monitoring and high degree of specificity and sensitivity are indicated. The major factor limiting the use of the HPLC in the clinical laboratory is the long (one to six hour) turnaround time.

The shortcomings of long turnaround time and procedural complexity for chromatographic methods for clinical use have been overcome by two methods with acceptable clinical specificity and sensitivity and short analysis times. The homogeneous enzyme immunoassay provides for rapid measurement of lidocaine concentrations.[145,146] It is based on a competitive antibody system where lidocaine in biological sample competes with enzyme-labeled drug that converts NAD to NADH. Enzyme activity is directly proportional to drug concentration in clinical samples.

For lidocaine concentrations, this method has been shown to correlate well with GLC procedures.[145,147] Advantages of this system include small sample requirements (<100 µL), rapid analysis time (one to two minutes per sample), and a low coefficient of variation (<5% at 3 µg/mL). Disadvantages include inability to quantitate lidocaine metabolites and the high cost of reagents.

A second rapid analytical technique is the fluorescence polarization immunoassay.[148] This technique shares the advantages and disadvantages of the enzyme immunoassay method, but has the added advantage of being completely automated. The fluorescence polarization immunoassay is highly sensitive (100 ng/mL) with coefficients of variation of less than 5% at 1.5 and 3.0 µg/mL.

PROSPECTUS

Lidocaine has been and will undoubtedly continue to be the drug of choice for the treatment and prevention of ventricular arrhythmias. The drug is characterized, however, by substantial interpatient pharmacokinetic variability, and its clearance is altered by a number of drug and disease factors commonly present in patients who require lidocaine. Intrasubject variability in lidocaine disposition also appears to be significant in many patients over the course of an infusion regimen. This variability in lidocaine pharmacokinetics, coupled with the relatively narrow therapeutic range, suggests pharmacokinetic-based dosage individualization would be highly useful.

While several forecasting methods have been published and are widely touted, their clinical applications have been limited. Although lidocaine has been available for 40 years, the knowledge and technology currently used in the clinical setting often fail to individualize lidocaine therapy as effectively as is possible for some other drugs. The need for this knowledge and technology should serve as a stimulus for continued clinical and basic research to provide enhanced treatment of the patient requiring lidocaine.

APPENDIX

In the first edition of *Applied Pharmacokinetics*, a detailed approach for using a two-compartmental model to plan lidocaine dosage regimens was described. This appendix summarizes that approach.

Sample Lidocaine Dosage Calculations

A 65-year-old male was admitted to the coronary care unit with a three-hour history of severe, crushing substernal chest pain radiating down both arms and an electrocardiogram consistent with an anterior myocardial infarction. Frequent multifocal ventricular ectopies and a short run of symptomatic ventricular tachycardia were documented shortly after admission. The clinical estimate of cardiac index was 60% of normal (see Table 21-7). Lidocaine was ordered, and a dosage regimen was calculated to achieve a plasma concentration of 3.0 µg/mL.

I. Loading Infusion to be Given over Five Minutes

$$
\begin{aligned}
k_O^L &= C_{ss} \cdot V_c \\
&= (3.0 \text{ mg/L}) \, (40 \text{ L}) \\
&= (120 \text{ mg @ } 24 \text{ mg/min}) \qquad\qquad \text{(Eq. 21-4)}
\end{aligned}
$$

II. Maintenance Infusion

$$
\begin{aligned}
\text{a)} \quad k_{10}^{adj} &= F \, (0.032 - 0.000178 \times \text{Age}) \\
&= 0.6 \, (0.032 - 0.000178 \times 65) \\
&= 0.01226 \text{ min}^{-1}
\end{aligned}
$$

$$
\begin{aligned}
\text{b)} \quad k_O^M &= (C_{SS}) \, (k_{10}^{adj}) \, (V_C) \\
&= (3) \, (0.01226) \, (40) \\
&= 1.5 \text{ mg/min} \qquad\qquad \text{(Eq. 21-5)}
\end{aligned}
$$

III. Additional Lidocaine to be Administered within First Three Half-Lives if Arrhythmia Not Controlled

$$
\begin{aligned}
\text{a)} \quad \beta &= \left(k_{10}^{adj} \right) \left[\frac{k_{21}}{\alpha} \right] \\
\beta &= (0.01226) \left(\frac{0.035}{0.12} \right) \\
\beta &= 0.00358 \\
t\tfrac{1}{2}_\beta &= \left(\frac{0.693}{0.00358} \right) = 194 \text{ minutes}
\end{aligned}
$$

$$b) \quad X_p^{ss} = \frac{(k_{12})\,(k_O^M)}{(k_{21})\,(k_{10})}$$

$$= \frac{(0.07)\,(1.5)}{(0.035)\,(0.01226)} = 245 \text{ mg}$$

(Eq. 21-6)

The 245 mg calculated here represents an estimate of the patient's lidocaine deficit immediately after the loading dose. Up to 75% of this amount can be administered in the first three half-lives without adjustment in the maintenance infusion.

Table 21-7. *Estimation of Cardiac Function Index Based on Clinical Criteria[a]*

Clinical criteria

1.	Degree of heart failure	Points	
	S_3 present	1	
	Pulmonary congestion		
	1+ to 2+ Rales	1	
	3+ Rales	2	
	Pulmonary edema	3	
	Jugular venous distention		
	1–3 cm	2	
	> 3 cm	3	
	Peripheral edema		
	1+	1	
	2+ to 4+	2	
	Pre-renal azotemia	2	

Total points	Percent subtracted from 100% normal
If total ÷ 5 is less than 0.2 then subtract	0%
If total ÷ 5 is 0.2 to 0.49 then subtract	5%
If total ÷ 5 is 0.5 to 0.9 then subtract	10%
If total ÷ 5 is 1.0 to 1.49 then subtract	15%
If total ÷ 5 is 1.5 to 1.99 then subtract	20%
If total ÷ 5 is more than 2.0 then subtract	25%

2.	Blood pressure:	Normal	0%
		Low	10%
		Palpable only	15%
3.	Rhythm:	Normal sinus; rate < 110	0%
		Normal sinus; rate > 110	5%
		Supraventricular tachycardia; rate < 110	10%
		Supraventricular tachycardia; rate > 110	15%
4.	Urine Output:	Normal (> 25 mL/hr)	0%
		Oliguria (<25 mL/hr)	10%
5.	Peripheral vasoconstriction present		5%
6.	Acute myocardial infarction when #1 to #5 normal		10%

[a] To determine the cardiac function index, add the percent indicated in the right-hand column for each of the clinical criteria present on the left-hand side of the table. Subtract total from 100%. Maximum reduction in cardiac function index should not exceed 50%.

IV. **Interim Adjustment of Lidocaine Regimen.** Ten minutes after the end of the loading dose of lidocaine, another short run of ventricular tachycardia occurred, and it was decided additional lidocaine was needed.

a) An additional dose of 50 mg was given by increasing the infusion rate from the maintenance rate of 1.5 mg/min to 11.5 mg/min for five minutes.

b) A second 50 mg was given by changing the infusion rate to 2.5 mg/min for 50 minutes.

c) After 50 minutes at 2.5 mg/min, the maintenance rate was returned to 1.5 mg/min.

REFERENCES

1. Zipes DP. Management of cardiac arrhythmias. In: Braunwald E, ed. Heart Disease: A Textbook of Cardiovascular Medicine, 2nd ed. Philadelphia: WB Saunders; 1984:653–56.
2. Bigger JT, Hoffman BF. Antiarrhythmic drugs. In: Gilman AG et al, eds. The Pharmacological Basis of Therapeutics, 6th ed. New York: MacMillan Publishing; 1980:779–81.
3. Anon. Cardiac arrhythmias. In: Sokolow M, McIlroy MB, eds. Clinical Cardiology, 3rd ed. LOs Altos: Lange Medical Publications; 1981:561–82.
4. Harrison DC et al. The relationship of blood levels, infusion rates and metabolism of lidocaine to its antiarrhythmic action. In: Sandoe E et al, eds. Symposium on Cardiac Arrhythmias. Sweden: AB Astra; 1970:427–47.
5. Hsiek Y et al. Pharmacology of cardiovascular drugs. In: Hurst JW, ed. The Heart, 4th ed. New York: McGraw-Hill; 1978:1942–958.
6. Gianelly R et al. Effect of lidocaine on ventricular arrhythmias in patients with coronary heart disease. N Eng J Med. 1967;277:1215–219.
7. Aiderman EL et al. Evaluation of lidocaine resistance in man using intermittent large-dose infusion techniques. Am J Cardiol. 1974;34:342–49.
8. Zenner JC et al. Blood lidocaine levels and kinetics following high-dose intramuscular administration. Circulation. 1973;48:984–87.
9. Pieper JA et al. Lidocaine clinical pharmacokinetics. Drug Intell Clin Pharm. 1981;16:291–94.
10. Rowland M et al. Disposition kinetics of lidocaine in normal subjects. Ann NY Acad Sci. 1971;179;383–98.
11. Tucker GT, Boas RA. Pharmacokinetic aspects of regional anesthesia. Anesthesiology. 1971;34:538–49.
12. Harrison DC, Alderman EL. The pharmacology and clinical use of lidocaine as an antiarrhythmic drug. Mod Treat. 1972:9:139.
13. Benowitz NO, Meister W. Clinical pharmacokinetics of lidocaine. Clin Pharmacokinet. 1978:3:177–201.
14. Collinsworth KA et al. Clinical pharmacology of lidocaine as an antiarrhythmic drug. Circulation. 1974:50;1217–230.
15. Thomson PD et al. Lidocaine pharmacokinetics in advanced heart failure, liver disease and renal disease in humans. Ann Intern Med. 1973:78;499–508.
16. Zito RA, Reid PA. Lidocaine pharmacokinetics predicted by indocyanine green clearance. N Engl J Med. 1978;298:1160–163.
17. Lie KI et al. Lidocaine in the prevention of primary ventricular fibrillation. N Engl J Med. 1974:291:1324–326.
18. Deglin SM et al. Rapid serum lidocaine determination in the coronary care unit. JAMA. 1980:244;571–73.
19. Boyes RN et al. Pharmacokinetics of lidocaine in man. Clin Pharmacol Ther. 1971;12:105–16.
20. Zito RA et al. Variability of early lidocaine levels in patients. Am Heart J. 1977;94:292–96.

21. Stargel WW et al. Clinical comparison of rapid infusion and multiple injection methods of lidocaine loading. Am Heart J. 1981;102:872–76.
22. Sawyer DR et al. Continuous infusion of lidocaine in patients with cardiac arrhythmias. Unpredictability of plasma concentrations. Arch Intern Med. 1981;141:43–5
23. McNamara PJ et al. Factors influencing the serum free fraction of lidocaine in man. Clin Pharmacol Ther. 1980;27:271.
24. Pieper JA et al. Lidocaine toxicity. Effects of total versus free lidocaine concentrations. Circulation. 1980;62;181.
25. Routledge PA et al. Lidocaine plasma protein binding. Clin Pharmacol Ther. 1980;27:247–51.
26. Lelorier J et al. Pharmacokinetics of lidocaine after prolonged intravenous infusions in uncomplicated myocardial infarction. Ann Intern Med. 1977:87;700–2.
27. Keenaghan JB, Boyes RN. The tissue distribution, metabolism and excretion of lidocaine in rats, guinea pigs, dogs, and man. J Pharmacol Exp Ther. 1972;180:454–63.
28. Bennett PN et al. Pharmacokinetics of lidocaine and its deethylated metabolite. Dose and time dependency studies in man. J Pharmacokinet Biopharm. 1982;10:265–81.
29. Huet M et al. Bioavailability of lidocaine in normal volunteers and cirrhotic patients. Clin Pharmacol Ther. 1979;25:230.
30. Ryden L et al. Comparison between effectiveness of intramuscular and intravenous lidocaine on ventricular arrhythmia complicating acute myocardial infarction. Br Heart J. 1973;35:1124–131.
31. Bellet S et al. Intramuscular lidocaine in the therapy of ventricular arrhythmias. 1971;27:291–93.
32. Fehmers M, Dunning A. Intramuscularly and orally administered lidocaine in the treatment of ventricular arrhythmias in acute myocardial infarction. Am J Cardiol. 1972;29:514–19.
33. Perucca E, Richens E. Reduction of oral bioavailability of lidocaine by induction of first pass metabolism in epileptic patients. Br J Clin Pharmacol. 1979;8:21–31.
34. Schwartz ML et al. Antiarrhythmic effectiveness of intramuscular lidocaine. Influence of different injection sites. J Clin Pharmacol. 1974;15:77–83.
35. Cohen LS et al. Plasma levels of lidocaine after intramuscular administration. Am J Cardiol. 1972;29:520–23.
36. Ryden L et al. Blood levels of lidocaine after intramuscular administration to patients with proven or suspected acute myocardial infarction. Br Heart J. 1972;34:1012–17.
37. Meyer MB, Zelechowski K. Intramuscular lidocaine in normal subjects. In: Scott, Julian, eds. Lidocaine in the Treatment of Ventricular Arrhythmias. Edinburgh: Livingstone; 1971:161.
38. Valentine PA et al. Lidocaine in the prevention of sudden death in the pre-hospital phase of acute infarction. N Engl J Med. 1974;291:1327–331.
39. Lie KI et al. Efficacy of lidocaine in preventing ventricular fibrillation within one hour after a 300 mg intramuscular injection. Am J Cardiol 1978;42:486–88.
40. Scott DB et al. Factors affecting plasma levels of lignocaine and pilocarpine. Br J Anesth. 1972;44:1040–48.
41. Mather LE et al. The effects of adding adrenalin to etidocaine and lignocaine in extradural anesthesia. II. Pharmacokinetics. Br J Anaesth. 1976;48:989–93.
42. Jones DA et al. Plasma concentrations of lignocaine and its metabolites during fiberoptic bronchoscopy. Br J Anaesth. 1982:54:853–56.
43. de Boer AG et al. Rectal bioavailability of lidocaine in man. Partial avoidance of "first pass" metabolism. Clin Pharmacol Ther. 1979;26:701–9.
44. Wyman MG et al. Multiple bolus technique for lidocaine administration during the first hours of a myocardial infarction. Am J Cardiol. 1978;41:313–17.
45. Routledge PA et al. Increased alpha$_1$-acid glycoprotein and lidocaine disposition in myocardial infarction. Ann Intern Med. 1980;93:701–4.
46. Benowitz N et al. Lidocaine disposition kinetics in monkey and man. I. Prediction by perfusion model. Clin Pharmacol Ther. 197;16:87–8.
47. Benowitz N et al. Lidocaine disposition kinetics in monkey and man. II. Effects of hemorrhage and sympathomimetic drug administration. Clin Pharmacol Ther. 1974;16:99–109.
48. Ahmad K, Medzihradsky F. Distribution of lidocaine in blood and tissues after single doses and steady infusion. Res Commun Chem Pathol Pharmacol. 1971;2:813–28.

49. Nation RL et al. Lidocaine kinetics in cardiac patients and aged subject. Br J Clin Pharmacol. 1977;4:439–48.
50. Bauer LA et al. Influence of long-term infusions on lidocaine kinetics. Clin Pharmacol Ther. 1982;31:433–37.
51. Abernathy DA, Greenblatt DJ. Lidocaine disposition in obesity. Am J Cardiol. 1984;53:1183–186.
52. Abernathy DR, Greenblatt DJ. Impairment of lidocaine clearance in elderly male subjects. J Cardiovas Pharmacol. 1983;5:1093–96.
53. Williams RL et al. Influence of aviral hepatitis on the disposition of two compounds with high hepatic clearance: Lidocaine and indocyanine green. Clin Pharmacol Ther. 1976;20:290–99.
54. Gillette JR. Factors affecting drug metabolism. Ann NY Acad Sci. 1971;179:43–66.
55. Wilkinson GR, Shand DG. A physiologic approach to hepatic drug clearance. Clin Pharmacol Ther. 1975;18:377–90.
56. Stargel WW et al. Importance of blood collection tubes in plasma lidocaine determinations. Clin Chem. 1979;24:617–19.
57. Shnider SM, Way EL. The kinetics of transfer of lidocaine (Xylocaine) across the human placenta. Anesthesiology. 1968;29:944–50.
58. Tucker GT et al. Binding of anilide-type local anestheties in human plasma. I. Relationships between binding, physiochemical properties and anesthetic activity. Anesthesiology. 1979;33:287–302.
59. Burney RG et al. Effects of pH on protein binding of lidocaine. Anesth Analg. 1978;57:478–80.
60. McNamara PJ et al. Effect of smoking on the binding of lidocaine to human serum proteins. J Pharm Sci. 1980;69:749–51.
61. Piafsky K, Knoppert D. Binding of local anesthetics to α_1-acid glycoprotein. Clin Res. 1978;26:836A.
62. Routledge PA et al. Relationship between α_1-acid glycoprotein and lidocaine disposition in mycardial infarction. Clin Pharmacol Ther. 1981;30:154–57.
63. Routledge PA et al. Lidocaine disposition in blood and epilepsy. Br J Clin Pharmacol. 1981;12:663–66.
64. Piafsky KM et al. Increased plasma protein binding of propranolol and chlorpromazine mediated by disease-induced alterations of plasma α_1-acid glycoprotein. N Engl J Med. 1978;299:1435–439.
65. Routledge PA et al. Sex-related difference in the plasma protein binding of lidocaine and diazepam. Br J Clin Pharmacol. 1981;11:245–50.
66. Johansson BG et al. Sequential changes of plasma proteins after myocardial infarction. Scand J Clin Lab Invest. 1972;29:117–26.
67. Rodman JH et al. Clinical studies with computer assisted initial lidocaine therapy. Arch Int Med. 1984;144:703–9.
68. Stenson RE et al. Interrelationships of hepatic blood flow, cardiac output and blood levels of lidocaine in man. Circulation. 1971;48:205–11.
69. Strong JM et al. Pharmacologic activity, metabolism and pharmacokinetics of glycinexylidide. Clin Pharmacol Ther. 1975;17:184–94.
70. Nelson SD et al. Quantification of lidocaine and several metabolites using chemical-ionization mass spectrometry and stable isotope labeling. J Pharm Sci. 1977;66:1180–189.
71. Mather LE, Thomas J. Metabolism of lidocaine in man. Life Sci. 1972;11:915–19.
72. Pang KS, Rowland M. Hepatic clearance of drugs. II. Experimental evidence for acceptance of the "well-stirred" model over the "parallel tube" model using lidocaine in the perfused rat liver in situ preparation. J Pharmacokinet Biopharm. 1977;5:655–80.
73. Beckett AH et al. The metabolism and excretion of lidocaine in man. J Pharm Pharmacol. 1966;18:765–815.
74. Strong JM et al. Identification of glycinexylidide in patients treated with intravenous lidocaine. Clin Pharmacol Ther. 1973;14:67–72.
75. Wing LMH et al. Lidocaine disposition—sex differences and effects of cimetidine. Clin Pharmacol Ther. 1984;35:695–701.
76. Halkin H et al. Influence of congestive heart failure on blood levels of lidocaine and its active monodeethylated metabolite. Clin Pharmacol Ther. 1975;17:669–76.

77. Collinsworth KA et al. Pharmacokinetics and metabolism of lidocaine in patients with renal failure. Clin Pharmacol Ther. 1975;18:59–64.

78. Narang PY et al. Lidocaine and its active metabolite. Clin Pharmacol Ther. 1978;24:654–62

79. Drayer DE et al. Plasma levels, protein binding and elimination data of lidocaine and active metabolites in cardiac patients of various ages. Clin Pharmacol Ther. 1983;34:14–22.

80. Pang KS, Rowland M. Hepatic clearance of drugs. III. Additional experimental evidence supporting the "well-stirred" model; using metabolite (AMGX) generated from lidocaine under varying hepatic blood flow rate and linear conditions in the perfused rat liver in situ preparation. J Pharmacokinet Biopharm. 1977;5:681–99.

81. Burney RG et al. Antiarrhythmic effects of lidocaine metabolites. Am Heart J. 1974;88:765–69.

82. Prescott LF et al. Impaired lidocaine metabolism in patients with myocardial infarction. Br Med J. 1976;1:939–41.

83. Aps C et al. Logical approach to lidocaine therapy. Br Med J. 1975;1:13–5.

84. Lalka D et al. Lidocaine pharmacokinetics and metabolism in acute myocardial infarction patients. Clin Res. 1980;28:329A.

85. Bax NDS et al. Lidocaine and indocyanine green kinetics in patients following myocardial infarction. Br J Clin Pharmacol. 1980;10:353–61.

86. Forrest JA et al. Antipyrine, paracetamol and lidocaine elimination in chronic liver disease. Br Med J. 1977;1:1384–387.

87. Feely J et al. Effect of hypotension on liver blood flow and lidocaine disposition. N Engl J Med. 1982;307:866–69.

88. Elvin AT et al. Effect of food on lidocaine kinetics. Mechanism of food-related alteration in high intrinsic clearance drug elimination. Clin Pharmacol Ther. 1981;30:455–60.

89. Grossman R et al. Quantification of portosystemic shunting from the splanchnic and mesenteric beds in alcoholic liver disease. Am J Med. 1972;53:715–22.

90. Conrad KA et al. Lidocaine elimination: Effects of metoprolol and of propranolol. Clin Pharmacol Ther. 1983;33:133 38.

91. Ochs HR et al. Reduction in lidocaine clearance during continuous infusion and by co-administration of propranolol. N Engl J Med. 1980;303:373–77.

92. Feely J et al. Increased toxicity and reduced clearance of lidocaine by cimetidine. Ann Intern Med. 1982;96:592–94.

93. Feely J, Guy E. Lack of effect of ranitidine on the disposition of lidocaine. Br J Clin Pharmacol. 1983;15:378–79.

94. Wiklind L. Human hepatic blood flow and its relation to systemic circulation during intravenous infusion of lidocaine. Acta Anaesthesid Scand. 1977;21:148–60.

95. Binnion PF et al. Relation between plasma lidocaine levels and induced hemodynamic changes. Br Med J. 1969;3:390–92.

96. Schumaker RR et al. Hemodynamic effects of lidocaine in patients with heart disease. Circulation. 1968;38:965–72.

97. Hansson L et al. Hemodynamic effects of acute and prolonged beta adrenergic blockage in essential hypertension. Acta Med Scand. 1974;196:27–34.

98. Weiss YA et al. (+)-Propranolol clearance, an estimation of hepatic blood flow in man. Br J Clin Pharmacol. 1978;5:457–60.

99. Greenblatt DJ et al. Impairment of antipyrine clearance in human by propranolol. Circulation. 1978;57:1161–164.

100. Bax NDS et al. Inhibition of antipyrine metabolism by beta adrenoreceptor antagonists. Br J Clin Pharmac. 1981;12:779–84.

101. Sheridan DJ et al. Antiarrhythmic action of lidocaine in early myocardial infarction. Lancet. 1977;1:824–25.

102. Lalka D et al. Procainamide accumulation kinetics in the immediate post-myocardial infarction period. J Clin Pharmacol. 1978;18:397–401.

103. Foldes FF et al. Comparison of toxicity of intravenously given local anesthetic agents in man. JAMA. 1960;172:1493–498.

104. Buckman K et al. Lidocaine efficacy and toxicity assessed by a new rapid method. Clin Pharmacol Ther. 1980;28:177–81.

105. Pfeifer HJ et al. Clinical use and toxicity of intravenous lidocaine. A report from the Boston Collaborative Drug Surveillance Program. Am Heart J. 1976;92:168–73.

106. Pitt A et al. Lidocaine given prophylactically to patients with acute myocardial infarction. Lancet. 1971;1:612–16.

107. Wikinski JA et al. Mechanism of convulsions elicited by local anesthetic agents. Anesth Analg. 1970;49:504–10.

108. Davison R et al. Excessive serum lidocaine levels during maintenance infusions: Mechanisms and prevention. Am Heart J. 1982;104:203–8.

109. Greenblatt DJ et al. Pharmacokinetic approach to the clinical use of lidocaine intravenously. JAMA. 1976;236:273–77.

110. Ridell JG et al. A new method for constant plasma drug concentrations: Applications to lidocaine. Ann Intern Med. 1984;100:25–8.

111. Salzer LB et al. A comparison of methods of lidocaine administration in patients. Clin Pharmacol Ther. 1981;29:617–24.

112. Stargel WW et al. Clinical comparison of rapid infusion and multiple injection methods for lidocaine loading. Am Heart J. 1981;102:872–76.

113. Sebaldt RJ et al. Lidocaine therapy with an exponentially declining infusion. Ann Intern Med. 1984;101:632–34.

114. Wyman MG, Hammersmith L. Comprehensive treatment plan for the prevention of primary ventricular fibrillation in acute myocardial infarction. Am J Cardiol. 1974;33:661–67.

115. Routledge PA et al. Control of lidocaine therapy. New perspectives. Ther Drug Monit. 1982;4:265–70.

116. Joel SE et al. Kinetic predictive techniques applied to lidocaine therapeutic drug monitoring. Ther Drug Monit. 1983;5:271–77.

117. Vozeh S et al. Rapid prediction of individual dosage requirements for lidocaine. Clin Pharmacokinet. 1984;9:354–63.

118. Rodman J et al. Clinical evaluation of a pharmacokinetic model and computer program for improving lidocaine dosage regimens. Clin Pharmacol Ther. 1979;25:245.

119. Fredricks DS, Boersma RB. Lidocaine infusions; Effect of duration and method of discontinuation on recurrence of arrhythmias and pharmacokinetic variables. Am J Hosp Pharm. 1979;36:778–81.

120. Barchowsky A et al. On the role of α_1-acid glycoprotein in lidocaine accumulation following myocardial infarction. Br J Clin Pharmacol. 1982;13:411–15.

121. LeLorier J et al. Effect of duration of infusion on the disposition of lidocaine in dogs. J Pharmacol Exp Ther. 1977;203;507–11.

122. Vicuna N et al. Dose-dependent pharmacokinetic behavior of lidocaine in the conscious dog. Res Commun Chem Pathol Pharmacol. 1978;22:485–91.

123. Chiou WL et al. Method for the rapid estimation of the total body drug clearance and adjustment of dosage regimens in patients using a constant rate intravenous infusion. J Pharmacokinet Biopharm. 1978;6:135–51.

124. Sheiner LB et al. Forecasting individual pharmacokinetics. Clin Pharmacol Ther. 1979;26:294–305.

125. Stargel WW et al. Importance of blood collection tubes in plasma lidocaine determinations. Clin Chem. 1979;25:617–19.

126. Borga O et al. Plasma protein binding of basic drugs. 1. Selective displacement from α_1-acid glycoprotein by tris (2-butoxyethyl) phosphate. Clin Pharmacol Ther. 1977;22:539–44.

127. Way El et al. The absorption, distribution and excretion of d,1 methadone. J Pharmacol Exp Ther. 1949;97:222–28.

128. McMahon FG, Woods LA. Further studies on the metabolism of lidocaine (Xylocaine) in the dog. J Pharmacol Exp Ther. 1951;103:354–58.

129. Sung CY, Truant AP. The physiological disposition of lidocaine and its comparison in some respects with procaine. J Pharmacol Exp Ther. 1954;112:432–42.

130. Beckett AH et al. Determination of lidocaine in blood and urine in human subjects undergoing local anesthetic procedures. Anesthesiology. 1965;20:294–300.
131. Svinhuford G et al. The estimation of lidocaine and prilocaine in biological material by gas chromatography. Scand J Clin Lab Invest. 1965;17;162.
132. Keenaghan JB. The determination of lidocaine and prilocaine in whole blood by gas chromatography. Anesthesiology. 1968;29:110–12.
133. Tucker GT. Determination of bupivacaine and other anilide-type local anesthetics in human blood and plasma by gas chromatography. Anesthesiology. 1970;32:255–60.
134. DiFazio CA, Brown RE. The analysis of lidocaine and its postulated metabolites. Anesthesiology. 1972;34:86–8.
135. Nation RL et al. Gas chromatographic method for the quantitative determination of lidocaine and its metabolite monethylglycinexylidide in plasma. J Chromatog. 1976;116:188–93.
136. Rosseel MT, Bogaert MG. Determination of lidocaine and its desethylated metabolites in plasma by capillary column gas-liquid chromatography. J Chromatog. 1978;154:99–102.
137. Adjepon-Yamoah KK, Prescott LF. Gas liquid chromatographic estimation of lidocaine, ethylglycinexylidide, glycinexylidide, and 4-hydroxylidine in plasma and urine. J Pharm Pharmacol. 1974;26:889–93.
138. Strong JM, Atkinson AJ. Simultaneous measurement of lidocaine and its desethylated metabolite by mass fragmentography. Anal Chem. 1972;44:2287–290.
139. Abernathy DR, Greenblatt DJ. Lidocaine determination in human plasma with application to single low-dose pharmacokinetic studies. J Chromatog. 1982;232:180–85.
140. Massoud AM et al. Simultaneous determination of lidocaine and thiopental in plasma using high pressure liquid chromatography. J Liquid Chromatog. 1978;1:607–16.
141. Nation RL et al. High pressure liquid chromatographic method for simultaneous determination of lidocaine and its N-dealkylated metabolites in plasma. J Chromatog. 1979;162:466–73.
142. Hill J et al. High pressure liquid chromatographic determination of lidocaine and its active deethylated metabolites. J Pharm Sci. 1980;69:1341–343.
143. Flood JG et al. Simultaneous liquid chromatographic determination of three antiarrhythmic drugs; Disopyramide, lidocaine and quinidime. Clin Chem. 1980;26:197–200.
144. Narang PK et al. Lidocaine and its active metabolites. Clin Pharmacol Ther 1978;24:654–62.
145. Cobb ME et al. Homogenous enzyme immunoassay for lidocaine in serum. Clin Chem. 1977;23;1161.
146. Wahlberg CB. Lidocaine by enzyme immunoassay. J Analyt Toxicol. 1978.2:121–23.
147. Jain S, Johnston A. The measurement of lidocaine at low concentrations in plasma. A comparison of gas liquid chromatography with enzyme inmunoassay. Br J Clin Pharmacol. 1979;8:598–99.
148. Jolley ME. Fluorescence polarization immunoassay for determination of therapeutic drug levels in human plasma. J Anal Toxicol 1981;5:236–40.
149. Kruger Theimer E. Continuous intravenous infusion and multicompartment accumulation. Eur J Pharmacol. 1968;4:317–24.
150. Jelliffe RW et al. An improved MAP Bayesian computer program for adaptive control of lidocaine therapy. Clin Pharmacol Ther. 1983;33:255.
151. Wyman MG et al. Multiple bolus technique for lidocaine in acute ischemic heart disease. II. Treatment of refractory ventricular arrhythmias and the pharmacokinetic significance of severe left ventricular failure. J Am Coll Cardiol. 1983;2:764–69.
152. Pomier-Layrargues G et al. Effect of portocaval shunt on drug disposition in patients with cirrhosis. Gastroenterology. 1986;91:163–67.
153. Lerman J et al. Effects of age on the serum concentration of α_1-acid glycoprotein and the binding of lidocine in pediatric patients. Clin Pharmacol Ther. 1989;46:219–25.
154. Nattel et al. Therapeutic blood lidocaine concentrations after local anesthesia for cardiac electrophysiologic studies. N Engl J Med. 1979;301:418–20.
155. Schwartz ML et al. Blood levels of lidocaine following subcutaneous administration prior to cardiac catheterization. Am Heart J. 1974;88:721–23.

156. Estes NAM et al. Therapeutic serum lidocaine and metabolite concentrations in patients undergoing electrophysiologic study after discontinuation of intravenous lidocaine infusion. Am Heart J. 1989;117:1060–64.

157. Thomson AH et al. The pharmacokinetics and pharmacodynamics of lignocaine and MEGX in healthy subjects. J Pharmacokinet Biopharm. 1987;15:101–15.

158. Davies RF et al. Perioperative variability of binding of lidocaine, quinidine, and propranolol after cardiac operations. J Thorac Cardiovasc Surg. 1988;96:634–41.

159. Bargetzi MJ et al. Lidocaine metabolism in human liver microsomes by cytochrome P450IIIA4. Clin Pharmacol Ther. 1989;46:521–27.

160. Pang KS et al. An enzyme-distributed system for lidocaine metabolism in the perfused rat liver preparation. J Pharmacokinet Biopharm. 1986;14:107–30.

161. Bennett PD et al. Competition between lidocaine and one of its metabolites, glycylxylidide, for cardiac sodium channels. Circulation. 1988;78:692–700.

162. Oellerich M et al. Lignocaine metabolite formation as a measure of pre-transplant liver function. Lancet. 1989;1:640–42.

163. Burdelski M et al. A novel approach to assessment of liver function in donors. Transplant Proc. 1988;20(Suppl. 1):591–93.

164. Oellerich M et al. Lidocaine metabolite formation as a measure of liver function in patients with cirrhosis. Ther Drug Monit. 1990;12:219–26.

165. Schroeder TJ et al. Lidocaine metabolism as an index of liver function in hepatic transplant donors and recipients. Transplant Proc. 1989;21:229–301.

166. Littlefield M e tal. MEGX determined by flourescence polarization immunoassay (FPIA) as a liver function test. Clin Chem. 1988;34:1159.

167. Thomson AH et al. The pharmacokinetics and pharmacodynamics of lignocaine and MEGX in healthy subjects. J Pharmacokinet Biopharm. 1987;15:101–15.

168. Finholt DA et al. Lidocaine pharmacokinetics in children during general anesthesia. Anesth Analg. 1986;65:279–82.

169. Bauer LA et al. Cimetidine-induced decrease in lidocaine metabolism. Am Heart J. 1984;108:413–15.

170. Jackson JE et al. Effects of histamine-2 receptor blockade on lidocaine kinetics. Clin Pharmacol Ther. 1985;37:544–48.

171. Knapp AB et al. The lidocaine-cimetidine interaction. An Intern Med. 1983;98:174–77.

172. Powell JR et al. Effect of duration of lidocaine infusion and route of cimetidine administration on lidocaine pharmacokinetics. Clin Pharm. 1986;5:993–98.

173. Beach CL et al. Clinical assessment of a two-compartment bayesian forecasting method for lidocaine. Ther Drug Monit. 1988;10:74–9.

174. Thomson AH et al. Changes in lidocaine disposition during long-term infusion in patients with acute ventricular arrhythmias. Ther Drug Monit. 1987;9:283–91.

175. Vozeh S et al. Computer-assisted individualized lidocaine dosage: clinical evaluation and comparison with physician performance. Am Heart J. 1987;113:928–33.

176. Vozeh S, Steiner C. Estimates of the population pharmacokinetic parameters and performance of bayesian feedback: a sensitive analysis. J Pharmacokinet Biopharm. 1987;15:511–28.

177. Uematsu T et al. Prediction of individual dosage requirements for lignocaine: a validation study for bayesian forecasting in japanese patients. Ther Drug Monit. 1989;11:25–31.

178. Tam YK et al. Mechanisms of lidocaine kinetics in the isolated perfused rat liver I. Effects of continuous infusion. Drug Metab Disp. 1987;15:12–6.

179. Lennard MS et al. Time-dependent kinetics of lignocaine in the isolated perfused rat liver. J Pharmacokinet Biopharm. 1983;11:165–82.

180. Suzuki T et al. Precursor-metabolite interaction in the metabolism of lidocaine. J Pharm Sci. 1984;73:136–38.

181. Beach CL et al. Clinical assessment of a two-compartment bayesian forecasting method for lidocaine. Ther Drug Monit. 1988;10:74–9.

182. Thomson AH et al. Changes in lidocaine disposition during long-term infusion in patients with acute ventricular arrhythmias. Ther Drug Monit. 1987;9:283–91.

183. Vozeh S et al. Computer-assisted individualized lidocaine dosage: clinical evaluation and comparison with physician performance. Am Heart J. 1987;113:928–33.

184. Vozeh S, Steiner C. Estimates of the population pharmacokinetic parameters and performance of bayesian feedback: a sensitive analysis. J Pharmacokinet Biopharm. 1987;15:511–28.

Chapter 22

Procainamide

James D. Coyle and John J. Lima

Procainamide (PA), a class 1A antiarrythmic agent, is effective in the treatment of a variety of supraventricular and ventricular arrhythmias. Its use is moderated by the relatively high incidence of drug-induced lupus erythematosus associated with chronic therapy.[2-5] Koch-Weser established the importance of therapeutic drug monitoring to the rational use of PA when he demonstrated a poor relationship between PA dose and plasma concentration (see Figure 22-1), a relatively good relationship between plasma PA concentration and antiarrhythmic response (see Figure 22-2), and a relatively narrow therapeutic index.[1,7] This chapter reviews our current understanding of PA pharmacokinetics and pharmacodynamics as it relates to therapeutic drug monitoring.

CLINICAL PHARMACOKINETICS

The pharmacokinetics of PA and its major metabolite, N-acetylprocainamide (NAPA), have been studied extensively and are summarized in Table 22-1 on page 22-4. We will first review what is known regarding the pharmacokinetics of the parent compound and then briefly review the pharmacokinetics of its metabolite.

Absorption

Absorption of orally administered PA appears to be a first-order process[7,8] which can occur equally well at all levels of the small intestine.[9] Absorption is relatively rapid with an average absorption half-life of about 20 minutes.[7,8] However, the rate of absorption varies considerably among individuals. Following the administration of 500 mg PA HCl capsules (Pronestyl), the absorption half-life ranged from 8 to 154 minutes in 11 healthy volunteers.[8] The absorption characteristics of a generic, immediate-release PA capsule (Ascot) were similar to those observed for Pronestyl in patients under steady-state conditions.[145]

The mean peak plasma PA concentration in five normal subjects receiving a single mean oral dose of 12.6 mg/kg was 4.2 ± 0.3 mg/L.[10] In the same study,

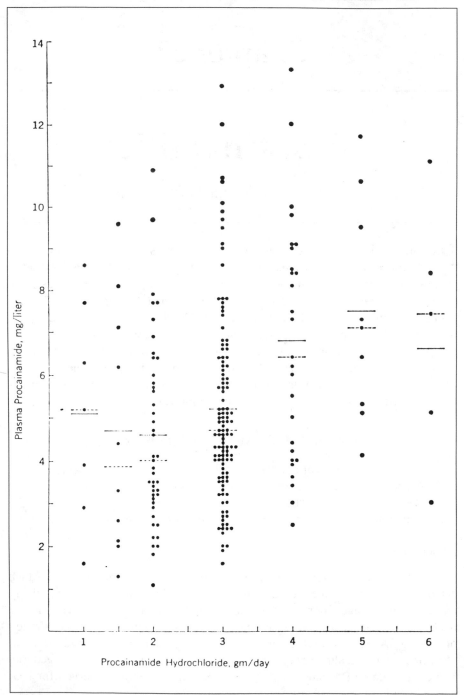

Figure 22-1. *Average steady-state plasma PA concentration as a function of daily oral PA dose in 186 patients as reported by Koch-Weser. The mean (——) and median (- - - -) plasma concentrations are given for each dosage. The poor relationship between plasma concentration and dose resulted from significant interpatient differences in PA pharmacokinetics (reproduced with permission from reference 198).*

five cardiac patients received a mean oral dose of 9.4 mg radiolabeled PA per kg in place of their normal maintenance dose. The mean peak concentration of radiolabeled drug was 7.1 ± 1.4 mg/L.

Peak concentrations generally occur within one hour in normal volunteers,[7] but peak time is variable among patients. Lima reported that the peak concentration occurred at the time of the next dose in 8 of 31 cardiac patients.[11] Koch-Weser has reported similar variability in 15 acute myocardial infarction patients.[7] Variable peak times may result from absorption time lags of up to 1.5 hours,[7,8] decreased rates of absorption, and intersubject differences in PA distribution and elimination.

The bioavailability of PA from immediate-release capsules (Pronestyl) averaged 83% ± 16% (range: 66% to 113%) in 11 healthy volunteers.[8] Grasela and Sheiner,[12] using a Bayesian approach, estimated that 85% of PA was bioavailable from Pronestyl capsules in their cardiac patients. Koch-Weser[7] reported that 75% to 95% of a PA dose was bioavailable in most of his patients; however, approximately 10% of his patients had lower bioavailabilities; less than 50% of the dose reached the systemic circulation in about 2% of patients. Limited data suggest that presystemic (first-pass) metabolism is a major factor in the less-than-complete bioavailability of PA.[13]

Food does not appear to decrease the extent of PA absorption from immediate-release capsules, although it may affect the rate of absorption.[14] Adequate absorption of oral PA (as judged by therapeutic effect and minimum steady-state PA concentrations ≥4 mg/L at a dose of 500 mg every four hours) has been reported following the resection of all but 26 centimeters of the small intestine in a patient

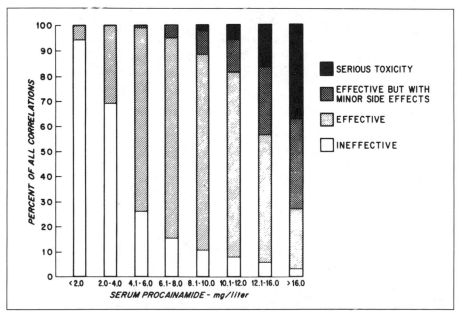

Figure 22-2. *Relationship between plasma PA concentrations and its antiarrhythmic efficacy and toxicities in 306 patients as reported by Koch-Weser. The data suggest a therapeutic range of about 4 to 10 mg/L (reproduced with permission from reference 199).*

Table 22-1. *Summary of Procainamide and NAPA Pharmacokinetic Parameters*

	Population averages ± 1 SD (Normal renal and hepatic function)		
	Adults[a]	Children[142]	Neonates[143]
Procainamide			
CL_S (mL/min/kg)	8.6 ± 1.9 (34, 35, 37, 40, 54)	19.4 ± 2.0	—
CL_R (mL/min/kg)	4.5 ± 1.1 (34, 35, 37, 40, 54)	—	0.20
CL_{NR} (mL/min/kg)	4.1 ± 1.4 (34, 35, 37, 40, 54)	—	—
V_1 (L/kg)	0.67 ± 0.13 (8, 34, 37, 38)	2.2 ± 0.3	—
V_{ss} (L/kg)	2.0 ± 0.42 (8, 34, 35, 37, 38, 54)	—	—
F (oral)	0.83 ± 0.16 (8)	—	—
ka (min^{-1})	0.0336 ± 0.0325 (8)	—	—
% excreted in urine as			
PA	52 ± 11 (10, 13, 60)	—	—
NAPA	16 ± 6.7 (10, 13, 60)	—	—
$t\frac{1}{2}_{\lambda 1}$ (hr)	0.091 ± 0.031 (34)	0.17 ± 0.057	—
$t\frac{1}{2}_{\lambda 2}$ (hr)	3.3 ± 0.64 (34, 35, 37, 40, 54)	1.7 ± 0.1	13.5
NAPA			
CL_S (mL/min/kg)	3.28 ± 0.52 (35)	—	—
CL_R (mL/min/kg)	2.79 ± 0.33 (35)	—	—
CL_{NR} (mL/min/kg)	0.49 ± 0.21 (35)	—	—
V_{ss}	Similar to PA (35)	—	—
$t\frac{1}{2}_{\lambda 2}$ (hr)	6.2 ± 0.67 (35)	—	—
% excreted unchanged in urine	85.5 ± 4.05 (35)	—	—

a   References are listed in parentheses.

with small bowel infarction.[15] Somogyi and Bochner[16] suggested that ranitidine significantly decreases the extent of PA absorption in a dose-dependent fashion. However, this observation needs to be confirmed using both intravenous and oral doses of PA.

Two sustained-release PA tablets are currently being marketed in the United States. Procan-SR is a wax matrix tablet containing PA HCl which is slowly released from the matrix as it passes through the gastrointestinal tract.[17] Release of PA HCl from the other product, Pronestyl-SR, is controlled by the tablet coating during the first 30 to 60 minutes after ingestion and then by dissolution of drug from a gummy, nondisintegrating matrix core which is formed in the gastrointestinal tract when the two core polymers come in contact with water.[144]

The average bioavailability of PA from Procan-SR tablets is similar to that from an immediate-release capsule (Pronestyl) based on crossover studies using normal subjects[18] and patients.[19,20,146] These studies revealed no statistically significant differences in relative bioavailability using such indices as area under the plasma-concentration time curve (AUC) and average plasma concentration at steady state. In contrast, Grasela and Sheiner[12] used a Bayesian approach to demonstrate significantly reduced bioavailability (0.68 versus 0.85, p <0.005) of PA from Procan-SR in a non-crossover study involving 39 cardiac patients. It is not apparent whether this difference is real or an artifact of the methodology used by the investigators. From a clinical standpoint, it is important to recognize that two of these studies reported significant interpatient variation in relative bioavailability, with ranges of 0.59 to 1.27[19] and 0.53 to 1.44.[20] This variability should be considered when patients are switched from immediate-release PA capsules to Procan-SR or vice versa.

The absorption characteristics of Procan-SR and Pronestyl-SR are generally similar.[147,148] The highest plasma concentrations of PA were observed 2.2 and 3.8 hours (p <0.05) following administration of Procan-SR and Pronestyl-SR, respectively, suggesting that PA was absorbed from the latter formulation more slowly.[147] Although the extent of absorption from both formulations was similar,[147,148] patients who crossed over from Procan-SR to Pronestyl-SR required 25% more Pronestyl-SR to maintain targeted serum concentrations.[148] Despite the similarity in mean steady-state AUC values, interpatient variability in relative bioavailability was considerable,[148] as has been noted in other studies of immediate- and sustained-release formulations.[19,20] The antiarrhythmic activity of both formulations is similar,[148] and additional evidence of Pronestyl-SR's effectiveness in treating premature ventricular depolarizations has been published.[21]

The presence of broken or intact wax matrices in the feces of patients taking Procan-SR is usually not an indication of a bioavailability problem.[17,22] However, poor absorption (presence of matrices with significant amount of PA remaining) has been reported in a patient with diarrhea[23] and in colostomy patients.[17] Normally, parts of tablet cores also may be found in the feces of patients taking Pronestyl-SR.[144] Although food prolongs the gastric emptying time, it only slightly increases the PA AUC (relative to the fasting state) following administration of a single dose of Procan-SR.[149] Studies evaluating sustained-release preparations available outside the United States have been published.[24–29]

A potential problem with the bioavailability of PA administered intravenously in 5% dextrose in water (D5W) has been demonstrated.[30,150] PA complexes with glucose[31-33] resulting in the "loss" of PA in a solution stored at room temperature for various periods of time.[30,150] Gupta[32,33] has examined various factors affecting complex formation and has demonstrated that the complexed PA may be released *in vitro* by treatment with 5N HCl. It is not known whether PA is decomplexed *in vivo*. Until this question is resolved, PA diluted in D5W should be infused within 8 to 12 hours of preparation. Alternatively, PA for intravenous administration may be diluted in 0.9% sodium chloride if this diluent is not contraindicated in the patient. Adjusting the pH of the dextrose solution to 7.5 with sodium bicarbonate will also minimize or avoid the "loss" of PA.[150]

The absorption of PA after intramuscular administration is usually rapid (absorption half-life 9.9 to 17 minutes) and complete.[1] Peak concentrations generally occur within 25 minutes and are about 30% higher than peak concentrations after the same dose given orally.[7] Absorption may be delayed when cardiac output or arterial pressure is significantly depressed.[7]

Distribution

As previously discussed,[11] two-compartment models are usually adequate to describe the disposition of PA following intravenous infusions. The initial rapid decline of plasma PA concentrations is generally complete within 30 minutes ($t\frac{1}{2}$ = five minutes).[34] Others have used a three-compartment model to describe PA and NAPA disposition.[35,36] Stec and Atkinson adapted a distribution clearance model to a three-compartment model.[36] By employing measured red blood cell (RBC) to plasma concentration ratios for PA and NAPA, they calculated central volumes of distribution of 5.5 and 6.0 L, respectively, which are numerically close to blood volume. The potential advantage of this model over more conventional pharmacokinetic ones lies in its ability to better predict the effects of hemodynamic changes on the kinetics of drug distribution.[36]

The reported volume of the central compartment is 0.67 ± 0.13 L/kg.[8,34,37,38] The mean volume of distribution at steady state (V_{ss}) is 2.0 ± 0.42 L/kg.[8,34,37,38] This V_{ss} suggests that PA distributes extensively into tissues with approximately 70% of the total amount of drug in the body being in the tissue compartment at steady state. PA is about 15% bound to plasma proteins at plasma PA concentrations up to at least 100 mg/mL.[1,39] (Lima, unpublished data)

Christoff et al.[40] compared the distribution of PA in obese volunteers [actual body weight (ABW) >1.4 × ideal body weight (IBW)] to volunteers of normal body weight (ABW = IBW $\pm$ 20%). PA V_{ss} was similar in both groups (158 $\pm$ 33 L in obese versus 150 $\pm$ 26 L in normal). This finding suggests that PA distributes poorly into fat tissue and that estimates of PA V_{ss} should be based on ideal body weight.

The PA plasma:erythrocyte concentration ratio has been reported to be 1.58,[1] 1.05,[41] and 0.66.[36,96] The reason for this disparity is not apparent to us after examination of the studies. The metabolism of PA by red blood cells[42,43] is a potential source of error in all three investigations.

Several investigators have examined the effect of disease states on PA distribution. The V_{ss} in cardiac patients[12,34] and patients with renal impairment[37,44] was similar to that in normal subjects. Koch-Weser[7] suggested that PA volume of distribution was reduced in patients with abnormally low cardiac outputs (1.48 to 1.78 L/kg versus 1.74 to 2.22 L/kg). However, distribution volume was calculated by the back-extrapolation method following oral doses of PA; hence, it is impossible to be certain that the observed difference reflects actual V_{ss} changes.

Metabolism

Figure 22-3 summarizes the metabolic pathways for PA in humans. Acetylation of the arylamine group results in the formation of N-acetylprocainamide (NAPA), a major PA metabolite. N-dealkylation (desethylation) of the aliphatic amine results in desethylprocainamide (DEPA) formation. Desethyl-N-acetylprocainamide (DENAPA) is formed by the acetylation of DEPA and the desethylation of NAPA. Acetylation of DEPA is quantitatively the more important of the two pathways.[45] Hydrolysis of the amide linkage of PA results in the formation of p-aminobenzoic acid (PABA). The extent of PA hydrolysis is controversial, with estimates ranging from 0% to 10% of a PA dose being recovered in the urine as PABA and its conjugates.[10,39,46,47] Less than 4% of NAPA is deacetylated to reform PA.[48,49,193] Another putative route of PA metabolism is a pathway which involves the formation of a reactive, hydroxylamine intermediate and a nitroso compound that may be involved in PA-induced lupus erythematosus.[50–53,176] The formation of PA hydroxylamine by rat and human liver microsomes has been reported.[175]

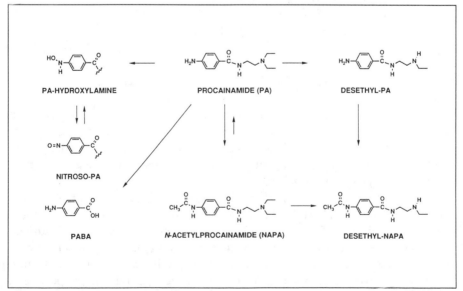

Figure 22-3. Known pathways of PA metabolism. Approximately 10% to 40% of a PA dose is recovered in the urine as NAPA. Less than 3% of NAPA is deacetylated to reform PA. Urinary excretion of the desethyl metabolites accounts for only about 1% of a PA dose. The contribution of PA hydrolysis to PABA is controversial. The hydroxylamine and nitroso metabolites may be involved in the induction of PA-induced lupus.

PA metabolic pathways accounted for 46% ± 6.8% (range 32.2% to 55.3%) of PA total body clearance in normal subjects.[35,37,40,54] The nonrenal clearance of PA in these subjects averaged 4.34 ± 1.38 mL/min/kg ABW (range 2.45 to 7.69 mL/min/kg). Lima et al.[34] have demonstrated a similar (3.8 ± 1.6 mL/min/kg) nonrenal PA clearance in cardiac patients.

Acetylation. Acetylation of PA is mediated by N-acetyltransferase (NAT),[55,56] an enzyme which is found in the liver and in extrahepatic sites such as the intestines,[57] lung, kidney,[58,59] and red blood cells.[42,43] The contribution of extrahepatic acetylation to acetylation clearance in humans is not known, although evidence from five animal species suggests that the contribution of these sites is small.[58]

The metabolism of PA by NAT is bimodally distributed.[47,55,60–63] Approximately 50% of both the black and white population of the United States are fast acetylators; the other 50% are slow acetylators of PA and other drugs including isoniazid, sulfamethazine, dapsone, and sulfapyridine.[57] Work with isoniazid[64] and sulfamethazine[65,66] suggests that there may be a third intermediate acetylator phenotype which is a subset of the fast acetylator group.

Acetylator phenotyping with PA has been based on either the ratio of serum NAPA concentration to serum PA concentration at a specific time or the ratio of NAPA to PA in urine collected over a specified interval. While these NAPA:PA indices appear to be valid in individuals with normal renal function, they are invalid in individuals with renal impairment. This is because NAPA is eliminated by the kidneys to a greater extent than PA (85% versus 50%). Consequently, NAPA accumulates to a greater extent as renal function deteriorates. Lima and Jusko derived an expression for the apparent acetylation clearance (CL_{AP}) which is relatively independent of renal function:

$$CL_{AP} = \frac{ER_{NAPA}}{C_{PA}}$$

(Eq. 22-1)

where ER_{NAPA} is the NAPA urinary excretion rate at steady state and C_{PA} is the steady-state plasma PA concentration.[63] In their group of cardiac patients, CL_{AP} rates less than 80 mL/min appeared to indicate a slow acetylator phenotype, and CL_{AP} rates greater than 120 mL/min were associated with the fast acetylator phenotype. Patients with severe renal impairment may be incorrectly phenotyped by CL_{AP} because the assumption that renal NAPA clearance is much greater than nonrenal NAPA clearance is not valid in these patients.

Fast acetylators of PA have higher acetylation clearances and excrete a larger fraction of a PA dose as NAPA relative to slow acetylators. Lima et al.[34] estimated acetylation clearances of 3.17 ± 1.33 mL/min/ kg and 1.08 ± 0.22 mL/min/kg in fast and slow acetylating cardiac patients with no renal impairment, respectively. In these patients, the fraction of a PA dose eliminated by metabolism to NAPA would average 0.33 and 0.20 in fast and slow acetylators, respectively. These data are similar to those published by other investigators.[35,37,67,68]

N-Dealkylation (Desethylation). Metabolism of drugs by N-dealkylation is mediated by the microsomal mixed-function oxidases.[69] The existence of this pathway of PA metabolism has been known for a number of years,[70,71] although the contribution it makes to PA elimination is unknown. Urinary excretion of DEPA and DENAPA accounted for an average of only 0.58% and 0.53%, respectively, of intravenous PA doses administered to six normal volunteers.[177] Ruo et al.[71] measured the steady-state plasma concentrations of PA, NAPA, and DEPA, and DENAPA in a group of ten patients treated with PA. In the nine patients who were not on chronic hemodialysis (renal function implied to be normal to slightly impaired), PA, NAPA, DENAPA concentrations were 11.5 ± 6.5, 12.8 ± 8.8, and 1.6 ± 1.3 (range 0.4 to 3.9) mg/L, respectively. DEPA concentrations in eight of these nine patients were less than the limit of detection (0.5 mg/L) for the analytical method used, and in one patient the concentration was 0.8 mg/L. The patient on hemodialysis in this group had plasma PA, NAPA, DEPA, and DENAPA concentrations of 2.6, 43.6, less than 0.5, and 11.9 mg/L, respectively. Based on these relatively low concentrations and their weak antiarrhythmic activity,[71] the desethyl metabolites do not appear to be therapeutically important except, perhaps, in the renal failure patient who may achieve potentially significant plasma DENAPA concentrations.

Factors Affecting the Metabolism of PA. Our understanding of PA pharmacokinetics is based on the assumption that its distribution and clearance are linear at therapeutic concentrations. However, there is increasing evidence that nonrenal and total PA clearance are concentration-dependent. Studies of isoniazid[72] and sulfamethazine[73,74] acetylation in normal volunteers suggest that the acetylation of these compounds is concentration-dependent. Tilstone and Lawson[67] reported that both apparent acetylation clearance and total clearance of PA were concentration-dependent in a group of seven slow acetylator patients. Coyle et al.[54] examined the pharmacokinetics of PA in four normal volunteers, each of whom received intravenous doses of about 3 and 12 mg PA/kg/ABW. The nonrenal clearance of PA decreased with the higher dose in all four subjects: the average change was 36% (range 31% to 43%) (p <0.05). Total PA clearance decreased by an average of 24% (range 4.6% to 46%) (p <0.05). Changes in PA renal clearance, V_{ss}, and half-life were not statistically significant. While these nonrenal and total clearance changes appear to be of sufficient magnitude to be clinically significant, quantitative extrapolation of these data to the patient care situation is difficult because the clearances are concentration-averaged parameters.

The effects of disease on nonrenal PA clearance have received little attention. *Chronic liver disease* (postnecrotic or Laennec's cirrhosis) has been reported to impair the acetylation and hydrolysis of PA while enhancing the acetylation of PABA.[75] However, the validity of these conclusions is questionable because PA was administered orally, metabolic indices that are dependent on renal function were used, and the control group was less than one-half the age of the treatment groups. Another study that examined the effects of chronic heart failure, chronic respiratory failure, and chronic renal failure on PA metabolism has the same design problems.[76]

Grasela and Sheiner[12] reported an 11% decrease in PA acetylation clearance in their cardiac patients with *congestive heart failure*, most of whom were in Class I by New York Heart Association criteria. Consistent with this observation, Bauer et al.[151] reported a decreased total PA clearance in patients with heart failure compared to patients without heart failure (3.4 versus 6.4 mL/min/kg, p <0.05); however, it is uncertain this difference in total clearance reflects a decreased nonrenal PA clearance because the investigators did not measure renal PA clearance. In contrast, acute myocardial infarction and congestive heart failure had no effect on the pharmacokinetics of PA in a study of 37 patients and ten control patients.[152] This apparent discrepancy may be explained by the fact that blood samples in the pharmacokinetic study of Kessler et al.[152] were collected for only six hours after the start of a PA infusion, and a one-compartment model was used to describe plasma concentrations. Consistent with this explanation, PA clearances were higher and half-lives were shorter in this study than those reported in similar patient populations.[34,151] Thus, limited available data suggest that heart failure decreases the nonrenal clearance of PA.

Gibson et al.[37] have reported that nonrenal PA clearance is decreased in patients with *end-stage renal failure*. Nonrenal PA clearance in their four normal subjects was 4.04 ± 0.89 mL/min/kg (range 2.79 to 4.88 mL/min/kg) whereas in the four anephric patients it was 1.47 ± 0.24 mL/min/kg (range 1.13 to 1.68 mL/min/kg) (p <0.01). In contrast, Lima et al.[34] did not observe a statistically significant effect of renal impairment on acetylation clearance in 15 cardiac patients. The apparent difference in these observations may be due to the difference in the degree of renal impairment in the two study populations, the different causes of renal impairment in the two populations, and/or the difference in clearance parameters measured (i.e., total nonrenal clearance versus acetylation clearance). The possibility of decreased nonrenal PA clearance should be considered in patients with renal impairment, particularly those with end-stage renal disease.

Drug-induced changes in nonrenal PA clearance have also been reported. Olsen and Morland[77] examined the effect of ethanol on PA pharmacokinetics using two different protocols. In both studies, PA half-life was decreased, whereas total clearance, the percentage of NAPA in blood and urine, and the $AUC_{NAPA\ to}\ AUC_{PA}$ ratio were all increased by coadministration of ethanol. The effect of ethanol on total PA clearance was significantly greater in slow acetylators than in fast acetylators. PA volume of distribution and the renal clearances of both PA and NAPA were not affected. These data suggest that ethanol induces the acetylation of PA. There is some evidence which suggests that cimetidine[78,155] and ranitidine[16,153] may decrease PA nonrenal clearance. These observations are suspect because an oral rather than an intravenous PA administration route was used. Amiodarone may decrease the nonrenal clearance of PA in rats;[156] however, whether nonrenal clearance changes contribute to the decreased total PA clearance observed with amiodarone coadministration in humans[163,164] is unknown. DuSouich and Courteau[79] provided evidence that acetylation was induced in rabbits by complete Freund's adjuvant (a water-in-oil emulsion of killed mycobacteria used in this study to stimulate reticuloendothelial system activity) and high-dose hydrocortisone (150 mg/kg/day for ten days, used to inhibit reticuloendothelial system activity). We are not aware of any human data on the effects of steroids on acetylation capacity. Tilorone, a synthetic interferon inducer, increased the urinary excretion of NAPA, apparently increased the NAPA AUC, and had no effect on NAPA renal clearance or total PA clearance in rats.[154] This suggests that this immunomodulating agent, and possibly others, may increase acetylation. Hydralazine has been reported to decrease the acetylation of PA in animal studies;[80] however, this interaction was not observed when human subjects were given usual therapeutic doses of the two drugs.[81] Finally, clofibrate was reported to increase or decrease N-acetyltransferase-mediated acetylation of PA in the hepatic cytoplasm of rats, depending on the concentrations of PA and acetyl-CoA used.[168]

Coadministration of PABA and PA increased plasma PA concentrations and decreased plasma NAPA concentrations in one patient.[157] In further studies of five patients taking PA, 1.5 gm of PABA (potassium salt) every six hours for 24 hours also increased PA concentrations and decreased NAPA concentrations. PABA decreased the NAPA:PA plasma concentration ratio from 1.6 to 0.95 (p <0.05), had no effect on PA and NAPA renal clearances, and decreased the apparent acetylation clearance of PA from 98 mL/min to 63 mL/min (p <0.05).[158] This drug interaction may be clinically useful, particularly in patients with moderate to severe renal impairment. NAPA:PA plasma concentration ratios following PA administration are considerably higher in patients with renal impairment compared to patients with no renal impairment because the total clearance of NAPA is more dependent on renal elimination than PA.[34] It is possible that renally impaired patients may experience adverse effects resulting from excessive accumulation of NAPA and yet fail to achieve therapeutic concentrations of PA. By decreasing acetylation clearance, PABA administration will result in an increase in PA concentrations and a decrease in NAPA concentrations. This potentially beneficial drug interaction requires further study.

Excretion

In normal subjects, renal clearance accounts for approximately 40% to 60% of PA total body clearance and averages 5.0 ± 1.0 mL/min/kg.[35,37,40,54] PA renal clearance in seven cardiac patients with no gross renal impairment was 3.8 ± 1.4 mL/min/kg.[34] Since PA renal clearance:creatinine clearance ratios average 2 to 3 in adults,[55,82] proximal tubular secretion as well as glomerular filtration are involved in the elimination of PA by the kidneys. Distal tubular reabsorption appears to be insignificant, since changes in urine pH[55,82] and flow rate[82] do not affect PA renal clearance.

Several factors that do affect the renal clearance of PA have been identified. The influence of the most obvious factor, *renal impairment*, has been reviewed by Lima[11] and Karlsson.[83] Briefly, PA renal clearance decreases with decreasing renal function and, since PA volume of distribution is unchanged, PA half-life increases. PA half-life in one study of four surgically or physiologically anephric patients was 13.9 ± 4.5 hours as compared to 3.1 ± 0.5 hours in four normal subjects.[37]

That *age* affects PA renal clearance is not surprising since renal function generally declines with age, but evidence suggests that the effect is greater than would be expected on the basis of the age-related decrease in glomerular filtration rate. Reidenberg et al.[84] examined the relationship between the PA renal clearance:creatinine clearance ratio and the age of a total of 46 patients who were receiving PA for the treatment of arrhythmias. They found that children and young adults (less than 30 years) generally had ratios ranging between 4:1 and 5:1 and that this ratio gradually declined to between 1:1 and 3:1 in elderly patients. They suggested that this finding reflects a decreasing contribution of tubular secretion relative to glomerular filtration with increasing age. Bauer et al.[151] reported that age, renal impairment, and heart failure decreased PA clearance and further concluded that the effects of age and renal function on PA clearance were independent of each other. The relative effect of aging on glomerular filtration and tubular secretion needs to be examined using a more reliable index of glomerular filtration rate, such as inulin or iothalamate renal clearance.

Impaired cardiac function with poor perfusion of the kidneys probably affects PA renal clearance, but little information is available. Lima et al.[85] and Koch-Weser[7] both reported increased steady-state PA concentrations in patients with severely decreased cardiac output. Lalka et al.[86] suggested that decreased renal perfusion might explain the decrease in total PA clearance they observed in five post-myocardial infarction patients. However, the patient with the severest degree of heart failure in this study had the highest PA clearance. Grasela and Sheiner[12] reported an 11% decrease in PA renal clearance in their cardiac patients with congestive heart failure (mostly Class I by the New York Heart Association criteria). The paucity of data makes it impossible to assess the relationship between heart failure and PA renal clearance.

Obesity has been reported to influence PA renal clearance. Christoff et al.[40] examined the disposition of PA in seven obese and seven non-obese subjects following the IV administration of 300 mg of PA over one hour. Creatinine clearances were not statistically significantly different in the two groups. However, PA renal clearance was 514 ± 119 mL/min in the obese group and 352 ± 102 mL/min in the non-obese group (p <0.05). PA renal clearance per kg ideal body weight revealed similar differences; however, PA renal clearance per kg actual body weight was the same in the two groups (5.35 ± 1.81 versus 5.32 ± 1.07 mL/min/kg ABW). Total PA clearance, the physiologic determinant of average steady-state PA concentration, was also not significantly different between the groups when corrected for actual body weight [8.72 ± 1.61 versus 10.1 ± 2.7 mL/min/kg ABW in obese and non-obese subjects, respectively (p >0.20)]. These data suggest that PA maintenance doses may be based on actual weight in obese persons. These findings may not apply to morbidly obese patients since the study of Christoff et al.[40] did not include such subjects.

Cimetidine and *ranitidine* have both been shown to affect PA renal clearance. Somgoyi et al.[41] reported that PA AUC increased by 44%, PA renal clearance decreased by 43%, and PA half-life increased by 26% in six volunteers after coadministration of cimetidine (400 mg one hour before the PA dose and then 200 mg every four hours for three doses). Similar data have been reported by others.[78,155] Single 200 and 400 mg oral doses of cimetidine decreased PA renal clearance 31% and 40%, respectively, in seven healthy volunteers.[159] NAPA renal clearance was decreased 16% by the 400 mg dose. These data, combined with evidence that cimetidine does not affect glomerular filtration rate,[87] strongly suggest that cimetidine inhibits the tubular secretion of PA in humans and that the effect may be clinically important. The competition of organic bases—including PA, cimetidine, and NAPA—for secretion by the proximal tubules of rabbit kidneys is well established.[88,89]

The clinical significance of an interaction between ranitidine and procainamide is uncertain. Somogyi et al.[16] reported that 150 mg of ranitidine administered every 12 hours beginning 13 hours before PA dosing increased the AUC of PA and NAPA by 13.9% and 12.7%, respectively, and decreased renal clearances by 18.6% and 10.1%, respectively. Administration of 300 mg of ranitidine one hour before the PA dose followed by 150 mg every four hours for three doses resulted in a 20.8% increase in PA AUC and a 35% decrease in PA renal clearance. In contrast, Rodvold et al.[155] reported that 150 mg of ranitidine given every 12 hours for four days had no effect on the AUC and renal clearances of PA and NAPA following four days of treatment with Procan-SR, 500 mg every six hours. Rocci et al.[153] reported that 150 mg of ranitidine given every 12 hours for three days had no effect on the AUC and renal clearances of PA and NAPA following the administration of a single 1 gm dose of PA (immediate-release formulation). In summary, the data from these studies suggest that: 1) usual therapeutic doses of ranitidine (300 mg/day) affect PA renal clearance less than do usual therapeutic doses of cimetidine; 2) the interaction between usual therapeutic doses of ranitidine and PA is probably not clinically significant; and 3) the dose of PA may require adjustment when doses of ranitidine exceed 300 mg/day.

Five days of treatment with famotidine, a H_2-receptor antagonist which undergoes renal tubular secretion, had no effect on the pharmacokinetics of PA and NAPA.[160]

Other drugs may also alter renal PA clearance. Trimethoprim increased plasma concentrations of PA and NAPA by decreasing renal clearance of both compounds by 47% and 13%, respectively; the acetylation clearance of PA may also be increased.[161,162] Amiodarone increased plasma concentrations of PA and NAPA from 6.8 to 11 mg/L and 6.9 to 9.1 mg/L, respectively, in patients receiving an average PA dose of 3.7 gm/day.[163] The mechanism of this interaction was studied in eight patients by comparing the pharmacokinetics of intravenous PA alone and following one to two weeks of amiodarone treatment.[164] Amiodarone treatment decreased the average total PA clearance from 0.43 to 0.33 L/hr/kg, increased the mean half-life from 3.8 to 5.2 hours, and had no effect on the volume of distribution (V_{area}). PA renal clearance was determined in two of the eight patients and was shown to be decreased by amiodarone. Although limited, the data suggest that the increase in PA (and NAPA) concentrations seen with amiodarone coadministration is due to a decrease in the secretion clearance of PA and NAPA. This putative mechanism for the decrease in PA clearance is unusual because very little amiodarone is found in urine.[165] It is possible that amiodarone competes with PA for active tubular secretion, but is then reabsorbed. Intravenous infusions of NAPA achieving average steady-state concentrations of 8.4 mg/L prolonged the elimination half-life of PA from 4.6 to 5.7 hours (p <0.01), decreased the renal clearance of PA from 267 to 137 mL/min (p = 0.055), and had no effect on V_{ss}.[166] The propensity of NAPA to reduce the total clearance of PA was inversely related to the initial PA clearance. Finally, in one case report, 324 mg of Quinaglute given every eight hours increased steady-state plasma concentrations of PA from 9.1 to 15.4 mg/L; NAPA concentrations increased from 5.8 to 7.4 mg/L.[167]

The *dialyzability* of PA and NAPA by several methods has been reported, including hemodialysis,[44,90–93] chronic ambulatory peritoneal dialysis (CAPD),[169–171] hemoperfusion,[173] and combined hemodialysis and hemodilution.[174] The replacement dose (RD) of PA as a consequence of dialysis by any of these methods may be estimated by

$$RD = (C_{ss})\,(V_{ss}) \left[1 - e^{-\left(\frac{Cl_d + CL_o}{V_{ss}}\right)(t_d)} \right] \left[\frac{CK_d}{Cl_d + Cl_o} \right]$$

where C_{ss} is the PA plasma concentration at steady state; V_{ss} is the PA volume of distribution at steady state; Cl_d is the "dialysance" clearance; Cl_o is the "other" clearance (sum of the body's renal and nonrenal clearances) for PA; and t_d is the dialysis time. The clearance of PA by CAPD is very low (1 to 7 mL/min),[169–171] and no replacement dose is necessary. The clearance of PA by hemodialysis averages 68 mL/min (range: 25 to 91.2 mL/min, n = 27);[44,90–93] whether or not a replacement dose is required in patients being hemodialyzed is not clear. The need for and size of post-dialysis replacement doses should be based on plasma PA concentrations observed before and after dialysis, recognizing that of a time-dependent redistribution of PA from the peripheral compartment occurs,[92] and clinical judgment. Atkinson et al.[93] reported that hemodialysis doubled PA clearance and quadrupled NAPA clearance in a patient with severe PA toxicity.

NAPA Pharmacokinetics

The pharmacokinetic characteristics of NAPA are of considerable interest because NAPA concentrations frequently equal or exceed those of PA and because NAPA possesses both toxic and antiarrhythmic activity. The steady-state volume of distribution of NAPA is similar to that of PA.[35] NAPA is approximately 10% bound to plasma protein at concentrations of 1 to 16 mg/L in normal subjects.[55] The renal clearance of NAPA is 2.51 ± 0.26 mL/min/kg in normal subjects;[48] this accounts for approximately 87% of NAPA total body clearance in fast acetylators[48,193] and 77% of NAPA total body clearance in slow acetylators.[193] NAPA is therefore more dependent on renal function for elimination than PA and accumulates to a greater extent than PA in patients with renal failure.[94] Like PA, NAPA is secreted by the proximal tubules, although the contribution of secretion to renal clearance appears to be less for NAPA.[35] The nonrenal clearance of NAPA is reported to be lower in fast acetylators than in slow acetylators (2.2 versus 3.9 L/hr, p = 0.012) and inversely correlated with percentage sulfapyridine acetylation.[193] In contrast to their findings with PA, Christoff et al. did not observe a significant difference in NAPA renal clearance between obese and non-obese subjects.[40] NAPA half-life in normal subjects ranges from 5.1 to 7.7 hours,[35,48,95,193] while in anephric patients it is 41.5 ± 7.8 hours.[37] Peritoneal dialysis and CAPD are not efficient means of dialyzing NAPA.[169–171] The hemodialysis clearance of NAPA is similar to or slightly less than that of PA and is useful in the treatment of NAPA intoxication.[44,91–93,96] Dialysis clearance of NAPA in renally impaired patients by hemoperfusion, continuous hemofiltration, and hemodiafiltration have been reported to be higher than hemodialysis and have been preferred over hemodialysis in NAPA-intoxicated patients.[172–174] The pharmacokinetics of NAPA have been extensively reviewed by others.[97,194]

PHARMACODYNAMICS

Therapeutic Response

Procainamide Concentrations. The largest study of the relationship between plasma PA concentrations and its effects was conducted by Koch-Weser et al.[1,7,98,99] They evaluated the therapeutic and toxic effects of PA in 306 patients being treated for ventricular arrhythmias associated with myocardial infarction (63%), chronic coronary heart disease (24%), or other heart diseases (11%). PA was the only antiarrhythmic agent used in each patient, although details of other therapy were not provided. Each patient's therapy was guided by his physician who had no knowledge of plasma PA concentrations. PA efficacy was based on the physician's judgment that the arrhythmia was "satisfactorily controlled." Side-effects were considered serious if PA was discontinued, and minor if therapy was continued. The temporal relationship of blood sampling to PA dose was not specified. PA therapy was ineffective in a majority of patients with plasma PA concentrations of less than 4 mg/L. PA therapy was effective in 85% of patients with plasma PA concentrations of 4 to 8 mg/L without any serious toxicities. Increasing the concentration to 8 to 12 mg/L produced a satisfactory response in an additional 10% of patients who had not responded to lower levels; however, serious toxicities were noted in approximately 5% of patients at these concentrations. Concentrations greater than 12 mg/L were rarely effective if lower concentrations were not and were associated with a progressively increasing incidence of serious toxicities. Koch-Weser[98,99] therefore concluded that the therapeutic range for the treatment of ventricular arrhythmias was 4 to 10 mg/L.

Although several investigators have reported therapeutic ranges similar to that of Koch-Weser,[100–104] several groups have reported the need for higher plasma PA concentrations. Lima et al.[85] examined the plasma PA concentration-effect relationship in 34 patients receiving continuous intravenous infusions of PA for the treatment of lidocaine-resistant ventricular arrhythmias. Ten of eleven patients (91%) with plasma PA concentrations greater than 8 mg/L responded to treatment, whereas only 15 of 23 patients (65%) with concentrations less than 8 mg/L responded. The investigators suggested that plasma PA concentrations in excess of 8 mg/L were required to treat some patients with ventricular arrhythmias. The apparent discrepancy between this finding and that of Koch-Weser may be due to the use of lidocaine-resistant patients by Lima et al. and the high percentage (74%) of patients with ventricular tachycardia in their group. Treatment of ventricular tachycardia may require higher plasma concentrations of PA than, for example, those required for the suppression of premature ventricular contractions (PVCs) following acute myocardial infarction.

Giardina et al.[21] examined the PA concentration-effect relationship in 22 patients on a sustained-release PA preparation (Pronestyl-SR). All patients had chronic cardiac disease, had more than 10 PVCs per hour, and had responded to PA therapy during a previous acute dose-ranging study with a greater than 75% reduction in PVCs. The average minimum steady-state plasma PA concentration in these patients was 6.8 ± 4.5 mg/L (range 1.8 to 17.0 mg/L). Five of the 22 patients (23%) required plasma PA concentrations greater than 10 mg/L (range 12.3 to 17.0 mg/L). Although dosage requirements may have been overestimated because of rapid dosage adjustments, the presence of chronic cardiac disease as the cause of the arrhythmias in these patients may also account for the higher plasma PA concentrations required.

Greenspan et al.[105] studied a series of 16 patients with recurrent, sustained ventricular tachycardia or ventricular fibrillation who were treated with PA. In 14 of these patients, the arrhythmia could be reproduced by programmed electrical stimulation (PES). Each of the 14 received 1000 mg PA intravenously over 20 minutes; attempts were made to induce arrhythmias and blood samples were drawn for determination of plasma PA concentrations 5 to 15 minutes after the end of the infusion. Additional 250 mg doses of PA were administered until the arrhythmias were no longer inducible. In the remaining two patients, the ventricular tachycardia was incessant and was suppressed by intravenous PA infusion before electrophysiologic testing. A chronic dosing regimen was then designed for each of the 16 patients to maintain plasma PA concentrations above the level shown to be effective during PES studies. Fourteen patients tolerated the oral doses of PA and after three days, therapy was demonstrated to be effective (PES studies) and to have resulted in trough PA levels equal to or greater than the level previously demonstrated to be effective. Two patients did not tolerate the initial oral regimens—one tolerated a lower dose which was shown by PES to be effective and the other did not tolerate any dose which suppressed his tachycardia. The effective PA concentration during acute dose adjustment was 13.6 ± 8.6 mg/L (range 4.3 to 32.3 mg/L); 9 of the 15 patients (60%) for whom plasma concentration data were reported required concentrations greater than 10 mg/L. The average effective PA concentration associated with chronic dosing was 13.1 ± 6.8 mg/L (range 6.0 to 35.0 mg/L); 11 of 15 patients (73%) had plasma PA concentrations greater than 10 mg/L.

It is possible that effective PA concentrations were overestimated by Greenspan et al. as a result of their acute drug testing protocol. Available data suggest that PA's electrophysiologic effects may occur in a peripheral compartment in many normal subjects[38,178] and arrhythmia patients.[106,179,180] The rate of PA distribution into the effect compartment probably decreases with increasing ischemia.[107] Determination of therapeutic plasma PA concentrations under the nonequilibrium conditions[181] of this acute drug testing protocol may therefore be inaccurate. In addition, while the protocol defines *an* effective plasma PA concentration, it does not necessarily define the *minimum* effective concentration.[182] However, Greenspan et al. followed their patients for 19 ± 14 months (range: 4 to 48 months). Of the 15 patients who were arrhythmia-free upon release from the hospital, ten continued their oral regimen and remained arrhythmia-free. The five patients in whom the dosage was decreased all developed ventricular tachycardia or fibrillation. Two of these five patients died suddenly, while arrhythmias in the other three were abolished when their original dosage regimen was resumed. These follow-up data argue against a major overestimation of effective plasma PA concentrations in this study. Again, the need for high-dose PA in these patients may be related to the nature of the patient population (recurrent ventricular tachycardia associated with significant coronary artery disease in most patients).

Myerburg et al.[108] have examined the PA concentration-effect relationship in 18 patients: six with PVCs associated with acute myocardial infarction (MI), six with PVCs associated with stable chronic ischemic heart disease (CIHD), and six with recurrent symptomatic ventricular tachycardia (VT) with chronic PVCs between VT episodes. After a two-hour baseline period of Holter monitor recording in MI and CIHD patients, five 100 mg intravenous doses of PA were administered, each over one minute and at five-minute intervals. Each patient then received a 500 mg oral dose of PA 4.5 hours after the initial infusion. Holter monitoring continued for at least seven hours after the initial infusion. PA concentrations were determined in plasma samples drawn approximately five minutes, 35 minutes, two hours, four hours, and six hours after the last infusion. PVC frequency was measured from the Holter recording for the 30 minute periods nearest to each blood sampling time. Dosing in patients with VT was not as well controlled because of the more serious nature of the arrhythmia. In these patients, dosing was based on "clinical indications," and the effective plasma level was defined as the minimum plasma PA concentration required to suppress VT for at least 48 hours. The plasma PA concentration-effect data from this study are shown in Table 22-2. While this study involved very select groups of patients and is subject to the same concerns with respect to a plasma concentration-effect time lag (see discussion of Greenspan et al. above), it strongly suggests that the plasma PA concentration required to treat an arrhythmia is dependent on the type of arrhythmia. The effective PA concentration in the MI and CIHD groups were within the 4 to 10 mg/L defined by Koch-Weser in all 12 patients, although the concentrations in the CIHD group were significantly higher and at the upper end

Table 22-2. *Plasma Procainamide Concentration – Effect Data from Myerburg et al.[108]*

Group	Plasma PA concentration[a] required for 85% suppression of PVCs	Plasma PA concentration required to suppress spontaneous VT (mg/L)
MI	5.0 ± 0.5 (4.3–5.7)	—
CIHD	9.3 ± 0.7 (8.0–10.0)	—
VT	14.9 ± 3.8 (9.3–18.8)	9.1 ± 3.4 (5.5–14.9)

[a] Mean $\pm$ SD (range).
[b] MI = Myocardial infarction; CIHD = Chronic ischemic heart disease; VT = Ventricular tachycardia; PVCs = Premature ventricular contractions.

of this therapeutic range. Plasma concentrations required for 85% suppression of PVCs were above this therapeutic range in five of six VT patients. With ventricular tachycardia suppressions used as the endpoint, two of six patients required PA concentrations greater than 10 mg/L.

Myerburg et al.[109] have also provided evidence that maintenance of therapeutic plasma PA concentrations (i.e., 4 to 8 mg/L) may affect the long-term therapeutic outcome in cardiac arrest patients. Six of their patients with stable, therapeutic PA concentrations remained free of cardiac arrest during a minimum of 12 months follow-up. In contrast, eight of ten patients who had variable, subtherapeutic PA concentrations experienced recurrent cardiac arrests. Data from this study also suggest that the complete suppression of complex PVC activity is not required to prevent recurrent cardiac arrests. This observation is consistent with their later data[108] demonstrating that lower PA concentrations were required to suppress VT than to suppress chronic PVCs in their VT patients.

Morady et al.[182] examined procainamide's acute antiarrhythmic effects during programmed electrical stimulation studies of 31 patients with inducible, sustained, monomorphic ventricular tachycardia. Twenty-six patients had a history of coronary artery disease and acute myocardial infarction. Cumulative, intravenous loading doses of 7.5, 15, 22.5, and 30 mg/kg were administered at a rate of 50 mg/min, and each loading dose was followed by a 2 mg/min infusion. Repeat programmed electrical stimulation was begun five minutes after the end of each loading dose and required 5 to 20 minutes for completion. Plasma procainamide and N-acetylprocainamide concentrations were measured at the end of each stimulation protocol in all patients. The mean ($\pm$ SD) plasma procainamide concentrations resulting from the incremental doses were 5.5 ± 1.2, 9.0 ± 1.6, 12.6 ± 2.2, and 16.3 ± 3.2 mg/L. Induction of ventricular tachycardia was suppressed in 8 of the 31 patients following the administration of the 7.5 mg/kg dose. Plasma procainamide concentrations in these eight patients ranged from 3.6 to 6.4 mg/L. When higher doses of PA were given, ventricular tachycardia was suppressed in only two additional patients whose plasma procainamide concentrations were 12 and 12.4 mg/L. Interestingly, a therapeutic window appeared to exist for PA's antiarrhythmic effect in three of the ten patients in whom ventricular tachycardia was suppressed. Finally, six of the eight patients who responded after the 7.5 mg/kg dose underwent repeat testing while on oral procainamide therapy. Plasma procainamide concentrations at the time of repeat testing were within 0.5 to 2.1 mg/L of the effective concentration defined by acute drug testing, and in all six patients ventricular tachycardia could not be induced.

In summary, 4 to 10 mg/L appears to be a generally useful therapeutic range for PA when it is used to treat ventricular arrhythmias. A large majority of patients who respond to PA do so within this range of plasma concentrations. However, a select group of patients, particularly those experiencing ventricular tachycardia associated with chronic heart disease, may require and tolerate higher PA concentrations. Most of these patients respond to concentrations of 10 to 20 mg/L if PA therapy is going to be successful.[85,105,108]

NAPA Concentrations. Application of this general therapeutic range for PA to the individual patient is complicated by the presence of NAPA, an active metabolite whose plasma concentration frequently equals or exceeds that of the parent drug.[110–119,126–128] Early studies suggested that PA and NAPA were equally efficacious and potent.[116–117] Thus, it has been recommended that the sum of plasma PA and NAPA concentrations be used to guide PA therapy, with a suggested therapeutic range of 5 to 30 mg PA + NAPA/L.[11,120,121,195] In our opinion, the following evidence suggests that this "summed" approach is not justified. First, current data suggest that the potency of NAPA is lower than that of PA. Although they are of similar potency in the mouse chloroform-induced fibrillation model,[110,116] NAPA is only one-third to one-sixth as potent an antiarrhythmic agent as PA in other animal models.[112,113,125] In keeping with this lower potency, the therapeutic range for NAPA in humans is generally considered to be approximately 10 to 30 mg/L.[195] Secondly, because NAPA produces electrophysiologic effects that are different from PA,[112,114,115,122,123] their antiarrhythmic actions are unlikely to be additive for all, if any, types of arrhythmias. In fact, Roden et al.[124] have demonstrated that response to one of these drugs does not predict response to the other. In 23 patients with chronic, high-frequency PVCs, four of the seven patients who responded to NAPA did not respond to PA, and 11 of 15 patients who responded to PA did not respond to NAPA. Finally, Funck-Brentano et al.[166] have studied the antiarrhythmic interactions of PA and NAPA in nine patients with frequent PVCs. Each patient received intravenous infusions of PA, NAPA, or both PA and NAPA on three different occasions, and the effect of each treatment on PVC frequency was assessed. PA alone was effective (greater than 85% reduction in single PVC frequency) in six patients. NAPA alone was effective in suppressing single PVCs in only one patient at the concentration used in this study. (Note that the target NAPA concentration used in this study, 8 mg/L, was below the therapeutic range for NAPA alone but was chosen to simulate the clinical situation of a patient without significant renal impairment being treated with procainamide.) Most importantly, the addition of NAPA at a targeted concentration of 8 mg/L had little, if any, effect on the antiarrhythmic response to PA.

Because of the significant body of data supporting the use of PA concentrations alone for therapeutic drug monitoring purposes, the uncertainty concerning NAPA's contribution to the antiarrhythmic activity of administered PA, and the additional cost involved in monitoring both PA and NAPA concentrations (in most labs the cost is doubled), we generally recommend the use of plasma PA concentrations alone in helping to make decisions regarding the efficacy of PA in patients with ventricular arrhythmias. This approach has also been recommended by others.[98,129,130] Nevertheless, one must recognize that in any given patient, NAPA may contribute to or even be entirely responsible for the efficacy of PA therapy as suggested by the data of Roden et al. described above.[124] This is particularly likely in patients with severe renal impairment who respond to PA administration. These patients tend to have relatively high plasma NAPA concentrations (e.g., 15 to 30 mg/L) with relatively low plasma PA concentrations (e.g., 2 to 5 mg/L). The use of plasma NAPA concentrations alone, or the sum of plasma PA and NAPA concentrations to guide efficacy decisions may be justified in these patients, although supporting data are very limited. We do routinely recommend monitoring both plasma PA and NAPA concentrations in patients with moderate to severe renal impairment to identify patients at increased risk for toxicity as described below.

Toxic Concentrations

Koch-Weser examined the concentration-adverse effect relationship for PA (see Figure 22-2).[1,7,98,99] The incidence of both minor side effects (e.g., gastrointestinal disturbances, weakness, malaise, mean arterial pressure decrements greater than 20%, and prolongation of P-R, QRS, and Q-T intervals by 10% to 30%) and serious adverse effects (e.g., mean arterial pressure decrements greater than 20%, prolongation of P-R, QRS, and Q-T intervals by greater than 30%, development of new arrhythmias, and cardiac arrest) increased with increasing PA concentrations. In this study, minor side effects were observed in approximately 10% of patients with plasma PA concentrations of 8.1 to 10.0 mg/L, whereas serious toxicities were seen in only 2% of patients. At plasma PA concentrations of 12.1 to 16.0 mg/L, minor and serious adverse effects were observed in 27% and 16% of patients, respectively. At higher concentrations, serious adverse effects were seen in approximately 35% of all patients, with minor toxicities observed in an additional 35%.

More recent studies with high-dose PA[85,105,108] suggest that many patients tolerate PA concentrations between 10 and 20 mg/L better than would be expected from Koch-Weser's results. Accumulation of high NAPA concentrations in Koch-Weser's patients may explain the differences,[11] but this explanation is speculative since Koch-Weser did not measure NAPA concentrations nor did he describe the renal function of his patients. Since NAPA administration has been associated with many of the same adverse effects as PA administration,[117,118,122,124,126,127] the potential contributions of NAPA to toxicity must be considered, particularly in patients with severe renal impairment. Vlasses et al.[131] suggested that excessive accumulation of NAPA (serum concentrations = 42 to 59.4 mg/L) may have contributed to the deaths of four patients who were being treated with PA (serum concentrations = 6.2 to 13.3 mg/L) in the presence of severe renal impairment.

Lima et al.[85] provided evidence that the risk of toxicity is increased when the sum of PA and NAPA concentrations exceeds 25 to 30 mg/L. Analysis of data presented by Giardina et al.[21] supports this guideline. In their study of 22 patients receiving chronic sustained-release PA therapy for the treatment of PVCs, seven patients experienced adverse effects. Six of these seven patients (86%) had maximum PA plus NAPA concentrations greater than 25 mg/L, whereas only three of the remaining 15 patients (20%) had maximum summed concentrations greater than 25 mg/L. Minimum summed concentrations in the adverse-effect group were greater than 25 mg/L in three of seven patients (43%), whereas none of the patients in the other group had a minimum summed concentration greater than 25 mg/L. Although PA and NAPA concentrations greater than 25 to 30 mg/L are neither sufficient nor necessary for adverse effects to occur,[21,132] they do appear to identify patients at increased risk of toxicity.

Reports[6,133–135,183,184] have associated a sustained-release PA preparation (Procan-SR) with an apparently increased incidence of PA-induced granulocytopenia. This increased number of granulocytopenia cases appears to reflect an increased use of PA or an increased awareness of this adverse effect[136,185] rather than a particular propensity of the Procan-SR formulation to cause granulocytopenia.[186] It is important to counsel patients to report signs and symptoms of neutropenia (fever, malaise, sore throat, or other symptoms of infections) and to periodically have their complete blood count checked during the first three months of therapy. Cases of pure red cell aplasia,[187,188] thrombocytopenia,[189] and pancytopenia[190,191] have also been reported.

CLINICAL APPLICATION OF PHARMACOKINETIC DATA

Intravenous Dosing

Lima et al.[11,85,137] have described a two-infusion technique for intravenous administration of PA (see Figure 22-4). This technique is designed to rapidly (approximately 15 minutes) and safely achieve and maintain plasma PA concentrations in the range of 4 to 8 mg/L. The loading dose is 17 mg PA HCl/kg IBW infused at a constant rate over one hour. This is immediately followed by a maintenance infusion of 2.8 mg PA HCl/kg ABW/hr. The maintenance infusion rate should be reduced by one-third in patients with moderately impaired renal function or cardiac output and by two-thirds in patients with severe renal or cardiac output impairment. The loading dose should be decreased to 12 mg/kg in patients with severely impaired renal function or cardiac output.

If it is necessary to increase the rate of administration because of inadequate plasma concentrations or response, additional loading doses of 2 mg PA HCl/kg IBW can be administered for each 1 mg/L increase in plasma concentration desired. The maintenance infusion may be increased without an additional loading dose if rapid achievement of the new steady-state concentration is not necessary. The appropriate maintenance dose for the desired plasma concentration can be calculated based on the plasma concentration produced by the initial maintenance infusion. Aggressive dosage changes (e.g., doubling or tripling the dose rate) generally should be avoided because of the potential for disproportionate increases in plasma PA concentration and toxicity.

Giardina et al.[100] recommend a different approach to initial intravenous PA therapy. They suggest that 100 mg of PA HCl be administered as a two-minute infusion at five-minute intervals until the arrhythmia is controlled, a cumulative dose of 1 gm is reached, or toxicity develops. While this method is frequently used, we prefer the two-infusion technique described above for routine clinical use because it is relatively simple and plasma PA concentrations of 4 to 8 mg/L are rapidly achieved and maintained.

Under certain circumstances, it may be desirable to achieve and maintain one or more targeted plasma PA concentrations even more rapidly than is possible using the two-infusion technique described above. The use of PA for acute drug testing during human electrophysiology studies is an example of such a situation.

Krüger-Thiemer developed the theoretical basis for accomplishing this for multi-compartment drugs using exponentially declining infusions.[196] Coyle et al.[138] have developed a computer-based infusion system which is capable of rapidly (within five to ten minutes) achieving and maintaining one or more targeted plasma PA concentrations using a modification of Krüger-Thiemer's exponentially declining infusion approach. The system was tested in four dogs with targeted plasma PA

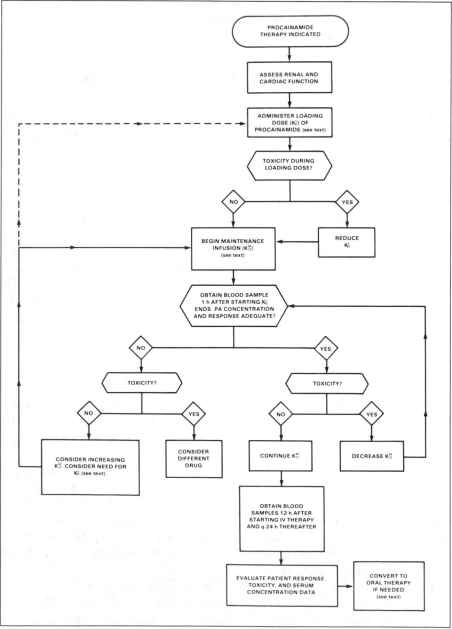

Figure 22-4. *Algorithm for treatment of patients with PA using the two-infusion technique.*

concentrations of 4, 8, and 12 mg/L. The resulting mean plasma concentration versus time data is shown in Figure 22-5. There were no statistically significant differences in concentrations during each of the "steady states" and no significant differences between the targeted concentrations and those actually achieved (p >0.05). This infusion system is currently being evaluated in patients.

Oral Dosing

Lima[11] has previously discussed the selection of an oral PA dose if the patient is being treated with an intravenous PA infusion and steady state has been achieved. The daily oral dose may be calculated by:

$$\text{Daily Dose} = \frac{\left(C_{SS}^{PO} \right)\left(\dfrac{K_O}{C_{SS}^{iv}} \right)(24)}{F} \tag{Eq. 22-2}$$

where C_{SS}^{PO} is the desired average steady-state concentration during oral therapy, C_{SS}^{iv} is the observed steady-state concentration during IV therapy, k_o is the maintenance IV infusion rate in mg/hr, and F is the bioavailability of the oral preparation (assumed to be 0.83). One-fourth of this daily dose can then be administered every six hours using a sustained-release PA preparation. Every three-to-four-hour

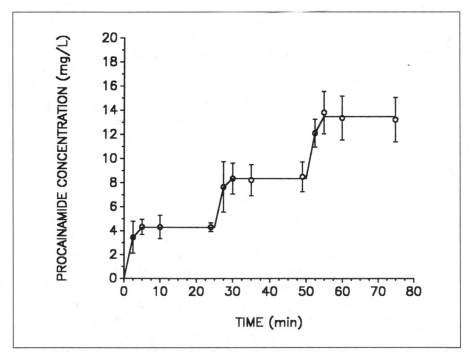

Figure 22-5. *Mean plasma PA concentration versus time in four dogs receiving PA infusions using a new exponentially declining infusion system developed by one of the authors (JDC). The error bars represent one standard deviation unit. The line connects consecutive data points during the loading doses and represents the mean concentration during plateau. The targeted plasma concentrations were 4, 8, and 12 mg/L.*

dosing is required with immediate-release products unless the patient has sufficient renal impairment to significantly prolong the PA half-life. It is important to
check the pre-dose ("trough") PA concentration after steady state has been reached
(12 to 18 hours if renal function is normal; 48 to 72 hours if significant renal
impairment exists) since PA bioavailability may vary considerably from the
assumed value.

Initiation of oral PA therapy in patients who have not previously been treated
with IV PA therapy is more difficult. We believe that an initial maintenance dose
of 50 mg PA HCl/kg ABW/day as recommended by Koch-Weser and Klein[1] and
two manufacturers[138] is appropriate for the treatment of ventricular arrhythmias in
patients with normal renal and cardiac function. Others have recommended
somewhat lower doses,[139,140] but in one study[139] the recommended dose resulted in
trough plasma PA concentrations less than 4 mg/L in 5 of 14 patients. The oral
maintenance dose should be decreased as described above for IV dosing in patients
with renal or cardiac impairment. An initial dose of twice the maintenance dose
(e.g., a 1 gm loading dose if maintenance dose is 500 mg every three hours) may
be used to more rapidly achieve therapeutic levels.

Timing of Samples for Therapeutic Drug Monitoring

The measurement of plasma PA concentration is a valuable tool in guiding PA
therapy. PA concentrations provide important information which assists in therapeutic decision making when they are appropriately measured and evaluated in
the context of the patient's therapeutic and toxicologic response.

When PA is administered using the two-infusion technique, we recommend
obtaining samples for plasma PA concentrations 2 and 12 hours after the beginning
of therapy and at 24-hours intervals thereafter. Two hours is selected for the first
sample because the concentration at this time is within 95% of the steady-state
concentration in most patients. Adjustment of these sample times may be necessary if therapeutic response is inadequate, if toxicity develops, or if dosage
adjustments are made. We recommend measuring plasma NAPA concentrations
only when moderate to severe renal impairment exists and then only as an index
of toxicity. In these cases, it should be remembered that the half-life of NAPA
may be as long as 40 hours in functionally anephric patients. NAPA may therefore
continue to accumulate for as long as one week, depending on the severity of renal
impairment.

Selection of appropriate sampling times for patients on oral PA therapy is more
difficult. The variability of peak times makes it impossible to accurately measure
peak concentrations without multiple (three or more) samples within a dosing
interval. Although this might be of value in selected patients, the cost of this
approach argues against its routine use. We recommend measuring pre-dose
("trough") steady-state PA concentrations during oral PA therapy. Steady-state
PA concentrations should be achieved within 12 to 18 hours in patients with
normal renal function and within 48 to 72 hours in patients with severe renal
impairment. Again, NAPA should generally only be measured (as an index of
toxicity) in patients with significant renal impairment.

Red blood cells metabolize PA *in vitro*.[42,43] Chen et al.[43] have demonstrated NAPA appearance rates of approximately 0.05 and 0.10 mg/L/hr in heparinized blood stored at 5 °C and 25 °C, respectively. A second, unidentified metabolite was also formed. No metabolism occurred when similar studies were conducted using plasma instead of blood. These data suggest that heparinized blood samples should be centrifuged and separated promptly to avoid artifactual changes in the plasma concentrations of PA and its metabolites. The significance of red cell metabolism in samples that are not anticoagulated has not been reported.

ANALYTICAL METHODS

Numerous methods have been developed to analyze PA and/or NAPA in biological fluids. These include the following: spectrophotometric (SP), spectro-fluorophotometric (SPF), gas chromatographic (GC), high-performance liquid chromatographic (HPLC), thin layer chromatographic (TLC) assays, and competitive binding immunoassays (CBI) [including fluorescence polarization immunoassays (TDx), enzyme immunoassays (EMIT), fluoroimmunoassays (TDA), and radioimmunoassay (RIA)]. These methods have been reviewed by Lima[11] and are compared in Table 22-3. For clinical laboratories, the nonradiolabeled CBI systems are probably the methods of choice. Our group has evaluated the TDA and Emit Qst PA and NAPA analyses and found them to be suitable for therapeutic drug monitoring.[141,197] Differences among the systems, including automation,

Table 22-3. Comparison of Assay Methods for Procainamide and NAPA[a]

Analytical method[b]	Limit of sensitivity	Assayable samples			Minimum sample volume required	Analysis time	Comments
		Plasma/serum	Urine	Saliva			
SP	3	3	3	3	3	3	NAPA not assayable simultaneously
SPF	3	3	3	3	3	3	NAPA not assayable simultaneously
HPLC	1	1	1	1	1	1	
GC	1	1	1	1	1	1	
TLC	1	1	1	1	1	1	
CBI (TDx, TDA, EMIT)	3	1	?	?	1	1	Separate test for NAPA available
RIA	3	1	?	?	2	1	Does not measure NAPA

[a] Arbitrary ranking scale of 1 (Excellent) to 5 (Poor) with a score of 3 being average or nominal.
[b] SP = Spectrophotometry; SPF = Spectrofluorophotometry; HPLC = High performance liquid chromatography; GC = Gas chromatography; TLC = Thin layer chromatography; CBI = Competitive binding immunoassays; TDx = Fluorescence polarization immunoassays; TDA = Fluoroimmunoassays; EMIT = Enzyme immunoassay; RIA = Radioimmunoassay.

precision, accuracy, analytical time, and cost, should be carefully examined before deciding upon the one which best suits the needs of a particular laboratory. A more sensitive method for measuring concentrations of PA and NAPA in plasma, serum, and urine (as low as 0.1 to 2.0 µg/mL) using EMIT has been published.[192]

PROSPECTUS

Although PA has been in use for over 30 years, major gaps still exist in our understanding of its pharmacokinetics and pharmacodynamics. These include the following:

- **Definition of Therapeutic Range.** Optimum use of PA requires a thorough understanding of the contribution of NAPA to its antiarrhythmic activity. Our recommendation to use PA concentrations alone to monitor drug therapy reflects the inadequacy of our current knowledge in this area.
- **Characterization of Concentration-Dependent PA Disposition.** The clinical significance of nonlinear PA clearance remains to be established.
- **Dose-Dependent Indices of Acetylator Phenotype.** The concentration-dependence of PA nonrenal clearance strongly suggests that PA acetylation clearance is concentration-dependent. This, in turn, suggests that indices of acetylator phenotype such as NAPA:PA ratios in serum or urine and CL_{AP} may be dependent on the dose of PA (or other test drug) administered and the resulting plasma PA concentration. The significance of this question is increased by the varying doses of PA used in several studies of PA acetylation polymorphism.
- **Effect of Disease States on PA Kinetics.** Our understanding of the effect of disease states on PA pharmacokinetics is based on a very small number of studies. More studies in this area are important to the selection of appropriate loading and maintenance dosing regimens.

REFERENCES

1. Koch-Weser J, Klein SW. Procainamide dosage schedules, plasma concentrations, and clinical effects. JAMA. 1971;215:1454–460.
2. Griesemer, DA. Procainamide-induced lupus. Johns Hopkins Med J. 1976;138:289–95.
3. Weinstein A. Drug-induced lupus erythematosus. Prog Clin Immunol. 1980;4:1–21.
4. Alorcon-Segovia D. Drug-induced antinuclear antibodies and lupus syndromes. Drugs. 1976;12:69–77.
5. Uetrecht JP, Woosley RL. Acetylator phenotype and lupus erythematosus. Clin Pharmacokinet. 1981;6:118–34.
6. Gabrielson RM. Procainamide and neutropenia. Ann Intern Med. 1984;100:766.
7. Koch-Weser J. Pharmacokinetics of procainamide in man. Ann N Y Acad Sci. 1971;179:370–82.
8. Manion CV et al. Absorption kinetics of procainamide in humans. J Pharm Sci. 1977;66:6981–984.
9. Weliky I, Neiss ES. Absorption of procainamide from the human intestine. Clin Pharmacol Ther. 1975;17:248. Abstract.
10. Giardina EGV et al. Metabolism of procainamide in normal and cardiac subjects. Clin Pharmacol Ther. 1976;19:339–51.
11. Lima JJ. Procainamide. In: Evans WE et al, eds. Applied Pharmacokinetics. Principles of Therapeutic Drug Monitoring. Vancouver, WA: Applied Therapeutics;1980:404–35.

12. Grasela TH, Sheiner LB. Population pharmacokinetics of procainamide from routine clinical data. Clin Pharmacokinet. 1984;9:545–54.

13. Graffner C et al. Pharmacokinetics of procainamide intravenously and orally as conventional and slow-release tablets. Clin Pharmacol Ther. 1975;17:414–23.

14. McKnight WD, Murphy ML. The effect of food on procainamide absorption. South Med J. 1976;69:851–52.

15. Felser J, Hui KK. Procainamide absorption in short bowel syndrome. JPEN. 1983;7:154–55.

16. Somogyi A, Bochner F. Dose and concentration dependent effect of ranitidine on procainamide disposition and renal clearance in man. Br J Clin Pharmacol. 1984;18:175–81.

17. Flanagan, AD. Pharmacokinetics of a sustained release procainamide preparation. Angiology. 1982;33:71–77.

18. Smith TC, Kinkel AW. Plasma levels of procainamide after administration of concentrional and sustained-release preparations. Curr Ther Res. 1980;27:217–28.

19. Kuehl P, Arquin P. Steady-state (SS) bioavailability (F) of a sustained-release (SR) procainamide (PCM) preparation. Drug Intell Clin Pharm. 1982;16:475–76. Abstract.

20. Vlasses PH et al. Immediate-release and sustained-release procainamide. Bioavailability at steady-state in cardiac patients. Ann Intern Med. 1983;98:613–14.

21. Giardina EGV et al. Efficacy, plasma concentrations and adverse effects of a new release procainamide preparation. Am J Cardiol. 1980;46:855–62.

22. Sramek JJ, Kajawall A. Carcass of a pill: no cause for alarm. N Engl J Med. 1981;305:231. Letter.

23. Woosley RL et al. Antiarrhythmic therapy; clinical pharmacology update. J Clin Pharmacol. 1984;24:295–305.

24. Birkhead J et al. Sustained-release procainamide in patients with myocardial infarction. Br Heart J. 1976;38:77–80.

25. Bauer GE et al. The assessment of an antiarrhythmic agent, sustained-release procainamide, with the aid of Holter monitoring. Med J Aust. 1977;2:733–35.

26. Hore P et al. A pharmacokinetic comparison of two sustained-release oral procainamide preparations. Br J Clin Pharmacol. 1979;8:267–71.

27. Cunningham T et al. Procainamide blood levels after administration of a sustained-release preparation. Med J Aust. 1977;1:370–72.

28. Shaw TRD et al. Procainamide absorption studies to test the feasibility of using a sustained-release preparation. Br J Clin Pharmacol. 1975;2:515–19.

29. Ihlen H, Ditlefsen EML. Procainamide in acute myocardial infarction: a study of two different tablet preparations of sustained-release type. Curr Ther Res. 1975;18:720–26.

30. Kirschenbaum HL et al. Stability of procainamide in 0.9% sodium chloride or dextrose 5% in water. Am J Hosp Pharm. 1979;36:1464–465.

31. Baaske DM et al. Stability of procainamide hydrochloride in dextrose solutions. Am J Hosp Pharm. 1980;37:1050–52. Letter.

32. Gupta VD. Complexation of procainamide with dextrose. J Pharm Sci. 1982;71:994–96.

33. Gupta VD. Complexation of procainamide with hydroxide-containing compounds. J Pharm Sci. 1983;72:205–207.

34. Lima JJ et al. Clinical pharmacokinetics of procainamide infusions in relation to acetylator phenotype. J Pharmacokinet Biopharm. 1979;7:69–85.

35. Dutcher JS et al. Procainamide and N-acetylprocainamide kinetics investigated simultaneously with stable isotope methodology. Clin Pharmacol Ther. 1977;22:447–57.

36. Stec GP, Atkinson AJ Jr. Analysis of the contributions of permeability and flow to intercompartmental clearance. J Pharmacokinet Biopharm. 1981;9:167–80.

37. Gibson TP et al. Kinetics of procainamide and N-acetylprocainamide in renal failure. Kidney Int. 1977;12:422–29.

38. Galeazzi RL et al. Relationship between the pharmacokinetics and pharmacodynamics of procainamide. Clin Pharmacol Ther. 1976;20:278–89.

39. Mark LC et al. The physiological disposition and cardiac effects of procainamide. J Pharmacol Exp Ther. 1951;102:5–15.

40. Christoff PB et al. Procainamide disposition in obesity. Drug Intell Clin Pharm. 1983;17:516–22.
41. Somogyi A et al. Cimetidine-procainamide pharmacokinetic interaction in man: evidence of competition for tubular secretion of basic drugs. Eur J Clin Pharmacol. 1983;25:339–45.
42. Drayer DE et al. *In vitro* acetylation of drugs by human blood cells. Drug Metab Dispos. 1974;2:499–505.
43. Chen ML et al. Pharmacokinetics of drugs in blood III: metabolism of procainamide and storage effect of blood samples. J Pharm Sci. 1983;72:572–74.
44. Nattel S et al. Procainamide acetylation and disposition in dialysis patients. Clin Invest Med. 1979;2:5–11.
45. Ruo TI et al. Plasma concentrations of desethyl N-acetylprocainamide in patients treated with procainamide and N-acetylprocainamide. Ther Drug Monit. 1981;3:231–37.
46. Dreyfuss J et al. Metabolism of procainamide in rhesus monkey and man. Clin Pharmacol Ther. 1972;13:366–71.
47. DuSouich P, Erill E. Patterns of acetylation of procainamide and procainamide-derived p-Aminobenzoic acid in man. Eur J Clin Pharmacol. 1976;10:283–87.
48. Strong JM et al. Pharmacokinetics in man of the N-acetylated metabolite of procainamide. J Pharmacokinet Biopharm. 1975;3:223–35.
49. Stec GP et al. Kinetics of N-acetylprocainamide deacetylation. Clin Pharmacol Ther. 1980;28:659–66.
50. Freeman RW et al. Evidence for the biotransformation of procainamide to a reactive metabolite. Toxicol Appl Pharmacol. 1979;50:9–16.
51. Uetrecht JP et al. Metabolism of procainamide in the perfused rat liver. Drug Metab Dispos. 1981;9:183–87.
52. Uetrect JP et al. The implications of procainamide metabolism to its inductions of lupus. Arthritis Rheum. 1981;24:994–1003.
53. Uetrecht JP et al. Metabolism of procainamide to hydroxylamine by rat and human hepatic microsomes. Drug Metab Dispos. 1984;12:77–81.
54. Coyle JD et al. Concentration-dependent clearance of procainamide in normal subjects. Biopharm Drug Dispos. 1985;159–65.
55. Reidenberg MM et al. Polymorphic acetylation of procainamide in man. Clin Pharmacol Ther. 1975;17:722–30.
56. Hein DW et al. Biochemical evidence for the coexistence of monomorphic and polymorphic N-acetyltransferase activities on a common protein in rabbit liver. J Pharmacol Exp Ther. 1982;220:1–7.
57. Lunde PKM et al. Disease and acetylation polymorphism. Clin Pharmacokinet. 1977;2:182–97.
58. Litterst CL et al. Comparison of *in vitro* drug metabolism by lung, liver and kidney of several common laboratory species. Drug Metab Dispos. 1975;259–65.
59. Berkersky I, Colburn WA. Acetylation of sulfisoxazole by isolated perfused rat kidney. J Pharm Sci. 1980;69:1359.
60. Gibson TP et al. Acetylation of procainamide in man and its relationship to isonicotinic acid hydrazide acetylation phenotype. Clin Pharmacol Ther. 1974;17:395–99.
61. Karlsson E, Molin L. Polymorphic acetylation of procainamide in healthy subjects. Acta Med Scand. 1975;197:299–302.
62. Frislid K et al. Comparison of the acetylation of procainamide and sulfadimidine in man. Eur J Clin Pharmacol. 1976;9:433–38.
63. Lima JJ, Jusko WJ. Determination of procainamide acetylator status. Clin Pharmacol Ther. 1978;23:25–29.
64. Chapron DJ et al. Evidence for a trimodal pattern of acetylation of isoniazid in uremic subjects. J Pharm Sci. 1978;67:1018–19.
65. Chapron DJ et al. Kinetic discrimination of three sulfamethazine acetylation phenotypes. Clin Pharmacol Ther. 1980;27:104–13.
66. Lee EJD, Lee LKH. A simple pharmacokinetic method for separating the three acetylation phenotypes: a preliminary report. Br J Clin Pharmacol. 1982;13:375–78.

67. Tilstone WJ, Lawson DH. Capacity-limited elimination of procainamide in man. Res Commun Chem Pathol Pharmacol. 1978;21:343–46.
68. Ylitalo P et al. Significance of acetylator phenotype in pharmacokinetics and adverse effects of procainamide. Eur J Clin Pharmacol. 1983;25:791–95.
69. Williams DA. Drug metabolism. In: Roye WO, ed. Principles of Medical Chemistry. Philadelphia: Lea & Febiger; 1974;107.
70. Taber DF et al. N-desethylacecainide is a metabolite of procainamide in man; convenient method for the preparation of an N-dealkylated drug metabolite. Drug Metab Dispos. 1979;7:346.
71. Ruo TI et al. Identification of desethyl procainamide in patients: a new metabolite of procainamide. J Pharmacol Exp Ther. 1981;216:357–62.
72. Ellard GA, Gammon PT. Pharmacokinetics of isoniazid metabolism in man. J Pharmacokinet Biopharm. 1976;4:83–113.
73. Olson W et al. Dose-dependent changes in sulfamethazine kinetics in rapid and slow isoniazid acetylators. Clin Pharmacol Ther. 1978;23:204–11.
74. DuSouich P et al. Mechanisms of nonlinear disposition kinetics of sulfamethazine. Clin Pharmacol Ther. 1979;25:172–83.
75. DuSouich P, Erill S. Metabolism of procainamide and p-aminobenzoic acid in patients with chronic liver disease. Clin Pharmacol Ther. 1977;22:588–95.
76. DuSouich P, Erill S. Metabolism of procainamide in patients with chronic heart failure, chronic respiratory failure and chronic renal failure. Eur J Clin Pharmacol. 1978;14:21–27.
77. Olsen H, Morland J. Ethanol-induced increase in procainamide acetylation in man. Br J Clin Pharmacol. 1982;13:203–208.
78. Christian CD Jr et al. Cimetidine inhibits renal procainamide clearance. Clin Pharmacol Ther. 1984;36:221–27.
79. DuSouich P, Courteau H. Induction of acetylating capacity with complete Freund's adjuvant and hydrocortisone in the rabbit. Drug Metab Dispos. 1981;9:279–83.
80. Schneck DW et al. The effect of hydralazine and other drugs on the kinetics of procainamide acetylation by rat liver and kidney. N-acetyltransferase. J Pharmacol Exp Ther. 1978;204:212–18.
81. Schneck DW et al. Plasma levels of free and acid-labile hydralazine: effects of multiple dosing and of procainamide. Clin Pharmacol Ther. 1978;24:714–19.
82. Galeazzi RL et al. The renal elimination of procainamide. Clin Pharmacol Ther. 1975;19:55–62.
83. Karlsson E. Clinical pharmacokinetics of procainamide. Clin Pharmacokinet. 1978;3:97–107.
84. Reidenberg MM et al. Aging and renal clearance of procainamide and acetylprocainamide. Clin Pharmacol Ther. 1980;28:732–35.
85. Lima JJ et al. Safety and efficacy of procainamide infusions. Am J Cardiol. 1979;43:98–105.
86. Lalka D et al. Procainamide accumulation kinetics in the immediate post-myocardial infarction period. J Clin Pharmacol. 1978;18:397–401.
87. Larrson R et al. The effect of cimetidine, a new histamine H_2-receptor antagonist, on renal function. Acta Med Scand. 1979;205:87–89.
88. McKinney TD, Speeg KV Jr. Cimetidine and procainamide secretion by proximal tubules *in vitro*. Am J Physiol. 1982;242:F672–80.
89. McKinney TD. Procainamide uptake by rabbit proximal tubules. J Pharmacol Exp Ther. 1983;224:302–306.
90. Gibson TP et al. Elimination of procainamide in end-stage renal disease. Clin Pharmacol Ther. 1975;17:321–29.
91. Gibson TP et al. Artificial kidneys and clearance calculations. Clin Pharmacol Ther. 1976;20:720–26.
92. Gibson TP et al. N-acetylprocainamide levels in patients with end-stage renal failure. Clin Pharmacol Ther. 1976;19:206–12.
93. Atkinson AJ Jr et al. Hemodialysis for severe procainamide toxicity: clinical and pharmacokinetic observations. Clin Pharmacol Ther. 1976;20:585–92.
94. Drayer DE et al. Cumulation of N-acetylprocainamide, an active metabolite of procainamide, in patients with impaired renal function. Clin Pharmacol Ther. 1977;22:63–79.

95. Wierzchowiecki M et al. Pharmacokinetic studies of procainamide (PA) in patients with impaired renal function. Clin Pharmacol Ther. 1980;18:272–76.
96. Stec GP et al. N-acetylprocainamide pharmacokinetics in functionally anaphric patients before and after perturbation by hemodialysis. Clin Pharmacol Ther. 1979;26:618–28.
97. Connolly SJ, Kates RE. Clinical pharmacokinetics of N-acetylprocainamide. Clin Pharmacokinet. 1982;7:206–20.
98. Koch-Weser J. Serum procainamide levels as therapeutic guides. Clin Pharmacokinet. 1977;2:389–402.
99. Koch-Weser J. Clinical application of the pharmacokinetics of procainamide. Cardiovasc Clin. 1974;6:63–75.
100. Giardina EGV et al. Intermittent intravenous procainamide to treat ventricular arrhythmias. Correlation of plasma concentration with effect on arrhythmia, electrodiagram, and blood pressure. Ann Intern Med. 1973;78:183–93.
101. Gey GO et al. Plasma concentration of procainamide and prevalence of exertional arrhythmias. Ann Intern Med. 1974;80:718–22.
102. Bellet S et al. The intramuscular use of pronestyl (procainamide). Am J Med. 1952;13:145.
103. Enselberg CD, Lipkin M. The intramuscular administration of procainamide. Am Heart J. 1952;44:781.
104. Bigger JT, Heissenbuttel RH. The use of procainamide and lidocaine in the treatment of cardiac arrhythmias. Prog Cardiovasc Dis. 1969;11:515.
105. Greenspan AM et al. Large-dose procainamide therapy for ventricular tachyarrhythmia. Am J Cardiol. 1980;46:453–62.
106. Giardina EGV, Bigger JT Jr. Procainamide against re-entrant ventricular arrhythmias. Circulation. 1973;48:959–70.
107. Wenger TL et al. Procainamide delivery to ischemic canine myocardium following rapid intravenous administration. Circ Res. 1980;46:789–95.
108. Myerburg RJ et al. Relationship between plasma levels of procainamide, suppression of premature ventricular complexes and prevention ventricular complexes and prevention of recurrent ventricular tachycardia. Circulation. 1981;64:280–90.
109. Myerburg RJ et al. Antiarrhythmic drug therapy in survivors of pre-hospital cardiac arrest: comparison of effects on chronic ventricular arrhythmias and recurrent cardiac arrest. Circulation. 1979;146:358–63.
110. Drayer DE et al. N-acetylprocainamide: an active metabolite of procainamide. Proc Soc Exp Biol Med. 1974;146:358–63.
111. Refsum H et al. Effects of N-acetylprocainamide as compared with procainamide in isolated rate atria. Eur J Pharmacol. 1975;33:47–52.
112. Minchin RF et al. Antiarrhythmic potency of procainamide and N-acetylprocainamide in rabbits. Eur J Pharmacol. 1978;47:51–56.
113. Bagwell EE et al. Correlation of the electrophysiological and antiarrhythmic properties of the N-acetyl metabolite of procainamide with plasma and tissue drug concentrations in the dog. J Pharmacol Exp Ther. 1976;197:38–48.
114. Dangman KH, Hoffman BF. *In vivo* and *in vitro* antiarrhythmic and arrhythmogenic effects of N-acetylprocainamide. J Pharmacol Exp Ther. 1981;217:851–62.
115. Jaillon P, Winkle RA. Electrophysiologic comparative study of procainamide and N-acetylprocainamide in anesthetized dogs: concentration-response relationships. Circulation. 1979;60:1385–394.
116. Elson J et al. Antiarrhythmic potency of N-acetylprocainamide. Clin Pharmacol Ther. 1975;17:134–40.
117. Lee WK et al. Antiarrhythmic efficacy of N-acetylprocainamide in patients with premature ventricular contractions. Clin Pharmacol Ther. 1976;19:508–14.
118. Atkinson AJ Jr et al. Dose-ranging trials of N-acetylprocainamide in patients with premature ventricular contractions. Clin Pharmacol Ther. 1977;21:575–87.
119. Lertora JJL et al. Long-term antiarrhythmic therapy with N-acetylprocainamide. Clin Pharmacol Ther. 1979;25:273–82.

120. Atkinson AJ Jr et al. Impact of active metabolites on monitoring plasma concentrations of therapeutic drugs. Ther Drug Monit. 1980;2:19–27.

122. Jailon P et al. Electrophysiologic effects of N-acetylprocainamide in human beings. Am J Cardiol. 1981;47:1134–140.

123. Sung RJ et al. Electrophysiologic properties and antiarrhythmic mechanisms of intravenous N-acetylprocainamide in patients with ventricular dysrhythmias. Am Heart J. 1983;105:811–19.

124. Roden DM et al. Antiarrhythmic efficacy, pharmacokinetics and safety of N-acetylprocainamide in human subjects: comparison with procainamide. Am J Cardiol. 1980;46:463–68.

125. Reynolds RD et al. Comparison of antiarrhythmic effects of procainamide, N-acetylprocainamide, and p-hydroxy-n-(3-dietthylaminoprophyl) benzamide (41325). Proc Soc Exp Biol Med. 1982;169:156–60.

126. Winkle RA et al. Clinical pharmacology and antiarrhythmic efficacy of N-acetylprocainamide. Am J Cardiol. 1981;47:123–30.

127. Klunger J et al. Long-term antiarrhythmic therapy with acetylprocainamide. Am J Cardiol. 1981;48:1124–132.

128. Rodman JH et al. N-acetylprocainamide kinetics and clinical response during repeated dosing. Clinical Pharmacol Ther. 1982;32:378–86.

129. Follath F et al. Reliability of antiarrhythmic drug plasma concentration monitoring. Clin Pharmacokinet. 1983;8:63–82.

130. Kates RE. Plasma level monitoring of antiarrhythmic drugs. Am J Cardiol. 1983;52:8c–13c.

131. Vlasses PH et al. Lethal accumulation of procainamide metabolite in renal insufficiency. Drug Intell Clin Pharm. 1984;18:493–94. Abstract.

132. Bocardo D et al. Adverse reactions and efficacy of high-dose procainamide therapy in resistant tachyarrhythmias. Am Heart J. 1981;102:797–98.

133. Ellrodt AG et al. Severe neutropenia associated with sustained-release procainamide. Ann Intern Med. 1984;100:197–201.

134. Berger BE, Hauser DJ. Agranulocytosis due to new sustained-release procainamide. Am Heart J. 1983;105:1035–36.

135. Christensen DJ et al. Agranulocytosis, thrombocytopenia, and procainamide. Ann Intern Med. 1984;100:918. Letter.

136. Nagesh KG et al. Procainamide-induced agranulocytosis. J Kans Med Soc. 1980;81:18–24.

137. Lima JJ et al. Pharmacokinetic approach to intravenous procainamide therapy. Eur J Clin Pharmacol. 1978;13:303–308.

138. Coyle JD et al. Initial *in vivo* evaluation of a computer-based infusion system for achieving and maintaining multiple, sequential, constant serum concentrations of procainamide. Pharmacotherapy. 1991;11:96. Abstract.

139. Shaw TRD et al. Use of plasma levels in evaluation of procainamide dosage. Br Heart J. 1974;36:265–70.

140. Treatment of cardiac arrhythmias. The Medical Letter 1983;25:21–28.

141. MacKichan JJ et al. Fluoroimmunoassays for procainamide and N-acetylprocainamide compared with a liquid-chromatographic method. Clin Chem. 1984;30:768–73.

142. Singh et al. Procainamide elimination kinetics in pediatric patients. Clin Pharmacol Ther. 1982;32:607–11.

143. Lima JJ et al. Fetal uptake and neonatal disposition of procainamide and its acetylated metabolite: a case report. Pediatrics. 1978;61:491–93.

144. Christian S. Personal communication. Squibb.

145. Kasmer RJ et al. Comparable steady-state bioavailability between two preparations of conventional-release procainamide hydrochloride. Drug Intell Clin Pharm. 1987;21:183–86.

146. Reed WE et al. Sustained-release procainamide: use of serum concentrations to determine dose. South Med J. 1985;78:1190–193.

147. Baker BA et al. Comparative bioavailability of two oral sustained-release procainamide products. Clin Pharm. 1988;7:135–38.

148. Hilleman DE et al. Comparative bioequivalence and efficacy of two sustained-release procainamide formulations in patients with cardiac arrhythmias. Drug Intell Clin Pharm. 1988;22:554–58.

149. Rocci ML et al. Food-induced gastric retention and absorption of sustained-release procainamide. Clin Pharmacol Ther. 1987;42:45–49.

150. Raymond GG et al. Stability of procainamide hydrochloride in neutralized 5% dextrose injection. Am J Hosp Pharm. 1988;45:2513–517.

151. Bauer LA et al. Influence of age, renal function, and heart failure on procainamide clearance and n-acetylprocainamide serum concentrations. Int J Clin Pharmacol Ther Toxicol. 1989;27:213–16.

152. Kessler KM et al. Procainamide pharmacokinetics in patients with acute myocardial infarction or congestive heart failure. J Am Coll Cardiol. 1986;7:1131–139.

153. Rocci ML et al. Ranitidine-induced changes in the renal and hepatic clearance of procainamide are correlated. J Pharmacol Exp Ther. 1989;248:923–28.

154. Svennson CK et al. Effect of the immunomodulator tolerance on the *in vivo* acetylation of procainamide in the rat. Pharmaceutical Res. 1989;6:477–80.

155. Rodvold KA et al. Interaction of steady-state procainamide with H_2-receptor antagonists cimetidine and ranitidine. Ther Drug Monit. 1987;9:378–83.

156. Liu LL et al. Effect of amiodarone on the disposition of procainamide in the rat. J Pharm Sci. 1988;77:662–65.

157. Nylen ES et al. Reduced acetylation on procainamide by para-aminobenzoic acid. J Am Coll Cardiol. 1986;7:185–87.

158. Cohen AL et al. Unpublished data.

159. Lai MY et al. Dose-dependent effect of cimetidine on procainamide disposition in man. Int J Clin Pharmacol Ther Tox. 1988;26:118–201.

160. Klotz U et al. Famotidine, a new H_2-receptor antagonist, does not affect hepatic elimination of diazepam or tubular secretion of procainamide. Eur J Clin Pharmacol. 1985;28:671–75.

161. Kosoglou T et al. Trimethoprim alters the disposition of procainamide and N-acetylprocainamide. Clin Pharmacol Ther. 1988;44:467–77.

162. Vlasses PH et al. Trimethoprim inhibition of the renal clearance of procainamide and N-acetylprocainamide. Arch Intern Med. 1989;149:1350–353.

163. Saal AK et al. Effect of amiodarone on serum quinidine and procainamide levels. Am J Cardiol. 1984;53:1264–267.

164. Windle J et al. Pharmacokinetic and electrophysiologic interaction of amiodarone and procainamide. Clin Pharmacol Ther. 1987;41:603–10.

165. Mason JW. Amiodarone. N Eng J Med. 1987;316:455–65.

166. Funck-Brentano C et al. Pharmacokinetic and pharmacodynamic interaction of N-acetyl-procainamide and procainamide in humans. J Cardiovasc Pharmacol. 1989;14:364–73.

167. Hughes B et al. Increased procainamide plasma concentrations caused by quinidine: a new drug interaction. Am Heart J. 1987;114:908–909.

168. Kang ES et al. Procainamide N-acetyltransferase: modulation by clofibrate and a microsomal form. Gen Pharmacol. 1989;20:223–27.

169. Raehl CL et al. Procainamide administration during continuous ambulatory peritoneal dialysis. Am Heart J. 1985;110:1306–308.

170. Raehl CL et al. Procainamide pharmacokinetics in patients on continuous ambulatory peritoneal dialysis. Nephron. 1986;44:191–94.

171. Sica DA et al. Pharmacokinetics of procainamide in continuous ambulatory peritoneal dialysis. Int J Clin Pharmacol Ther Toxicol. 1988;26:59–64.

172. Domoto D et al. Removal of toxic levels of N-acetylprocainamide with continuous arteriovenous hemofiltration or continuous arteriovenous hemodiafiltration. Ann Intern Med. 1987;106:550–52.

173. Braden G et al. Hemoperfusion for treatment of N-acetylprocainamide intoxication. Ann Intern Med. 1986;105:64–65.

174. Rosansky SJ et al. Procainamide toxicity in a patient with acute renal failure. Am J Kid Dis. 1986;VII:502–506.

175. Budinsky RA et al. The formation of procainamide hydroxylamine by rat and human liver microsomes. Drug Met Disp. 1987;15:37–43.
176. Adams LE et al. Immunodulatory effects of procainamide metabolites: their implications in drug-related lupus. J Lab Clin Med. 1989;113:482–92.
177. Coyle JD et al. Reversed-phase liquid chromatography method for measurement of procainamide and three metabolites in serum and urine: percent of dose excreted as desethyl metabolites. J Pharm Sci. 1987;76:402–405.
178. Boudoulas H et al. Pharmaockinetic-pharmacodynamic relationships of intravenous procainamide in normals. J Clin Pharmacol. 1985;25:474. Abstract.
179. Liem LB et al. Pharmacodynamics of procainamide in patients with ventricular tachyarrhythmias. J Clin Pharmacol. 1988;28:984–89.
180. Schienman MM et al. Electrophysiologic effects of procaine amide in patients with intraventricular conduction delay. Circulation. 1974;49:522–29.
181. Morady F et al. Pharmacodynamics of intravenous procainamide as used during acute electropharmacologic testing. Am J Cardiol. 1988;61:93–98.
182. Morady F et al. Effects of incremental doses of procainamide on ventricular refractoriness, intraventricular conduction, and induction of ventricular tachycardia. Circulation. 1986;74:1355–364.
183. Fleet S. Agranulocytosis, procainamide, and phenytoin. Ann Intern Med. 1984;100:616–17. Letter.
184. Hoyt RE. Severe neutropenia due to sustained-release procainamide. South Med J. 1987;80:1196.
185. Freed JS et al. Septic complications of procainamide-induced agranulocytosis: report of two cases. Mt Sinai J Med. 1988;55:194–97.
186. Meyers DG et al. Severe neutropenia associated with procainamide: comparison of sustained-release and conventional preparations. Am Heart J. 1985;109:1393–395.
187. Agudelo CA et al. Pure red cell aplasia in procainamide-induced systemic lupus erythematosus. Report and review of the literature. J Rheumatol. 1988;15:1431–432.
188. Giannone L et al. Pure red cell aplasia associated with administration of sustained-release procainamide. Arch Intern Med. 1987;147:1179–180.
189. Meisner DJ et al. Thrombocytopenia following sustained-release procainamide. Arch Intern Med. 1985;145:700–702.
190. Shields AF et al. Procainamide-associated pancytopenia. Am J Hematol. 1988;27:299–301.
191. Gill KS et al. Another case of procainamide-induced pancytopenia. Am J Hematol. 1989;31:298. Letter.
192. Henry PR et al. More-sensitive enzyme-multiplied immunoassay technique for procainamide and N-acetylprocainamide in plasma, serum, and urine. Clin Chem. 1988;34:957–60.
193. Coyle JD et al. Acecainide pharmacokinetics in normal subjects of known acetylator phenotype. Biopharm Drug Dispos. 1991;12:599–612.
194. Atkinson AJ Jr et al. Pharmacokinetics of N-acetylprocainamide. Angiology. 1986;37:959–67.
195. Atkinson AJ Jr et al. Comparison of the pharmacokinetic and pharmacodynamic properties of procainamide and N-acetylprocainamide. Angiology. 1988;39:655–67.
196. Krüger-Thiemer E. Continuous intravenous infusion and multicompartment accumulation. Eur J Pharmacol. 1968;4:317–24.
197. Carnes CA, Coyle JD. Evaluation of very rapid Emit Qst Methods for measuring serum procainamide and N-acetylprocainamide concentrations. Pharmacotherapy. 1992;12:40–44.
198. Koch-Weser J, Klein SW. JAMA. 1971;215:1454–460.
199. Koch-Weser. J Cardiovasc Clin. 1974;6 (II):63–75.

Chapter 23

Quinidine

Clarence T. Ueda

Quinidine has been used in the treatment of ventricular and supraventricular arrhythmias for over half a century, and it is the prototype antiarrhythmic to which others are compared. Over the years, it has been recognized that patient response to treatment with quinidine varies markedly.[1-3] In part, this is due to large patient-to-patient variations in quinidine bioavailability, distribution, and elimination and the effects of various diseases on quinidine disposition. Because quinidine has a low therapeutic index[3-6] and a highly variable patient response, and because therapeutic and toxic effects can generally be related to plasma and serum concentrations,[3-5,7,8] it has become increasingly apparent that quinidine dosage should be determined on an individual patient basis by use of serum or plasma quinidine concentrations.

CLINICAL PHARMACOKINETICS

Absorption

Quinidine sulfate, gluconate, and polygalacturonate are all given by mouth in solid dosage forms. The quinidine base content of these salts is 83%, 62%, and approximately 60%, respectively. For intramuscular and intravenous administration, quinidine gluconate is used almost exclusively. Following oral administration, the absolute bioavailability (F) of quinidine is about 0.70, but it varies widely (0.45 to 1.0) between patients.[9-12] The remaining drug appears to be cleared presystemically by the liver.[9-11] This agrees with the observation that less than 5% of a given dose is detected in the feces after oral administration.[1,13]

Quinidine is a weak base; therefore, gastrointestinal absorption of quinidine is optimal in the small intestine. Following the ingestion of conventional quinidine sulfate tablets and capsules, peak plasma drug concentrations are reached in one to three hours.[1,4,12,14-18] Drug absorption from sustained-release quinidine sulfate tablets (Quinidex Extentabs) is slower and more protracted.[19,20] Quinidine polygalacturonate tablets (Cardioquin) and conventional quinidine sulfate tablets and capsules are bioequivalent in their rate and extent of quinidine absorption.[18,21]

Quinidine gluconate for oral use is available only in the form of sustained-release tablets, and significant differences in bioavailability have been observed with these preparations.[18,22,23]

Following the administration of conventional tablets and capsules, plasma quinidine concentrations are generally higher and appear earlier when the drug is given on an empty stomach.[24,25] With these preparations, meals tend to reduce the rate of absorption of quinidine but not the extent of drug availability.[26-28] With sustained-release quinidine preparations, on the other hand, the effect of food on quinidine absorption appears to depend on the nature or composition of the meal.[27,29] While some foods have no effect on the absorption of quinidine from sustained-release products,[27] low and high fat meals have been found to increase the absorption rate and availability of quinidine from the gluconate preparation.[29] High fat meals increased the availability of the drug only.[29]

With the exception of aluminum hydroxide gel,[16,28,30] the absorption of oral quinidine may be adversely affected by the various antacid and antidiarrheal preparations that are given concomitantly to combat quinidine-induced diarrhea.[31-34] In addition, it has been suggested that when coadministered with cimetidine, the availability of quinidine may be reduced.[35]

In patients with congestive heart failure[36,37] the rate of oral quinidine absorption is diminished, probably as a result of a reduction in splanchnic blood flow rate. The extent of quinidine absorption, however, is not altered in these patients.[37]

After intramuscular injection, quinidine absorption can be erratic, unpredictable, and incomplete.[10] Protracted absorption for over four hours has been seen following intramuscular quinidine administration.[14] These observations are probably due to the precipitation of quinidine at the injection site. This aspect would also explain the intense pain and muscle damage that are reported following injection of this drug.

Mason et al.[14] observed no differences in the rates of quinidine absorption when given by intramuscular injection or orally in conventional tablets and capsules, and an aqueous solution. They did show, however, that the availability of quinidine is greater after intramuscular injection.

Distribution

Quinidine distribution in the body is rapid and primarily extravascular. It is described by a two-compartment, open pharmacokinetic model with a half-life for the α, or distribution, phase of about seven minutes and an overall volume of distribution (V_d) of 3 L/kg.[10,11,38-40] The central compartment volume, V_1, is approximately 0.7 L/kg.[10,38,40]

In the patient with congestive heart failure, V_1 and V_d are reduced.[36,39,40] It has been suggested that V_d may also be reduced in uremic patients,[41] but increased in patients with cirrhosis.[42]

In the plasma concentration range generally considered to be therapeutic (2 to 5 µg/mL),[6,43] quinidine binding to plasma proteins is moderate in both affinity and extent. The important binding proteins appear to be albumin and α_1-acid glycoprotein.[44] Approximately 70% to 90% of the drug is plasma protein bound with an average apparent association constant of 10^4 M^{-1}.[44–54] Quinidine plasma protein binding is diminished in patients with liver disease,[42,50–52] patients with cyanotic congenital heart disease,[55] patients receiving heparin anticoagulant treatment,[54,56] and in neonates and infants less than 18 months of age.[57] Quinidine binding has been shown to increase following trauma,[44] surgery,[58] cardiac arrest,[59] and during an acute myocardial infarction.[60] Further, in children, it has been reported to increase from the neonatal period through 11 years of age.[55] However, the binding of quinidine in plasma of patients with poor renal function,[47,50] congestive heart failure,[6] respiratory insufficiency,[52] or hyperlipoproteinemia[53] is not altered.

On the basis of results obtained in healthy volunteers,[61] V_d and unbound plasma quinidine fractions do not appear to change with age.

Quinidine readily diffuses into the red blood cell. Hughes et al.[62] found a value of 0.82 for the red cell:plasma partition ratio, which corresponds to a blood:plasma quinidine concentration ratio of 0.92.

Quinidine also distributes into the saliva and cerebrospinal fluid (CSF). Marked intra- and interpatient variations in the ratio of saliva:serum quinidine have been observed.[63–66] Therefore, the use of saliva quinidine concentrations for therapeutic drug monitoring should be on an individual patient basis. The concentrations of quinidine in the CSF are lower than the corresponding concentrations of unbound drug in the serum.[67] CSF concentrations are approximately 16% of the unbound serum quinidine concentrations and only 3% of the total serum concentrations.

Metabolism

The major route of quinidine elimination appears to be via metabolism in the liver, since renal excretion of intact drug accounts for only 10% to 20% of a given dose.[9,38–40] The mean value for the elimination half-life of quinidine is six to seven hours.[6,9–11,38–40] However, this value, as well as the other quinidine disposition constants, is known to vary considerably between patients.[6,9–11,38–40] Ochs et al.[61] reported that the elimination half-life of quinidine is greater in the elderly person (greater than 60 years of age) than in the younger subject (less than 35 years of age). In contrast, the serum half-life of quinidine is reportedly shorter (two to three hours) in children less than 12 years old.[68] It has been suggested that patients with cirrhosis have a significantly longer quinidine half-life of nine hours.[42] The elimination half-life does not appear to be altered in patients with congestive heart failure (CHF)[6,36,39,40] or poor renal function.[6,69]

Total body quinidine clearance is about 4.5 mL/min/kg with wide patient-to-patient variation.[11,38–40] In comparison to adolescent children and young adults who were found to possess similar clearances, Szefler et al.[68] observed that the clearance of quinidine was faster in children less than 12 years old. Quinidine clearance is reduced in patients with CHF,[39,40] elderly subjects,[61,70] and possibly patients with uremia.[41] Clearance does not appear to be altered in patients with liver dysfunction.

Several drugs have been reported to alter the elimination kinetics of quinidine when taken together. The elimination half-life of quinidine is shorter when administered with the enzyme-inducing agents phenobarbital, phenytoin, and rifampin.[71–73] This alteration is most likely due to an increase in the metabolic clearance of quinidine. The concomitant administration of quinidine with cimetidine, amiodarone, or verapamil has resulted in a reduction in quinidine clearance and prolongation of its elimination half-life.[74–78] Although it has been suggested that propranolol decreases the clearance of quinidine with no change in its elimination half-life,[42] kinetic interaction between the two drugs was not seen by others.[79–81] Similarly, caffeine or diltiazem coadministration,[82,83] like smoking,[84] does not appear to affect the disposition kinetics of quinidine.

An interesting interaction with quinidine has been observed with nifedipine.[85–88] Nifedipine has been shown to suppress the serum concentrations of quinidine when the two drugs are given together. At this time, however, the nature and relevance of this interaction, which has been observed in a small number of subjects, have not been established.

As discussed in Chapter 7: Genetic Polymorphisms of Drug Metabolism, quinidine is a potent inhibitor of the genetically regulated polymorphic drug metabolizing enzyme, debrisoquine hydroxylase.[89–92] Quinidine itself, however, is not a substrate for this polymorphic enzyme.[93,94] Instead, the oxidation of quinidine to its 3-hydroxy and N-oxide metabolites appears to be catalyzed by the liver microsomal cytochrome P450 enzyme that has been termed, $P450_{NF}$ or nifedipine oxidase.[93]

Quinidine metabolites (see Figure 23-1) that have been identified include 3-hydroxyquinidine, 2'-quinidinone (or 2-oxoquinidinone), quinidine-N-oxide, quinidine 10,11-dihydrodiol, and O-desmethylquinidine.[95–100] Palmer et al.[101] have suggested the existence of various conjugated drug species. Additionally, lactic acid conjugates of both quinidine and the 3-hydroxy metabolite have been proposed.[102]

Very little is known about the relative contribution of each metabolite to the overall removal of quinidine by drug metabolism. The 3-hydroxyquinidine and 2'-quinidinone metabolites are generally considered to be the principal products of drug metabolism. Approximately 10% of a dose appears to be metabolized to the 3-hydroxy metabolite, an additional 3% to quinidine 10,11-dihydrodiol, and 1% to quinidine-N-oxide.[100] Another 1% to 2% is converted to the O-demethylated derivative.[103]

The disposition characteristics of several quinidine metabolites have been described following the administration of quinidine and after direct administration of the metabolite.[100,104–107] The results of these studies indicate that for 3-hydroxyquinidine,[104] its elimination half-life is significantly longer than the parent drug. After direct administration, a mean terminal serum half-life of 12.4 ± 2.9 hours was observed, and it was suggested that the metabolite is eliminated primarily by renal excretion. The renal clearance of 3-hydroxyquinidine was 16.0 ± 2.6 L/hr. The elimination half-life of quinidine-N-oxide, however, is considerably shorter than quinidine (less than three hours).[105] The following values were observed for total body clearance, volume of distribution, and renal clearance of the N-oxide metabolite after direct oral administration: 9.3 ± 2.8 L/hr, 30.2 ± 6.3 L, and 1.28 ± 0.30 L/hr, respectively.

The following values for renal clearance, apparent volume of distribution, and elimination half-life were observed for quinidine 10,11-dihydrodiol following the administration of quinidine: 0.11 L/hr/kg, 0.43 L/kg, and 1.96 hours, respectively.[100] The plasma protein binding characteristics of the quinidine metabolites are summarized in Table 23-1.

On a qualitative basis, there is little doubt that some of the quinidine metabolites possess antiarrhythmic activity. Quantification of this activity, particularly as it relates to their effectiveness in humans, is much more difficult to ascertain. In various animal preparations, 3-hydroxyquinidine, 2'-quinidinone, quinidine-N-oxide and O-desmethylquinidine have all been shown to possess some antiarrhythmic activity.[103,111–116] Of the quinidine metabolites that have been investigated for their effects in humans, 3-hydroxyquinidine appears to possess the greatest amount of antiarrhythmic activity.[104,110,117] When compared to quinidine, the relative potency of the 3-hydroxy metabolite was approximately 60%,[104] and it has been suggested that the antiarrhythmic effects of 3-hydroxyquinidine and quinidine are additive following quinidine therapy.[110,115] Studies[105,114–117] suggest that quinidine-N-oxide possesses little, if any, quinidine-like antiarrhythmic activity. Similarly, it is very unlikely that 2'-quinidinone contributes to the therapeutic effects observed after the quinidine administration.[116]

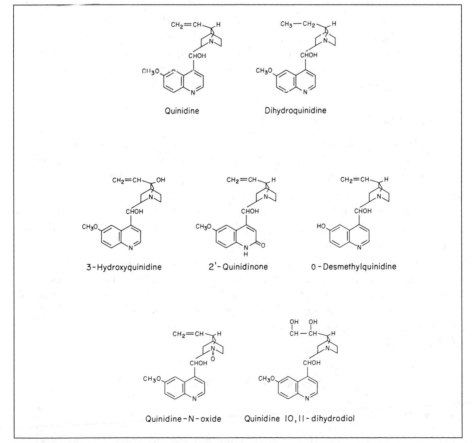

Figure 23-1. *Structures of quinidine, dihydroquinidine, and various metabolites.*

Table 23-1. Plasma Protein Binding for Various Quinidine Metabolites

Metabolite	Bound fraction
3–Hydroxyquinidine	44%–74%[103,106,108–110]
Quinidine-N-oxide	93%–96%[105,108]
2'–Quinidinone	46%–47%[103,108]
0–Desmethylquinidine	≥ 90%[108]

Excretion

The excretion of quinidine by the kidneys accounts for 10% to 20% of an administered dose.[9,38–40] Renal excretion occurs by glomerular filtration and is dependent upon the pH of the urine. Renal quinidine clearance has been shown to diminish with increased urine pH.[118,119] Drug clearance by the kidneys is lower in the elderly person and is positively correlated with creatinine clearance.[61] Quinidine is poorly dialyzable by both peritoneal dialysis[120,121] and hemodialysis.[122,123]

Renal excretion accounts for the elimination of approximately 10%, 3% and 1% of an intravenous quinidine dose in the forms of 3-hydroxyquinidine, quinidine 10,11-dihydrodiol, and quinidine-N-oxide, respectively.[100] Another 1% to 2% is excreted in the urine as O-desmethylquinidine.[103] Rakhit et al.[100] observed non-linear renal excretion kinetics with 3-hydroxyquinidine. Quinidine is also excreted in breast milk.[124] (See Table 23-2 for a summary of the important quinidine pharmacokinetic constants.)

Dose-Dependent Pharmacokinetics

It has been suggested that the disposition kinetics of quinidine are dose-dependent.[125] However, the available evidence is inconclusive on this point. Bolme and Otto[125] based their conclusion on the observation that the relationship between steady-state plasma quinidine concentration and daily dose was nonlinear in five healthy volunteers. Others[11,126] seem to agree with this contention, although Russo et al.[126] observed no changes in total body clearance with the two quinidine dosage regimens they investigated. In contrast, Fremstad et al.[127] detected no concentration-dependent quinidine disposition kinetics when the drug was given by a constant intravenous infusion at two different rates. Using doses of quinidine gluconate of 5, 10, and 15 mg/kg, Gey et al.[128] found that the relationship between plasma quinidine concentration and dose was generally linear. With these divergent observations, the issue of whether the disposition kinetics of quinidine is dose-dependent is difficult to assess.

PHARMACODYNAMICS

Clinical Response

While it is widely recognized that the antiarrhythmic effects of quinidine are achieved within a relatively narrow range of drug concentrations,[3–5,7,8] the definition of therapeutically effective plasma (or serum) concentrations for quinidine is highly dependent on the specificity of the assay used and complicated by the presence of active metabolite(s), and to a lesser extent by dihydroquinidine, in the blood. Commercial quinidine preparations usually contain less than 10% dihydroquinidine as an impurity, but the levels can be as high as 20% of the dose.[129] Dihydroquinidine has antiarrhythmic[116,130-132] and pharmacokinetic[133,134] properties that are similar to those of quinidine. The presence of dihydroquinidine, however, which probably partially accounts for the lack of a better correlation between plasma quinidine concentrations and drug effect(s)[135-137] does not offset the value, usefulness, and importance of monitoring the effects of quinidine with plasma or serum drug concentrations.[138]

The therapeutic plasma range for quinidine when determined with a relatively nonspecific assay is generally higher and wider than the ranges determined with more specific procedures. For example, with the protein precipitation method[139] quinidine concentrations of about 3 to 8 µg/mL are considered therapeutic.[4,5,140] As assay specificity improves, therapeutic drug effects are generally associated with lower plasma or serum concentrations. With the double extraction procedure of Cramer and Isaksson,[141] antiarrhythmic effects are achieved with plasma or serum quinidine concentrations between 2 and 5 µg/mL.[6,43] When assays that are specific for quinidine are used (e.g., thin layer or high performance liquid chromatographic methods), therapeutic effects without overt toxicity can be expected when the plasma concentrations are within the range of 1 to about 3 to 4 µg/mL.[103,136,142] However, higher plasma quinidine concentrations (up to 6 µg/mL) may be required for the treatment of some arrhythmias.[136]

Adverse Effects

Two major types of adverse effects are relatively common with quinidine. They are gastrointestinal side effects (primarily quinidine-induced diarrhea) and hypersensitivity reactions. Patients have been known to discontinue the drug because of intolerable nausea, diarrhea, and/or vomiting. These effects, however, are

Table 23-2. *Summary of Pharmacokinetic Parameters*

Parameter	Population averages ± SD
CL_S (mL/min/kg)	4.72 ± 1.69
CL_R (mL/min/kg)	0.93 ± 0.52
CL_{NR} (mL/min/kg)	3.26 ± 1.74
V_1 (L/kg)	0.66 ± 0.38
V_β (L/kg)	2.61 ± 1.10
F (oral)	0.71 ± 0.16
Urinary quinidine excretion (%)	19.50 ± 7.77
$t\frac{1}{2}_\alpha$ (min)	6.69 ± 4.03
$t\frac{1}{2}_\beta$ (hr)	6.44 ± 1.63

generally not related to the concentrations of quinidine in the plasma or serum. In this regard, a noteworthy idiosyncratic reaction to quinidine is the life-threatening torsades de pointes.[108]

Toxic effects of quinidine, such as cinchonism or arrhythmias, like other adverse effects, vary extensively between patients. These differences are due to many factors, including patient differences in physical status[143] and the route and rate by which the drug is given.[5,143,144] Some patients have survived plasma and serum quinidine concentrations in excess of 20 µg/mL.[145–147] However, most studies[145,146,148,149] suggest that regardless of the quinidine assay method used, plasma or serum quinidine concentrations above 10 µg/mL will almost assuredly produce toxic drug effects and may even be fatal.

In perhaps the most extensive study designed to delineate the relationship between serum quinidine concentrations and response, Sokolow and Ball,[5] using a single extraction assay procedure, showed that in 177 patients the incidence of important myocardial toxicity was only 1.6% when the drug concentrations were less than 6 µg/mL. Myocardial toxicity was never seen with drug concentrations below 3 µg/mL, the lower limit of the therapeutic range. The incidence of toxicity increased to 12% with serum quinidine concentrations between 6 and 8 µg/mL, 30% at concentrations between 8 and 10 µg/mL, 45% at 12 to 13 µg/mL, and 65% when quinidine concentrations exceeded 14 µg/mL. Although this information on toxicity was obtained with a single assay procedure, it serves as a good guideline for extrapolation to other analytical methods.

CLINICAL APPLICATION OF PHARMACOKINETIC DATA

Dosing

For a number of reasons discussed above[9–11,38–40,150] (e.g., narrow therapeutic window, large interpatient variations in pharmacokinetics, differences in assay specificities, presence of active metabolites and possible nonlinear pharmacokinetics) quinidine dosing should be approached conservatively. That is, the initial dosage regimen should be directed toward achieving serum quinidine concentrations at the lower end of the therapeutic range. Additionally, the requirements for quinidine can differ substantially between patients depending on the nature of their arrhythmias. The following dosing recommendations can be used in the initiation of quinidine therapy. Adjustments in these dosing schedules may be necessary once steady-state conditions have been achieved and the patient's arrhythmia status has been re-evaluated.

The daily dosage requirements for quinidine can be estimated from the following relationship:

$$\text{Daily Dosage} = \frac{C_{av} \cdot CL \cdot 1440}{F}$$

(Eq. 23-1)

where C_{av} is the average plasma or serum quinidine concentration desired at steady state, CL is total body clearance in mL/min/kg, and F is the bioavailability factor. The constant 1440 is the number of minutes in a day.

A treatment schedule with quinidine should achieve an average steady-state plasma (or serum) drug concentration of about 2 µg/mL as determined by a specific drug assay. From Equation 23-1, the daily dosage requirement to reach this level would be:

$$\text{Daily Dosage} = \frac{(2\ \mu g/mL)\ (4.7\ mL/min/kg)\ (1440\ min/day)}{0.70}$$

$$= \frac{13\ mg/kg/day}{0.70}$$

$$\approx 19\ mg/kg/day\ \text{of quinidine base} \hspace{2cm} \text{(Eq. 23-2)}$$

Since quinidine sulfate, gluconate, and polygalacturonate contain 83%, 62%, and 60% of active drug, respectively, the daily dosage with quinidine sulfate should be 23 mg/kg/day [(19 mg/kg/day)/0.83] given in divided doses (e.g., every six hours). For a 70-kg patient, this dosage would be 400 mg of quinidine sulfate every six hours. With quinidine gluconate, the daily dosage requirement is 30 mg/kg/day [(19 mg/kg/day)/0.62] in divided doses (e.g., every eight hours). With increasing use of sustained-release quinidine preparations, it is important to emphasize that because of the difference in base content between the sulfate and gluconate salts, the commercially available sustained-release product containing quinidine sulfate is not interchangeable with a similar preparation containing gluconate.[151,152] On a tablet-for-tablet basis, quinidine gluconate products will produce lower serum drug concentrations.

The use of a less specific quinidine assay has the following effects on the dosing of quinidine using pharmacokinetic principles. In addition to affecting the definition of the therapeutic plasma concentration range, since plasma or serum quinidine concentration-time data [i.e., area under the curve (AUC) values] are used to assess F and CL, these assays tend to overestimate F and underestimate CL.[140] Greenblatt and colleagues[10,150] obtained average values for F and CL of 0.81 to 0.84 and 3.85 mL/min/kg, respectively. With their assay and assuming a therapeutic plasma quinidine concentration range of 2 to 5 µg/mL, a desirable C_{av} might be 3 µg/mL. Substituting these values for C_{av}, F, and CL into Equation 23-1, the calculated daily dose of quinidine sulfate is 24 mg/kg/day, which for a 70-kg patient amounts to giving the same dose that was indicated by a quinidine-specific assay, (i.e., quinidine sulfate 400 mg every six hours).

In young adults (less than 30 years of age) and children (less than 12 years of age) in whom CL might be more rapid,[61,68] larger daily doses may be required to obtain the desired C_{av}.

For a given dosage regimen, Equation 23-3 can be used to provide an estimate of the average quinidine concentration at steady state, or total body clearance when C_{av} can be assessed.

$$C_{av} = \frac{F \cdot Dose}{CL \cdot \tau}$$

(Eq. 23-3)

where F and CL were defined previously and τ is the dosing interval.

In addition to patient-to-patient differences in quinidine disposition kinetics, oral drug availability may vary quite widely due to presystemic clearance of quinidine by the liver.[9-11] This first-pass effect has been shown to account for the removal of from 5% to 55% of an orally administered quinidine dose. Therefore, major discrepancies that may be seen between the computed or predicted and observed plasma or serum quinidine concentrations are probably due to patient variations in disposition kinetics, first-pass effect, or both. The variability in CL between patients is greater than the variation in F. However, both are reasonably constant in a given patient.

CHF and possibly cirrhosis are presently the only disease states that may require an adjustment in the quinidine dosage regimen. CHF patients may need smaller quinidine doses due to their smaller volumes of distribution.[40] Cirrhotic patients reportedly possess longer elimination half-lives.[42] Therefore, less frequent dosing (e.g., every eight hours) or a smaller quinidine dose may be required in patients with cirrhosis.

Although quinidine has been administered parenterally in acute situations by intramuscular injection, this mode of administration is no longer recommended. In these situations, the drug can be given by **slow** intravenous infusion.[143,144] For intravenous administration, a quinidine gluconate dose of 5 to 8 mg/kg diluted in 40 mL of 5% dextrose in water and infused at a constant rate over 20 to 25 minutes has been shown to be safe and effective.[144] Using this procedure, peak plasma quinidine concentrations of about 3 to 4 μg/ mL are obtained at the time of cessation of drug input. After an initial rapid fall-off, the plasma drug concentrations decline slowly on termination of the infusion. In patients with CHF, the infused dose of quinidine gluconate should be reduced 25%.

On a milligram-for-milligram basis, an intramuscular dose of quinidine gluconate produces serum quinidine concentrations at steady state that are similar to the levels reached with the same dose of quinidine sulfate given orally.[153]

Algorithm

It is widely recognized that when standard quinidine dosages (e.g., 200 mg every six hours) are used, patient-to-patient variations in plasma or serum quinidine concentrations can be extensive. Interpatient plasma or serum quinidine concentration differences are reduced when the dosage is adjusted for body weight (i.e., mg/kg). Other factors such as the coexistence of CHF, cirrhosis and patient age must also be considered when designing the quinidine dosage regimen.

The algorithm shown in Figure 23-2 provides a rational approach for treating arrhythmias with quinidine. On the basis of mean patient data obtained with specific quinidine assays, it is appropriate to initiate quinidine therapy with a dosage regimen of 19 mg/kg/day of quinidine base in divided doses. With this dosage, the predicted or expected value of C_{av} would be 2 μg/mL, and the plasma quinidine concentrations should be within the therapeutic drug concentration

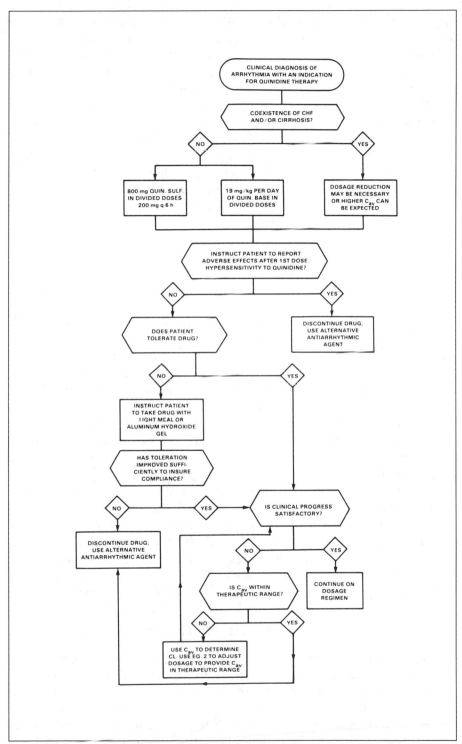

Figure 23-2. *Algorithm for the treatment of arrhythmias with quinidine. "Therapeutic range" is between 1 and 3 to 4 μg/mL, or between 2 and 5 μg/mL, depending on the specificity of the assay method used (see text).*

range between doses. In patients with CHF, it is not unlikely for C_{av} to be higher than 2 μg/mL with this dosage regimen because of the lower clearance of quinidine in these patients; therefore, it would be appropriate to lower the dose given. In young adult cardiac patients (less than 30 years old), however, a larger daily dose of quinidine may be required because of the patient's greater systemic clearance.

After a minimum of two to three days on the dosage regimen and if the drug is adequately tolerated by the patient, the status of the arrhythmia should be re-evaluated and, if necessary, blood sample(s) collected to obtain an estimate of C_{av}. With conventional quinidine sulfate tablets and capsules and an every-six-hour dosing schedule, samples should be obtained approximately four hours post-dose to estimate C_{av} (i.e., midway between the maximum and minimum plasma or serum drug concentrations in the dosing interval). For quinidine gluconate given every eight hours, samples should be obtained at about five to six hours after the dose.

If the arrhythmia is controlled and no adverse drug effects are observed, quinidine administration should be continued on the same dosing schedule. For these patients, although it is not absolutely essential, it is frequently desirable to obtain an estimate of C_{av} for baseline information in the event that there is a change in the arrhythmia status.

An estimate of C_{av} should be obtained if arrhythmias are uncontrolled in a compliant patient. If therapeutic drug concentrations have not been achieved, the quinidine dosage should be increased in an attempt to control the arrhythmia. One can use the C_{av} estimate with Equation 23-3 to provide an approximation of CL for the patient and then, resubstituting this value into the equation, determine the new quinidine dosage based on the desired C_{av}.

If therapeutic quinidine concentrations have been reached without any apparent control of the arrhythmia, it is unlikely that increasing the dose will result in an antiarrhythmic effect without producing adverse effects. In these cases, it is advisable to use an alternate antiarrhythmic agent.

Gastrointestinal side effects are the chief complaints following oral quinidine administration. Quinidine gluconate may be better tolerated than the sulfate salt in some patients, probably as a result of the effects of the dosage form. Thus, in patients who are unable to tolerate quinidine sulfate, a comparable daily dose of the gluconate salt should be tried before quinidine therapy is abandoned.

For routine therapeutic drug monitoring, it is desirable to obtain pre-dose or trough plasma quinidine concentrations to evaluate arrhythmia control.

ANALYTICAL METHODS

Over the years, a number of methods have been used to assay quinidine in various biological media. More recently, newer immunologically based methods such as the Emit, TD_x, and TDA quinidine assays have been developed with greater specificity for quinidine than the majority of the previously used procedures and with significantly reduced analysis time. An added advantage of the newer assay methods is that they are easily automated and readily available in this form.

The majority of the more established quinidine assays fall into one of the following categories: spectroscopic (fluorescence, ultraviolet, and visible) or chromatographic (gas, liquid, and thin-layer). The principal difference between these procedures is their specificity for quinidine. In general, most of these methods do not separate and/or distinguish quinidine from dihydroquinidine (a known impurity in drug-grade quinidine, see Figure 23-1) or drug metabolites and are therefore nonspecific. This is particularly the case for the fluorometric quinidine assays, which may still be employed in some laboratories.

Assay specificity for quinidine is improved when the method includes an extraction and/or separation procedure before the detection step. This procedure removes or minimizes the effect of extraneous endogenous and exogenous substances such as drug metabolites that would normally interfere with the quinidine determination. The most specific quinidine assays incorporate both an extraction and a chromatographic separation procedure in the assay method.

Table 23-3 summarizes the advantages and disadvantages of the various methods that are available for the determination of quinidine in biological materials. The type of quinidine assay that should be employed depends upon the requirements of the determination. Pharmacokinetic studies of quinidine require a much higher degree of specificity and sensitivity for the drug than that required for routine clinical drug monitoring and therefore take longer to perform. However, for therapeutic drug monitoring a short turn-around time that may necessitate a sacrifice in assay specificity is of more importance.

A number of reports[195–205] have compared the various quinidine assays. In terms of specificity, sensitivity, efficiency, and rapidity of the assay procedure, quinidine analysis by high performance liquid chromatography is the preferred method because of its versatility (e.g., simultaneous determination of active metabolites, applicability to various biological specimens) and ease of operation. Although the commercial quinidine immunoassays do not differentiate between quinidine and dihydroquinidine and may cross-react with some metabolites (e.g., O-desmethylquinidine), these assays are acceptable for therapeutic drug monitoring.

PROSPECTUS

Despite the introduction of several new antiarrhythmic agents, quinidine remains a mainstay drug for the treatment of cardiac rhythm disorders. While much is known about the pharmacokinetics and pharmacodynamics of quinidine and the antiarrhythmic activities of several quinidine metabolites, very little is known about the formation and disposition characteristics of the metabolites following the administration of the parent drug in cardiac patients and factors that affect the fate and time-course of these drug entities in the body. The elucidation of this information for the quinidine metabolites represents the principal challenges for quinidine therapeutic monitoring programs in the future.

Table 23-3. Comparison of the Relative Advantages and Disadvantages of the Various Quinidine Assay Methods[a]

Analysis method	Specificity for quinidine	Sensitivity	Metabolite analysis	Dihydroquinidine analysis	Assayable Samples				Minimum sample volume	Analysis time	Analysis cost	Instrument and equipment costs	Specialized operator training	References
					Plasma/serum	Urine	Saliva	Others						
Spectroscopic														
Fluorometric														
Protein precipitation	5	3	No	No	X				3	2	3	3	None	139
Extraction	3–4	3	No	No	X	X	X	X	3	2	3	3	None	10,141,154–161
Ultraviolet	3	3	No	No	X	X	X	?	3	3	3	3	None	162
Colorimetric	4	4	No	No	X	X	X	?	3	3	3	3	None	163
Chromatographic														
Gas-liquid	2	2	No	No	X	X	X	X	2	2	2–3	3	None	164–167
Liquid	1	2	Yes	Yes	X	X	X	X	2	2	2–3	4	None	39,168–184
Thin-layer	1	2	Possible	Yes	X	X	X	X	3	4	3	3–4	Some	9,185–189
Others														
Mass spectrometry	1	1	?	No	X	?	?	?	3	3	5	5	Yes	190
Emit	2	2	No	No	X				1	1	2–4[b]	3–4	None	191
TDA	2	2	No	No	X				1	1	3	4	None	192
TDx	2	2	No	No	X				1	1	3	4	None	193
ICS	3	2	No	No	X				1	1	3	4	None	194

[a] Arbitrary ranking scale of 1 (excellent) to 5 (poor) with a score of 3 being average or nominal.
[b] Analytical costs decrease as sample numbers per run increase.

REFERENCES

1. Yount EH, Rosenblum M. Studies of plasma quinidine levels in relation to therapeutic effect and toxic manifestations. South Med J. 1950;43:324–29.
2. Weisman SA. Review and evaluation of quinidine therapy for auricular fibrillation. JAMA. 1953;152:496–99.
3. Gaughan CE et al. Acute oral testing for determining antiarrhythmic drug efficacy I: quinidine. Am J Cardiol. 1976;38:677–84.
4. Sokolow M, Edgar AL. Blood quinidine concentrations as a guide in the treatment of cardiac arrhythmias. Circulation. 1950;1:576–92.
5. Sokolow M, Ball RE. Factors influencing conversion of chronic atrial fibrillation with special reference to serum quinidine concentration. Circulation. 1956; 14:568–83.
6. Kessler KM et al. Quinidine elimination in patients with congestive heart failure or poor renal function. N Engl J Med. 1974;290:706–9.
7. Heissenbuttel RH, Bigger JT. The effect of oral quinidine on intraventricular conduction in man: Correlation of plasma quinidine with changes in QRS duration. Am Heart J. 1970;80:453–62.
8. Fieldman A et al. The effect of quinidine sulfate on QRS duration and QT and systolic time intervals in man. J Clin Pharmacol. 1977;17:134–39.
9. Ueda CT et al. Absolute quinidine bioavailability. Clin Pharmacol Ther. 1976;20:260–65.
10. Greenblatt DJ et al. Pharmacokinetics of quinidine in humans after intravenous, intramuscular and oral administration. J Pharmacol Exp Ther. 1977;202:365–78.
11. Guentert TW et al. Quinidine pharmacokinetics in man: choice of a disposition model and absolute bioavailability studies. J Pharmacokinet Biopharm. 1979;7:315–30.
12. Guentert TW et al. Gastrointestinal absorption of quinidine from some solutions and commercial tablets. J Pharmacokinet Biopharm. 1980;8:243–55.
13. Houston AB, Perry WF. The plasma concentration of quinidine after oral administration and its effect on auricular fibrillation. Can Med Assoc J. 1950;36:56–60.
14. Mason WD et al. Comparative plasma concentrations of quinidine following administration of one intramuscular and three oral formulations to 13 human subjects. J Pharm Sci 1976;65:1325–29.
15. Strum JD et al. Comparative bioavailability of four commercial quinidine sulfate tablets. J Pharm Sci. 1977;66:539–42.
16. Romankiewicz JA et al. The non-interference of aluminum hydroxide gel with quinidine sulfate absorption: An approach to control quinidine-induced diarrhea. Am Heart J. 1978;96:518–20.
17. Covinsky JO et al. Relative bioavailability of quinidine gluconate and quinidine sulfate in healthy volunteers. J Clin Pharmacol. 1979;19:261–69.
18. McGilveray IJ et al. Bioavailability of 11 quinidine formulations and pharmacokinetic variation in humans. J Pharm Sci. 1981;70:524–29.
19. Sawyer WT et al. Bioavailability of a commercial sustained-release quinidine tablet compared to oral quinidine solution. Biopharm Drug Dispos. 1982;3:301–10.
20. Gibson DL et al. Relative bioavailability of a standard and a sustained-release quinidine tablet. Clin Pharm. 1982;1:366–68.
21. Soeterbock AM, Van Thiel M. Serum quinidine levels after chronic administration of four different quinidine formulations. J Int Med Res. 1976;4:393–401.
22. Sirois G et al. Relative bioavailability of three commercial quinidine dosage forms. Biopharm Drug Dispos. 1980;1:167–77.
23. Meyer MC et al. Serious bioavailability problems with a generic prolonged-release quinidine gluconate product. J Clin Pharmacol. 1982;22:131–34.
24. Hiatt EP. Plasma concentrations following the oral administration of single doses of the principal alkaloids of cinchona bark. J Pharmacol Exp Ther. 1944;81:160–63.
25. Ditlefsen EML. Concentrations of quinidine in blood following oral, parenteral and rectal administration. Acta Med Scand. 1953;146:81–92.
26. Woo E, Greenblatt DJ. Effect of food on enteral absorption of quinidine. Clin Pharmacol Ther. 1980;27:188-93.
27. Spenard J et al. Influence of food on the comparative bioavailability of a fast- and slow-release dosage form of quinidine gluconate. Int J Clin Pharmacol Ther Toxicol. 1983;21:1–9.

28. Ace LN et al. Effect of food and an antacid on quinidine bioavailability. Biopharm Drug Dispos. 1983;4:183–90.
29. Martinez MN et al. Effect of dietary fat content on the bioavailability of a sustained release gluconate tablet. Biopharm Drug Dispos. 1990;11:17–29.
30. Mauro VF et al. Effect of aluminum hydroxide gel on quinidine gluconate absorption. DICP Ann Pharmacother. 1990;24:252–54.
31. Remon JP et al. Interaction entre antiarythmiques, antiacides et antidiarrheiques III. Influence d'antiacides et d'antidiarrheiques sur la resorption *in vitro* de sels de quinidine. Pharm Acta Helv. 1979;54:19–22.
32. Bucei AJ et al. *In vitro* interaction of quinidine with kaolin and pectin. J Pharm Sci. 1981;70:999–1002.
33. Moustafa MA et al. Decreased bioavailability of quinidine sulphate due to interactions with adsorbent antacids and antidiarrhoeal mixtures. Int J Pharm. 1987;34:207–11.
34. Ponzillo JJ et al. Effect of diphenoxylate with atropine sulfate on the bioavailability of quinidine sulfate in healthy subjects. Clin Pharm. 1988;7:139–42.
35. MacKichan JJ et al. Effect of cimetidine on quinidine biovailability. Biopharm Drug Dispos. 1989;10:121–25.
36. Crouthamel WG. The effect of congestive heart failure on quinidine pharmacokinetics. Am Heart J. 1975;90:335–39.
37. Ueda CT, Dzindzio BS. Bioavailability of quinidine in congestive heart failure. Br J Clin Pharmacol. 1981;11:571–77.
38. Ueda CT et al. Disposition kinetics of quinidine. Clin Pharmacol Ther. 1976;19:30–6.
39. Conrad KA et al. Pharmacokinetic studies of quinidine in patients with arrhythmias. Circulation. 1977;55:1–7.
40. Ueda CT, Dzindzio BS. Quinidine kinetics in congestive heart failure. Clin Pharmacol Ther. 1978;23:158–64.
41. Cutler RE et al. Pharmacokinetic studies in chronic renal disease and hemodialysis. Proceedings of Tenth Annual Contractors' Conference of the Artificial Kidney Program. National Institute of Arthritis and Metabolic Diseases. 1977;45–7.
42. Kessler KM et al. Quinidine pharmacokinetics in patients with cirrhosis or receiving propranolol. Am Heart J. 1978;96:627–35.
43. Warner H. Therapy of common arrhythmias. Med Clin North Am. 1974;58:995-1017.
44. Edwards DJ et al. Factors affecting quinidine protein binding in humans. J Pharm Sci. 1984;73:1264–67.
45. Conn HL, Luchi PJ. Ionic influences of quinidine-albumin interaction. J Pharmacol Exp Ther. 1961;133:76–83.
46. Conn HL, Luchi PJ. Some quantitative aspects of the binding of quinidine and related quinoline compounds by human serum albumin. J Clin Invest. 1961;40:509–16.
47. Skuterud B et al. Serum protein binding of quinidine and diphenylhydantoin in healthy human volunteers and in patients with chronic renal failure. In: Symposium: basis of drug therapy in man. 5th Int. San Francisco, CA: Congr Pharmacol;1972:79–80.
48. Ueda CT, Makoid MC. Quinidine and dihydroquinidine interactions in human plasma. J Pharm Sci. 1979;68:448–50.
49. Woo E, Greenblatt DJ. Pharmacokinetic and clinical implications of quinidine protein binding. J Pharm Sci. 1979;68:466–70.
50. Reidenberg MM, Affrime M. Influence of disease on binding of drugs to plasma proteins. Ann NY Acad Sci. 1973;226:115–26.
51. Affrime M, Reidenberg MM. The protein binding of some drugs in plasma from patients with alcoholic liver disease. Eur J Clin Pharmacol. 1975;8:267–69.
52. Perez-Mateo M, Erill S. Protein binding of salicylate and quinidine in plasma from patients with renal failure, chronic liver disease and chronic respiratory insufficiency. Eur J Clin Pharmacol. 1977;11:225–31.
53. Kates RE et al. Binding of quinidine to plasma proteins in normal subjects and in patients with hyperlipoproteinemias. Clin Pharmacol Ther. 1978;23:30–5.

54. Kessler KM et al. Blood collection techniques, heparin and quinidine protein binding. Clin Pharmacol Ther. 1979;25:204–10.
55. Pickoff AS et al. The effect of age and cyanosis on the protein binding of quinidine in the pediatric patient. Am J Cardiol. 1981;47:440.
56. Kessler KM, Perez GO. Decreased quinidine plasma protein binding during hemodialysis. Clin Pharmacol Ther. 1981;30:121–26.
57. Pickoff AS et al. Age-related differences in the protein binding of quinidine. Dev Pharmacol Ther. 1981;3:108–15.
58. Fremstad D et al. Increased plasma binding of quinidine after surgery: a preliminary report. Eur J Clin Pharmacol. 1976;10:441–44.
59. Kessler KM et al. Abnormal quinidine binding in survivors of prehospital cardiac arrest. Am Heart J. 1984;107:665–69.
60. Kessler KM et al. The clinical implication of changing unbound quinidine levels. Am Heart J. 1989;118:63–9.
61. Ochs HR et al. Reduced quinidine clearance in elderly persons. Am J Cardiol. 1978;42:481–85.
62. Hughes IE et al. The distribution of quinidine in human blood. Br J Clin Pharmacol. 1975;2:521–25.
63. Jaffe JM et al. Relationship between quinidine plasma and saliva levels in humans. J Pharm Sci. 1975;64:2028–29.
64. Yosselson-Superstine S et al. Relationship between quinidine concentrations measured in saliva and erythrocytes, and in serum. Int J Clin Pharmacol Ther Toxicol. 1982;20:181–86.
65. Narang PK et al. Quinidine saliva concentrations: absence of correlation with serum concentrations at steady state. Clin Pharmacol Ther. 1983;34:695–702.
66. Ueda CT et al. Relationship between saliva and serum quinidine concentrations and suppression of ventricular premature beats. Ther Drug Monit. 1984;6:43–9.
67. Ochs HR et al. Entry of quinidine into cerebrospinal fluid. Am Heart J. 1980;100:341–46.
68. Szefler SJ et al. Rapid elimination of quinidine in pediatric patients. Pediatrics. 1982;70:370–75.
69. Levy R et al. Quinidine pharmacokinetics in anephric and normal subjects. Clin Res. 1976;24:85A.
70. Drayer DE et al. Prevalence of high (3S)-3-hydroxyquinidine/quinidine ratios in serum, and clearance of quinidine in cardiac patients with age. Clin Pharmacol Ther. 1980;27:72–5.
71. Data JL et al. Interaction of quinidine with anticonvulsant drugs. N Engl J Med. 1976;294:699–702.
72. Twum-Barima Y, Carruthers SG. Quinidine-rifampin interaction. N Engl J Med. 1981;304:1466–69.
73. Bussey HI et al. The influence of rifampin on quinidine and digoxin. Arch Intern Med. 1984;144:1021–23.
74. Hardy BG et al. Effect of cimetidine on the pharmacokinetics and pharmacodynamics of quinidine. Am J Cardiol. 1983;52:172–75.
75. Saal AK et al. Effect of amiodarone on serum quinidine and procainamide levels. Am J Cardiol. 1984;53:1264–67.
76. Lavoie R et al. The effect of verapamil on quinidine pharmacokinetics in man. Drug Intell Clin Pharm. 1986;20:457.
77. Trohman RG et al. Increased quinidine plasma concentrations during administration of verapamil: a new quinidine-verapamil interaction. Am J Cardiol. 1986;57:706–7.
78. Hardy BG, Schentag JJ. Lack of effect of cimetidine on the metabolism of quinidine: effect on renal clearance. Int J Clin Pharmacol Ther Toxicol. 1988;26:388–91.
79. Ochs HR et al. Effect of propranolol on pharmacokinetics and acute electrocardiographic changes following intravenous quinidine in humans. Pharmacology. 1978;17:301–6.
80. Kates RE, Blanford MF. Disposition kinetics of oral quinidine when administered concurrently with propranolol. J Clin Pharmacol. 1979;19:378–83.
81. Fenster P et al. Kinetic evaluation of the propranolol-quinidine combination. Clin Pharmacol Ther. 1980;27:450–53.
82. Zeller FP et al. Effect of caffeine on the oral absorption and disposition of quinidine. Clin Pharm. 1984;3:72–5.

83. Matera MG et al. Quinidine-diltiazem: pharmacokinetic interaction in humans. Curr Ther Res. 1986;40:653–56.

84. Edwards DJ et al. Lack of effect of smoking on the metabolism and pharmacokinetics of quinidine in patients. Br J Clin Pharmacol. 1987;23:351–54.

85. Green JA et al. Nifedipine-quinidine interaction. Clin Pharm. 1983;2:461–5.

86. Farringer JA et al. Nifedipine-induced alterations in serum quinidine concentrations. Am Heart J. 1984;108:1570–72.

87. Van Lith RM, Appleby DH. Quinidine-nifedipine interaction. Drug Intell Clin Pharm. 1985;19:829–30.

88. Munger MA et al. Elucidation of the nifedipine-quinidine interaction. Clin Pharmacol Ther. 1989;45:411–16.

89. Otton SV et al. Competitive inhibition of sparteine oxidation in human liver by beta-adrenoceptor antagonists and other cardiovascular drugs. Life Sci. 1984;34:73–80.

90. Inaba T et al. Quinidine: potent inhibition of sparteine and debrisoquine oxidation *in vivo*. Br J Clin Pharmacol. 1986;22:199–201.

91. Funck-Brentano C et al. Genetically-determined interaction between propafenone and low dose quinidine: role of active metabolites in modulating net drug effect. Br J Clin Pharmacol. 1989;27:435–44.

92. Brinn R et al. Sparteine oxidation is practically abolished in quinidine-treated patients. Br J Clin Pharmacol. 1986;22:194–97.

93. Guengerich FP et al. Oxidation of quinidine by human liver cytochrome P-450. Mol Pharmacol. 1986;30:287–95.

94. Mikus G et al. Pharmacokinetics and metabolism of quinidine in extensive and poor metabolisers of sparteine. Eur J Clin Pharmacol. 1986;31:69–72.

95. Carroll FI et al. Carbon-13 magnetic resonance study. Structure of the metabolites of orally administered quinidine in humans. J Med Chem. 1974;17:985–87.

96. Beermann B et al. The metabolism of quinidine in man: structure of a main metabolite. Acta Chem Scand B. 1976;30:465.

97. Drayer DE et al, Active quinidine metabolites. Clin Res. 1976;24:623A.

98. Guentert TW et al. Isolation, characterisation and synthesis of a new quinidine metabolite. Eur J Drug Metab Pharmacokinet. 1982;7:31–8.

99. Leroyer R et al. Metabolites plasmatiques de la quinidine chez l'insuffisant renal chronique. Therapie. 1983;38:621–26.

100. Rakhit A et al. Pharmacokinetics of quinidine and three of its metabolites in man. J Pharmacokinet Biopharm. 1984;12:1–21.

101. Palmer KH et al. The metabolic fate of orally administered quinidine gluconate in humans. Biochem Pharmacol. 1969;18:1845–860.

102. Leferink JG et al. A novel quinidine metabolism in a suicide case with quinidine sulphate detected by gas chromatography mass spectrometry. J Anal Toxicol, 1977;1:62–5.

103. Drayer DE et al. Steady-state serum levels of quinidine and active metabolites in cardiac patients with varying degrees of renal function. Clin Pharmacol Ther. 1978;24:31–9.

104. Vozeh S et al. Kinetics and electrocardiographic changes after oral 3-OH-quinidine in healthy subjects. Clin Pharmacol Ther. 1985;37:575–81.

105. Ha HR et al. Kinetics and dynamics of quinidine-N-oxide in healthy subjects. Clin Pharmacol Ther. 1987;42:341–45.

106. Ackerman BH et al. Disposition of 3-hydroxyquinidine in patients receiving initial intravenous quinidine gluconate for electrophysiology testing of ventricular tachycardia. DICP Ann Pharmacother. 1989;23:275–78.

107. Wooding-Scott RA et al. The pharmacokinetics and pharmacodynamics of quinidine and 3-hydroxyquinidine. Br J Clin Pharmacol. 1988;26:415–21.

108. Thompson KA et al. Plasma concentrations of quinidine, its major metabolites, and dihydroquinidine in patients with torsades de pointes. Clin Pharmacol Ther. 1988;43:636–42.

109. Wooding-Scott RA et al. Total and unbound concentrations of quinidine and 3-hydroxyquinidine at steady state. Am Heart J. 1987;113:302–6.

110. Vozeh S et al. Pharmacodynamics of 3-hydroxyquinidine alone and in combination with quinidine in health persons. Am J Cardiol. 1987;59:681–84.

111. Nwangwu PU et al. The antiarrhythmic activities of 6'-hydroxycinchonine, 6'-benzyloxycinchonine and 6'-allyloxycinchonine compared with quinidine in mice. J Pharm Pharmacol. 1979;31:488–89.

112. Rakhit A et al. Pharmacokinetics and pharmacodynamics of quinidine N-oxide, a major quinidine metabolite. APhA:Acad Pharm Sci;1981:11(1):74. Abstract.

113. Juliard JM et al. Comparaison des effets electrophysiologiques cardiaques de la quinidine, de la 3-hydroxy-quinidine et de la 3-hydroxy-hydroquinidine chez le chien anesthesie, etude des relations effets-concentrations plasmatiques. Arch Mal Coeur. 1983;76:670–78.

114. Uematsu T et al. Relative electrophysiological potencies of quinidine, 3-OH quinidine and quinidine-N-oxide in guinea-pig heart. Arch Int Pharmacodyn. 1989;297:29–38.

115. Vozeh S et al. Antiarrhythmic activity of two quinidine metabolites in experimental reperfusion arrhythmia: relative potency and pharmacodynamic interaction with the parent drug. J Pharmacol Exp Ther. 1987;243:297–301.

116. Thompson KA et al. Comparative *in vitro* electrophysiology of quinidine, its major metabolites and dihydroquinidine. J Pharmacol Exp Ther. 1987;241:84–90.

117. Kavanagh KM et al. Contribution of quinidine metabolites to electrophysiologic responses in human subjects. Clin Pharmacol Ther. 1989;46:352–58.

118. Conn HL, Luchi RJ. Some cellular and metabolic considerations relating to the action of quinidine as a prototype antiarrhythmic agent. Am J Med. 1964;37:685–99.

119. Gerhardt RE et al. Quinidine excretion in aciduria and alkaluria. Ann Intern Med. 1969;71:927–33.

120. Chin TWF et al. Quinidine pharmacokinetics in continuous ambulatory peritoneal dialysis. Clin Exp Dialysis Apheresis. 1981;5:391–97.

121. Hall K et al. Clearance of quinidine during peritoneal dialysis. Am Heart J. 1982;104:646–47.

122. Woie L, Oyri A. Quinidine intoxication treated with hemodialysis. Acta Med Scand. 1974;195:237–39.

123. Gibson TP. Dialyzability of common therapeutic agents. Dialysis Transplant. 1979;8:24–40.

124. Hill LM, Malkasian GD. The use of quinidine sulfate throughout pregnancy. Obstet Gynecol. 1979;54:366–68.

125. Bolme P, Otto U. Dose-dependence of the pharmacokinetics of quinidine. Eur J Clin Pharmacol. 1977;12:73–6.

126. Russo J et al. Assessment of quinidine gluconate for nonlinear kinetics following chronic dosing. J Clin Pharmacol. 1982;22:264–70.

127. Fremstad D et al. Pharmacokinetics of quinidine related to plasma protein binding in man. Eur J Clin Pharmacol. 1979;15:187–92.

128. Gey GO et al. Quinidine plasma concentration and exertional arrhythmia. Am Heart J. 1975;90:19–24.

129. The United States Pharmacopeia. 21st ed. Rockville: United States Pharmacopeial Convention. 1985.

130. Lewis T et al. Observations upon the action of certain drugs upon fibrillation of the auricles. Heart. 1922;9:207–67.

131. Alexander F et al. The relative value of synthetic quinidine, dihydroquinidine, commercial quinidine, and quinine in the control of cardiac arrhythmias. J Pharmacol Exp Ther. 1947;90:191–201.

132. Model W et al. Relative potencies of various cinchona alkaloids in patients with auricular fibrillation. Fed Proc. 1949;8:320–21.

133. Ueda CT et al. Disposition kinetics of dihydroquinidine following quinidine administration. Res Commun Chem Path Pharmacol. 1976;14:215–25.

134. Ueda CT, Dzindzio BS. Pharmacokinetics of dihydroquinidine in congestive heart failure patients after intravenous quinidine administration. Eur J Clin Pharmacol. 1979;16:101–5.

135. Edwards IR et al. Correlation between plasma quinidine and cardiac effect. Br J Clin Pharmacol. 1974;1:455–59.

136. Carliner NH et al. Relation of ventricular premature beat suppression to serum quinidine concentration determined by a new and specific assay. Am Heart J. 1980;100:483–89.

137. Holford NHG et al. The effect of quinidine and its metabolites on the electrocardiogram and systolic time intervals: concentration-effect relationships. Br J Clin Pharmacol. 1981;11:187–95.

138. Halkin H et al. Steady-state serum quinidine concentration: role in prophylactic therapy following acute myocardial infarction. Israel J Med Sci. 1979;15:583–87.

139. Brodie BB, Udenfriend S. The estimation of quinidine in human plasma with a note on the estimation of quinidine. J Pharmacol Exp Ther. 1943;78:154–58.

140. Guentert TW et al. Divergence in pharmacokinetic parameters of quinidine obtained by specific and nonspecific assay methods. J Pharmacokinet Biopharm. 1979;7:303–11.

141. Cramer G, Isaksson B. Quantitative determination of quinidine in plasma. Scand J Clin Lab Invest. 1963;15:553–56.

142. Dzindzio BS et al. Unpublished data.

143. Woo E, Greenblatt DJ. A re-evaluation of intravenous quinidine. Am Heart J. 1978;96:829–32.

144. Hirschfeld DS et al. Clinical and electrophysiological effects of intravenous quinidine in man. Br Heart J. 1977;39:309–16.

145. Kalmansohn RW, Sampson JJ. Studies of plasma quinidine content II. Relation to toxic manifestations and therapeutic effect. Circulation. 1950;1:569–75.

146. Ditlefsen EML, Knutsen B. Quinidine treatment in chronic auricular fibrillation I. Conversion to sinus rhythm, related to quinidine serum concentration. Acta Med Scand. 1956;156:1–14.

147. Bailey DJ. Cardiotoxic effects of quinidine and their treatment. Arch Intern Med. 1960;105:13–22.

148. Kalmansohn RW, Sampson JJ. Studies of plasma quinidine content in relation to single dose administration, toxic manifestations and therapeutic effect. Am J Med. 1949;6:393–94.

149. Ditlefsen EML. Concentrations of quinidine in blood following oral, parenteral and rectal administration. Acta Med Scand. 1953;146:81–92.

150. Ochs HR et al. Single and multiple dose pharmacokinetics of oral quinidine sulfate and gluconate. Am J Cardiol. 1978;41:770–77.

151. Wright GJ et al. Comparative quinidine plasma profiles at steady state of two controlled-release products and quinidine sulfate in solution. Biopharm Drug Dispos. 1987;8:159–72.

152. Mahon WA et al. Comparative bioavailability of study of three sustained release quinidine formulations. Clin Pharmacokinet. 1987;13:118–24.

153. Griggs DE et al. Therapeutic use of quinidine. Med Clin North Am. 1952;26:1025–34.

154. Edgar AL, Sokolow M. Experiences with the photofluorometric determination of quinidine in blood. J Lab Clin Med. 1950;36:478–84.

155. Gelfman N, Seligson D. Quinidine. Am J Clin Pathol. 1961;36:390–92.

156. Hartel G, Harjanne A. Comparison of two methods for quinidine determination and chromatographic analysis of the difference. Clin Chim Acta. 1969;23:289–94.

157. Byrne-Quinn E, Wing AJ. Maintenance of sinus rhythm after DC reversion of atrial fibrillation: a double-blind controlled trial of long-acting quinidine bisulphate. Br Heart J. 1970;32:370–76.

158. Brodie BB et al. The estimation of basic organic compounds in biological material II. Estimation of fluorescent compounds. J Biol Chem. 1947;168:311–18.

159. Brodie BB et al. The estimation of basic organic compounds in biological material I. General principles. J Biol Chem. 1947;168:299–309.

160. Armand J, Badinand A. Dosage de la quinidine (ou de la quinine) dans les milieux biologiques. Ann Biol Clin. 1972;30:599–604.

161. Broussand LA. Fluorometric determination of quinidine. Clin Chem. 1981;27:1929–30.

162. Josephson ES et al. The estimation of basic organic compounds in biological material VI. Estimation by ultraviolet spectrophotometry. J Biol Chem. 1947;168:341–44.

163. Brodie BB, Udenfriend S. The estimation of basic organic compounds and a technique for the appraisal of specificity: application to the cinchona alkaloids. J Biol Chem. 1945;158:705–14.

164. Midha KK, Charette C. GLC determination of quinidine from plasma and whole blood. J Pharm Sci. 1974;63:1244–47.

165. Valentine JL et al. GLC determination of quinidines in human plasma. J Pharm Sci. 1976;65:96–8.

166. Moulin MA, Kinsun H. A gas-liquid chromatographic method for the quantitative determination of quinidine in blood. Clin Chim Acta. 1977;75:491–95.

167. Kessler KM et al. Simultaneous quantitation of quinidine, procainamide, and N-acetylprocainamide in serum by gas-liquid chromatography with a nitrogen-phosphorus selective detector. Clin Chem. 1982;28:1187–90.

168. Guentert TW et al. Determination of quinidine and its major metabolites by high-performance liquid chromatography. J Chromatogr. 1976;162:59–70.

169. Drayer DE et al. Specific determination of quinidine and (3S)-3-hydroxyquinidine in human serum by high-pressure liquid chromatography. J Lab Clin Med. 1977;90:816–22.

170. Crouthamel WG et al. Specific serum quinidine assay by high-performance liquid chromatography. Clin Chem. 1977;23:2030–33.

171. Achari RG et al. Rapid determination of quinidine in human plasma by high-performance liquid chromatography. J Chromatogr Sci. 1978;16:271–73.

172. Powers JL, Sadee W. Determination of quinidine by high-performance liquid chromatography. 1978;24:299–302.

173. Peat MA, Jennison TA. High-performance liquid chromatography of quinidine in plasma, with use of a microparticulate silica column. Clin Chem. 1978;24:2166–68.

174. Sved S et al. The estimation of quinidine in human plasma by ion pair extraction and high-performance liquid chromatography. J Chromatogr. 1978;145:437–44.

175. Kates RE et al. Rapid high-pressure liquid chromatographic determination of quinidine and dihydroquinidine in plasma samples. J Pharm Sci. 1978. 67:269–70.

176. Bonora MR et al. Determination of quinidine and metabolites in urine by reverse-phase high-pressure liquid chromatography. Clin Chim Acta. 1979;91:277–84.

177. Kline BJ et al. Determination of quinidine and dihydroquinidine in plasma by high performance liquid chromatography. Anal Chem. 1979;51:449–51.

178. Weidner N et al. A high-pressure liquid chromatography method for serum quinidine and (3S)-3-hydroxyquinidine. Clin Chim Acta. 1979;91:7–13.

179. Reece PA, Peikert M. Simple and selective high-performance liquid chromatographic method for estimating plasma quinidine levels. J Chromatogr. 1980;181:207–17.

180. Guentert TW et al. An integrated approach to measurements of quinidine and metabolites in biological fluids. J Chromatogr. 1980;183:514–18.

181. Pershing LK et al. A HPLC method for the quantitation of quinidine and its metabolites in plasma: an application to a quinidine-phenytoin drug interaction study. J Anal Toxicol. 1982;6:153–56.

182. Leroyer R. Specific determination of quinidine and metabolites in biological fluids by reversed-phase high-performance liquid chromatography. J Chromatogr. 1982;228:366–71.

183. Rakhit A et al. Improved liquid-chromatographic assay of quinidine and its metabolites in biological fluids. Clin Chem. 1982;28:1505–9.

184. Leroyer R et al. Reverse-phase liquid chromatography and pharmacokinetic study of two hydroxylated analogues of quinidine in dogs. J Pharm Sci. 1984;73:844–46.

185. Hartel G, Korhonen A. Thin-layer chromatography for the quantitative separation of quinidine and quinidine metabolites from biological fluids and tissues. J Chromatogr. 1968,37:70–5.

186. Steyn JM, Hundt HYL. A thin-layer chromatographic method for the quantitative determination of quinidine in human serum. J Chromatogr. 1975;111:463–65.

187. Christiansen J. Quantitative *in situ* thin-layer chromatography of quinidine and salicylic acid in capillary blood. J Chromatogr. 1976;123:57–63.

188. Wesley-Hadzija B, Mattocks AM. Specific thin-layer chromatographic method for the determination of quinidine in biological fluids. J Chromatogr. 1977;144:223–30.

189. Kelner M, Bailey DN. Micro-analysis for quinidine in serum by thin-layer chromatography followed by fluorescence densitometry. Clin Chem. 1983;29:2100–102.

190. Garland WA, Trager WF. Direct (non-chromatographic) quantification of drugs and their metabolites from human plasma utilizing chemical ionization mass spectrometry and stable isotope labeling: quinidine and lidocaine. Biomed Mass Spec. 1974;1:124–29.

191. Syva Co. Emit Quinidine Assay. Product information. Palo Alto, CA: 1984 February.

192. Ames Division, Miles Laboratories. Ames TDA Quinidine Assay. Product information. Elkhart, IN: 1984 December.

193. Abbott Laboratories. TDx Quinidine. Product information. North Chicago, IL: 1984 April.

194. Beckman Instruments. ICS Quinidine Assay. Product information. Brea, CA: 1986 September.

195. Guentert TW, Riegelman S. Specificity of quinidine determination methods. Clin Chem. 1978;24:2065–66.

196. Edelbroek PM, de Wolff FA. The quinidine-fluorometry dilemma. Clin Chem. 1981;27:1778–79.

197. Greenblatt DJ, Woo E. The specificity of the extraction fluorescence assay for serum or plasma quinidine. J Clin Pharmacol. 1981;21:333–36.

198. Drayer DE et al. Liquid chromatography and fluorescence spectroscopy compared with a homogeneous enzyme immunoassay technique for determining quinidine in serum. Clin Chem. 1981;27:308–10.

199. Ha HR et al. Quinidine determination in serum: enzyme immunoassay (EIA) V HPLC. Br J Clin Pharmacol. 1981;11:312–14.

200. Dextraze PG et al. Comparison of an enzyme immunoassay and a high performance liquid chromatographic method for quantitation of quinidine in serum. Clin Toxicol. 1981;18:291–97.

201. Smith GH, Levy RH. serum quinidine determination: comparison of mass-spectrometric and extraction-fluorescence methods. Drug Intell Clin Pharm. 1982;16:693–95.

202. Vasiliades J, Finkel JM. Determination of quinidine in serum by spectrofluorometry, liquid chromatography and fluorescence scanning thin-layer chromatography. J Chromatogr. 1983;278:117–32.

203. Bridges RR et al. Comparison of quinidine by fluorescence polarization immunoassay and high pressure liquid chromatography. J Anal Toxicol. 1984;8:161–63.

204. Bottorff MB et al. Comparison of high pressure liquid chromatography and fluorescence polarization immunoassay to assess quinidine pharmacokinetics. Biopharm Drug Dispos. 1987;8:213–21.

205. Wooding-Scott RA et al. Comparison of assay procedures used to measure total and unbound concentrations of quinidine. DICP Ann Pharmacother. 1989;23:999–1004.

Chapter 24

Beta Blockers

David J. Kazierad, Karen D. Schlanz,
and Michael B. Bottorff

The beta blockers are among the most widely prescribed classes of drugs in clinical practice in the United States. Although these agents produce their pharmacologic actions by selective antagonism of β-adrenergic receptors of the autonomic nervous system, their pharmacokinetic and pharmacologic properties are varied and sometimes quite dissimilar. In addition to preferential antagonism of β-receptors, newer agents have been designed to selectively inhibit β_1-receptors, block α_1-receptors, or act as partial β-receptor agonists. Table 24-1 lists the pharmacologic properties of currently available beta blockers.

Beta blockers differ from most other classes of drugs included in this book. Presently, monitoring plasma concentrations for beta blockers is unnecessary since the clinical response to these agents is easily assessed by such hemodynamic parameters as heart rate or blood pressure. In addition, there is large interpatient variability in concentration-effect relationships due to variation in pharmacokinetics and intrinsic sensitivity to beta-blockade. This class of agents has a wide therapeutic index and concentration determinations do not necessarily predict all beta blocker responses. However, because they are used so extensively, an understanding of their disposition and pharmacodynamics is important in clinical practice.

Chemically, all beta blockers exist as stereoisomers, and in general are administered as a racemic mixture of the active levorotatory (l) and inactive dextrorotatory (d) isomers (also referred to as enantiomers). Timolol and penbutolol are exceptions to this in that they are commercially available in their pure active l-isomer form. Enantiomers can have different pharmacokinetic properties which may result in unequal concentrations of each isomer at the β-receptor. Pharmacokinetic parameters derived from assays which quantify only the total concentration of all isomers may not correlate well with the disposition of the active isomer. When evaluating serum concentration measurements of racemic beta blockers, it is imperative to differentiate between total and individual isomer concentrations.

This chapter describes in detail the pharmacokinetic characteristics of the prototype beta-blocking compound, propranolol. In addition, the pharmacokinetic properties

Table 24–1. Pharmacologic Properties of Beta Blockers

Drug	Receptor blocking activity	Partial agonist activity	N-octanol buffer[a] partition coefficient	Beta blocking plasma concentrations (ng/mL)
Acebutolol	β_1	+	0.70	200–2000
Atenolol	β_1	0	0.02	200–500
Betaxolol	β_1	0	3.9	20–50
Esmolol	β_1	0		150–1000
Labetalol	$\beta_1, \beta_2, \alpha_1$	0	11.5	700–3000
Metoprolol	β_1	0	0.98	50–100
Nadolol	β_1, β_2	0	0.07	50–100
Penbutolol	β_1, β_2	+		1–200
Pindolol	β_1, β_2	++	0.82	5–15
Propranolol	β_1, β_2	0	20.2	50–100
Timolol	β_1, β_2	0	1.2	5–10

[a] pH 7.4 at 37° C.

of each of the other currently marketed beta blockers will be summarized and compared to those of propranolol. Table 24-2 presents the major pharmacokinetic parameters of the beta blockers discussed in this chapter.

Many beta blockers, specifically those that are lipophilic in nature, undergo polymorphic metabolism through the debrisoquine pathway. The population can be divided into those who are extensive metabolizers (EMs) and poor metabolizers (PMs) of these drugs. This chapter also describes the effects of polymorphic metabolism on the pharmacokinetics and pharmacodynamics of the beta blockers (see Chapter 7: Genetic Polymorphisms of Drug Metabolism for a more extensive discussion of this concept).

The pharmacodynamic relationships of the beta blockers have been studied to a lesser extent than the pharmacokinetic characteristics. This chapter reviews the information available about the concentration/effect relationships (i.e., beta-blockade, antihypertensive, antianginal, antiarrhythmic, and negative inotropic effects) of specific β-adrenergic antagonists, data that are necessary for the rational use of these drugs. Patient factors that may influence the pharmacodynamic response to beta blockers are also discussed.

CLINICAL PHARMACOKINETICS

Propranolol

Propranolol is most commonly taken orally on a chronic basis, although an intravenous form is available for acute administration. The commercial product is a racemic mixture of d- and l-stereoisomers.[1] Since the l-isomer of propranolol is approximately 100 times more potent than d-propranolol, it is responsible for essentially all of the clinical effects.

Absorption. Propranolol is almost completely absorbed from the gastrointestinal tract, with less than 5% of the administered dose recovered in the feces.[2,3] The high degree of absorption is due to the high lipid solubility of the drug. For conventional-release tablets, the rate of absorption is rapid with peak plasma concentrations occurring within two hours.[4,5] Peak plasma concentrations following administration of sustained-release capsules occur four to six hours after the dose.[5]

First Pass Metabolism. Although propranolol is completely absorbed following oral administration, its bioavailability is low due to a high hepatic extraction ratio and significant first-pass metabolism (see Propranolol: Metabolism). The high variability (25% to 70%) in the systemic availability of oral propranolol among patients can be attributed to many factors, including differences in dose, dosage form (conventional versus sustained-release), age, disease, and concomitant administration of other drugs or food. In normal volunteers, systemic bioavailability is 30% to 40% under steady-state conditions.[6] High-protein meals[7,8] and hydralazine[9] increase hepatic blood flow and reduce first-pass extraction thereby increasing the bioavailability by 20% to 50%.

Because first-pass removal of propranolol following oral administration is a saturable process, its bioavailability increases with the dose.[13,14] Wagner[15] has suggested that Michaelis-Menten first-pass removal is evident following oral

Table 24–2. Pharamacokinetic Parameters of Beta Blockers

Drug	Bioavailability (%)	Protein binding (%)	Total Clearance (L/hr/kg)	V_d (L/kg)	$t\frac{1}{2}$ (hr)	Major route of elimination[a]	Drug accumulation in renal disease
Acebutolol	35–40	15	0.29	1.2	11	HM/RE (≈40% unchanged)	Yes (Diacetolol)
Atenolol	50–60	<5	0.16	1.2	6.9	RE	Yes
Betaxolol	80–90	55	0.28	8.7	14	HM	No
Esmolol	N/A	55	17	3.4	0.15	Esterases in RBCs	No
Labetalol	30–40	50	1.3	5.6	4	HM	No
Metoprolol	40–50	12	0.97	4.2	2.8–7.6	HM	No
Nadolol	30–50	20	0.1	2.0	20	RE	Yes
Penbutolol	95	90–95	0.34	0.6	18–27	HM	No
Pindolol	87	40–60	0.46	2.0	2–4	HM/RE (40% unchanged)	No
Propranolol	30–40	90	0.9	3.3	3–6	HM	No
Timolol	75	10	0.46	2.0–2.5	4	HM	No

[a] RE = Renal excretion; HM = Hepatic metabolism; RBCs = Red blood cells.

administration of compounds with high hepatic extraction ratios such as propranolol, resulting in enzyme saturation and increased bioavailability. This phenomenon may partially explain why the bioavailability of sustained-release propranolol preparations is only about 50% that of the same dose administered as regular propranolol tablets.[5,16,17] Reduced first-pass metabolism is also evident as the doses of regular-release propranolol are increased. Silber et al. gave oral propranolol in daily doses of 40 to 320 mg and noted that average steady-state plasma propranolol concentrations increased disproportionately as the dose increased.[18] Over this range of daily propranolol doses at steady state, there was an average 56% reduction in intrinsic clearance and a 175% increase in propranolol half-life. The formation clearances of three major propranolol metabolites (propranolol glucuronide, 4-hydroxypropranolol glucuronide, and naphthoxylactic acid) were saturable with increasing doses, as was the formation clearance of other unidentified metabolic pathways (accounting for approximately 45% of the propranolol dose).

Saturable first-pass metabolism and propranolol bioavailability is best illustrated by considering the partial metabolic clearances of the metabolites. Walle et al.[19] gave propranolol to seven male volunteers in single oral doses of 80 mg and measured propranolol in serum and 14 propranolol metabolites in urine. Oral clearance varied threefold (27.5 to 71.4 mL/min/kg); however, there was little variation in the clearance through glucuronidation (range 6.8 to 9.9 mL/min/kg). Moderate variation was observed in clearance by side chain oxidation (10.9 to 25.8 mL/min/kg), and the highest variability was seen with clearance through ring oxidation (7.5 to 41.8 mL/min/kg). Thus, it appears that most of the variability in propranolol bioavailability following oral administration is due to activity of ring oxidation to the 4-hydroxypropranolol, 4-hydroxypropranolol glucuronide, and 4-hydroxypropranolol sulfate metabolites.

Another interesting aspect of propranolol pharmacokinetics is the apparent increase in bioavailability that occurs with chronic oral dosing. Several studies have documented an increase in the ratio of the AUC following single oral doses compared to the AUC_{0-t} at steady state.[5,6,11,12,16] Using simultaneous administration of unlabeled oral and tritiated intravenous propranolol, Wood et al. found that bioavailability increased from 22% after single doses to 34% at steady state.[6] There was also a small, but statistically insignificant, reduction in systemic clearance and a concomitant increase in half-life from 4.3 hours to 5.4 hours.

The degree of accumulation to steady state appears similar for both regular-release (49% increase) and sustained-release (68% increase) products.[5] As noted for other drugs with high hepatic extraction ratios, propranolol exhibits nonlinear accumulation with chronic oral dosing. This is apparently caused by a reduction in intrinsic clearance that increases bioavailability. However, the increased plasma concentrations do not significantly alter the degree or duration of beta-blocking effects.[5,20]

As noted earlier, most of the pharmacologic effect attributed to propranolol is due to the more potent l-isomer. It has been suggested that there is no stereoselective difference in the presystemic metabolism of propranolol isomers, since no differences were observed in the oral bioavailability of l-propranolol and racemic propranolol (40.7% versus 42.4%, respectively).[21] When evaluated separately, however, clearance of the l-isomer is relatively slower; this observation is consistent with *in vitro* and *in vivo* data (see Propranolol: Metabolism). The nonlinear accumulation associated with chronic dosing to steady state occurs to a similar degree for both d- and l-propranolol. In a study of normal volunteers, Lalonde et al.[22] showed that the AUC for d-propranolol increased by 42% from single doses to steady state. The AUC of l-propranolol increased by 28%, resulting in an AUC l to d ratio of 1.52 for single doses and 1.32 at steady state.

Distribution. Propranolol is widely distributed throughout the body and has an apparent volume of distribution of 150 to 260 L.[14,23] Because of high octanol:water partitioning, propranolol accumulates rapidly in highly vascularized tissues such as the brain, adipose tissue, and muscle.[24] Animal studies evaluating the time course of drug concentrations in various tissues have substantiated the association between rate of drug distribution and lipid solubility.[25,26]

The influence of lipid solubility on the extent and rate of drug distribution is most notable in tissues for which permeability rather than flow is the rate-limiting determinant of drug distribution, such as in the central nervous system (CNS). Studies with propranolol in various animals have shown the time course of drug concentrations in the brain to be similar to the time course of drug concentrations in serum (see Figure 24-1). Although propranolol has the highest octanol:water partition ratio, all beta blockers taken on a chronic basis penetrate the CNS and may elicit near-maximal CNS pharmacologic response.[27,28] Thus, lipid solubility may predict overall distribution characteristics of a beta blocker, but may be of limited value in predicting the intensity of pharmacologic effect.

The serum protein binding of propranolol cannot be solely accounted for by binding to serum albumin.[13] Like many other weak bases, propranolol also binds significantly to acute phase reactant proteins such as α_1-acid glycoprotein (AAG).[29,30]

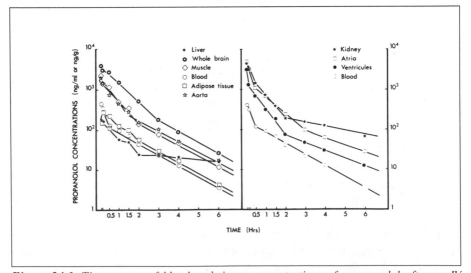

Figure 24-1. *Time course of blood and tissue concentrations of propranolol after an IV administration of 2 mg/kg in the rat. Points represent mean values for three animals (reprinted with permission from reference 223).*

Because the concentration of AAG changes acutely in many disease states, the binding and free fraction of propranolol (and other beta blockers) may be altered in several pathophysiologic conditions.[31]

In humans, propranolol is extensively bound to serum proteins, with reported free fractions in serum ranging from 5% to 12% (mean about 10%).[32,33] Binding of propranolol is strongly correlated with serum AAG concentration and appears to remain constant over the range of serum propranolol concentrations observed clinically (see Figure 24-2).[33] Approximately 25% to 30% of the drug is bound to serum albumin with 50% to 70% of total concentrations bound to AAG.[29]

Currently there is little objective clinical data to support the hypothesis that the unbound concentration of propranolol is a better clinical indicator of pharmacologic response. This may reflect the fact that: 1) the determination of unbound concentrations of propranolol (and other beta blockers) is too difficult and time consuming for clinical purposes; and 2) the variability in protein binding appears less significant than variability in dose-response relationships (variable pharmacokinetics and intrinsic sensitivity to beta-blockade).[20] Nonetheless, using isoproterenol stimulation to estimate the propranolol affinity constant (K_a) for β-receptors *in vivo*, McDevitt et al.[34] have shown that the K_a for free drug correlated better with beta-blockade than total propranolol serum concentrations. As such, conditions that dramatically alter AAG concentrations and thus, protein binding of propranolol in serum (e.g., myocardial infarction),[35] could potentially alter the pharmacodynamic response to propranolol. Given the difficulty in measuring unbound propranolol concentrations in patient care conditions, some investigators have proposed a method for estimating the unbound percentage of propranolol using an inverse relationship with AAG concentrations.[31,36] As proposed by Routledge and Shand:

$$\% \, F \; = \; \frac{100}{B/F \; + 1}$$

$$B/F \; = \; 0.0654 \, AAG \; + \; 1.72$$

where %F is the percent propranolol concentration unbound, AAG is the concentration of α_1-acid glycoprotein, and B:F is the binding molar ratio of bound to unbound drug in the plasma.

Propranolol binding to serum proteins exhibits stereoselectivity. The ratio of the unbound fraction of l-propranolol to d-propranolol in the serum of normal volunteers averages 0.72 to 0.86, indicating a stereoselective preference for binding of the l-enantiomer.[37,38] With respect to the individual binding proteins in serum, the l:d unbound ratio is 0.79 for AAG and 1.07 for albumin, indicating the preferential binding of l-propranolol to AAG and d-propranolol to albumin.[37] The magnitude of this stereoselective binding is relatively small, and thus can be considered to have negligible clinical significance in most cases. However, Walle et al.[37] noted that the unbound l:d-propranolol ratio decreased from 0.93 to 0.81

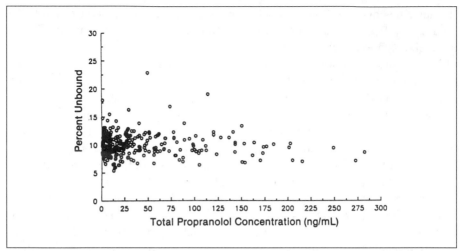

Figure 24-2. *Percent unbound concentration in serum as a function of total propranolol concentration, showing a lack of saturable protein binding in the range of concentrations seen clinically (reprinted with permission from reference 33).*

as the overall protein binding of propranolol increased. This may result in less availability of the active l-enantiomer in clinical conditions associated with extreme elevations of AAG.

Metabolism. Propranolol is almost completely eliminated from plasma via hepatic metabolism. The metabolic pathways involved are part of the cytochrome P450 mixed function oxidase system, the sum of which results in a high intrinsic clearance (CL_{int}). Thus, propranolol metabolism following intravenous administration is highly dependent on hepatic blood flow. Clearance after oral administration (CL_{oral}) is directly proportional to CL_{int}. Hence, propranolol metabolism is commonly used as a marker for drugs with a high intrinsic clearance and the literature is abundant with articles on propranolol metabolism and pharmacokinetics (see Chapter 6: Influence of Hepatic Disease on Pharmacokinetics for more detailed discussions on hepatic drug metabolism).

The total body clearance of propranolol is directly related to liver blood flow and intrinsic clearance; thus, a change in either will alter the pharmacokinetic profile.[14] Cytochrome P450 mediated reactions are responsible for the majority of propranolol metabolism, and it has been demonstrated that the amount of P450 found in liver biopsies correlates well with the magnitude of propranolol oral clearance.[39] The high-affinity enzyme system for propranolol can become saturated, presenting the possibility of dose-dependent and nonlinear pharmacokinetics. This was initially suggested when early investigators discovered that serum concentrations of propranolol were not detected after 30 mg single doses of the drug.[3] The hypothesis was that larger doses were needed to saturate the enzyme system and allow for greater bioavailability. Any increase in serum concentrations would then be the result of diminished or saturated hepatic metabolism, providing for an increase in calculated bioavailability via the equation: $F = 1 - E$ (where F represents bioavailability and E the hepatic extraction ratio).

When propranolol is administered chronically, it exhibits nonlinear accumulation. This phenomenon may result from the ability of propranolol to inhibit its own metabolism, either by impairing intrinsic clearance[40-42] or by reducing cardiac output and attenuating hepatic blood flow.[43] Propranolol and other beta blockers are known to inhibit the metabolism of antipyrine, a low clearance marker compound whose hepatic elimination is essentially dependent on CL_{int} and the metabolic activity of the cytochrome P450 mixed function oxidase system.[41,42] Since nonlinear accumulation of orally administered propranolol should (according to the well-stirred model of hepatic drug metabolism)[44] result from reductions in intrinsic clearance, the most likely cause of the nonlinear accumulation is inhibition of hepatic enzyme activity with repeated dosing. This may partially account for the unexpectedly long time required to reach steady state relative to that which would have been predicted using the half-life of propranolol observed following single-dose studies.[6]

Because of wide patient variability in the parameters responsible for hepatic metabolism (e.g., liver blood flow, intrinsic clearance, genetic differences), propranolol serum concentrations may vary by four- to twenty-fold following oral doses.[4,34,45] This variability may be related to dose, patient characteristics, concomitant medications, and other factors. Walle et al. have suggested that less variability may be seen at higher doses, because enzymes responsible for propranolol elimination are more likely to be saturated.[46] In patients with hypertension and/or coronary artery disease, propranolol serum concentrations were linearly related to doses of 160 to 960 mg/day and increased in a nonlinear fashion at doses between 40 to 160 mg/day. There was a threefold difference in propranolol concentrations among patients taking 40 to 160 mg/day and only a 1.3-fold variation among patients taking 160 to 960 mg/day. The smaller degree of variability observed in this study relative to others may have been due to a more specific assay (gas chromatography-mass spectrometry) and controlled dosing conditions to prevent noncompliance. This suggests that propranolol pharmacokinetics may not be as variable as previously thought, and that the intrinsic response to beta-blockade may be more responsible for the wide difference in propranolol dose needed to achieve the appropriate therapeutic response (see pharmacodynamics below).[47-49]

The elimination half-life of propranolol at steady state ranges from three to six hours, with an average of approximately four hours.[6,14] As the dose increases, the half-life is likely to be longer due to saturation of metabolic enzymes. For example, Thadani and Parker found that the half-life of propranolol was 3.5 hours at doses of 160 mg/day and 6.4 hours at doses of 320 mg/day.[4] Walle et al. have noted that when propranolol is discontinued at steady state, there is a terminal propranolol elimination half-life of 16 to 24 hours, which is presumably due to prolonged elimination of propranolol glucuronide and deconjugation to propranolol.[50] The pharmacodynamic half-life of propranolol is considerably longer than the elimination half-life, indicating a nonlinear relationship between effect and serum concentrations.[20] This explains why once- or twice-a-day dosing of regular-release propranolol formulations is effective in patients with either hypertension or angina.[4,51-53] The longer pharmacodynamic half-life also may reflect prolonged elimination of propranolol from target organs.[54]

Propranolol is extensively metabolized in the liver to at least 22 metabolites. Walle et al.[55] have accounted for essentially all of an administered dose of propranolol, resulting in the proposed metabolic scheme shown in Figure 24-3. The three major metabolic routes are ring oxidation (4-hydroxypropranolol and its glucuronide/sulfate conjugates), side chain oxidation (naphthoxylactic acid, propranolol glycol and its glucuronide, desisopropylpropranolol and its glucuronide), and glucuronidation of propranolol itself. The products of these pathways and their percent recovery in urine are shown in Table 24-3.[56] At least four of these metabolites have pharmacologic activity[57,58] and may provide some contribution, albeit small, to the overall pharmacologic response to propranolol.[59,60]

The most widely researched metabolite is 4-hydroxypropranolol. The amount of 4-hydroxypropranolol produced is proportional to the dose of the parent drug, although the serum concentration ratio of 4-hydroxypropranolol to propranolol decreases from 1.07 at daily doses of 40 mg to 0.09 at doses of 640 mg due to nonlinear increases in serum propranolol concentrations.[12] The 4-hydroxypropranolol metabolite is produced by naphthalene ring oxidation by a high-affinity, low-capacity system, which is subject to polymorphic expression in most white populations (see below and Chapter 7: Genetic Polymorphisms of Drug Metabolism). It was originally thought that 4-hydroxypropranolol was produced only after oral administration;[2] however, Walle et al.[12] have demonstrated its production following single intravenous doses. The concentrations of 4-hydroxypropranolol

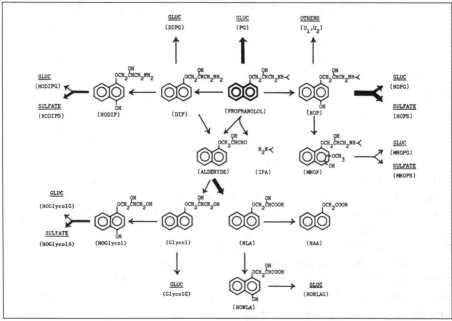

Figure 24-3. *Propranolol Metabolism in Man. HOP = Hydroxypropranolol; DIP = N-desisopropylpropranolol; glycol = propranolol glycol; NLA = χ-maphthoxyacetic acid; HODIP = ring-hydroxylated N-desisopropylpropranolol; HO-glycol = ring-hydroxylated propranolol glycol; HONLA = ring-hydroxylated χ-maphthoxylactic acid; MHOP = methoxyhydroxypropranolol; IPA = isopropylamine; G = glucuronide conjugate; S = sulfate conjugate. Reprinted with permission from reference 55.*

Table 24-3. *Stereochemical Composition of Propranolol Metabolites in Urine*[56]

Metabolite[a]	(−)/(+)-enantiomer ratio[b]		Metabolites in urine (%)[c]		
	Mean ± s.e. mean	Range	(±)-racemate[d]	(+)-enantiomer	(−)-enantiomer
Unchanged propranolol	1.50 ± 0.10[e]	1.35–1.81 (1.41)	0.4	0.16	0.24
Propranolol glucuronide	1.76 ± 0.10[e]	1.63–2.04 (1.65)	15.0	5.4	9.6
Side-chain oxidation					
NLA	1.45 ± 0.10[e]	1.31–1.60 (1.47)	19.4	7.9	11.5
GI	1.56 ± 0.13[e]	1.16–2.00 (1.64)	0.4	0.16	0.24
GIG	5.84 ± 0.33[e]	5.02–7.24 (5.41)	1.4	0.2	1.2
DIPG	3.81 ± 0.65[e]	2.24–5.81 (3.40)	1.0	0.2	0.8
Sum			22.2	8.5	13.7
Ring oxidation					
HOP	1.04 ± 0.17	0.47–1.48 (0.87)	1.0	0.5	0.5
HOPG	1.78 ± 0.19[e]	1.56–2.35 (1.56)	10.9	3.9	7.0
HOPS	0.27 ± 0.03[e]	0.21–0.35 (0.30)	19.2	15.1	4.1
Sum			31.1	19.5	11.6
Total metabolites			68.7	33.5	35.2

[a] GI = Propranolol glycol; other abbreviations are defined in Figure 24-3.
[b] Numbers within parentheses from subject given reverse-labeled pseudoracemates.
[c] Expressed as percent of total recovery of propranolol and metabolites in the 0–24 hr urine.
[d] Mean values from [4'-^{3}H] propranolol in similar subjects.
[e] Significantly different from unity; $p < 0.01$ (Student's t-test).

were lower following intravenous doses compared to oral doses that produced similar propranolol serum concentrations, suggesting significant presystemic formation of this and other propranolol metabolites. At the time of peak propranolol serum concentrations (0.5 to 1.5 hours post-dose), the concentration ratio of 4-hydroxypropranolol:propranolol approaches unity, but declines thereafter due to the shorter elimination half-life of 4-hydroxypropranolol compared to propranolol.[2,12,61] The main route of 4-hydroxypropranolol elimination is through O-glucuronidation. Following chronic oral dosing, 4-hydroxypropranolol concentrations do not accumulate; in contrast, propranolol-O-glucuronide concentrations do accumulate in an exponential fashion and exceed propranolol concentrations in the serum (see Figure 24-4).[12] Propranolol-O-glucuronide is subsequently eliminated by urinary excretion; it has a renal clearance (CL_R) of approximately 40 mL/min and a serum elimination half-life of approximately three hours.[2,12]

The beta-blocking potency of 4-hydroxypropranolol is similar to that of the parent compound;[60] however, it most likely does not significantly contribute to the overall pharmacologic response of propranolol, particularly during chronic oral dosing.[62] Lalonde et al.[5] have shown that the ratios for 4-hydroxypropranolol to propranolol AUCs were 0.074 after single doses of the regular-release dosage form and 0.037 at steady state. Thus, it is unlikely that 4-hydroxypropranolol contributes substantially to the beta-blocking effect at steady state. The concentrations of 4-hydroxypropranolol were essentially undetectable following sustained-release propranolol administration. In summary, it is doubtful that 4-hydroxypropranolol contributes much to the overall pharmacodynamic response to propranolol, since 1) serum concentrations are small compared to propranolol; 2) there is no hyster-

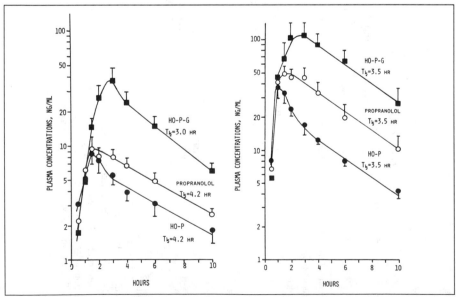

Figure 24-4. *Plasma concentration-time curves for propranolol, 4-hydroxypropranolol (HO-P) and 4-hydroxypropranolol glucuronide (HO-P-G) following a single 20 mg oral dose (panel A) and an 80 mg single oral dose (panel B) of propranolol to six normal subjects. The levels are expressed as mean ± SEM (reprinted with permission from reference 12).*

esis in time-connected propranolol concentration-effect curves; and 3) the E_{max} model adequately describes the pharmacodynamic relationship between propranolol serum concentrations and a reduction in exercise heart rate without considering 4-hydroxypropranolol concentrations.[20] (See Chapter 4: Pharmacodynamics for explanation of the E_{max} model.)

Following oral administration, serum concentrations of l-propranolol exceed those of d-propranolol by 40% to 90%, because there is a stereospecific preference for hepatic clearance of the d-enantiomer.[63–65] This difference reflects a lower intrinsic hepatic clearance for l-propranolol as supported by *in vitro* data,[66] and may also be due to higher plasma protein binding of the levo form (see Propranolol: Distribution). The half-life of each enantiomer in man is similar, suggesting there is no significant difference in flow-dependent systemic clearance.[22] Different results are seen when the enantiomers are administered separately; d-propranolol in this case has a shorter half-life than l-propranolol.[67] However, when coadministered in a racemic formulation, l-propranolol reduces hepatic blood flow and therefore the systemic clearance of d-propranolol.

As shown in Figure 24-5, most of the stereoselective metabolism of d-propranolol is due to ring oxidation, leading to greater bioavailability of the more active l-enantiomer.[56] L-propranolol subsequently undergoes preferential metabolism by side-chain oxidation and glucuronidation. Thus, most of the enantiomeric selectivity in propranolol metabolism appears to result from differences in the catalytic activity of the P450 isozymes involved in ring oxidation. These data are of clinical importance and help explain why similar total (d + l) concentrations of propranolol were more than two to three times more potent after oral versus intravenous administration.[59]

Elimination. Because propranolol is so extensively metabolized in the liver, very little is excreted unchanged in the urine. Urinary recovery of unchanged drug is less than 1% of the administered dose.[46] Walle et al.[55] have accounted for most

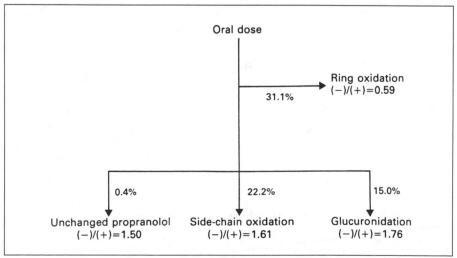

Figure 24-5. *Stereoselective metabolism of propranolol through the primary metabolic pathways (reprinted with permission from reference 56).*

of the by-products of propranolol metabolism through urinary recovery of metabolites. Approximately 90% of a radioactive dose of propranolol can be recovered in the urine, 83% within 24 hours. Of the radioactivity excreted in urine, recovery is primarily as propranolol glucuronide (17%), naphthoxylactic acid (21%), 4-hydroxypropranolol sulfate (22%), and 4-hydroxypropranolol glucuronide (12%). Naphthoxylactic acid and propranolol glucuronide may exhibit capacity-limited renal elimination.[12,68] The accumulation of propranolol metabolites is directly related to dose and renal function, resulting in serum metabolite concentrations that are several times higher than those of the parent compound.[69,70] Propranolol glucuronide may accumulate in patients with renal dysfunction and serve as a pool for elevated propranolol serum concentrations, due to tissue or blood deconjugation.[50] 4-hydroxypropranolol concentrations are not elevated, since this metabolite is removed through conjugation mechanisms that are unimpaired in renal dysfunction.[69,70] Figure 24-6 shows the disposition of propranolol and four major metabolites in patients with renal failure. Altered pharmacokinetic parameters for propranolol in renal insufficiency are summarized in Table 24-4.[71] Some authors have observed increased bioavailability[72] resulting in propranolol serum concentrations[71] that are two to three times higher in patients with chronic renal failure compared to dialysis patients. However, the half-life of propranolol is not significantly changed in any degree of renal insufficiency.

These alterations in propranolol and metabolite kinetics in patients with renal insufficiency do not warrant dosage adjustments in this patient population. Al-

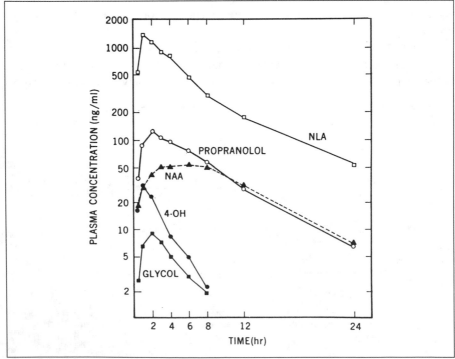

Figure 24-6. *Mean (n = 6) plasma propranolol levels and metabolites after 160 mg propranolol (reprinted with permission from reference 224).*

though concentrations of most metabolites are increased, they appear to contribute little to the pharmacologic and/or toxicologic effects. The kinetics of 4-hydroxy-propranolol are not altered in patients with declining renal function. However, reports of increased bioavailability suggest that patients who are not on dialysis should be started on lower doses initially and then titrated to the desired clinical response.

Acebutolol

Absorption. Acebutolol is a cardioselective beta blocker with partial agonist activity (PAA). The drug is rapidly absorbed after oral administration with peak plasma concentrations occurring within two hours for acebutolol and four hours for the metabolite, diacetolol.[73] The rate of absorption, peak concentration, and AUC of acebutolol are slightly decreased by food; however, the AUC of diacetolol is decreased significantly.[74] The absolute bioavailability of acebutolol is approximately 35% to 40%, which is greater than most other beta blockers.[75,76]

Distribution. Acebutolol has the lowest volume of distribution of all beta blockers. Following intravenous administration, the mean apparent volume of distribution at steady state (V_{ss}) is approximately 1.2 L/kg.[77] *In vitro*, acebutolol and diacetolol are approximately 11% to 19% and 6% to 9% protein bound, respectively.[78] Acebutolol is approximately 50% bound to erythrocytes.[79] The drug and its metabolite cross the placenta and significant amounts are distributed into milk.[80] Acebutolol also enters the cerebrospinal fluid, but concentrations are much lower than in plasma.[81]

Metabolism. Acebutolol is metabolized by hydrolysis to form acetolol, which is subsequently converted via N-acetylation to diacetolol. The extent of metabolism appears to be independent of the genetic acetylator phenotype of the patient.[82] Diacetolol is equipotent to acebutolol and has a similar pharmacokinetic profile.[83] Following single oral doses, there is a greater than proportional increase in AUC with increasing oral dose. There is also an increase in the steady-state AUC compared to single doses, indicating drug accumulation with multiple dosing.[75] The accumulation of the acetyl metabolite is even more pronounced than the parent compound; mean concentrations are 2.5 times greater after multiple dosing than after a single dose.[75] These effects may be attributed to a combination of saturation of hepatic uptake and metabolism, resulting in nonlinear metabolism at higher doses.

Table 24-4. *Pharmacokinetics of Propranolol in Various Degrees of Renal Function*[71]

	V_d (L/kg)	$t\frac{1}{2}$ (hr)	CL (L/min/m^2)
Healthy volunteers	3.3 = 0.2	3.1 = 0.3	42.1 ± 0.07
Chronic renal failure	3.0 = 0.4	3.8 = 0.09	28.3 ± 0.52
Dialysis	3.5 = 0.4	2.6 = 0.2	46.9 ± 0.30

[a] Mean ± SD.

Elimination. Acebutolol and its metabolites are excreted in urine and in the feces by biliary secretion.[84] Large biliary to plasma ratios suggest acebutolol is actively secreted into bile and may undergo significant enterohepatic circulation.[85] Plasma concentrations appear to decline in a biphasic manner with a mean distribution half-life of about three hours and a mean elimination half-life of 11 hours with a range of 6 to 12 hours.[73] In patients with various degrees of renal dysfunction, the pharmacokinetic disposition of acebutolol is not significantly different from that found in healthy volunteers.[86] However, there is considerable accumulation of diacetolol resulting in a several-fold increase in AUC and a doubling of elimination half-life in patients with creatinine clearances of less than 10 mL/min. Daily dose should be halved in patients with a creatinine clearance less than 30 mL/min and reduced by 75% if clearance is less than 10 mL/min.[86] It appears that the percentage of acebutolol eliminated by nonrenal clearance increases with decreasing renal function. The drug and its metabolite are removed by hemodialysis; however, nothing is known about its removal by peritoneal dialysis.[87]

The total clearance of acebutolol is decreased in geriatric patients resulting in twofold increases in drug concentrations. This may be a result of decreased renal function in the elderly or an increase in bioavailability. The apparent V_d is also decreased in geriatric patients.[88]

The pharmacokinetics of acebutolol and diacetolol were not significantly affected by liver disease following a single 400 mg dose.[89]

Atenolol and Nadolol

Absorption. Nadolol and atenolol are the most hydrophilic of the currently available beta blockers. Generally, the more hydrophilic compounds are less well absorbed than the lipophilic beta blockers. Approximately 50% of nadolol and atenolol are absorbed following oral administration.[90,91] Coadministration with food does not affect the rate or extent of absorption of either drug.

Distribution. As the lipid solubility of beta blockers decreases, there is a reduction in both the extent and rate of distribution. Atenolol is negligibly bound to plasma proteins,[29] while nadolol is over 20% bound.[90]

Metabolism and Elimination. Both atenolol and nadolol are primarily eliminated by urinary excretion. Hepatic metabolism contributes little or nothing to the overall clearance of either drug. Following oral or intravenous administration of nadolol, an average of 15% to 20% is recovered unchanged in urine and 70% to 85% in feces.[90,92] Biliary secretion has been shown to account for up to 41% of a dose.[93] Approximately 40% to 50% of an oral dose of atenolol is excreted unchanged in the urine, with the remainder eliminated in the feces. Biliary secretion of atenolol is significant, with the urine:bile ratio of parent drug and metabolites being 9:1.[94] Although nonrenal elimination of atenolol is small, metabolites are produced, including a hydroxylated metabolite and glucuronic acid conjugates.[94] Even though atenolol is hydroxylated, its metabolism is completely independent of debrisoquine polymorphism.[95]

As expected, both atenolol and nadolol accumulate in patients with renal impairment, and the total clearance of both drugs correlates well with creatinine clearance.[96,97] The elimination half-life of nadolol has been reported to exceed 50 hours in patients with creatinine clearances of less than 10 mL/min.[94] Nadolol is effectively removed from serum by hemodialysis with a mean half-life of 4.4 hours.[94]

The mean half-life of atenolol in patients with severe renal failure [glomerular filtration rate (GFR) <10 mL/min] ranges between 50 and 73 hours.[98,99] Flouvar et al.[99] studied atenolol removal in hemodialysis patients and found that the half-life declined from 73 hours to 7.5 hours during the procedure. McAnish et al.[97] have generated the nomogram shown in Table 24-5 to aid in dosing atenolol in patients with differing degrees of renal function.

Betaxolol

Absorption. Betaxolol is well absorbed from the gastrointestinal tract with peak concentrations occurring two to four hours following oral administration.[100,101] Coadministration of betaxolol with food does not alter the extent or rate of absorption of the drug.[102] Relative to other beta blockers, there appears to be less intersubject and intrasubject variability in betaxolol plasma levels. When compared to atenolol, intersubject variance was one-fourth as much with betaxolol, and intrasubject variability was one twenty-fifth that of atenolol.[103]

Distribution. Betaxolol is extensively distributed and has an apparent volume of distribution of 4.9 to 9.8 L/kg.[100,101] The drug distributes into the fetal circulation as well as into breast milk.[102] Betaxolol is approximately 55% bound to plasma proteins.[102]

Metabolism. Although betaxolol is lipid soluble, it does not undergo extensive first-pass metabolism like propranolol. The bioavailability of the drug is relatively high for beta blockers, ranging from 80% to 90%.[101,104] Betaxolol is metabolized primarily by O-dealkylation, followed by aliphatic hydroxylation. The major metabolites of betaxolol are not active, although one of the minor metabolites is believed to possess about 50% the activity of the parent drug.[105] There is no accumulation of betaxolol upon dosing to steady state, and concentrations increase proportionally with rising doses.[104] Unlike other hepatically metabolized beta blockers like propranolol, betaxolol clearance is not affected by concomitant cimetidine therapy.[106]

Elimination. After both oral and intravenous administration, the mean elimination half-life of betaxolol is 14 hours.[101] Approximately 12% to 16% of betaxolol is eliminated unchanged in the urine.[101,105] No significant change in total body clearance has been noted in patients with renal dysfunction; however, those on dialysis experienced a reduction in clearance of 31% to 42%.[107]

Table 24-5. Atenolol Nomogram

Recommended daily dosage	Creatinine clearance
100 mg	35–125 mL/min/1.73 m^2
50 mg	15–35 mL/min/1.73 m^2
25 mg	less than 15 mL/min/1.73 m^2

Esmolol

Absorption. Esmolol is the first beta blocker marketed with an extremely short half-life, making the drug useful only in an intravenous form for clinical situations requiring beta-blockade with rapid onset and virtually immediate offset of action should side effects occur. The main features of esmolol are cardioselectivity and an ultra short duration of action, with a relative potency of 0.02 compared to propranolol (propranolol = 1.0).

Distribution and Metabolism. Structurally, esmolol consists of main beta blocker nucleus onto which an ester is attached. This results in rapid hydrolysis by esterases found in red blood cell cytosol.[108] Because these esterases are not inhibited by cholinesterase inhibitors, no notable drug interactions with esmolol have been described. Hydrolysis results in the formation of clinically insignificant amounts of methanol and the acid metabolite, ASL-8123, which is devoid of beta-blocking activity.[109] In a study by Sum et al., intravenous infusions of esmolol of 400 µg/kg/min, resulted in an elimination half-life of about nine minutes and a total body clearance of 285 mL/min/kg, indicating extensive extrahepatic clearance.[108] The apparent volume of distribution was 3.4 L/kg. Approximately 82% of esmolol appears to be metabolized to the acid metabolite, which has an elimination half-life of 3.7 hours.[108]

Elimination. Although acid metabolite concentrations accumulate twofold in patients with renal dysfunction, overall esmolol pharmacokinetics are unaltered in patients with either renal or hepatic dysfunction; therefore, no dosage changes are necessary in these patient populations.[110,111]

Labetalol

Absorption. Labetalol is a nonselective β-adrenergic blocker and a selective α_1-adrenergic antagonist. Following oral administration, labetalol is rapidly and completely absorbed with peak concentrations occurring within one to two hours in the fasting state.[112–114] The presence of food delays absorption, and increases the absolute bioavailability of labetalol possibly by decreasing first-pass metabolism and/or affecting hepatic blood flow.[115,116]

Distribution. Following intravenous administration, labetalol is widely distributed into extravascular space and has a mean apparent volume of distribution at steady state of 9.4 L/kg.[117] Labetalol is approximately 50% bound to plasma proteins.[118] It crosses the placenta with small and variable amounts distributing into milk; however, no adverse effects have been noted in feeding infants.[119,120]

Metabolism. Following oral administration, labetalol is extensively metabolized by the liver and possibly in the GI mucosa.[116,118] There is considerable interindividual variability in the amount of an oral dose reaching the systemic circulation. Comparing oral to intravenous doses, McNeil et al. found that bioavailability ranged from 11% to 86% with a mean of 33%.[121] Similar results have been demonstrated by other groups.[117,122] Following multiple-dose oral administration, there is a linear increase in the steady-state AUC over a dosage range of 200 mg to 1200 mg daily.[123] Because labetalol accumulates with chronic dosing, acute administration does not predict steady-state concentrations.[124]

The plasma clearance of labetalol exceeds the rate of hepatic blood flow,[115] which may reflect some extra-hepatic clearance. Alternatively, since red blood cell concentrations of labetalol exceed those in plasma, plasma clearance may overestimate blood clearance.[125]

Oxidative metabolism may also be an important route of labetalol elimination.[126] Labetalol has been shown to decrease the clearance of antipyrine, suggesting that it may inhibit oxidative drug metabolism.[41] Enzyme induction by glutethimide has been shown to decrease systemic availability of labetalol by 43%, although there were no significant changes in heart rate or blood pressure.[127] Enzyme inhibition by cimetidine has resulted in large decreases in the oral clearance and increased systemic availability of labetalol, although no significant pharmacodynamic changes were observed.[126,127]

There are conflicting results on the effect of age on the pharmacokinetic disposition of labetalol. An early study demonstrated that the bioavailability of labetalol strongly correlated with age in a group of ten hypertensive patients.[113] Other investigators have not observed an effect of age on bioavailability, but have demonstrated a prolongation in the elimination half-life, greater peak concentrations, and reduced systemic clearance of labetalol in ten hypertensive patients with a mean age of 67 years.[112] Rocci et al. found no difference in these pharmacokinetic parameters between young and elderly hypertensive patients.[128]

In patients with impaired hepatic function, the apparent V_d of labetalol is decreased and bioavailability is twice that seen in normal age-matched controls.[129] The elimination half-life is not affected in this patient population.

Elimination. Within 24 hours, about 55% to 60% of a dose is excreted in urine primarily as glucuronide conjugates, with less than 5% excreted as unchanged drug. Fecal samples collected over four days contained less than 30% of the total dose.[118] The distribution and elimination kinetics of labetalol are similar in patients with severe renal failure (CL_{cr} <10 mL/min) and in normal controls, requiring no dosage modification.[130] Labetalol is not appreciably removed (less than 1% of dose) by hemodialysis or peritoneal dialysis.[131]

Metoprolol

Absorption. The pharmacokinetic profile of metoprolol strongly correlates with debrisoquine oxidative phenotype.[132,133] Following oral administration, absorption of metoprolol from the gastrointestinal tract is essentially complete.[134] However, like propranolol, the drug undergoes extensive first-pass metabolism before reaching the systemic circulation resulting in considerable intersubject variation in bioavailability.[7,135] Food increases the bioavailability of metoprolol but has no effect on the time to reach peak plasma concentrations.[7,136,137]

Distribution. Compared to propranolol, metoprolol is moderately lipophilic and much less protein bound, with only about 12% of the drug bound to plasma proteins.[138]

Metabolism. Metoprolol is extensively metabolized in the liver (see Figure 24-7), with approximately 85% of the administered dose recovered in urine as α-hydroxymetoprolol (10%), unchanged metoprolol (10%), and the amphoteric metabolite (65%).[95] These metabolites have substantially less beta-blocking activity than the parent compound and, therefore, make no important contribution to the pharmacodynamics of metoprolol.[134] The α-hydroxy pathway has been shown to closely cosegregate with that of debrisoquine 4-hydroxylation, such that poor metabolizers (PMs) of debrisoquine have higher urinary metoprolol:α-hydroxy-metoprolol ratios.[95] Since this pathway represents only 10% of the overall elimination of metoprolol, the PM phenotype alone cannot explain the large difference in pharmacokinetics seen between extensive metabolizers (EMs) and PMs. The amphoteric metabolite formation may also be reduced in PMs, suggesting some degree of cosegregation with this metabolic pathway and the PM debrisoquine phenotype.[139]

Evidence also supports an *in vivo* and *in vitro* stereoselective effect for the metabolism of metoprolol by the debrisoquine 4-hydroxylase isozyme.[95,140,141] In fact, stereoselective differences in EMs and PMs resulted in altered pharmacodynamics, with EMs having more pronounced beta-blockade at a given total metoprolol plasma concentration, which may be explained by relatively higher levels of the active l-enantiomer in EMs than PMs (l-isomer:d-isomer AUC ratios 1.4 in EMs and 0.9 in PMs).[141] These data suggest that the stereoselectivity of the oral clearance of metoprolol in EMs is virtually eliminated in PM subjects.

It has also been shown that PM subjects experience more intense and prolonged beta-blocking effects following administration of metoprolol.[132] PM:EM AUC

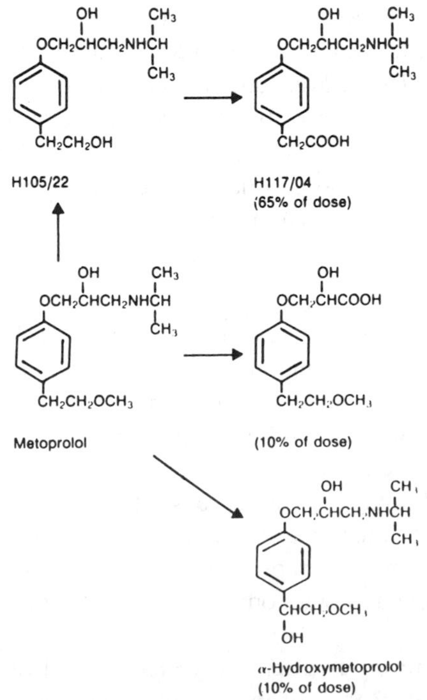

Figure 24-7. Metoprolol metabolism (reprinted with permission from reference 225).

ratios are approximately 5.8, with PMs also having a threefold increase in metoprolol elimination half-lives (7.6 hours versus 2.8 hours in EMs) and a threefold increase in peak serum concentration.

Elimination. Metoprolol is extensively metabolized in the liver with approximately 10% of an administered dose excreted unchanged in the urine. Therefore, there appears to be no need for dosage adjustment in patients with renal impairment.[142]

Penbutolol

Absorption. Penbutolol is commercially available as the pure active l-isomer. It is rapidly and almost completely absorbed (95%) after oral administration.[143] Absorption from the gastrointestinal tract is not dose-dependent and it appears that no first-pass effect occurs.[144] Although the presence of food delays peak plasma concentrations from one hour after administration in the fasting state to 2.25 hours, there is no effect on the extent of absorption.[145-147]

Distribution. Similar to propranolol, penbutolol is extensively bound to plasma proteins (90% to 95%) and is highly lipid soluble.[148,149] Volume of distribution estimates range from 32.4 to 42.5 L.[150]

Metabolism. Penbutolol is extensively metabolized by glucuronidation and hydroxylation.[143] Although evidence suggests that one or more of the metabolites may have pharmacologic activity, the identity of an active metabolite has not been established.[143,145] Penbutolol AUC varies linearly and in proportion to the dose administered.[144]

Elimination. Less than 4% to 6% of the parent drug is excreted unchanged in the urine in patients with normal renal function.[144,146] The mean elimination half-life of penbutolol is 18 to 27 hours in normal volunteers.[143,144,151] In patients with renal insufficiency, Bernard et al. observed no accumulation of penbutolol after 30 days of treatment.[143] However, the serum concentrations of the glucuronide metabolites increased slightly during this time.

Pindolol

Pindolol was the first beta blocker marketed in the United States to possess partial agonist activity. As such, it is necessary to separate the uniqueness of this particular pharmacologic property (with questionable clinical significance) from differences between the pharmacokinetics of pindolol and the prototype beta blocker propranolol.

Absorption. Pindolol is almost completely absorbed following oral administration, producing peak plasma concentrations in about two hours.[152] Compared to propranolol, pindolol has a relatively low hepatic extraction ratio of approximately 23%; therefore, pindolol does not exhibit dose-dependent bioavailability and does not accumulate upon chronic dosing to steady state.[153] Bioavailability is reduced from 86% to 52% in patients with uremia.[153] Plasma concentrations vary fourfold in subjects with normal renal function; however, this variability is similar following intravenous and oral administration, and therefore does not reflect variability in bioavailability.[154]

Distribution. Pindolol is more hydrophilic than propranolol, and thus possesses a more limited apparent volume of distribution. However, pindolol does cross the blood-brain barrier and can induce CNS side effects similar to propranolol.[155] The drug is approximately 40% to 60% bound to plasma albumin and AAG.[154]

Metabolism and Elimination. Pindolol is eliminated through a combination of hepatic metabolism and renal excretion. Serum half-life averages approximately two to four hours in patients with normal renal function and increases to about five hours in patients with significant renal impairment.[152–154,156] The identified metabolites are primarily glucuronide and sulfate conjugates and have no measurable beta-blocking activity.[157]

The presence of moderate-to-severe renal impairment reduces total body clearance by one-half (from 538 to 252 mL/min) and can be almost completely explained by a reduction in renal clearance.[156] The renal clearance of pindolol exceeds creatinine clearance in normal subjects, indicating possible tubular secretion.[153] However, this was not observed in patients with impaired renal function, where renal clearance was directly related to creatinine clearance.[155]

Timolol

Absorption. Timolol differs from most other commercially available beta blockers in that it is marketed as the active l-isomer rather than a racemic mixture. The drug is rapidly and nearly completely absorbed (90%) with peak plasma concentrations occurring one to two hours after oral administration.[158] The absorption and fate of timolol are not influenced by the presence of food.[159]

Distribution. Timolol is not extensively bound to plasma proteins (10%) and is less lipid soluble than propranolol.[160] Timolol is distributed into breast milk, but this is unlikely to be clinically significant.[161]

Metabolism. Timolol is extensively metabolized through the cytochrome P450 mixed function oxidase system, by hydrolytic cleavage of the morpholine ring and subsequent oxidation.[158,162] Else et al.[163] reported a minimal first-pass effect with a bioavailability of 75% when comparing oral and intravenous doses. Approximately 80% of an administered dose of timolol is cleared hepatically.[158,164]

Because timolol exhibits linear kinetics,[165,166] the AUC varies proportionally to the dose administered. Furthermore, there is no accumulation or alteration in the pharmacokinetic parameters that occurs with chronic administration.[165] The metabolism of timolol is under genetic control and has been shown to cosegregate with the 4-hydroxylation of debrisoquine.[167,168] Therefore, mean AUCs are two to four times higher in PMs than in EMs.

Elimination. Up to 20% of a timolol dose is excreted unchanged in the urine.[158,164] Two major metabolites account for 40% and minor metabolites account for approximately another 10% to 20% of the radioactivity collected in urine after 72 hours.[164] It is not known whether these metabolites possess pharmacologic activity.

The disposition of timolol is minimally affected by renal failure. There is no significant change in the half-life, C_{max}, or nonrenal clearance of timolol when administered to patients with varying degrees of renal insufficiency.[169]

There is no significant difference in the plasma clearance, half-life, or volume of distribution of intravenous timolol in patients with acute myocardial infarction versus healthy volunteers.[170]

POLYMORPHIC DRUG METABOLISM

Recent evidence strongly supports that most of the hepatically metabolized beta blockers are, to varying degrees, dependent on the debrisoquine 4-hydroxylase isozyme for removal from the body.[133,171] Polymorphic drug metabolism is extensively discussed in Chapter 7: Genetic Polymorphisms of Drug Metabolism. Generally speaking, the lipophilic beta blockers are more likely to exhibit clinically important differences in pharmacokinetics and pharmacodynamics between EMs and PMs of debrisoquine. In contrast, the hydrophilic beta blockers exhibit no such differences. In theory, beta blockers metabolized by debrisoquine hydroxylase should exhibit an increased oral bioavailability, prolonged elimination time, and an extended duration of action in patients with the PM phenotype. On the other hand, it is virtually impossible to prospectively identify a patient as being an EM or a PM. Furthermore, wide interpatient variability in pharmacokinetics[34,46] and β-receptor sensitivity[172,173] can obscure the identification of genetically-determined alterations in metabolism as the main determinant of pharmacodynamic response. Nevertheless, the clinical implications for PMs of beta blockers are an increased duration of action and, according to β-receptor theory, no alteration in magnitude of effect.[133,174,175]

Table 24-6 summarizes the significant pharmacokinetic differences in beta blockers whose metabolism cosegregates with that of debrisoquine. The largest pharmacokinetic differences are seen with metoprolol, whose metabolism to α-hydroxy is catalyzed by debrisoquine hydroxylase.[176,177] Although this metabolite only accounts for 10% of metoprolol metabolism in EMs, O-demethylation, accounting for approximately 65% of metoprolol metabolism, is at least partially catalyzed by debrisoquine hydroxylase. EMs of metoprolol preferentially O-demethylate the d-isomer of metoprolol, whereas the α-hydroxylation pathway is nonstereoselective. This is confirmed by *in vivo* evidence that EMs more rapidly

Table 24-6. *Phenotypic Differences in Pharmacokinetics between EMs and PMs of the Debrisoquine Pathway*[134]

Drug	Oral AUC ratio PM/EM	Peak plasma concentration ratio PM/EM	Elimination t½ (hr) PM	Elimination t½ (hr) EM
Metoprolol	6	3	2.8	7.6
Timolol	2–4	2	3.2	5.5
Propranolol	1	1	4.0	4.4
Atenolol	1	1	6.7	6.4

clear d-metoprolol.[178] Thus, at any given total (d + 1) serum concentration of metoprolol, EMs will have relatively higher concentrations of the active 1-isomer and more pronounced beta-blocking effects (see Figure 24-8). Stereoselective differences in polymorphic metabolism for metoprolol are shown in Figure 24-9.

Few pharmacokinetic or pharmacodynamic differences are observed in EMs and PMs of propranolol.[179,180] The production of 4-hydroxypropranolol depends on the debrisoquine hydroxylase pathway; however, because this is a relatively minor pathway for overall propranolol elimination, no change is seen in overall propranolol pharmacokinetics or beta-blocking response. Recent evidence suggests that metabolism of propranolol to naphthoxylactic acid is reduced by 55% in PMs of mephenytoin.[181] Again, propranolol oral clearance was not different between EMs and PMs of mephenytoin; however, propranolol oral clearance was reduced by approximately 50% (for both propranolol enantiomers) and half-life increased twofold in one subject who was a PM for both the debrisoquine and mephenytoin phenotypes.

PHARMACODYNAMICS

β-adrenergic blocking drugs exert their cardiovascular effects predominantly through competitive antagonism of β-receptors resulting in alterations in myocardial contractility and rate. Reduction of these parameters is the primary mechanism by which most beta blockers produce their therapeutic effects in conditions like

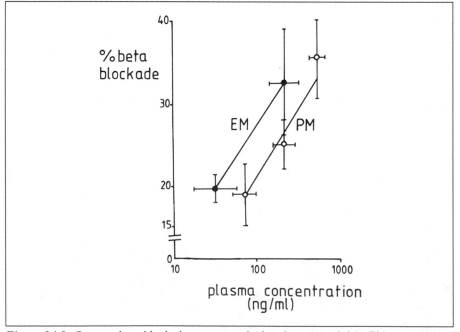

Figure 24-8. Percent beta-blockade versus total (d + 1) metoprolol in EMs and PMs of debrisoquine (reprinted with permission from reference 178).

angina and hypertension. Some beta blockers, however, combine other pharmacologic actions with β-receptor blockade (partial β-receptor agonism, α_1-receptor
antagonism) to produce their therapeutic effects.

The use of serum concentrations to predict physiologic response with beta
blockers began after early studies showed a poor correlation between the dose
administered and the measured therapeutic effect.[182-184] Much of the variability
between dose and response may result from the considerable interindividual differences in the pharmacokinetics of the beta blockers resulting in unpredictable
serum concentrations. The relationship between plasma concentration and β-receptor blockade is best understood by considering the concentration dependence
of binding to a saturable receptor site. Because the number of β-receptors is
limited, usual doses of beta blockers produce near maximal binding to β-receptors.
Therefore, further increases in plasma concentrations would not be expected to
produce greater effects.

The potency and pharmacodynamic response of beta blockers are assessed by
the relative degree of beta-blockade produced by a specific concentration of the
drug. Beta-blockade refers to the reduction in heart rate caused by β-adrenergic
antagonists after a controlled pharmacologic or physiologic stimulus. The chronotropic stimulus used in comparative investigations (i.e., exercise versus isoproterenol) must be noted, since these two methods do not always yield equivalent
results.

Another consideration in comparing the pharmacodynamics of beta blockers is
that a lower dose of isoproterenol is required to augment heart rate after administration of a selective versus a nonselective beta blocker. Because there is relative

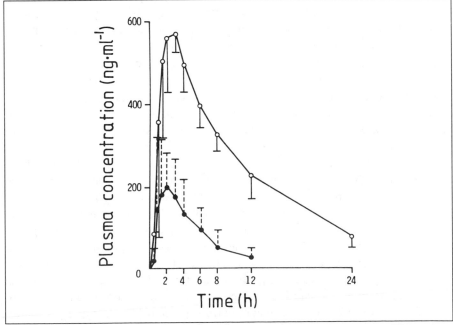

Figure 24-9. *Plasma metoprolol concentration versus time in EMs (●) and PMs (○). Reprinted
with permission from reference 132.*

sparing of peripheral β_2-receptors, cardioselective beta blockers may not block isoproterenol-induced vasodilation. Vasodilation will then contribute to an accelerated heart rate via autonomic reflex activity. This is one example of how specific differences in beta blocker pharmacology can affect pharmacodynamic relationships.

In the absence of heightened sympathetic tone, there is a poor correlation between beta blocker serum concentration and the reduction of resting heart rate.[45,185,186] This lack of correlation is not surprising since resting heart rate is predominately regulated by the parasympathetic system, whereas heart rate during exercise is almost exclusively under adrenergic control. Therefore, a good correlation exists between serum concentrations and reduction in augmented heart rates.[166,182,187–191] This correlation is maintained for beta blockers with partial agonist activity (PAA) even though these agents have little effect on resting heart rate.[191]

There is wide variation in beta blocker serum concentrations required to produce maximal beta-blockade. In studies with propranolol, Hager et al.[185] reported that subjects who demonstrated maximum reduction in heart rate required concentrations above 200 ng/mL, whereas Mullane et al.[192] found that concentrations greater than 80 ng/mL failed to further increase the percentage reduction in heart rates. Maximum inhibition of heart rate with timolol has been shown to occur at 30 ng/mL,[165] while Conway et al.[187] observed maximum beta-blockade with atenolol at 0.5 ng/mL. The concentrations associated with maximum beta-blockade may, therefore, vary with any drug in a given population. The reasons for this wide variation may relate to altered receptor sensitivity or density,[193,194] post-receptor changes,[195] and/or differential binding to the receptor.[196]

One attempt to explain some of the intersubject variability in response to beta-blockade has been to compare bound and unbound serum concentrations. McDevitt et al.[34] found no correlation between total propranolol concentrations and the dose of isoproterenol required to cause a specified increase in heart rate; however, free propranolol concentrations correlated to a statistically significant degree. However, Lalonde et al.,[20] using an exercise technique to produce tachycardia, showed similar model fits between total and unbound concentrations of propranolol within each subject, indicating that protein binding did not account for the intersubject variability in response.

All beta blockers demonstrate sustained hemodynamic effects beyond those predicted from the serum-concentration profile. As a result, the half-life of the measured effect often does not correlate with the elimination half-life of the drug. Several investigators have attempted to explain this phenomenon. Based on classical receptor theory, McDevitt and Shand[197] demonstrated that when response is measured by antagonism of isoproterenol using dose ratio -1, then plasma concentrations and efficacy decline in parallel. However, when the stimulus is exercise-induced tachycardia, the percent reduction in heart rate does not parallel drug concentrations; instead it is a function of the log plasma concentrations. Therefore, according to the log-linear pharmacodynamic model, drug concentrations decline exponentially with time (first order), while drug effects fall linearly with time (zero order), explaining why the drug's effects appear to last longer than the elimination half-life of the drug. One problem with the log-linear model is that biologic responses have a maximum and minimum effect such that increasing or decreasing concentrations no longer produce a linear relationship. Nonlinearity occurs below 20% and above 80% of the maximum effect. For this reason, Holford and Sheiner argue that the E_{max} model should be considered the basic pharmacodynamic model.[198] Using the E_{max} model, Lalonde et al.[20] have simulated the time course of pharmacologic effect (see Chapter 4: Pharmacodynamics, Figure 4-4). At concentrations well above the EC_{50}, inhibition of heart rate remains relatively constant with time as concentrations decline. At concentrations below 0.25 times the EC_{50}, effects decline in parallel with concentrations (first order), while between these two ranges, effects decline linearly with time (zero order).[20] Using pindolol as an example, Galeazzi et al.[199] have offered the explanation that the reason effects last longer than the apparent presence of drug in plasma may be a result of dissociation constants that are much smaller than the detection limit of the assays used to measure the drug.

Antihypertensive Effect

In contrast to the significant correlation between serum concentrations of beta blockers and their effect on augmented heart rate, a poor correlation exists between concentration and their hypotensive effects.[183,184,189,200,201] Some investigators, however, have shown a good association.[202]

The dose of beta blocker needed to produce a maximum blood pressure response is lower than the dose needed to produce a maximal reduction in heart rate.[200,201] This suggests that the drug's effects on blood pressure are not directly dependent upon its effects on heart rate. The blood pressure dose-response curve is relatively flat, with high and low doses producing similar hypotensive effects.

As with other effects of beta blockers, the antihypertensive effects persist well beyond the time serum concentrations are still measurable, suggesting that these drugs may be dosed less frequently than predicted on the basis of their elimination half-life.[52]

Antianginal Effect

The antianginal action of beta blockers is related to their ability to reduce two major determinants of myocardial oxygen demand: heart rate and contractility. However, whether they alter contractility to a significant extent is speculative since changes in this parameter are difficult to assess.

Several investigators have found a correlation between concentration and a reduction in anginal frequency or an increase in exercise tolerance.[190,203,204] Two independent groups have shown that the antianginal efficacy of propranolol begins at concentrations of 30 ng/mL.[186,204] Pine et al.[186] determined that the maximum therapeutic response with propranolol occurred between 64% and 98% of total beta-blockade, corresponding to serum concentrations ranging from 14 to 90 ng/mL. This study demonstrates that there is less variability when relating therapeutic response to the percent reduction in heart rate during maximal exercise, than when relating it to either dose or concentration.

As with other pharmacodynamic effects, duration of action is sustained longer than predicted from the elimination half-life.[4,203]

Antiarrhythmic Effects

The antiarrhythmic effects of the beta blockers are believed to be related to their antiadrenergic activity, since catecholamines are arrhythmogenic and the membrane-stabilizing effects of beta blockers are only seen at concentrations higher than those normally obtained clinically. The antiarrhythmic effect of beta blockers occurs over a wide range of serum concentrations. One group reported that 32 patients responded with 70% to 100% premature ventricular contraction (PVC) suppression at propranolol concentrations ranging between 12 and 1100 ng/mL.[205]

There does not appear to be a good correlation between serum concentrations and arrhythmia suppression.[206,207] However, Woosley et al. have noted that effective doses and concentrations of propranolol needed for arrhythmia suppression are much higher than those needed for beta-blockade.[205]

Because of the tremendous natural variation in ventricular ectopy, it is difficult to determine the duration of the antiarrhythmic effect over a short time period. No investigation has specifically addressed the question of how long beta blockers can suppress arrhythmias, although once-daily and twice-daily propranolol schedules have been effective.

Inotropic Effects

Correlation between the negative inotropic effect and beta blocker concentration has not been well studied. Using linear regression analysis, Morris et al.[208] compared medium-dose (160 mg/day) and high-dose (480 mg/day) propranolol therapy and found that changes in ejection fraction and wall motion score were not significantly correlated with serum concentrations. In contrast, Boudoulas et al.[209] showed that the negative inotropic effects of propranolol, measured echocardiographically, paralleled serum concentrations. Data from this study also demonstrated that plasma concentrations below 2.5 ng/mL produced no significant negative inotropic effect, and that the negative inotropic effect had a shorter duration than the negative chronotropic effect. Measuring aortic flow velocities, Clifton et al.[210] demonstrated a direct relationship between l-propranolol concentrations and reduction in systolic function during exercise using the E_{max} and sigmoid E_{max} models. By comparing EC_{50} values, this study demonstrated that propranolol has a more potent effect on heart rate than on systolic function. However, the maximum reduction in systolic function (E_{max}) from baseline was 47% which was significantly greater than the 30% reduction in heart rate. These results suggest that there is not a proportional reduction in heart rate and inotropic response with propranolol administration and that the presence of a reduction in heart rate does not necessarily imply that a negative inotropic effect is also achieved. Since the end point of therapy with beta blockers is often determined by titrating the dose to a specific heart rate response, this may be an important factor in treating disease states such as angina pectoris in which a negative chronotropic and inotropic response are desired.

Pharmacodynamics of Adverse Effects

Concentration-dependent adverse effects of the beta blockers are uncommon because of their wide therapeutic range. The value of beta blocker serum concentrations in predicting adverse events is limited because side effect profiles of the beta blockers are more patient specific than concentration dependent. Adverse effects are more common in disease states or conditions which are sensitive to reductions in sympathetic stimulation. For example, these drugs may exacerbate congestive heart failure at relatively small doses (low serum concentrations), because this population depends upon augmented sympathetic tone for the maintenance of cardiac output. In contrast, similar concentrations would not be expected to produce cardiac decompensation in a population with normal myocardial function.

Selectivity for the β_1-receptor is a concentration-dependent effect.[203] Therefore, cardioselective beta blockers are more likely to affect β_2-receptors at increased concentrations. This may become clinically important in the case of a drug like metoprolol administered to a poor metabolizer. These patients will have much higher concentrations than extensive metabolizers, thereby losing cardioselectivity and increasing the risk of bronchospasm in poor metabolizers.

Special Populations

There are many patient factors which may be important in evaluating the pharmacodynamic response to beta blockers. It is well established that β-adrenergic receptor affinity is reduced with advancing age.[193,212] The sensitivity of the β-receptor is decreased for both agonist and antagonists in the elderly, such that plasma concentrations of unbound propranolol required to produce a given shift in the isoproterenol dose response curve increase with age.[193,213] The heart rate response to labetalol has also been shown to be less sensitive in the elderly at a given plasma concentration.[111] However, Klein et al.[195] demonstrated that although the elderly were less sensitive to a β-agonist, their response to timolol was equal to that seen in a group of young subjects. They suggest that differences observed with propranolol may be due to age-related changes in stereoselective metabolism or protein binding, and that differences in β-receptor response are a result of post-receptor alterations occurring in the elderly. Attempting to account for stereoselective metabolism and protein binding, Tenero et al.[213] studied the β-adrenergic sensitivity and protein binding of l-propranolol (the active isomer) in a group of young and elderly volunteers. They concluded that the elderly have a greater apparent dissociation constant for unbound l-propranolol than younger subjects, indicating decreased β-receptor sensitivity.

Racial differences may also contribute to variability in response to beta blockers. A difference in the predicted E_{max} was observed in a study comparing the effects of metoprolol in a group of black and white subjects. At similar metoprolol concentrations, there was a rightward shift in the change in heart rate versus dose of isoproterenol curve among white subjects, suggesting increased β-receptor sensitivity in black subjects.[172] Measuring the reduction in heart rate and blood pressure during treadmill exercise testing, Zhou et al.[173] demonstrated that Chinese subjects had at least a twofold greater sensitivity to the beta-blocking effects of propranolol than did white subjects.

There is also evidence that smokers may not respond as well to beta blockers as nonsmokers.[214] This may be due to a decreased β-receptor density in cigarette smokers.[215]

CLINICAL APPLICATION OF PHARMACOKINETIC DATA

Serum concentrations of beta blockers are not routinely monitored for a variety of reasons. There is a broad range of serum concentrations which produce pharmacologic effect, resulting in a wide therapeutic index based on population estimates. Additionally, the large degree of interpatient variability in concentration-effect relationships makes it difficult to define a therapeutic range. Furthermore, serum concentrations do not necessarily predict all beta blocker responses. It has also been demonstrated that pharmacologic effects persist beyond those predicted by the serum concentration-time profiles.[216,217] In addition, the beta blockers have easily measurable responses (blood pressure and heart rate). Therefore, the advantages of obtaining serum concentrations over clinical assessment are not clearly evident.

Although routine monitoring of beta blocker serum concentrations has little clinical utility, an understanding of the pharmacokinetic and pharmacodynamic characteristics of these drugs is important in clinical pharmacology. As previously stated, the beta blockers are among the most extensively prescribed classes of drugs in this country. There is wide variability in their pharmacokinetic and pharmacologic properties. Additionally, appropriate pharmacokinetic studies and reliable data are vital to the drug development process and the use of generic products of these agents. Furthermore, numerous assays are available for measuring their serum concentrations, making them useful examples for models of stereoisomers, high-clearance drugs, exploring pharmacodynamic relationships, and for the examining processes such as polymorphic drug metabolism. For these reasons, this chapter has been included in this text as a basis for comprehension of the pharmacokinetic and pharmacodynamic attributes of the beta blockers.

ANALYTICAL METHODS

Numerous published assays abound for the quantification of the various beta blockers. The most common approach involves the use of high performance liquid chromatography (HPLC). Originally, achiral methods for measuring total concentrations of beta blockers in diverse biologic fluids were developed.

All beta blockers have at least one asymmetric carbon or chiral center in their side chain, and except for timolol and penbutolol, are used clinically as racemic mixtures. Diverse HPLC approaches have been used to resolve and quantify the isomers of beta blockers. The most common approach had been the conversion of isomers into diastereomers using an enantiomerically pure derivatizing agent followed by chromatography on an achiral HPLC system.[218] The determination of enantiomeric purity through the synthesis and separation of diastereomeric derivatives entails the danger of inaccurate results due to possible enantiomeric contamination of the derivatizing agent. The reagent may rapidly racemize during storage. An additional complication is that enantiomers may have quite different rates and/or equilibrium constants when they react with the derivatizing agent, resulting in the generation of diastereomeric products differing in proportion from the starting enantiomeric composition. These problems can be avoided by directly resolving the enantiomers using chiral chromatography.

The enantiomers of a number of beta blockers have been resolved using HPLC with chiral stationary phase (HPLC-CSP). With one based on (R)-N-(3,5-dinitrobenzoyl)phenylglycine, Wainer et al.[219] resolved propranolol. It was first converted to an oxazolidone derivative and then chromatographed using a hexane/2-propanol mobile phase. Metoprolol can be stereochemically resolved without derivatization on a cyclodextrin-based chiral stationary phase (CSP).[220] Many beta blockers have also resolved on a CSP based upon α_1-acid glycoprotein, as oxazolidone derivatives or underivatized.[221,222] Problems can be encountered with the CSP columns because they tend to be unstable and degrade quickly. In addition, they tend to be rather costly.

Recently, a new HPLC-CSP based upon cellulose-tris(3,5- dimethylphenyl-carbamate) coated on macroporous silica (OD-CSP) has been developed. The OD-CSP can resolve the underivatized enantiomers of a number of beta blockers with relatively high efficiency and short retention times. In addition, it tends to be more stable than previously developed HPLC-CSPs. However, it is higher in price.

PROSPECTUS

Since the introduction of propranolol over 20 years ago, β-adrenergic blockers have achieved an important role in treating a wide variety of cardiovascular and noncardiovascular disorders including hypertension, angina pectoris, migraine, and glaucoma. Continued refinement of this class of agents has resulted in a group of drugs which are selective antagonists for β_1-receptors, have partial β-agonist activity, and others which combine antagonist effects on both β- and α-receptors. Presently, there are over ten beta blockers available on the United States market and several others on the world market or under clinical investigation.

One important observation regarding beta blockers is the large degree of intersubject variability in their pharmacokinetics and pharmacodynamics. Some of the recently explored explanations for this variability include stereoselective metabolism and protein binding, genetic polymorphic metabolism, and receptor sensitivity.

Until recently, the relationship between concentration and response of beta blockers was evaluated using total concentrations of active and inactive isomers. It is clear that the more lipophilic beta blockers like propranolol exhibit stereoselective oral clearance such that certain individuals preferentially metabolize the inactive d-isomer to a greater extent than the active l-isomer. Monitoring only total concentrations will not indicate the ratio of active to inactive isomers, making it difficult to correlate concentration and effect. Some of the variability in response to beta blockers may be minimized by the use of easier-to-perform and more reliable assays for separating stereoisomers. Another mechanism to potentially minimize variability in response is to evaluate concentration-response relationships for beta blockers which are available as the active l-isomer (e.g., timolol) or to use beta blockers which are less lipophilic and not subject to hepatic metabolism.

Clinically, beta blockers have been used primarily for the management of hypertension and angina pectoris. Monitoring drug concentrations has been unnecessary for these two disease states because the measurement of blood pressure and heart rate are very good endpoints of therapy. More recently, the use of beta blockers in the management of congestive heart failure has received attention in the clinical literature. Although the mechanism is unknown, several possibilities have been proposed. The beneficial effects of beta blockers may be related to up-regulation of β-receptors and increased receptor density, protection against the cardiotoxic effects of catecholamines, or through antiarrhythmic mechanisms. Although most of the research in this area has been done with metoprolol, the most appropriate drug is unknown. What is even more unclear is the starting dose and how the dose should be titrated. With new evidence supporting the hypothesis that the negative chronotropic and inotropic effects of the beta blockers occur at different concentrations, simply monitoring heart rate in heart failure patients may not be the most appropriate method of dose titration. If better relationships between l-isomer concentrations and inotropic effects can be established for beta blockers, it may become important to monitor drug concentrations in this population of patients.

Another area of clinical research which may support the use of serum concentrations for monitoring beta blocker therapy is in post-myocardial infarction and the prevention of sudden cardiac death. Presently, beta blockers are one of the most effective adjunctive therapies for reducing mortality and reinfarction. Recent data have presented an unfavorable view for the use of antiarrhythmic drugs in this group of patients which may expand the clinical use of beta blocker therapy. Presently, both acebutolol and propranolol have approved indications as antiarrhythmic agents. Since neither drug has a clearly defined therapeutic range, doses are chosen based on adverse effects and heart rate response. The use of more appropriate pharmacodynamic models may result in defining a better therapeutic range for these drugs based on active isomer concentrations.

Future research efforts need to continue to focus on stereoselective and genetic differences in beta blockers, as well as examine active isomer concentration-response relationships in areas beyond the effects on beta-blockade. Better correlations of concentration and effect may be achieved through the use of more appropriate pharmacodynamic models.

REFERENCES

1. Barrett AM, Cullum VA. The biological properties of the optical isomers of propranolol and their effects on cardiac arrhythmias. Br J Pharmacol. 1968;34:43–55.
2. Paterson JW et al. The pharmacodynamics and metabolism of propranolol in man. Pharmacol Clin. 1970;2:127–33.

3. Shand DG, Rangno RE. The disposition of propranolol. I: Elimination during oral absorption in man. Pharmacology 1972;7:159–68.

4. Thadani U, Parker JO. Propranolol in the treatment of angina pectoris: comparison of duration of action in acute and sustained oral therapy. Circulation 1979;59:571–79.

5. Lalonde RL et al. Propranolol pharmacokinetics and pharmacodynamics after single doses and at steady-state. Eur J Clin Pharmacol. 1987;315–18.

6. Wood AJJ et al. Direct measurement of propranolol bioavailability during accumulation to steady-state. Br J Clin Pharmacol Ther. 1978;6:345–50.

7. Melander A et al. Enhancement of the bioavailability of propranolol and metoprolol by food. Clin Pharmacol Ther. 1977;22:108–12.

8. McLean AJ et al. Reduction of first pass hepatic clearance of propranolol by food. Clin Pharmacol Ther. 1981;30:31–34.

9. McLean AJ et al. Interaction between oral propranolol and hydralazine. Clin Pharmacol Ther. 1980;27:726–32.

10. Walle T et al. Presystemic and systemic glucuronidation of propranolol. Clin Pharmacol Ther. 1979;26:167–72.

11. Walle T et al. Naphthoxylactic acid after single and long-term doses of propranolol. Clin Pharmacol Ther. 1979;26:548–54.

12. Walle T et al. 4-hydroxypropranolol and its glucuronide after single and long-term doses of propranolol. Clin Pharmacol Ther. 1980;27:22–31.

13. Evans GH, Shand DG. Disposition of propranolol: independent variation in steady-state circulating drug concentrations and half-life as a result of plasma drug binding in man. Clin Pharmacol Ther. 1973;14:494–500.

14. Kornhauser DM et al. Biological determinants of propranolol disposition in man. Clin Pharmacol Ther. 1978;23:165–74.

15. Wagner JG. Propranolol: pooled Michaelis-Menten parameters and the effect of input rate on bioavailability. Clin Pharmacol Ther. 1985;37:481–87.

16. Garg DC et al. Comparative pharmacokinetics and pharmacodynamics following single and multiple doses of conventional and long-acting propranolol. Clin Pharmacol Ther. 1984;35:242. Abstract.

17. Ohashi K et al. Clinical pharmacokinetics and pharmacologic actions of a long-acting formulation of propranolol. Arzneimittelforschung 1984;507–12.

18. Silber BM et al. Dose-dependent elimination of propranolol and its major metabolites in humans. J Pharm Sci. 1983;72:725–32.

19. Walle T et al. Partial metabolic clearances as determinants of the oral bioavailability of propranolol. Br J Clin Pharmacol. 1986;22:317–23.

20. Lalonde RL et al. Propranolol pharmacodynamic modeling using unbound and total concentrations in healthy volunteers. J Pharmacokinet Biopharm. 1987;15:569–82.

21. Jackman GP et al. No stereoselective first-pass hepatic extraction of propranolol. Clin Pharmacol Ther. 1981;30:291–96.

22. Lalonde RL et al. Nonlinear accumulation of propranolol enantiomers. Br J Clin Pharmacol. 1988;26:100–102.

23. Evans GH et al. The disposition of propranolol III. Decreased half-life and volume of distribution as a result of plasma protein binding in man, monkey, dog, and rat. J Pharmacol Exp Ther. 1973;186;114–22.

24. Bianchetti G et al. Kinetics of distribution of dl-propranolol in various organs and discrete brain areas of the rat. J Pharmacol Exp Ther. 1980;214:682–87.

25. Garvey HL, Ram N. Comparative antihypertensive effects and tissue distribution of beta-adrenergic blocking drugs. J Pharmacol Exp Ther. 1975;194:220–33.

26. Tocco DJ et al. Uptake of propranolol and timolol by rodent brain: relationship to central pharmacologic actions. J Cardiovasc Pharmacol. 1980;2:133–43.

27. Laverty R, Taylor KM. Propranolol uptake into the central nervous system and the effect on rat behavior and amine metabolism. J Pharm Pharmacol. 1968;20:605–609.

28. Salem SA, McDevitt DG. Central effects of beta-adrenoreceptor antagonists. Clin Pharmacol Ther. 1983;33:52–57.
29. Belpaire FM et al. Binding of beta-adrenoreceptor blocking drugs to human serum albumin and alpha-1-acid glycoprotein and human serum. Eur J Clin Pharmacol. 1982;22:253–56.
30. Piafsky KM, Borga O. Plasma protein binding of basic drugs II: importance of alpha-1-acid glycoprotein for interindividual variation. Clin Pharmacol Ther. 1977;22:545–49.
31. Piafsky KM et al. Increased plasma protein binding of propranolol and chlorpromazine mediated by disease induced elevations of plasma alpha-1-acid glycoprotein. N Engl J Med. 1978;299:1435–439.
32. Sager G et al. Variable binding of propranolol in human plasma. Biochem Pharmacol. 1979;28:905–11.
33. Straka RJ et al. Nonlinear accumulation of unbound propranolol after oral administration. J Pharm Sci. 1987;76:521–24.
34. McDevitt DG et al. Plasma binding and affinity of propranolol for a beta receptor in man. Clin Pharmacol Ther. 1976;20:152–57.
35. Routledge PA et al. Increased plasma propranolol binding in myocardial infarction. Br J Clin Pharmacol. 1980;9:438–40.
36. Routledge PA, Shand DG. Propranolol. In: Evans, Jusko, Schentag, eds. Applied Pharmacokinetics. Spokane, WA: Applied Therapeutics; 1980;465–85.
37. Walle UK et al. Stereoselective binding of propranolol to human plasma, alpha-1-acid glycoprotein, and albumin. Clin Pharmacol Ther. 1983;34:718–23.
38. Lalonde RL et al. Effects of age on the protein binding and disposition of propranolol stereoisomers. Clin Pharmacol Ther. 1990;47:447–55.
39. Sotaniemi EA et al. Plasma clearance of propranolol and sotalol and hepatic drug-metabolizing enzyme activity. Clin Pharmacol Ther. 1979;26:153–61.
40. Schneck DW, Pritchard JF. The inhibitory effect of propranolol pretreatment on its own metabolism in the rat. J Pharmacol Exp Ther. 1981;218:575–81.
41. Daneshmend TK, Roberts CJC. The short-term effects of propranolol, atenolol and labetalol on antipyrine kinetics in normal subjects. Br J Clin Pharmacol. 1982;13:817–20.
42. Bax NDS et al. Inhibition of antipyrine metabolism by beta-adrenoreceptor antagonists. Br J Clin Pharmacol. 1981;12:779–84.
43. Nies AS et al. The hemodynamic effects of beta adrenergic blockade on the flow-dependent hepatic clearance of propranolol. J Pharmacol Exp Ther. 1973;184:716–20.
44. Wilkinson GR, Shand DG. A physiologic approach to hepatic drug clearance. Clin Pharmacol Ther. 1975;18:377–90.
45. Vervloet E et al. Propranolol serum levels during twenty-four hours. Clin Pharmacol Ther. 1977;22:853–57.
46. Walle T et al. The predictable relationship between plasma levels and dose during chronic propranolol therapy. Clin Pharmacol Ther. 1978;24:668–77.
47. Nies AS, Shand DG. Clinical pharmacology of propranolol. Circulation 1975;52:6–15.
48. Prichard BNC, Gillam PMS. Treatment of hypertension with propranolol. Br Med J. 1969;1:7–16.
49. Zacharias FJ et al. Propranolol in hypertension: a study of long-term therapy, 1964–1970. Am Heart J. 1972;83:755–61.
50. Walle T et al. Propranolol glucuronide cumulation during long-term propranolol therapy: a proposed storage mechanism for propranolol. Clin Pharmacol Ther. 1979;26:686–95.
51. Leaman DM et al. Persistence of biologic activity after disappearance of propranolol from the serum. J Thorac Cardiovasc Surg. 1976;72:67–72.
52. Wilson M et al. The effect on blood pressure of beta-adrenoceptor blocking drugs administered once daily and their duration of action when therapy is ceased. Br J Clin Pharmacol. 1976;3:857–61.
53. Wilcox EG. Randomized study of six beta blockers and a thiazide diuretic in essential hypertension. Br Med J. 1978;2:383–85.
54. Plachetka JR et al. Persistent myocardial propranolol levels in man. Am J Cardiol. 1981;47:430. Abstract.

55. Walle T et al. Quantitative account of propranolol metabolism in urine of normal man. Drug Metab Dispos. 1985;13:204–209.
56. Walle T et al. Stereoselective ring oxidation of propranolol in man. Br J Clin Pharmacol. 1984;18:741–47.
57. Ishizaki T et al. Cardiovascular actions of a new metabolite of propranolol: isopropylamine. J Pharmacol Exp Ther. 1974;189:626–32.
58. Saelens DA et al. Studies on the contribution of active metabolites to the anticonvulsant effects of propranolol. Eur J Pharmacol. 1977;42:39–46.
59. Coltart DJ, Shand DG. Plasma propranolol levels in the quantitative assessment of beta-adrenergic blockade in man. Br Med J. 1970;3:731–34.
60. Fitzgerald JD, O'Donnell SR. Pharmacology of 4-hydroxypropranolol, a metabolite of propranolol. Br J Pharmacol. 1971;43:222–35.
61. Wong L et al. Plasma concentrations of propranolol and 4-hydroxypropranolol during chronic oral propranolol therapy. Br J Clin Pharmacol. 1979;24:3–12.
62. Cleaveland CR, Shand DG. Effect of route of administration on the relationship between beta-adrenergic blockade and plasma propranolol level. Clin Pharmacol Ther. 1972;13:181–85.
63. Olanoff LS et al. Food effects on propranolol systemic and oral clearance: support for a blood flow hypothesis. Clin Pharmacol Ther. 1986;40:408–14.
64. Walle T et al. Stereoselective delivery and actions of beta receptor antagonists. Biochem Pharmacol. 1988;37:115–24.
65. Silber B et al. Stereoselective disposition and glucuronidation of propranolol in humans. J Pharm Sci. 1982;71:699–703.
66. Von Bahr C et al. Oxidation of (R)- and (S)-propranolol in human and dog liver microsomes. Species differences in stereoselectivity. J Pharmacol Exp Ther. 1982;222:458–62.
67. George CF et al. Pharmacokinetics of dextro-, levo- and racemic propranolol in man. Eur J Clin Pharmacol. 1972;4:74–76.
68. Walle T et al. Steady-state plasma concentrations and urinary excretion of propranolol-o-glucuronide and propranolol in patients during chronic oral propranolol therapy. Fed Proc. 1976;35:665. Abstract.
69. Stone WJ, Walle T. Massive propranolol metabolite retention during maintenance hemodialysis. Clin Pharmacol Ther. 1980;28:449–55.
70. Schneck DW et al. Effect of dose and uremia on plasma and urine profiles of propranolol metabolites. Clin Pharmacol Ther. 1980;27:744–55.
71. Bianchetti G et al. Pharmacokinetics and effects of propranolol in terminal uraemic patients and in patients undergoing regular dialysis treatment. Clin Pharmacokinet. 1976;1:373–84.
72. Lowenthal DT et al. Pharmacokinetics of oral propranolol in chronic renal disease. Clin Pharmacol Ther. 1974;16:761–69.
73. Gulaid AA et al. The pharmacokinetics of acebutolol in man, following the oral administration of acebutolol HCl as a single (400 mg) and during and after repeated oral dosing (400 mg, b.d.) Biopharm Drug Dispos. 1981;2:103–14.
74. Zaman R et al. The effect of food and alcohol on the pharmacokinetics of acebutolol and its metabolite, diacetolol. Biopharm Drug Dispos. 1984;5:91–95.
75. Meffin PJ et al. Dose-dependent acebutolol after oral administration. Clin Pharmacol Ther. 1978;24:542–47.
76. Roux A et al. Systemic bioavailability of acebutolol in man. Biopharm Drug Dispos. 1983;4:293–97.
77. Meffin PJ et al. Acebutolol disposition after intravenous administration. Clin Pharmacol Ther. 1977;22:557–67.
78. Coombs TJ et al. Blood plasma binding of acebutolol and diacetolol in man. Br J Clin Pharmacol. 1980;9:395–97.
79. Roux A et al. Pharmacokinetics of acebutolol in patients with all grades of renal failure. Eur J Clin Pharmacol. 1980;17:339–48.
80. Bianchetti G et al. Placental transfer and pharmacokinetics of acebutolol and N-acetyl acebutolol in the newborn. Br J Pharmacol. 1981;72:135P–36P.

81. Zaman R et al. The penetration of acebutolol and its major metabolite, diacetolol, into human cerebrospinal fluid and saliva. Br J Clin Pharmacol. 1981;12:427–29.

82. Gulaid AA et al. Lack of correlation between acetylator status and the production of the acetyl metabolite of acebutolol in man. Br J Clin Pharmacol. 1978;5:261–62.

83. Basil B, Jordan R. Pharmacological properties of diacetolol (M&B 16,942), a major metabolite of acebutolol. Eur J Pharmacol. 1982;80:47–56.

84. Collins RF, George CF. Studies on the disposition and fate of [^{14}C]-acebutolol in man and dog. Br J Clin Pharmacol. 1976;3:346P.

85. Kaye CM, Oh VMS. The biliary excretion of acebutolol in man. J Pharm Pharmacol. 1976;28:449–50.

86. Kirch W et al. The influence of renal function on plasma levels and urinary excretion of acebutolol and its main N-acetyl metabolite. Clin Nephrol. 1982;18:88–94.

87. Smith RS et al. Acebutolol pharmacokinetics in renal failure. Br J Clin Pharmacol. 1983;16:253–58.

88. Roux A et al. A pharmacokinetic study of acebutolol in aged subjects as compared to young subjects. Gerontology 1983;29:202–208.

89. Zamen R et al. Lack of effect of liver disease on the pharmacokinetics of acebutolol and diacetolol: a single-dose study. Biopharm Drug Dispos. 1985;6:131–37.

90. Dreyfuss J et al. Pharmacokinetics of nadolol, a beta receptor antagonist: administration of therapeutic single and multiple-dosage regimens to hypertensive patients. J Clin Pharmacol. 1979;19:712–20.

91. Mason WD et al. Kinetics and absolute bioavailability of atenolol. Clin Pharmacol Ther. 1979:25;408–15.

92. Dreyfuss J et al. Metabolic studies in patients with nadolol: oral and intravenous administration. J Clin Pharmacol. 1977;17:300–307.

93. Dusouich P et al. Enhancement of nadolol elimination by activated charcoal and antibiotics. Clin Pharmacol Ther. 1983;33:585–90.

94. Reeves PR et al. Metabolism of atenolol in man. Xenobiotica 1978;8:313–20.

95. Lennard MS et al. The polymorphic oxidation of beta-adrenoceptor antagonists. Clin Pharmacokinet. 1986;11:1–17.

96. Herrera J et al. Elimination of nadolol by patients with renal impairment. Br J Clin Pharmacol. 1979;7:227S–31S.

97. McAnish J et al. Atenolol kinetics in renal failure. Clin Pharmacol Ther. 1980;28:302–309.

98. Kirch W et al. Single intravenous dose kinetics and accumulation of atenolol in patients with renal failure and on hemodialysis. Arch of Toxicol. 1980;4(Suppl.):366–69.

99. Flouvar B et al. Pharmacokinetics of atenolol in patients with terminal renal failure and influence of hemodialysis. Br J Clin Pharmacol. 1980;9:379–85.

100. Giudicelli J et al. Beta-adrenoceptor blocking effects and pharmacokinetics of betaxolol (SL 75212) in man. Br J Clin Pharmacol. 1980;10:41–49.

101. Warrington SJ et al. Blood concentrations and pharmacodynamic effect of SL 75212, a new beta adrenoceptor antagonist, after oral and intravenous administration. Br J Clin Pharmacol. 1980;10:449–52.

102. Beresford R, Heel RC. Betaxolol. Drugs 1986;31:6–28.

103. Kunka RL et al. Steady-state fluctuation and variability of betaxolol and atenolol blood levels. Ther Drug Monit. 1989;11:523–27.

104. Ludden TM et al. Absolute bioavailability and dose proportionality of betaxolol in normal healthy subjects. J Pharm Sci. 1988;77:779–83.

105. Ferrandes B et al. Pharmacokinetics and metabolism of betaxolol in various animal species and man. In Morselli PL et al, eds. L.E.R.S. Monograph Series. Vol. 1. New York: Raven Press; 1983;51–64.

106. Jammet P et al. Interaction between cimetidine and beta-blockers propranolol and betaxalol. J Pharmacol. 1984;15:549.

107. Morselli PL et al. Comparative pharmacokinetics of several beta-blockers in renal and hepatic insufficiency. In Morselli PL et al, eds. L.E.R.S. Monograph Series. Vol. 1. New York: Raven Press; 1983;233–41.

108. Sum CY et al. Kinetics of esmolol, an ultra-short-acting beta-blocker, and of its major metabolite. Clin Pharmacol Ther. 1983;34:427–34.
109. Gorczynski RJ. Basic pharmacology of esmolol. Am J Cardiol. 1985;56:3F–13F.
110. Flaherty JF et al. Pharmacokinetics of esmolol and ASL-8123 in renal failure. Clin Pharmacol Ther. 1989;45:321–27.
111. Buchi KN et al. Pharmacokinetics of esmolol in hepatic disease. J Clin Pharmacol. 1987;27:880–84.
112. Abernethy DR et al. Comparison in young and elderly patients of pharmacodynamics and disposition of labetalol in systemic hypertension. Am J Cardiol. 1987;60:697–702.
113. Kelly JG et al. Bioavailability of labetalol increases with age. Br J Clin Pharmacol. 1982;14:304–305.
114. Maronde RF et al. Study of single and multiple dose pharmacokinetic/pharmacodynamic modeling of the antihypertensive effects of labetalol. Am J Med. 1983;75:40–46.
115. Daneshmend TK, Roberts CJC. The influence of food on oral and intravenous pharmacokinetics of a high clearance drug: a study with labetalol. Br J Clin Pharmacol. 1982;14:73–78.
116. Mantyla R et al. Effect of food on the bioavailability of labetalol. Br J Clin Pharmacol. 1980;9:435–37.
117. Kanto J et al. Pharmacokinetics of labetalol in healthy volunteers. Int J Clin Pharmacol Ther Toxicol. 1981;19:41–44.
118. Martin LE et al. Metabolism of labetalol by animals and man. Br J Clin Pharmacol. 1976;3(Suppl.3):695–710.
119. Lunell NO et al. Transfer of labetalol into amniotic fluid and breast milk in lactating women. Eur J Clin Pharmacol. 1985;28:597–99.
120. Michael CA. Use of labetalol in the treatment of severe hypertension during pregnancy. Br J Clin Pharmacol. 1979;8(Suppl.2):211S–15S.
121. McNeil JJ et al. Pharmacokinetics and pharmacodynamic studies of labetalol in hypertensive subjects. Br J Clin Pharmacol. 1979;8:157S–61S.
122. Awni WM et al. Interindividual and intraindividual variability in labetalol pharmacokinetics. J Clin Pharmacol 1988,28:344–49.
123. Chung M et al. Rising multiple-dose pharmacokinetics of labetalol in hypertensive patients. J Clin Pharmacol. 1986;26:248–52.
124. McNeil JJ et al. Labetalol steady-state pharmacokinetics in hypertensive patients. Br J Clin Pharmacol. 1982;13(Suppl.1):75S–80S.
125. Lalonde RL et al. Labetalol pharmacokinetics and pharmacodynamics: evidence of stereoselective disposition. Clin Pharmacol Ther. 1990;48:509–19.
126. O'Rear TL et al. Effects of enzyme inhibition on labetalol pharmacokinetics and pharmacodynamics. Clin Pharmacol Ther. 1990;47:172.
127. Daneshmend TK, Roberts CJC. The effects of enzyme induction and enzyme inhibition on labetalol pharmacokinetics. Br J Clin Pharmacol. 1984;18:393–400.
128. Rocci ML et al. Pharmacokinetics and pharmacodynamics of labetalol in elderly and young hypertensive patients following single and multiple doses. Pharmacotherapy 1990;10:92–99.
129. Homeida M et al. Decreased first-pass metabolism of labetalol in chronic liver disease. Br Med J. 1978;2:1048–1050.
130. Wood AJ et al. Elimination kinetics of labetalol in severe renal failure. Br J Clin Pharmacol. 1982;13(Suppl.1):81S–86S.
131. Halstenson CE et al. The disposition and dynamics of labetalol in patients on dialysis. Clin Pharmacol Ther. 1986;40:462–68.
132. Lennard MS et al. Oxidative phenotype—a major determinant of metoprolol metabolism and response. N Engl J Med. 1982;307:1558–560.
133. Dayer P et al. Interindividual variation of beta-adrenoceptor blocking drugs, plasma concentration and effect: influence of genetic status on behavior of atenolol, bopindolol, and metoprolol. Eur J Clin Pharmacol. 1985;28:149–53.
134. Borg KO et al. Metabolism of metoprolol-(^{3}H) in man, the dog, and the rat. Acta Pharmacol Toxicol. 1975;36(Suppl.5):125–35.
135. Johnsson G et al. Combined pharmacokinetic and pharmacodynamic studies in man of the adrenergic β_1-receptor antagonist metoprolol. Acta Pharmacol Toxicol. 1975;36(Suppl.5):31–44.

136. Lundborg P, Steen B. Plasma levels and effect on heart rate and blood pressure of metoprolol after acute administration in 12 geriatric patients. Acta Med Scand. 1976;200:397–402.

137. Kendall MJ et al. Plasma metoprolol concentrations in young, old, and hypertensive subjects. Br J Clin Pharmacol. 1977;4:497–99.

138. Johnsson G, Regardh C-G. Clinical pharmacokinetics of β-adrenoreceptor blocking drugs. Clin Pharmacokinet. 1976;1:233–63.

139. McGourty JC et al. Metoprolol metabolism and debrisoquine oxidation polymorphism-population and family studies. Br J Clin Pharmacol. 1985;20:555–66.

140. Meyer UA et al. The molecular mechanisms of two common polymorphisms of drug oxidation—evidence for functional changes in cytochrome P450 isozymes catalyzing bufurolol and mephenytoin oxidation. Xenobiotica 1986;16:449–64.

141. Lennard MS et al. Differential stereoselective metabolism of metoprolol in extensive and poor debrisoquine metabolizers. Clin Pharmacol Ther. 1983;34:732–37.

142. Jordo L et al. Pharmacokinetic and pharmacodynamic properties of metoprolol in patients with impaired renal function. Clin Pharmacokinet. 1980;5:169–80.

143. Bernard N et al. Pharmacokinetics of penbutolol and its metabolites in renal insufficiency. Eur J Clin Pharmacol. 1985;29:215–19.

144. Jun HW et al. Plasma level profiles and clinical response of penbutolol after three different single oral doses in man. J Clin Pharmacol. 1979;19:415–23.

145. Giudicelli JF et al. Comparative β-adrenoceptor blocking effects and pharmacokinetics of penbutolol and propranolol in man. Br J Clin Pharmacol. 1977;4:135–40.

146. Vallner JJ et al. Plasma levels studies of penbutolol after oral dose in man. J Clin Pharmacol. 1977;17:231–36.

147. Sharma SD et al. Effect of food on the bioavailability of penbutolol. Curr Ther Res. 1980;27:576–83.

148. Gottschalk R, Sistovaris N. Protein binding studies of furosemide and penbutolol. Arzneimittelforschung 1985;35:899–902.

149. Hajdu P, Damm D. Physicochemical and analytical studies of penbutolol. Arzneimittelforschung 1979;29:602–606.

150. Vedin JA, et al. Pharmacodynamic and pharmacokinetic study of oral and intravenous penbutolol. Eur J Clin Pharmacol. 1983;25:529–34.

151. Spahn H et al. Penbutolol pharmacokinetics: the influence of concomitant administration of cimetidine. Eur J Clin Pharmacol. 1986;29:555–60.

152. Gugler R, Bodem G. Single- and multiple-dose pharmacokinetics of pindolol. Eur J Clin Pharmacol. 1978;13:13–16.

153. Lavene D et al. Pharmacokinetics and hepatic extraction ratio of pindolol in hypertensive patients with normal and impaired renal function. J Clin Pharmacol. 1977;17:501–508.

154. Gugler R et al. Pharmacokinetics of pindolol in man. Eur J Clin Pharmacol. 1974;7:17–24.

155. Taylor EA et al. Cerebrospinal fluid concentrations of propranolol, pindolol and atenolol in man: evidence for central actions of beta-adrenoceptor antagonists. Br J Clin Pharmacol. 1981;12:549–59.

156. Chau NP et al. Pindolol availability in hypertensive patients with normal and impaired renal function. Clin Pharmacol Ther. 1977;22:505–10.

157. Ohnhaus EE et al. Pharmacokinetics of unlabelled and ^{14}C-labelled pindolol in uraemia. Eur J Clin Pharmacol. 1974;7:25–29.

158. Tocco DJ et al. Physiological disposition and metabolism of timolol in man and laboratory animals. Drug Metab Dispos. 1975;3:361–70.

159. Mantyla R et al. Pharmacokinetic interactions of timolol with vasodilating drugs, food and phenobarbitone in healthy human volunteers. Eur J Clin Pharmacol. 1983;24:227–30.

160. Baer JE, Stone CA. Physiological disposition and metabolism of MK-950. Report for the Merck Institute for Therapeutic Research. 1974;S-1.

161. Fidler J et al. Excretion of oxprenolol and timolol in breast milk. Br J Obstet Gynecol. 1983;90:961–65.

162. Tocco DJ et al. Timolol metabolism in man and laboratory animals. Drug Metab Dispos. 1980;8:236–40.
163. Else OF et al. Plasma timolol levels after oral and intravenous administration. Eur J Clin Pharmacol. 1978;14:431–34.
164. Tocco DJ et al. Electron-capture GLC determination of timolol in human plasma and urine. J Pharm Sci. 1975;64:1879–881.
165. Bobik A et al. Timolol pharmacokinetics and effects on heart rate and blood pressure after acute and chronic administration. Eur J Clin Pharmacol. 1979;16:243–49.
166. Singh BN et al. Plasma timolol levels and systolic time intervals. Clin Pharmacol Ther. 1980;28;159–66.
167. Lewis RV et al. Timolol and atenolol: relationship between oxidation phenotype, pharmacokinetics and pharmacodynamics. Br J Clin Pharmacol. 1985;19:329–33.
168. Lennard MS et al. Timolol metabolism and debrisoquine oxidation polymorphism: a population study. Br J Clin Pharmacol. 1989;27:429–34.
169. Lowenthal DT et al. Timolol kinetics in chronic renal insufficiency. Clin Pharmacol Ther. 1978;23:606–15.
170. Vedin JA et al. Pharmacokinetics of intravenous timolol in patients with acute myocardial infarction and in healthy volunteers. Eur Clin Pharmacol. 1982;23:43–47.
171. Smith RL. Polymorphic metabolism of the beta-adrenoreceptor blocking drugs and its clinical relevance. Eur J Clin Pharmacol. 1985;28(Suppl.):77–84.
172. Rutledge DR et al. Racial differences in drug response: isoproterenol effects on heart rate following intravenous metoprolol. Clin Pharmacol Ther. 1989;45:380–86.
173. Zhou HH et al. Altered sensitivity to and clearance of propranolol in men of Chinese descent as compared with American whites. N Engl J Med. 1989;320:565–70.
174. Schlanz KD et al. Metoprolol pharmacodynamics and quinidine-induced inhibition of polymorphic drug metabolism. Pharmacotherapy 1990;10:232. Abstract.
175. McGourty JC et al. Pharmacokinetics and beta-blocking effects of timolol in poor and extensive metabolizers of debrisoquine. Clin Pharmacol Ther. 1985;38:409–13.
176. Lennard MS et al. Metoprolol oxidation by rat liver microsomes. Inhibition by debrisoquine and other drugs. Biochem Pharmacol. 1986;35:2757–761.
177. Otton SV et al. Use of quinidine inhibition to define the role of the sparteine/debrisoquine cytochrome P450 in metoprolol oxidation by human liver microsomes. J Pharmacol Exp Ther. 1988;247:242–47.
178. Lennard MS et al. Differential stereoselective metabolism of metoprolol in extensive and poor debrisoquine metabolizers. Clin Pharmacol Ther. 1983;34:732–37.
179. Raghuram TC et al. Polymorphic ability to metabolize propranolol alters 4-hydroxypropranolol levels but not beta-blockade. Clin Pharmacol Ther. 1984;36:51–56.
180. Lennard MS et al. The relationship between debrisoquine oxidation phenotype and the pharmacokinetics and pharmacodynamics of propranolol. Br J Clin Pharmacol. 1984;17:679–85.
181. Ward SA et al. Propranolol's metabolism is determined by both mephenytoin and debrisoquin hydroxylase activities. Clin Pharmacol Ther. 1989;45:72–79.
182. Zacest R and Koch-Weser J. Relation of propranolol plasma level to beta-blockade during oral therapy. Pharmacology 1972;7:178–84.
183. von Bahr C et al. Plasma levels and effects of metoprolol on blood pressure, adrenergic beta-receptor blockade and plasma renin activity in essential hypertension. Clin Pharmacol Ther. 1976;20:130–37.
184. Lehtonen A et al. Plasma concentrations of propranolol in patients with essential hypertension. Eur J Clin Pharmacol. 1977;11:155–57.
185. Hager WD et al. Assessment of beta-blockade with propranolol. Clin Pharmacol Ther. 1981;30:283–90.
186. Pine M et al. Correlation of plasma propranolol concentration with therapeutic response in patients with angina pectoris. Circulation 1975;52:886–93.
187. Conway FJ et al. Human pharmacokinetic and pharmacodynamic studies on atenolol, a new cardioselective beta-adrenoreceptor blocking drug. Br J Clin Pharmacol. 1976;3:267–72.

188. Kendall MJ et al. Pharmacokinetic and pharmacodynamic studies of single oral doses of metoprolol in normal volunteers. Eur J Drug Metab Pharmacokinet. 1977;2:73–80.

189. Amery A et al. Relationship between blood level of atenolol and pharmacologic effect. Clin Pharmacol Ther. 1977;21:691–99.

190. Jackson G et al. Atenolol: once-daily cardioselective beta-blockade for angina pectoris. Circulation 1980;61:555–60.

191. Gugler R et al. The effect of pindolol on exercise-induced cardiac acceleration in relation to plasma levels in man. Clin Pharmacol Ther. 1975;17:127–33.

192. Mullane JF et al. Propranolol dosage, plasma concentration and beta-blockade. Clin Pharmacol Ther. 1982;32:692–700.

193. Vestal RE et al. Reduced B-adrenoreceptor sensitivity in the elderly. Clin Pharmacol Ther. 1979;26:181–86.

194. Zhou H et al. Interindividual differences in β-adrenoceptor density contribute to variability in response to β-adrenoceptor antagonists. Clin Pharmacol Ther. 1989;45:587–92.

195. Klein C et al. Beta-adrenergic receptors in the elderly are not less sensitive to timolol. Clin Pharmacol Ther. 1986;40:161–64.

196. Steinberg SF, Bilezikian JP. Total and free propranolol levels in sensitive and resistant patients. Clin Pharmacol Ther. 1983;33:163–67.

197. McDevitt DG, Shand DG. Plasma concentrations and the time course of beta-blockade due to propranolol. Clin Pharmacol Ther. 1975;18:708–13.

198. Holford NH, Sheiner LB. Kinetics of pharmacologic response. Pharmacol Ther. 1982;16:143–66.

199. Galeazzi RL et al. Constant kinetics and constant concentration effect relationship during long-term beta-blockade with pindolol. Clin Pharmacol Ther. 1983;33:733–40.

200. Myers MG, Thiessen JJ. Metoprolol kinetics and dose response in hypertensive patients. Clin Pharmacol Ther. 1980;27:756–62.

201. Myers MG et al. Atenolol in essential hypertension. Clin Pharmacol Ther. 1976;19:502–507.

202. Esler M et al. Pathophysiologic and pharmacokinetic determinants of the antihypertensive response to propranolol. Clin Pharmacol Ther. 1977;22:299–308.

203. Thadani U, Parker JO. Propranolol in angina pectoris. Duration of improved exercise tolerance and circulatory effects after acute oral administration. Am J Cardiol. 1979;44:118–25.

204. Alderman EL, Davies RO, Crowley JJ et al. Dose response effectiveness of propranolol for the treatment of angina pectoris. Circulation 1975;51:964–75.

205. Woosley RL et al. Suppression of chronic ventricular arrhythmias with propranolol. Circulation 1979;60:819–24.

206. Pratt CM et al. Evaluation of metoprolol in suppressing complex ventricular arrhythmias. Am J Cardiol. 1983;52:73–78.

207. Morganroth J. Short-term evaluation of atenolol in hospitalized patients with chronic ventricular arrhythmias. Drugs 1983;25:181–85.

208. Morris KG et al. Comparison of high-dose and medium-dose propranolol in the relief of exercise-induced myocardial ischemia. Am J Cardiol. 1983;52:7–13.

209. Boudolas H et al. Pharmacodynamics of inotropic and chronotropic responses to oral therapy with propranolol. Chest 1978;73:146–53.

210. Clifton GD et al. Pharmacodynamics of propranolol on left ventricular function: assessment by doppler echocardiography. Clin Pharmacol Ther. 1990;48:431-38.

211. McDevitt DG. Clinical significance of cardioselectivity; state of the art. Drugs 1983;25 (Suppl.2):219–26.

212. Feldman RD et al. Alterations in leukocyte β-receptor affinity with aging: a potential explanation for altered β-adrenergic sensitivity in the elderly. N Engl J Med. 1984;310:815–19.

213. Tenero DM et al. Altered beta-adrenergic sensitivity and protein binding to l-propranolol in the elderly. J Cardiovasc Pharmacol. 1990;16:702–707.

214. Penny WJ, Mir MA. Cardiorespiratory response to exercise before and after acute beta-adrenoceptor blockade in non-smokers and chronic smokers. Int J Cardiol. 1986;11:293–304.

215. Laustiola KE et al. Decreased β-adrenergic receptor density and catecholamine response in male cigarette smokers: a study of monozygotic twin pairs discordant for smoking. Circulation 1988;78:1234–240.

216. Boudoulas H et al. Time course of the blockade effect of propranolol on sinus node and atrioventricular node. J Clin Pharmacol. 1979;19:95–99.

217. Levenson LW et al. Propranolol: disparity between hemodynamic actions and biologic half-life. Circulation 1974;50:III-78.

218. Hermansson J. Simultaneous determination of d- and l-propranolol in human plasma by high-performance liquid chromatography. J Chromatog. 1980;221:109–17.

219. Wainer IW, Doyle TD. The direct enantiomeric determination of (-) and (+)-propranolol in human serum by high-performance liquid chromatography on a chiral stationary phase. J Chromatog. 1984;306:405–11.

220. Armstrong DW et al. Separation of drug stereoisomers by formation of β-cyclodextrin inclusion complexes. Science 1986;232:1132–135.

221. Hermansson J. Resolution of racemic aminoalcohols beta blockers, amines, and acids as enantiomeric derivatives using a chiral α_1-acid glycoprotein column. J Chromatog. 1985;325:379–84.

222. Schill G et al. Chiral separations of cationic and anionic drugs on an α_1-acid glycoprotein-bonded stationary phase. J Chromatog. 1986;365:73–88.

223. J Pharmacol Exp Ther. 1980;214:682–870.

224. Clin Pharmacol Ther. 1980;27:744–55.

225. Clinical Pharmacokinet. 1986;11:1–17.

Chapter 25

Phenytoin

Thomas N. Tozer and Michael E. Winter

Phenytoin (Dilantin, formerly diphenylhydantoin; chemical name 5,5-diphenyl-2,4-imidazolidinedione) is a drug whose plasma concentration is frequently monitored; yet the concentration of phenytoin is unquestionably the most difficult to interpret pharmacokinetically. Although these statements appear to be contradictory, they are related by a lack of predictability of the phenytoin plasma concentration-time profile.

Table 25-1 shows how phenytoin concentrations vary among patients treated chronically with 300 mg/day. Because concentrations associated with optimal therapy are usually between 10 and 20 mg/L, it is apparent that there is a high incidence of concentrations for which subtherapeutic responses are probable and, at the same time, there is about a 16% incidence of concentrations at which toxic responses are probable.

The poor correlation between plasma concentration and the rate of phenytoin administration in chronic therapy is further demonstrated by the data in Figure 25-1. Clearly, there is no dosage at which the incidence of both subtherapeutic concentrations and potentially toxic concentrations is not high. These interindividual differences are explained, in large part, by capacity-limited metabolism. This mechanism also explains why the dosage adjustment required to achieve a

Table 25-1. *Distribution of Phenytoin Concentrations in Plasma Among 100 Ambulant Patients Chronically Treated with 300 mg of Phenytoin Sodium Daily[a]*

Plasma phenytoin concentration (mg/L)	% of patients
0–5	27
5–10	30
10–20	29
20–30	10
>30	6

[a] Data abstracted from Figure 2 of reference 1.

therapeutic concentration in an individual patient is often quite small—that is, small relative to the required change in concentration. Needless to say, this mechanism makes evaluation and interpretation of phenytoin concentrations difficult.

This chapter explores the clinical pharmacokinetics and pharmacodynamics of phenytoin. Particular emphasis is given to the mechanism and consequences of capacity-limited metabolism and to the information needed for monitoring plasma phenytoin concentrations.

CLINICAL PHARMACOKINETICS

Absorption

The oral and parenteral routes of administration each present problems that primarily relate to the low solubility of phenytoin acid, 14 mg/L at room temperature,[2] and the relatively high pKa, 8.3.

Oral Administration

Three dosage forms are available for oral administration, as listed in Table 25-2. Capsules of the sodium salt are by far the most commonly used. The content of this dosage form is expressed in milligrams of phenytoin sodium. The fraction of this amount which is phenytoin itself is 0.92; this fraction is referred to as the **salt form factor**, S.

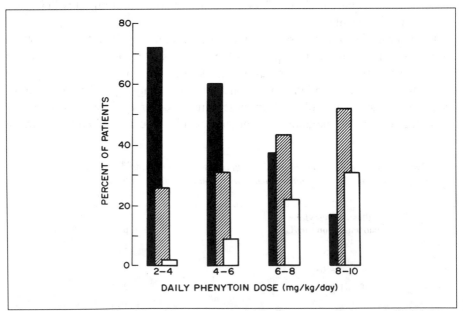

Figure 25-1. *The percentage of patients with plasma phenytoin concentrations either below (dark bars) or above (light bars) the usual therapeutic concentration range of 10 to 20 mg/L is large compared to the percentage within the range (shaded bars), regardless of the daily phenytoin dose even when normalized to body weight. Adapted from Figure 15 of reference 2.*

The tablet, containing phenytoin acid, is "chewable" and thus is a convenient pediatric dosage form. Phenytoin suspensions of the acid, available in two concentrations, have limited utility for two reasons. First, unless well-dispersed, precipitation of the drug in the bottle gives rise to doses lower-than-expected initially and higher-than-expected as the container is emptied. Second, the usual methods for measurement of liquids, especially with teaspoons, are inexact. When the phenytoin suspension is put into a unit-dose package, it is important to state on the label whether or not rinsing of the container is needed to ensure proper delivery of the intended dose. In addition, because two concentrations of suspensions are available, there is a potential for error. The most dangerous is the mistaken administration of the 125 mg/5 mL preparation in place of the pediatric suspension containing 30 mg/5 mL.

The bioavailability of phenytoin has been reviewed,[3] and several studies have shown substantial differences among these products in general use. The salt is readily soluble in water, but in the acidic medium of the stomach, it precipitates after dissolving. The size of the acid crystals, aggregates, or particles entering the intestine is probably the critical factor in determining the rate and extent of absorption. Thus, whether the acid or the sodium salt is administered, the absorption of the drug depends upon product formulation.

Bioavailability of phenytoin is difficult to determine by conventional methods because clearance is concentration-dependent. The area under the plasma concentration-time curve (AUC) is less after oral than after intravenous administration.[4] However, after correcting for the nonlinear elimination, Jusko et al.[5] demonstrated that the bioavailability of high quality products approaches 1.0. Nonetheless, changes in dosage form or manufacturer should be avoided once a patient's dosage requirements have been established, as a relatively small decrease or increase in bioavailability can greatly alter the steady-state plasma concentration during chronic administration.[6]

The rate of absorption varies considerably among dosage forms. The time at which the concentration peaks is three to twelve hours after a single oral dose of a capsule or tablet.[4,7] However, for some preparations and in some individuals, the time to peak may be more than 12 hours. This slow absorption and the relatively slow elimination of the drug have led to the recommendation of once-daily

Table 25-2. Phenytoin Dosage Forms

	Oral			Parenteral
	Tablets	**Capsules**	**Suspension**	**Solution**
Phenytoin acid	50 mg[a]		30 mg/5 mL[a]	
			125 mg/5 mL	
Phenytoin sodium[b] (92% phenytoin)		30 mg		50 mg/mL
		100 mg		

[a] Pediatric dosage forms.
[b] The content is given in mg of phenytoin sodium.

administration. The Food and Drug Administration, however, has cautioned against the use of any product other than Dilantin Kapseals for once-a-day use[8] because many generic preparations are more rapidly absorbed and may produce an intolerable fluctuation in the plasma phenytoin concentration. It should be pointed out that the average steady-state plasma concentrations for the more rapidly absorbed dosage forms are virtually the same as those achieved by the more slowly absorbed products[9] as long as the bioavailability is unchanged.[10]

The time to reach the maximum phenytoin plasma concentration after a single oral dose increases with the dose as shown in Table 25-3. Thus, after an oral loading dose, several hours may be required to reach the peak value, and the greater the dose, the longer the time to reach the peak. The prolonged absorption also tends to diminish the fluctuations expected on a fixed regimen at higher doses.

The greatly increased peak time with dose is probably a consequence of two mechanisms. One is the relatively low solubility of the drug which may lead to prolonged input at a rate determined, in large part, by the low concentration (i.e., saturated solution) in the diffusion layer around drug particles. The other is the capacity-limited metabolism the drug undergoes. Even in the presence of first-order absorption, the peak time increases with dose when elimination is saturable.[11]

Although not thoroughly studied, the bioavailability of phenytoin may be reduced in gastrointestinal diseases, particularly those associated with increased intestinal motility. The relatively slow absorption of drug suggests this possibility. Thus, in cases of severe diarrhea, malabsorption syndrome, or gastric resection, decreased bioavailability should be considered, even with products known to be well absorbed.

The absorption of phenytoin is impaired when given concurrently to patients receiving continuous nasogastric feedings.[12] The steady-state plasma concentration is drastically reduced. The most likely mechanism is a reduced bioavailability due to rapid gastrointestinal transit. A number of approaches to resolve this problem have been suggested. They usually include dividing the daily dose and withholding the administration of the nutritional supplement for one to two hours before and after each phenytoin dose. This approach may not correct the problem completely, and it compromises the patient's nutritional supplementation. For these reasons, parenteral administration in divided daily doses is probably preferred for these patients, especially when they have a high risk of seizure.

Table 25-3. Time at Which Phenytoin Concentration Peaks after Administering a Single Oral Dose[10]

Dose (mg)	Peak time (hr)
400	8.4
800	13.2
1600	31.5

Parenteral Administration

Phenytoin sodium is given both intravenously and intramuscularly to patients who cannot receive the drug orally or who require a rapid onset of drug effects. However, both of these routes of administration have limitations.

The major disadvantage of the intravenous route is the requirement for slow administration of the 40% propylene glycol and 10% alcohol diluent which is adjusted to pH 12 with sodium hydroxide. This vehicle is required to maintain phenytoin in solution at a concentration of 50 mg of the sodium salt per milliliter. Cardiovascular collapse and central nervous system depression are the major toxicities which have been associated with intravenous administration. These reactions may be primarily due to the propylene glycol. To reduce or avoid these problems, the rate of administration should never exceed 50 mg/min.

Because of the inconvenience of administering the drug slowly, there is often a desire to give phenytoin with other intravenous fluids. This is not recommended because it is insoluble and may precipitate as phenytoin acid.[13] If phenytoin admixtures are to be used, they should be carefully monitored for crystal growth, and the infusion should be started immediately after preparation. Only normal saline or Lactated Ringer's Solution should be used. The acid pH of dextrose solutions has been a particular problem. Admixtures with all other drugs should be avoided to prevent pH-related precipitation.

The intramuscular route of administration should be avoided because phenytoin precipitates at the site of injection. The tissue buffers the injection solution, and the propylene glycol-alcohol solvent is absorbed from the injection site, resulting in the deposition of phenytoin crystals. Consequently, absorption from this site tends to be erratic and slow, often continuing for five days or more.[14] Figure 25-2

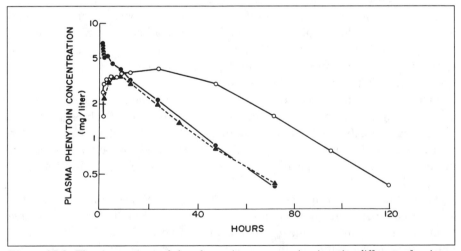

Figure 25-2. The time course of the phenytoin concentration is quite different after intra-muscular administration (500 mg, ○) compared to that after either intravenous (250, ●) or oral (300, ▲) administration. The points shown are the averages of 12 subjects (IM and IV) and six subjects (oral). Intramuscular and intravenous data from reference 14; oral data from reference 4.

shows the prolonged plasma phenytoin concentration-time curve resulting from intramuscular administration relative to those resulting from intravenous and oral administration.

A major problem is encountered when the route of administration is changed from oral to intramuscular, or the reverse.[15] Because only 50% to 75% of an intramuscular dose is absorbed within 24 hours; the conversion from oral to intramuscular administration at the same dose results in a drop in the plasma phenytoin concentration. Because of interindividual and intersite variability in phenytoin absorption, the intramuscular route should probably be avoided or, at the least, carefully monitored. In addition, this route of administration is painful and can cause muscle damage.[16]

Distribution

The rate and extent of phenytoin distribution are of therapeutic importance for entirely different reasons.

Time for Tissue Equilibration. Following an intravenous dose, phenytoin rapidly distributes to the tissues, with distribution equilibrium being achieved in 30 to 60 minutes.[14,17,18] The elevated concentration observed initially and the rapid distribution can be seen in Figure 25-2. The time required for attainment of distribution equilibrium partially explains why phenytoin should not be administered as a bolus dose, but rather infused at a rate not exceeding 50 mg/min. Thus, a loading dose of 1000 mg for a rapid antiarrhythmic or anticonvulsant response should not be administered over less than 20 minutes and is probably more safely administered over at least 30 to 60 minutes. Bigger et al.[18] have suggested that, in the treatment of cardiac arrhythmias, 100 mg (50 mg/min) can be administered every six minutes until the arrhythmia is controlled. The total intravenous dose should probably not exceed 1000 mg (14 mg/kg).

The drug rapidly distributes to the brain,[19,20] and the concentration in the brain is equal to or slightly higher than that in plasma within ten minutes after a ten-minute infusion.[20] The rapid distribution phase in plasma is not observed in either brain tissue or cerebrospinal fluid. This fact suggests that the central nervous system effects initially observed when a dose of phenytoin is given too rapidly by the intravenous route may be associated with the propylene glycol vehicle and not with the drug itself. The concentration of phenytoin in the cerebrospinal fluid, which has virtually no protein, is similar to that unbound in plasma when distribution equilibrium is achieved.[21] The concentrations in the various parts of the brain correlate with the lipid content, a consequence of high affinity for phospholipids.[22]

Volume of Distribution. The initial dilution space of phenytoin is difficult to assess because of the requirement for short-term infusion of the parenteral dosage form and the nonlinear kinetics of the drug. Except for situations of rapid intravenous infusion, the distribution of phenytoin can be considered to be uni-compartmental. This is particularly the case for oral and intramuscular administration.

Once distribution equilibrium is achieved, within two hours of a 10- to 20-minute infusion, the drug appears to be diluted into a space comparable to the total body water, 0.6 to 0.7 L/kg. This value is deceptive, however, in that the drug is highly bound to both plasma proteins and tissue components. The concentration in the brain is comparable to that in plasma, and the concentration in cerebrospinal fluid is the same as that in plasma water, suggesting that the percent bound in brain and plasma are the same.

Plasma Protein Binding. Phenytoin binds primarily to albumin in plasma, and under normal conditions the fraction unbound is 0.1. At therapeutic concentrations the fraction unbound (f_{up}) is related to the affinity constant, K_a, and the concentration of sites on albumin available for binding (P):[23]

$$f_{up} = \frac{1}{1 + K_a \cdot P}$$ (Eq. 25-1)

At the usual concentrations of albumin, 4.3 gm/dL, f_{up} is equal to 0.1. At phenytoin concentrations less than 20 mg/L, (P) is approximately equal to the serum albumin concentration; thus, the value of K_a must equal 2.1 dL/gm for f_{up} to equal 0.1. The expected relationship[24] between the fraction unbound and the serum albumin (Alb) is then:

$$f_{up} = \frac{1}{1 + 2.1 \cdot Alb}$$ (Eq. 25-2)

A change in the albumin concentration alters the fraction unbound and the apparent volume of distribution. Based on the principles of protein binding and the assumption that tissue binding is unaltered, the volume of distribution (V_d) can be roughly estimated (Winter and Tozer, unpublished data) from the serum albumin as follows:

$$V_d \text{ (in L/kg)} = \frac{2.8}{Alb \text{ (in grams/dL)}}$$ (Eq. 25-3)

This equation applies to situations in which only the albumin concentration is altered (i.e., in the presence of normal renal function and no displacing drugs).

Equations 25-1 to 25-3 are based on the assumption that there is only one binding site on albumin and that only a small fraction of the sites available for binding are occupied. The typical concentration of albumin in serum is 4.3 gm/dL or 0.6 mmol (molecular weight = 67,000). When phenytoin concentrations approach this value, the fraction unbound increases because of a decrease in available binding sites. As a general rule, if the phenytoin concentration is below 0.1 mmol (25 mg/L for a drug with a molecular weight of 250), the fraction unbound is reasonably constant. The presence of other drugs that bind to the same site on albumin can displace phenytoin if they are at total concentrations of 0.1 mmol or more.

Distribution in Various Clinical States. In the presence of certain disease states or certain other drugs (see Table 25-4), the affinity of albumin for phenytoin is altered; in virtually all circumstances, the binding is decreased. The fraction unbound is increased two- to threefold in uremia.[25-30] Part of this change is accounted for by a decrease in serum albumin, but the majority of the decreased binding is caused by another mechanism. An altered albumin molecule or a decreased apparent affinity for albumin due to the accumulation of a substance which displaces the drug has been suggested.[28-30] The value of K_a in uremia is usually about 1 dL/gm, so that the fraction unbound is approximately:

$$f_{up}' = \frac{1}{1 + Alb}$$

(Eq. 25-4)

where f_{up}' is the fraction unbound in renal disease and Alb is the serum albumin in gm/dL.[24]

Tissue binding does not appear to be affected by renal failure.[25] Thus, the apparent volume of distribution increases essentially in proportion to the increase in the fraction unbound,

$$V_d \ (L/kg) = \frac{f_{up}'}{f_{up}} \ (0.65)$$

(Eq. 25-5)

where f_{up} is the fraction unbound (0.1) when renal function is normal. From Equations 25-4 and 25-5, the volume of distribution can be estimated (Winter and Tozer, unpublished data) in a patient with severe renal function impairment:

$$V_d \ (L/kg) = \frac{6.5}{1 + Alb}$$

(Eq. 25-6)

The value of V_d in renal failure is, then, on average, about 1 to 2 L/kg, depending on the serum albumin concentration.

The affinity of albumin for phenytoin is decreased about twofold in patients with creatinine clearances below 10 mL/min. There is also a decrease in the affinity in patients with creatinine clearances between 10 and 25 mL/min;[31] here, however, there is a higher degree of variability in the affinity and in the fraction unbound.

A decrease in plasma protein binding, and hence an increase in volume of distribution, also occurs in chronic hepatic disease.[30,32] The changes here are

Table 25-4. *Examples of Conditions in Which Plasma Protein Binding of Phenytoin is Decreased[24]*

↓ in serum albumin concentration	Apparent ↓ in affinity for serum albumin
Burns	Renal failure[a]
Hepatic cirrhosis	Jaundice (severe)[a]
Nephrotic syndrome	Other drugs (displacers)
Pregnancy	
Cystic fibrosis	

[a] ↓ serum albumin concentration also commonly present.

primarily a result of a reduction in serum albumin, although an increased concentration of bilirubin with associated displacement may also contribute. Estimates of the volume of distribution can therefore be approximated using Equation 25-3, except perhaps in severely jaundiced patients. The same applies to other conditions, such as nephrotic syndrome, burns, injury, and pregnancy, in which the serum albumin concentration is decreased. The changes produced in volume of distribution by altered binding to plasma proteins are meaningful with respect to the interpretation of phenytoin (total) concentrations. However, the changes probably have little or no therapeutic consequences in terms of either loading or maintenance dosage requirements.

Unbound Concentrations. Theoretically, the unbound concentration is a better correlate of phenytoin's efficacy and toxicity than the total plasma concentration, and should therefore be a better guide to therapy. However, the current methods available for separating the unbound drug are not commonly used in clinical practice.

One alternative method is measurement of the drug in saliva.[33-35] The concentration in saliva is about equal to that unbound in plasma. There is, however, considerable variability in the ratio of concentrations in saliva and unbound in plasma. Although some of this variability is due to error in the measurement of plasma protein binding, the actual error is unknown, and the routine use of saliva concentration measurements is not recommended.

Metabolism

Metabolic Fate. Elimination of phenytoin occurs primarily by biotransformation to several inactive hydroxylated metabolites.[36,37] Figure 25-3 shows the structures of phenytoin and several of its reported metabolites. Some of these metabolites, notably 5-(p-hydroxyphenyl)-5-phenylhydantoin (p-HPPH), are further metabolized by conjugation with glucuronic acid. The urinary recovery of p-HPPH and its glucuronide accounts for 60% to 90% of an oral dose of phenytoin.[4,15,38]

The metabolites, p-HPPH and the diol (see IV in Figure 25-3), are excreted in the urine primarily as the S isomers. This is a consequence of stereoselective formation of an epoxide on one of the phenyl rings by an arene oxidase enzyme.[39] This formation of optically active metabolites shows a specificity of about 10:1 for p-HPPH in humans.[40] It is presently unknown whether there are separate R- and S-specific arene oxidases or if the operational one lacks total specificity.

Capacity-Limited Metabolism. The rate of any enzymatically mediated reaction is expected to have an upper limit as the concentration of the substrate is increased; the enzyme has a limited capacity. For most drugs, the rate of metabolism is well below this limit at the concentrations associated with therapy. For such drugs, the rate of metabolism is, therefore, directly proportional to the plasma concentration. This is not the case for phenytoin. At therapeutic concentrations, the rate of metabolism is close to the limit and, therefore, the process is said to be **capacity-limited** or to show **saturability**.

Evidence for the capacity-limited metabolism of phenytoin is observed in many ways. For example, Figure 25-4 shows the semilogarithmic decline of plasma phenytoin concentration with time following the discontinuation of drug administration. The convex curvature indicates an increase in the fractional rate of elimination as the concentration decreases. This increase is consistent with capacity-limited metabolism, but other explanations are possible.

Perhaps the most compelling evidence for saturable metabolism is the disproportionate increase in the plasma phenytoin concentration at steady state as the rate of administration is increased. Figure 25-5 shows this relationship for each of several patients. The consequence of this kind of elimination is apparent: for each individual the dosage required to achieve a steady-state concentration above 20 mg/L is not much greater than that required for a concentration of 10 mg/L.

To explain the kinetic behavior of phenytoin and to aid in predicting and evaluating dosage requirements and plasma concentrations, a model for phenytoin disposition is useful (see Figure 25-6). In this model, metabolism is assumed to occur enzymatically to give an unstable intermediate, an epoxide, which is further metabolized to other products. The only other route of phenytoin elimination is renal excretion. The latter pathway contributes only about 1% to 5% and is thus usually ignored.

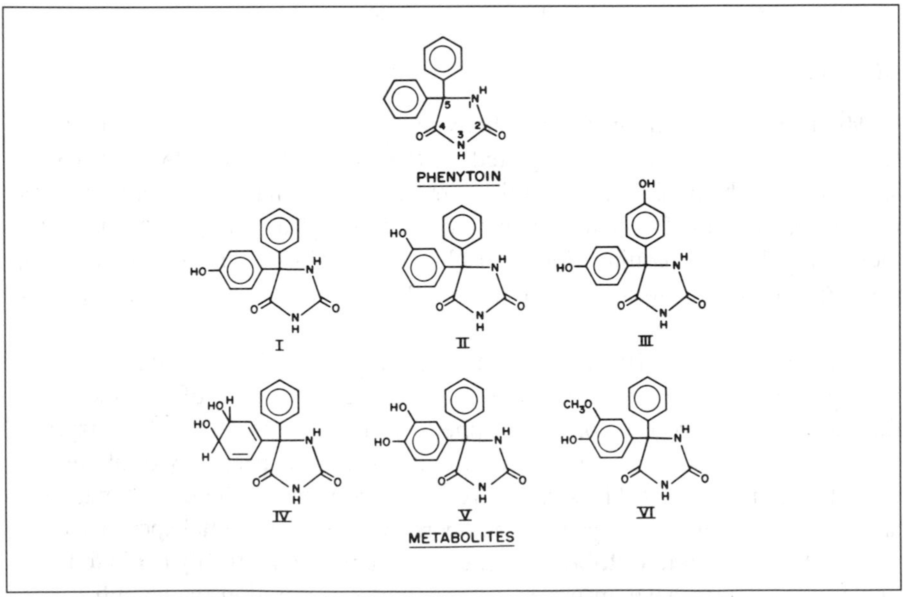

Figure 25-3. Structures of phenytoin and some of its metabolites: I. 5-(p-hydroxyphenyl)-5-phenylhydantoin; II. 5-(m-hydroxyphenyl)-5-phenylhydantoin; III. 5,5–bis-(p-hydroxyphenyl)hydantoin; IV. 5-(3,4-dihydroxy-2,5-cyclohexadiene)-5-phenylhydantoin; V. 5-(3,4-dihydroxyphenyl)-5-phenylhydantoin; VI. 5-(3-methoxy-4-hydroxyphenyl)-5-phenylhydantoin.

The rate-limiting enzymatic reaction is assumed to follow typical Michaelis-Menten kinetics in which the rate of the reaction depends upon the substrate concentration in plasma (C_p) as follows:

$$\text{Rate} = \frac{V_{max} \cdot C_p}{K_m + C_p}$$

(Eq. 25-7)

where V_{max} is the maximum rate of metabolism (metabolic capacity), in mg per day, and K_m (units of mg/L) is a constant with a value equal to the plasma concentration at which the rate of metabolism is one-half the maximum.

Parameter Values. Values of V_{max} and K_m usually vary in adults from 100 to 1000 mg/day and 1 to 15 mg/L or more, respectively.[42–51] Our estimates of the average values in epileptic patients are about 500 mg/day or, expressed relative to body weight, 7 mg/day/kg and 4 mg/L, respectively. These values are based on the patients for whom an analysis of phenytoin kinetics was undertaken. Admittedly, this may have been a biased sample in that the kinetics were often pursued in patients with problems in controlling their therapy. Problem patients have a tendency toward lower values of K_m, and our bias may be in this direction.

There is less information on the parameter values in children.[52–55] The value of V_{max} (mg/day/kg) in children (less than six years of age) is greater than in older children (7 to 16 years of age), which is greater than that in adults. Using these data, we suggest V_{max} values of 10 to 13 mg/day/kg for children six months through

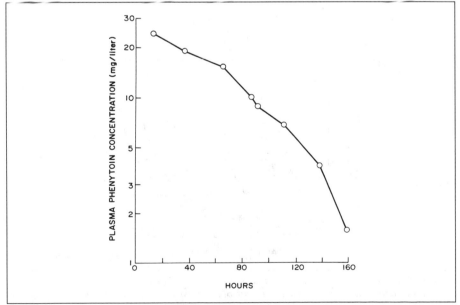

Figure 25-4. The plasma phenytoin concentration declines convexly on a semilogarithmic plot when a daily dose of 7.9 mg/kg is discontinued in an individual subject. This nonlinearity is evidence of dose-dependent kinetics. Data from reference 41.

six years of age and 8 to 10 mg/day/kg for those 7 through 16 years of age. The estimates of K_m are highly variable in children. Some authors[52-54] have suggested levels of 2 to 3 mg/L, and others[55] suggest values in the range of 6 to 8 mg/L.

Steady-State Concentration. The consequences of capacity-limited metabolism are most readily observed under steady-state conditions—that is, when the drug is chronically administered at a fixed rate (Dose/τ) until the rate of elimination and the average rate of absorption are equal. Assuming conditions simulating an intravenous infusion, the rate of input, R_{in} (S · F · Dose/τ) must then be equal to the rate of elimination; thus,

$$R_{in} = \frac{V_{max} \cdot C_{SS}}{K_m + C_{SS}}$$

(Eq. 25-8)

where C_{ss} is the steady-state or plateau concentration; S is the salt form factor, and F is the bioavailability.

If this relationship is rearranged to express the steady-state concentration as a function of the rate in, the effect of capacity-limited metabolism is clear.

$$C_{SS} = \frac{K_m \cdot R_{in}}{V_{max} - R_{in}}$$

(Eq. 25-9)

or

$$\frac{C_{SS}}{K_m} = \frac{R_{in}}{V_{max} - R_{in}}$$

(Eq. 25-10)

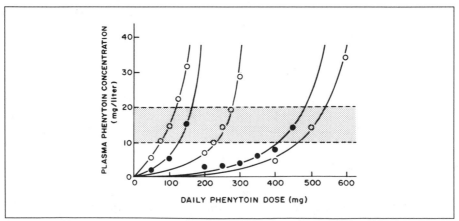

Figure 25-5. *For each patient the plasma phenytoin concentration at steady state increases disproportionately with an increase in the rate of administration. In all patients, the daily dose required to achieve a steady-state concentration of 20 mg/L is not much greater than that required to achieve a value of 10 mg/L, within the therapeutic concentration range. These patients show differences that are greater than those expected in random samples. Selection here was to show the kinetic behavior in patients in whom several dosage adjustments were required. The lines are computer fits of the data using the model in Figure 25-6. Adapted from reference 42.*

When the rate of absorption approaches the maximum rate of metabolism, the steady-state concentration increases disproportionately toward infinity. Values of R_{in} greater than V_{max} are not applicable, because steady state cannot occur under these conditions. Equation 25-10 shows that when the steady-state concentration is comparable to or greater than the value of K_m, the value of R_{in} approaches V_{max}. For phenytoin, therapeutic concentrations almost always exceed the value of K_m; thus, capacity-limited metabolism is evident.

Equation 25-8 can be rearranged to give the following:

$$R_{in} = V_{max} - K_m \left[\frac{R_{in}}{C_{SS}} \right]$$

(Eq. 25-11)

This is one of the linearizations of the Michaelis-Menten equation. The value of R_{in}/C_{SS} is conventionally called clearance because it is the parameter that relates the rate of elimination to the plasma concentration. A plot of R_{in}/C_{SS} gives a straight line with a y-intercept of V_{max} and a slope of $-K_m$. It is one of the more useful methods of assessing steady-state concentrations obtained with two or more rates of administration and will be discussed below and shown in Figure 25-13.

Expressing the last relationship as

$$V_{max} = R_{in} + K_m \left[\frac{R_{in}}{C_{SS}} \right]$$

(Eq. 25-12)

and treating V_{max} and K_m as variables, we find that an infinite number of sets of V_{max} and K_m values are consistent with a given steady-state concentration when the drug is administered at rate R. On plotting V_{max} versus K_m, the y-intercept is R_{in}

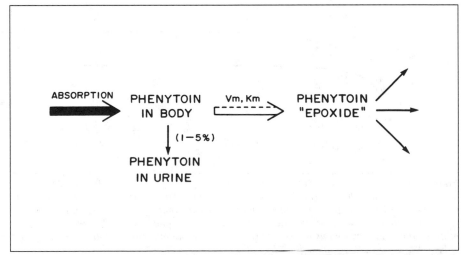

Figure 25-6. *Pharmacokinetically, phenytoin elimination appears to be rate-limited by a single metabolic step, presumably to an epoxide intermediate, and characterized by the Michaelis-Menten enzyme kinetic parameters K_m and V_{max}. Some elimination occurs by renal excretion, but its contribution is usually negligible.*

and the x-intercept is $-C_{ss}$. This relationship is the basis of the methods described below (B, C, and D) for estimating the values of the pharmacokinetic parameters, V_{max} and K_m.

Concentration During and After an Infusion

Time to Plateau. Because of phenytoin's nonlinear elimination, the time required to reach a steady-state concentration varies with the rate of administration and depends upon the values of V_{max} and K_m.[56,57] For a constant rate of infusion of phenytoin, in which case the net rate of change of phenytoin in the body ($V_d \cdot dC/dt$) is the difference between the rates in and out, then:

$$V_d \cdot dC/dt = R_{in} - \frac{V_{max} \cdot C}{K_m + C}$$

(Eq. 25-13)

which, on integration, is equal to:

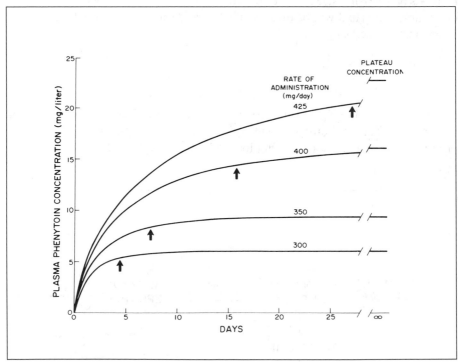

Figure 25-7. *On administration of the drug at constant rates of 300, 350, 400, and 425 mg/day, the plasma concentration approaches steady-state values of 6, 9.3, 16, and 22.7 mg/L, respectively. Not only is the steady-state concentration disproportionately increased, but so is the time required to approach the plateau. The arrows indicate the time required to reach 90% of the plateau value. An intravenous infusion is simulated in a patient with the following parameter values: K_m, 4 mg/L; V_{max}, 500 mg/day; V_d, 50 L.*

$$\frac{K_m \cdot V_{max}}{(V_{max} - R_{in})} \ln \left[\frac{R_{in} \cdot K_m - (V_{max} - R_{in}) \cdot C_1}{R_{in} \cdot K_m - (V_{max} - R_{in}) \cdot C_2} \right]$$

$$+ C_1 - C_2 = \frac{(V_{max} - R_{in})}{V_d} \cdot t \qquad \text{(Eq. 25-14)}$$

where C_1 is the concentration at zero time and C_2 is the concentration at time t. When C_1 is zero, the time $t_{90\%}$ required to achieve 90% of the steady-state value (i.e., C_2 equals 90% of C_{ss}) is:

$$t_{90\%} = \frac{K_m \cdot V_d}{(V_{max} - R_{in})^2} (2.3 \cdot V_{max} - 0.9 \cdot R_{in}) \qquad \text{(Eq. 25-15)}$$

The time increases dramatically as the value of R_{in} approaches V_{max}. If it equals or exceeds V_{max}, steady state is never achieved.

Using values of 4 mg/L, 50 L and 500 mg/day for K_m, V_d, and V_{max}, respectively, the approach to plateau is shown in Figure 25-7. The higher the rate of administration, the longer it takes to approach steady state and, as one would expect, the steady-state concentration is increased disproportionately. Note that for steady-state concentrations of 10 to 20 mg/L, the values of $t_{90\%}$ are about 8 and 21 days for the parameter values given.

The time needed to reach a given plateau concentration varies with the values of K_m and V_{max}. Table 25-5 lists the times to achieve 90% of a plateau of 16 mg/L. The smaller the value of K_m, the longer it takes to reach the same plateau concentration. Indeed, for patients with a small value of K_m (2 mg/L or less), several weeks of accumulation are required to achieve therapeutic steady-state concentrations, and the rate of administration required to maintain a concentration within the therapeutic range is close to the maximum rate of metabolism.

For monitoring a plasma phenytoin concentration, it is critical to know if the observed level represents a steady-state value. This judgment can be made from general information on the time required to achieve a given concentration when the patient is on a fixed daily dose. Substituting Equation 25-12 into Equation

Table 25-5. *Time to Accumulate to 90% of a Plateau Concentration of 16 mg/L as a Function of the V_{max} and K_m Values[a]*

Situations	k_m (mg/L)	V_{max} (mg/day)	$t_{90\%}$ (days)
1	1	425	50
2	2	450	27
3	4	500	16
4	8	600	10
5	12	700	8

[a] Calculated from Equations 25-12 and 25-15, using a daily dose of 400 mg of phenytoin acid and a value of 50 L for V_d.

25-15 and taking the conservative approach of using a K_m of 2 mg/L and a V_d of 50 L, we find the time $t_{90\%}$ required for the observed concentration to represent 90% of the steady-state value on the dosage regimen is:

$$t_{90\%} = \frac{(115 + 35 \cdot C)C}{R_{in}}$$

(Eq. 25-16)

The daily dose is normalized to 70 kg. For example, if a concentration of 8 mg/L were measured 14 days after a 50-kg patient started a regimen of 200 mg phenytoin sodium twice daily, the calculated $t_{90\%}$ is 6.1 days. Thus, one can conclude that the observed concentration value is essentially a steady-state value.

Note that the intent of Equation 25-15 differs from that of Equation 25-16. The former is a prediction of the time to approach steady state; the latter is an evaluation of whether a measured concentration is likely to represent a steady-state value.

Decline of Concentration on Discontinuing Drug. The rate of decline of the phenytoin concentration is important when toxic effects (or high-concentrations) are observed. In this situation, discontinuance of drug administration is desirable to achieve the usual therapeutic concentrations most rapidly. The decline with time may be calculated from the following relationship:

$$K_m \cdot \ln\left(\frac{C_1}{C_2}\right) + C_1 - C_2 = \frac{V_{max}}{V_d} \cdot t$$

(Eq. 25-17)

Figure 25-8 shows the decline in the plasma phenytoin concentration from an initial value of 50 mg/L when administration is discontinued. At concentrations greater than 12 mg/L, the rate of metabolism is greater than 75% of the metabolic capacity, V_{max} (see Equation 25-7). The decline of the plasma concentration (solid line) is therefore approximately equal to V_{max}/V_d (dashed line). This measurement of the rate of decline is often a reasonable method of estimating the value of V_{max}/V_d. The value can be more closely obtained from:

$$\frac{V_{max}}{V_d} = \frac{C_1 - C_2 + K_m \cdot \ln\left(\frac{C_1}{C_2}\right)}{t}$$

(Eq. 25-18)

by assuming a typical value for K_m. Values for K_m can be calculated accurately (see Equation 25-17) only if several levels are measured, including one or more below the value of Km. This is an unlikely situation in the usual course of therapeutic monitoring.

When a high concentration is observed and a decision is made to withhold the drug, knowledge of the time required for the level to decline to 20 mg/L is desirable. The primary information needed is an estimation of V_{max}/V_d. Although it may seem appropriate to use the average value of 500 mg/day/50 L, a more cautious approach is to decide first why the concentration is high. If the concentration is high because the patient's metabolic capacity (V_{max}) is less than the rate of administration, then a decreased estimate of V_{max}/V_d is in order. For an overdose of the drug, the average may be appropriate. Measurement of a plasma concentration one to two days later may be helpful; however, the possibility of absorption continuing after the first sample is obtained must be considered.

Changes in Salt Form or Bioavailability

Because of capacity-limited metabolism, a small change in the input due to a change in the dosage form or bioavailability can produce a dramatic change in the steady-state concentration. To illustrate this point, consider a patient who has a steady-state concentration of 14 mg/L on a dose of 400 mg/day and whose K_m and V_{max} values are 4 mg/L and 473 mg/day, respectively. With a change from a sodium phenytoin dosage form with a salt form factor (S) of 0.92 to a suspension with an S of 1, the steady-state concentration increases (see Equation 25-9) from 14 to 22 mg/L—a 60% increase in the concentration with only a 9% increase in the rate of input. Differences in bioavailabilities of dosage forms or differences resulting

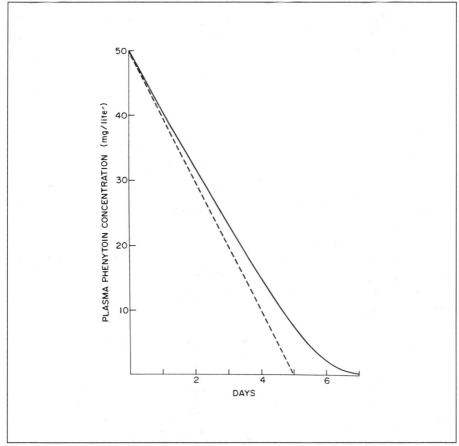

Figure 25-8. *The decline of the plasma phenytoin concentration (——) following discontinuation of the drug, when a concentration of 50 mg/L is present, appears to be almost linear and to approach the rate expected if the drug is continually eliminated at the maximum rate of metabolism, V_{max} (- - - - -). The parameter values in Figure 25-7 are used in the simulation.*

from various disease states (especially gastrointestinal diseases) are clearly of therapeutic importance. Although the change in concentration may be considerable, a long time may be required to go from one steady state to another when either the salt form or the bioavailability is altered.

Clearance and Half-life

Clearance is the parameter that relates rate of elimination to the plasma concentration. From Equation 25-7, it can be seen that the clearance (CL) of phenytoin is a function of the plasma concentration:

$$CL = \frac{V_{max}}{K_m + C}$$

(Eq. 25-19)

Because phenytoin clearance depends on concentration, it is of limited utility and probably should never be used. Furthermore, measurement of bioavailability using the area under the curve is also inappropriate, because clearance is not constant.

Half-life (t½) is another parameter that has little utility for phenytoin. The half-life depends both upon how readily a drug is removed from plasma (CL) and upon how it is distributed (V_d):

$$t½ = 0.693 \frac{V_d}{CL}$$

(Eq. 25-20)

It follows from Equations 25-19 and 25-20 that

$$t½ = 0.693 \frac{V_d}{V_{max}} (K_m + C)$$

(Eq. 25-21)

The half-life is a function of plasma concentration. It is not the time required to eliminate one-half of the drug in the body, but is rather an "instantaneous" value for the time required to eliminate half of the drug present, if the fractional rate of elimination were to continue at that value. Since clearance and half-life are first-order pharmacokinetic parameters, and phenytoin obeys Michaelis-Menten kinetics, these terms should not be used for phenytoin. The most useful parameters are V_{max}, K_m, and V_d.

Table 25-6. *Selected Conditions in Which the Metabolism of Phenytoin Is Altered*

	Condition or disease	Example
V_{max} ↑	Enzyme induction	Concurrent administration of phenobarbital or carbamazepine.
V_{max} ↓	Hepatic cirrhosis	↓ enzyme activity is assumed to be the major effect.
K_m ↑	Competitive inhibition	Concurrent administration of cimetidine or chloramphenicol.
K_m ↓	↓ plasma protein binding	↓ serum albumin or presence of displacers such as valproic acid or salicylate.

Consequences of Altered Metabolism

There are many conditions in which the metabolism of phenytoin is altered. Table 25-6 lists examples of such conditions. The kinetic consequences of alterations in phenytoin metabolism are most meaningful under steady-state conditions, as shown in Figure 25-9. An increase in the value of K_m, as in the presence of a competitive inhibitor, produces a proportional increase in the steady-state concentration for a given dosage regimen. This is also apparent from Equation 25-9. An increase or a decrease in the value of V_{max} can have a dramatic effect on the steady-state level. If the maximum rate of metabolism is reduced to a value less than R_{in}, the plasma concentration will climb toward infinity. If V_{max} is increased, the steady-state concentration is reduced by a factor greater than that by which V_{max} was increased.

Renal Excretion

Only 1% to 5% of a dose is recovered unchanged in the urine[58,59] when renal function is normal. The percentage is greater at high concentrations than at low concentrations because of capacity-limited metabolism. The recovery is also

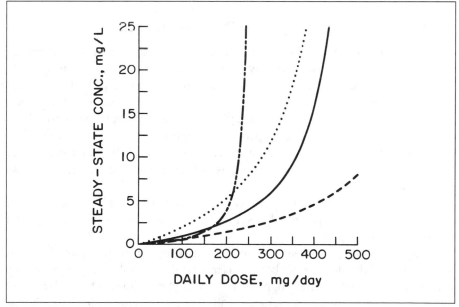

Figure 25-9. The consequence of altered metabolism depends on the mechanism of the alteration. The relationship between steady-state plasma concentration and daily dose (———) in a typical patient (V_{max} = 500 mg/day, K_m = 4 mg/L, V_d = 50 L) is altered as follows: V_{max} is increased by induction to 750 mg/day (- - - - -); K_m is increased by competitive inhibition to 8 mg/L (.......); V_{max} is reduced to 250 mg/day; and K_m is decreased to 1 mg/L by concurrent effects of hepatic cirrhosis and displacement from plasma protein binding sites (— - - — - -). For each alteration, note the differences in the steady-state concentrations observed on a fixed dose of 300 mg/day.

greater at high urine flow rates because the renal clearance is urine-flow dependent.[59] In most clinical situations, however, the renal excretion of phenytoin is minor and can be neglected.

The major phenytoin metabolite, p-HPPH-glucuronide, is actively secreted[59] into the renal tubule. Because its elimination is rate-limited by its formulation from phenytoin, the rate of excretion of the metabolite is an index of the rate of metabolism of phenytoin. Because this metabolite accounts for 60% to 90% of the total elimination, it can be used to assess compliance and bioavailability. For example, when a low phenytoin concentration is observed, measurement of the 24-hour total p-HPPH excretion allows one to conclude whether the drug is being absorbed or not.[60] If the excretion is low (less than 50% of dose) and bioavailability is not believed to be reduced, then noncompliance is a likely explanation. A high urinary output of the metabolite in spite of a low phenytoin concentration confirms rapid metabolism.

Because p-HPPH-glucuronide is renally eliminated, it accumulates in patients with compromised renal function. This accumulation appears to be unimportant, since the metabolite is inactive. Except for patients with severe renal failure, the recovery of the metabolite can be used to test for drug input, regardless of renal function, as the compound is eliminated only by renal excretion.

Hemodialysis, Hemoperfusion, and Plasmapheresis

Only 2% to 4% of the phenytoin initially in the body is removed during an eight-hour period of hemodialysis by conventional methods.[61] Administration of the drug therefore does not have to be altered because a patient undergoes intermittent (every two to three days) hemodialysis. Because of a low serum albumin concentration and renal failure, plasma protein binding is decreased. This requires an adjustment of the "therapeutic" concentration range but has little effect on the dosage requirements of these patients. Because of the small percentage removed by hemodialysis, the method is not useful for detoxification of an overdosed patient.

A typical period of hemoperfusion can effectively remove phenytoin from the body[62] and is therefore potentially useful but seldom required for detoxifying a severely overdosed patient.

Phenytoin is also removed to a limited extent by plasmapheresis. Approximately 10% of the drug in the body is removed during a 4.4-hour, two-plasma volume exchange procedure.[63] In patients on phenytoin who also have diseases in which plasmapheresis is used therapeutically, the loss of drug by the procedure is probably not of major importance unless the patient undergoes the procedure frequently.

PHARMACODYNAMICS

Clinical Response

The usually accepted therapeutic range for plasma phenytoin concentrations is 10 to 20 mg/L. These concentrations are usually effective in controlling both seizure disorders and cardiac arrhythmias.[2,18,19,64,65] In the treatment of seizure disorders the response to phenytoin is graded, with 50% of patients showing a decreased frequency at concentrations greater than 10 mg/L and 86% at concentrations greater than 15 mg/L.[66] Occasionally, there are patients who are seizure-free with concentrations below 10 mg/L;[67] thus, clinical evaluation of the patient should accompany monitoring of the plasma concentration. Recent studies suggest that when phenytoin concentrations are optimized, the necessity for additional anticonvulsant agents is decreased.[68]

When phenytoin is used as an antiarrhythmic agent, 90% of the patients who are successfully treated have plasma concentrations below 18 mg/L, with the majority having concentrations between 10 and 18 mg/L.[18] Serious consideration should be given to adding or changing to another antiarrhythmic or anticonvulsant agent if a satisfactory therapeutic response is not achieved with a phenytoin concentration of 20 mg/L.

Adverse Effects

Phenytoin side effects, such as hypertrichosis, gingival hypertrophy, thickening of facial features, carbohydrate intolerance, folic acid deficiency, peripheral neuropathy, vitamin D deficiency, osteomalacia, and systemic lupus erythematosus, do not appear to be readily related to the plasma phenytoin concentration. This may, in part, be due to the fact that many of these side effects occur over a prolonged time period and infrequently monitored plasma concentrations may not represent the true average phenytoin concentration to which the patient is exposed.

Central nervous system side effects, such as nystagmus, ataxia, and decreased mentation, have been associated with elevated phenytoin concentrations, with more severe symptoms occurring at higher concentrations. Far-lateral nystagmus occurs in the majority of patients at concentrations exceeding 20 mg/L, and nystagmus at a 45° lateral gaze, as well as ataxia, usually occurs at concentrations exceeding 30 mg/L. Significantly diminished mental capacity and ataxia are usually apparent when phenytoin concentrations are above 40 mg/L (see Figure 25-10).[69]

Elderly patients appear to have greater mental changes than do younger patients at the same concentration.[69] Decreased plasma protein binding with age may partially account for this observation.

Nystagmus is usually accepted as the first sign of elevated phenytoin concentrations because it is probably the most frequent objective symptom that can be documented. Nystagmus, however, does not always occur first, and phenytoin toxicity should be considered in patients with unusual involuntary muscular movements, mental symptoms, or ataxia, even if nystagmus is not present.[67,69,70] Seizure activity and the induction of involuntary movements have also been described in patients with phenytoin concentrations above 20 mg/L.[71-73]

In addition to these side effects associated with phenytoin, additional precautions must be observed when the drug is given intravenously because the propylene glycol diluent is potentially a cardiac depressant.[74] Symptoms associated with rapid intravenous injections of phenytoin include bradycardia, hypotension, and widening of the QRS and QT intervals on an electrocardiogram. These symptoms can be diminished or avoided by injecting the drug slowly as discussed previously.

Therapeutic Window

Adjustment of Parameters versus Measured Concentration. The usually accepted therapeutic or "target" concentration of 10 to 20 mg/L has been established in patients with normal plasma protein binding ($f_{up} = 0.1$). It follows that the therapeutic unbound phenytoin concentration is approximately 1 to 2 mg/L and can be calculated using the following formula:

$$C_u = f_{up} \cdot C \qquad\qquad \text{(Eq. 25-22)}$$

where C is the total drug concentration, C_u is the unbound concentration, and f_{up} is the fraction of the total in plasma that is unbound.

In the clinical setting, it is the total phenytoin concentration that is measured and reported. Therefore, an adjustment in either the therapeutic range or the reported concentration is required in patients with altered phenytoin binding. One approach is to use the measured or reported phenytoin concentration and adjust the expected therapeutic range, V_d, and K_m values for that patient. While this

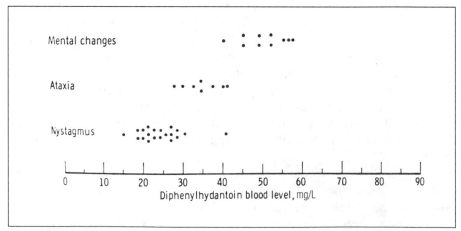

Figure 25-10. *The onset of central nervous system side-effects is related to the phenytoin concentration. Far-lateral nystagmus is most frequently observed with a concentration exceeding 20 mg/L; however, this symptom may be first observed at much lower or higher concentrations. Ataxia and gross mental changes are usually evident at concentrations greater than 30 to 40 mg/L, respectively (reproduced with permission from reference 69).*

approach is workable, most of the available nomogram and dosing adjustment aids require the use of total phenytoin concentrations that represent normal binding (i.e., an unbound fraction of 0.1).

The second and preferred approach is to adjust the reported phenytoin concentration to that which would have been observed had plasma protein binding been normal. This allows one to use the available nomograms and equations and the average parameter values for normal binding.

Adjustment for Serum Albumin. In patients with hypoalbuminemia the fraction unbound is increased. To allow use of total phenytoin concentrations and the usual therapeutic range of 10 to 20 mg/L in these patients, the observed concentration can be adjusted by using the following equation (derived from equation in reference 75):

$$C_{normal} = \frac{C_{observed}}{0.2 \cdot Alb + 0.1} \qquad \text{(Eq. 25-23)}$$

where $C_{observed}$ is the measured phenytoin concentration, Alb is the patient's albumin concentration in gm/dL, and C_{normal} is the phenytoin concentration that would have been observed if the patient's albumin concentration had been normal (4.4 gm/dL). This equation can be approximated by using the ratio of the normal value, 4.4 gm/dL, to the patient's serum albumin.

$$C_{normal} = C_{observed} \frac{4.4}{Alb \ (in \ gm/dL)} \qquad \text{(Eq. 25-24)}$$

Adjustment in Renal Disease. In patients with renal failure, it appears that the unbound fraction is increased approximately two- to threefold.[25,26] When the fraction unbound is doubled in a uremic patient, the expected therapeutic effect of a measured phenytoin concentration would be equivalent to that of an approximately doubled concentration. Alternatively, one could reduce the usual therapeutic range by one-half to a target or desired phenytoin concentration of 5 to 10 mg/L.

Plasma protein binding changes rapidly following a change in renal function. In patients who develop acute renal failure, the plasma protein binding is clearly decreased within a few days.[76] In patients with end-stage renal disease (ESRD), plasma protein binding appears to return to near normal within two days of a successful kidney transplant.[77]

Patients with moderately decreased renal function show a trend toward decreased plasma protein binding; however, as long as the creatinine clearance is greater than 25 mL/min, the changes are minimal and adjustment of the measured phenytoin concentration is probably not necessary. Patients with a creatinine clearance of 10 to 25 mL/min appear to be in a borderline range; in them a decrease in phenytoin binding is likely but is difficult to predict.[31] Some patients with creatinine clearances near 10 mL/min have relatively normal binding, while others with a creatinine clearance close to 20 mL/min have binding characteristics similar to patients with ESRD. This variability in binding should be kept in mind when evaluating phenytoin concentrations in patients with creatinine clearances in the range of 10 to 25 mL/min.

Many patients with ESRD (i.e., creatinine clearance of less than 10 mL/min) who are undergoing dialysis also have a low serum albumin. For this reason, it is frequently necessary to adjust the measured phenytoin concentration for both renal function and altered serum albumin.

In such patients, the following equation (adapted from reference 75) can be used to adjust the measured or observed phenytoin concentrations:

$$C_{normal\ binding} = \frac{C_{observed}}{0.1 \cdot Alb + 0.1} \qquad \text{(Eq. 25-25)}$$

where $C_{normal\ binding}$ is the phenytoin concentration one would expect to measure if protein binding were normal and $C_{observed}$ is the concentration observed or measured by the assay. The value which should be used when comparing the phenytoin concentration to the usual therapeutic range of 10 to 20 mg/L is $C_{normal\ binding}$.

Adjustment for Displacement by Other Drugs. Many of the drugs which have been shown to displace phenytoin from its albumin binding sites are weak acids, including phenylbutazone,[78] salicylic acid,[26] valproic acid,[79] and sulfisoxazole.[78] Displacement of phenytoin from albumin by such drugs in the clinical setting is difficult to predict because knowledge of not only the binding affinity, but also the displacing drug's concentration, is required. As a general rule, phenytoin displacement is unimportant unless the displacing drug is highly bound to serum albumin and is present in concentrations exceeding 25 mg/L.

In patients receiving phenytoin and valproic acid concurrently, the degree of displacement depends upon the time of sampling relative to the time of the last valproic acid dose. Obtaining samples just before the next valproic acid dose minimizes the problem of phenytoin displacement, as predose valproic acid concentrations are frequently about 25 mg/L. In most cases, data on affinity constants and concentration at the time of sampling of a displacer are seldom known. For these reasons, evaluation of phenytoin concentrations in the presence of a displacing drug usually requires an empiric approach, in which target concentration adjustments are made when an unusual relationship between concentration and patient response is encountered. Saliva and erythrocyte phenytoin concentrations have been suggested as a means to estimate the unbound plasma concentration.[42,80] Neither of these methods has been used extensively for routine patient care, possibly because of inconvenience in performing the erythrocyte drug concentration and the necessary calculations, or in the case of saliva concentrations, the variability from patient to patient in the ratio of free drug to salivary drug concentration.[34]

CLINICAL APPLICATION OF PHARMACOKINETIC DATA

Loading Dose

When phenytoin therapy is initiated, rapid achievement of therapeutic concentrations may be necessary. A loading dose (D_L) can be calculated using the following equation:

$$D_L = \frac{V\,(C_{desired} - C_{observed})}{S \cdot F}$$ (Eq. 25-26)

where $C_{desired}$ is the target concentration, $C_{observed}$ is the concentration before administration of the loading dose, V_d is the apparent volume of distribution, and F is the bioavailability, which is assumed to be 1. The salt form factor (S) is 0.92 for the sodium salt form and 1 for the acid form. If no phenytoin has been administered previously, $C_{observed}$ is assumed to be zero.

If the values of $C_{desired}$ and V_d are assumed to be 20 mg/L and 0.65 L/kg,[38,74] respectively, the loading dose for achieving 20 mg/L is approximately 14 mg/kg or 1000 mg for the average 70 kg patient.

If the loading dose is to be given by the intravenous route, it should be administered slowly to avoid the cardiac toxicities associated with the propylene glycol diluent.[18,74] If the loading dose is to be given orally, it should be divided and administered at two-hour intervals to avoid the gastrointestinal distress associated with large doses of phenytoin.[10,81] Following administration of an oral loading dose, the peak level does not occur for several hours, and it is substantially lower than the expected peak concentration following intravenous administration.[81,82] When large oral doses are administered, the peak level may not be achieved for 30 hours (see Table 25-3) and the observed concentration is usually about half of that estimated from Equation 25-26.[10,83] The lower concentration can be explained, in part, by metabolism of some of the absorbed drug. In addition, at the time of the peak following oral administration, not all of the dose has been absorbed.

To increase the peak concentration and decrease the time required to achieve the peak, large doses of phenytoin should be administered in divided doses of 200 to 400 mg every two to three hours. If rapid achievement of a therapeutic concentration is required, the intravenous route should be used. If a patient has a known or estimated phenytoin concentration before the administration of the loading dose, that value $(C_{observed})$ should be subtracted from the desired concentration $(C_{desired})$ and the adjusted loading dose calculated from Equation 25-26.

Confusion often arises about the need for a change in the loading dose when binding to albumin is altered. Little or no change is required because the volume of distribution and the therapeutic concentration range are inversely related. For example, when the serum albumin concentration is reduced, the volume of distribution is increased (see Equation 25-3) and the target concentration is decreased (see Equation 25-22) by virtually the same factor, resulting in little or no change in the loading dose, as calculated from Equation 25-26.

Maintenance Dose

Individualization of phenytoin dosage is difficult. Capacity-limited metabolism results in a relatively narrow therapeutic dosage range for each patient. The most commonly prescribed dosage is 300 mg/day, even though the majority of patients on this regimen appear to have phenytoin concentrations less than 10 mg/L.[64,84] This average maintenance dose may have been derived empirically since a high percentage of patients develop side effects or toxicities on 400 mg/day and a large number of adult patients are not therapeutically controlled on 200 mg/day (see Figure 25-1).

There have been reports that the drug may be administered once daily because of slow absorption characteristics following oral administration.[85] As stated previously, once-daily dosing should be reserved for Dilantin Kapseals at the present time. Even with Dilantin Kapseals, it would seem reasonable to administer the drug more frequently when the total daily dose exceeds 6 mg/kg.

When a patient varies significantly from the average weight of 70 kg, some adjustment in the customary daily maintenance dose of 300 mg is likely to be required. Frequently, 5 mg/kg/day is used to determine doses for small adult or pediatric patients. This approach tends to underdose these patients, in whom the measured phenytoin concentrations are usually lower than those seen in the adult population.[86,87]

The V_{max} for children appears to be in the range of 8 to 13 mg/kg/day.[54,55] Depending on the K_m value, phenytoin maintenance doses of 7 to 12 mg/kg/day would not be unusual. There are some data to suggest that pediatric patients tend to have a K_m value that is lower than that in the average adult.[52,54] Dosing patients with K_m values much lower than the therapeutic range tends to be difficult on a chronic basis. Here, the daily dose required to maintain steady-state concentration within the therapeutic range is very close to V_{max}, and small increases in daily dose result in markedly disproportionate increases in steady-state concentration.

Not all studies support the hypothesis that children have K_m values that are lower than the average adult.[55] It is possible that much of the current pediatric literature is biased towards patients with a low K_m.

Body surface area (BSA) or weight raised to a power of 0.6 to 0.7 has been used to adjust maintenance doses (D_M) of phenytoin:[54,88,89]

$$\frac{\text{Patient's } D_M}{\text{(in mg/day)}} = \left(\frac{\text{Usual Adult } D_M}{\text{(in mg/day)}} \right) \left(\frac{\text{Patient's BSA (in m}^2)}{1.73 \text{ m}^2} \right) \quad \text{(Eq. 25-27)}$$

and

$$\frac{\text{Patient's } D_M}{\text{(in mg/day)}} = \left(\frac{\text{Usual Adult } D_M}{\text{(in mg/day)}} \right) \left(\frac{\text{Patient's Weight (in kg) 0.7}}{70 \text{ kg}} \right) \quad \text{(Eq. 25-28)}$$

because weight to the 0.7 power is approximately proportional to body surface area.

When maintenance doses are calculated (see Equation 25-8) from a desired plasma concentration and assumed values for V_{max} and K_m, it should be recognized that the higher the selected steady-state concentration, the greater the chance of overshooting the desired concentration. For this reason, a steady-state concentration of 10 to 12 mg/L is probably a more reasonable target than 15 to 20 mg/L.

After selection and initiation of a maintenance dose, patients should be evaluated for efficacy and toxicity. In this evaluation it is important to remember that one to two weeks or longer may be required for steady state to be achieved.[8,56] Moreover, the higher a measured plasma concentration, the less likely that steady state has been achieved.

A patient's response is evaluated by recording seizure frequency, watching for adverse reactions, and obtaining phenytoin plasma concentrations. The maintenance dose can then be adjusted, but care should be taken to avoid manipulating the dose based on the plasma phenytoin concentration without considering the clinical response of the patient. Because of the capacity-limited metabolism, dose adjustments of less than 100 mg/day are frequently required, and adjustments of more than 100 mg/day should be undertaken with caution.

Plasma Concentration Monitoring and Dosage Adjustment

Data Collection. A complete evaluation of a plasma phenytoin concentration requires an accurate history of the phenytoin dosing regimen and the other drugs a patient is receiving, as well as pertinent laboratory data. Important laboratory data include serum creatinine, or a measurement of the creatinine clearance, and the serum albumin; these factors are associated with altered plasma protein binding. If renal failure or hypoalbuminemia is present, the measured phenytoin concentration will require adjustment (see Pharmacodynamics: Therapeutic Window). Additional laboratory data, such as serum bilirubin, liver enzymes, and prothrombin time, may give some indication of hepatic function. In severe chronic hepatic disease, a decreased ability to metabolize phenytoin is anticipated, as is diminished plasma protein binding. The latter is primarily a consequence of the hypoalbuminemia associated with chronic liver disease.

The sensitive relationship between daily dose and steady-state concentration of phenytoin makes even relatively slight modifications in either absorption or elimination clinically significant. Compliance and bioavailability are more critical than usual. Drugs such as chloramphenicol, isoniazid, diazoxide, disulfiram, and cimetidine have been shown to increase phenytoin concentrations.[64,90–92] As would be expected with capacity-limited metabolism, those patients with the highest initial phenytoin concentrations are likely to be the most affected.[93] The current data would suggest that there is little or no inhibition of phenytoin metabolism by ranitidine.[94] Carbamazepine and, occasionally, phenobarbital have been associated with a reduction in phenytoin concentration, presumably because of enzyme induction resulting in an increase in the maximum metabolic rate V_{max}.[64,90,95]

It has been well-documented that phenytoin concentrations are decreased in some patients when folic acid is added to their regimen.[96] Data indicate that the decrease in phenytoin concentration is due to a decrease in the K_m, with V_{max} being relatively unchanged.[97,98]

Serum phenytoin concentrations are decreased during pregnancy, presumably due to enzyme induction,[99,100] but diminished serum albumin may also contribute. Dosage requirements during pregnancy are difficult to predict, but an increase may be necessary to avoid the increased frequency of seizures observed in pregnant epileptic women.[100]

Care should be taken to identify any concurrent drug therapy that could be associated with plasma protein displacement (see Pharmacodynamics: Therapeutic Window).

The monitoring of ambulatory patients is particularly difficult because compliance is always difficult to assess. Even in a controlled environment, care should be taken to ensure that all doses are administered.

Time of Sampling. A strong case can be made for monitoring phenytoin concentrations in all patients. This is based on the difficulties encountered in estimating appropriate dosage regimens and distinguishing some of the central nervous system side effects of phenytoin from those of other anticonvulsant drugs or from symptoms of the disease state itself. At a minimum, patients who have not achieved optimal seizure control or who have developed symptoms consistent with phenytoin toxicity should have phenytoin concentrations measured.

The average steady-state concentration is important for determining the pharmacokinetic parameters V_{max} and K_m. It is also required when a nomogram is used to adjust the maintenance dose. When a patient has achieved steady state on an oral dosing regimen, the fluctuation in phenytoin concentration is relatively small. Thus, it makes little difference when a plasma sample is obtained, and it can be assumed that the trough concentration approximates the average concentration. The relative error in assuming the trough to be the average concentration is greater and potentially important when the drug is given once daily and the trough concentration is less than 5 mg/L or when the dose is more than 400 mg (5.7 mg/kg) per day.

If the drug is given by an intermittent short-term intravenous infusion, the average concentration at steady state (C_{ss}) can be estimated with the following equation:

$$C_{ss} = \frac{S \cdot F \cdot Dose}{2\ V_d} + Trough\ Concentration$$

(Eq. 25-29)

This equation assumes steady state has been achieved and that the average concentration is approximately halfway between the peak and trough concentrations. When Dilantin Kapseals are given orally, the average concentration may be approximated by the following equation:

$$C_{ss} = \frac{S \cdot F \cdot Dose}{4\ V_d} + Trough\ Concentration$$

(Eq. 25-30)

This approximation is based on the observation of a fluctuation at steady state following oral dosing is about half that observed with intravenous administration. In general, most patients receiving 300 mg of phenytoin orally, once daily, have an average concentration that is 1 to 2 mg/L higher than the trough. If given in divided doses, the fluctuation is negligible.

The time required to achieve steady state is often a critical question which can be answered by use of Equation 25-15. Frequently, however, the question is whether or not a measured phenytoin level is likely to be a steady-state value. In this case, Equation 25-16 can be used (see Clinical Pharmacokinetics: Time to Plateau). An alternative approach is to use the nomogram developed by Vozeh and Follath.[101]

Revision of Parameter Values

Estimation of V_{max} and K_m for phenytoin usually requires that steady state has been achieved and that the average concentration (C_{ss}) during a dosing interval is known or can be approximated. Changes in clinical status, rate or route of administration, or concurrent drug therapy, frequently preclude the assumption of steady state in the acute-care setting.

The long-term stabilities of V_{max} and K_m have not been studied. Judgment must be applied when using pharmacokinetics as an aid to phenytoin dose adjustment. In most cases, the calculated parameter and subsequent dose adjustments should be viewed as a "rational approach" rather than the "correct answer."

It should also be remembered that most approaches require normal plasma protein binding ($f_{up} = 0.1$). If abnormal binding is present, a correction should be made so that the adjusted concentration represents the total phenytoin concentration that would be observed if binding were normal (see Equations 25-23 and 25-25).

CASE HISTORIES

One Steady-State Level

Case History: 1a. *R.J., a 37-year-old, 70 kg male, has been receiving 300 mg of sodium phenytoin once daily at bedtime for several months. He has noted a decreased seizure frequency but still has one or more per week. He has no symptoms that might be associated with an elevated phenytoin concentration. His serum albumin and renal function are normal, as are his liver function tests. He is receiving no other medications. A steady-state phenytoin concentration of 8 mg/L was obtained. What maintenance dose of phenytoin would be appropriate for achieving a steady-state concentration of 15 mg/L?*

There are a number of approaches that can be used to solve this problem; all of them, however, require certain assumptions.

Method A. Equation 25-12 can be used to calculate V_{max}, if the value of K_m is assumed or known. In this equation, the phenytoin dose and V_{max} are in units of mg/day and K_m and C_{ss} are in mg/L. Using the average value of 4 mg/L for K_m, the estimated value of V_{max} would be:

$$V_m = (0.92)(1)(300 \text{ mg/day}) + 4 \text{ mg/mL} \left[\frac{(0.92)(1)(300 \text{ mg/day})}{8 \text{ mg/mL}} \right] = 414 \text{ mg/day}$$

(Eq. 25-31)

With the estimates of V_{max} and K_m, a new maintenance dosing rate can be calculated using Equation 25-8.

$$R = \frac{V_{max} \cdot C_{SS}}{S \cdot F [K_m + C_{SS}]} = \frac{326 \text{ mg/day}}{S \cdot F}$$

(Eq. 25-32)

Note that this maintenance dose of 326 mg/day of phenytoin acid (chewable tablets or suspension) is equivalent to 355 mg/day of sodium phenytoin (capsules or injectable).

Adjustment of the maintenance dose to this specific calculated value would be inappropriate, as the values of K_m are V_{max} are only estimates. The most reasonable dose to administer is approximated with 300 and 400 mg on alternate days. Taking a more conservative approach, a K_m value below 4 mg/L could have been selected. The calculated maintenance dose to achieve 15 mg/L would then have been less than 326 mg/day.

Because some time may be required to achieve steady state on the new maintenance dose of 350 mg/day, it may be desirable to administer a small loading dose (D_L) to increase the present level of 8 mg/L rapidly to a desired target concentration. This can be accomplished using Equation 25-26.

$$D_L = \frac{(0.65 \text{ L/kg})(70 \text{ kg})(15 \text{ mg/L} - 8 \text{ mg/L})}{(0.92)(1)}$$

$$D_L = 345 \text{ or } 350 \text{ mg}$$

(Eq. 25-33)

It is important to remember that oral absorption is slow and the target level of 15 mg/L may not be achieved when the loading dose is given orally. The IV route would be used only if rapid attainment of the new level were critical. The loading dose is used in addition to the new maintenance dose, so that the total dose for that day would be 700 mg.

Method B: "Orbit Graph." An alternative method is shown in Figure 25-11. This method allows estimation of the most probable values of V_{max} and K_m for the individual patient, based upon information previously obtained in a patient population. If the procedure outlined in Figure 25-11 is followed, the most probable estimates of V_{max} and K_m are 6.4 mg/day/kg (451 mg/day/70 kg) and 5 mg/L, respectively. A new maintenance dose can be determined using Equation 25-4 or Figure 25-11. For this case, 4.7 mg/day/kg or 364 mg/day/70 kg of sodium phenytoin is obtained. Again, a daily dose of 350 mg (300 and 400 mg on alternate days) of sodium phenytoin would probably be prescribed because of convenience and the uncertainty that exactly 364 mg/day is required.

In addition to methods A and B there is a nomogram that can be used to adjust phenytoin doses.[103] The nomogram is similar to the first approach, in that the author has selected a representative K_m value. In general, the nomogram approach is reasonably satisfactory, but it does not allow the clinician to adjust the K_m value. If a more conservative dose adjustment is desired, a lower steady-state phenytoin concentration can be selected.

Two or More Steady-State Observations

Dose adjustments based on two or more steady-state levels are more likely to yield accurate and patient-specific data. Caution should still be exercised in assuring that, for both levels, protein binding is normal, steady state is achieved, and there is patient compliance.

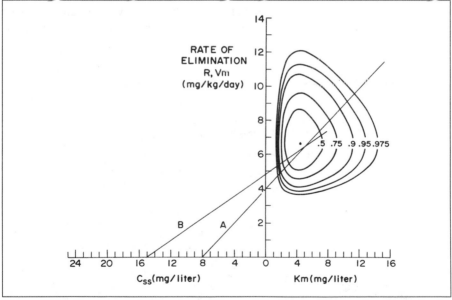

Figure 25-11. *The most probable values of V_{max} and K_m for a patient may be estimated using a single steady-state phenytoin concentration and a known dosing regimen. The eccentric circles or "orbits" represent the fraction of the sample patient population whose K_m and V_{max} values are within that orbit. Use of graph: 1. Plot the daily dose of phenytoin (mg/day/kg) on the vertical line (rate of elimination). 2. Plot the steady-state concentration (C_{ss}) on the horizontal line. 3. Draw a straight line connecting C_{ss} and daily dose through the orbits (line A). 4. The coordinates of the midpoint of the line crossing the innermost orbit through which the line passes are the most probable values for the patient's V_{max} and K_m. 5. To calculate a new maintenance dose, draw a line from the point determined in step 4 to the new desired C_{ss} (line B). The point at which line B crosses the vertical line (rate of elimination) is the new maintenance dose (mg/day/kg). The line A represents a C_{ss} of 8 mg/L on 276 mg/day of phenytoin acid (300 mg/day of sodium phenytoin) for a 70 kg patient. Line B was drawn assuming the new desired C_{ss} was 15 mg/L. The original figure (from reference 102) is modified so that R (equivalent to R_{in}) and V_{max} are in mg/day/kg of phenytoin acid.*

Case History: 1b. *The daily dose of 300 mg (previous C_{ss} of 8 mg/L) was increased to 350 mg/day (sodium phenytoin). Two months later, R.J. returned to the clinic with excellent seizure control, but complained of an inability to concentrate. A phenytoin concentration was obtained and reported to be 20 mg/L. How should his dosage be adjusted to achieve a phenytoin concentration of 14 mg/L?*

Method C. Figure 25-12 demonstrates a method for multiple steady-state phenytoin concentrations.[104] The values for V_{max} and K_m, satisfying both observations, are 5.6 mg/day/kg (392 mg/day/70 kg) and 2.5 mg/L. Substituting these parameter values into Equation 25-8 yields a new maintenance dose of 333 mg, to obtain a steady-state concentration of 14 mg/L. Using the alternative approach of constructing line B gives the same value, 4.8 mg/day/kg, for the maintenance dose.

Although a daily dose of 333 mg is not convenient, the two steady-state values indicate the need for a fine dosage adjustment to achieve a target concentration of 14 mg/L. If 325 mg were prescribed, the expected C_{ss} would be about 12 mg/L as calculated from Equation 25-9.

Note that R and V_{max} are in the units of the salt form. In this case, a plot of the daily doses of sodium phenytoin yielded a V_{max} of 392 mg/day of sodium phenytoin per 70 kg. If the daily doses were converted to phenytoin acid, the V_{max} would be

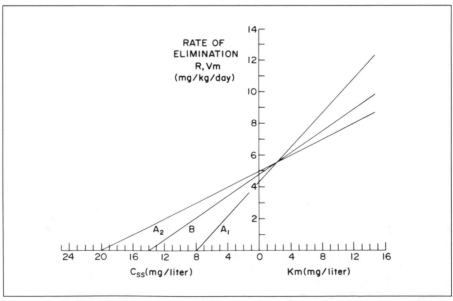

Figure 25-12. *Determination of V_{max} and K_m values for a patient for whom phenytoin C_{ss} on two or more dosing regimens are known. Use of graph: 1. Draw lines A_1 and A_2 using steps 1 through 3 in Figure 25-11 for two separate dosing regimens and corresponding C_{ss}. The points of intersection for lines A_1 and A_2 are the coordinates for V_{max} and K_m of the patient. 2. Draw a line from the point of intersection to the desired C_{ss} (line B) to estimate the required dosage rate (mg/day/kg). This rate is where line B crosses the vertical line (rate of elimination). Line A_1 represents a C_{ss} of 8 mg/L on 300 mg/day, and line A_2 represents a C_{ss} of 20 mg/L on 350 mg/day for a 70 kg patient. Line B was drawn assuming the new desired C_{ss} was 14 mg/L.*

92% of the value above. In both cases the K_m value is 2.5 mg/L. Both administration rates must represent either the acid or sodium salt, and the salt form should be considered when calculating new dosing regimens.

If more than two dosing regimens and corresponding steady-state concentrations are obtained and plotted on Figure 25-12, multiple points of intersections are likely. These discrepancies may be the result of assay error, noncompliance, changes in the pharmacokinetic parameters, or the use of concentrations which are not truly at steady state.

Method D. Figure 25-13 shows another approach for obtaining information from two or more steady-state levels. The method involves plotting the daily maintenance dose of phenytoin (R_{in}) versus the phenytoin clearance [daily maintenance dose divided by the steady-state concentration (R_{in}/C_{ss})].[46,47,51]

By calculation, the values of R/C_{ss} for the daily doses of 300 mg and 350 mg are 37.5 L/day and 17.5 L/day, respectively. When the daily doses are plotted versus these values on Figure 25-13, a V_{max} of 390 mg/day is obtained. A value of 2.5 mg/L for K_m is obtained from the slope of the line. Using the V_{max} and K_m values derived from Figure 25-13, a new dosing regimen of 331 mg/day can be calculated

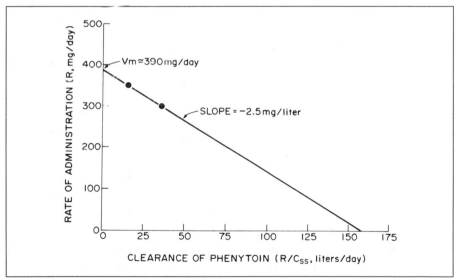

Figure 25-13. *An alternative method for determination of* V_{max} *and* K_m *values from steady-state concentrations on two or more dosing regimens. Use of graph: 1. Plot the rate of administration (mg/day) versus clearance of phenytoin (L/day) for two or more steady-state concentrations. 2. Draw a straight line of best fit through the points plotted. The intercept on the rate of administration axis is* V_{max} *(mg/day), and the slope of the line (where* R_1 *and* R_2 *are the respective dosing rates)*

$$\frac{R_1 - R_2}{\dfrac{R_1}{C_{ss_1}} - \dfrac{R_2}{C_{ss_2}}}$$

is the negative value of K_m.

from Equation 25-8 to achieve a steady-state concentration of 14 mg/L. As in method C, the units of V_{max} are consistent with the dose administered, and adjustments should be made if the alternative dosage form is used (i.e., sodium phenytoin versus phenytoin acid).

The approaches used in Methods C and D are essentially the same; any differences in the estimates of the pharmacokinetic parameters or dosing regimens are due to errors in plotting or interpreting the data. If more than two steady-state concentrations are obtained, the line of best fit should be used to approximate the parameter values.

Non-Steady-State Observations

Non-steady-state concentrations of phenytoin are difficult to evaluate, and in most cases it is not possible to derive pharmacokinetic parameters (V_{max}, K_m) accurately when phenytoin concentrations are changing with time. One exception to this rule is when a high phenytoin concentration is allowed to decline with no additional doses being given. In this case, the decline in concentration depends on the amount metabolized each day and the volume of distribution. For example, consider a patient whose phenytoin concentration of 50 mg/L decreases by 10 mg/L each day (i.e., 50 mg/L on day one, 40 mg/L on day two, and 30 mg/L on day three). Assuming that the concentrations of 50 to 30 mg/L were well above K_m, the amount of phenytoin metabolized per day is close to the value of V_{max}, and, using the value of 50 liters for V_d, the amount metabolized is 500 mg/day (50 L $\times$ 10 mg/L/day). The accuracy of this method depends on the errors in the concentration difference and in the value assumed for the volume of distribution. Also of importance is whether or not absorption is essentially complete by the time the first observation (50 mg/L) is made. If absorption continues into the observed decay phase, V_{max} is underestimated. As has been pointed out earlier, large oral doses of phenytoin may continue to be absorbed for prolonged periods of time. In patients who accidentally or intentionally become overdosed, absorption can continue for several days, even when no further drug is administered.[105,106] When absorption continues, the value of V_{max} is underestimated because actual rate of drug elimination is greater than calculated.

In the clinical setting, K_m can seldom be accurately estimated from a phenytoin decay curve as concentrations above and below K_m are needed. Most patients have K_m values that are below the therapeutic range,[45,46,51] and a maintenance dose is usually reinstituted before concentrations below K_m are achieved.

A more complex situation is one in which phenytoin concentrations are rising or falling toward steady state while the patient receives a fixed daily dose.

Case History 2. *Now consider L.S., a 70 kg patient who received 400 mg/day (suspension) following a loading dose which achieved an initial concentration of 10 mg/L. Nine days later L.S. had a phenytoin level of 20 mg/L. Is the level of 20 mg/L likely to be a steady-state value? What dose is required to maintain a level between 10 and 20 mg/L?*

The first question can be answered by using Equation 25-16.

$$t_{90\%} = \frac{[115 + 35 \ (20)] \ [(20)]}{(0.92) \ (1) \ (400)}$$

$$t_{90\%} = 44 \text{ days}$$

Since L.S. has been receiving the maintenance dose for less than 44 days, the level of 20 mg/L is not likely to represent steady state. Although L.S. had an initial level of 10 mg/L, the time required to achieve that level on 400 mg/day is only a small proportion of the 44 days.

The second question can be answered by considering how much phenytoin had been administered and the apparent change (Δ) in the amount in the body over the nine days.

$$R_{in} - \frac{\Delta \ (\text{Amount in Body})}{t} = \frac{\text{Amount Eliminated}}{t} \qquad \text{(Eq. 25-34)}$$

Note that phenytoin is at steady state when there is no change in the amount in the body. If we substitute the change-in-concentration times the volume of distribution, $[(C_2 - C_1) \ V_d]$ for the change in the amount in the body, we have:

$$R_{in} - \left[\frac{(C_2 - C_1) \ (V_d)}{t} \right] = \frac{\text{Amount Eliminated}}{t} \qquad \text{(Eq. 25-35)}$$

Based on the patient's daily dose and the measured levels, the amount eliminated per day is:

$$400 \text{ mg/day} - \left[\frac{(20 \text{ mg/L} - 10 \text{ mg/L} \ (45 \cdot 5 \text{ L})}{9 \text{ days}} \right] = 350 \text{ mg/day} \qquad \text{(Eq. 25-36)}$$

Because 350 mg/day was the average rate of elimination when the phenytoin level rose from 10 to 20 mg/L, a daily replacement dose of about 350 mg should result in steady-state levels somewhere between 10 and 20 mg/L. Because of potential assay errors and the uncertainty in the volume of distribution estimate, this maintenance dose may require future adjustments.

This approach is most reliable when the actual amount of drug absorbed is known, the change in concentration is small, and the time interval is optimal. As a general guideline, the phenytoin concentration should not be more than doubled if it is increasing nor less than halved if it is declining. Although the optimal time interval is difficult to define, it should be at least two to three days, but not so long that C_2 approaches the new steady state. If the desired concentration is greater or less than the measured concentrations, V_{max} can be approximated by substituting into Equation 25-12 a plausible value for K_m, the average of C_1 and C_2 for C_{ss} and the calculated value of amount eliminated/t for $S \times F \times R$. A new maintenance dose to achieve the desired C_{ss} can then be approximated by using the new value of V_{max} and the assumed value of K_m in Equation 25-8.

Pediatric Case

Case History 3. *V.B. is a 30 kg, 8-year-old child with uncontrolled grand mal seizures. A steady-state phenytoin concentration of 5 mg/L was measured follow-ing long-term therapy with 150 mg/day of phenytoin as the chewable tablets in three divided doses. What would be a reasonable dose to achieve a new steady-state level of 10 mg/L?*

There are few pharmacokinetic aids available for pediatric dosing of phenytoin. The orbit graph, Figure 25-11, is not appropriate. The R, V_{max} scale is in mg/kg and does not represent the pediatric population. The most reasonable approach is to use Method A (see Case History 1a), which assumes an average value for K_m. The difficulty lies in what should be chosen as the average K_m. For purposes of illustration, we will use a conservatively low value of 2 mg/L.

Equation 25-12 indicates that V_{max} for V.B. is 210 mg/day.

$$V_{max} = 1 \cdot 1 \cdot 150 + \left[(2) \left(\frac{1 \cdot 1 \cdot 150}{5} \right) \right]$$

$$V_{max} = 150 + 60$$

$$V_{max} = 210 \text{ mg/day}$$

Based on this value and the assumed value of K_m, 2 mg/L, the maintenance dose required to achieve a steady-state level of 10 mg/L is 175 mg/day of phenytoin acid [or 190 mg of sodium phenytoin (see Equation 25-8)]:

$$R_{in} = \frac{(210 \text{ mg/day}) (10 \text{ mg/L})}{2 \text{ mg/L} + 10 \text{ mg/L}}$$

$$\frac{\text{Dose}}{\tau} = \frac{175 \text{ mg/day}}{S \cdot F}$$

$$\frac{\text{Dose}}{\tau} \text{ of Phenytoin Acid} = \frac{175}{(1)(1)}$$

$$= 175 \text{ mg/day}$$

$$\frac{\text{Dose}}{\tau} \text{ of Sodium Phenytoin} = \frac{175}{(0.92)(1)}$$

$$= 190 \text{ mg/day}$$

Figure 25-14 is an algorithm summarizing the principal steps in monitoring phenytoin therapy. Both the pharmacologic effects (therapeutic and toxic) and the plasma phenytoin concentrations are considered. When an adjustment in dosage is required, pharmacokinetic analysis is helpful for estimating the values of V_{max} and K_m in an individual patient.

ANALYTICAL METHODS

Phenytoin has been analyzed using spectrophotometric, colorimetric (with derivation), gas chromatographic, high-performance liquid chromatographic and immunologic methods. Examples are given in Table 25-7. High-performance liquid chromatography and immunologic methods are the most common procedures for routine clinical monitoring.

The immunologic methods include enzyme immunoassay [enzyme multiplied immunoassay technique (EMIT) and enzyme-linked immunosorbent assay (ELISA)], substrate-labeled fluorescent immunoassay (SLIFA), fluorescence polarization immunoassay (FPIA), apoenzyme reactive immunoassay system (ARIS), and enzyme immunochromatography (ACCULEVEL).[107]

The immunologic methods are generally specific; however, cross-reactivity with compounds similar to phenytoin can occur. In patients with uremia there have been reports of phenytoin levels being substantially higher when measured by the EMIT procedure than when determined by GLC or HPLC procedures,[108] presumably because of accumulation of phenytoin metabolites. Interference by metabolites has been shown to be essentially eliminated in the fluorescence polarization immunoassay.[109,110]

Both chromatographic and immunologic techniques can be accurately performed with coefficients of variation of less than 10% at concentrations within the therapeutic range. They are, in general, specific and sensitive to a concentration of 1 mg/L or less. Unfortunately, these assays have been shown[111,112] to be improperly handled in many laboratories in the past. Inadequate attention to quality control was probably in large part responsible for the wide interlaboratory variability reported.[111]

The user of plasma phenytoin concentrations must be cognizant of assay error when interpreting measured values. An allowance of $\pm$ 10% is often in order. For example, a measured value of 20 mg/L can be considered to be 18 to 22 mg/L. Calculations of the pharmacokinetic parameters V_{max} and K_m for these limits permit dosages to be adjusted based on the more conservative estimate.

PROSPECTUS

There are a number of areas of research and technical development that need to be addressed to improve therapy with phenytoin. Protein binding is one such area. Theoretically, the unbound concentration in plasma is preferred over the total plasma concentration, but such measurements are not routinely performed clinically. The usefulness of the unbound concentration needs to be evaluated with respect to the additional cost of obtaining it. Research is needed to better define the conditions for which the additional measurement is indicated, and to develop a practical means to increase accuracy and decrease the cost of determining the unbound concentration.

A major area requiring attention, and perhaps requiring new approaches for data treatment, is the stability of the values of V_{max}, K_m, and V_d with time. There is a general perception that the intrasubject values of these parameters remain constant. We know that a number of factors influence phenytoin absorption and disposition, but how the values change with time within an individual needs further examina-

Table 25-7. *Comparison of the Relative Advantages and Disadvantages of the Various Plasma Phenytoin Assay Methods*[a]

Analytical method[b]	Specificity for phenytoin	Limit of sensitivity	Metabolite analysis	Minimum sample volume required for plasma/serum (mL)	Analysis time	Analysis costs			Comments
						Estimated reagent costs	Tech. cost per assay	Initial equipment cost	
HPLC	1	1	c	0.2	2	2	3	3	Requires high-level of practical skills.
GC									
On column methylation	1	1	c	0.5	2	2	3	3	Method used in much of older literature.
Pre-column methylation	1	1	c	0.5	3	2	3	3	
EMIT	2	1	—	0.2	1	4	1	2	Rapid, minimal training required.
FPIA	2	1	—	0.2	1	4	1	2	Rapid, automated, minimal training required.

[a] Arbitrary Ranking Scale of 1 (excellent / a lot) to 5 (poor/very little) with a score of 3 being average or nominal.

[b] HPLC = High performance liquid chromatography; GC = Gas chromatography; EMIT = Enzyme immunoassay; FPIA = Fluorescence polarization immunoassay.

[c] Hydrolysis and separate assay required.

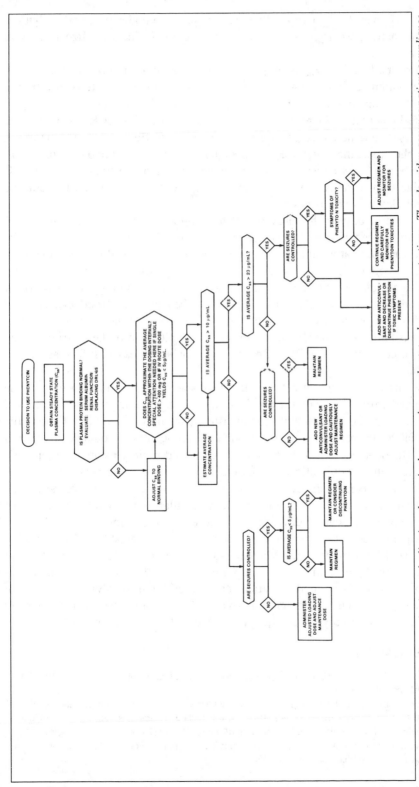

Figure 25-14. Algorithm for monitoring and adjusting phenytoin therapy using steady-state plasma concentrations. The algorithm assumes patient compliance, achievement of steady state, constant bioavailability, no change in the patient's clinical condition (e.g., renal function), and no other drug therapy. It can be used to monitor additional steady-state concentrations obtained subsequent to a dose adjustment or monitoring period.

tion. As we identify the temporal changes in phenytoin absorption, distribution, and elimination, we may be able to more accurately individualize phenytoin therapy.

In enzyme kinetics, V_{max} is proportional to the amount of enzyme present and K_m is a parameter indicating the concentration at which the rate of reaction is one-half the maximum value. Applying this model *in vivo*, one would expect enzyme induction to increase V_{max}, but to have no effect on K_m. Competitive inhibitors should increase the value of K_m, but have no effect on V_{max}. Furthermore, one might expect the value of K_m (especially if based on the unbound concentration) to be relatively constant because it depends on a property of the enzyme. If the value truly varies as much as current data treatments indicate, it would be helpful to know why this is so.

We are now only at the threshold of learning about the pharmacokinetics of phenytoin in pediatric and geriatric populations. This is particularly true for neonates and premature infants. Although this information is difficult to obtain, it has the potential to greatly assist in adjusting dosage for these patients. Another area that needs work is that of the absorption of phenytoin in a variety of gastrointestinal diseases. Phenytoin is known to be slowly absorbed, especially in large doses as previously noted in healthy volunteers. Whenever the gastrointestinal transit time is shortened, or in conditions in which part of the gastrointestinal tract is resected, bioavailability of phenytoin may be decreased. Information here is lacking.

The current approach of establishing a satisfactory phenytoin regimen is one of trial and error. Even with the application of the nonlinear principles discussed in this chapter, several concentration measurements may be required. Frequently, the initial dosage regimen results in a phenytoin concentration outside the desired range. The development of a method which would rapidly establish a patient's parameter values would allow for optimal maintenance dosage early in therapy. There are a number of approaches, ranging from intensive evaluation of the decline of a plasma concentration and metabolite accumulation to the administration of stable isotopes, that can be developed to resolve this problem.

The pharmacokinetic behavior of phenytoin is well established and readily summarized by a model with Michaelis-Menten elimination. We now need to develop clinical tools and educational programs that will allow the kinetic principles to be routinely applied to patient care. In addition, resolving some of the uncertainty in the characterization and variability of patient-specific parameters will improve our ability to use phenytoin effectively in the clinical setting.

REFERENCES

1. Koch-Weser. The serum level approach to individualization of drug dosage. Eur J Clin Pharmacol. 1975;9:1–8.
2. Lund L. Effects of phenytoin in patients with epilepsy in relation to its concentration in plasma. In: David DS, Prichard BNC, eds. Biological Effects of Drugs in Relation to Their Concentration in Plasma. Baltimore: University Park Press; 1972;227–39.
3. Neuvonen PJ. Bioavailability of phenytoin; clinical pharmacokinetic and therapeutic implications. Clin Pharmacokinet. 1979;4:91–103.

4. Gugler R et al. Phenytoin: pharmacokinetics and bioavailability. Clin Pharmacol Ther. 1976;19:135–42.
5. Jusko WJ et al. Nonlinear assessment of phenytoin bioavailability. J Pharmacokinet Biopharm. 1976;4:327–36.
6. Sawchuck RJ et al. Rapid and slow release phenytoin in epileptic patients at steady state: Assessment of relative bioavailability utilizing Michaelis-Menten parameters. J Pharmacokinet Biopharm. 1982;10:383–91.
7. Dill WA et al. Studies on 5, 5-diphenylhydantoin (Dilantin) in animals and man. J Pharmacol Exp Ther. 1956;118:270–79.
8. Food and Drug Administration New prescribing directions for phenytoin. FDA Drug Bull. 1978;8:27–8.
9. Sawchuck RJ, Rector TS. Steady-state plasma concentrations as a function of the absorption rate and dosing interval for drugs exhibiting concentration-dependent clearance: consequences for phenytoin therapy. J Pharmacokinet Biopharm. 1979;7:543–55.
10. Jung D et al. Effect of dose on phenytoin absorption. Clin Pharmacol Ther. 1980;28:479–85.
11. McCauley DL et al. Time for phenytoin concentration to peak: consequences of first-order or zero-order absorption. Ther Drug Monitor. 1989;11:540.–42
12. Bauer LA. Interference of oral phenytoin absorption by continuous nasogastric feedings. Neurology (NY). 1982;32:570–72.
13. Bauman JL et al. Phenytoin crystallization in intravenous fluids. Drug Intell Clin Pharm. 1977;11:646–49.
14. Kostenbauder HB et al. Bioavailability and single-dose pharmacokinetics of intramuscular phenytoin. Clin Pharmacol Ther. 1975;18:449–56.
15. Wilder BJ et al. A method for shifting from oral to intramuscular diphenylhydantoin administration. Clin Pharmacol Ther. 1974;16:507–13.
16. Serrano EE, Wilder BJ. Intramuscular administration of diphenylhydantoin. Histologic follow up. Arch Neurol. 1974;31:276–78.
17. Suzuki T et al. Kinetics of diphenylhydantoin disposition in man. Chem Pharm Bull. 1970;18:405–11.
18. Bigger T et al. Relationship between the plasma level of diphenylhydantoin sodium and its cardiac antiarrhythmic effects. Circulation. 1968;38:363–74.
19. Vajda F et al. Human brain cerebrospinal fluid, and plasma concentrations of diphenylhydantoin and phenobarbital. Clin Pharmacol Ther. 1974;15:597–603.
20. Wilder BJ et al. Efficacy of intravenous phenytoin in the treatment of status epilepticus; kinetics of central nervous system penetration. Ann Neurol. 1977;1:511–18.
21. Sironi VA et al. Antiepileptic drug distribution in cerebral cortex, Ammon's horn, and amygdala in man. J Neurosurg. 1980;52:686–92.
22. Goldberg MA. Phenytoin: binding. Adv Neurol. 1980;27:323–37.
23. Shoeman DW, Azarnoff DL. The alteration of plasma proteins in uremia as reflected in their ability to bind digitoxin and diphenylhydantoin. Pharmacology. 1971;7:169–77.
24. Tozer TN. Implication of altered plasma protein binding in disease states. In: Benet LZ et al., eds. Pharmacokinetic Basis for Drug Treatment. New York: Raven Press; 1984.
25. Odar-Cederlof I, Borga O. Kinetics of diphenylhydantoin in uremic patients: consequences of decreased plasma protein binding. Eur J Clin Pharmacol. 1974;7:31–7.
26. Odar-Cederlof I, Borga O. Impaired protein binding of phenytoin in uremia and displacement effects of salicylic acid. Clin Pharmacol Ther. 1976;20:36–47.
27. Odar-Cederlof I. Plasma binding of phenytoin and warfarin in patients undergoing renal transplantation. Clin Pharmacokinet. 1977;2:147–53.
28. Suoholm I et al. Protein binding of drugs in uremia and normal serum: The role of endogenous binding inhibitors. Biochem Pharmacol. 1976;25:1205–213.
29. Boobis SW. Alteration of plasma albumin in relation to decreased drug binding in uremia. Clin Pharmacol Ther. 1977;22:147–53.
30. Hooper WD et al. Plasma protein binding of diphenylhydantoin. Effects of sex hormones, renal, and hepatic disease. Clin Pharmacol Ther. 1974;15:276–82.

31. Liponi DL et al. Renal function and therapeutic concentrations of phenytoin. Neurology. 1984;34:395–97.
32. Wallace S, Brodie MJ. Decreased drug binding in serum from patients with chronic hepatic disease. Eur J Clin Pharmacol. 1976;9:429–32.
33. Bochner F et al. Diphenylhydantoin concentrations in saliva. Arch Neurol (Chicago). 1974;31:57–9.
34. Reynolds F et al. Salivary phenytoin concentrations in epilepsy and in chronic renal failure. Lancet. 1976;2:384–86.
35. Paxton JW et al. Phenytoin concentrations in mixed parotid and submandibular saliva and serum measured by radioimmunoassay. Br J Clin Pharmacol. 1977;4:185–92.
36. Glazko AJ. Antiepileptic drugs: biotransformation, metabolism, and serum half-life. Epilepsia. 1975;16:367–91.
37. Witkin KM et al. Determination of 5-(hydroxyphenyl)-5-phenylhydantoin and studies relating to the disposition of phenytoin in man. Ther Drug Monit. 1979;1:11–34.
38. Glasko AJ et al. Metabolic disposition of diphenylhydantoin in normal human subjects following intravenous administration. Clin Pharmacol Ther. 1969;10:498–504.
39. Maguire JH et al. Absolute configurations of the dihydrodiol metabolites of 5,5-diphenylhydantoin (phenytoin) from rat, dog, and human urine. Drug Metab Dispos. 1980;8:325–31.
40. Butler TC et al. Studies of the metabolism of 5,5-diphenylhydantoin relating principally to the stereoselectivity of the hydroxylation reactions in man and the dog. J Pharmacol Exp Ther. 1976;199:82–92.
41. Arnold K, Gerber N. The rate of decline of diphenylhydantoin in human plasma. Clin Pharmacol Ther. 1970;11:121–34.
42. Richens A, Dunlop A. Serum phenytoin levels in the management of epilepsy. Lancet. 1975;2:247–48.
43. Eadie MJ et al. The elimination of phenytoin in man. Clin Exp Pharmacol Physiol. 1976;3:217–24.
44. Houghton GW et al. Effect of age, height, weight, and sex on serum phenytoin concentration in epileptic patients. Br J Clin Pharmacol. 1975;2:251–56.
45. Mawer GE et al. Phenytoin dose adjustment in epileptic patients. Br J Pharmacol. 1974;1:163–68.
46. Ludden TM et al. Individualization of phenytoin dosage regimens. Clin Pharmacol Ther. 1977;21:287–93.
47. Martin E et al. The clinical pharmacokinetics of phenytoin. J Pharmacokinet Biopharm. 1977;5:579–96.
48. Allen JP et al. Phenytoin cumulation kinetics. Clin Pharmacol Ther. 1979;26:445–48.
49. Gerber N, Wagner JG. Explanation of dose-dependent decline of diphenylhydantoin plasma levels by fitting to the integrated form of the Michaelis-Menten equation. Res Commun Chem Pathol Pharmacol. 1972;3:455–66.
50. Vozeh S et al. Predicting individual phenytoin dosage. J Pharmacokinet Biopharm. 1981;9:131–46.
51. Lambie DG et al. Therapeutic and pharmacokinetic effects of increasing phenytoin in chronic epileptics on multiple drug therapy. Lancet. 1976;2:386–89.
52. Garrettson LK, Jusko WJ. Diphenylhydantoin elimination kinetics in overdosed children. Clin Pharmacol Ther. 1975;17:481–91.
53. Chiba K et al. Michaelis-Menten pharmacokinetics of diphenylhydantoin and application in the pediatric age patient. J Pediatr. 1980;96:479–84.
54. Grasela TH et al. Steady-state pharmacokinetics of phenytoin from routinely collected patient data. Clin Pharmacokinet. 1983;8:355–64.
55. Bauer LA, Blouin RA. Phenytoin Michaelis-Menten pharmacokinetics in Caucasian pediatric patients. Clin Pharmacokinet. 1983;8:545–49.
56. Ludden TM et al. Rate of phenytoin accumulation in man: a simulation study. J Pharmacokinet Biopharm. 1978;6:399–415.
57. Wagner JG. Time to reach steady state and prediction of steady-state concentrations for drugs obeying Michaelis-Menten elimination kinetics. J Pharmacokinet Biopharm. 1978;6:209–25.
58. Karlen B et al. Assay of diphenylhydantoin (phenytoin) metabolites in urine by gas chromatography. Metabolite pattern in humans. Eur J Clin Pharmacol. 1975;8:359–63.

59. Bochner F et al. The renal handling of diphenylhydantoin and 5-(p-hydroxyphenyl) 5-phenylhydantoin. Clin Pharmacol Ther. 1973;14:791–96.

60. Kutt H et al. Some causes of ineffectiveness of diphenylhydantoin. Arch Neurol. 1966;14:489–92.

61. Martin E et al. Removal of phenytoin by hemodialysis in uremic patients. JAMA. 1977;238:1750–753.

62. Pond S et al. Pharmacokinetics of hemoperfusion for drug overdose. Clin Pharmacokinet. 1979;4:329–54.

63. Liu E, Rubenstein M. Phenytoin removal by plasmapheresis in thrombotic thrombocytopenic purpura. Clin Pharmacol Ther. 1982;31:762–65.

64. Lund L. Anticonvulsant effects of diphenylhydantoin relative to plasma levels: an prospective three year study in ambulant patients with generalized epileptic seizures. Arch Neurol. 1974;31:289–94.

65. Vajda FJE et al. The possible effects of long-term high plasma levels of phenytoin on mortality after acute myocardial infarction. Eur J Clin Pharmacol. 1973;5:138–44.

66. Buchthal F et al. Clinical and electroencephalographic correlations with serum levels of diphenylhydantoin. Arch Neurol. 1960;2:624–30.

67. Lascelles PT et al. The distribution of plasma phenytoin levels in epileptic patients. J Neurol Neurosurg Psychiatry. 1970;33:501–5.

68. Reynolds EH et al. Phenytoin monotherapy for epilepsy: a long-term prospective study, assisted by serum level monitoring, in previously untreated patients. Epilepsia. 1981;22:485–88.

69. Kutt H et al. Diphenylhydantoin metabolism, blood levels and toxicity. Arch Neurol. 1964;11:642–48.

70. Ahmand S et al. Involuntary movements caused by phenytoin intoxication in epileptic patients. J Neurol Neurosurg Psychiatry. 1975;38:225–31.

71. Levy L, Fenichel GM. Diphenylhydantoin activated seizures. Neurol. 1969;15:716–22.

72. Shuttleworth E et al. Choreoathetosis and diphenylhydantoin intoxication. JAMA. 1974;230:1179–181.

73. Chalhub EG et al. Phenytoin-induced dystonia and choreoathetosis in two retarded epileptic children. Neurol. 1975;26:494–98.

74. Louis S et al. The cardiovascular changes caused by intravenous Dilantin and its solvent. Am Heart J. 1967;74:523–29.

75. Sheiner LB, Tozer TN. Clinical pharmacokinetics: The use of plasma concentrations of drugs. In: Melmon KL, Morrelli HF, eds. Clinical Pharmacology: Basic Principles in Therapeutics. New York: MacMillan; 1978;71–109.

76. Andreasen F, Jakobsen P. Determination of furosemide in blood and its binding to proteins in normal plasma and in plasma from patients with acute renal failure. Acta Pharmacol Toxicol. 1974;35:49–57.

77. Levy G et al. Effect of renal transplantation on protein binding of drugs in serum of donor and recipient. Clin Pharmacol Ther. 1976;20:512–16.

78. Lunde PKM et al. Plasma protein binding of diphenylhydantoin in man: Interactions with other drugs and the effect of temperature and plasma dilution. Clin Pharmacol Ther. 1970;11:844–55.

79. Mattson RH et al. Valproic acid in epilepsy: Clinical and pharmacological effects. Ann Neurol. 1978;3:20–5.

80. Kurata D, Wilkinson GR. Erythrocyte uptake and plasma binding of diphenylhydantoin. Clin Pharmacol Ther. 1974;16:355–62.

81. Wilder BJ et al. Plasma Phenytoin levels after loading and maintenance doses. Clin Pharmacol Ther. 1973;14:797–801.

82. Hvidberg E, Dam M. Clinical pharmacokinetics of anticonvulsants. Clin Pharmacokinet. 1976;1:161–88.

83. Record KE et al. Oral phenytoin loading in adults: rapid achievement of therapeutic plasma levels. Ann Neurol. 1979;5:268–70.

84. Wilson JT, Wilkinson CR. Delivery of anticonvulsant drug therapy in epileptic patients assessed by plasma level analysis. Neurology. 1979;24:614–23.

85. Standjord RE, Johannessen SI. One daily dose of diphenylhydantoin for patients with epilepsy. Epilepsia. 1974;15:317–27.

86. Borofsky LG et al. Diphenylhydantoin: efficacy, toxicity and dose-serum level relationship in children. Ped Pharmacol Ther. 1972;81:995–1002.

87. Svensmark O, Buchthal F. Diphenylhydantoin and phenobarbital. Am J Dis Child. 1964;108:82–7.

88. Richens A. Clinical pharmacokinetics of phenytoin. Clin Pharmacokinet. 1979;4:153–69.

89. Barot MH et al. Individual variation in daily dosage requirements for phenytoin sodium in patients with epilepsy. Br J Clin Pharmacol. 1978;6:267–71.

90. Kutt H. Interactions of antiepileptic drugs. Epilepsia. 1975;16:393–402.

91. Roe TF et al. Drug interactions: Diazoxide and diphenylhydantoin. J Pediatr. 1975;87:480–84.

92. Bartle WR et al. Dose-dependent effect of cimetidine on phenytoin kinetics. Clin Pharmacol Ther. 1983;33:649–55.

93. Phillips P, Hansky J. Phenytoin toxicity secondary to cimetidine administration. Med J Aust. 1984;141:602.

94. Mitchard M et al. Ranitidine drug interactions—a literature review. Pharmacol Ther. 1987;32:293–325.

95. Molholm-Hansen J. Carbamazepine-induced acceleration of diphenylhydantoin and warfarin metabolism in man. Clin Pharmacol Ther. 1971;12:539–43.

96. Makki KA et al. Metabolic effects of folic acid replacement therapy in folate deficient epileptic patients. In: Johannessen SI et al, eds. Antiepileptic Therapy: Advances in Drug Monitoring. New York: Raven Press; 1980;391–96.

97. Berg MJ et al. Phenytoin and folic acid. Individualized drug-drug interaction. Ther Drug Monit. 1983;5:395–99.

98. Berg MJ et al. Phenytoin and folic acid interaction: a preliminary report. Ther Drug Monit. 1983;5:589–94.

99. Dam M et al. Antiepileptic drugs: metabolism in pregnancy. Clin Pharmacokinet. 1979;4:53–62.

100. Knight AH, Phind EG. Epilepsy and pregnancy: a study of 153 pregnancies in 59 patients. Epilepsia. 1975; 16:99–110.

101. Vozeh S, Follath F. Assessment of serum phenytoin level. Eur J Clin Pharmacol. 1980;17:33–5.

102. Vozeh S et al. Predicting individual phenytoin dosage. J Pharmacokinet Biopharm. 1981;9:131–46.

103. Rambeck B et al. Predicting phenytoin dose: a revised nomogram. Ther Drug Monit. 1981;1:325–54.

104. Mullen RW. Optimal phenytoin therapy: a new technique for individualizing dosage. Clin Pharmacol Ther. 1978;23:228–32.

105. Chaikin P et al. Unusual absorption profile of phenytoin in a massive overdose case. Clin Res. 1979;27:541A. Abstract.

106. Wilder BJ et al. Correlation of acute diphenylhydantoin intoxication with plasma levels and metabolite excretion. Neurology. 1973;23:1329–332.

107. Glazko AJ. Phenytoin: chemistry and methods of determination. In: Levy RH et al, eds. Antiepileptic Drugs. 3rd ed. New York: Raven Press; 1989:159–76.

108. Flachs H, Rasmussen JM. Renal Disease may increase apparent phenytoin in serum as measured by enzyme-multiplied immunoassay. Clin Chem. 1980;26:361. Letter.

109. Green PJ et al. Phenytoin can be measured reliably in uremic patients by immunoassay. Clin Chem. 1983;29:737.

110. Sirgo MA et al. Interpretation of serum phenytoin concentration in uremia is assay-dependent. Neurology. 1984;34:1250–251.

111. Pippenger CE et al. Interlaboratory variability in determination of plasma antiepileptic drug concentration. Arch Neurol. 1976;33:351–55.

112. Richens A. Drug level monitoring—quantity and quality. Br J Clin Pharmacol. 1978;5:285–88.

Chapter 26

Carbamazepine, Valproic Acid, Phenobarbital, and Ethosuximide

René H. Levy, Alan J. Wilensky, and Gail D. Anderson

The introduction of valproic acid and carbamazepine in the 1970s was a major advance in the development of anticpileptic drugs. The structures of these drugs and the spectra of their antiseizure activity opened new horizons in the pharmacotherapy of epilepsy. In conjunction with the introduction of new drugs, neurologists, clinical pharmacists, and epileptologists increased their sophistication in therapeutic monitoring. They revised a number of former notions regarding the use of antiepileptic drugs, particularly the relative merits of monotherapy and polytherapy. In addition to valproic acid and carbamazepine, which have become primary agents, this chapter addresses ethosuximide and phenobarbital. With phenytoin, these four drugs are those most used in antiepileptic drug treatment worldwide.

CLINICAL PHARMACOKINETICS

Carbamazepine

Carbamazepine (see Table 26-1) is available in both tablet and oral suspension formulations. A large body of data indicates that the absorption of carbamazepine from regular tablets is generally slow and irregular.[1] Time to peak concentration varies from four to eight hours or longer because of the very low water solubility (< 200 µg/mL) of this drug and its dissolution-rate-limited absorption. In fact, it has been suggested that the rate and extent of its absorption may be dose-dependent. A recent study has suggested that carbamazepine undergoes both first-order and zero-order absorption, with approximately 35% of a dose absorbed by zero-order kinetics.[2] Evidence that the dissolution rate of tablets can be affected by moisture has been put forth.[3] Absorption of the suspension is more rapid, resulting in peak concentrations in one to three hours.[4] The absolute bioavailability of carbamazepine has not been measured. Measurements based on both radioactivity data and comparison of tablets to nonaqueous solutions suggest greater than 75% bioavailability.

Since an intravenous preparation of carbamazepine is not available for human use, carbamazepine volume of distribution values are inferred from studies of oral administration. Carbamazepine has a relatively large volume of distribution (0.8 to 2.0 L/kg), and is found in cerebrospinal fluid, amniotic fluid, and breast milk. Brain-to-plasma ratios in patients on chronic therapy range between 0.8 and 1.6. Cerebrospinal fluid:plasma concentration ratios ranging from 0.17 to 0.31 are consistent with the extent of plasma protein binding. Likewise, salivary concentrations predictably reflect unbound plasma concentrations, and measurements of carbamazepine in saliva can become a useful tool in therapeutic monitoring. Breast milk to maternal serum ratios of carbamazepine concentration are approximately 0.4. Distribution of carbamazepine into breast milk results in carbamazepine concentrations of approximately 1 μg/mL in 11 of 12 nursed infants studied.[5] In one infant, plasma concentration of carbamazepine reached 4.7 μg/mL. However, no adverse reactions could be attributed to carbamazepine in this study.

Carbamazepine binds to both albumin and α_1-acid glycoprotein (α_1-AGP) with a free fraction ranging from 16.9% to 31.8% that varies inversely with α_1-AGP concentrations. Carbamazepine binding is not appreciably affected by other drugs. However, physiological conditions (e.g., pregnancy, hepatic disease) associated with low serum albumin can result in elevated free fractions.

The distribution characteristics of carbamazepine-10,11-epoxide (CBZ-epoxide) have been studied because of this metabolite's anticonvulsant properties and its potential contribution to the therapeutic and toxic effects of the parent drug.[6] The epoxide metabolite is less bound than carbamazepine, and its free fraction in plasma is twice that of the parent drug. Therefore, free concentrations of CBZ-epoxide may be equal to free concentrations of carbamazepine. Concentrations of

Table 26-1. Summary of Pharmacokinetic Parameters (Carbamazepine)

	Population Averages (± SD) (Normal renal and hepatic function)				
		Adults			
	Single dose in normals	Chronic monotherapy	Chronic polytherapy	Children	Neonates
CL_S (mL/hr/kg)	21 ± 5	25 ± 16	108 ± 39		
V_{ss} (L/kg)	0.8–2.0				
F (oral)	>0.70	>0.70	>0.70		
k_a (hr^{-1})	0.4	0.4	0.4	0.4	0.5
% excreted in urine as					
parent drug	2		1	<1	
metabolites	21	30	51		
$t^{1}\!/_{2}{}^{\lambda}N$ (hr): (i.e., $t^{1}\!/_{2\beta}$)	25–40	15–25	6–14	2.5–15	8–37

the epoxide in cerebrospinal fluid, saliva, and breast milk represent 50%, 40%, and 40% of the corresponding plasma concentrations, respectively. Thus, the distribution of the epoxide in those fluids is consistent with its extent of plasma binding.

The major metabolites of carbamazepine are shown in Figure 26-1.[7] The most important (quantitatively) pathway represents epoxidation in the 10,11-position (hepatic monooxygenases) followed by hydrolysis of the epoxide to the corresponding 10,11-transdiol through microsomal epoxide hydrolase. A fraction of the 10,11-dihydrodiol is found in urine in the form of glucuronide. Two other pathways are shown in Figure 26-1: N-glucuronidation and ring hydroxylation leading to a number of mono- and di-hydroxy metabolites. A total of 33 metabolites of carbamazepine have been described. The quantitative importance of the epoxide-diol pathway is affected by the presence of other antiepileptic drugs. This pathway accounts for 25% of a carbamazepine dose in monotherapy and 40% to 50% of the dose in polytherapy. In a previous study,[8] 80% to 90% of a dose of epoxide was converted to the transdiol.

Although the plasma clearance of carbamazepine is greater than that of other antiepileptic drugs, its extraction ratio is still less than 0.2. A striking feature of the plasma clearance of carbamazepine is its variability. For a given dose, plasma concentrations may vary five- to sevenfold. Over the last ten years, several studies have attempted to define the elusive serum concentration:dose ratio (or concentration:dose relationship) of carbamazepine. Recently, it has become apparent that

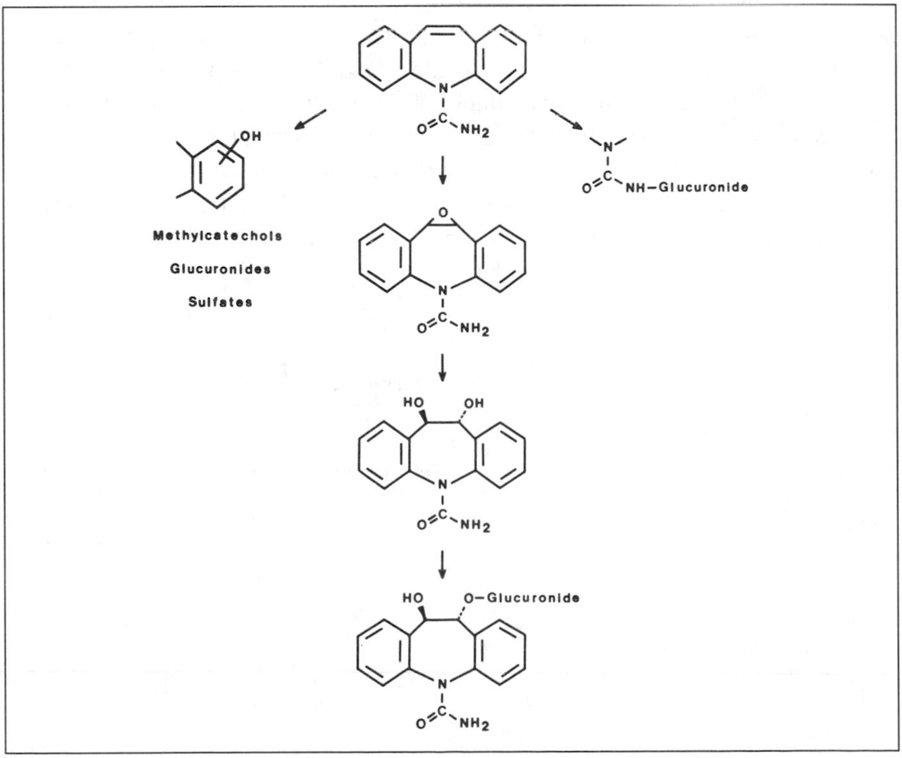

Figure 26-1. *Metabolic scheme for carbamazepine.*

the clearance of carbamazepine is affected primarily by two factors: age and poly-therapy. The concentration:dose ratio of carbamazepine increases linearly with age. Within each age group, the concentration:dose ratio decreases by 30% to 50% whenever one or two other antiepileptic drugs (phenytoin, phenobarbital, primidone) are co-administered.[9] Two recent studies[10,11] have shown that the large variability in carbamazepine clearance can be completely explained by induction of its metabolism through the epoxide-diol pathway. What has been described for the clearance of carbamazepine is also applicable to its half-life. Studies in normal volunteers show that the half-life of carbamazepine is 33 hours in single-dose studies and 15 to 25 hours in subchronic dosing studies. When carbamazepine half-life was measured by stable isotope methodology in adult patients on poly-therapy, the half-life ranged between 5 and 13 hours. The shortest half-lives were obtained in children receiving polytherapy. Studies which evaluated the variability in steady-state plasma concentrations in epileptic patients found that the oscilla-tions were twice as large in patients on polytherapy. Intermittent side effects of carbamazepine can be shown to be correlated with fluctuations in plasma concen-trations.[12] Consequently, the potential utility of a sustained-release formulation of carbamazepine is being assessed.[13]

Valproic Acid

Valproic acid (see Table 26-2) is a branched-chain fatty acid which is rapidly and completely absorbed.[14] It is available in a number of forms in various countries: acid in capsule or enteric-coated tablet, syrup, sodium salt, and divalproex sodium. A "sprinkle" capsule form containing coated particles of valproate exists and an intravenous formulation will be available. Valproate is rapidly absorbed once it is released from its formulation. The time required to reach a peak concentration is less than two hours for the acid or the regular sodium-salt formulations and three to eight hours for the enteric-coated tablets. Meals can have a profound effect on the time to peak concentration for the enteric-coated tablets; however, the long

Table 26-2. *Summary of Pharmacokinetic Parameters (Valproate)*

	Population Averages (± SD) (Normal renal and hepatic function)			
	Adults		**Children**	**Neonates**
	Monotherapy	Polytherapy		
CL_S (mL/hr/kg)	7–11	15–18	13–28	10–18
V_{ss} (L/kg)	0.12–0.23			
F (oral)	1.00	1.00	1.00	1.00
k_a (hr^{-1})	17 ± 16			
% excreted in urine as				
parent drug	1–3			
metabolites	>90			
$t^1/_2{}^\lambda 1$ (hr)	4.1 ± 2.6			
$t^1/_2{}^\lambda N$ (hr): (i.e., $t^1/_2{}_\beta$)	9–18	6–12	8–11	10–67

peak times represent delayed, rather than prolonged, absorption. The "sprinkle" capsule delivers valproic acid at a slower rate than the enteric-coated tablet, resulting in smaller peak-to-trough fluctuations. Time to peak concentration occurs within one hour.[15]

The absolute bioavailability of sodium valproate was measured by comparing the areas under the curve (AUC) obtained after oral and intravenous administration. In spite of differences in populations (healthy volunteers or epileptic patients) and formulations (oral solution, rapid-release, or enteric-coated tablets), the absolute bioavailability of valproate is consistently close to unity. This observation indicates that valproate is not subject to a first-pass effect which is consistent with its low metabolic clearance.

As expected from its acidic structure and extensive plasma binding, valproic acid's volume of distribution is small, ranging from 0.12 to 0.23 L/kg. In epileptic patients and in healthy adult volunteers, the free fraction of valproate ranges from 6% to 10%. Valproate binding is concentration-dependent and varies twofold within the therapeutic range. It is also affected by albumin concentration and disease state. Valproate free fraction increases to 18% in renal failure patients and to 29% in patients with alcoholic cirrhosis. Valproate free fraction also increases in the presence of salicylate and free fatty acids. Determination of valproate free fraction may be affected by increases in free fatty acids that occur in sera kept at 37 °C. The concentration of valproate in other body fluids is also consistent with its extensive plasma binding. In cerebrospinal fluid, valproate concentration is 10% of that in plasma. The concentration ratio of breast milk to plasma concentration is 0.07. The saliva concentration of valproate ranges from 0.4% to 6% of the plasma concentration, but the correlation between concentrations in both fluids is poor.

Valproic acid has an unusual metabolic pathway that is related to its fatty-acid structure (see Figure 26-2). In addition to glucuronidation and oxidative pathways such as ω and ω_1 oxidation, it also is metabolized by β-oxidation, probably through the mitochondrial fatty-acid enzyme system. Another metabolic pathway produces the 3-ene, 4-ene, and diene metabolites. Plasma concentrations of valproate metabolites are much lower than those of the parent drug. Of all valproate metabolites, 3-keto valproate reaches the highest plasma concentration, which is only 10% to 30% that of the parent drug. Unsaturated metabolites of valproate have anticonvulsant properties. Although their plasma concentrations represent less than 5% of those of valproate, they may contribute to the effects of the parent drug by selective accumulation in the brain.

Valproic acid is eliminated mostly by metabolism; the fraction of dose recovered unchanged in urine is less than 5%. The total-body plasma clearance of valproate is low, and its extraction ratio (after conversion of plasma to blood clearance) is less than 5%. The clearance of valproate changes drastically from 7 to 11 mL/hr/kg during monotherapy to 15 to 18 mL/hr/kg when valproate is administered with other antiepileptic drugs.[14] This effect is so pronounced that therapeutic levels cannot be achieved in some patients on polytherapy. In children, total plasma clearance ranges from 10 to 20 mL/hr/kg during monotherapy to 20 to 40 mL/hr/kg on polytherapy.[16] In some children, very high clearances (>40 mL/hr/kg) have been reported, resulting in dose requirements of up to 105 mg/kg/day.[17]

Hepatic disease has two opposing effects on valproate clearance. Clearance is increased due to a higher free fraction in the serum and decreased due to diminished drug-metabolizing activity. Although free serum levels are increased, the total serum levels of valproate are not altered in this situation. Valproate clearance is also affected by the concentration-dependence of valproate binding. Several studies have found that the serum concentration:dose relationship is curvilinear (i.e., the concentration to dose ratio decreases with increasing doses). This effect is attributed principally to an increase in valproate free fraction at higher concentrations (>70 µg/mL).

Although valproate exhibits biexponential behavior after intravenous administration to volunteers, the alpha phase is so rapid that most studies report the terminal half-life. The effect of polytherapy on clearance is reflected in the effect of other drugs on valproate half-life. The half-life ranges from 8 to 18 hours with monotherapy and decreases to 4 to 12 hours with polytherapy. Consistent with this effect, the variability in steady-state serum levels is greater in patients on polytherapy. Valproate half-life also appears to be age-dependent. In newborns and in

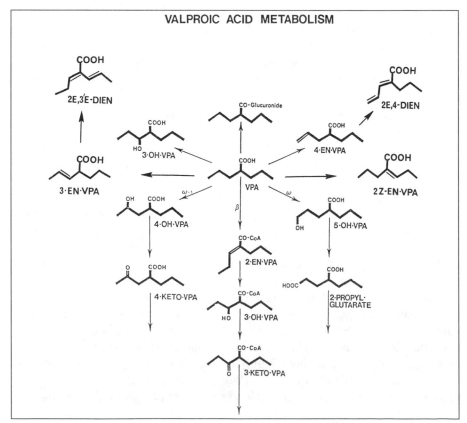

Figure 26-2. *Metabolic scheme for valproic acid.*

infants up to the age of two months, valproate half-life is 10 to 67 hours, much longer than in adults. However, valproate half-life in epileptic children is not appreciably different from that in adults.

Renal excretion does not represent an important pathway of elimination for valproic acid (2% to 3% of the dose). The fact that renal clearance of free valproate (2 to 4 mL/min) is small relative to glomerular filtration rate suggests that valproate is significantly reabsorbed and that renal insufficiency should not affect the plasma levels of this drug.

Phenobarbital

Early work on the rate and extent of absorption of phenobarbital (see Table 26-3) indicated the potential for dissolution-rate-limited absorption. More recent studies[18] have found that phenobarbital (acid, tablets) is absorbed rapidly and completely. The time required to reach peak serum concentration ranges from 0.5 to 4 hours. The rate of absorption of phenobarbital after oral administration is not appreciably different from its rate of absorption after intramuscular administration. The absolute bioavailability of phenobarbital was measured relative to availability following intramuscular and intravenous administration and found to be close to unity.

The distribution characteristics of phenobarbital can be separated into an early phase and a late phase. Initially, phenobarbital distributes into the well-perfused organs, with the exception of the brain. Phenobarbital appears to penetrate the brain slowly, and when it is used to treat status epilepticus, an immediate effect is not expected. A few hours after administration, phenobarbital is found in nearly equal concentrations in all tissues of the body. The steady-state volume of distribution is 0.6 ± 0.05 L/kg. Phenobarbital distributes into cerebrospinal fluid, saliva, and breast milk. The cerebrospinal fluid to plasma concentration ratio

Table 26-3. Summary of Pharmacokinetic Parameters (Phenobarbital)

	Population Averages ($\pm$ SD) (Normal renal and hepatic function)		
	Adults	Children	Neonates
CL_S (mL/hr/kg)	3.7 ± 0.7		
CL_R (mL/hr/kg)	~ 1.5		
CL_{NR} (mL/hr/kg)	~ 2.2		
V_1 (L/kg)	0.3 ± 0.09		
V_{ss} (L/kg)	0.6 ± 0.05		~ 1.0
F (oral)	1.00 ± 0.11	~ 1.00	<1.00
k_a (hr^{-1})	2.21 ± 0.57		
% excreted in urine as parent drug metabolites	20–40 45–65		~ 20
$t^{1/2}_{\lambda 1}$ (hr)	0.28 ± 0.23		
$t^{1/2}_{\lambda N}$ (hr): (i.e., $t^{1/2}_{\beta}$)	75–126	37–73	45–500

(0.47) is close to the free fraction of phenobarbital in plasma (0.40). Breast milk to maternal serum concentration ratios are approximately 0.4[18] which can result in both therapeutic serum concentrations and clinical signs of toxicity in the nursed infant.[19,20] The drug is bound mainly to plasma albumin, and its free fraction increases in hypoalbuminemia.

Metabolism represents an important route of elimination (45% to 65% of the dose). Two major metabolic pathways are shown in Figure 26-3: parahydroxylation on the phenyl ring and formation of an N-glucoside.[21] A significant fraction of the parahydroxy metabolite is glucuronidated. Together these pathways account for 30% to 50% of a dose. Other minor metabolites include formation of a dihydrodiol as well as aliphatic hydroxylation on the ethyl side-chain.

The total body clearance of phenobarbital is 3.7 ± 0.7 mL/hr/kg. The renal clearance (1.5 mL/hr/kg) is urine-flow as well as pH-dependent. The influence of water excretion is explained by the high degree of tubular reabsorption, while the pH-dependence is totally consistent with the pH partition hypothesis.

Of all antiepileptic drugs, phenobarbital exhibits the longest elimination half-life. The half-life in adults (75 to 126 hours) is shorter than in neonates and longer than in children.

Ethosuximide

Ethosuximide (see Table 26-4) is relatively water soluble and is rapidly absorbed from tablets.[22] The time required to reach peak serum concentration is less than three hours. In light of its very low clearance, no first-pass effect is expected. Ethosuximide appears to distribute in total body water in a manner analogous to that of antipyrine, and its volume of distribution is very close to the volume of total body water. Since ethosuximide is not bound to plasma proteins, its concen-

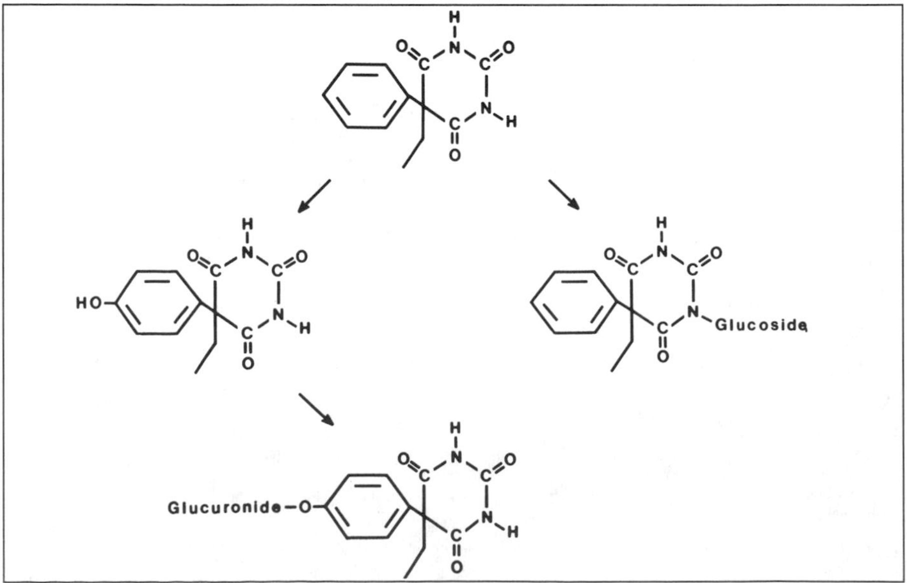

Figure 26-3. *Metabolic scheme for phenobarbital.*

tration in cerebrospinal fluid, saliva, and breast milk approximates that in plasma. Distribution of ethosuximide into breast milk results in an ethosuximide plasma concentration in the nursed infant that is approximately equal to the maternal serum concentration.[23] A metabolic scheme for ethosuximide is shown in Figure 26-4. All ethosuximide metabolites result from hydroxylation. Hydroxylation of the ethyl side-chain at the C-1 position yields the major metabolite (30% to 50% of the dose). Approximately 20% of a dose is excreted unchanged in urine. The total body clearance of ethosuximide is very small (11 ± 2.4 mL/min/kg), while its half-life is relatively long and age-dependent (40 to 60 hours in adults and 25 to 35 hours in children).

PHARMACODYNAMICS

Carbamazepine

Optimal serum carbamazepine concentrations vary considerably among patients. A more refined therapeutic range might be constructed by taking into account concentrations of the epoxide metabolite and protein binding, but this has not been accomplished.

Shorvon et al.[24] treated 25 newly diagnosed patients with generalized tonic-clonic and/or partial seizures with carbamazepine using a target concentration range of 4 to 8 µg/mL. Seizures were completely controlled in 17 patients with levels within the targeted range; seizures remained uncontrolled in three patients despite serum concentrations of 4 to 8 µg/mL. Seizures also were completely controlled in five other patients in spite of carbamazepine serum concentrations of less than 4 µg/mL. In a double-blind comparison with phenytoin, Troupin et al.[25] used either carbamazepine or phenytoin monotherapy to treat 47 patients with long-term poorly controlled seizures. Twenty-five patients with a mean carbamazepine serum concentration of 9.9 µg/mL (range, 6 to 12 µg/mL) had a better

Table 26-4. *Summary of Pharmacokinetic Parameters (Ethosuximide)*

	Population Averages ($\pm$ SD) (Normal renal and hepatic function)	
	Adults	Children
CL_S (mL/hr/kg)	11 ± 2.4	
CL_R (mL/hr/kg)	2.8 ± 0.7	
CL_{NR} (mL/hr/kg)	8.2 ± 2.2	
V_{ss} (L/kg)	0.62–0.67	0.69
F (oral)	~ 1.00	~ 1.00
% excreted in urine as		
parent drug	12–20	
metabolites	40–60	
$t^{1/2}_{\lambda}N$ (hr): (i.e., $t^{1/2}_{\beta}$)	40–60	26–36

response to carbamazepine than to phenytoin. Thus, a therapeutic range of 4 to 12 µg/mL is reasonable. Patients with uncontrolled, severe epilepsy are more likely to require serum carbamazepine concentrations at the upper end of this range.

A few patients have intolerable carbamazepine side effects even at very low serum levels (<4 µg/mL), especially if initial dosing is increased too rapidly. Dulled mentation is the common complaint. Most of these patients are never able to attain adequate serum levels for seizure control. Careful studies[12,26] of intermittent carbamazepine side effects, including hourly serum level monitoring, suggest that the threshold for common side effects such as diplopia, drowsiness, and headache is approximately 8 µg/mL for most patients. Peak serum concentrations are closely associated with the appearance of side effects, and dosing schedules should be rearranged to aim for lower peak concentrations that may eliminate the side effects. At levels above 12 µg/mL, the frequency and severity of side effects increases dramatically, usually without any improvement in seizure control.[27] Persistently high serum levels may result in an increase in the number of seizures and a change in clinical characteristics of the seizures. Massive overdosage results in serum levels greater than 20 µg/mL (sometimes lasting for several days) with initial agitation followed by stupor and, in severe cases, coma.[28]

Valproic Acid

A carefully controlled study by Gram et al.[29] demonstrated a 75% reduction in seizure frequency in a group of 13 adult patients on polytherapy with various seizure disorders, when trough valproate serum levels were no lower than 39 to 49 µg/mL. Further studies[30] supported 40 µg/mL as the minimum threshold for definite antiepileptic activity in most patients. Rowan and co-workers[31] intensively

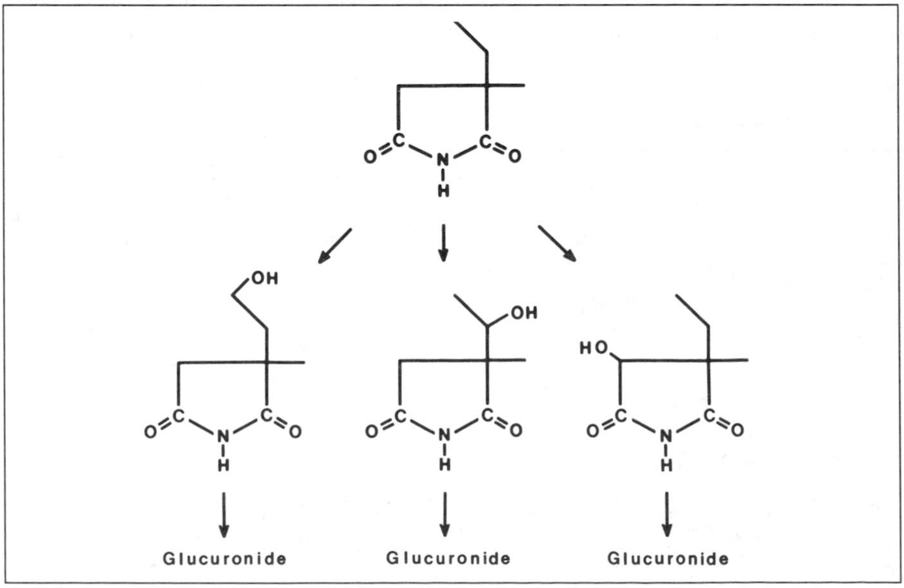

Figure 26-4. Metabolic scheme for ethosuximide.

monitored electroencephalograms (EEGs) and measured serum valproate levels hourly to demonstrate that some patients require peak serum concentrations greater than 100 µg/mL for maximum benefit. More recent studies have demonstrated that some patients require serum levels in the 125 to 150 µg/mL range before achieving seizure control. This is especially true for patients with complex partial seizures. There is a time component to valproate pharmacodynamics in that it may take several weeks at a given serum concentration for full therapeutic effects to develop; these effects may persist for several days after the drug has been discontinued and serum levels are below detectable limits.[32]

Gastrointestinal side effects (e.g., nausea, vomiting, gastrointestinal distress) and drowsiness commonly occur on initiation of valproate therapy. Initiating therapy with small doses and increasing the dose gradually until tolerance is achieved can alleviate many of these symptoms. Enteric-coated tablets and "sprinkle" capsules reduce nausea. In monotherapy patients, dose-related adverse effects of valproate (e.g., tremor, confusion) begin to appear when serum concentrations of valproate are approximately 80 µg/mL; they occur in a majority of patients when serum concentrations exceed 100 µg/mL.[33] Excessive weight gain (>4 kg) occurs in approximately 50% of patients and is occasionally sufficiently severe to require discontinuation of valproate. Alopecia has also been reported. Although dose reduction is occasionally helpful for both weight gain and alopecia, the dose dependency of these adverse effects has not been clearly established. Asymptomatic hyperammonemia commonly occurs and has been shown to be directly related to valproate plasma concentration. Hyperammonemia is greater in patients on polytherapy.

A transient elevation in liver enzymes occurs in 40% of patients and is not accompanied by symptoms of hepatic dysfunction. However, a rare, fatal, valproate-induced hepatotoxicity can occur. A retrospective analysis of the literature indicates that the overall prevalence is 1/10,000, with most cases occurring in children less than two years old, especially when they are receiving polytherapy.[34]

Coma, pulmonary edema, and death from massive valproate overdosage associated with a serum concentration of 1970 µg/mL has been reported.[35] Other patients with similar serum concentrations have recovered following supportive treatment and hemodialysis.[36]

Phenobarbital

In 1968, Buchthal and co-workers[37] reported that a mean serum phenobarbital concentration of 10 µg/mL reduced the incidence of paroxysmal activity in the EEG by 90%, and seizure control was improved in 11 hospitalized patients with generalized tonic-clonic seizures when serum concentrations of 10 to 25 µg/mL were reached. These observations were supported by a recent study[38] of phenobarbital monotherapy in 13 patients with previously untreated epilepsy. In children with febrile convulsions, phenobarbital serum concentrations of 16 µg/mL or greater resulted in a six-month recurrence rate of 4%, compared with a 21% recurrence rate in untreated children. The recurrence rate was 21% in children with levels of 15 µg/mL or less.[39]

Sedation and ataxia occur in chronically treated patients at phenobarbital serum concentrations of 35 to 80 μg/mL. Coma with intact reflexes has occurred in habituated patients at serum concentrations of 65 to 117 μg/mL, and coma without reflexes is associated with levels greater than 100 μg/mL.[40] Tolerance to phenobarbital appears to be a true pharmacodynamic tolerance.[41] In our own studies in naive volunteers, considerable drowsiness occurred after administration of single doses that resulted in phenobarbital serum concentrations of 4 to 5 μg/mL, whereas patients who were treated chronically and who had serum levels five or more times higher did not complain of sedation.[42]

There is a growing concern about the detrimental effects of chronic administration of phenobarbital on cognition and behavior. Detailed neuropsychological studies[43,44] in children and adults taking phenobarbital chronically have shown a positive correlation between phenobarbital serum concentration and memory impairment, even at concentrations within the therapeutic range.[45] Cognitive impairment may occur independently of the better-known idiosyncratic reactions such as hyperactivity and tantrums in children. Theodore and Porter[46] reviewed the literature and advocated gradual removal of phenobarbital from antiepileptic regimens, with compensatory adjustments in dosage of nonsedating antiepileptic agents, in order to reduce toxicity.

Ethosuximide

In 23 of 29 patients with absence seizures, Browne and co-workers[47] demonstrated a 75% or greater reduction in seizure frequency when serum concentrations of ethosuximide were greater than 40 μg/mL. Only three of six patients improved similarly with levels less than 40 μg/mL. Sherwin and co-workers[48] reported that in their prospective study of absence seizures, 91% of patients who became seizure-free had ethosuximide concentrations greater than 40 μg/mL, 9% had levels from 30 to 40 μg/mL, and none had levels less than 30 μg/mL. Thus, there is general agreement that the minimum effective ethosuximide serum concentration is on the order of 40 μg/mL.

There is no obvious correlation between serum ethosuximide concentration and clinical side effects. A provisional upper limit to the therapeutic range is 100 μg/mL, but a few patients require higher levels for maximum seizure control.

CLINICAL APPLICATION OF PHARMACOKINETIC DATA

General Considerations

The goal of antiepileptic drug therapy is the best possible seizure control with minimal side effects. To achieve this, the least amount of antiepileptic drug necessary to control the patient's seizures is used. The first step is to select an antiepileptic medication appropriate for the individual patient's seizure type. Then, a dosing regimen is designed based on the drug's pharmacokinetics and pharmacodynamics and the patient's individual characteristics. The final dosing regimen will depend upon the patient's response to the drug.

Therapeutic ranges for individual drugs developed from clinical trials are based on population characteristics, and often the populations upon which they are based are not large. Pharmacokinetic parameters are also often based on limited data. Individual patients vary widely from reported averages with respect to absorption, metabolism, and response to these drugs. Thus, it is not unusual for patients to become seizure-free when serum drug concentrations are well above the upper end of the usual therapeutic range. Similarly some patients may be very sensitive to a given medication and develop side effects when serum drug concentrations are well within the therapeutic range. The goal is not to obtain a serum drug level in the middle of the therapeutic range; it is, rather, to obtain a patient who is seizure-free without side effects.

After therapy has been initiated with a rational drug regimen, the regimen must be adjusted according to the patient response. If seizures are controlled with no side effects, no adjustments should be made. If seizures are controlled but side effects are present, then the dosage should be decreased. If seizures are not controlled and there are no side effects, the dose should be increased until either seizures are controlled or side effects occur. When side effects cannot be eliminated and seizures are not controlled, the medication is not ideal for the patient. At this point, a decision has to be made whether to maintain the patient on current medication and accept less than optimal seizure control or to change medications in an attempt to achieve control of seizures.

A rational program of drug dosing adjustment can be carried out only through the use of appropriate serum-level monitoring that is based on known pharmacokinetic and pharmacodynamic data. Intervals between doses should be as long as possible since patients are more compliant when they do not have to take medications more than once or twice daily. However, a regimen that involves giving larger doses less frequently may have to be abandoned if drug absorption is rapid enough to produce a brief period of toxicity. Instead, the dosing interval may have to be shortened and smaller doses given. After a dosing change, one should not evaluate the effect of that change until a new steady-state concentration has been reached (i.e., about four to five half-lives). Then one can compare the effect of the dosage change on the serum drug concentration with its effect on the patient's clinical status. Knowledge of the therapeutic range is used to assess the likelihood of a particular response to a dosage change. Thus, when serum drug concentrations are at the upper end of the usual therapeutic range in patients whose seizures are uncontrolled but who are free of drug side effects, the next increase in dose might be expected to produce drug toxicity. The clinician must take this into account in deciding the amount or advisability of the dose increase. Conversely, a patient with a serum drug concentration at the lower end of or below the therapeutic range whose seizures are uncontrolled would be expected to tolerate a dose increase without toxicity.

Because of the wide interpatient variation in the metabolism of antiepileptic drugs, some patients on high doses will have low drug levels despite reliable drug intake; this situation can be detected only by measuring serum concentrations. In addition, patient complaints that may be due to drug toxicity can be assessed rationally only in light of serum drug levels. When a patient is taking more than one antiepileptic drug, one cannot identify the drug causing the toxicity solely on the basis of clinical findings. Drug concentrations should also be measured when a drug interaction is suspected. Antiepileptic drugs interact widely with other medications, and toxicity (or decreased efficacy due to decrease in free serum concentration) can occur whenever other medications are taken by patients. In an individual patient, the magnitude of drug-drug interactions is unpredictable. It is possible that unexpected or disappointing results of therapy are secondary to a drug interaction.

One final point needs to be considered in devising medication changes in patients with epilepsy. Patients tend to have more seizures when undergoing changes from one medication to another. Also, withdrawing an antiepileptic drug too rapidly when adding a new medication can result in withdrawal seizures and/or status epilepticus. This is particularly true for the barbiturates and probably also true for carbamazepine. All drug crossovers must be designed to minimize the likelihood of these seizures. Serum concentrations of the new drug must be adequate before the old drug or drugs are withdrawn entirely. Problems with toxicity may also develop during the crossover, necessitating changes in the planned dosing regimen. Thus, drug crossovers will, for clinical reasons, tend to take longer than expected on the basis of pharmacokinetics alone.

Carbamazepine

Because carbamazepine induces its own metabolism, and since its metabolism can be induced by other antiepileptic drugs, three patient groups must be considered when treatment with this medication is initiated. The first of these consists of patients who have not received previous medication and whose livers have not been chronically exposed to enzyme-inducing drugs. The second group of patients are those who have previously taken other antiepileptic drugs and are switching to carbamazepine alone. The patients in this group have had previous exposure to enzyme-inducing drugs and carbamazepine metabolism may be partially enhanced even upon initial exposure to this drug. However, in these patients one does not have to address problems of drug interactions. The third group of patients are those already taking other antiepileptic drugs who will add carbamazepine to their drug regimen. Metabolism in this group of patients will be at least partially induced, and carbamazepine metabolism may also be affected by drug interactions with other medications. The general pattern of use of carbamazepine under each of these three conditions must be adjusted for the characteristics of the individual patient. The primary factor to be taken into account is the patient's age: younger patients tend to require larger doses per kilogram weight than do older patients to achieve a given serum concentration. However, the wide interindividual variations among patients (even of the same age, gender, and size) in the metabolism of and response to carbamazepine make it necessary to individualize the final dosing regimen.

Carbamazepine therapy should be initiated slowly in all patients to avoid gastrointestinal side effects. However, this is particularly important in patients who have taken no antiepileptic medications previously since they will have a prolonged carbamazepine half-life and excessive serum concentrations may develop if usual doses are prescribed initially. These patients also have to be given time to develop tolerance to the pharmacodynamic effects of the drug. Carbamazepine is supplied as 100 mg and 200 mg tablets and as a suspension. Depending on the patient's age and size, start with either 100 or 200 mg once a day in the evening. This dose can then be increased by an additional 100 to 200 mg per day every six days. Before each dose increase, the patient's status should be reviewed to assess seizure activity and the extent of potential side effects. The process continues until a suitable maintenance dose is reached. The usual range of daily maintenance doses is 10 to 50 mg/kg in children and 10 to 20 mg/kg in adults. Medication should be given a minimum of twice a day. Although the half-life of carbamazepine tends to be longer than 24 hours initially, autoinduction of metabolism decreases the half-life and twice-daily dosing ultimately will be required. In adults, since carbamazepine half-life seldom is less than 12 hours, the twice-daily regimen should be acceptable for most patients. Nevertheless, many patients will require dosing at least three times a day to avoid the sharp carbamazepine absorption peaks which occur one to two hours after a dose; some patients may experience transient dose-related toxicity at this time. Since many adults ultimately take 1000 mg or more of carbamazepine per day, and since some may not tolerate more than 400 mg of carbamazepine in a single dose, three divided doses may be needed. Children need relatively larger doses and smaller, more frequent dosing intervals (three to four times/day) because their clearance rate is greater and the corresponding half-life of carbamazepine is decreased.

Due to the autoinduction of carbamazepine, patients beginning carbamazepine therapy must be closely monitored. Once these patients are stabilized on a suitable maintenance dose of carbamazepine, serum concentrations should be monitored and dosages adjusted upward if needed to compensate for enzyme induction. Although a linear relationship between dose and serum level can be found within a given patient, the increase in serum level associated with any given dose increment is less than proportional. This is probably due to increased enzyme induction even in those patients whose hepatic metabolizing enzymes were thought to be operating at maximum capacity.[49,50]

It is possible to rapidly load critically ill patients with carbamazepine suspension using nasogastric or nasoduodenal tubes.[51] Loading doses (7.4 to 10.4 mg/kg) produce therapeutic concentrations within one to two hours. Rectal administration of the carbamazepine suspension may be useful to provide maintenance doses if oral dosing is interrupted. Rectally administered carbamazepine is absorbed too slowly to be useful in status epilepticus.[3,52]

When carbamazepine is substituted for another antiepileptic medication with known enzyme-inducing capabilities, the half-life will be relatively short initially. In this situation, the carbamazepine dose can be increased more rapidly; adult patients often are started on 200 mg of carbamazepine twice a day, for example. Since carbamazepine has a shorter half-life than phenytoin and phenobarbital, it will reach steady state before those medications are completely cleared from the body. Serum levels should be monitored after carbamazepine reaches steady state, and after the antiepileptic drug that has been discontinued has been completely cleared. The clearance of carbamazepine may decrease when the influence of other enzyme-inducing antiepileptic drugs is absent.

When carbamazepine is added to an existing antiepileptic drug regimen, it may be difficult to achieve carbamazepine therapeutic serum concentrations because the other drugs may stimulate its hepatic metabolism. Despite large doses of carbamazepine, on the order of 30 mg/kg/day in adults, serum levels may remain low. The most frequent interaction occurs between phenytoin and carbamazepine; phenytoin levels may increase if carbamazepine is added to the patient's drug regimen. There is good evidence that CBZ-epoxide levels are higher than usual in these patients and contribute to the overall antiepileptic effect. Unless epoxide levels are monitored, the contribution of the epoxide to the effective treatment of the patient cannot be rationally evaluated. The problem is particularly prominent when carbamazepine and valproic acid are used together. Valproic acid inhibits the epoxide hydrolase resulting in epoxide accumulation, and patients may present with toxicity despite low carbamazepine levels. Carbamazepine epoxide serum concentrations (usually 1 to 2 µg/mL) may be as high as 7 to 8 µg/mL. The tendency for carbamazepine concentrations to remain low in patients taking other antiepileptic drugs must be recognized and should not be attributed to non-compliance.[10] It may be necessary to discontinue the other antiepileptic drugs in order to obtain high enough levels of carbamazepine to be able to assess whether or not they will control the patient's seizure disorder. Other clinically important drug interactions can occur; for example, both propoxyphene and erythromycin inhibit carbamazepine metabolism.

Valproic Acid

It is difficult to establish a clinically rational dosing regimen for valproic acid based on pharmacokinetic data. Although a therapeutic range has been delineated for valproic acid, there is some evidence that this drug exhibits both a delayed onset of action and continued action after it is undetectable in serum.[32] Difficulties in developing a pharmacokinetically based dosing regimen, as opposed to a clinically based one, are also compounded by the short half-life of this drug, which results in wide fluctuations in serum drug levels. Unless serum concentrations are taken at a set time relative to dosing, they are not strictly comparable. Furthermore, valproic acid is highly protein bound. As a result, at high drug levels, the free drug concentration may be increased without a corresponding increase in the total drug serum concentration. The data available for establishing the therapeutic range are based on total drug serum concentrations, rather than free drug concentrations, and may be misleading.

Valproic acid is the medication of choice for myoclonic and atonic seizures, as well as for reflex seizures such as those caused by light. It is as effective as ethosuximide in controlling absence seizures and is very effective in the control of primary generalized tonic-clonic seizures. There is also increasing evidence of a degree of effectiveness in all forms of partial seizures. Because of valproic acid's broad spectrum of activity, its use is increasing rapidly. Since it is also effective in patients with seizure types that are difficult to control (e.g., atonic and myoclonic seizures), it is frequently given in conjunction with other medications. This tendency to use polytherapy for patients taking valproic acid increases the chance of drug interactions.

Theoretically, valproic acid should be administered at least three, and preferably four, times a day because of its short half-life. However, two- or three-times-a-day dosing is the general rule. Even once-daily dosing has been shown to be as effective clinically as divided daily doses.[53] Nevertheless, daily divided doses are required in many patients because of gastrointestinal side effects and drowsiness associated with the large single daily dose. The clinical effectiveness of once-daily dosing appears to be related to the discordance between clinical effects and serum drug concentrations and may be due to antiepileptic activity of some of valproic acid's many long-lasting metabolites.[54]

In order to avoid gastrointestinal side effects, patients are started on 25% to 30% of the minimum 15 mg/kg/day maintenance dose, and the dose is increased approximately every seven days until the maintenance dose is reached. In patients who are not taking any other antiepileptic drugs, 15 mg/kg will produce a serum concentration at the lower end of the "therapeutic range." Because of the drug's short half-life, steady state is reached in three to four days, and the dose can be increased by 5 to 10 mg/kg weekly according to the clinical status of the patient. Despite fluctuations in serum drug levels, monitoring valproic acid serum concentrations can be useful to evaluate compliance and to guide dosing in a patient who is not responding as expected. However, since serum valproic acid concentrations may vary by as much as 100% over a single dosing interval,[31] care must be taken to sample always at the same time relative to drug dosing. The optimal time is just prior to the first morning dose (i.e., at trough level). However, this is frequently impractical.

Due to a high degree of protein binding and a shift to a larger free fraction at higher drug levels, total serum concentrations of valproic acid, especially when high, do not accurately reflect the amount of drug to which the brain is exposed. Furthermore, when valproic acid is used in conjunction with other anticonvulsants, serum valproate concentrations may not increase with an increase in dose. The lack of correlation between a change in dose and a change in serum drug concentration may be due to an increase in the free fraction rather than to an absolute increase in the total serum concentration or to induction of valproic acid metabolism. Therefore, the free serum concentration of valproic acid should be measured in patients who are not controlled following a dose increase.[55]

Because of its many interactions with other drugs, valproic acid is easier to use alone rather than in combination with other anticonvulsants. European investigators[30] have reported that in patients on multiple anticonvulsants, including valproic acid, serum concentrations of valproic acid could not be raised as high as desired. In children on monotherapy mean daily doses of 40 mg/kg/day produced mean peak serum levels of 91 µg/mL; in children on polytherapy, mean doses of 76 mg/kg resulted in mean peak concentration of 114 µg/mL.[56] After all other medications were discontinued, serum valproic acid concentrations could be increased resulting in improved seizure control. These results are consistent with the known pharmacokinetic and pharmacodynamic characteristics and interactions of valproic acid. They also support the general principle of monotherapy. Even if the pharmacokinetic effects of drug interactions are known, it is usually more efficient and of greater clinical benefit to avoid them, rather than to try to compensate for them.

Phenobarbital

Phenobarbital, the oldest of the current antiepileptic drugs, is used widely in infants and children as a sole anticonvulsant, but in adolescents and adults it is used more commonly as an adjunct in combination with one other major antiepileptic drug. As noted above, the pharmacokinetic properties of phenobarbital are well understood. There is little evidence that phenobarbital metabolism is induced by itself or by other medications.[42] In general, when phenobarbital is used with other agents, the metabolism of the other drugs is usually enhanced. The primary exception to this rule is the interaction between valproic acid and phenobarbital: phenobarbital metabolism is inhibited in this situation and serum phenobarbital concentrations increase if phenobarbital doses are not decreased.[57] Chloramphenicol has been reported to produce a similar effect.[58]

For an individual patient, a change in the dose of phenobarbital predictably affects the phenobarbital serum concentration. Nevertheless, phenobarbital serum concentrations should be monitored, especially when therapy is initiated. Phenobarbital has a long serum half-life of about 96 hours and can be administered as a single daily dose. In the majority of patients, phenobarbital doses of 1 to 3 mg/kg for adults and a somewhat higher dose for children will result in therapeutic serum drug levels. With time, most patients become tolerant to the sedative properties of phenobarbital; however, excessive sedation can be minimized by gradually increasing the phenobarbital dose over a period of several weeks when initiating therapy. The usual practice is to begin with about 25% of the final planned daily dose each evening for approximately five to seven days. The dose may then be increased to about 50% of the final dose after five to seven days. If this is well tolerated, the dose is increased to about 75% of the final dose for another five to seven days, and finally, the total daily dose can be administered once a day by the fourth week of therapy. Serum concentrations of phenobarbital will reach steady state about 20 to 30 days after initiation of the full dosage. At that time, serum levels should be checked and the patient reassessed to see if the desired therapeutic effect, without toxicity, has been obtained. If necessary, the dose may then be increased or decreased. Although it is best to measure the serum concentration of anticonvulsant medications just prior to each daily dose, phenobarbital's half-life is so long that serum phenobarbital concentrations seldom fluctuate during the day. Consequently, the serum phenobarbital concentration may be measured at any convenient time.[59]

Once a patient is stabilized on phenobarbital, dosage adjustments are relatively simple. Due to the linear nature of phenobarbital pharmacokinetics, any percentage change in dosage is reflected by a similar percentage change in serum drug level.

Loading doses of phenobarbital (10 mg/kg) administered at a rate of 100 mg/min can be used to treat status epilepticus. Even though maximum brain-to-plasma ratios of phenobarbital occur only after 60 minutes, effective brain concentrations are achieved within three minutes.[59]

Problems arise only when phenobarbital is administered with valproic acid which inhibits phenobarbital metabolism. In a patient who is already taking valproic acid, the initial dose of phenobarbital should be approximately one-half the usual dose. Once steady state is reached, the serum concentrations can be checked and the dose adjusted. When valproic acid is added to the drug regimen of a patient already taking phenobarbital, it is imperative to immediately halve the dose of phenobarbital to prevent its accumulation. This usually results in maintenance of a fairly constant phenobarbital level. Since the degree of inhibition of metabolism in any individual cannot be predicted with great accuracy, patients must be observed closely and phenobarbital serum concentrations adjusted as necessary once steady state is reached.

Ethosuximide

Ethosuximide is used to treat absence (petit mal) seizures and is the drug of choice for patients whose seizures consist solely of absence attacks. Two important factors which must be taken into account when administering ethosuximide are the difference in half-lives between children and adults (approximately 30 and 60 hours, respectively), and the need to increase the dose in children as they grow. An initial dose of 15 to 20 mg/kg in children under the age of ten will usually produce serum drug levels in the range of 50 µg/mL. In adolescents and adults, a similar dose will produce a somewhat higher serum drug level of 60 to 80 µg/mL. Although ethosuximide's relatively long half-life is compatible with once-a-day dosing, it is usually given in divided doses with or shortly after meals to avoid gastric upset.

To minimize gastric upset, the initial ethosuximide dose of one capsule after the evening meal should be gradually increased by one capsule every three to five days until the projected maintenance dose is reached. Steady state will be reached in approximately seven to ten days after the maintenance dose has been attained. The serum level and clinical status of the patient can be evaluated and the dose adjusted accordingly. Because of the linear nature of ethosuximide kinetics, a given percentage change in a dose will produce a corresponding change in the serum drug concentration.

Ethosuximide has a wide therapeutic range: 40 to 100 µg/mL. Therapy is usually initiated at a relatively low dose, since many patients respond to ethosuximide levels at the low end of the therapeutic range. If the initial dose does not produce complete seizure control, it should be increased until control is achieved. Although the upper end of the therapeutic range is reported to be 100 µg/mL, many patients with absence seizures respond at concentrations in the 125 to 150 µg/mL range without adverse effects. The ethosuximide dosage should be based upon seizure control or clinical status of these patients rather than on serum drug concentration.[60] Absence seizures begin in childhood, are most common in children and adolescents, frequently occur without the patient's being aware of them, and are not life-threatening. As a result, non-compliance to drug therapy is a major problem in the management of this seizure disorder. Therefore, a regular schedule of serum drug concentration monitoring should be instituted in order to evaluate compliance on the part of the patient. Therapeutic drug monitoring is also important because changes in body size and metabolism occur as children grow and enter adolescence. Ethosuximide dosage can then be adjusted to maintain serum drug concentrations at the level which has proved ideal for the individual patient. In patients with a good therapeutic response who are not undergoing rapid changes in body weight or passing through puberty, serum drug-concentration monitoring every four to six months may be sufficient. If there are complicating factors, serum concentration should be checked more frequently.

The only drug interaction which may be of some clinical significance is with valproic acid. Since ethosuximide is frequently given in combination with valproic acid, one must be aware that the addition of valproic acid may result in a modest increase in ethosuximide levels, probably by inhibiting ethosuximide metabolism.[61] If this occurs, it may be necessary to slightly reduce the ethosuximide dose.

ANALYTICAL METHODS

Carbamazepine

Carbamazepine (see Table 26-5) undergoes partial thermal degradation during gas-liquid chromatography (GLC). Although numerous GLC procedures have been developed which measure either the intact drug or a variety of derivatives or degradation products, none is entirely satisfactory.[62] The best approach to analyzing the intact compound is to use 13-C carbamazepine as an internal standard, but this approach requires mass-spectrometric detection.[63]

Reversed-phase high-performance liquid chromatography (HPLC) with 50% methanol-water mobile phase, a C18 column, and detection at 212 nm allows quantitative analysis of carbamazepine and its epoxide metabolite in serum or plasma.[64] Because the epoxide is acid-labile, extraction is performed at neutral pH.[8]

Enzyme multiplied immunoassay (EMIT) and fluorescence polarization immunoassay (FPIA) are widely used for carbamazepine analysis. The epoxide metabolite cannot be measured separately, but does cross-react in both assays to the extent of approximately 15% of the response achieved for an equivalent concentration of the parent drug.

Free carbamazepine can be analyzed using a commercially available ultrafiltration system with EMIT and specially prepared calibrators. HPLC assay of ultrafiltrates permits analysis of the epoxide as well.[65]

Valproic Acid

GLC analysis of valproate (see Table 26-6) is performed without derivative formation using column packings designed for free fatty acid work, such as 5%

Table 26-5. Comparison of the Relative Advantages and Disadvantages of the Various Carbamazepine Assays

Analytical[a] method	Specificity for carbamazepine[b]	Limit of sensitivity µg/mL (free levels)	Metabolite analysis	Assayable samples					Minimum sample volume required	Speed		Analysis cost[c]		Specialized operator training[d]	Preference & rank[e]			Comments
				Plasma/serum	Free levels	Urine	Saliva	CFS		1–10 samples	10–100 samples	Estimated reagent and tech. cost/assay	Initial equipment costs		Small service	Large service	Research	
GLC	1	0.5	Y	Y	Y	Y	Y	Y	0.5 mL	4 hr	20/day	4	2	4	5	4	4	CV ≤ 10%
HPLC	1	0.5	Y	Y	Y	Y	Y	Y	0.5 mL	4 hr	20/day	4	3	3	3	3	1	CV ≤ 5%[f]
EMIT																		
Manual	2	2.0 (0.5)	N	Y	Y	N	Y	Y	50 µL	1 hr	50/day	3	1	2	1	2	3	CV < 10%
Automated	2	2.0 (0.5)	N	Y	Y	N	Y	Y	50 µL	<1 hr	100/day	2	4	2	2	1	3	CV < 10%
FPIA	2	0.5	N	Y	Y	N	?	?	50 µL	<1 hr	100/day	2	5	2	2	1	3	CV < 4%

[a] GLC = Gas-liquid chromatography; HPLC = High performance liquid chromatography; EMIT = Enzyme multiplied immunoassay; FPIA = Fluorescence polarization immunoassay.

[b] Arbitrary Rating Scale of 1 (Excellent) to 5 (Poor).

[c] 1 = least expense.

[d] 1 = least training.

[e] 1 = preferred method.

[f] Simultaneous analysis of phenytoin, primidone, and phenobarbital possible.

Free Fatty Acid Packing (FFAP) on Gas Chrom Q 80 to 100 mesh. The drug may be extracted from serum or plasma by acidification and mixing with a small volume of chloroform. After centrifugation, an aliquot of the lower chloroform bead is injected into the chromatograph.[66] Alternatively, extraction with a larger volume of chloroform, followed by partial evaporation, may be performed. In this case a small volume of isoamyl acetate is added to the chloroform to protect against complete evaporation, which could result in loss of drug.[67] Injection of even small amounts of chloroform results in contamination of flame ionization detectors which then require frequent cleanings.

Valproate analyses by EMIT or FPIA are satisfactory, although there is some cross-reaction with unsaturated metabolites. Either serum or heparinized plasma may be used, but plasma treated with other anticoagulants should be avoided, because of potential cross-reaction.

Free valproate should be measured only in serum which is fresh or has been stored frozen. Ultrafiltration is preferred over equilibrium dialysis. Analysis is easiest by EMIT, but also possible by GLC.[65]

Phenobarbital

GLC analysis of phenobarbital (see Table 26-7) may be performed on the unchanged drug or its alkylated derivatives. GLC of the unchanged drug is difficult because of its interaction with the packing solid support.[68] On-column alkylation is very convenient and allows simultaneous analysis of phenytoin. However, alkaline hydrolysis occurs to varying degrees, and the choice of an appropriate internal standard with similar breakdown characteristics is critical.[69] If methylation is used, phenobarbital and mephobarbital form the same derivatives. Precolumn alkylation is an alternative.[70] The demethylated metabolite of mephenytoin is a common cause of interference in GLC procedures.

HPLC analysis of phenobarbital may be performed using the same assay configuration as for carbamazepine.[71] Potential interferences are carbamazepine epoxide and the demethylated metabolite of mephenytoin.

EMIT and FPIA perform well for phenobarbital, but the potential exists for cross-reaction with co-administered barbiturates (specifically mephobarbital in EMIT and phenobarbital in FPIA). A "dip-stick" phenobarbital assay, using homogeneous enzyme immunoassay technology but requiring no instrumentation, is also commercially available through Syntex Diagnostics (Acculevel).

Ethosuximide

The most sensitive analysis for ethosuximide (see Table 26-8) is by GLC with flame-ionization detection. Extraction is with chloroform, and a small volume of isoamyl acetate is added prior to evaporation of most, but not all of the organic phase in order to reduce drug losses due to volatility.[72] Injection of even small amounts of chloroform results in detector contamination, and frequent cleanings are necessary.

Ethosuximide can be analyzed in an HPLC panel that includes a number of other antiepileptic drugs.[73] Its relatively poor ultraviolet (UV) absorbance at 195

Table 26-6. Comparison of the Relative Advantages and Disadvantages of the Various Valproic Acid Assays

Analytical[a] method	Specificity for valproic acid[b]	Limit of sensitivity µg/mL (free levels)	Metabolite analysis	Assayable samples					Minimum sample volume required	Speed		Analysis cost[c]		Specialized operator training[d]	Preference & rank[e]			Comments
				Plasma/serum	Free levels	Urine	Saliva	CFS		1–10 samples	10–100 samples	Estimated reagent and tech. cost/assay	Initial equipment costs		Small service	Large service	Research	
GLC (Packed column)	1	0.8	Y	Y	Y	Y	Y	Y	0.2 mL	3 hr	30/day	4	2	4	4	4	1	CV ≤ 5%[f]
EMIT																		
Manual	2	10(2)	N	Y	Y	N	Y	Y	50 µL	1 hr	50/day	3	1	2	1	2	2	CV < 10%
Automated	2	10(2)	N	Y	N	N	Y	Y	50 µL	<1 hr	100/day	2	4	2	2	1	2	CV < 10%
FPIA	2	0.7	N	Y	N	N	N	Y	50 µL	<1 hr	100/day	2	5	2	2	1	2	CV < 4%

a GLC = Gas-liquid chromatography; EMIT = enzyme multiplied immunoassay, FPIA = fluorescence polarization immunoassay.
b Arbitrary Rating Scale of 1 (Excellent) to 5 (Poor).
c 1 = least expense.
d 1 = least training.
e 1 = preferred method.
f Simultaneous analysis of ethosuximide possible.

Table 26-7. Comparison of the Relative Advantages and Disadvantages of the Various Phenobarbital Assay

Analytical[a] method	Specificity for phenobarbital[b]	Limit of sensitivity μg/mL (free levels)	Metabolite analysis	Assayable samples				Minimum sample volume required	Speed		Analysis cost[c]		Specialized operator training[d]	Preference & rank[e]			Comments
				Plasma/serum	Urine	Saliva	CFS		1–10 samples	10–100 samples	Estimated reagent and tech. cost/assay	Initial equipment costs		Small service	Large service	Research	
GLC																	
Alkylation	2	0.5	Y	Y	Y	Y	Y	0.5 mL	4 hr	20/day	4	2	4	3	3	1	CV ≤ 5%[f]
No derivative	1	2.5	N	Y	Y	Y	Y	1.0 mL	4 hr	20/day	4	2	4	5	5	5	CV ≤ 10%[f]
HPLC	1	0.5	Y	Y	Y	Y	Y	0.5 mL	4 hr	20/day	3	3	3	3	3	1	CV ≤ 5%[f]
EMIT																	
Manual	2	5.0	N	Y	N	Y	Y	50 μL	1 hr	50/day	2	1	2	1	2	3	CV < 10%
Automated	2	5.0	N	Y	N	Y	Y	50 μL	< 1 hr	100/day	2	4	2	4	1	3	CV < 10%
FPIA	2	0.5	N	Y	N	N	N	50 μL	< 1 hr	100/day	2	5	2	4	1	3	CV < 2%

[a] GLC = Gas-liquid chromatography; HPLC = High performance liquid chromatography; EMIT = Enzyme multiplied immunoassay; FPIA = Fluorescence polarization immunoassay.

[b] Arbitrary Rating Scale of 1 (Excellent) to 5 (Poor).

[c] 1 = least expense.

[d] 1 = least training.

[e] 1 = preferred method.

[f] Simultaneous analysis of phenytoin, primidone, and carbamazepine possible.

***Table 26-8.** Comparison of the Relative Advantages and Disadvantages of the Various Ethosuximide Assays*

Analytical method[a]	Specificity for ethosuximide[b]	Limit of sensitivity μg/mL (free levels)	Metabolite analysis	Assayable samples				Minimum sample volume required	Speed		Analysis cost[c]		Specialized operator training[d]	Preference & rank[e]			Comments
				Plasma/serum	Urine	Saliva	CFS		1–10 samples	10–100 samples	Estimated reagent and tech. cost/assay	Initial equipment costs		Small service	Large service	Research	
GLC	1	0.1	Y	Y	Y	Y	Y	0.1 mL	3 hr	30/day	4	2	4	4	4	1	CV ≤ 5%[f]
HPLC	1	2	?	Y	Y	Y	Y	0.5 mL	4 hr	20/day	3	3	3	3	3	2	CV ≤ 5%
EMIT																	
Manual	2	10	N	Y	N	Y	Y	50 μL	1 hr	50/day	3	1	2	1	2	3	CV < 10%
Automated	2	10	N	Y	N	Y	Y	50 μL	<1 hr	100/day	2	4	2	2	1	3	CV < 10%

a GLC = Gas-liquid chromatography; HPLC = High performance liquid chromatography; EMIT = Enzyme multiplied immunoassay.

b Arbitrary Rating Scale of 1 (Excellent) to 5 (Poor).

c 1 = least expense.

d 1 = least training.

e 1 = preferred method.

f Simultaneous analysis of valproic acid possible.

to 215 nm is somewhat offset by the high plasma concentrations encountered clinically. Some of the HPLC assays utilize a simple precipitation of proteins with acetonitrile or acetone, followed by injection of the supernatant. Although rapid, these methods suffer from relatively poor sensitivity and short column life. Conversely, if extraction is used, the precautions concerning evaporation described above also apply here.

The EMIT assay for ethosuximide is sensitive to only 10 µg/mL, but is used widely in clinical laboratories and performs well in interlaboratory quality control surveys. Desmethyl methsuximide interferes with the EMIT assay. An FPIA assay is now available.

PROSPECTUS

In spite of the progress made in the last two decades in the rational use of antiepileptic drugs, the seizures of a significant proportion of patients with epilepsy remain uncontrolled. Evidence for this consensus comes from the fact that several new anticonvulsants (i.e., felbamate, lamatrogine, nafimidone, stiripentol, zonisamide, vigabatrin) have reached the clinical phases of development. The literature available to date indicates that even for these new drugs a knowledge of the clinical pharmacological properties will be necessary to optimize clinical use.

REFERENCES

1. Morselli PL. Carbamazepine: absorption, distribution and excretion. In: Levy RH et al, eds. Antiepileptic Drugs. 3rd ed. New York: Raven Press; 1989:473–90.
2. Riad LE et al. Simultaneous first- and zero-order absorption of carbamazepine tablets in humans. J Pharm Sci. 1986;75:897.
3. Wang JT et al. Effects of moisture on dissolution of carbamazepine tablets. Pharm Res. 1989;6(Suppl):S-176.
4. Graves NM et al. Relative bioavailability of rectally administered carbamazepine suspension in humans. Epilepsia. 1985;26:429–33.
5. Kuhnz W et al. Carbamazepine and carbamazepine-10,11-epoxide during pregnancy and postnatal period in epileptic mothers and their nursed infants: pharmacokinetics and clinical effects. Pediatr Pharmacol. 1983;3:199–208.
6. Kerr BM, Levy RH. Carbamazepine: carbamazepine epoxide. In: Levy RH et al, eds. Antiepileptic Drugs. 3rd ed. New York: Raven Press; 1989:505–20.
7. Faigle JW, Feldmann KF. Carbamazepine: biotransformation. In: Levy RH et al, eds. Antiepileptic Drugs. 3rd ed. New York: Raven Press; 1989:491–504.
8. Tomson T et al. Single dose kinetics and metabolism of carbamazepine-10,11-epoxide. Clin Pharmacol Ther. 1983;33:58–65.
9. Levy RH, Kerr BM. Clinical pharmacokinetics of carbamazepine. J Clin Psychiatry. 1988;49(Suppl):58–61.
10. Bourgeos BFD, Wad N. Carbamazepine-10,11-diol steady state serum levels and renal excretion during carbamazepine therapy in adults and children. Ther Drug Monit. 1984;6:259–65.
11. Eichelbaum M et al. Carbamazepine metabolism in man: induction and pharmacogenetic aspects. Clin Pharmacokinet. 1985;10:80–90.
12. Tomson T. Interdosage fluctuations in plasma carbamazepine concentration determine intermittent side effects. Arch Neurol. 1984;41:830–4.
13. Larkin JG et al. A double-blind comparison of conventional and controlled-release carbamazepine in healthy subjects. Br J Clin Pharmacol. 1989;27:313–22.

14. Levy RH, Shen DD. Valproate: absorption, distribution, and excretion. In: Levy RH et al, eds. Antiepileptic Drugs. 3rd ed. New York: Raven Press; 1989:583–99.
15. Carrigan PJ. Absorption characteristics of a new valproate formulation: Divalproex sodium-coated particles in capsules (Depakote Sprinkle). J Clin Pharmacol. 1990;30:743–7.
16. Cloyd JC et al. Valproic acid pharmacokinetics in children. II. Discontinuation of concomitant antiepileptic drug therapy. Neurology. 1985;35:1623–7.
17. Kriel RL et al. Valproic acid pharmacokinetics in children: III. Very high dosage requirements. Pediatr Neurol. 1986;2:202–8.
18. Rust RS, Dodson WE. Phenobarbital: absorption, distribution, and excretion. In: Levy RH et al, eds. Antiepileptic Drugs. 3rd ed. New York: Raven Press; 1989:293–304.
19. Kaneko S et al. The problems of antiepileptic medication in the neonatal period: is breast-feeding advisable? In: Janz D et al, eds. Epilepsy, Pregnancy, and the Child. New York: Raven Press; 1982:343.
20. Nau H et al. Placental transfer and pharmacokinetics of primidone and its metabolites pheno-barbital, PEMA and hydroxyphenobarbital in neonates and infants of epileptic mothers. Eur J Clin Pharmacol. 1980;18:31–42.
21. Anderson G. Phenobarbital: biotransformation. In: Levy RH et al, eds. Antiepileptic Drugs. 3rd ed. New York: Raven Press; 1989:305–12.
22. Chang T. Ethosuximide: absorption, distribution, and excretion. In: Levy RH et al, eds. Antiepileptic Drugs. 3rd ed. New York: Raven Press; 1989:671–8.
23. Koup JR et al. Ethosuximide pharmacokinetics in a pregnant patient and her newborn. Epilepsia. 1978;19:535–9.
24. Shorvon SD et al. One drug for epilepsy. Br Med J. 1978;1:474–6.
25. Troupin AS et al. Carbamazepine - A double-blind comparison with phenytoin. Neurology. 1977;27:511–9.
26. Hoppener RJ et al. Correlation between daily fluctuations of carbamazepine serum levels and intermittent side effects. Epilepsia. 1980;21:341–50.
27. Kutt H. Clinical pharmacology of carbamazepine. In: Pippenger CE et al, eds. Antiepileptic Drugs: Quantitative Analysis and Interpretation. New York: Raven Press; 1978:297–305.
28. Weaver DF et al. Massive carbamazepine overdose: clinical and pharmacologic observations in five episodes. Neurology. 1988;38:755–9.
29. Gram L et al. Sodium valproate, serum level and clinical effect in epilepsy: a controlled study. Epilepsia. 1979;20:303–12.
30. Henriksen O, Johannessen SI. Clinical pharmacokinetic observations on sodium valproate - 5-year follow-up study in 100 children with epilepsy. Acta Neurol Scand. 1982;65:504–23.
31. Rowan AJ et al. Sodium valproate: serial monitoring of EEG and serum levels. Neurology. 1979;29:1450–9.
32. Lockard JS, Levy RH. Valproic acid: reversibly acting drug? Epilepsia. 1976;17:477–9.
33. Turnbull DM et al. Correlation between dose, plasma concentration and clinical effect during sodium valproate monotherapy. Br J Clin Pract. 1983;29(Suppl):53–5.
34. Dreifuss FE. Valproate: toxicity. In: Levy RH et al, eds. Antiepileptic Drugs. 3rd ed. New York: Raven Press; 1989:643–51.
35. Schmidt D. Adverse effects of valproate. Epilepsia. 1984;25(Suppl. 1):S44–49.
36. Mortensen PB et al. Biochemical investigations and hemodialysis treatment. Int J Clin Pharmacol Ther Toxicol. 1983;21:64–8.
37. Buchthal F et al. Relation of EEG and seizures to phenobarbital in serum. Arch Neurol. 1968;19:567–72.
38. Feely M et al. Phenobarbitone in previously untreated epilepsy. J Neurol Neurosurg Psychiatry. 1980;43:365–8.
39. Faero O et al. Successful prophylaxis of febrile convulsions with phenobarbital. Epilepsia. 1972;13:279–85.
40. Penry JK, Newmark ME. The use of antiepileptic drugs. Ann Int Med. 1979;90:207–18.

41. Butler TC. Some quantitative aspects of the pharmacology of phenobarbital. In: Pippenger CE et al, eds. Antiepileptic Drugs: Quantitative Analysis and Interpretation. New York: Raven Press; 1978:261–71.

42. Wilensky AJ et al. Kinetics of phenobarbital in normal subjects and epileptic patients. Eur J Clin Pharmacol. 1982;23:87–92.

43. MacLeod CM et al. Memory impairment in epileptic patients: selective effects of phenobarbital concentration. Science. 1978;202:1102–4.

44. Camfield CS et al. Side effects of phenobarbital in toddlers; behavior and cognitive aspects. J Pediatr. 1979;95:361–5.

45. Farwell JR et al. Phenobarbital for febrile seizures–effects on intelligence and on seizure recurrence. N Engl J Med. 1990;322:364–9.

46. Theodore WH, Porter RJ. Removal of sedative-hypnotic antiepileptic drugs from the regimens of patients with intractable epilepsy. Ann Neurol. 1983;13:320–4.

47. Browne TR et al. Ethosuximide in the treatment of absence (petit mal) seizures. Neurology. 1975;25:515–24.

48. Sherwin AL et al. Improved control of epilepsy by monitoring plasma ethosuximide. Arch Neurol. 1973;28:178–81.

49. Richens A. Clinical pharmacology and medical treatment. In: Laidlaw J, Richens A, eds. A Textbook of Epilepsy. 2nd ed. Edinburgh: Churchill Livingstone; 1982:292–347.

50. Henriksen O et al. How to use carbamazepine. In: Morselli PL et al, eds. Antiepileptic Drug Therapy in Pediatrics. New York: Raven Press; 1983:237–43.

51. Miles MV et al. Rapid loading of critically ill patients with carbamazepine suspension. Pediatrics. 1990;86:263–66.

52. Graves NM, Kriel RL. Rectal administration of antiepileptic drugs in children. Pediatr Neurol. 1987;3:321–6.

53. Covanis A, Jeavons PM. Once-daily sodium valproate in the treatment of epilepsy. Dev Med Child Neurol. 1980;22:202-4.

54. Löscher W et al. Comparative evaluation of anticonvulsant and toxic potencies of valproic acid and 2-envalproic acid in different animal models of epilepsy. Eur J Pharmacol. 1984;99:211–8.

55. Levy RH. Monitoring of free valproic acid levels? Ther Drug Monit. 1980;2:199–201.

56. Cloyd JC et al. Valproic acid pharmacokinetics in children. II. Discontinuation of concomitant antiepileptic drug therapy. Neurology. 1985;35:1623–7.

57. Patel IH et al. Phenobarbital-valproic acid interaction in normal man. Clin Pharmacol Ther. 1980;27:515–21.

58. Kutt H. Phenobarbital: interactions with other drugs. In: Levy RH et al, eds. Antiepileptic Drugs. 3rd ed. New York: Raven Press; 1989:313–27.

59. Painter MJ. Phenobarbital: clinical use. In: Levy RH et al, eds. Antiepileptic Drugs. 3rd ed. New York: Raven Press; 1989:329–40.

60. Sherwin AL. How to use ethosuximide. In: Morselli PL et al, eds. Antiepileptic Drug Therapy in Pediatrics. New York: Raven Press; 1983:229–36.

61. Mattson RH, Cramer JA. Valproate: interactions with other drugs. In: Levy RH et al, eds. Antiepileptic Drugs. 3rd ed. New York: Raven Press; 1989:621–32.

62. Kutt H. Carbamazepine: chemistry and methods of determination. In: Levy RH et al, eds. Antiepileptic Drugs. 3rd ed. New York: Raven Press; 1989:457–71.

63. Trager WF et al. Simultaneous analysis of carbamazepine and carbamazepine-10,11-epoxide by GC/CI/MS, a stable isotope methodology. Analyt Lett. 1978;1:119–33.

64. Sawchuck RJ, Cartier LL. Simultaneous liquid chromatographic determination of carbamazepine and its epoxide metabolite in plasma. Clin Chem. 1982;28:2127–30.

65. Levy RH et al. Filtration for free drug level monitoring: carbamazepine and valproic acid. Ther Drug Monit. 1984;6:67–76.

66. Levy RH et al. GLC determination of valproic acid in plasma. Analyt Lett. 1978;1:257–67.

67. Kupferberg HJ. Gas-liquid chromatographic quantitation of valproic acid. In: Pippenger CE et al, eds. Antiepileptic Drugs: Quantitative Analysis and Interpretation. New York: Raven Press; 1978:147–51.

68. Johannessen SI. Phenobarbital: chemistry and methods of determination. In: Levy RH et al, eds. Antiepileptic Drugs. 3rd ed. New York: Raven Press; 1989:283–92.

69. Dudley KH et al. Gas chromatographic on-column methylation technique for the simultaneous determination of antiepileptic drugs in blood. Epilepsia. 1977;18:259–76.

70. Kapetanovic IM, Kupferberg HJ. Stable isotope methodology and gas chromatography mass spectrometry in pharmacokinetic study of phenobarbital. Biomed Mass Spectrom. 1980;7:47-52.

71. Sawchuck RJ, Cartier LL. Liquid chromatographic method for the simultaneous determination of phenytoin and 5- (4-hydroxyphenyl)-5-phenylhydantoin in plasma and urine. Clin Chem. 1980;26:835–9.

72. Glazko AJ, Dill WA. Ethosuximide: Chemistry and methods for determination. In: Woodbury DM, Penry JK, Schmidt RP, eds. Antiepileptic Drugs 1st ed. New York: Raven Press; 1972:413–15.

73. Chang T. Ethosuximide: chemistry and methods of determination. In: Levy RH et al, eds. Antiepileptic Drugs. 3rd ed. New York: Raven Press; 1989:663–9.

Chapter 27

Corticosteroids

William J. Jusko and Elizabeth A. Ludwig

Corticosteroids, while a relatively old class of drugs, remain important for immunosuppression and as anti-inflammatory agents. The major problems that persist with these drugs is the empiricism in arriving at therapeutic doses and the considerable toxicity which often occurs with chronic therapy even when dosages appear reasonable. For example, a strong correlation exists between the frequency of side effects and the mean daily prednisone dose and serum albumin concentration.[1] The minimum incidence of adverse effects was 12% in the low dose/normal albumin group but rose to 62% in the high dose/low albumin group. The side effects in 43 patients included cushingoid features (n = 14), hemorrhage (n = 12), psychoses (n = 10), hyperglycemia (n = 6), and myopathy (n = 1). More chronic effects such as osteoporosis are also of concern. These problems reflect the ability of glucocorticoids to adversely affect numerous tissue and organ systems. The increased frequency of side effects in patients with low serum albumin concentrations may be due to altered protein binding and reduced hepatic function.

This chapter addresses the important clinical pharmacokinetic properties of the major glucocorticoids and presents efforts made to quantitate their pharmacodynamics.

CORTICOSTEROID ABSORPTION AND DISPOSITION

Comparative Properties

The primary glucocorticoids employed for systemic therapy are cortisol (or cortisone), prednisone (or prednisolone), methylprednisolone, and dexamethasone. Their structures are shown in Figure 27-1. Cortisone and prednisone are prodrugs (and metabolites) of the active compounds, cortisol and prednisolone.

A comparison of the major pharmacokinetic properties of the corticosteroids is given in Table 27-1.[2–19] The bioavailability of these compounds is generally high from the brand-name tablet dosage forms. However, in the case of prednisone and prednisolone, bioavailability data do not exist for most of the generic products.[20–23]

The incomplete systemic availability may be partly due to a first-pass effect, at least in the case of cortisol.[4] The average bioavailability for retention enemas is 63% for cortisol[4] and 44% for prednisolone.[24]

The corticosteroids are poorly water-soluble and must be formulated as sodium salts of 21-phosphate or 21-succinate esters for intravenous administration. These two esters are rapidly hydrolyzed in the liver to their free alcohol forms yielding at least 92% availability of the active corticosteroid.[6,12,25,26]

The pharmacokinetics of prednisone and prednisolone,[27] various corticosteroids,[28] and dexamethasone[29] have been reviewed. This chapter summarizes the important properties of these drugs and addresses more recent findings. Earliest comparisons of the major corticosteroids lacked the insights brought about by improvements since 1979 in analytical specificity via high performance liquid chromatography (HPLC) and the recognition that protein binding of prednisolone is dose related.[6]

As shown in Table 27-1, there is only a 2.5-fold range of clearances (CL) and steady-state volumes of distribution (V_{ss}) among these compounds. Cortisol has the shortest half-life (t½) (about 1.7 hours) because of its larger CL and smaller V_{ss}. Dexamethasone, conversely, has a lower CL, a larger V_{ss}, and thus, the longest half-life (4.2 hours). The half-life is an important determinant of corticosteroid pharmacodynamics because the duration of action is determined by how long plasma concentrations are maintained above the IC_{50} (concentration causing 50% inhibition) for various responses. Cortisol and prednisolone exhibit dose-dependent CL and V_{ss} because their binding to transcortin is nonlinear.[6] All of the glucocorticoids are extensively metabolized by the liver and kidney and 3% to 30% of doses are excreted unchanged in urine.[6,27,28.]

Prednisolone

The pattern of prednisone and prednisolone plasma concentrations after an oral dose (20 mg) of prednisone and an intravenous dose (20 mg) of prednisolone (as the prednisolone sodium phosphate ester) is shown in Figure 27-2. Absorption of

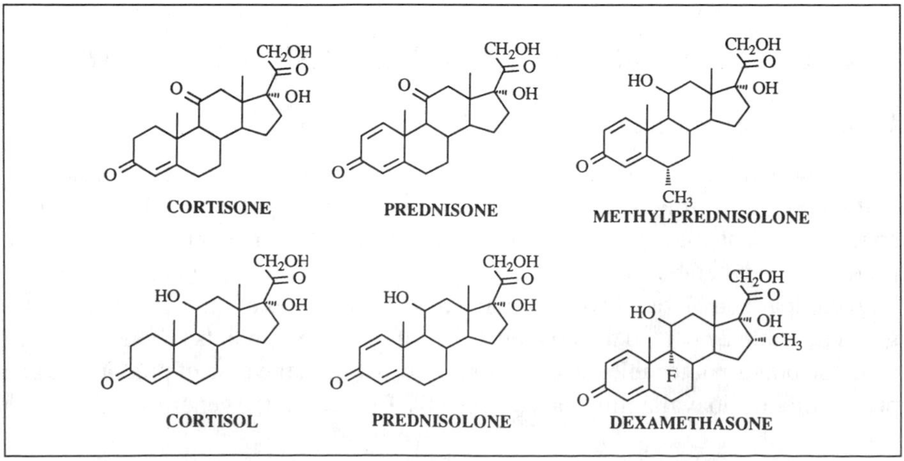

Figure 27-1. *Chemical structures of the major corticosteroids used systemically.*

Table 27-1. *Pharmacokinetic Properties of the Major Systemic Corticosteroids*[a]

Corticosteroid	K_{pb}	F (%)	t½ (hr)	V_{ss} (L/kg)	CL (mL/kg/hr)	References
Cortisol	35.7	56–71	1.7 (1.3–1.9)	0.5 (0.3–0.8)	340 (310–440)	2–4
Prednisone	41.4	60–100	2.9 (2.3–3.5)	0.7 (0.3–0.8)	140 (60–170)	5–10
Methylprednisolone	70.7	74–99	2.7 (2.0–2.8)	1.2 (0.8–1.4)	265 (230–420)	11–15
Dexamethasone	67.8	62–78	4.2 (2.4–4.7)	1.2 (0.7–1.4)	180 (140–250)	16–19

[a] Typical values (range among studies and doses).
[b] Octanol:water partition coefficient.

prednisone is rapid, and peak concentrations are attained within two hours. Extensive first-pass conversion of prednisone to prednisolone occurs as indicated by the immediate, high concentrations of the latter. After intravenous (IV) administration of prednisolone phosphate, ester hydrolysis is extremely rapid producing most of the free alcohol form of the steroid within 15 to 30 minutes. Prednisolone concentrations then decline biexponentially with a half-life of about three hours. Prednisone and prednisolone undergo interconversion with the active compound typically dominating by a 5 to 10:1 area under the concentration-time curve (AUC) ratio.[6,10,30] Cortisol, methylprednisolone, and dexamethasone also undergo hydroxy-keto reversible metabolism at the ll position (see Figure 27-1). The keto forms of the steroids are inactive.

For prednisolone, about 2% of the dose is excreted in urine as prednisone and 20% as prednisolone.[31] Other metabolic routes include 6-hydroxylation (about 5% to 18% of the dose),[32] reduction of the 20-keto group of both prednisolone and prednisone to form the C-20 alcohols (12% for prednisolone and less than 1% for prednisone are found in urine),[31] cleavage of the dihydroxyacetone side chain to give a C-17 ketone, and reduction of the A-ring double bonds. Some of these phase-I metabolites are then conjugated to form their glucuronides.[33] As directly found in rats, both the liver[34] and kidney[35] are probably major metabolic organs in man.

Numerous studies in humans have demonstrated dose-dependent disposition of cortisol[2] and prednisolone.[6-9] Both the apparent CL and V_{ss} increase twofold between the dose levels of 5 and 40 mg of prednisolone. Because $t\frac{1}{2}$ depends on the ratio of V_{ss} to CL, the half-life remains constant with dose.

Prednisolone binding to plasma proteins is nonlinear. Figure 27-3 shows prednisolone binding as a function of both drug and plasma protein concentration.[36] Binding occurs primarily to transcortin and albumin,[1,6,36] and slightly to α_1-acid glycoprotein.[37] Transcortin occurs in plasma at very low concentrations

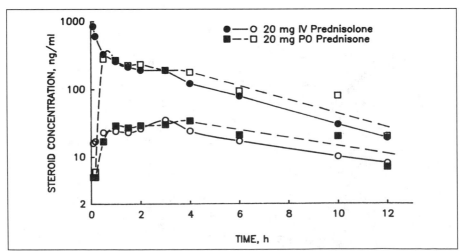

Figure 27-2. *Plasma prednisolone (upper curves) and prednisone (lower curves) concentra-tions observed after a single oral dose of 20 mg prednisone (■—□) and an intravenous dose of 20 mg prednisolone phosphate (●—○) to a healthy male volunteer.*

$(8 \times 10^{-7}$ M), but binds prednisolone (and cortisol) with high affinity $(K_A = 2 \times 10^7$ M^{-1}). In contrast, albumin has a high plasma concentration $(7 \times 10^{-4}$ M), but low affinity $(K_A = 1.4 \times 10^3$ M^{-1}) for prednisolone. At very low prednisolone concentrations, binding is typically maximal at 90% to 95%, but saturation readily occurs to produce about 60% binding at prednisolone plasma concentrations of 500 ng/mL or greater (i.e., doses of 20 mg or higher; see Figure 27-2). Prednisone also binds to transcortin, but ten times more weakly $(K_A = 4.3 \times 10^6$ M^{-1}), while it binds similarly to albumin $(K_A = 1 \times 10^3$ M^{-1}).[38] Cortisol and prednisolone bind similarly to both proteins and are, in fact, competitive inhibitors of each other's binding.[39] The nonlinear binding of prednisolone complicates adjustment of doses below 20 mg because the increased fraction bound to transcortin makes less drug available for distribution to receptor sites.

The traditional approach of adjusting pharmacokinetic parameters for nonlinear protein binding based on unbound drug concentrations for low clearance drugs is appropriate for prednisolone. The CL and V_{ss} values become nearly constant with dose indicating linear kinetics with respect to free drug.[6] This procedure has since become the norm for assessing the elimination and distribution kinetics of prednisolone in various studies of drug and disease interactions. However, it should be noted that very high doses (1200 mg) such as those used to treat shock produce a lower prednisolone clearance that is probably caused by saturable metabolism.[40]

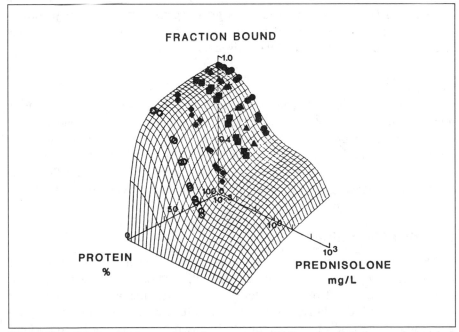

Figure 27-3. *Relationship between the plasma protein binding of prednisolone, unbound drug concentrations, and protein concentrations of 100%, 87.5%, 75%, 50%, and 25% of normal. The curved surface was fitted to the experimental data assuming steroid binding to transcortin and albumin (reprinted with permission from reference 36).*

Over the oral (but not IV) dose range of 0.2 to 0.8 mg/kg of prednisone or prednisolone, the AUC of unbound prednisolone increases by less than fourfold indicating some nonlinearity in systemic availability.[41]

Of potential value in patient monitoring are observations that a linear relationship exists between prednisolone clearance and a six-hour plasma prednisolone concentration following oral or IV doses.[42] This single sample allows one to rapidly identify those patients who may have unusually high or low rates of metabolism or incomplete absorption.

Methylprednisolone

Methylprednisolone and methylprednisone differ from prednisolone and prednisone only by the addition of the 6α-methyl group (see Figure 27-1). This structure blocks the specific binding of these corticosteroids to transcortin. Instead, the 6α-methyl compounds are primarily bound (75% to 82%) to albumin, and the extent of binding is constant.[43] The nonspecific binding of various glucocorticoids correlates well with their octanol-water partition coefficients.[43] The absence of nonlinear transcortin binding partly accounts for the linear pharmacokinetics of methylprednisolone in the 5 to 40 mg dose range.[13] However, large intravenous doses (10 mg/kg) yield a reduced total CL of methylprednisolone.[12]

Methylprednisolone has a larger V_{ss} (1.2 L/kg) than does prednisolone (0.7 L/kg) partly due to the lack of transcortin binding and its larger partition coefficient (see Table 27-1). This results in considerably greater penetration of methylprednisolone into bronchoalveolar fluids[44] and may create a therapeutic advantage for this steroid in the treatment of pulmonary diseases.

Dexamethasone

Dexamethasone is not bound to transcortin and its plasma protein binding in humans is in the range of 68%[45] to 75%.[46] The AUC of dexamethasone does not increase in proportion to oral doses of 0.5 to 1.5 mg,[19] but CL appears to be linear up to larger IV doses of 1.5 mg/kg.[47] Dexamethasone has been used extensively over the past ten years as the Dexamethasone Suppression Test (DST), a psychoendocrinological probe for endogenous depression, a condition which produces adrenal hyperactivity.[29]

Reversible Metabolism

The ll-keto/hydroxy interconversion that takes place between prednisone and prednisolone (see Figure 27-1) as catalyzed by llβ-hydroxy steroid dehydrogenase in various tissues is also a characteristic of cortisol, methylprednisolone, and dexamethasone.[48] Similarly, reversible metabolism occurs for numerous estrogens, androgens, and other compounds.[48] This process distorts the traditional meaning of CL = Dose/AUC and may invalidate the noncompartmental calculation of V_{ss} from Dose AUMC/AUC^2, where AUMC is the area under the moment curve. Calculation of the true clearances for interconversion (CL_{12} and CL_{21}) and elimination of drug (CL_{10}) and metabolite (CL_{20}) requires IV administration of both drug and metabolite and measurement of their four resultant AUC values.[48,49] Equations based on moment analysis allow generation of all CL and volume values, residence time, and recycling characteristics of reversible drug/metabolite systems.[48,49] Conventional analysis yields CL terms which underestimate the "true" values by up to 30% and volume terms which err by 10% to 61% for methylprednisolone in the rabbit, a species which handles this steroid similarly to humans. Most of the CL and V_{ss} values in the literature for corticosteroids were generated by conventional methods and should be viewed as "apparent" values. However, they remain of value when interconversion is slight and in assessing net steroid behavior in comparative studies.

While the corticosteroids, especially cortisol, are eliminated relatively rapidly, interconversion allows for efficient removal of high concentrations of the active drug; however, conservation of drug in the body occurs in metabolite form. Thus, reversibility augments biological exposure to steroids by serving as a dampening "compartment" that reduces fluctuations in serum concentrations and prolongs the half-life because of such recycling.

The reversible metabolism of prednisolone and prednisone in humans is a nonlinear process because the AUC ratio of the two compounds increases with dose[6] as does their steady-state concentration ratio during prednisolone infusion.[7]

Physiological Factors Affecting Disposition

Circadian. Serum cortisol concentrations are governed by a circadian rhythm; maximum concentrations (acrophase) occur in the early morning hours and episodic bursts of adrenal secretion occur randomly throughout the 24-hour period.[50] Thus, it is important to examine other chronobiological aspects of corticosteroid disposition. Transcortin binding capacity for prednisolone is minimal at 8 a.m. (10.65 µg bound/dL) and greatest at midnight (17.54 µg bound/dL) in healthy subjects.[51] Cortisol CL also appears to exhibit circadian variation with higher values found from 5 to 11 a.m. (149 versus 91 L/m²/dL) when plasma cortisol concentrations are usually maximal.[52]

Oral doses of 0.2 mg/kg prednisone were given to normal subjects at 6 a.m., 12 noon, 6 p.m., 12 midnight, and AUC values of unbound prednisolone of 110, 100, 70, and 90 ng × hr/mL were found.[53] Intravenous doses of 0.075 mg/kg prednisolone were given at 6 a.m. and 6 p.m., and free prednisolone CL was 14% lower in the morning.[9] No differences occurred with larger doses (1.5 mg/kg) of prednisolone. The apparently high prednisolone CL and/or low bioavailability of prednisone occurring at 6 p.m. differs from the behavior of cortisol. These possible circadian effects need further study.

The pharmacodynamics of corticosteroids are strongly linked to circadian factors. Evening administration produces greater adrenal suppression than morning doses of corticosteroids.[54] The effectiveness of methylprednisolone in allergic asthma appears optimal when the largest amounts of steroid are present in the morning and early afternoon.[55] Methylprednisolone CL is 28% greater when dosed at 4 p.m. (versus 8 a.m.), but no differences were found in three dynamic markers of steroid responsiveness in normal volunteers.[188]

Intrasubject Variation. Prednisolone does not cause induction of its own metabolism; thus, its kinetics are fairly stable in patients on long-term prednisone treatment. The average coefficient of variation (CV) of prednisolone AUC values in ten patients studied on two occasions separated by 45 to 325 days was only 5%.[56] However, kinetics may differ between daily and alternate-day therapy. Free prednisolone CL was 20% lower during daily therapy compared to a pretreatment phase and differed by 17% between "on" and "off" days of alternate-day therapy in a group of Japanese patients.[57] Fewer cushingoid effects were found during the intermittent regimen.

Genetics. Pharmacogenetics are a partial determinant of corticosteroid disposition. A moderate degree of co-variance exists in prednisolone and dexamethasone CL; 14 subjects given both steroids exhibited a correlation coefficient of 0.55 in CL values.[18] No differences in 6β-hydroxycortisol excretion occur between good and poor metabolizers of sparteine.[58] Prednisolone CL and 6β-hydroxyprednisolone excretion appeared normal in a single poor debrisoquine metabolizer.[32] Enzyme inducers such as rifampin increase hepatic levels of cytochrome CYP3A which is responsible for cortisol 6β-hydroxylase activity[59] and presumably that of prednisolone 6-hydroxylation. The array of prednisolone disposition studies in normal subjects does not reveal any polymorphism which might be exhibited as outlying CL values.[5-10]

Age and Gender. Children with asthma in the age range of 8 to 12 years exhibit somewhat greater total prednisolone CL than adults (245 ± 33 versus 201 ± 54 mL/min/1.73 m^2).[60] The same study showed no gender differences of CL in asthmatic children and healthy adults.[60,61] However, the unbound prednisolone CL has been found to be approximately 20% greater in females compared to male adult subjects (see Figure 27-4).[9,32]

A significant inverse relationship was found between the CL and age for both prednisolone and methylprednisolone in asthmatic patients.[42] For prednisolone, children less than 12 years of age had a 49% higher CL/kg than patients over 12 years. In an evaluation of dexamethasone pharmacokinetics in patients of various ages, newborns exhibited higher peak and 12-hour serum concentrations.[62]

Compared to younger patients, the elderly have a high prevalence of adverse effects (40%), including osteoporosis (16%) and hypertension (12%), when treated with long-term corticosteroids.[63] Old age causes a modest shift in the circadian pattern of serum cortisol concentrations[64] and resistance to cortisol suppression was found (using the dexamethasone suppression test) in the aged.[65] The elderly have a 38% reduction in unbound prednisolone CL and a 24% smaller unbound V_{ss}.[66] A slower decline in cortisol concentrations occurred after IV prednisolone, probably reflecting slower cortisol CL rather than less adrenal suppression *per se*.

Pregnancy. During pregnancy, dexamethasone elimination is increased 2.3-fold compared to nonpregnant women.[17] Pregnancy causes increased 6β-hydroxycortisol excretion indicating that a state of enzyme induction may exist.[67]

Clinical Drug Interactions

The corticosteroids are sensitive to an array of induction and inhibitory drug interactions. These, as well as non-interactions found in the literature, are listed in Table 27-2.[68–95]

Induction. All of the corticosteroids are susceptible to enzyme induction by anticonvulsants, an interaction which has had severe clinical consequences. Reports exist of loss of corticosteroid efficacy in treatment of asthma,[68–70] rheumatoid arthritis,[71] and renal transplantation[96] in patients in whom anticonvulsants or rifampicin were added.

An in-depth assessment of the anticonvulsant interaction with prednisolone was carried out in healthy subjects before and after treatment with 300 mg phenytoin per day for six to eight days.[32] The findings are depicted in Figure 27-4. Phenytoin increased the total and nonrenal CL of unbound prednisolone by 48% in females and 49% in males. The corresponding values for the nonrenal (metabolic) CL were

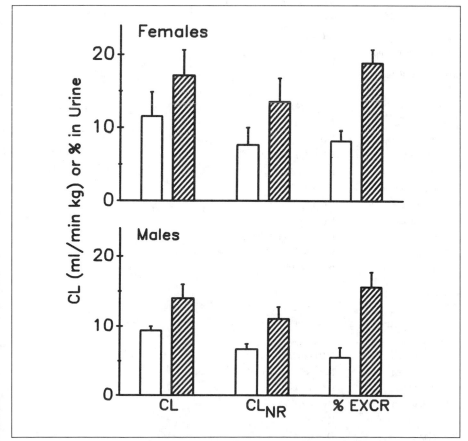

Figure 27-4. *Effect of phenytoin on total clearance of unbound prednisolone (CL), nonrenal clearance (CL_{NR}), and percent excretion of 6β-hydroxyprednisolone in urine (% EXCR). Male and female subjects were given 0.8 mg/kg IV prednisolone before (hollow bars) and after (hatched bars) treatment with 300 mg phenytoin daily for six to eight days (from Frey and Frey, reference 32).*

77% in females and 65% in males. The prednisolone metabolite, 6β-hydroxy-prednisolone, was particularly sensitive to the inductive effect with increases in percent urinary recovery of 130% (females) and 183% (males). This behavior is analogous to that of 6β-hydroxycortisol, a useful marker of enzyme induction.[97]

Non-Interactions. Several important non-interactions occur. The absence of effects of theophylline,[75] azathioprine,[77] and tobacco smoking[18] facilitate clinical use of the corticosteroids. While cimetidine has a slight inhibitory effect on prednisolone[79] and dexamethasone[80] disposition, these interactions are probably of no consequence. Similarly, the small effects of cyclosporine[84–86] are probably

Table 27-2. Metabolic Drug Interactions Affecting Corticosteroids[a,b]

Induction

Phenobarbital	P (+25%),[68] MP (+86%),[11] D (+87%)[68]
Phenytoin	C (+37%),[69] P (+49%),[32] P (+77%),[70] MP (+130%),[11] D (+140%)[72]
Rifampicin	P (+143%)[73]
Carbamazepine	P (+42%)[74]
Ephedrine	D (+42%)[75]
Cyclophosphamide	D (+43%)[76]

No or Slight Effect

Theophylline	D (−11%)[75]
Diazepam	MP (+3%)[11]
Azathioprine	P (0, −5%)[77]
Cortisol	P (+9%)[78]
Cimetidine	P (−14%),[79] D (−8%)[80]
Ranitidine	P (−0.5%)[79]
Troleandomycin	P (−9%)[81]
Ketoconazole	P (−6%)[82]
Methotrexate	P (+7%)[83]
Tobacco	P (+3, +13%),[18] D (18%)[18]
Cyclosporine	P (−1%),[84] P (−22%),[85] MP (+2%)[86]
Tenidap	P (−10%)[190]

Inhibition

Oral contraceptives	P (−39, −24%),[87] P (−38%)[88]
Conjugated estrogens	P (−25%)[89]
Troleandomycin	MP (−60%)[90]
Erythromycin	MP (−46%)[91]
Ketoconazole	MP (−60%),[92] P (−50%)[93]
Glycyrrhizin	P (−31%)[191]
Indomethacin	P (−40%)[94]
Naproxen	P (−35%)[94]
Isoniazid	D (−27%)[95]

[a] C = Cortisol; P = Prednisolone; MP = Methylprednisolone; D = Dexamethasone.
[b] Number in parentheses denotes direction and average change in clearance of the designated corticosteroid.

inconsequential. The use of low dose methotrexate reduces steroid requirements in steroid-dependent asthma patients,[189] but this is not due to a pharmacokinetic interaction.[83]

Inhibition. The effects of oral contraceptives (OCs) on prednisolone disposition are of interest because the interaction is appreciable and because of its dual nature (see Figure 27-5). The OCs cause two hepatic effects: a reduction in unbound prednisolone CL (by 38%) and an increase in serum transcortin concentrations (by 80%).[88] Both effects raise total serum prednisolone concentrations, making it especially important to assess unbound steroid. Conjugated estrogens also decrease free prednisolone CL (by 25%) in older women.[89]

The antibiotics, troleandomycin (TAO)[90] and erythromycin,[91] and the antifungal agent, ketoconazole,[92] markedly inhibit methylprednisolone CL. Interestingly, TAO[81] and probably ketoconazole[82] do not disturb prednisolone disposition. While there is consistency among the corticosteroids in sensitivity to enzyme induction (see Table 27-2), the converse occurs in metabolic inhibition. The TAO-methylprednisolone interaction offers a positive patient benefit because TAO therapy produces a "steroid-sparing" effect in asthma. This permits steroid tapering, improved therapeutic efficacy and/or reduced adverse effects.[90,98] This effect is only partly due to the diminished CL and extended time-course of methylprednisolone serum concentrations. The ketoconazole-prednisolone interaction needs clarification. Our studies of 16 mg prednisolone doses show no kinetic or dynamic interactions with ketoconazole,[82] while another study shows a 50% lower unbound CL of a larger steroid dose (0.8 mg/kg).[93]

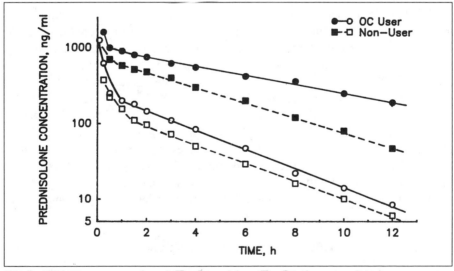

Figure 27-5. *Time-course of total (■—●) and free (□—○) plasma prednisolone concentrations following 40 mg IV doses to women who were oral contraceptive (OC) users (○—●) and non-OC-users (□—■) (from Boekenoogen et al., reference 88).*

Glycyrrhizin, a saponin of licorice root, is a strong inhibitor of the 11β-dehy-drogenase enzyme and markedly reduces the unbound CL of prednisolone (by 31%).[191] This interaction is probably of concern for licorice itself and for the anti-ulcer drug, carbenoxolone, as well.

The effects of anticonvulsant therapy on methylprednisolone disposition were assessed with and without TAO treatment in three patients.[81] TAO substantially offsets the induction effect of phenytoin and phenobarbital.

A reduced unbound prednisolone CL (by 35% to 40%) was found in the presence of naproxen and indomethacin, which is potentially important when these drugs are used to treat patients with rheumatic disease.[94] The new anti-inflamma-tory agent, tenidap, has no overall effect on prednisolone CL (unbound), but reduces its renal clearance by 44%.[190] These studies should be extended to the numerous other NSAIDS.

Bioavailability. Potential drug interactions in relation to corticosteroid absorp-tion have been assessed. Cholestyramine[99] and antacids[100,101] do not affect *predni-solone* bioavailability. However, two types of antacids (magnesium and aluminum hydroxides) reduced the bioavailability of prednisolone from *prednisone* tablets by 20% to 43% in healthy subjects and liver disease patients.[102]

Effects of Other Drugs. Corticosteroids are frequently coadministered with other drugs and their reverse interactions are important. Cyclosporine and predni-solone or methylprednisolone are used concurrently in renal and liver transplant patients. While cyclosporine may have a slight inhibitory effect on prednisolone CL (see Table 27-2), modest to marked increases (135%) in cyclosporine plasma concentrations occur following high-dose methylprednisolone treatment.[103] Theo-phylline and corticosteroids are used for asthma, but these drugs have little or no interaction.[104,105] Moderate single or chronic doses of cortisol or prednisolone do not appear to generally affect hepatic metabolism or function[106] as determined by their lack of influence on theophylline,[104,105] antipyrine,[106] hexobarbital,[108] tolbuta-mide[108] and BSP[106] disposition. However, both acute and chronic oral doses of prednisone increase ethanol elimination by about 10%.[192]

Caution is needed when adding or deleting corticosteroids in rheumatoid arthritis patients on salicylate therapy. Corticosteroids increase salicylate renal clearance sufficiently to cause problematic changes in serum salicylate concentra-tions.[109] Chronic doses of corticosteroids produce an average of 20% increase in inulin clearance, apparently by increasing glomerular plasma flow.[110] Single doses of sodium salicylate were not affected, however, before and during chronic dosing with oral prednisone.[111]

Pathophysiological Effects on Steroid Disposition

Obesity. Prednisolone pharmacokinetics were compared in healthy obese and normal subjects after a 40 mg IV dose of prednisolone.[112] The uncorrected V_{ss} of total prednisolone was 20% greater in obese subjects (36.7 and 44.1 L). Uptake of prednisolone into adipose tissue is limited, as reflected by the partition value of 0.09 into excess body weight. Uncorrected (absolute) total and free prednisolone CL were increased in obesity (11.1 and 8.3 L/hr total; 65.4 and 44.6 L/hr free).

Free prednisolone CL correlated strongly (r = 0.80) with the degree of obesity expressed as TBW:IBW (total to ideal body weight). Thus, prednisolone dosing and parameter adjustment to TBW is most appropriate.

Oral doses of dexamethasone produce a 44% increase in AUC and a 22% longer half-life when given to obese versus normal-weight subjects.[113] While these differences were not statistically significant, more subjects may yield meaningful differences since similar effects occur for methylprednisolone. Methylprednisolone disposition was assessed after 0.6 mg/kg doses in healthy obese and non-obese males. Uptake of methylprednisolone into adipose tissue was limited because the V_{ss}/kg TBW was substantially lower in the obese. Methylprednisolone protein binding was identical in both groups (78%). In contrast to prednisolone, methylprednisolone half-life was prolonged and CL was significantly reduced in the obese subjects (38%) even when corrected for body weight (see Figure 27-6). Thus, methylprednisolone should be dosed based on IBW and less frequent dosing may be necessary in obese subjects due to their decreased CL values. Interestingly, obese subjects exhibit no differences in sensitivity (IC_{50}) to adrenal suppression and to basophil and T-helper cell trafficking.

Hepatic Disease. Concern that corticosteroid interconversion and metabolism may be impaired in chronic liver disease (CLD) has led to numerous investigations which have primarily focused on prednisone/prednisolone. The most extensive assessment involved administration of 0.8 mg/kg doses of oral prednisone and IV prednisolone in 22 patients (decompensated cirrhotics and stable renal transplant recipients) with a broad range of liver function.[115] After oral prednisone the AUC ratio of prednisolone to prednisone declined slightly with decreasing galactose elimination capacity (GEC), a measure of cytosolic liver enzyme activity. This

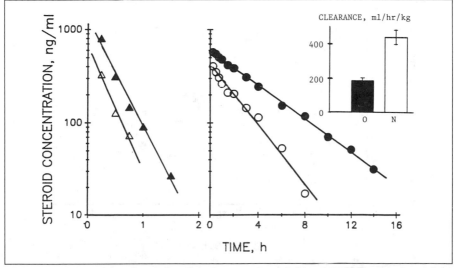

Figure 27-6. *Disposition of methylprednisolone succinate (left) and methylprednisolone (right) after administration of IV methylprednisolone as its succinate ester (0.6 mg/kg) to normal (△—○) and obese (▲—●) subjects. The insert shows mean clearance (± SD) in the normal (N) and obese (O) groups (adapted from from reference 114),*

suggests some impaired conversion of prednisone to prednisolone. Steroid exposure (AUC of unbound prednisolone) decreased with increasing serum albumin concentrations (see Figure 27-7). This is largely attributable to the good relationship observed between free prednisolone CL and GEC. The V_{ss} of prednisolone was independent of liver function. Dose reduction may be necessary in CLD patients since exposure to biologically active unbound prednisolone is increased.

Dexamethasone pharmacokinetics were examined after a 1 mg IV dose in CLD patients and normal subjects.[117] The mean dexamethasone CL was substantially reduced (72%) and the mean half-life prolonged (5.9 versus 3.5 hours) in the CLD patients. Methylprednisolone disposition was assessed in six stable CLD patients and compared to healthy men following a single IV dose of methylprednisolone.[118] Interestingly, mean parameters were similar in both groups for CL (about 360 L/hr/kg IBW), V_{ss} (about 1.4 L/kg), and t½ (about 2.5 hours). This indicates that methylprednisolone may offer a pharmacokinetic advantage relative to prednisolone in CLD.

Renal Diseases. Renal disease-induced alterations in steroid pharmacokinetics are related to the specific pathology.

The effect of hypoalbuminemia on prednisolone disposition was studied in six patients with nephrotic syndrome after 0.8 mg/kg IV doses.[119] Relative to healthy controls, the unbound fraction of prednisolone was higher in the nephrotic patients and was inversely related to albumin concentrations (r = 0.92), thus indicating a relationship between protein binding and disease activity. The mean unbound drug CL was similar to control values, and the V_{ss} of total but not unbound prednisolone

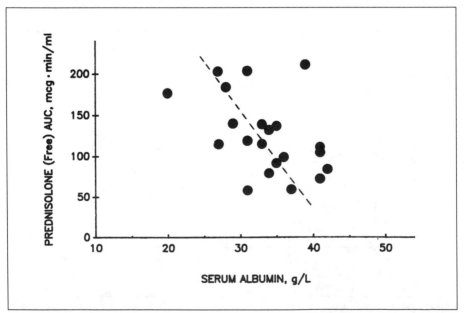

Figure 27-7. *Area-under-the-curve of unbound prednisolone in relation to serum albumin concentrations in a group of kidney transplant and cirrhotic patients given an IV bolus dose of 0.8 mg/kg prednisolone (from reference 115).*

was larger. In contrast, another study found free prednisolone CL to be substantially reduced (75%) in 11 nephrotic children compared to controls.[120] This condition needs further evaluation with respect to prednisolone disposition.

The disposition of methylprednisolone was examined after the administration of 12 to 20 mg/kg doses of methylprednisolone sodium succinate in 14 patients with nephrosis. The kinetics of large doses were similar to low-dose (0.5 to 1 mg/kg) data from asthmatic patients; the mean CL was about 0.4 L/hr/kg, V_{ss} was about 1.2 L/kg, and there was reasonable consistency among the patients.[121]

Chronic renal disease patients were compared to healthy controls after a 20 mg IV dose of prednisolone. The free fraction of prednisolone was greater at all concentrations, most likely a combined result of hypoalbuminemia and competitive binding of uremic substances. The mean free prednisolone CL was 40% lower in the uremics. The isolated perfused rat kidney[35] reveals excretion as well as extensive metabolism of unchanged prednisolone, processes likely to be impaired with renal dysfunction.

Metabolic differences were observed[117] after simultaneous administration of 1 mg IV doses of prednisolone, cortisol, and dexamethasone to 16 patients with chronic renal failure. Interestingly, total prednisolone CL was higher (37%), cortisol CL was slightly lower (15%), and the dexamethasone CL was substantially higher (69%) than the controls. These results require further verification due to the drug mixture, low doses, and short duration of blood sampling. Since only modest changes in cortisol protein binding have been described in uremia,[123] cortisol disposition in chronic renal disease may not be significantly affected. Similarly, a small reduction (69% versus 77%) in dexamethasone protein binding occurs in uremic versus normal serum occurs.[45] No alternations in dexamethasone pharmacokinetics were found in chronic renal failure patients after oral doses.[124] The mean CL of methylprednisolone was reduced (47%) in uremic subjects compared to normals after 0.5 mg/kg IV doses.[125]

In seven patients undergoing hemodialysis, prednisolone free fraction was similar to controls (12.1%) after prednisolone 15 mg IV; however, the AUC of free prednisolone was 29% greater than in healthy subjects.[126] The hemodialysis CL of total prednisolone is concentration-dependent while unbound prednisolone CL is constant (76 mL/min); removal of only 7% to 17% of the dose occurs.[127] Appreciable hemodialysis removal of methylprednisolone results in a shortened (32%) plasma half-life relative to normals.[128] Peritoneal dialysis (CAPD) produces a dialysate removal rate of unbound cortisol that is similar to the urinary free cortisol excretion rate in normal subjects.[129]

The total CL of prednisolone was linearly related to creatinine clearance in 113 kidney transplant recipients after 10 mg oral prednisolone doses as shown in Figure 27-8.[130] In this and another study,[131] cushingoid patients exhibited a lower total CL of prednisolone, suggesting there is a relationship between the biologic effect of prednisolone (relative steroid exposure) and renal function.[131] Further, 28 stable renal transplant patients (with normal liver function tests) exhibited a lower GEC than controls at one month and one year after transplantation.[132] Correspondingly, the mean unbound prednisolone clearance was 31% (one month) and 40% (one year) lower, indicating impairment of both cytosolic and microsomal liver function in such patients.

Oral prednisone and prednisolone bioavailability were compared in nine renal transplant patients after their usual daily doses (12.5 to 22.5 mg).[131] Mean prednisolone bioavailability from oral prednisone and prednisolone relative to IV doses was 84.5% and 95.5% (not significant) using unbound concentrations; the conversion of prednisone to prednisolone occurred rapidly. Both oral corticosteroids should thus provide similar immunosuppressive effects in these patients.

Methylprednisolone disposition was studied[86] in nine renal transplant recipients receiving 10 to 60 mg daily doses in addition to cyclosporine and azathioprine. The mean CL of methylprednisolone in patients (379 mL/hr/kg) was not different from normal volunteers (373 mL/hr/kg) but varied appreciably (range, 105 to 672). The influence of cyclosporine on methylprednisolone CL cannot be excluded. These findings may partially explain why renal transplant patients respond variably to standardized dosage regimens.

Thyroid Disease. Eight patients with hyperthyroidism were given 0.8 mg/kg doses of IV prednisolone and oral prednisone before and after treatment with carbimazole.[133] The hyperthyroid state produced a modest increase in the mean

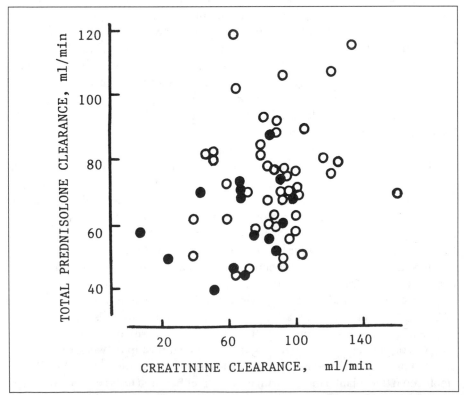

Figure 27-8. *Apparent clearances of total prednisolone in renal transplant patients maintained on 10 mg/day doses of oral prednisolone. Symbols denote cushingoid (●) and non-cushingoid (○) patients (adapted from reference 130).*

free prednisolone CL (22%), and a reduction in V_{ss} for unbound prednisolone (0.98 versus 1.45 L/kg). The systemic availability of unbound prednisolone after prednisone was markedly reduced (34%). Higher doses of prednisolone are warranted in hyperthyroid patients. Only a small reduction in methylprednisolone CL (17%) was observed in six hyperthyroid adults.[134] As with prednisolone, the V_{ss} of methylprednisolone was lower (70 versus 102 L).

Cystic Fibrosis. Prednisolone pharmacokinetics were evaluated in eight cystic fibrosis (CF) patients after 40 mg/1.73 m^2 doses of oral prednisone and IV prednisolone.[135] When compared to data from age-matched asthmatics, the total prednisolone CL was greatly increased (53%) in the CF patients; all drug and metabolites excreted in the urine exhibited proportional increases. The V_{ss} was also larger (49%), but the plasma protein binding was only minimally affected in the CF patients. Bioavailability was complete. More frequent doses of prednisolone and methylprednisolone[136] may be necessary in the treatment of CF patients due to the marked increases in clearance.

Asthma. Variability of prednisolone requirements and clinical response in steroid-dependent asthmatics does not appear to be a consequence of altered disposition. No difference in unbound prednisolone CL (about 200 mL/min/1.73 m^2) or V_{ss} (about 50 L/1.73 m^2) was found in adult asthmatics compared to healthy controls. Another study confirmed complete bioavailability of oral prednisolone in steroid-resistant asthmatics, with CL and V_{ss} values that were similar to those of healthy subjects.[140] However, occasional patients absorb prednisone or methylprednisolone incompletely.[42] Pharmacokinetic parameters obtained after IV prednisolone doses of 40 mg in responsive and relatively resistant pediatric patients (8 to 12 years of age) were similar to adult data.[60] Similarly, methylprednisolone CL in adult asthmatics did not differ from that of controls.[13,81]

Leukemia. The pharmacokinetics of oral prednisolone were studied in six children with acute lymphoblastic leukemia (ALL) after 10 to 20 mg doses.[143] A fourfold variation was observed in CL with a mean value (15 mL/min/kg); this is considerably higher than that observed in pediatric asthmatics (3 to 7 mL/min/kg).[60] Previous use of cytotoxic agents in the leukemics,[76] as well as their younger age,[42] may have produced these results. The effects of other neoplastic diseases on corticosteroid disposition need further study.

Surgery. Significant changes in corticosteroid pharmacokinetics have been reported in the perioperative period. A marked increase in cortisol CL (135%) and V_{ss} (181%) occurred during major surgery compared to preoperative values in four normal subjects.[144] Methylprednisolone sodium succinate (total doses 1.7 to 2.4 gm) was given in the cardioplegia solution of six patients undergoing cardiopulmonary bypass.[145] Because the total CL of the ester was fivefold lower in these patients relative to healthy volunteers, the appearance of methylprednisolone was slower. The mean CL of methylprednisolone was about 50% that of healthy subjects, whereas the V_{ss} was similar in both groups, resulting in reasonably high methylprednisolone concentrations. Thus, full or enhanced availability of methylprednisolone is expected in these patients despite the severe surgical or pathological changes that occur.

Other Diseases. Inflammatory bowel disease does not impair the absorption or disposition of prednisolone.[137–139] Further studies are needed of the effects of rheumatic diseases on corticosteroid pharmacokinetics,[141] but no changes in plasma protein binding occur.[142] More rapid dexamethasone clearance and/or reduced bioavailability occur in depressed patients who do not respond to the DST.[146,147] Dexamethasone kinetics return to normal upon remission of the depressive symptoms.[147]

CORTICOSTEROID DYNAMICS

Mechanisms of Action

The corticosteroids have immunosuppressive, anti-inflammatory, and lympholytic effects at pharmacologic doses and affect numerous biochemical processes. Reviews of the major steps and mechanisms of corticosteroid effects are available.[148–151]

The binding of steroid to cytosolic receptors present in numerous tissues is the major initiating event in producing most, if not all, pharmacodynamic effects (see Figure 27-9). Unbound steroid in plasma diffuses into cells to bind with the intracellular receptor with considerable specificity and affinity. The equilibrium dissociation constant (K_D) is approximately equal to physiologic concentrations of free hormone in plasma (1 to 10 ng/mL). After binding, the steroid-bound receptor is then activated. This process is thought to involve either dissociation of an oligomer (HSP90) or a change in conformation to expose the DNA-binding

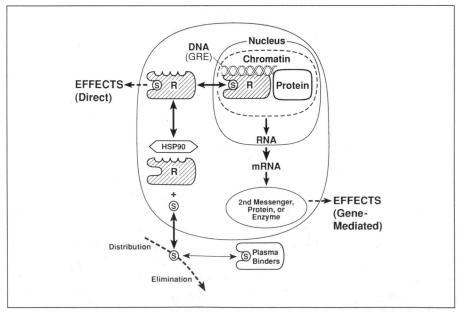

Figure 27-9. Receptor (R)-mediated mechanisms of corticosteroid (S) hormone effects in steroid sensitive cells. HSP90 refers to the 90 KD heat shock protein and GRE are glucocorticoid response elements of DNA.

site.[149] In any case, the activated receptor is able to rapidly translocate into the nucleus, presumably by a facilitated transport mechanism. The activated receptor associates with specific sequences in the genome known as glucocorticoid response elements (GRE). These regulate and usually increase the transcription of specific genes, thereby modulating mRNA concentrations and affecting synthesis of various specific proteins, second messengers, or enzymes. For example, there is a mRNA responsible for increasing synthesis of the tyrosine aminotransferase (TAT) enzyme in the liver. Two elements are needed for gene-mediated effects of steroids in various tissues: the glucocorticoid receptor and the biochemical machinery for synthesis of particular mRNA and proteins or factors responsible for specific steroid actions.

Mathematical models for the gene-mediated action of corticosteroids have been developed for cell culture[152] and *in vivo* rat systems.[153-154] These models allow quantitation of the role of pharmacokinetic, receptor, and post-receptor events in controlling steroid effects and an improved understanding of how dosage regimens can affect steroid responses.[155]

Dynamics

Some effects of corticosteroids (including changes in plasma cortisol concentrations, circulating cells in blood, and the appearance of various other compounds or enzymes in blood) appear to be compatible on a kinetic basis with a "direct" mechanism of action.[151] In essence, the effects of the corticosteroids begin to occur nearly immediately on administration and disappear slowly as the steroid concentrations in plasma fall below the K_D value.

The effects of increasing doses of IV methylprednisolone on basophils in blood, measured as whole blood histamine, are shown in Figure 27-10.[156] The kinetics of methylprednisolone were linear, monoexponential, and exhibited a half-life averaging 2.4 hours in normal men. The blood basophils were essentially constant in number on the baseline day. After methylprednisolone, blood basophils began to fall immediately. This was due to their movement into extravascular sites as the return process was inhibited. When methylprednisolone concentrations fall below the IC_{50} value of about 2 ng/mL, the cells return to the blood, gradually reattaining the baseline levels. It is noteworthy that larger doses of steroids primarily extend the duration of the effect rather than the maximum intensity of the response. Because of this, frequency of dosing may be more important than size of doses administered. Simple and realistic models in terms of blood/extravascular structure were used to fit basophil data from all dose levels simultaneously. The IC_{50} is similar to actual values of K_D for methylprednisolone/receptor binding.[157]

A generalized type of dose-response profile that occurs for corticosteroids is shown in Figure 27-11.[158,159] The net effect (AUC of Effect) is related to steroid exposure (AUC) in a linear/log fashion but without an asymptote. Larger doses produce progressively greater intensity and duration of effects.[158,159] A linear relationship between log methylprednisolone dose and AUC of Effect for fasting blood sugar, blood lymphocytes, and blood "segmented cells" for steroid doses of 16 to 1000 mg has been found[160] which is similar to that in Figure 27-11. Pred-

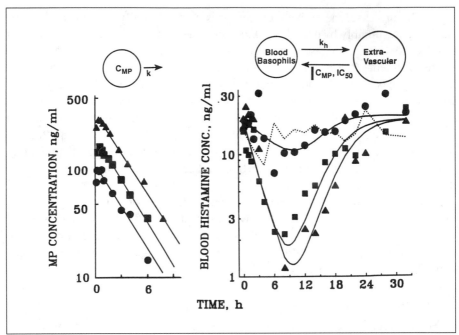

Figure 27-10. *The top panels represent the pharmacokinetic (left) and two-compartment cell distribution and direct suppression model for basophils (whole blood histamine) (right) in relation to methylprednisolone (C_{MP}) concentrations where IC_{50} is the C_{MP} producing 50% inhibition of basophil return to blood. The lower panels show methylprednisolone concentrations (left) and blood basophils as whole blood histamine concentrations versus time in a normal male subject at baseline (.........) and after 10 (●), 20 (■), and 40 (▲) mg of intravenous methylprednisolone (as the sodium succinate salt). Solid lines depict least-squares values based on simultaneous fitting of data from all dose levels to the kinetic/dynamic models (from Kong et al., reference 156).*

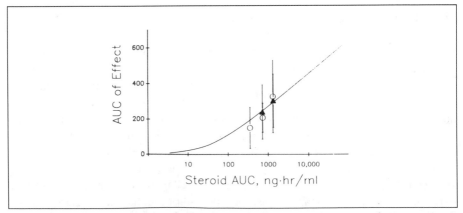

Figure 27-11. *The area between the baseline and effect curve, a measure of net response, is plotted versus the log of methylprednisolone AUC. The solid line depicts the model expectations over a broad range of steroid doses. Symbols show average (± SD) data from two studies: ○[156] and ▲[159] (adapted from reference 158).*

nisolone effects on T-suppressor (OKT3 or CD8⁺) and T-helper (OKT4 or CD4⁺) lymphocytes is similar to the data in Figures 27-10 and 27-11.[161] The direct suppression model can describe the baseline circadian rhythm of T-helper cells to account for the fall and rise of such cells in blood along with steroid-induced movements of cells in and out of the blood compartment.[114] It is notable that the T-helper cell response measured *in vivo* is directly proportional to the mixed lymphocyte response obtained as an *in vitro* bioassay to quantitate steroid effects.[162]

The scheme in Figure 27-12 is useful for summarizing the major factors affecting the gene-mediated determinants of corticosteroid responses.[151] The profile also pertains to the "direct effects" of steroids when alterations of blood cell distribution and the synthesis and degradation of compounds in plasma are considered.

A feature of corticosteroid pharmacodynamics is a slow onset and slow dissipation of effects.[151] Such a pattern is found in examining various pulmonary function tests after prednisolone is given to asthmatic patients.[163] For prednisone or prednisolone, the maximum effect is usually seen at six to eight hours after the dose with a gradual return to baseline by 24 to 36 hours, depending on the dose. Dexamethasone produces a more prolonged response in both its adrenal suppression[164] and gene-mediated effects.[165]

Table 27-4 summarizes the primary pharmacodynamic properties of the four systemic corticosteroids.[157,164,166,167] Potency is related directly to receptor affinity (K_D) for all of the steroids. The overall duration of biological effects is partly explained pharmacokinetically by the time that steroid concentrations are maintained above IC_{50} or K_D values following individual dosages. Thus, the steroids

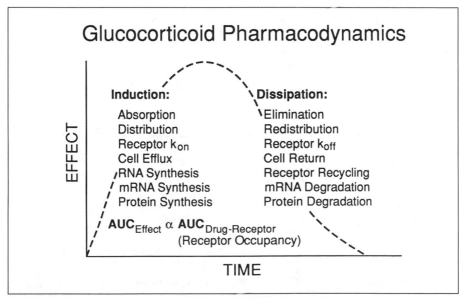

Figure 27-12. Schematic depiction of major determinants of the time-course of onset and dissipation of corticosteroid effects as well as the overall area-under-the-curve (AUC) of effect (from Jusko, reference 151).

with larger $t\frac{1}{2}$ values have longer responses. However, the remaining effect profiles are further related to the subsequent time that it takes for receptors and/or biological factors to recycle or return to baseline values (see Figure 27-12).

Mixed Lymphocyte Reaction. The Mixed Lymphocyte Reaction (MLR) is an index of immunosuppressive activity which has been shown to be of value in predicting survival of human renal allografts.[168] The reaction is a type of bioassay which measures the capacity of drug in patient plasma to inhibit incorporation of tritiated thymidine into the DNA of cultured, normal mononuclear lymphocytes over a three-day incubation period. Its greatest value in relation to corticosteroid disposition has been in demonstrating that it is the unbound, rather than the total, serum concentrations of prednisolone that best describe the MLR-versus-concentration relationship.[169] Enzyme induction with phenytoin[170] and metabolic inhibi-

Table 27-3. *Pathophysiological Factors Affecting Corticosteroid Disposition*[a]

Abnormality	Steroid	Pharmacokinetic observations
Obesity	P[112]	47% ↑ abs CLf; 47% ↑ abs V_{ss}f; $-t\frac{1}{2}$
	D[113]	44% ↓ abs CLt; 22% ↑ $t\frac{1}{2}$
	MP[114]	38% ↓ abs CLt; 14% ↓ abs V_{ss}t; 32% ↑ $t\frac{1}{2}$
Liver disease	P[115,116]	↓ CLf; 47% ↓ CLt
	D[117]	72% ↓ CLt; 69% ↑ $t\frac{1}{2}$
	MP[118]	8% ↓ CLt; $-V_{ss}$t; 29% ↑ $t\frac{1}{2}$
Renal diseases		
Nephrotic syndrome	P[119,120]	6% ↓ CLf; 11% ↑ V_{ss}f; 75% ↓ CLf
	MP[121]	3% ↓ CLt; 21% ↑ V_{ss}t; 22% ↑ $t\frac{1}{2}$
Chronic renal failure (CRF)	P[112,117]	40% ↓ CLf; 54% ↑ $t\frac{1}{2}$; 37% ↓ CLt
	C[117]	15% ↓ CLt
	D[117,124]	69% ↑ CLt; $-$CLt
CRF with dialysis	P[126]	35% ↓ CLf
Transplantation	P[130]	$-$F
	MP[86]	$-$CLt
Hyperthyroidism	P[133]	22% ↑ CLf; 32% ↓ V_{ss}f; 34% ↓ F
	MP[134]	17% ↓ CLt; 31% ↓ V_{ss}t; 8% ↓ $t\frac{1}{2}$
Cystic fibrosis	P[135]	53% ↑ CLt; 49% ↑ V_{ss}t; 12% ↓ $t\frac{1}{2}$; $-$F
Inflammatory bowel disease	P[137]	16% ↓ CLf; 20% ↑ V_{ss}t; 8% ↑ $t\frac{1}{2}$; $-$F
	P[138]	8% ↑ CLf; $-$F
	P[139]	33% ↑ CLt; 40% ↑ V_{ss}; 3% ↑ $t\frac{1}{2}$; $-$F
Asthma	P[61,140]	$-$CLf; $-V_{ss}$f; $-t\frac{1}{2}$; $-$F
	MP[13,81]	$-$CLt
Rheumatic disease	P[141]	Variable plasma concentrations;
	P[142]	No plasma protein binding changes
Leukemia (ALL)	P[60,143]	↑ CLt, ↓ $t\frac{1}{2}$
Surgery	C[144]	135% ↑ CLt; 181% ↑ V_{ss}t, 20% ↑ $t\frac{1}{2}$
	MP[145]	49% ↓ CLt; 5% ↓ V_{ss}t, 233% ↑ $t\frac{1}{2}$
Depression	D[147]	43% ↑ CLt; 14% ↓ $t\frac{1}{2}$

[a] C = Cortisol; P = Prednisolone; MP = Methylprednisolone; D = Dexamethasone; f = Free drug;
t = Total drug; abs = Absolute.

Table 27-4. *Pharmacodynamic Properties of the Major Systemic Corticosteroids*

| Drug | Relative potency[164,166,167] | | | | Relative receptor affinity[a] | | Duration of biological effects (hr) |
	Anti-inflammatory	Adrenal suppressive	Lymphocyte suppression	Metabolic	Lung	Synovial	
Cortisol	1	1	1	1	9	11	8–12
Prednisolone	4	4	0.3	4	16	14	12–36
Methylprednisolone	5	3	9	5	42	27	12–36
Dexamethasone	25	52	0.8	17	100	100	24–48

[a] Measurements of human lung and synovial tissue.[157]

tion with oral contraceptives[171] do not affect the unbound concentration/MLR response curves, indicating that altered microsomal enzyme activity does not change the plasma concentration of prednisolone metabolites with agonistic or antagonistic activity. An unexplained finding is the marked shift of the MLR-free prednisolone concentration profile observed in serum from patients with nephrotic syndrome; this indicates an unusual sensitivity to the steroid.[171]

Adverse Effects Related to Clearance

The clinical effects of the corticosteroids are diverse. Single or acute doses seldom cause problems other than occasional effects such as gastrointestinal disturbances, hyperglycemia, and psychiatric reactions such as psychosis or euphoria.[1] Chronic therapy can cause disturbances of numerous organ systems that often limit therapy. These include cushingoid effects, osteoporosis, and muscle wasting. Doses are typically established empirically and specific regimens are often recommended for each clinical situation. The ultimate goal is to taper the dose and switch to alternate-day therapy.

The corticosteroids are cleared from the body rapidly so that most dosage regimens produce variable serum concentrations (i.e., a steady state is not attained). Thus, it has been necessary to examine entire serum concentration profiles in the search to relate "blood levels" to either efficacy or toxicity.

The report by Kozower and co-workers in 1974 remains relevant.[172] They administered doses of 0.3 mg/kg of prednisolone phosphate and determined CL in normal volunteers and in patients receiving prednisone for various illnesses. Patients who had developed side effects had lower clearances. However, when examining drug efficacy, no difference in CL existed between those who did and did not respond to prednisone therapy. Also, neither greater toxicity nor increased efficacy occurred in patients receiving comparatively higher maintenance doses.

Intravenous and oral prednisolone disposition was assessed in six noncushingoid and six cushingoid kidney transplant patients on similar daily doses of prednisone (mean of 19 mg).[173] The noncushingoid patients had a higher plasma clearance (147 mL/min) than did the cushingoid group (CL = 82 mL/min).

Subsequent studies have been mixed in supporting these early observations. Renal transplant patients were examined after IV prednisolone, and slightly lower unbound CL values were observed in patients with cushingoid side effects.[174] An extensive study of 35 renal transplant patients assessed the value of measuring prednisolone kinetics following 30 mg oral doses to predict graft survival and the occurrence of adverse effects from long-term treatment with prednisolone.[175] The incidence of rejection was similar in patients with high (>0.2 L/kg/hr) and low CL (<0.2 L/kg/hr); however, rejection more frequently resulted in graft loss in the high CL group. Patients with and without cushingoid side effects had similar prednisolone CL and maintenance doses, and no differences existed in peak and AUC values of cortisol. However, they also examined the incidence of serious complications (such as virus infections, steroid diabetes, and osteonecrosis) occurring within one year after renal transplantation. In patients with high CL (≥0.16 L/kg/hr) 5 of 15 developed severe problems. In those with low CL (<0.16 L/kg/hr),

12 of 20 developed severe complications. This study would have been augmented by measurements of serum protein binding to assess the AUC of unbound prednisolone. However, it supports the tendency for patients with low CL values to be more susceptible to adverse reactions.

Prednisolone pharmacokinetics and protein binding were studied in 16 cushingoid and 46 noncushingoid long-term kidney transplant patients on 10 mg oral maintenance doses of prednisolone or prednisone.[131] The cushingoid patients had lower creatinine clearances (67 versus 90 mL/min) and lower unbound prednisolone CL values (319 versus 367 mL/min) than the noncushingoid patients. There was a weak but significant correlation (r = 0.273) between total prednisolone CL and creatinine CL (see Figure 27-8).

Renal and/or hepatic disease are associated with reductions in unbound prednisolone CL, and patients with cushingoid or other adverse effects are likely to have a diminished metabolic rate for prednisolone. Both situations call for vigilance in the use of corticosteroids and a reduction in the maintenance dose if control of disease symptoms or transplanted organ function can be suitably retained.

Adrenal Suppression

Cortisol concentrations in plasma are controlled by the hypothalmic-pituitary-adrenal axis and exhibit a circadian rhythm with a period of 24 hours.[50] Maximum cortisol values of 100 to 160 ng/mL typically occur between 6 and 10 a.m. Superimposed on this profile are episodic bursts of cortisol secretion stimulated by ACTH which cause rapid fluctuations in serum concentrations over brief (0.2 to 2-hour) intervals. A pharmacodynamic model consisting of a cosinor biorhythmic control, a switch function for episodic secretion, and a one-compartment system with a secondary circadian CL mechanism has been used for endogenous cortisol secretion and disposition.[50]

The exogenous corticosteroids suppress cortisol secretion in general correlation with their other potencies (see Table 27-4). Therapeutic doses of prednisolone and methylprednisolone cause adrenal suppression for 12 to 18 hours with serum cortisol usually recovering within 24 hours. Dexamethasone, in oral doses of 0.5 to 1.5 mg, causes suppression for 24 to 36 hours; normal morning values are reattained by 48 hours.[19] Potency ratios of the various corticosteroids have been assessed in terms of their extent and duration of cortisol suppression.[164] The cortisol AUC in the presence and absence of the exogenous steroid better quantitates the net time course of adrenal suppression.[92] Optimally, pharmacokinetic/pharmacodynamic modeling should allow separation of variables and the generation of an IC_{50} value that reflects adrenal suppression by the administered steroids.[156] Such an IC_{50} value for methylprednisolone is similar to the K_D value for steroid-receptor binding.[157]

The goal in chronic corticosteroid therapy is to maintain adequate clinical effects while minimizing extended adrenal suppression. Monitoring serum cortisol facilitates this aim and lends itself to pharmacodynamic quantitation.

ANALYTICAL METHODS

Corticosteroids are commonly measured in plasma or other biological fluids by high performance liquid chromatographic (HPLC) or radioimmunoassay (RIA) methods. Prednisone, prednisolone, and cortisol can be determined simultaneously by sensitive and selective HPLC methods with UV detection to quantitation limits in plasma of about 10 ng/mL.[176,177] Various RIA methods allow greater sensitivity (<1 ng/mL) for cortisol (e.g., Diagnostic Products Corporation) or for prednisolone,[30,178] but there is usually concern for cross-reactivity between these steroids when they are present together. Methylprednisolone, methylprednisone, and cortisol can be jointly determined by HPLC to concentrations of 10 ng/mL.[90,179] Methylprednisolone sodium succinate can similarly be measured.[180] Methylprednisolone can interfere with commercial RIAs for cortisol, producing values that average 80% higher than true cortisol concentrations.[159] HPLC can be used to assess the disposition of large doses of dexamethasone (to 1 ng/mL),[181] but RIA is needed for the conventional 1 mg doses as used in the DST where 20 pg/mL can be quantitated.[182] Commercial RIA methods for dexamethasone are available (e.g., IgG Corporation). Several hydroxylated metabolites of prednisolone in urine can be determined by HPLC.[31] Quantitation of urinary 6β-hydroxycortisol for use as an index of enzyme induction can be done by HPLC[183] or immunoassay[184] methods.

The plasma protein binding of prednisone,[38] prednisolone,[36] cortisol,[39] methylprednisolone,[43] methylprednisone,[43] and dexamethasone[45] has usually been measured by equilibrium dialysis. However, complexities such as radioisotopic impurities, fluid shifts, and nonlinear drug binding require careful use of this method.[36] More recently, ultrafiltration (e.g., Centrifree, Amicon) has proven to be a simpler and easier method for determining cortisol,[185] prednisolone,[57] and methylprednisolone[156] plasma protein binding. Traditionally, transcortin or corticosteroid-binding-globulin (CBG) concentrations have been obtained in drug disposition studies by calculation from nonlinear binding graphs (see Figure 27-3).[36] More recently, radioimmunoassay[186] and enzyme-linked immunoassay (ELISA)[187] methods for CBG have been published, some antibodies are now commercially available (e.g., Medgenix, Ratingen, Germany).

PROSPECTUS

The systemic corticosteroids are usually well absorbed and eliminated at a moderate rate (half-life = two to five hours), principally by biotransformation to a variety of inactive hydroxylated metabolites. Bioavailability problems occur occasionally but are not common. Nonlinear plasma protein binding and reversible metabolism complicate the pharmacokinetics of cortisol and prednisolone.

All of the corticosteroids are sensitive to enzyme-induction interactions with rifampin and the anticonvulsants; numerous agents (e.g., cimetidine, tobacco) have no effects; selected metabolic inhibitors are of concern (oral contraceptives, erythromycin, TAO, ketoconazole, naproxen). Prednisolone and methylprednisolone have differing sensitivities to drug and disease interactions. Moderate doses of corticosteroids seldom affect the disposition of other drugs except for chronic salicylates. Physiologic factors of concern for altered steroid disposition include young age, old age, and pregnancy. Pathophysiologic factors of importance for some steroids include obesity, thyroid disorders, cystic fibrosis, major surgery, and hepatic and renal impairment. The rapid elimination of steroids has commonly required complete plasma concentration versus time profiles in patients to assess possible altered absorption or disposition, but recent use of a single-dose, single-point (six-hour) method for prednisolone offers promise of facilitated patient evaluation.

Corticosteroids produce numerous debilitating adverse effects with chronic use which tend to occur more frequently in patients with low clearances. On the other hand, loss of efficacy has been reported in patients receiving enzyme inducers. The corticosteroids produce their immunosuppressive and anti-inflammatory effects by receptor-mediated mechanisms with a slow onset, delayed maximum, and slowly dissipating response pattern. Recognition of such profiles, the role of the limited quantity of receptors, and the requirement for receptor recycling may allow further improvements in rational selection of the steroid and dosage regimen for optimal patient therapy.

Acknowledgements

Manuscript assistance from Ms. Sandra M. Wheaton and Ms. Suzanne M. Jusko and review by Dr. Stanley J. Szefler are appreciated. Supported by Grant No. 24211 from The National Institutes of General Medical Sciences, NIH.

REFERENCES

1. Lewis GP et al. Prednisone side-effects and serum-protein levels. Lancet 1971;2:778–81.
2. Toothaker RD, Welling PC. Effect of dose size on the pharmacokinetics of intravenous hydrocortisone during endogenous hydrocortisone suppression. J Pharmacokinet Biopharm. 1981;10:147–56.
3. Toothaker RD et al. Effect of dose size on the pharmacokinetics of oral hydrocortisone suspension. J Pharm Sci. 1982;71:1182–185.
4. Lima JJ, Jusko WJ. Bioavailability of hydrocortisone retention enemas in relation to absorption kinetics. Clin Pharmacol Ther. 1980;28:262–69.
5. Rose JQ et al. Bioavailability and disposition of prednisone and prednisolone from prednisone tablets. Biopharm Drug Dispos. 1980;1:247–58.
6. Rose JQ et al. Dose dependent pharmacokinetics of prednisone and prednisolone in man. J Pharmacokinet Biopharm. 1981;9:389–417.
7. Legler UF et al. Prednisolone clearance at steady state in man. J Clin Endocrinol Metab. 1982;55:762–67.
8. Bergrem H et al. Pharmacokinetics and protein binding of prednisolone after oral and intravenous administration. Eur J Clin Pharmacol. 1983;24:415–19.
9. Meffin PJ et al. Alterations in prednisolone disposition as a result of time of administration, gender, and dose. Br J Clin Pharmacol. 1984;17:395–404.
10. Ferry JJ et al. Relative and absolute bioavailability of prednisone and prednisolone after separate oral and intravenous doses. J Clin Pharmacol. 1988;28:81–87.
11. Stjernholm MR, Katz FH. Effects of diphenylhydantoin, phenobarbital, and diazepam on the metabolism of methylprednisolone and its sodium succinate. J Clin Endocrinol Metab. 1975;41:887–93.

12. Derendorf H et al. Kinetics of methylprednisolone and its hemisuccinate ester. Clin Pharmacol Ther. 1985;37:502–507.
13. Szefler SJ et al. Methylprednisolone versus prednisolone pharmacokinetics in relation to dose in adults. Eur J Clin Pharmacol. 1986;30:323–29.
14. Antal EJ et al. Influence of route of administration on the pharmacokinetics of methylprednisolone. J Pharmacokinet Biopharm. 1983;11:561–76.
15. Al-Habet SMH, Rogers HJ. Comparative pharmacokinetics of methylprednisolone phosphate and hemisuccinate in high doses. Pharm Res. 1988;5:509–13.
16. Duggan DE et al. Bioavailability of oral dexamethasone. Clin Pharmacol Ther. 1975;18:205–209.
17. Tsuei SE et al. Disposition of synthetic glucocorticoids. I: Pharmacokinetics of dexamethasone in healthy adults. J Pharmacokinet Biopharm. 1979;7:249–64.
18. Rose JQ et al. Effect of smoking on prednisone, prednisolone, and dexamethasone pharmacokinetics. J Pharmacokinet Biopharm. 1981;9:1–14.
19. Loew D et al. Dose-dependent pharmacokinetics of dexamethasone. Eur J Clin Pharmacol. 1986;30:225–30.
20. Sullivan TJ et al. Comparative bioavailability: eight commercial prednisone tablets. J Pharmacokinet Biopharm. 1976;4:157–72.
21. Tembo AV et al. Bioavailability of prednisolone tablets. J Pharmacokinet Biopharm. 1977;5:257–70.
22. Sugita ET, Niebergall PJ. Bioavailability monograph: prednisone. J Am Pharm Assoc. 1975;NS15:529–32.
23. Thiessen JJ et al. Bioavailability monograph: prednisolone. J Am Pharm Assoc. 1976; NS16:143–46.
24. Lee DAH et al. Plasma prednisolone levels and adrenocortical responsiveness after administration of prednisolone-21-phosphate as a retention enema. Gut 1979;20:349–35.
25. Derendorf H et al. Pharmacokinetics of prednisolone after high doses of prednisolone hemisuccinate. Biopharm Drug Dispos. 1985;6:423–32.
26. Greenberger PA et al. Comparison of prednisolone kinetics in patients receiving daily or alternate-day prednisone for asthma. Clin Pharmacol Ther. 1986;39:163–8.
27. Frey BM, Frey FJ. Clinical pharmacokinetics of prednisone and prednisolone. Clin Pharmacokinet. 1990;19:126–46.
28. Gustavson LE, Benet LZ. Pharmacokinetics of natural and synthetic glucocorticoids. In: Anderson DC, Winter JSD, eds. Adrenal Cortex. Cornwall, England: Butterworth and Co., Ltd.;1985;11:235–81.
29. Lowy MT, Meltzer HY. Dexamethasone bioavailability: implications for DST research. Biol Psychiatry 1987;22:373–85.
30. Meikle AW et al. Kinetics and interconversion of prednisolone and prednisone studied with new radioimmunoassays. J Clin Endocrinol Metab. 1975;41:717–21.
31. Garg V, Jusko WJ. Simultaneous analysis of prednisone, prednisolone, and their major hydroxylated metabolites in urine by high-performance liquid chromatography. J Chromatogr. 1991;567:39–47.
32. Frey FJ, Frey BM. Urinary 6β-hydroxyprednisolone excretion indicates enhanced prednisolone catabolism. J Lab Clin Med. 1983;101:593–604.
33. Vermeulen A. The metabolism of 4-^{14}C-prednisolone. J Endocrinol. 1959;18:278–91.
34. Morais JA, Wagner JG. Steroid metabolism in isolated rat hepatocytes. Eur J Drug Metab Pharmacokinet. 1985;10:295–307.
35. Rocci ML et al. Prednisolone metabolism and excretion in the isolated perfused rat kidney. Drug Metab Dispos. 1981;9:177–82.
36. Boudinot FD, Jusko WJ. Fluid shifts and other factors affecting plasma protein binding of prednisolone by equilibrium dialysis. J Pharm Sci. 1984;73:774–80.
37. Milsap RL, Jusko WJ. Binding of prednisolone to α1-acid glycoprotein. J Steroid Biochem. 1983;18:191–94.
38. Boudinot FD, Jusko WJ. Plasma protein binding interaction of prednisone and prednisolone. J Steroid Biochem. 1984;21:337–39.

39. Rocci ML et al. Prednisolone binding to albumin and transcortin in the presence of cortisol. Biochem Pharmacol. 1982;31:289–92.
40. Derendorf H et al. Pharmacokinetics of prednisolone after high doses of prednisolone hemisuccinate. Biopharm Drug Dispos. 1985;6:423–32.
41. Frey FJ et al. The dose-dependent systemic availability of prednisone: one reason for the reduced biological effect of alternate-day prednisone. Br J Clin Pharmacol. 1986;21:183–89.
42. Hill MR et al. Monitoring glucocorticoid therapy: a pharmacokinetic approach. Clin Pharmacol Ther. 1990;48:390–98.
43. Ebling WF et al. 6α-Methylprednisolone and 6α-methylprednisone plasma protein binding in humans and rabbits. J Pharm Sci. 1986;75:760–63.
44. Vichyanond P et al. Penetration of corticosteroids into the lung: evidence for a difference between methylprednisolone and prednisolone. J Allergy Clin Immunol. 1989;84:867–73.
45. Tsuei SE et al. Disposition of synthetic glucocorticoids. II: Dexamethasone in parturient women. Clin Pharmacol Ther. 1980;28:88–98.
46. Cummings DM et al. Characterization of dexamethasone binding in normal and uremic human serum. DICP Ann Pharmacother. 1990;24:229–31.
47. Rohdewald P et al. Pharmacokinetics of dexamethasone and its phosphate ester. Biopharm Drug Dispos. 1987;8:205–12.
48. Ebling WF, Jusko WJ. The determination of essential clearance, volume, and residence time parameters of recirculating metabolic systems: the reversible metabolism of methylprednisolone and methylprednisone in rabbits. J Pharmacokinet Biopharm. 1986;14:557–99.
49. Wagner JG et al. Reversible metabolism and pharmacokinetics: application to prednisone and prednisolone. Res Commun Chem Pathol Pharmacol. 1981;32:387–405.
50. Jusko WJ et al. Partial pharmacodynamic model for the circadian-episodic secretion of cortisol in man. J Clin Endocrinol Metab. 1975;40:278–89.
51. Angeli A et al. Diurnal variation of prednisolone binding to serum corticosteroid-binding globulin in man. Clin Pharmacol Ther. 1978;23:47–53.
52. de Lacerda L et al. Diurnal variation of the metabolic clearance rate of cortisol. Effect on measurement of cortisol production rate. J Clin Endocrinol Metab. 1973;36:1043–49.
53. English J et al. Diurnal variation of prednisolone kinetics. Clin Pharmacol Ther. 1983;33:381–85.
54. Nichols T et al. Diurnal variation in suppression of adrenal function by glucocorticoids. J Clin Endocrinol. 1965;25:343–49.
55. Reinberg A et al. Circadian changes in effectiveness of corticosteroids in eight patients with allergic asthma. J Allergy Clin Immunol. 1983;71:425–33.
56. Langhoff E et al. Intraindividual consistency of prednisolone kinetics during long-term prednisone treatment. Eur J Clin Pharmacol. 1984;26:651–53.
57. Yasuda K et al. Changes in the pharmacokinetics of plasma total and free prednisolone during daily and intermittent regimens. J Clin Endocrinol Metab. 1990;70:957–64.
58. Park BK et al. 6β-Hydroxycortisol excretion in relation to polymorphic N-oxidation of sparteine. Brit J Clin Pharmacol. 1982;13:737–40.
59. Ged C et al. The increase in urinary excretion of 6β-hydroxycortisol as a marker of human hepatic cytochrome P450IIIA induction. Br J Clin Pharmacol. 1989;28:373–87.
60. Rose JQ et al. Prednisolone disposition in steroid-dependent asthmatic children. J Allergy Clin Immunol. 1981;67:188–93.
61. Rose JQ et al. Prednisolone disposition in steroid-dependent asthmatics. J Allergy Clin Immunol. 1980;66:366–73.
62. Richter O et al. Pharmacokinetics of dexamethasone in children. Pediatric Pharmacol. 1983;3:329–37.
63. Thomas TPL. The complications of systemic corticosteroid therapy in the elderly. Gerontology 1984;30:60–65.
64. Sherman B et al. Age-related changes in the circadian rhythm of plasma cortisol in man. J Clin Endocrinol Metab. 1985;61:439–43.
65. Oxenkrug GF et al. Aging and cortisol resistance to suppression by dexamethasone: a positive correlation. Psychiatry Res. 1983;10:125–30.

66. Stuck AE et al. Kinetics of prednisolone and endogenous cortisol suppression in the elderly. Clin Pharmacol Ther. 1988;43:354–62.

67. Ohkita C, Goto M. Increased 6-hydroxycortisol excretion in pregnant women: implication of drug-metabolizing enzyme induction. DICP Ann Pharmacother. 1990;24:814–16.

68. Brooks SM et al. Adverse effects of phenobarbital on corticosteroid metabolism in patients with bronchial asthma. N Engl J Med. 1972;286:1125–128.

69. Evans PJ et al. Anticonvulsant therapy and cortisol elimination. Br J Clin Pharmacol. 1985;20:129–32.

70. Petereit LB, Meikle AW. Effectiveness of prednisolone during phenytoin therapy. Clin Pharmacol Ther. 1977;22:912–16.

71. Brooks PM et al. Effects of enzyme induction on metabolism of prednisolone, clinical and laboratory study. Ann Rheum Dis. 1976;35:339–43.

72. Haque N et al. Studies of dexamethasone metabolism in man: effect of diphenylhydantoin. J Clin Endocrinol Metab. 1972;34:44–50.

73. McAllister WAC et al. Rifampicin reduces effectiveness and bioavailability of prednisolone. Br Med J. 1983;286:923–25.

74. Olivesi A. Modified elimination of prednisolone in epileptic patients on carbamazepine monotherapy, and in women using low-dose oral contraceptives. Biomed Pharmacother. 1986; 40:301–308.

75. Brooks SM et al. The effects of ephedrine and theophylline on dexamethasone metabolism in bronchial asthma. J Clin Pharmacol. 1977;17:308–18.

76. Moore MJ et al. Rapid development of enhanced clearance after high-dose cyclophosphamide. Clin Pharmacol Ther. 1988;44:622–28.

77. Frey FJ et al. A single dose of azathioprine does not affect the pharmacokinetics of prednisolone following oral prednisone. Eur J Clin Pharmacol. 1981;19:209–12.

78. Meffin PJ et al. Cortisol does not inhibit prednisolone clearance. Br J Clin Pharmacol. 1985;20:414–16.

79. Sirgo MA et al. Effects of cimetidine and ranitidine on the conversion of prednisone to prednisolone. Clin Pharmacol Ther. 1985;37:534–38.

80. Peden NR et al. Cortisol and dexamethasone elimination during treatment with cimetidine. Br J Clin Pharmacol. 1984;18:101–103.

81. Szefler SJ et al. Steroid-specific and anticonvulsant interaction aspects of troleandomycin-steroid therapy. J Allergy Clin Immunol. 1982;69:455–60.

82. Yamashita SK et al. Lack of pharmacokinetic and pharmacodynamic interactions between ketoconazole and prednisolone. Clin Pharmacol Ther. 1991;49:558–70.

83. Glynn-Barnhart A et al. Effect of low-dose methotrexate on the disposition of glucocorticoids and theophylline. J Allergy Clin Immunol. 1991;88:180–86.

84. Frey FJ et al. Evidence that cyclosporine does not affect the metabolism of prednisolone after renal transplantation. Transplantation 1987;43:494–98.

85. Rocci ML Jr et al. The effect of cyclosporine on the pharmacokinetics of prednisolone in renal transplant patients. Transplantation 1988;45:656–60.

86. Tornatore KM et al. Methylprednisolone disposition in renal transplant recipients receiving triple-drug immunosuppression. Transplantation 1989;48:962–65.

87. Meffin PJ et al. Alterations in prednisolone disposition as a result of oral contraceptive use and dose. Br J Clin Pharmacol. 1984;17:655–64.

88. Boekenoogen SJ et al. Prednisolone disposition and protein binding in oral contraceptive users. J Clin Endocrinol Metab. 1983;56:702–709.

89. Gustavson LE et al. Impairment of prednisolone disposition in women taking oral contraceptives or conjugated estrogens. J Clin Endocrinol Metab. 1986;62:234–37.

90. Szefler SJ et al. The effect of troleandomycin on methylprednisolone elimination. J Allergy Clin Immunol. 1980;66:447–51.

91. LaForce CF et al. Inhibition of methylprednisolone elimination in the presence of erythromycin therapy. J Allergy Clin Immunol. 1983;72:34–39.

92. Glynn AM et al. Effects of ketoconazole on methylprednisolone pharmacokinetics and cortisol secretion. Clin Pharmacol Ther. 1986;39:654–59.

93. Zurcher RM et al. Impact of ketoconazole on the metabolism of prednisolone. Clin Pharmacol Ther. 1989;45:366–72.

94. Rae SA et al. Alternation of plasma prednisolone levels by indomethacin and naproxen. Br J Clin Pharmacol. 1982;14:459–61.

95. Santoso B et al. The influence of isoniazid pre-treatment on the elimination of dexamethasone. Eur J Clin Pharmacol. 1989;36S:A268.

96. Wassner SJ et al. The adverse effect of anticonvulsant therapy on renal allograft survival. J Pediatrics 1976;88:134–37.

97. Ohnhaus EE, Park BK. Measurement of urinary 6β- hydroxycortisol excretion as an *in vivo* parameter in the clinical assessment of the microsomal enzyme-inducing capacity of antipyrine phenobarbitone and rifampicin. Eur J Clin Pharmacol. 1979;11:139–45.

98. Wald JA et al. An improved protocol for the use of troleandomycin (TAO) in the treatment of steroid-requiring asthma. J Allergy Clin Immunol. 1979;78:36–43.

99. Audetat V, Bircher J. Bioavailability of prednisolone during simultaneous treatment with cholestyramine. Gastroenterology. 1976;71:1110-111.

100. Bergrem H et al. Absorption of prednisolone. I: The effect of fasting food and food combined with antacids. Scand J Urol Nephrol Suppl. 1981;64:167–73.

101. Albin H et al. Effect of aluminium phosphate on the bioavailability of cimetidine and pred-nisolone. Eur J Clin Pharmacol. 1984;26:271–73.

102. Uribe M et al. Decreased bioavailability of prednisone due to antacids in patients with chronic active liver disease and in healthy volunteers. Gastroenterology. 1981;80:661–65.

103. Klintmalm G, Sawe J. High dose methylprednisolone increases plasma cyclosporin levels in renal transplant recipients. Lancet. 1984:731.

104. Leavengood DC et al. The effect of corticosteroids on theophylline metabolism. Ann Allergy. 1983;50:249–51.

105. Fergusson RJ et al. Effect of prednisolone on theophylline pharmacokinetics in patients with chronic airflow obstruction. Thorax. 1987;42:195–98.

106. Weiersmuller A et al. The influence of prednisolone on hepatic function in normal subjects. Effects on galactose elimination capacity, sulfobromophthalein transport maximum and storage capacity and d-glucaric acid output. Am J Dig Dis. 1977;22:424–28.

107. Downie WW et al. The effect of prednisolone on the metabolic handling of antipyrine. Eur J Drug Metab Pharmacokinet. 1978;2:99–101.

108. Breimer DD et al. Influence of corticosteroid on hexobarbital and tolbutamide disposition. Clin Pharmacol Ther. 1978;24:208–12.

109. Klinenberg JR, Miller F. Effect of corticosteroids on blood salicylate concentration. JAMA. 1965;194:601–4.

110. Baylis C, Brenner BM. Mechanisms of the glucocorticoid-induced increase in glomerular filtration rate. Am J Physiol. 1978;234:F166–F170.

111. Day RO et al. Interaction of salicylate and corticosteroids in man. Br J Clin Pharmacol. 1988;26:334–37.

112. Milsap RL et al. Prednisolone disposition in obese men. Clin Pharmacol Ther. 1984; 36:824–31.

113. Lamiable D et al. Pharmacocinetique de la dexamethasone par voie orale chez le sujet obese. Therapie 1990;45:311–14.

114. Dunn T et al. Comparative pharmacokinetics and pharmacodynamics of methylprednisolone in obese and non-obese men. Clin Pharmacol Ther. 1990;47:181.

115. Renner E et al. Effect of liver function on the metabolism of prednisone and prednisolone in humans. Gastroenterol. 1986;90:819–28.

116. Madsbad S et al. Impaired conversion of prednisone to prednisolone in patients with liver cirrhosis. Gut. 1980;21:52–6.

117. Kawai S et al. Differences in metabolic properties among cortisol, prednisolone and dexameth-asone in liver and renal diseases: accelerated metabolism of dexamethasone in renal failure. J Clin Endocrinol Metab. 1985;60:848–54.

118. Ludwig EA et al. Pharmacokinetics of methylprednisolone hemisuccinate and methylprednisolone in chronic liver disease. Pharmacotherapy. 1989;9:191.
119. Frey FJ, Frey BM. Altered prednisolone kinetics in patients with the nephrotic syndrome. Nephron 1982;32:45–48.
120. Miller PFW et al. Pharmacokinetics of prednisolone in children with nephrosis. Arch Dis Child. 1990;65:196–200.
121. Assael BM et al. Disposition of pulse dose methylprednisolone in adult and paediatric patients with the nephrotic syndrome. Eur J Clin Pharmacol. 1982;23:429–33.
122. Bergrem H. The influence of uremia on pharmacokinetics and protein binding of prednisolone. Acta Med Scand. 1983;213:333–37
123. Rosman PM et al. Cortisol binding in uremic plasma. II: Decreased cortisol binding to albumin. Nephron 1984;37:229–31.
124. Workman RJ et al. Dexamethasone suppression testing in chronic renal failure, pharmacokinetics of dexamethasone and demonstration of a normal hypothalamic-pituitary-adrenal axis. J Clin Endocrinol Metab. 1986;63:741–46.
125. Brier ME et al. Bioavailability of methylprednisolone in patients with renal insufficiency. Clin Pharmacol Ther. 1985;37:184.
126. Bergrem H. Pharmacokinetics and protein binding of prednisolone in patients with nephrotic syndrome and patients undergoing hemodialysis. Kidney Int. 1983;23:876–81.
127. Frey FJ et al. Nonlinear plasma protein binding and haemodialysis clearance of prednisolone. Eur J Clin Pharmacol. 1982;23:65–74.
128. Sherlock JE, Letteri JM. Effect of hemodialysis on methylprednisolone plasma levels. Nephron 1977;18:208–11.
129. Zager PG et al. Dialysance of adrenocorticoids during continuous ambulatory peritoneal dialysis. J Clin Endocrinol Metab. 1988;67:110–15.
130. Bergrem H et al. Prednisolone pharmacokinetics in cushingoid and non-cushingoid kidney transplant patients. Kidney Int. 1985;27:459–64.
131. Gambertoglio JG et al. Prednisone and prednisolone bioavailability in renal transplant patients. Kidney Int. 1982;21:621–26.
132. Frey FJ et al. Impaired liver function in stable renal allograft recipients. Hepatology 1989;9:606–13.
133. Frey FJ et al. Altered metabolism and decreased efficacy of prednisolone and prednisone in patients with hyperthyroidism. Clin Pharmacol Ther. 1988;44:510–21.
134. Hill M et al. Methylprednisolone pharmacokinetics in patients with thyroid disease. Pharmacotherapy 1989;9:191.
135. Dove AM et al. Altered prednisolone pharmacokinetics in patients with cystic fibrosis. J Pediatr. 1992. [In Press.]
136. Green CG et al. Rapid methylprednisolone clearance in a patient with cystic fibrosis. Drug Intell Clin Pharm. 1988;22:876–78.
137. Milsap RL et al. Effect of inflammatory bowel disease on absorption and disposition of prednisolone. Dig Dis Sci. 1983;28:161–68.
138. Olivesi A. Normal absorption of oral prednisolone in children with active inflammatory bowel disease including cases with proximal to distal small bowel involvement. Gastroenterol Clin Biol. 1985;9:564–71.
139. Elliott PR et al. Prednisolone absorption in acute colitis. Gut 1980;21:49–51.
140. Mortimer O et al. Bioavailability of prednisolone in asthmatic patients with a poor response to steroid treatment. Eur J Respir Dis. 1987;71:372–79.
141. Hayes M et al. Plasma prednisolone studies in rheumatic patients. Ann Rheum Dis. 1983; 42:151–54.
142. Agabeyoglu IT et al. Plasma protein binding of prednisolone in normal volunteers and arthritic patients. Eur J Clin Pharmacol. 1979;16:399–404.
143. Choonara I et al. Pharmacokinetics of prednisolone in children with acute lymphoblastic leukaemia. Cancer Chemother Pharmacol. 1989;23:392–94.
144. Kehlet H, Binder CHR. Alterations in distribution volume and biological half-life of cortisol during major surgery. J Clin Endocrinol Metab. 1973; 36:330–33.

145. Kong A-N et al. Pharmacokinetics of methylprednisolone sodium succinate and methylprednisolone in patients undergoing cardiopulmonary bypass. Pharmacotherapy. 1990;10:29–34.
146. Carson SW et al. Cortisol suppression per nanogram per milliliter of plasma dexamethasone in depressive and normal subjects. Biol Psychiatry 1988;24:569–77.
147. Maguire KP et al. Dexamethasone kinetics in depressed patients before and after clinical response. Psychoneuroendocrinology 1990;15:113–23.
148. Baxter JD, Funder JW. Hormone receptors. N Engl J Med. 1979;301:1149–1161.
149. Distelhorst CW. Recent insight into the structure and function of the glucocorticoid receptor. J Lab Clin Mcd. 1989;113:404–12.
150. Munck A et al. Glucocorticoid receptors and actions. Am Rev Resp Dis. 1990;141:S1–S10.
151. Jusko WJ. Corticosteroid pharmacodynamics: models for a broad array of receptor-mediated pharmacologic effects. J Clin Pharmacol. 1990;30:303–10.
152. Munck A, Holbrook NJ. Steroid hormone antagonism and a cyclic model of receptor kinetics. J Steroid Biochem. 1987;26:173–79.
153. Boudinot FD et al. Receptor-mediated pharmacodynamics of prednisolone in the rat. J Pharmacokinet Biopharm. 1986;14:469–93.
154. Nichols AI et al. Second generation model for prednisolone pharmacodynamics in the rat. J Pharmacokinet Biopharm. 1989;17:209–27.
155. Nichols AI, Jusko WJ. Receptor mediated prednisolone pharmacodynamics in rats: model verification using a dose-sparing regimen. J Pharmacokinet Biopharm. 1990;18:189–208.
156. Kong A-N et al. Pharmacokinetics and pharmacodynamic modeling of direct suppression effects of methylprednisolone on serum cortisol and blood histamine in human subjects. Clin Pharmacol Ther. 1989;46:616–28.
157. Portner M et al. Glucocorticoid receptors in human synovial tissue and relative receptor affinities of glucocorticoid-21-esters. Pharmaceut Res. 1988;5:623–27.
158. Wald JA et al. Two-compartment basophil cell trafficking model for methylprednisolone pharmacodynamics. J Pharmacokinet Biopharm. 1991;19:521–36.
159. Reiss WG et al. Steroid dose sparing: pharmacodynamic responses to single versus divided doses of methylprednisolone in man. J Allergy Clin Immunol. 1990;85:1058–66.
160. Derendorf H et al. Pharmacodynamics of methylprednisolone phosphate after single intravenous administration to healthy volunteers Pharmaceut Res. 1991;8:263–68.
161. Oosterhuis B et al. Prednisolone concentration-effect relations in humans and the influence of plasma hydrocortisone. J Pharmacol Exp Ther. 1986;239:919–26.
162. Oosterhuis B et al. Concentration-dependent effects of prednisolone on lymphocyte subsets and mixed lymphocyte culture in humans. J Pharmacol Exp Ther. 1987;243:716–22.
163. Ellul-Micallef R et al. The time-course of response to prednisolone in chronic bronchial asthma. Clin Sci Mol Med. 1974;47:105–17.
164. Meikle AW, Tyler FH. Potency and duration of action of glucocorticoids. Am J Med. 1977;63:200–207.
165. Izawa M et al. Dynamics of glucocorticoid receptor and induction of tyrosine aminotransferase in rat liver. Endocrinol Jpn. 1982;29:209–18.
166. Langhoff E, Ladefoged J. Relative potency of various corticosteroids measured in vitro. Eur J Clin Pharmacol. 1982;25:459–62.
167. Ponec M et al. Glucocorticoids: binding affinity and lipophilicity. J. Pharm Sci. 1986;75:973–75.
168. Cochrum KC et al. Correlation between MLC stimulation and graft survival in living relation and cadaver transplants. Ann Surg. 1974;180:617–22.
169. Frey BM et al. Prednisolone pharmacodynamics assessed by inhibition of the mixed lymphocyte reaction. Transplantation 1982;33:578–84.
170. Frey BM, Frey FJ. Phenytoin modulates the pharmacokinetics of prednisolone and the pharmacodynamics of prednisolone as assessed by the inhibition of the mixed lymphocyte reaction in humans. Eur J Clin Invest. 1984;14:1–6.
171. Frey BJ, Frey FJ. The effect of altered prednisolone kinetics in patients with the nephrotic syndrome and in women taking oral contraceptive steroids on human mixed lymphocyte cultures. J Clin Endocrinol Metab. 1985;60:361–69.

172. Kozower M et al. Decreased clearance of prednisolone: a factor in the development of corticosteroid side effects. J Clin Endocrinol Metab. 1974;38:407–12.
173. Gambertoglio JG et al. Prednisolone disposition in cushingoid and noncushingoid kidney transplant patients. J Clin Endocrinol Metab. 1980;51:561–65.
174. Frey FJ et al. Pharmacokinetics of prednisolone and endogenous hydrocortisone levels in cushingoid and noncushingoid patients. Eur J Clin Pharmacol. 1981;21:235–42.
175. Ost L et al. Clinical value of assessing prednisolone pharmacokinetics before and after renal transplantation. Eur J Clin Pharmacol. 1984;26:363–69.
176. Rose JQ, Jusko WJ. Corticosteroid analysis in biological fluids by high-performance liquid chromatography. J Chromatogr. 1979;162:273–80.
177. Frey FJ et al. Liquid-chromatographic measurement of endogenous and exogenous glucocorticoids in plasma. Clin Chem. 1979;25:1944–947.
178. Colburn WA, Buller RH. Radioimmunoassay for prednisolone. Steroids 1973;21:833–46.
179. Ebling WF et al. Analysis of cortisol, methylprednisolone and methylprednisolone hemisuccinate: absence of effects of troleandomycin on ester hydrolysis. J Chromatogr. 1984;305:271–80.
180. Kong A-N et al. Simultaneous analysis of methylprednisolone hemisuccinate, cortisol and methylprednisolone by normal-phase high-performance liquid chromatography in human plasma. J Chromatogr. 1988;432:308–14.
181. Lamiable D et al. High-performance liquid chromatographic determination of dexamethasone in human plasma. J Chromatogr. 1986;378:486–91.
182. Lo ES et al. Direct radioimmunoassay procedure for plasma dexamethasone with a sensitivity at the picogram level. J Pharm Sci. 1989;78:1040–44.
183. Roots I et al. Quantitative determination by HPLC of urinary 6β-hydroxycortisol, an indicator of enzyme induction by rifampicin and antiepileptic drugs. Eur J Clin Pharmacol. 1979;16:63–71.
184. Zhiri A et al. ELISA of 6-beta-hydroxycortisol in human urine: diurnal variations and effects of antiepileptic therapy. Clin Chim Acta. 1986;157:267–76.
185. MacMahon W et al. A simplified ultrafiltration method for determination of serum free cortisol. Clin Chim Acta. 1983;131:171–84.
186. Rosner W et al. Radioimmunoassay for human corticosteroid-binding globulin. Clin Chem. 1983;29:1389–391.
187. Fantl VE et al. Measurement of human corticosteroid binding globulin by enzyme-linked immunoassay. J Steroid Biochem. 1988;31:187–93.
188. Fisher LE et al. Pharmacokinetics and pharmacodynamics of methylprednisolone when administered at 8 am versus 4 pm. Clin Pharmacol Ther. 1992. [In Press.]
189. Dyer PD et al. Methotrexae in the treatment of steroid-dependent asthma. J Allergy Clin Immunol. 1991;88:208–12.
190. Garg V et al. Effect of the anti-inflammatory agent tenidap on the pharmacokinetics and pharmacodynamics of prednisolone. J Clin Pharmacol. 1992;32:222–30.
191. Chen MF et al. Effect of glycyrrhizin on the pharmacokinetics of prednisolone following low dosage of prednisolone hemisuccinate. Endocrinol Jpn. 1990;37:331–41.
192. Korri UM. The effect of glucocorticoids, beta-2-adrenoceptor agonists, theophylline and propranolol on the rate of ethanol elimination and blood acetate concentration in humans. Alcohol Alcohol. 1990;25:519–22.

Chapter 28

Cyclosporine

Gary C. Yee and Daniel R. Salomon

Cyclosporine (also called cyclosporin A [CSA]) is a cyclic peptide with immunosuppressive activity. The drug was discovered in 1969 when two new strains of fungi were isolated from soil samples.[1] A mixture of fungal metabolites was extracted from the fungus and tested for antifungal activity. CSA possessed only limited antifungal activity, but animal studies showed that it was unusually nontoxic. Additional pharmacological tests in 1972 showed that CSA had very potent immunosuppressive activity. After encouraging results in animal transplant models and the development of a suitable dosage form, CSA was first administered to patients in 1978.[1]

Chemically, CSA is a neutral, hydrophobic cyclic peptide of 11 amino acids, one of which is a novel amino acid.[2] The chemical structure of CSA has been elucidated by chemical degradation with X-ray crystallographic analysis. Synthesis of the CSA molecule also has been achieved recently.

CSA is used to prevent graft rejection in solid organ transplant recipients and graft-versus-host disease in marrow transplant recipients and to delay or prevent disease progression in patients with autoimmune diseases.[3] Studies in renal transplant patients show that CSA has improved early and probably long-term survival. The impact of CSA has been more dramatic in liver, heart, and heart-lung transplant patients in whom graft rejection is usually fatal. As a result, the number of liver and heart transplants has increased dramatically since the introduction of CSA. For example, in the year 1990, surgeons in the United States performed over 2000 heart transplants, compared to only 24 per year in 1976. Similarly, the number of liver transplants performed in the United States has increased from 14 per year to over 2500 per year during the same period. In marrow transplant recipients, CSA is one of the most effective single agents in the prevention of graft-versus-host disease.

CLINICAL PHARMACOKINETICS

Assay method and the biological fluid (or matrix) can affect estimates of pharmacokinetic parameters. Unless otherwise noted, all pharmacokinetic parameters are based on specific or relatively specific assay methods [high-performance liquid chromatography (HPLC) or monoclonal specific radioimmunoassay (MC-RIA)]. Since the polyclonal radioimmunoassay (PC-RIA) is no longer available, pharmacokinetic parameters based on this assay method will not be discussed in detail.

Absorption

CSA has been given by the oral, intramuscular, or intravenous route. The drug is incompletely absorbed after oral or intramuscular administration. After intramuscular administration, therapeutic serum CSA concentrations are rarely achieved, even when high single doses (17.5 to 20.0 mg/kg) are given.[4,5] Even after seven days of intramuscular CSA therapy, most patients have serum CSA concentrations of less than 200 ng/mL (PC-RIA).[5] These studies suggest that CSA is absorbed by capacity-limited processes after intramuscular administration. Bioavailability problems are the primary reason that the intramuscular preparation is no longer used.

CSA is available for oral administration as an olive oil solution and as a soft gelatin capsule. The solution must be further diluted in plain or chocolate milk, orange juice, or other liquid. CSA is erratically and incompletely absorbed after oral administration. About one-third of a dose is bioavailable after administration of the oral solution, with a range of less than 5% to 90% (see Table 28-1).[6–16] The absolute oral bioavailability of the soft gelatin capsule is not known, but studies in renal transplant recipients show that the AUC after administration of the soft gelatin capsule is similar to that after administration of the solution.[17,18] Although interpatient variability in oral bioavailability is greater than intrapatient variability, serial studies in healthy subjects and renal transplant recipients show that oral bioavailability can vary by more than twofold.[19,20] The AUC after oral CSA has been reported to gradually increase after several weeks of treatment in renal transplant recipients,[21,22] and this increase has been attributed to increased bioavailability or reduced clearance. Estimates of oral bioavailability depend on the assay method used to measure CSA concentration. Oral bioavailability based on CSA concentrations measured by PC-RIA are usually higher than those based on CSA concentrations based on MC-RIA or HPLC (see Table 28-1). One study has reported that oral CSA bioavailability decreases with increasing dose.[23] That same study also reported that CSA disposition, probably clearance, also changed with increasing dose. The two effects appeared to cancel each other, resulting in a linear increase in AUC with increasing oral dose.

After a lag time of 30 to 60 minutes, C_{max} is usually achieved two to six hours after administration of the oral solution or soft gelatin capsule. The absorption kinetics of CSA are complex and have been described as either zero-order[23,24] or a series of first-order[25] processes. In fasting healthy subjects given a single 10 mg/kg dose of the oral solution, mean plasma C_{max} values of 744 ng/mL are achieved.[25] In diabetic children and adolescents given a 7.5 mg/kg dose of the oral solution, mean blood C_{max} values of about 750 to 850 ng/mL were observed.[26] In fasting renal transplant recipients given daily doses of 9 to 22 mg/kg (mean 15), steady-state blood CSA concentrations of 1120 ng/mL are achieved.[27] In a study of healthy subjects, mean blood C_{max} values of 942 to 1274 ng/mL were achieved after a single 6 mg/kg dose of the soft gelatin capsule.[28] The same oral dose, when given as either the solution or as soft gelatin capsules, results in similar C_{max} values.[17,18]

Some studies have reported the occurrence of a second peak in plasma or whole blood CSA concentration after administration of the oral solution or capsule in 30% to 100% of normal healthy volunteers[16,19,23,25,28] or renal transplant recipients.[29,30] This second peak occurs about four to six hours after the first peak, and CSA concentrations reached during this second peak can sometimes exceed those achieved with the first peak. In one crossover study, all subjects exhibited double peaks at least once after oral CSA, and only one patient exhibited double peaks during both phases of the study.[16] These results suggest that most patients probably exhibit double peaks after some of their oral CSA doses. The reasons for this second peak are not clear. In one study, two peaks were observed when oral CSA capsules were taken with breakfast or with breakfast and bile acid tablets, but only one peak was observed when CSA was taken under fasting conditions.[28] It is

Table 28-1. *Summary of Oral Bioavailability Studies of Cyclosporine*[f,g]

No. of patients (type)	Dosage (mg/kg)	Assay	Food		Mean F (%)	References
5 (bone marrow)	NR	NR	NR		34	6
41 (renal)	6–22	HPLC	Yes		28	7
5 (renal)	17	HPLC	NR		73[a]	8
10 (renal)	15	HPLC MC-RIA PC-RIA	No		41 38 50	9
58 (renal)	15	HPLC PC-RIA	No		30 41	10
30 (renal)	14	HPLC PC-RIA	NR		36 44	11
8 (renal)	8	HPLC PC-RIA	NR		28 36	12
15 (liver)	9 6	HPLC	NR		<5–19[b] 27[c]	13
5 (cardiac)	346[d]	HPLC	NR		35	14
6 (cystic fibrosis)[e]	7.5	HPLC	No		11	15
8 (normal)	10	HPLC	Yes Yes	(LF) (HF)	21[a] 79[a]	16
			Yes Yes	(LF) (HF)	23 42	16

[a] Based on serum/plasma CSA concentrations.
[b] Children.
[c] Adults.
[d] Dose expressed in mg.
[e] Patients were candidates for heart-lung transplants.
[f] Except as noted, CSA concentrations were measured in whole blood.
[g] NR = Not reported; HPLC = High-performance liquid chromatography; MC-RIA = Monoclonal, specific radioimmunoassy; PC-RIA = Polyclonal, nonspecific radioimmunoassay; LF = Low-fat meal; HF = High-fat meal.

therefore possible that food stimulates bile acid production and gall bladder contraction, which results in resolubilization of CSA and subsequent absorption. Other possible explanations include enterohepatic reabsorption of unchanged drug or reconversion of metabolites to parent drug and subsequent reabsorption.

Many factors have been reported to influence oral CSA bioavailability. The vehicle used to dilute the oral solution does not appear to significantly affect oral CSA bioavailability.[31,32] In one study, dilution of CSA in water, orange juice, milk, or chocolate milk resulted in similar AUC and C_{max} values (PC-RIA).[32] Food has been reported to increase,[27] decrease,[33,34] or have no effect on[28,34-36] oral CSA bioavailability. The reasons for the conflicting results are unclear but may be related to either meal composition or the biologic fluid used to measure CSA concentration. Coadministration of a "standard hospital breakfast" increased bioavailability of the oral solution,[27] whereas coadministration of a light breakfast produced no significant change in bioavailability of the soft gelatin capsule.[28] It is therefore possible that differences in the fat content of the meals used in the various studies accounted for the divergent results. In support of that hypothesis, several studies have reported that coadministration of CSA with a high-fat meal increases oral CSA bioavailability compared with that observed with a low-fat meal.[16,37] Another interesting observation is that the increase in oral CSA bioavailability caused by a high-fat meal is greater when plasma rather than whole blood is used to measure CSA concentration.[16]

Other physiological factors also can influence the bioavailability of the oral solution. In marrow transplant recipients with diarrhea caused by chemoradiation-induced enteritis or acute graft-versus-host disease, oral CSA bioavailability can be impaired.[38] Mean serum C_{max} is reduced from about 900 ng/mL with no gastrointestinal disease to 350 and 125 ng/mL (PC-RIA) in patients with chemo-radiation enteritis or acute graft-versus-host disease of the gastrointestinal tract, respectively.[38] Diarrhea caused by viral gastroenteritis or other causes can also have similar effects on oral CSA bioavailability. Metoclopramide, a drug that increases gastric emptying, has been shown to increase oral CSA bioavailability in solid organ transplant recipients.[39] These observations may be clinically important in patients who are receiving metoclopramide for nausea and vomiting or for diabetic enteropathies. Finally, the estimated length of the small bowel has been reported to be an important determinant of the oral CSA dose in children after liver transplantation.[40] Patients with extensive intestinal resections (e.g., short gut syndromes) may therefore have reduced oral CSA bioavailability.

The mechanisms responsible for the erratic and incomplete bioavailability after oral administration remain unclear. The observation that metoclopramide, food, and diarrhea influence oral CSA bioavailability suggests that gastric emptying, bile acids, and gastrointestinal motility can influence oral CSA bioavailability.[260] Since bile acids facilitate the bioavailability of fat-soluble vitamins, some investigators have hypothesized that they also facilitate the oral bioavailability of CSA. This hypothesis is supported by the poor oral bioavailability of CSA after liver transplantation during the early postoperative period[13] and by the observation that the AUC after oral CSA increases significantly after T-tube clamping[41,42] or bile refeeding.[43] In addition, bile salts increase the *in vitro* solubility of CSA.[41] Liver transplant recipients with active bile drainage via a T-tube may therefore require higher CSA dosages to maintain therapeutic concentrations. Similarly, poor oral CSA bioavailability and a requirement for higher oral doses have been observed in heart-lung transplant candidates or recipients with cystic fibrosis, a disorder that has been associated with reduced bile acid output.[15,44] A trial of pancreatic enzyme supplementation in some of these patients did not improve oral CSA bioavailability.[15] Furthermore, some studies in healthy volunteers or renal transplant recipients have reported a higher AUC when CSA capsules are taken with a light breakfast and bile acid tablets compared with a light breakfast alone.[28,37] In another study, coadministration of oral CSA solution with a high-fat meal resulted in a similar AUC compared with a low-fat meal and bile acids.[37] The effect of food on oral CSA bioavailability also may be mediated by food-induced increases in bile acid secretion. However, coadministration of cholesytramine did not significantly alter the rate or extent of oral CSA bioavailability in cardiac transplant recipients.[35] Furthermore, coadministration of bile acids with oral CSA for one week did not significantly increase trough blood CSA concentrations in renal transplant recipients.[28] Therefore, it is possible that either bile acids or a high-fat meal are required for adequate CSA dissolution and subsequent absorption. The relative importance of each of these factors and their interactions as determinants of oral CSA bioavailability are complex and require further study.

Another interesting observation is that rat and human intestinal mucosa contain a high concentration of the specific cytochrome P450 enzyme that metabolizes CSA.[45] Watkins et al. have suggested that presystemic metabolism in the intestinal mucosa is responsible in part for the poor oral bioavailability of CSA.[46,47] This hypothesis would explain: 1) the apparent higher oral bioavailability of CSA based on the PC-RIA compared with HPLC (see Table 28-1); 2) the higher ratio of CSA concentration measured by PC-RIA to those measured by HPLC after oral administration compared with intravenous administration; 3) the higher ratio of CSA metabolite concentration to parent drug concentration after oral administration compared with intravenous administration; and 4) the apparent effect of erythromycin and possibly phenytoin on oral CSA bioavailability. Recently, CSA metabolites have been detected in portal venous blood in two patients during the anhepatic phase of liver transplantation.[261]

Distribution

CSA is highly tissue-bound, as evidenced by steady-state volume of distribution values that greatly exceed actual body weight (see Tables 28-2 and 28-3)[7–10,13,14,48–62] and by the observation that CSA is widely distributed in many tissues from patients postmortem.[63–65] Furthermore, CSA can be measured in tissues for at least two weeks after CSA therapy is discontinued.

Mean steady-state volume of distribution values based on blood CSA concentration are 4 to 6 L/kg in solid organ and marrow transplant recipients (see Table 28-2). Mean values in normal volunteers and cardiac transplant recipients appear to be slightly lower. Mean values based on CSA concentrations in serum/plasma separated at 37 °C are slightly lower while those based on CSA concentrations in serum/plasma separated at room temperature are higher (see Table 28-3). The volume of distribution based on serum/plasma concentration varies according to patient age.[62] Patients less than ten years old have the highest volume of distribution while those older than 40 years have the lowest volume of distribution values. Patients 11 to 20, 21 to 30, and 31 to 40 have similar volume of distribution values. Age-dependent changes in steady-state volume of distribution based on blood CSA concentration have not been observed,[54] although patients less than ten years old tend to have a higher volume of distribution than those for older patients. Hematocrit was not significantly different among patients in the different age groups.

Studies *in vitro* with radiolabelled CSA show that 10% to 20% of the drug distributes in the leukocyte fractions, 40% to 50% in the erythrocyte fraction, and 30% to 40% in the plasma fraction.[66] Binding of CSA to erythrocytes is saturable and dependent on temperature and hematocrit.[8,67–72] As temperature decreases or hematocrit increases, the proportion of CSA found in the cellular fraction increases. Studies by Agarwal et al. indicate that the drug may bind to an intra-erythrocytic protein similar in molecular size to calf thymus cyclophilin.[73]

In plasma, CSA is highly bound to lipoproteins, which comprise 10% to 15% of all plasma proteins.[57,66,67,74–76] The binding to lipoproteins *in vitro* is concentration-independent between the range of 25 to 500 ng/mL and temperature-depen-

Table 28-2. *Pharmacokinetic Parameters of Cyclosporine After IV Administration Based on Blood Concentration Data*

No. of patients (type)	Age (range)	Clearance (mL/min/kg)	Volume (L/kg)	t½ (hr)	References
5 (normal)	24 (20–34)	3.9	1.3	6.2	48
4 (renal failure)	48–61	6.1	3.5	15.8	49
30 (uremic)	39 (18–67)	8.4	NR	6.5	50
8 (liver failure)	NR	2.8	3.9	20.4	51
41 (renal)	31 (12–62)	5.7	4.5	10.7	7
7 (renal)	2–16	11.8	4.7	7.4	52
58 (renal)	50 (27–67)	5.7	3.6	15.1	10
10 (renal)	40–65	6.5	4.4	NR	9
8 (renal)	36 (25–61)	5.2	2.9	12.8	53
7 (liver)	36 (21–51)	5.5	NR	NR	13
9 (liver)	3.3 (0.6–5.6)	9.3	NR	NR	13
20 (bone marrow)	<10	13.1	8.1	NR	54
58 (bone marrow)	11–52	8.5–10.3	4.4–6.6	NR	54
9 (bone marrow)[b]	32	5.7	2.3	7.4	55
15 (cardiac)	25–62	5.1	NR	NR	56
4 (cardiac)	11–56	4.0	1.3	6.4	14

[a] Cyclosporine concentrations were measured by HPLC in all studies.
[b] Cyclosporine pharmacokinetics were studied pre-transplant.
[c] NR = Not reported.

dent.[66] At 20 °C, protein binding is higher (90% to 95%) than at 4 °C (70%). CSA appears to be associated primarily with high-density lipoproteins (HDL) and low-density lipoproteins (LDL), with smaller amounts associated with very-low-density lipoproteins (VLDL) and chylomicrons.[57,67,74-76] The fraction of drug unbound in plasma has been measured directly by equilibrium dialysis,[77] ultracentrifugation,[78] a partitioning method,[79] and estimated indirectly with a model.[22] Estimates of fraction unbound vary widely (see Table 28-4), which is probably related to technical difficulties in the methods. The fraction unbound in plasma shows wide inter- and intraindividual variability and is weakly correlated with lipoprotein concentrations.[8,19,80,81] Age-related differences in lipoprotein concentrations may explain in part the age-related differences in volume of distribution discussed above. In contrast to most plasma proteins, lipoprotein concentrations gradually increase with age. Increases in lipoprotein concentrations would result in a corresponding decrease in the fraction unbound in plasma. For drugs with a large volume of distribution (>100 L), such as CSA, a decrease in the fraction unbound in plasma would result in a lower volume of distribution.[82,83] In support of that hypothesis, one study found a highly significant correlation between volume of distribution, based on plasma concentrations, and fasting HDL cholesterol levels (r = 0.99).[55] In another study, however, no significant correlation was observed between age (between the range of 17 to 72) and fraction unbound in plasma.[81]

Table 28-3. *Pharmacokinetic Parameters of Cyclosporine After IV Administration Based on Serum/Plasma Concentration Data*[g]

No. of patients (type)	Age (range)	Clearance (mL/min/kg)	Volume (L/kg)	t½ (hr)[h]	References
7 (normal)[b]	24 (20–34)	7.8[d]	1.2	NR	57
		11.7[e]	1.9	NR	
8 (nephrotic syndrome)[c]	45 (27–66)	6.7	3.0	18.2	58
12 (renal)[b]	25–39	7.2–9.7	2.3–4.6	7.4	59
6 (renal)[b]	24–55	7.2–7.8	4.3	8.7	60
16 (bone marrow)[c]	30 (12–44)	9.8–12.8	3.5–4.3	6.7–12.7	61
12 (bone marrow)[c]	<10	82.2	34.4	NR	62
48 (bone marrow)[c]	10–40	43.0	20.5	NR	62
9 (bone marrow)[c]	>40	20.2	4.7	NR	62
9 (bone marrow)[b,f]	32	12.7	3.7	6.7	55

[a] Expressed as L/min.
[b] Serum/plasma was separated at 37 °C.
[c] Serum/plasma was separated at room temperature.
[d] IV cyclosporine was given after overnight fast.
[e] High-fat meals given before and after IV cyclosporine was given.
[f] Cyclosporine pharmacokinetics were studied pre-transplant.
[g] Cyclosporine concentrations were measured by HPLC in all studies.
[h] NR = Not reported.

The fraction of drug unbound in blood has not been measured experimentally but has been estimated indirectly with a model.[84] In that model, the fraction unbound in blood appears to be concentration-dependent, increasing as the steady-state blood concentration increases. These changes in the free fraction of CSA in blood are probably responsible for the changes in volume of distribution and total blood clearance observed during constant-rate infusion studies in rabbits.[85] In that study, when the free fraction in blood is increased from 0.11 to 0.20, steady-state volume of distribution would be predicted to increase from 3 to 5.4 L/kg.[84] Similar increases in steady-state volume of distribution were actually observed as the dosage or infusion rate was increased.[85] However, because binding of CSA in rabbit blood may be different from that in human blood, the clinical importance of these data is unclear.

Few studies have evaluated the effect of diet, other drugs, or various disease states on protein (or tissue) binding or the volume of distribution of CSA in humans. Many drugs that are commonly given to transplant patients, such as cephalosporins, gentamicin, trimethoprim-sulfamethoxazole, acyclovir, antihypertensive drugs, digoxin, and warfarin, have not been found to influence the fraction unbound of CSA.[81] However, the fraction unbound was higher during periods of benzylpenicillin or cloxacillin treatment and during periods of fever.[81] Diabetic patients have a significantly higher fraction unbound during the early post-transplant period compared with non-diabetic patients.[81] Another study has reported that high-fat meals increase the volume of distribution of CSA compared with ingestion of low-fat meals.[57] In that study, the mean steady-state volume of distribution, based on plasma CSA concentrations, was increased from 1.2 to 1.9 L/kg. A similar but less pronounced effect was also observed with volume of distribution values based on blood CSA concentrations.[16] The investigators had expected that high-fat meals would result in increased binding and a decreased fraction unbound, which would tend to decrease volume of distribution values. As a mechanism for the observations, the investigators postulated that, due to the increase in lipoprotein concentration caused by the high-fat meals, CSA is transported (bound to lipoproteins) into adipose tissue.

Table 28-4. *Summary of Studies to Measure Fraction of Cyclosporine Unbound in Plasma*[a]

No. of patients (type)	Method	Fraction unbound[b]	References
5 (renal)	UC	6.8 (4.3–12.2)	8, 80
7 (normal)	ED	1.6 (1.0–2.4)	19
66 (renal)	ED	1.4 (0.5–4.2)	81
8 (renal)	PM	9 (4–17)	79
5 (liver)		8 (6–10)	
4 (normal)		17 (14–20)	
21 (renal)	MP	2.9 (NR)	22

[a] UC = Ultracentrifugation; ED = Equilibrium dialysis; PM = Partitioning method; MP = Model-predicted; NR = Not reported.
[b] Mean (range), expressed as percentage.

The clinical importance of unbound CSA concentrations is unclear. Although pharmacokinetic simulations of low-clearance drugs, such as CSA, suggest that changes in the unbound fraction in plasma or blood can have marked effects on both total drug clearance and average steady-state drug concentration, these changes are unlikely to appreciably change unbound drug concentration at steady state.[82,86] Lindholm et al. have observed a significant correlation between fraction unbound in plasma and the onset of acute rejection in renal transplant recipients.[81] In that study, the mean percent unbound decreased from 1.59% one week before rejection to 1.34% one day before or on the day of diagnosis of the rejection episode. An association between high serum CSA concentrations (>1000 ng/mL [PC-RIA]) and hypertriglyceridemia has been observed in marrow transplant recipients.[87] None of the nine patients with high serum CSA concentration and hypertriglyceridemia developed acute renal dysfunction, but all of the patients developed acute graft-versus-host disease, which suggests that the fraction unbound was lower and that less unbound CSA was available to distribute to extravascular sites of action or toxicity. In support of this hypothesis, an unexpectedly high incidence of neurotoxicity after liver transplantation has been observed in CSA-treated patients with low cholesterol levels.[88]

Since CSA is a highly lipophilic drug, the effect of obesity on CSA distribution has been studied in renal and marrow transplant recipients.[54,89] There was no significant effect of obesity on CSA volume of distribution based on either serum or blood concentrations, which suggests that CSA distribution is limited primarily to lean body mass. In one study, however, the concentration of CSA in fat tissue obtained postmortem was usually higher than corresponding concentrations in other tissues.[65]

Metabolism

CSA is extensively metabolized, with subsequent biliary and, to a lesser extent, urinary elimination. At least 25 CSA metabolites have been isolated and identified from human bile, feces, blood, and urine;[65,90-96] they have been named according to a published nomenclature (see Table 28-5).[97] All of the metabolites identified thus far show that the cyclic oligopeptide structure is intact; most of the metabolites are either hydroxylated or N-demethylated, or both. The monohydroxylated metabolite, metabolite M1 (previously M17), appears to be the major metabolite in human blood.[22,65,90-92,95,98-102] In many patients, trough blood concentrations of this metabolite can exceed those of the parent drug. Liver transplant recipients have been reported to have a higher ratio of trough blood CSA M1 concentration to CSA concentration than renal or heart transplant recipients.[101] This ratio also has been reported to be higher after oral administration compared with intravenous administration.[98,102] Other oxidative metabolites that are present in appreciable concentrations in human blood are metabolites M9 (previously M1), M4N (previously M21), and M19 (previously M8). Two additional metabolites (not listed in Table 28-5) have been isolated and identified. The first is dihydro-M1, a novel reduced metabolite that is present in human blood and urine.[103] Since similar reactions are often mediated by endogenous reductases, it is possible that metabolism by enteric bacteria contributes to the poor oral bioavailability. The second is a sulfate conjugate which was isolated and identified from human bile and plasma.[104,105] Preliminary data show that this Phase II metabolic product is present in high concentrations in human plasma and has about 1000 times less immunosuppressive activity than the parent drug.[105]

Although CSA metabolites appear to be widely distributed in humans, their pharmacokinetics and distribution in human blood and tissues appear to differ from CSA. At steady state, the mean AUCs for blood concentrations of M1, M9, and M4N are about 70%, 21%, and 7.5% of the AUC for blood CSA concentrations, respectively.[22] Compared with CSA, the steady-state C_{max} for CSA metabolite M1 is about threefold lower while the elimination half-life is slightly longer. The longer half-life is one of the reasons that CSA metabolite M1 concentrations at the end of a dosing interval (i.e., trough) are nearly the same or higher than corresponding CSA concentrations. Conversely, the elimination half-lives for CSA metabolites M9 and M4N are slightly shorter compared with the parent drug.[22] In that study, the half-life of CSA significantly correlated with those of CSA metabolite M1 and M9, which suggests that the elimination of these metabolites is formation rate-limited. As with CSA, the blood-to-plasma distribution of CSA metabolites in human blood depends on temperature and hematocrit.[72,106] As

Table 28-5. *Nomenclature of Cyclosporine Metabolites According to the Position of Oxidation[a]*

New	Position of oxidation	Old
M1	1 beta (8')	M17
M1c	1 beta: 1 epsilon cyclized	M18
M4N	4-N-desmethylated	M21
M9	9-gamma	M1
M19	1 beta, 9-gamma	M8
M14N	1 beta, 4-N-desmethylated	M25
M49	4-gamma, 9-gamma	M10
M4N9	4-N-desmethylated, 9-gamma	M13
M69	6-gamma, 9-gamma	M16
M1c9	1 beta, 1 epsilon-cyclized, 9-gamma	M26
M4N69	4-N-desmethylated, 6-gamma, 9-gamma	M9
M1	1 beta	M17
M1A	1 beta oxidized to an acid	203–218
M1cAL	1 beta = CHO, 1 epsilon-cyclized	"biliary aldehyde"
M1cA	1 beta = COOH, 1 epsilon-cyclized	cyclic 203–218
MOX1	1 epsilon, tetra-oxirane = MOX (S) 1 + MOX (R)1	epoxide
M1OX	1 beta, 1 epsilon-tetra-oxirane = M1OX (S) + M1OX (R)	M17-epoxide
M1DI	MOX1 H_2O M1DI; 1 tetra, 1 beta = M1DI (6S, 7R) + M1DI (6R, 7S)	(dihydroxy) MeBmt[1]-CS

[a] Modified from a recently published nomenclature.[97] Other theoretical biotransformation products are not listed.

temperature decreases or hematocrit increases, a greater proportion of CSA metabolites is found in the cellular fraction. The major CSA metabolites (M1 and M9) appear to bind or partition more avidly to red blood cells than CSA.[22,72,106] Concentrations of CSA metabolite M1 in human kidney tissues and other tissues are often higher than those of the parent drug.[65,106]

The biological activity of the metabolites and their contribution to *in vivo* immunosuppression or renal toxicity are not clear.[97,107,262] In 1986, Rosano et al. reported the presence of CSA metabolites with immunosuppressive activity in the blood of renal transplant recipients.[99] Further studies indicated that CSA metabolites clearly had immunosuppressive activity and that, in some *in vitro* tests, the immunosuppressive activity of CSA metabolite M1 approached or was equal to that of the parent drug.[99,108] Since that initial report, many studies have evaluated the *in vitro* activity of CSA metabolites.[109–114] The results of these studies are conflicting; for example, some *in vitro* studies show that metabolite M1 has less than 10% of the immunosuppressive activity of the parent drug, while other studies show that this metabolite has nearly the same immunosuppressive activity of CSA. The variability in results is related to the use of different assays used to measure immunosuppression, the conditions of the assay in different studies, and the variable purity of the metabolites. It is not known which *in vitro* test is most predictive of clinical graft rejection in humans. Because the metabolic pathways in animals are different from those in humans, *in vivo* animal models may not be predictive of biological activity in humans. Although the renal toxicity of CSA metabolites is also controversial, *in vitro* and *in vivo* studies in animals suggest that the major CSA metabolites are not nephrotoxic.[109,115–117] It is possible, however, that an undetectable reactive intermediate is formed in kidney microsomes and causes renal toxicity. The contribution of CSA metabolites to nonrenal toxicities has not been studied. In one renal transplant recipient who developed suspected CSA-related neurotoxicity, an unusually high blood concentration of CSA metabolite M1 was measured, which the investigators suggested was responsible for the neurologic symptoms.[118]

The liver is probably the major site of CSA metabolism, as evidenced by metabolism in liver microsomes and the presence of numerous drug interactions with CSA and microsomal enzyme inducers or inhibitors. Recent studies with rabbit[119,120] and human microsomal enzymes[121–124] indicate that CSA metabolism is catalyzed by enzymes that are members of the cytochrome P450IIIA gene family. The human P450IIIA family is composed of at least four genes, which encode for four highly related proteins referred to as P450IIIA3 (HLp), P450IIIA4 (P450NF, hPCN1), P450IIIA5 (hPCN3, HLp3), and P450IIIA6 (HLp2, HFLa).[122,125–130] One study has demonstrated that enzymes in the family can differ in their ability to metabolize CSA to specific metabolites.[123] The molecular weight of these enzymes is about 52 kilodaltons (kD), and they are located in the centrilobular region of the liver and, as discussed earlier, in the intestinal mucosa. At least one of the members of the P450IIIA family appears to be polymorphically expressed.[130] Watkins et al. have recently developed a novel, noninvasive test of cytochrome P450IIIA activity that involves the administration of a small dose of radiolabeled erythromycin followed by measurement of the radiolabel in the breath.[131] The results of this breath test have been recently shown to correlate significantly with liver P450IIIA levels in patients awaiting liver transplantation.[263] The activity of cytochrome P450IIIA enzymes, as measured by the erythromycin breath test, has been shown to be predictive of trough CSA concentrations in psoriasis patients.[132] Many of the drugs that have been reported to interact with CSA are either inducers, inhibitors, or substrates for these same enzymes.[47,119–124, 126,128,131,133,134] Examples of such drugs include erythromycin, anticonvulsants, ketoconazole, rifampin, steroids, and several of the calcium channel blockers.

Blood CSA clearance is about 5 to 7 mL/min/kg in adult recipients of renal or liver allografts and about 8 to 10 mL/min/kg in adult recipients of marrow allografts (see Table 28-2). Based on these values, CSA can be classified as a low-to-intermediate extraction drug. Blood CSA clearance appears to be slightly lower in normal healthy volunteers and cardiac transplant recipients. Children less than ten years old have slightly higher blood clearance values (see Table 28-2). Blood CSA pharmacokinetics appear to be influenced by circadian rhythms,[135,136] and the results of one study suggest that blood CSA clearance is higher during the night than during the day.

When serum/plasma is separated at 37°C, serum/plasma CSA clearance of CSA is about 7 to 10 mL/min/kg in normal healthy adult volunteers and adult renal transplant recipients (see Table 28-3). When serum/plasma is separated at room temperature, serum/plasma clearance values are considerably higher. Serum/plasma clearance is age dependent. Patients less than ten years old have a significantly higher clearance than those 11 to 40 or greater than 40 years old.[62] The physiologic basis for the age-related changes in CSA clearance is not known, but may be related to age-related changes in binding of CSA to plasma proteins. In that study, median triglyceride concentrations were lowest in patients less than ten years old (62 mg/dL) and highest in those greater than 40 years old (191 mg/dL), with only minimal variation in patients 11 to 40 years old (140 to 158 mg/dL). In contrast to most plasma proteins, lipoprotein concentrations increase gradually with age. Increases in lipoprotein concentration would result in a corresponding decrease in fraction unbound in plasma. Since CSA is a low-to-intermediate extraction drug, decreases in fraction unbound would theoretically reduce hepatic clearance.[82] This theoretical model is supported by studies in rabbits in which a decrease in fraction unbound resulted in a decrease in CSA clearance[84] and by a study in humans that observed a significant correlation between plasma CSA clearance and lipoprotein concentrations.[137]

Most studies indicate that CSA concentrations decline in a biphasic manner, with mean terminal half-life values of 6 to 24 hours (see Tables 28-2 and 28-3). Blood sampling in most of these studies was limited to 12 to 24 hours. Because of the lipophilicity and extensive tissue distribution of CSA, the actual terminal phase half-life may be appreciably longer than 24 hours.

At the dosages used clinically, CSA appears to be metabolized via first-order processes. One study in rabbits reported nonlinear increases in total body clearance during constant-infusion studies.[85] In that study, the investigators suggested that changes in total body clearance were related to changes in the fraction unbound in blood rather than to changes in the intrinsic clearance of unbound drug.[85] But because binding in rabbits may be different from that in humans, the clinical importance of these data is unclear. In humans, one study reported nonlinear increases in steady-state plasma concentration as CSA dosage was increased.[59] In that study, steady-state plasma concentrations increased from 340 to 1010 ng/mL as the dosage given by continuous infusion was increased from 4 to 10 mg/kg/day. Mean clearance, calculated from steady-state concentrations, decreased from 0.58 L/hr/kg at a dosage of 4 mg/kg/day to 0.43 L/hr/kg at 10 mg/kg/day. Clearance at a dosage of 7 mg/kg/day was 0.54 L/hr/kg, which is nearly identical to the value at the lower dosage. This difference is not likely to be clinically important because transplant patients do not usually receive intravenous dosages as high as 7 mg/kg/day.

The presence of hepatic dysfunction has been reported to impair CSA metabolism.[51,138] In one study of marrow transplant recipients, CSA clearance (PC-RIA) after oral administration was delayed in patients with moderate hyperbilirubinemia.[138] Blood clearance in patients with biopsy-proven cirrhosis has been reported to be lower compared with solid organ transplant recipients (see Table 28-2).[51] In that study, the mean half-life was also longer than that reported in other studies. Some transplant recipients who develop acute viral hepatitis also have reduced CSA clearance. Conversely, blood clearance values in stable liver transplant recipients are similar to those in renal transplant recipients (see Table 28-3), which suggest that common biochemical tests of liver function, such as enzymes, bilirubin, or alkaline phosphatase, are not accurate measures of the ability of the liver to metabolize CSA.

Excretion

A relatively small amount of CSA is excreted unchanged in the urine, comprising less than 1% of an administered dose.[5,139] About 3% of the administered dose is excreted in the urine as CSA and CSA metabolites.[139] The major metabolites in urine are metabolites M1 (previously M17), M1c (previously M18), and M9 (previously M1);.[139] urinary concentrations of these metabolites are often higher than that of the parent drug. Renal clearance of CSA is about 2 mL/min based on blood CSA concentration data[22,139] and about 25 mL/min based on serum CSA concentration data.[140] Age has been reported to influence renal clearance; in that study, patients less than 25 years old had a twofold higher renal clearance value compared with older patients.[140] The presence of renal failure does not impair blood CSA clearance.[49] Although CSA concentrations in urine usually exceed those in blood or serum/plasma, it is not known whether the high urinary concentrations of CSA or CSA metabolites correlate with or contribute to the development of nephrotoxicity.

As expected from the molecular weight and lipophilic nature of CSA, biliary excretion is a major route of elimination for CSA and CSA metabolites. In animals, 24% and 48% of an administered dose of radiolabelled CSA were collected from 0 to 24 hour and 0 to 48 hour bile samples, respectively. Data from patients with a biliary T-tube in place suggest that biliary excretion is also a major route of elimination.[141] Biliary concentrations are much higher than concurrent blood or serum concentrations. Measurement of CSA concentrations in the bile shows that nearly all of the compounds eliminated in the bile are CSA metabolites rather than unchanged parent drug.[65,91,96,141] Enterohepatic recirculation of CSA or CSA metabolites, or both, probably occurs in some patients.

Drug Interactions

Many drugs have been reported to change CSA concentrations (see Table 28-6).[142,143] Most anticonvulsants and antituberculous therapy with rifampin-containing regimens can decrease CSA concentrations to levels that are at or below the limit of detection for most assays. In many cases, the rapid decrease in CSA concentration was associated with the onset of acute rejection. Because no pharmacokinetic interaction between valproate and CSA has been reported, valproate has been recommended for patients who require anticonvulsant therapy. Other drugs that have been reported to decrease CSA concentrations include sulfadimidine and trimethoprim, nafcillin, and octreotide.

Erythromycin, ketoconazole, and most calcium channel blockers have been clearly shown to increase CSA concentration. Other less well documented interactions have been reported with other macrolide antibiotics, other azole antifungal drugs, metoclopramide, fluoroquinolones, sulindac, imipenem/cilastin, oral contraceptives/danazol, methyltestosterone, colchicine, acetazolamide, ethanol, and cimetidine. Although the most commonly reported mechanism is inhibition of CSA metabolism, there is increasing evidence that erythromycin, metoclopra-

Table 28-6. *Drugs That Have Been Reported to Change Cyclosporine Concentration*[a]

↓ cyclosporine concentration	↑ cyclosporine concentration
Anticonvulsants	Acetazolamide
carbamazepine	Azole antifungal drugs
phenobarbital	fluconazole
phenytoin	itraconazole
Nafcillin	ketoconazole
Octreotide	Calcium antagonists
Rifampin	diltiazem
Sulfonamides and trimethoprim	nicardipine
	verapamil
	Cimetidine
	Colchicine
	Ethanol
	Imipenem/Cilastin
	Macrolide antibiotics
	erythromycin
	josamycin
	Metoclopramide
	Norfloxacin
	Steroid hormones
	methylprednisolone
	methyltestosterone
	oral contraceptives/danazol
	Sulindac

[a] Based on recently published review.[142,143]

mide, and probably other drugs increase oral CSA bioavailability. Nifedipine and nitrendipine are the calcium channel blockers that have not been reported to interact with CSA. High-dose methylprednisolone has been reported to increase or have no effect on trough CSA concentrations (depending on the assay method) and increase CSA clearance. Abrupt drug-induced increases in CSA concentration can result in acute renal impairment and occasional irreversible renal graft damage. Although diltiazem increases CSA concentration, renal impairment does not usually occur because of the apparent renal protective effect of diltiazem.

Because of deficiencies in study design, the mechanism of most of the interactions cannot be determined from the clinical reports. Since many of the drugs that have been reported to interact with CSA are either inducers, inhibitors, or substrates of cytochrome P450IIIA enzymes, it is likely that the primary mechanism for most of the drug interactions is altered metabolism of CSA.[47,119–124,126,128,131,133,134] Because high concentrations of cytochrome P450IIIA enzymes are found in human intestinal mucosa, changes in CSA metabolism could also alter oral CSA bioavailability.[45–47] In addition, other drugs could alter binding of CSA to lipoproteins, erythrocytes, or body tissues. With some drugs, more than one mechanism could be involved.

Further studies are needed to determine the mechanism of most of these pharmacokinetic interactions and whether closely related drugs in the same chemical class interact with CSA. Examples of important chemical classes include macrolide antibiotics, azole antifungal drugs, dihydropyridine calcium channel blockers, and fluoroquinolone antibiotics.

PHARMACODYNAMICS

When CSA was introduced into experimental clinical medicine in 1978, even crude pharmacodynamic relationships were not known. Drug concentrations of other immunosuppressive drugs are not usually monitored in transplant patients. The doses of conventional immunosuppressive drugs (prednisone, azathioprine, and antilymphocyte or antithymocyte globulin) are usually adjusted according to clinical evidence of graft rejection or adverse effects such as marrow suppression. Although this empiric method of adjusting CSA dosage was initially adopted by most transplant groups, it has become clear that CSA nephrotoxicity is often difficult to distinguish from inadequate immunosuppression in renal transplant recipients and that CSA dosage is not a useful guide in predicting systemic concentrations.

Most pharmacodynamic studies included relatively small numbers of patients and did not use multivariate statistical methods that adjusted for the presence of potentially confounding variables. For example, most transplant patients receive other immunosuppressive drugs in addition to CSA – usually glucocorticoids, azathioprine, and sometimes antilymphocyte antibodies. Thus, the pharmacodynamics of CSA may be influenced by the administration of other immunosuppressive drugs and other demographic factors such as the patient's clinical history and presentation. The clinical endpoints differed for different studies. For example, some studies defined graft rejection by clinical criteria alone without biopsy evidence while other studies required biopsy confirmation. It is interesting to note that, although the stated goal of most studies was to determine whether CSA concentrations correlated with the risk of graft rejection or nephrotoxicity, most of the investigators assumed that a therapeutic range existed and therefore adjusted CSA dosage to maintain CSA concentrations within that range.

Table 28-7 shows representative therapeutic ranges for different biological fluids and assays used by some of the major transplant groups. Most pharmaco-dynamic studies have used CSA concentration measured by either PC-RIA, HPLC, or polyclonal fluorescence polarization immunoassay (PC-FPIA). Other assay methods include the monoclonal, "specific" radioimmunoassay (MC-RIA); monoclonal, nonspecific radioimmunoassay; and, most recently, the monoclonal fluorescence polarization immunoassay (MC-FPIA).

Immunosuppression

The immunosuppressive activity of CSA is probably related to its inhibitory effect on interleukin or cytokine production, particularly interleukin-2 and gamma interferon.[144] At the molecular level, the drug appears to prevent the actual transcription of these cytokine genes.[145] As a result, graft rejection (or graft-ver-sus-host disease) cannot occur because the effector cells and the antibody response required to attack and destroy the tissue graft are not allowed to be fully expressed. Furthermore, there are some data that suggest that CD8 suppressor cells are relatively spared by CSA therapy,[146] which is consistent with the observation that suppressor cells require less interleukin-2 for proliferation and activity compared with CD4 helper cells.[147]

CSA appears to bind to a 17 kD cytoplasmic protein called cyclophilin,[148,149] which belongs to a family of cis-trans prolyl isomerases. This enzyme family appears to play an important role in altering the configuration of cytoplasmic proteins by acting on proline molecules present at the sites of bends in their tertiary structure. The resulting changes in configuration may activate or inhibit the

Table 28-7. *Therapeutic Ranges of Cyclosporine Concentration Measured in Different Biological Fluids and by Different Assay Methods[c]*

Assay	Biological fluid	
	Serum/plasma	Whole blood
Polyclonal radioimmunoassay[a]	100–250	200–800
Monoclonal radioimmunoassay[b]	50–125	150–400
Fluorescence polarization immunoassay (polyclonal)	150–400	200–800
Fluorescence polarization immunoassay (monoclonal)	50–125	150–400
High-performance liquid chromatography	50–125	150–400

[a] No longer available.
[b] Refers to monoclonal radioimmunoassay that is specific for parent drug.
[c] All therapeutic ranges are listed in ng/mL. All therapeutic ranges are approximate and may vary depending on institution.

activity of the target protein. It is also possible that a configuration change can affect the ability of a cytoplasmic signal protein to enter into the nucleus and influence gene transcription. Since CSA inhibits the isomerase activity of cyclophilin,[150] it may block the pathway of signals from the cytoplasm of activated T-cells and therefore block the transcription of cytokine genes in the nucleus. The new immunosuppressive drugs, FK 506 and rapamycin, also bind to a different member of the cytoplasmic cis-trans prolyl isomerase family.[151] However, differences in the effects of these drugs on cytokine gene transcription suggest that the role of this new enzyme family in immunosuppression has not been precisely defined.[152]

Clinical Studies. *Renal Transplantation.* Renal allograft recipients are the largest group of patients that receive CSA. Pharmacodynamic studies in this group of patients are difficult to interpret because of the difficulty in distinguishing between inadequate immunosuppression (graft rejection) and CSA-induced renal dysfunction.

The first study suggesting a relationship between CSA concentration and immunosuppressive activity in renal transplant recipients was reported by Keown and co-workers in 1981.[4] They showed that adequate immunosuppression, defined by mixed lymphocyte culture inhibition, was achieved *in vitro* with serum CSA concentrations of 200 to 400 ng/mL (PC-RIA). Since that study, other organ transplant groups have also reported that serum/plasma or whole blood trough CSA concentrations measured by PC-RIA correlate with the risk of graft rejection.[33,153–159] Other studies, however, have not observed a significant correlation between serum/plasma or whole blood trough concentrations measured by PC-RIA and the risk of graft rejection.[160–163]

Few pharmacodynamic studies have been reported with CSA concentrations measured by HPLC, MC-RIA, or PC-FPIA. One of the first studies to support the use of whole blood CSA concentrations measured by HPLC was an uncontrolled study by Moyer et al.[164] The investigators in that study reported a very low risk of graft rejection and nephrotoxicity and attributed their excellent results to careful monitoring of CSA concentrations and dosage adjustments to maintain concentrations within a therapeutic concentration range. Other studies, however, have not reported a significant correlation between CSA concentration measured by HPLC or MC-RIA and the risk of graft rejection.[157,161–163,165] In one study, the AUC for CSA concentration measured by HPLC correlated more accurately with the incidence of graft rejection than trough concentrations.[161] Two studies have reported that serum or whole blood trough CSA concentrations measured by PC-FPIA do not correlate with the risk of graft rejection.[157,163]

Pharmacodynamic studies that include CSA concentrations measured by both specific and nonspecific methods have been inconclusive. Two studies were unable to show a correlation between CSA concentration, measured by any method, and the risk of graft rejection.[162,163] One study found a correlation between CSA concentrations measured by PC-RIA and the risk of graft rejection but not with CSA concentrations measured by HPLC.[157] Another study has reported that whole blood CSA concentrations measured by a more specific method (MC-RIA) correlated with the incidence of graft rejection more accurately than those measured by PC-RIA.[156] In one study, patients who had acute graft rejection had lower ratios of whole blood CSA concentration measured by PC-RIA to those measured by HPLC than patients with normal graft function or CSA-induced nephrotoxicity.[162]

Bone Marrow Transplantation. In marrow transplant recipients, CSA is used to prevent or treat graft-versus-host disease, the T-cell mediated immune reaction of donor marrow cells against recipient organs. Moderate-to-severe (grades II to IV) acute graft-versus-host disease occurs in 25% to 50% of recipients of HLA-identical marrow grafts. The risk of acute graft-versus-host disease is higher in older patients and in recipients of HLA-nonidentical marrow grafts. Since treatment of established acute graft-versus-host disease is unsatisfactory, most marrow transplant teams give CSA and other immunosuppressive drugs as graft-versus-host disease prophylaxis.

One study has reported a relationship between serum trough concentrations (PC-RIA) and the risk of acute graft-versus-host disease.[166] In that study of 179 recipients of HLA-identical marrow grafts, trough concentration for a given week post-transplant was significantly associated with the risk that acute graft-versus-host disease would develop during the following week. When trough CSA concentration was modeled as a time-dependent covariate in a relative risk regression model, the relative risk for developing acute graft-versus-host disease was reduced as the CSA concentration increased. The relative risk was reduced by 30% (0.7) for each 100 ng/mL increase in trough CSA concentration. When patients were divided into arbitrary CSA concentration groups, the relative risks were 1.0, 0.6, and 0.2 for patients with trough concentrations of less than 100, 100 to 200, and greater than 200 ng/mL. Other covariates that significantly influenced the risk of acute graft-versus-host disease in that study were patient age, prophylaxis regimen, and year of transplantation. Two other studies have also reported a significant correlation between trough CSA concentrations (PC-RIA) and the risk of acute graft-versus-host disease.[167,168] Other studies, however, have not found a significant correlation between serum/plasma or whole blood trough CSA concentrations (PC-RIA) and the risk of acute graft-versus-host disease.[169-172]

Few studies have examined the relationship between trough CSA concentrations measured in whole blood or by other assay methods (HPLC, MC-RIA, or PC-FPIA) and the risk of acute graft-versus-host disease. One study in 29 marrow transplant recipients compared the correlation between trough CSA concentration measured by three assay methods (PC-RIA, HPLC, and PC-FPIA) and risk of acute graft-versus-host disease.[100] Although CSA concentrations measured by each of the assay methods tended to trend each other, CSA concentrations measured by the different assays did not correlate significantly with risk of acute graft-versus-host disease.

Liver and Heart Transplantation. Function of the newly grafted liver varies considerably during the first few weeks following transplantation. As a result, the ability of the liver to metabolize CSA and other drugs during this period can change rapidly, resulting in possible accumulation of CSA and CSA metabolites. Several studies have shown that the ratio of CSA concentration measured by PC-RIA to those measured by HPLC is higher and more variable in liver transplant recipients than in other solid organ transplant recipients.[173-178] Based on this observation, some investigators have recommended that CSA concentrations be measured by a specific assay method in this patient population. However, none of the studies has found a significant correlation between trough CSA concentrations (measured by PC-RIA, HPLC, or PC-FPIA) and the risk of graft rejection.[173,176,179] One possible explanation for the lack of a significant correlation is that early graft rejection could alter the metabolism of CSA or CSA metabolites resulting in changes in CSA concentration. Some investigators have attempted to correlate the ratio of CSA concentrations measured by two different methods to clinical events.[173,175,176,178,179] One of the studies reported that low ratios of CSA concentrations measured by PC-RIA to those measured by HPLC were associated with "good graft function."[173] None of these studies provide convincing evidence that this approach offers any advantage over monitoring CSA concentrations measured by one assay method.

Few studies have evaluated the relationship between CSA concentrations and clinical events after cardiac transplantation.[180,181] Based on a low incidence of rejection-related deaths in 49 cardiac transplant recipients, one study has reported that a target blood CSA concentration of 1000 ng/mL (PC-RIA) is appropriate.[180]

Renal Dysfunction

CSA-induced renal dysfunction occurs during the first few months of therapy in most patients receiving therapeutic dosages. Three clinical syndromes have been identified: 1) transient acute renal failure, 2) protracted acute renal failure, and 3) chronic nephropathy.[182-185] Transient acute renal failure is the most common form of renal dysfunction and is characterized by rapid reversal when the CSA dose is held or reduced. This syndrome is not usually associated with histopathologic abnormalities, which suggests that it is related to severe renal vasoconstriction. Repeated episodes of transient acute renal failure often result in the second syndrome, referred to as protracted acute renal failure. Recovery of renal function after this syndrome is usually not complete, even when CSA is withdrawn. Protracted acute renal failure can be associated with the development of thrombosis of glomerular arterioles or diffuse, interstitial fibrosis. Alternatively, CSA may exacerbate intravascular thrombus formation or may serve as a stimulus to interstitial cell proliferation. The third syndrome is a chronic, usually irreversible, nephropathy, which is often associated with mild proteinuria and tubular dysfunction. Renal biopsies in cardiac allograft patients with chronic CSA-related nephropathy showed tubulointerstitial abnormalities, sometimes with focal glomerular sclerosis.

The pathophysiology of acute CSA-induced renal dysfunction is primarily related to its effects on the renal vessels. Detailed studies of renal function show that CSA acutely reduces renal blood flow, with a corresponding increase in renal vascular resistance and reduction in glomerular filtration rate. Evidence for the vascular origin of acute CSA nephrotoxicity includes increased urinary excretion of vasoactive arachadonic acid metabolites such as thromboxane;[186] increased levels of atriopeptin, an endothelial-cell product with potent vasoconstrictive properties;[187] improved renal blood flow with thromboxane receptor antagonist administration;[188] presence of direct endothelial cell injury in cell culture;[189] and constriction of the afferent arteriole after CSA administration.[190]

The pathophysiology of chronic CSA-induced nephrotoxicity is less clear. Light and electron microscopic analyses of renal biopsies from renal allograft recipients have shown increased interstitial fibrosis and a nonspecific tubular vacuolization.[185] Similar pathologic findings have been observed in cardiac transplant recipients[191] and patients with autoimmune uveitis treated with CSA.[192] Although physiologic studies show that glomerular filtration rate and renal blood flow are reduced in patients receiving chronic CSA therapy, these changes may improve with time and standard dosage reductions.[193] Retrospective studies indicate that renal function stabilizes after the first year post-transplant, which suggests that chronic rejection rather than CSA-induced toxicity is the major cause of long-term renal dysfunction.[194,195]

Clinical Studies. *Renal Transplantation.* The major problem with the studies in renal allograft patients is the difficulty in distinguishing between acute or chronic graft rejection and CSA-induced renal dysfunction. Nephrotoxicity is usually a diagnosis of exclusion and is based on a biopsy that does not show graft rejection (if a biopsy is performed) and a decrease in serum creatinine when CSA dosage is decreased. Monitoring CSA concentrations is one of many techniques used to minimize the development of drug-induced nephrotoxicity. Keown et al. first reported that trough serum concentrations greater than 400 ng/mL (PC-RIA) preceded CSA nephrotoxicity in four patients.[4] This finding was later confirmed in a larger series.[33] Although other studies have also shown that high serum/plasma or whole blood trough CSA concentrations measured by PC-RIA correlate with the onset of renal dysfunction,[154,159,160,196–198] not all studies have reported a significant correlation with that assay method.[155–157,161,162]

Few studies have evaluated the correlation between CSA concentrations measured by HPLC, MC-RIA, or PC-FPIA and renal dysfunction. In most studies whole blood trough concentrations measured by HPLC were not predictive of nephrotoxicity.[157,161,162,165] But in an uncontrolled study, Moyer et al. concluded that careful maintenance of whole blood trough concentrations within 100 to 250 ng/mL minimized the incidence of nephrotoxicity.[164] In another study of stable renal transplant recipients 14 days to 4.5 years (average 1.5 years) post-transplant, nephrotoxic patients tended to have higher whole blood trough concentrations measured by HPLC than nontoxic patients.[163] Results of one study suggest that serum/plasma trough concentrations measured by HPLC also correlate with the onset of nephrotoxicity[199] while another study found no significant correlation.[163] Experience with CSA concentrations measured by PC-FPIA is limited and the results of pharmacodynamic studies have been inconclusive.[157,163] In one study of 334 renal transplant recipients, trough whole blood CSA concentrations of greater than 350 ng/mL (PC-FPIA) were associated with significantly better long-term graft function.[200] These data suggest that some nephrotoxicity may have to be tolerated in order to ensure adequate long-term immunosuppression.

Bone Marrow Transplantation. In marrow transplant recipients, renal dysfunction is a frequent problem because of the need to administer potentially nephrotoxic antibiotics during the period of granulocytopenia. Several studies have demonstrated that serum/plasma trough CSA concentrations (PC-RIA) correlate with the risk of renal dysfunction.[171,172,201,202] In one study, the median time of onset of renal dysfunction in patients with mean serum trough concentrations less than 150, 150 to 250, and greater than 250 ng/mL was 46, 29, and 20 days, respectively.[202] The relative risks of developing renal dysfunction were 1.0, 1.9, and 4.3 in patients with mean trough CSA concentrations of less than 150, 150 to 250, and greater than 250 ng/mL.[203] Exposure to nephrotoxic antibiotics was similar for the three groups. Other studies have failed to demonstrate a significant correlation between trough CSA concentration and risk of renal dysfunction.[170]

Few studies have evaluated the relation between CSA concentrations measured in whole blood or by HPLC, MC-RIA, or PC-FPIA and the risk of renal dysfunction. In one study, serum trough concentrations measured by PC-RIA correlated more accurately with the risk of renal dysfunction as compared with those measured by HPLC.[203] Another study in 29 marrow transplant recipients compared the correlation between trough plasma CSA concentration measured by PC-RIA or PC-FPIA or whole blood concentrations measured by HPLC and risk of renal dysfunction.[100] Although CSA concentration measured by each of the assay methods tended to trend each other, plasma concentrations measured by nonspecific assays (PC-FPIA or PC-RIA) were most strongly associated with the risk of renal dysfunction. Whole blood CSA concentrations measured by HPLC did not correlate with the risk of renal dysfunction. These data suggest that plasma CSA concentrations measured by nonspecific assays may more accurately correlate with renal dysfunction than whole blood concentrations measured by HPLC in marrow transplant recipients.

Liver and Heart Transplantation. The relationship between CSA concentration and risk of renal dysfunction after liver or heart transplantation is not clear. Some studies have not found a significant correlation between serum or whole blood trough CSA concentrations and the risk of renal dysfunction after liver transplantation.[176,179] Other studies, however, have reported that whole blood CSA concentrations measured by more specific assay methods (HPLC or MC-RIA) correlate with the onset of renal dysfunction.[173,178] These studies also found that whole blood CSA concentrations measured by PC-RIA were less predictive of the occurrence of renal dysfunction. Some investigators have attempted to correlate the ratio of CSA concentrations measured by two assay methods with the onset of renal dysfunction.[173,175,176,178,180] Although most of the studies failed to show a significant correlation between these ratios and the risk of renal dysfunction, Kohlhaw et al. reported that 11 of 12 patients with increased CSA metabolite levels (as measured by high ratios of CSA concentration measured by nonspecific assay methods to those measured by specific assay methods) had renal dysfunction at the same time or subsequent to the increase in metabolites.[175]

In *cardiac transplant* recipients, whole blood trough CSA concentrations do not correlate significantly with the risk of renal dysfunction.[180,181] It is interesting to note that some investigators have observed that cardiac transplant recipients can frequently tolerate higher trough CSA concentrations than renal transplant recipients. The reasons for this apparent difference are not known, but it may be related to a greater renal functional reserve in cardiac transplant recipients who have both kidneys intact or, alternatively, to the reduced ability of the denervated, transplanted kidney in renal transplant recipients to compensate for the CSA-induced effects on renal blood flow.

CLINICAL APPLICATION OF PHARMACOKINETIC DATA

While most clinicians agree that it is important to monitor CSA concentrations in all patients, the lack of definitive clinical studies precludes a general consensus on how to monitor them. Thus, many investigators have developed their own approaches, usually based on their clinical experience. This has led to considerable confusion and controversy in the transplantation community.[97,204–208]

Before CSA concentration data can be applied to patient care, it is important to understand that in most cases, CSA is used to *prevent* rather than to *treat* graft rejection or acute graft-versus-host disease. Unfortunately, there are no biochemical, histologic, or immunologic tests that reliably predict which patient will develop clinically important graft rejection or graft-versus-host disease. Therefore, we must depend on clinical and pathologic changes to definitively diagnose these immunosuppressive failures. Also, once graft rejection or acute graft-versus-host disease are evident clinically, they are not always easily reversible and can result in severe tissue injury and its associated morbidity and mortality.

Many pharmacodynamic studies show that CSA concentration influences the risk of graft rejection (or acute graft versus-host disease) or renal dysfunction. Based on these data, many investigators have recommended a specific therapeutic concentration range for a given transplant population. These studies, however, also illustrate the complexities associated with the use of a therapeutic concentration range. For example, a relatively low CSA concentration may be acceptable for patients who are at relatively low risk of developing graft rejection (or acute graft-versus-host disease). Examples of low-risk groups include recipients of HLA-identical grafts or those receiving combinations of immunosuppressive agents. Conversely, even high CSA concentrations may not be adequate for patients who are at high risk for developing graft rejection (or acute graft-versus-host disease). Examples of high-risk groups include recipients of cadaveric or mismatched grafts or those receiving CSA alone as immunosuppressive therapy.

Figure 28-1 shows a general algorithm for monitoring CSA concentrations. CSA concentrations should be monitored in nearly all patients, particularly if the drug is given orally. If it is important to rapidly attain therapeutic concentrations, or if poor oral bioavailability can be documented, then the intravenous preparation should be used. It is especially important to maintain therapeutic concentrations when the patient receives the graft and early in the post-grafting period when acute immunologic complications are most likely to occur.

After the drug has reached steady state, trough concentrations generally yield the most useful information for routine therapeutic monitoring. Because CSA pharmacokinetics have been reported to exhibit diurnal variation, blood samples should be obtained at approximately the same time of day.[135,136] Single "peak" concentrations after oral dosing are difficult to interpret because of the inter- and intrapatient variability in CSA bioavailability. Several blood samples between two to six hours after oral dosing can be obtained to minimize this variability, but this approach is inconvenient and expensive for routine monitoring. Other investigators have proposed the collection of eight to ten blood samples during a dosing interval to estimate AUC and average steady-state concentration.[161,208-210] Although this approach has certain advantages over monitoring of trough concentration and appears to reduce the number of required dosage adjustments, no studies have shown that this approach results in less graft rejection or nephrotoxicity compared with trough concentration monitoring. Another study suggests that measurement of plasma CSA concentration (PC-RIA) six hours after dosing provides more clinically useful information than trough concentrations.[211] CSA concentrations should be monitored two to three times a week during the first few weeks to months of therapy, and less often later in the post-transplant period. More frequent monitoring may be required if the patient has clinical problems that can change CSA pharmacokinetics (i.e., hepatic dysfunction, diarrhea) or begins therapy with a drug that potentially interacts with CSA.

Some investigators have evaluated a test-dose method or Bayesian approach to individualize CSA therapy. In the test-dose method, a single intravenous dose of CSA is given several days before transplant.[211-213] Estimated pharmacokinetics are then used to calculate a dosage regimen for an individual patient. Other investigators have used a Bayesian estimation of CSA clearance, based on population pharmacokinetic parameters.[214-215] The results of these studies suggest that both of these approaches can be helpful to individualize CSA therapy.

Although the most common indications for monitoring CSA concentration are to maintain adequate immunosuppression and minimize the risk of renal toxicity, there are also other indications. In renal transplant recipients, CSA concentrations can sometimes aid in distinguishing between graft rejection and drug-induced renal toxicity. Since transplant patients can sometimes experience nausea and vomiting, CSA concentrations can be used to determine if the drug is adequately absorbed. This is particularly a problem in marrow transplant patients, who receive high-dose chemotherapy either alone or combined with total body irradiation before transplant. It is important to closely monitor CSA concentrations when the route of administration is changed (i.e., when a patient changes from intravenous to oral therapy or vice-versa) or when the oral dosage form is changed (i.e., when a patient changes from the oral solution to the soft gelatin capsule). Finally, CSA concentrations can be used as a measure of patient compliance.[216]

There is controversy concerning the most appropriate biological fluid (plasma/serum or whole blood) and assay method (MC-RIA, PC-FPIA, MC-FPIA or HPLC) to monitor CSA concentration.[97,204-208] Because CSA binds to erythrocytes (and lipoproteins) in a temperature-dependent manner, some investigators have recommended whole blood as the most appropriate biological fluid. However, if serum or plasma is separated after equilibration at room or normal body temperature has occurred (one to two hours), either biological fluid can be used for routine monitoring or pharmacokinetic studies. If plasma is used, the type of anticoagulant (heparin versus EDTA) used in the blood collection tube has been reported to influence measured CSA concentration values.[217] Since the volume of whole blood

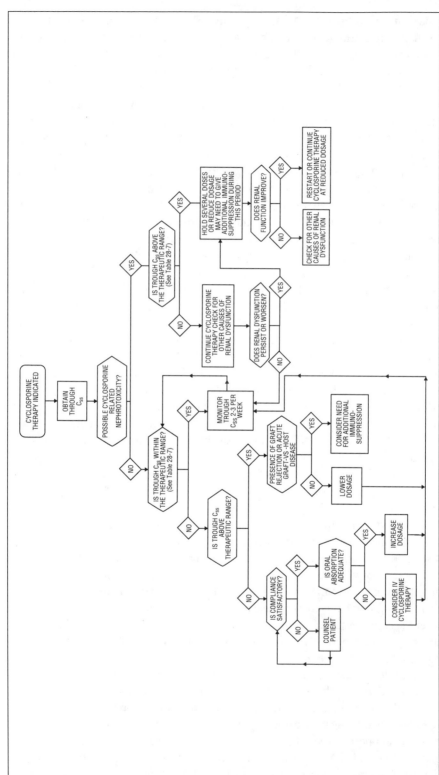

Figure 28-1. *Algorithm for Pharmacokinetic Monitoring of Cyclosporine Therapy in Transplant Patients.*

is about twice that of serum or plasma, whole blood concentrations are higher than serum/plasma concentrations and are therefore less often below the minimum detectable concentration of a given assay. Most institutions currently monitor CSA concentrations in whole blood.

Although most pharmacodynamic studies with large numbers of patients have measured CSA concentrations by PC-RIA, this assay method has not been available since 1988. Most pharmacodynamic studies have failed to show a significant correlation between whole blood CSA concentrations measured by HPLC and clinical events. Many laboratories measure serum/plasma or whole blood CSA concentrations by PC-FPIA or MC-FPIA because of the broad availability of TDx analyzers and their ease of use (discussed in detail below). Although few pharmacodynamic studies have included CSA concentrations measured by PC-FPIA, CSA concentrations measured by this method correlate with those measured by PC-RIA for most patients. Because of this close correlation, many laboratories that previously measured CSA concentrations by PC-RIA currently use the PC-FPIA. As discussed above, results of the few studies that have evaluated the correlation between CSA concentrations measured by more than one assay method and clinical events have been inconclusive and incomplete.

Based on the published pharmacodynamic studies, representative therapeutic concentration ranges used by many transplant centers are listed in Table 28-7. The ranges are usually similar for the major types of transplantation (renal, liver, cardiac, and bone marrow). Some institutions, however, recommend a different therapeutic concentration range for a specific transplant population (i.e., heart or liver transplant recipients). Because many transplant groups reduce the therapeutic concentration range with increasing time post-transplant, all ranges listed in the table are intended to be used during the early post-transplant period.

ANALYTICAL METHODS

Serum/plasma or whole blood CSA concentrations can be measured by specific or nonspecific assay methods (see Table 28-8).[97] To date, the only assay that is completely specific for the parent drug is HPLC. All of the immunoassays, including the monoclonal immunoassays, measure varying amounts of cross-reactive metabolites. Until 1988, only two assays were available: HPLC and the original PC-RIA developed by Sandoz. In 1988, Sandoz discontinued the PC-RIA and introduced two monoclonal RIA kits. One of the monoclonal RIA kits is relatively specific for the parent drug (MC-RIA) while the other is nonspecific and measures CSA and its metabolites. The latter monoclonal radioimmunoassay is not used by most clinical laboratories and will not be discussed in detail. Another company, Incstar, also has developed monoclonal RIA kits with the same monoclonal antibodies. The tracers, however, are labeled at different sites with different isotopes. Also in 1988, Abbott introduced a polyclonal nonspecific PC-FPIA for use on their TDx analyzer. More recently, Abbott introduced a monoclonal PC-FPIA that is more specific for the parent drug. All of the available im-

Table 28–8. Comparison of the Relative Advantages and Disadvantages of the Various Cyclosporine Assay Methods

Analytical method[a]	Specificity for cyclosporine[b]	Limit of sensitivity (ng/mL)	Metabolite analysis	Assayable samples			Minimum sample volume required (mL)	Speed[c]		Analysis costs[d]		Specialized operator training[e]	Preference and Rank[f]		
				Whole blood	Plasma/serum	Urine		1–10 Samples (hr)	10–100 Samples (hr)	Estimated reagent and tech. cost/assay	Initial equipment costs		Small service	Large service	Research
RIA-S	2	50	No	Yes	Yes	Yes	0.1	8	>24	2	2	1	2	2	2
RIA-NS	4	50	No	Yes	Yes	Yes	0.1	8	>24	2	2	1	2	2	3
FPIA-S	2	20	No	Yes	Yes	Yes	0.1	<1	<8	4	2	1	1	2	2
FPIA-NS	4	20	No	Yes	Yes	Yes	0.1	<1	<8	4	2	1	1	2	3
HPLC-E	1	50	Yes	Yes	Yes	Yes	1–2	8	>24	2	3	2	2	3	1
HPLC-CS	1	20	Yes	Yes	Yes	Yes	1	8	>24	3	4	4	4	1	1

a   HPLC = High-performance liquid chromatography with liquid-liquid extraction or extraction columns (E) or column switching (CS); RIA-S = Monoclonal, specific radioimmunoassay; RIA-NS = Monoclonal, nonspecific radioimmunoassay; FPIA-S = Monoclonal fluorescence polarization immunoassay; FPIA-NS = Polyclonal fluorescence polarization immunoassay.

b   Arbitrary ranking scale of 1 (excellent) to 5 (poor).

c   Assuming round-the clock scintillation counting or HPLC sample injection.

d   1 = Least expense.

e   1 = Least training.

f   1 = Preferred method; Small = <25 samples/week; Large = >100 samples/week.

munoassays can be used to measure both whole blood or plasma/serum CSA concentrations. Other immunoassays are being developed and tested and should be available in the near future.[218,219]

Monoclonal Radioimmunoassay (Sandoz)

All of the available monoclonal RIA kits can be used for serum/plasma or whole blood and are similar in performance and technical difficulty to the original PC-RIA. Based on two murine monoclonal antibodies developed at Sandoz,[220] two monoclonal RIA kits are available from Sandoz. One of the monoclonal RIA kits is relatively specific for parent drug (MC-RIA) while the other is nonspecific and measures CSA and its metabolites. The limit of sensitivity for these assays is about 50 ng/mL. Whole blood CSA concentrations measured by the more specific MC-RIA usually correlate reasonably well with those measured by HPLC. Although a few studies have reported excellent agreement between whole blood CSA concentrations measured by MC-RIA and those measured by HPLC,[221,222] most studies have reported that whole blood CSA concentrations measured by MC-RIA are about 5% to 30% higher than those measured by HPLC.[9,97,210,223–226] In one study, the ratio of whole blood trough CSA concentration measured by MC-RIA to those measured by HPLC was similar in children and adults and was highest in cardiac transplant recipients compared with renal, liver, and bone marrow transplant recipients.[224] The authors of that study speculated that elimination of CSA metabolites was impaired in cardiac transplant recipients because of their critical condition.

Most laboratories do not measure serum/plasma CSA concentrations by MC-RIA because the measured values are often near or below the limit of detection for the assay. Plasma CSA concentrations measured by MC-RIA appear to be nearly identical to or slightly higher than those measured by HPLC.[225,227]

The monoclonal, nonspecific RIA does not appear to have any advantages over the MC-RIA or other nonspecific immunoassays. Whole blood or plasma CSA concentrations measured by this method have been reported to be similar to or higher than those measured by PC-RIA.[223,228,229]

Monoclonal Radioimmunoassay (Incstar)

The monoclonal RIA kits available from Sandoz use a tritiated dihydro-CSA label and charcoal to separate bound from free drug. Because of the disadvantages associated with liquid scintillation counting and the charcoal separation step, Incstar developed a ^{125}I-CSA based RIA kit, initially for use with the polyclonal antibody and, more recently, for use with the two monoclonal antibodies developed by Sandoz.[230] CSA concentrations measured by this monoclonal RIA are reported to be nearly identical to those measured by MC-RIA.[230,231] As with the MC-RIA, whole blood CSA concentrations measured by this RIA method show an excellent correlation with those measured by HPLC. Most studies have reported that whole blood CSA concentrations measured by the Incstar monoclonal RIA kit are about 10% to 35% higher than those measured by HPLC.[97,230–232] Some studies, however, have reported nearly identical results between the Incstar monoclonal RIA and HPLC.[226] Although the monoclonal specific assay from Incstar appears to be comparable to the MC-RIA kit from Sandoz, some investigators have reported quality control problems with the standards included in the Incstar kit.[97,233]

Fluorescence Polarization Immunoassay (FPIA)

Both the polyclonal and monoclonal FPIA can be used for serum/plasma or whole blood and measure both CSA and a variable amount of CSA metabolites. The major advantages of the FPIA are excellent assay performance (i.e., accuracy and precision) and ease of use. Whole blood CSA concentrations measured by PC-FPIA correlate poorly with and are appreciably higher than those measured by HPLC. The mean ratio of whole blood CSA concentrations measured by PC-FPIA to those measured by HPLC ranges between 1.5 and 3, with considerable interpatient variability.[232,234–237] Whole blood or plasma CSA concentrations measured by PC-FPIA correlate reasonably well with those measured by the PC-RIA in most patients, with correlation coefficients usually exceeding 0.9. In serum/plasma, CSA concentrations measured by PC-FPIA are usually about 1.2 to 1.7 times higher than those measured by PC-RIA.[100,223,235,237–239] In whole blood, CSA concentrations measured by PC-FPIA are usually about 1.1 to 1.3 times higher than those measured by PC-RIA.[234–236] Transplant centers that measured whole blood CSA concentration by PC-RIA and switched to PC-FPIA would therefore have to increase slightly their therapeutic concentration range.

Because of its recent introduction in late 1990, few studies have evaluated in detail the MC-FPIA. The results of published studies suggest that whole blood CSA concentrations measured by MC-FPIA are nearly identical to those measured by MC-RIA and about 20% higher than those measured by HPLC.[240,241]

High-Performance Liquid Chromatography (HPLC)

Many HPLC methods for measurement of CSA concentration have been published.[242–250] The major disadvantage of all the procedures is that adequate resolution is achieved only if the column is heated to at least 60 °C. The extreme peak broadening at lower temperatures is related to the inability to resolve completely several conformers of CSA.[251] At these high temperatures, column life is shortened to several weeks when the columns are heated 30 to 40 hours per week. The second major disadvantage is that most of the present procedures cannot accurately measure CSA concentrations less than 50 ng/mL. The primary reason for the limited sensitivity is that many endogenous compounds and drugs absorb at the UV wavelength used to detect CSA (200 to 214 nm). Thus, sample clean-up requires laborious liquid-liquid extraction procedures which result in extraction efficiencies of 50% to 70%. Some laboratories have developed clean-up procedures that use small extraction columns rather than liquid-liquid extractions. The third major disadvantage of most of the methods is that, at concentrations of less than 100 ng/mL, the intra- and interday coefficient of variation is usually 10% to 20%.

The most novel and most technically difficult method uses two separate analytical columns and a column switching valve.[252-254] After minor sample preparation, CSA is extracted with the first column. The major advantage of this method is that there is no drug loss, and concentrations as low as 20 ng/mL can be easily detected, with a coefficient of variation of less than 5% (without an internal standard). With an auto-injector, laboratories can analyze about 50 samples daily. The major disadvantages of this method are the high initial equipment cost, complexity of the method, and, since two columns must be heated, the high cost of replacing columns.

Many HPLC methods to measure CSA metabolites have been developed.[99,255-258] One limitation in the development of these methods is the difficulty in obtaining pure standards of the proposed CSA metabolites. Most methods use laborious liquid-liquid extractions and require long chromatography times (45 to 60 minutes) to quantitate the large number of CSA metabolites in biological fluids. Many investigators also use only retention time to validate their method. It is therefore possible that a single peak represents more than one CSA metabolite. One column-switching HPLC method for measurement of the major CSA metabolites in blood has also been reported.[259]

Selection of an Analytical Method

Although specific analytical methods are usually preferable to nonspecific methods for therapeutic drug monitoring of most drugs, few studies have reported a significant correlation between whole blood CSA concentration measured by HPLC and clinical events. Furthermore, the practical limitations of present HPLC methods (e.g., cost, technical simplicity, speed) make nonspecific or relatively specific immunoassays an acceptable choice for many laboratories (see Table 28-8). For pharmacokinetic research, specific assay methods are preferred.

PROSPECTUS

Although CSA has been in clinical use for more than a decade, there are many unanswered questions concerning its pharmacokinetic and pharmacodynamic properties. With the development of sensitive and specific analytical methods, investigators have defined its basic pharmacokinetic profile and have identified many factors that can influence CSA pharmacokinetics such as age, hepatic function, hematocrit, and lipoprotein concentration. Many new CSA metabolites have been isolated and identified in humans. Although the major CSA metabolites are present in relatively high concentrations in human blood and have some immunosuppressive activity *in vitro*, their contribution to *in vivo* immunosuppression is not clear. Biochemical and molecular studies have identified the specific cytochrome P450 enzymes that metabolize CSA to its primary metabolites. Many new pharmacokinetic interactions between CSA and other drugs have been reported, and this knowledge has helped to elucidate the mechanism of many of these interactions.

The relationship between CSA concentrations measured by PC-RIA and therapeutic effect or toxicity has been established in several patient populations. This assay method, however, is no longer available. Few pharmacodynamic studies have reported a significant correlation between CSA concentrations measured by other assay methods and clinical outcome.

Although it is clear that CSA concentrations should be monitored in nearly all patients, there continues to be a general lack of consensus on how to apply CSA concentration data to patient care. Until rigorous pharmacodynamic studies are done, we will not know the most appropriate biological fluid or analytical method for routine monitoring. It may be that one method (or biological fluid) is preferred in specific situations (e.g., hepatic dysfunction) or in certain patient populations (e.g., liver transplant patients).

REFERENCES

1. Borel JF. The history of cyclosporin A and its significance. In: White DJG, ed. Cyclosporin A. New York: Elsevier;1982:5–18.
2. Von Wartburg A, et al. Cyclosporins, fungal metabolites with immunosuppressive activities. Prog Med Chem. 1988;25:1.
3. Kahan BD. Cyclosporine. N Engl J Med. 1989;321:1725.
4. Keown PA et al. Immunological and pharmacological monitoring in the clinical use of cyclosporine A. Lancet 1981;1:686.
5. Beveridge T et al. Cyclosporine A: pharmacokinetics after a single dose in man and serum levels after multiple dosing in recipients of allogeneic bone-marrow grafts. Curr Ther Res. 1981;30:5.
6. Wood AJ et al. Cyclosporine: pharmacokinetics, metabolism, and drug interaction. Transplant Proc. 1983;15:2409.
7. Ptachcinski RJ et al. Cyclosporine kinetics in renal transplantation. Clin Pharmacol Ther. 1985;38:296.
8. Legg B et al. Cyclosporin: pharmacokinetics and detailed studies of plasma and erythrocyte binding during intravenous and oral administration. Eur J Clin Pharmacol. 1988;34:451.
9. Speck RF et al. Cyclosporine kinetics in renal transplant patients as assessed by high-performance liquid chromatography and radioimmunoassay using monoclonal and polyclonal antibodies. Transplantation 1989;47:802.
10. Frey FJ et al. Trough levels and concentration time curves of cyclosporine in patients undergoing renal transplantation. Clin Pharmacol Ther. 1988;43:55.
11. Grevel J et al. Influence of demographic factors on cyclosporine pharmacokinetics in adult uremic patients. J Clin Pharmacol. 1989;29:261.
12. Morse GD et al. Comparison of cyclosporine assay methodology in the immediate postoperative period of renal transplantation. Ther Drug Monit. 1989;11:238.
13. Burckart GJ et al. Cyclosporine absorption following orthotopic liver transplantation. J Clin Pharmacol. 1986;26:647.
14. Venkataramanan R et al. Cyclosporine pharmacokinetics in heart transplant patients. Transplant Proc. 1986;18:768.
15. Cooney GF et al. Cyclosporine bioavailability in heart-lung transplant candidates with cystic fibrosis. Transplantation 1990;49:821.
16. Gupta SK et al. Effect of food on the pharmacokinetics of cyclosporine in healthy subjects following oral and intravenous administration. J Clin Pharmacol. 1990;30:643.
17. Nashan B et al. Effect of the application form of cyclosporine on blood levels: comparison of oral solution and capsules. Transplant Proc. 1988;20(Suppl.2):637.
18. Zehnder C et al. Cyclosporine A capsules: bioavailability and clinical acceptance in renal transplant patients. Transplant Proc. 1988;20(Suppl.2):641.

19. Lindholm A et al. Intraindividual variability in the relative systemic availability of cyclosporin after oral dosing. Eur J Clin Pharmacol. 1988;34:461.

20. Morse GD et al. Pharmacokinetics and clinical tolerance of intravenous and oral cyclosporine in the immediate postoperative period. Clin Pharmacol Ther. 1988;44:654.

21. Kahan BD et al. Pharmacokinetics of cyclosporine in human renal transplantation. Transplant Proc. 1983;15:446.

22. Awni WM et al. Long-term cyclosporine pharmacokinetic changes in renal transplant recipients: effects of binding and metabolism. Clin Pharmacol Ther. 1989;45:41.

23. Rcymond J et al. On the dose dependency of cyclosporin A absorption and disposition in healthy volunteers. J Pharmacokinet Biopharm. 1988;16:331.

24. Grevel J et al. Pharmacokinetics of oral cyclosporin A (Sandimmun) in healthy subjects. Eur J Clin Pharmacol. 1986;31:211.

25. Gupta SK, Benet LZ. Absorption kinetics of cyclosporine in healthy volunteers. Biopharm Drug Dispos. 1989;10:591.

26. Misteli C et al. Pharmacokinetics of oral cyclosporin A in diabetic children and adolescents. Eur J Clin Pharmacol. 1990;38:181.

27. Ptachcinski R et al. The effect of food on cyclosporine absorption. Transplantation 1985;40:174.

28. Lindholm A et al. The effect of food and bile acid administration on the relative bioavailability of cyclosporin. Br J Clin Pharmacol. 1990;29:541.

29. Henny FC et al. Pharmacokinetics and nephrotoxicity of cyclosporine in renal transplant rccipicnts. Transplantation 1985;40:261.

30. Phillips TM et al. Absorption profiles of renal allograft recipients receiving oral doses of cyclosporine: a pharmacokinetic study. Transplant Proc. 1988;20(Suppl.2):457.

31. Ota B. Administration of cyclosporine. Transplant Proc. 1983;15(Suppl.1):3111.

32. Johnston A et al. The effect of vehicle on the oral absorption of cyclosporin. Br J Clin Pharmacol. 1986;21:331.

33. Keown PA et al. The effects and side effects of cyclosporine: relationship to drug pharmacokinctics. Transplant Proc. 1982;14:659.

34. Wood AJ et al. Pharmacologic aspects of cyclosporine therapy: pharmacokinetics. Transplant Proc. 1985;17(Suppl.1):27.

35. Keogh A ct al. The effect of food and cholestryramine on the absorption of cyclosporine in cardiac transplant recipients. Transplant Proc. 1988;20:27.

36. Keown PA et al. The clinical relevance of cyclosporine blood levels as measured by radioimmunoassay. Transplant Proc. 1983;4:2438.

37. Shriner DA. Influence of dietary fat and bile salts on oral cyclosporine absorption in renal transplant patients. Pharmacotherapy. 1991;11:227.

38. Atkinson K et al. Oral administration of cyclosporine A for recipients of allogeneic marrow transplants: implications of clinical gut dysfunction. Br J Haematol. 1984;56:223.

39. Wadhwa NK et al. The effect of oral metoclopramide on the absorption of cyclosporine. Transplantation 1987;43:211.

40. Whitington PF et al. Small-bowel length and the dose of cyclosporine in children after liver transplantation. N Engl J Med. 1990;322:733.

41. Mehta MU et al. Effect of bile on cyclosporin absorption in liver transplant patients. Br J Clin Pharmacol. 1988;25:579.

42. Naoumov NV et al. Cyclosporin A pharmacokinetics in liver transplant recipients in relation to biliary T-tube clamping and liver dysfunction. Gut 1989;30:391.

43. Merion RM et al. Bile refeeding after liver transplantation and avoidance of intravenous cyclosporine. Surgery 1989;106:604.

44. Tan KKC et al. Altered pharmacokinetics of cyclosporin in heart-lung transplant recipients with cystic fibrosis. Ther Drug Monit. 1990;12:520.

45. Watkins PB et al. Identification of glucocorticoid-inducible cytochromes P450 in the intestinal mucosa of rats and man. J Clin Invest. 1987;80:1029.

46. Kolars JC et al. P450III metabolizes cyclosporin A in intestinal mucosa: observations in a novel rat model. Clin Res. 1989;37:933A.

47. Lucey MR et al. Cyclosporin toxicity at therapeutic blood levels and cytochrome P450IIIA. Lancet 1990;335:11.

48. Ptachcinski RJ et al. Cyclosporine kinetics in healthy volunteers. J Clin Pharmacol. 1987;27:243.

49. Follath F et al. Intravenous cyclosporine kinetics in renal failure. Clin Pharmacol Ther. 1983;34:638.

50. Reynolds KL et al. Cyclosporine pharmacokinetics in uremic patients: influence of different assay methods. Transplant Proc. 1988;20(Suppl.2):462.

51. Ptachcinski RJ et al. Clinical pharmacokinetics of cyclosporine. Clin Pharmacokinet. 1986;11:107.

52. Ptachcinski RJ et al. Cyclosporine pharmacokinetics in children following cadaveric renal transplantation. Transplant Proc. 1986;18:766.

53. Morse GD et al. Pharmacokinetics and clinical tolerance of intravenous and oral cyclosporine in the immediate postoperative period. Clin Pharmacol Ther. 1988;44:654.

54. Yee GC et al. Blood cyclosporine pharmacokinetics in patients undergoing marrow transplantation: influence of age, obesity, and hematocrit. Transplantation 1988;46:399.

55. Brunner LJ et al. Single-dose cyclosporine pharmacokinetics in various biological fluids of patients receiving allogeneic marrow transplantation. Ther Drug Monit. 1990;12:134.

56. Myre SA et al. Use of cyclosporine by constant-rate intravenous infusion immediately after heart transplantation. Transplant Proc. 1988;20(Suppl.3):316.

57. Gupta SK Benet LZ. High-fat meals increase the clearance of cyclosporine. Pharm Res. 1990;7:46.

58. Vernillet L et al. Pharmacokinetics of cyclosporine A in patients with nephrotic syndrome. Transplant Proc. 1988;20(Suppl.2):529.

59. Gupta SK et al. Pharmacokinetics of cyclosporin: influence of rate of constant intravenous infusion in renal transplant patients. Br J Clin Pharmacol. 1987;24:519.

60. Gupta SK et al. Pharmacokinetics of cyclosporin: influence of rate-duration profile of an intravenous infusion in renal transplant patients. Br J Clin Pharmacol. 1989;27:353.

61. Yee GC et al. Pharmacokinetics of intravenous cyclosporine in bone marrow transplant patients: comparison of two assay methods. Transplantation 1984;38:511.

62. Yee GC et al. Age-dependent cyclosporine pharmacokinetics in marrow transplant recipients. Clin Pharmacol Ther. 1986;40:438.

63. Ried M et al. Cyclosporine levels in human tissues of patients treated for one week to one year. Transplant Proc. 1983;15(Suppl.1):2434.

64. Atkinson K et al. Blood and tissue distribution of cyclosporine in humans and mice. Transplant Proc. 1983;15(Suppl.1):2430.

65. Lensmeyer GL et al. Deposition of nine metabolites of cyclosporine in human tissues, bile, urine, and whole blood. Transplant Proc. 1988;20(Suppl.2):614.

66. LeMaire M, Tillement JP. Role of lipoprotein and erythrocytes in the *in vitro* binding and distribution of cyclosporin A in the blood. J Pharm Pharmacol. 1982;34:715.

67. Niederberger W et al. Distribution and binding of cyclosporine in blood and tissues. Transplant Proc. 1983;15:2419.

68. Rosano TG. Effect of hematocrit on cyclosporine (cyclosporin A) in whole blood and plasma of renal-transplant patients. Clin Chem. 1985;31:410.

69. Agarwal RP et al. Assessment of cyclosporin A in whole blood and plasma in five patients with different hematocrits. Ther Drug Monit. 1985;7:61.

70. Agarwal RP et al. Temperature-dependent binding of cyclosporine to an erythrocyte protein. Clin Chem. 1987;33:481.

71. Legg B, Rowland M. Saturable binding of cyclosporin A to erythrocytes: estimation of binding parameters in renal transplant patients and implications for bioavailability assessment. Pharm Res. 1988;5:80.

72. Lensmeyer GL et al. Distribution of cyclosporin A metabolites among plasma and cells in whole blood: effect of temperature, hematocrit, and metabolite concentration. Clin Chem. 1989;35:56.

73. Agarwal RP et al. Evidence of a cyclosporine-binding protein in human erythrocytes. Transplantation 1986;42:627.

74. Mraz W et al. Distribution and transfer of cyclosporine among the various human lipoprotein classes. Transplant Proc. 1983;15:2426.

75. Gurecki J et al. The transport of cyclosporine in association with plasma lipoproteins in heart and liver transplant patients. Transplant Proc. 1985;17:1997.

76. Sgoutas D et al. Interaction of cyclosporin A with human lipoproteins. J Pharm Pharmacol. 1986;38:583.

77. Henricsson S. A new method for measuring the free fraction of cyclosporin in plasma by equilibrium dialysis. J Pharm Pharmacol. 1987;39:384.

78. Legg B, Rowland M. Cyclosporin: measurement of fraction unbound in plasma. J Pharm Pharmacol. 1987;39:599.

79. Zaghloul I et al. Blood protein binding of cyclosporine in transplant patients. J Clin Pharmacol. 1987;27:240.

80. Legg B et al. A model to account for the variation in cyclosporin binding to plasma lipids in transplant patients. Ther Drug Monit. 1988;10:20.

81. Lindholm A, Henricsson S. Intra- and interindividual variability in the free fraction of cyclosporine in plasma in recipients of renal transplants. Ther Drug Monit. 1989;11:623.

82. Gibaldi M, Koup JR. Pharmacokinetic concepts—drug binding, apparent volume of distribution and clearance. Eur J Clin Pharmacol. 1981;20:299.

83. Oie S, Tozer TN. Effect of altered plasma protein binding on apparent volume of distribution. J Pharm Sci. 1979;68:1203.

84. Awni WM, Sawchuk R. The pharmacokinetics of cyclosporine. II: Blood-plasma distribution and binding studies. Drug Metab Dispos. 1985;13:133.

85. Awni WM, Sawchuk R. The pharmacokinetics of cyclosporine. I: Single-dose and constant rate infusion studies in the rabbit. Drug Metab Dispos. 1985;13:127.

86. MacKichan JJ. Pharmacokinetic consequences of drug displacement from blood and tissue proteins. Clin Pharmacokinet. 1984;9(Suppl.1):32.

87. Nemunaitis J et al. High cyclosporin levels after bone marrow transplantation associated with hypertriglyceridaemia. Lancet 1986;2:744.

88. De Groen PC et al. Central nervous system toxicity after liver transplantation: the role of cyclosporine and cholesterol. N Engl J Med. 1987;317:861.

89. Yee GC et al. Effect of obesity on cyclosporine disposition. Transplantation 1988;45:649.

90. Maurer G. Metabolism of cyclosporine. Transplant Proc. 1985;17:19.

91. Maurer G et al. Disposition of cyclosporine in several animal species and man. I: Structural elucidation of its metabolites. Drug Metab Dispos. 1984;12:120.

92. Lensmeyer GL et al. Identification and analysis of nine metabolites of cyclosporine in whole blood by liquid chromatography. 2: Comparison of patient's results. Clin Chem. 1987;33:1851.

93. Wenger RM. Structures of cyclosporine and its metabolites. Transplant Proc. 1990;22:1104.

94. Christians U et al. Measurement of cyclosporine and 18 metabolites in blood, bile, and urine by high-performance liquid chromatography. Transplant Proc. 1988;20(Suppl.2):609.

95. Maurer G, Lemaire M. Biotransformation and distribution in blood of cyclosporine and its metabolites. Transplant Proc. 1986;18(Suppl.5):25.

96. Wang CP et al. Isolation of 10 cyclosporine metabolites from human bile. Drug Metab Dispos. 1989;17:292.

97. Various authors. Consensus document: Hawk's Cay meeting on therapeutic drug monitoring of cyclosporine. Transplant Proc. 1990;22:1357.

98. Yee GC et al. Measurement of blood cyclosporine metabolite concentrations with a new column-switching high-performance liquid chromatographic assay. Transplant Proc. 1988;20:585.

99. Rosano TG et al. Immunosuppressive metabolites of cyclosporine in the blood of renal allograft recipients. Transplantation 1986;42:262.

100. McGuire TR et al. Pharmacodynamics of cyclosporine in marrow transplant recipients: comparison of three assay methods. Transplantation. 1992. (In Press).

101. Wang CP et al. Cyclosporine metabolite concentrations in the blood of liver, heart, kidney, and bone marrow transplant patients. Transplant Proc. 1988;20(Suppl.2):591.

102. Wang CP et al. Cyclosporine metabolite profiles in the blood of liver transplant patients. Transplant Proc. 1988;20(Suppl.1):173.

103. Meier GP et al. Isolation and identification of a novel human metabolite of cyclosporin A: dihydro-CSA M17. Drug Metab Dispos. 1990;18:68.

104. Henricsson S. A sulfate conjugate of cyclosporin. Pharmacol Toxicol. 1990;

105. Johansson A et al. A novel sulfate conjugate of cyclosporine occurring in high concentrations *in vivo*. Transplantation 1990;49:619.

106. Rosano TG et al. Cyclosporine metabolites in human blood and renal tissue. Transplant Proc. 1986;18(Suppl.5):35.

107. Fahr A et al. Studies on the biologic activities of Sandimmun metabolites in humans and in animal models: review and original experiments. Transplant Proc. 1990;22:1116.

108. Freed BM et al. *In vitro* immunosuppressive properties of cyclosporine metabolites. Transplantation 1987;43:123.

109. Ryffel B et al. Nephrotoxic and immunosuppressive potentials of cyclosporine metabolites in rats. Transplant Proc. 1986;18(Suppl.5):41.

110. Wallemacq PE et al. Isolation, characterization, and *in vitro* activity of human cyclosporin A metabolites. Transplant Proc. 1989;21:906.

111. Zeevi A et al. Sensitivity of activated human lymphocytes to cyclosporine and its metabolites. Hum Immunol. 1988;21:143.

112. Schlitt HJ et al. Immunosuppressive activity of cyclosporine metabolites *in vitro*. Transplant Proc. 1987;19:4248.

113. Hartman NR, Jardine I. The *in vitro* activity, radioimmunoassay cross-reactivity, and molecular weight of thirteen rabbit cyclosporine metabolites. Drug Metab Dispos. 1987;15:661.

114. Copeland KR et al. Immunosuppressive activity of cyclosporine metabolites compared and characterized by mass spectroscopy and nuclear magnetic resonance. Clin Chem. 1990;36:225.

115. Donatsch P et al. Sandimmun metabolites: their potential to cause adverse reactions in the rat. Transplant Proc. 1990;22:1137.

116. Cole E et al. Toxic effects on renal cells in culture—a comparison of cyclosporin A and its metabolites. Transplant Proc. 1989;21:943.

117. Copeland KR et al. Toxicity of cyclosporine metabolites. Ther Drug Monit. 1990;12:525.

118. Kunzendorf U et al. Neurotoxicity caused by a high cyclosporine metabolite level. Transplantation 1989;48:531.

119. Fabre I et al. Metabolism of cyclosporin A. III: Interaction of the macrolide antibiotic, erythromycin, using rabbit hepatocytes and microsomal fractions. Drug Metab Dispos. 1988;16:296.

120. Bertault-Peres P et al. Metabolism of cyclosporine. II: Implication of the macrolide antibiotic inducible cytochrome P450 3c from rabbit liver microsomes. Drug Metab Dispos. 1987;15:391.

121. Kronbach T et al. Cyclosporine metabolism in human liver: identification of a cytochrome P450III gene family as the major cyclosporine-metabolizing enzyme explains interactions of cyclosporine with other drugs. Clin Pharmacol Ther. 1988;43:630.

122. Combalbert J et al. IV. Purification and identification of the rifampicin-inducible human liver cytochrome P450 (cyclosporin A oxidase) as a product of P450IIIA gene subfamily. Drug Metab Dispos. 1989;17:197.

123. Aoyama T et al. Cytochrome P450 hPCN3, a novel cytochrome P450IIIA gene product that is differentially expressed in adult human liver. J Biol Chem. 1989;264:10388.

124. Shaw PM et al. Purification and characterization of an anticonvulsant-inducible human cytochrome P450 catalyzing cyclosporin metabolism. Biochem J. 1989;263:653.

125. Nebert DW et al. The P450 superfamily: updated listing of all genes and recommended nomenclature for the chromosomal loci. DNA 1989;8:1.

126. Guengerich FP. Characterization of human microsomal cytochrome P450 enzymes. Ann Rev Pharmacol Toxicol. 1989;29:241.

127. Watkins et al. Identification of an inducible form of cytochrome P450 in human liver. Proc Natl Acad Sci. 1986;82:6310.

128. Guengerich FP et al. Characterization of rat and human liver microsomal cytochrome P450 forms involved in nifedipine oxidation, a prototype for genetic polymorphism in oxidative drug metabolism. J Biol Chem. 1986;261:5051.

129. Wrighton SA, VandenBranden M. Isolation and characterization of human fetal liver cytochrome P450HLp2: a third member of the P450III gene family. Arch Biochem Biophys. 1989;268:144.

130. Wrighton SA et al. Identification of a polymorphically expressed member of the human cytochrome P450III family. Mol Pharmacol. 1989;36:97.

131. Watkins PB et al. Erythromycin breath test as an assay of glucocorticoid-inducible liver cytochromes P-450: studies in rats and patients. J Clin Invest. 1989;83:688.

132. Watkins PB et al. The erythromycin breath test as a predictor of cyclosporine blood levels. Clin Pharmacol Ther. 1990;48:120.

133. Pichard L et al. Cyclosporin A drug interactions: screening for inducers and inhibitors of cytochrome P450 (cyclosporin A oxidase) in primary cultures of human hepatocytes and in liver microsomes. Drug Metab Dispos. 1990;18:595.

134. Watkins PB. The role of cytochromes P450 in drug metabolism and hepatotoxicity. Sem Liver Dis. 1990;10:235.

135. Cipolle RJ et al. Time-dependent disposition of cyclosporine after pancreas transplantation, and application of chronopharmacokinetics to improve immunosuppression. Pharmacotherapy 1988;8:47.

136. Venkataramanan R et al. Diurnal variation in cyclosporine kinetics. Ther Drug Monit. 1986;8:380.

137. Lithell H et al. Is the plasma lipoprotein pattern of importance for treatment with cyclosporine? Transplant Proc. 1986;18:50.

138. Yee GC et al. Effect of hepatic dysfunction on oral cyclosporine pharmacokinetics in marrow transplant patients. Blood 1984;64:1277.

139. Bleck JS et al. Urinary excretion of cyclosporin and 17 of its metabolites in renal allograft recipients. Pharmacology 1989;39:160.

140. Yee GC et al. Renal cyclosporine clearance in marrow transplant recipients: age-related variation. J Clin Pharmacol. 1986;26:658.

141. Venkataramanan R et al. Biliary excretion of cyclosporine in liver transplant patients. Transplant Proc. 1985;17:286.

142. Yee GC, McGuire TR. Pharmacokinetic drug interactions with cyclosporin (Part I). Clin Pharmacokinet. 1990;19:319.

143. Yee GC, McGuire TR. Pharmacokinetic drug interactions with cyclosporin (Part II). Clin Pharmacokinet. 1990;19:400.

144. Ryffel B. Pharmacology of cyclosporine. VI: Cellular activation: regulation of intracellular events by cyclosporine. Pharmacol Rev. 1989;41:407.

145. Kronke M et al. Cyclosporine A inhibits T-cell growth factor gene expression at the level of mRNA transcription. Proc Natl Acad Sci. 1984;81:5214.

146. Hess AD et al. The effect of cyclosporine A on T-lymphocyte subpopulations. In: White DJG, ed. Cyclosporin A. New York: Elsevier;1982:209–31.

147. Van Sickler J et al. Suppressor cells and T cell synergy in the primary MLR: interleukin-2 is required for maintenance of rat CD8+ suppressor cells. Cell Immunol. 1991;134:390.

148. Handschumacher RE et al. Cyclophilin: a specific cytosolic binding protein for cyclosporin A. Science 1984;226:544.

149. Fischer G et al. Cyclophilin and peptidyl-prolyl cis-trans isomerase are probably identical proteins. Nature 1989;337:476.

150. Takahashi N et al. Peptidyl-prolyl isomerase is the cyclosporine A-binding protein cyclophilin. Nature 1989;337:473.

151. Siekierka J et al. A cytosolic binding protein for the immunosuppressant FK-506 has peptidyl-prolyl isomerase activity but is distinct from cyclophilin. Nature 1989;341:755.

152. Rosen M et al. Inhibition of FKBP rotamase activity by immunosuppressant FK506: twisted amide surrogate. Science 1990;248:863.

153. Rogerson ME et al. Cyclosporine blood concentrations in the management of renal transplant recipients. Transplantation 1986;41:276.

154. Kahan BD et al. The value of serial serum trough cyclosporine levels in human renal transplantation. Transplant Proc. 1984;16(5):1195.

155. White DJG et al. Is the monitoring of cyclosporin-A serum levels of clinical value?. Transplant Proc. 1983;15:454.

156. Holt DW et al. Cyclosporine monitoring with polyclonal and specific monoclonal antibodies during episodes of renal allograft dysfunction. Transplant Proc. 1989;21:1482.

157. Lindholm A, Henricsson S. Simultaneous monitoring of cyclosporin in blood and plasma with four analytical methods: a clinical evaluation. Transplant Proc. 1989;21:1472.

158. Lindholm A et al. Influence of early cyclosporine dosage and plasma and whole blood levels on acute rejections in cadaveric renal allograft recipients. Transplant Proc. 1988;20:444.

159. Dunn F et al. The impact of steady-state cyclosporine concentrations on renal allograft outcome. Transplantation 1990;49:30.

160. Klintmalm G et al. Cyclosporine plasma levels in renal transplant patients. Transplantation 1985;39:132.

161. Kasiske BL et al. The relationship between cyclosporine pharmacokinetic parameters and subsequent acute rejection in renal transplant recipients. Transplantation 1988;46:716.

162. Veremis SA et al. Comparison of cyclosporine (CSA) blood levels and RIA/HPLC ratios among renal transplant patients with normal allograft function, CSA nephrotoxicity or rejection. Transplant Proc. 1989;21:1476.

163. Schroeder TJ et al. A comparison of the clinical utility of the radioimmunoassay, high-performance liquid chromatography, and TDx cyclosporine assays in outpatient renal transplant recipients. Transplantation 1989;47:262.

164. Moyer TP et al. Cyclosporine nephrotoxicity is minimized by adjusting dosage on the basis of drug concentration in blood. Mayo Clin Proc. 1988;63:241.

165. Ferguson RM et al. Cyclosporine blood level monitoring: the early post-transplant period. Transplant Proc. 1986;18(Suppl.1):113.

166. Yee GC et al. Serum cyclosporine concentration and risk of acute graft-versus-host disease after allogeneic marrow transplantation. N Engl J Med. 1988;319:65.

167. Santos GW et al. Cyclosporine plus methylprednisolone versus cyclophosphamide plus methylprednisolone as prophylaxis for graft-versus-host disease: a randomized double-blind study in patients undergoing allogeneic marrow transplantation. Clin Transplantation 1987;1:21.

168. Bandini G et al. Cyclosporin A: correlation of blood levels with acute graft-versus-host disease after bone marrow transplantation. Acta Haematol. 1987;78:6.

169. Barrett AJ et al. Cyclosporine A as prophylaxis against graft-versus-host disease in 36 patients. Br Med J. 1982;285:162.

170. Biggs JC, et al. The use of cyclosporine in human marrow transplantation: absence of a therapeutic window. Transplant Proc. 1985;17:1239.

171. Lindholm A et al. The role of cyclosporine dosage and plasma levels in efficacy and toxicity in bone marrow transplant recipients. Transplantation 1987;43:680.

172. Gratwohl A et al. Cyclosporine in human bone marrow transplantation: serum concentration, graft-versus-host disease, and nephrotoxicity. Transplantation 1983;36:40.

173. Tredger JM et al. Cyclosporine blood levels—an evaluation of radioimmunoassay with selective monoclonal or polyclonal antibodies and high-performance liquid chromatograpy in liver transplant recipients. Transplantation 1988;46:681.

174. Burckart G et al. Cyclosporine monitoring and pharmacokinetics in pediatric liver transplant patients. Transplant Proc. 1985;17:1172.

175. Kohlhaw K et al. Association of very high blood levels of cyclosporin metabolites with clinical complications after liver transplantation. Transplant Proc. 1989;21:2232.

176. Wallemacq PE et al. Cyclosporine monitoring by RIA and HPLC in liver transplantation: clinical correlation. Clin Transplantation 1987;1:132.

177. Burckart GJ et al. Cyclosporine trough concentration monitoring in liver transplant patients. Transplant Proc. 1986;18(Suppl.5):188.

178. Hamilton G et al. Cyclosporine A nephrotoxicity in liver graft recipients: determination of nephrotoxic cyclosporine blood concentrations in liver graft recipients as defined by the HPLC and RIA tests. Transplant Proc. 1987;19:4045.

179. Haven MC et al. Cyclosporine concentration in blood after liver transplantation: correlation of immunoassay results with clinical events. Clin Chem. 1989;35:564.

180. Griffith BP et al. Target blood levels of cyclosporine for cardiac transplantation. J Thorac Cardiovasc Surg. 1984;88:952.

181. Bennett WM et al. Renal consequences of a low dose cyclosporine triple therapy regimen in cardiac transplantation. Transplant Proc. 1989;21:2479.

182. Myers BD. Cyclosporine nephrotoxicity. Kidney Int. 1986;30:964.

183. Kopp JB et al. Cellular and molecular mechanisms of cyclosporine nephrotoxicity. J Am Soc Nephrol. 1990;1:162.

184. Mason J. Pharmacology of cyclosporine (Sandimmune). VII: Pathophysiology and toxicology of cyclosporine in humans and animals. Pharmacol Rev. 1989;42:423.

185. Mihatsch MJ et al. Cyclosporine nephrotoxicity. Adv Nephrol. 1988;17:303.

186. Perico N et al. Effect of short-term cyclosporine administration in rats on renin-angiotensin and thromboxane A_2. J Pharmacol Exp Ther. 1986;239:229.

187. Kon V et al. Cyclosporine causes endothelin-dependent acute renal failure. Kidney Int. 1990;37:298A.

188. Spurney RF et al. Thromboxane receptor blockade improves cyclosporine nephrotoxicity in rats. Protaglandins. 1990;29:135.

189. Zoja C et al. Cyclosporin-induced endothelial cell injury. Lab Invest. 1986;55:455.

190. English J et al. Cyclosporine-induced acute renal dysfunction in the rat. Transplantation. 1987;44:135.

191. Myers BD et al. Cyclosporine-associated chronic nephropathy. N Engl J Med. 1984;311:699.

192. Palestine AG et al. Renal histopathological alterations in patients treated with cyclosporine for uveitis. N Engl J Med. 1986;314:1293.

193. Bantle JP et al. Long-term effects of cyclosporine on renal function in organ transplant recipients. J Lab Clin Med. 1990;115:233.

194. Lewis R. Evolution of renal function in cardiac and renal allograft recipients receiving long-term cyclosporine. Literature Scan: Transplantation. 1990;6:1.

195. Brinker KR et al. A randomized trial comparing double-drug and triple-drug therapy in primary cadaveric renal transplants. Transplantation. 1990;50:43.

196. Holt DW et al. Blood cyclosporin concentrations and renal allograft dysfunction. Br Med J. 1986;293:1057.

197. Kahan BD et al. Multivariate analysis of risk factors impacting on immediate and eventual cadaver allograft survival in cyclosporine-treated recipients. Transplantation 1987;43:65.

198. Maiorca R et al. Cyclosporine toxicity can be minimized by careful monitoring of blood levels. Transplant Proc. 1985;17(Suppl.2):54.

199. Ubhi CS et al. Is there a therapeutic range for monitoring cyclosporin in renal allograft recipients? Nephrol Dial Transplant. 1988;3:814.

200. Salomon DR et al. Retrospective analysis of late renal graft dysfunction: correlation with mean cyclosporine levels and lack of evidence for chronic cyclosporine toxicity. Transplant Proc. 1991;23:1018.

201. Hows JM et al. Nephrotoxicity in bone marrow transplant recipients treated with cyclosporine A. Br J Haematol. 1983;54:69.

202. Kennedy MS et al. Correlation of serum cyclosporine concentration with renal dysfunction in marrow transplant recipients. Transplantation 1985;40:249.

203. Yee GC et al. Monitoring cyclosporine concentrations in marrow transplant recipients: comparison of two assay methods. Bone Marrow Transplant 1987;1:289.

204. Burckart GJ et al. Cyclosporine monitoring. Drug Intell Clin Pharm. 1986;20:649.

205. Shaw LM. Cyclosporine monitoring. Clin Chem. 1989;35:5.

206. Rodighiero V. Therapeutic drug monitoring of cyclosporin: practical applications and limitations. Clin Pharmacokinet. 1989;16:27.

207. NACB/AACC Task Force on Cyclosporine Monitoring: Critical issues in cyclosporine monitoring: report of the task force on cyclosporine monitoring. Clin Chem. 1987;33:1269.

208. Kahan BD, Grevel J. Optimization of cyclosporine therapy in renal transplantation by a pharmacokinetic strategy. Transplantation 1988;46:631.

209. Grevel J et al. Cyclosporine monitoring in renal transplantation: area under the curve monitoring is superior to trough-level monitoring. Ther Drug Monit. 1989;11:246.

210. Grevel J et al. Area-under-the-curve monitoring of cyclosporine therapy: performance of different assay methods and their target concentrations. Ther Drug Monit. 1990;12:8.

211. Cantarovich F et al. Cyclosporine plasma levels six hours after oral administration: a useful tool for monitoring therapy. Transplantation 1988;45:389.

212. Lokiec F et al. A safer approach to the clinical use of cyclosporine: the predose calculation. Transplant Proc. 1986;18(Suppl.5):194.

213. Bertault-Peres P et al. Clinical pharmacokinetics of cyclosporin A in bone marrow transplantation patients. Cancer Chemother Pharmacol. 1985;15:76.

214. Kahan BD et al. Application of Bayesian forecasting to predict appropriate cyclosporine dosing regimens for renal allograft recipients. Transplant Proc. 1986;18(Suppl.5):200.

215. Serre-Debeauvais F et al. Bayesian estimation of cyclosporine clearance in bone marrow graft. Ther Drug Monit. 1990;12:16.

216. Didlake RH et al. Patient noncompliance: a major cause of late graft failure in cyclosporine-treated renal transplants. Transplant Proc. 1988;20(Suppl.3):63.

217. Prasad R et al. A significant difference in cyclosporine blood and plasma concentrations with heparin or EDTA anticoagulant. Transplantation 1985;39:667.

218. Beresini M et al. EMIT cyclosporine assay for whole blood samples on the COBAS MIRA analyzer. Clin Chem. 1990;36:1034.

219. Hansen JB et al. A rapid and specific assay for the duPont aca discrete clinical analyzer, performed directly on whole blood. Transplant Proc. 1990;22:1189.

220. Quesniaux V et al. Potential of monoclonal antibodies to improve therapeutic monitoring of cyclosporine. Clin Chem. 1987;33:32.

221. Ball PE et al. Specific ^{3}H radioimmunoassay with a monoclonal antibody for monitoring cyclosporine in blood. Clin Chem. 1988;34:257.

222. Rosano TG et al. Selection of an optimal assay method for monitoring cyclosporine therapy. Transplant Proc. 1990;22:1125.

223. Lindholm A, Henricsson S. Comparative analyses of cyclosporine in whole blood and plasma by radioimmunoassay, fluorescence polarization immunoassay, and high-performance liquid chromatography. Ther Drug Monit. 1990;12:344.

224. Hirvisalo EL et al. Therapeutic cyclosporine monitoring: comparison of radioimmunoassay and high-performance liquid chromatography methods in organ transplant recipients. Ther Drug Monit. 1990;12:353.

225. Copeland KR, Yatscoff RW. Use of a monoclonal antibody for the therapeutic monitoring of cyclosporine in plasma and whole blood. Ther Drug Monit. 1988;10:453.

226. Wolf BA et al. Measurement of cyclosporine concentrations in whole blood: HPLC and radioimmunoassay with a specific monoclonal antibody and [3]H- or ^{125}I-labeled ligand compared. Clin Chem. 1989;35:120.

227. Vernillet L et al. Determination of cyclosporine in plasma: specific radioimmunoassay with a monoclonal antibody and liquid chromatography compared. Clin Chem. 1989;35:608.

228. Schran HF et al. Determination of cyclosporine concentrations with monoclonal antibodies. Clin Chem. 1987;33:2225.

229. Holt DW et al. Monoclonal antibodies for radioimmunoassay of cyclosporine: a multicenter comparison of their performance with the Sandoz polyclonal radioimmunoassay kit. Clin Chem. 1988;34:1091.

230. Wong PY, Ma J. Specific and nonspecific monoclonal ^{125}I-Incstar assays. Transplant Proc. 1990;22:1166.

231. Sgoutas DS, Hammarstrom M. Comparison of specific radioimmunoassays for cyclosporine. Transplantation 1989;47:668.

232. Blick KE et al. A validation study of selected methods routinely used for measurement of cyclosporine. Clin Chem. 1990;36:670.

233. Keown PA et al. Therapeutic monitoring of cyclosporine: impact of a change in standards on ^{125}I-monoclonal RIA performance in comparison with liquid chromatography. Clin Chem. 1990;36:804.

234. Strassman MJ et al. Three commercially available polyclonal immunoassays for cyclosporine in whole blood compared: 1. results with patient's specimens. Clin Chem. 1990;36:115.

235. Pesce AJ et al. An evaluation of cyclosporine monitoring by nonselective fluorescence polarization immunoassay. Transplant Proc. 1990;22:1171.

236. Plebani M et al. Fluorescence polarization immunoassay for cyclosporine A determination in whole blood. Ther Drug Monit. 1990;12:284.

237. Hayashi Y et al. Evaluation of fluorescence polarization immunoassay for determination of cyclosporin in plasma. Ther Drug Monit. 1990;11:205.

238. Sanghvi A et al. Abbott's fluorescence polarization immunoassay for cyclosporine and metabolites compared with the Sandoz "Sandimmune" RIA. Clin Chem. 1988;34:1904.

239. Wallemacq PE et al. Comparison of a fluorescence polarization immunoassay and a radioimmunoassay for the quantitation of cyclosporine A in organ transplantation. Transplant Proc. 1989;21:888.

240. Wang P et al. A monoclonal antibody fluorescent polarization immunoassay for cyclosporine. Transplant Proc. 1990;22:1186.

241. Yatscoff RW et al. Abbott TDx monoclonal antibody assay evaluated for measuring cyclosporine in whole blood. Clin Chem. 1990;36:1969.

242. Kahn GC et al. Routine monitoring of cyclosporine in whole blood and in kidney tissue using high performance liquid chromatography. J Anal Toxicol. 1986;10:28.

243. Carruthers SG et al. Simplified liquid-chromatographic analysis for cyclosporin A, and comparison with radioimmunoassay. Clin Chem. 1983;29:180.

244. Aravind MK et al. Measurement of cyclosporin by high-performance liquid chromatography following charcoal absorption from whole blood. J Chromatogr. 1985;344:428.

245. Sawchuk RJ, Cartier LL. Liquid-chromatographic determination of cyclosporin A in blood and plasma. Clin Chem. 1981;27:1368.

246. Garraffo R, Lapalus P. Simplified liquid chromatographic analysis for cyclosporin A in blood and plasma with use of rapid extraction. J Chromatogr. 1985;337:416.

247. Moyer TP et al. Cyclosporine: a review of drug monitoring problems and presentation of a simple, accurate liquid chromatographic procedure that solves these problems. Clin Biochem. 1986;19:83.

248. Yee GC et al. Liquid-chromatographic determination of cyclosporine in serum with use of a rapid extraction procedure. Clin Chem. 1982;28:2269.

249. Kates RE, Latini R. Simple and rapid high-performance liquid chromatographic analysis of cyclosporine in human blood and serum. J Chromatogr. 1984;309:441.

250. Plebani M et al. High-performance liquid chromatography for cyclosporin measurement: comparison with radioimmunoassay. J Chromatogr. 1989;476:93.

251. Bowers LD et al. Investigation of the mechanism of peak broadening observed in the high-performance liquid chromatographic analysis of cyclosporine. J Chromatogr. 1985;333:231.

252. Smith HT, Robinson WT. Semi-automated high-performance liquid chromatographic method for the determination of cyclosporine in plasma and blood using column-switching. J Chromatogr. 1984;305:353.

253. Gmur DJ et al. Modified column-switching high-performance liquid chromatographic method for the measurement of cyclosporine in serum. J Chromatogr. 1985;344:422.

254. Hosotsubo H et al. Determination of cyclosporin A in whole blood by high-performance liquid chromatography using automated column switching. J Chromatogr. 1986;383:349.

255. Bowers LD, Singh J. A gradient HPLC method for quantitation of cyclosporine and its metabolites in blood and bile. J Liq Chromatogr. 1987;10:411.

256. Shah AK, Sawchuk RJ. Improved liquid-chromatographic determination of cyclosporine and its metabolites in blood. Clin Chem. 1988;34:1467.

257. Christians U et al. Liquid-chromatographic measurement of cyclosporin A and its metabolites in blood, bile, and urine. Clin Chem. 1988;34:34.

258. Lensmeyer GL et al. Identification and analysis of nine metabolites of cyclosporine in whole blood by liquid chromatography. 1: Purification of analytical standards and optimization of the assay. Clin Chem. 1987;33:1841.

259. Gmur DJ et al. High-performance liquid chromatographic column-switching method for two cyclosporine metabolites in blood. J Chromatogr. 1988;425:343.

260. Honcharik N. The effect of food on cyclosporine absorption. Clin Biochem. 1991;24:89.

261. Kolars JC et al. First-pass metabolism of cyclosporin by the gut. Lancet. 1991;338:1488.

262. Yatscoff RW. The clinical significance of cyclosporine metabolites. Clin Biochem. 1991;24:23.

263. Lown K et al. The erythromycin breath test selectively measures P450IIIA in patients with severe liver disease. Clin Pharmacol Ther. 1992. [In Press.]

Chapter 29

Methotrexate

William R. Crom and William E. Evans

Methotrexate (MTX, amethopterin, 4-amino-N^{10}-methyl pteroylglutamic acid) is an analog of aminopterin, the folic acid antagonist introduced in 1948 by Farber for the treatment of acute leukemia. MTX is a weak dicarboxylic acid with pK_as of 4.8 and 5.5 and is essentially ionized and lipid insoluble at physiological pH. It differs from aminopterin by being methylated at the N^{10} position and has a molecular weight of 454.46.[1] MTX exerts its cytotoxic effects by competitively inhibiting dihydrofolate reductase (DHFR), the intracellular enzyme responsible for converting folic acid to reduced folate cofactors. Doses of MTX currently in clinical use range from 7.5 mg/m² to greater than 35,000 mg/m² with leucovorin rescue. This chapter focuses on various clinical, biological, and pharmacological factors which influence the dosage of MTX and provide a basis for the use of MTX serum concentrations to optimize MTX therapy in selected patients.

CLINICAL PHARMACOKINETICS

Absorption

A number of studies have been published[2-19] which document the relatively poor and unpredictable nature of MTX absorption from the gastrointestinal (GI) tract, as well as its dose-dependency. These studies show that the extent of absorption may be less than 50% even at relatively low doses (≤15 mg/m²) in contrast to older studies which demonstrated good absorption at low dosages.[20,21] These studies have taken on additional importance with the increasing use of oral MTX for treatment of nonmalignant diseases such as severe psoriasis, rheumatoid arthritis, and most recently, asthma.

Figure 29-1 summarizes the published studies of MTX oral absorption arranged according to the dosage (mg/m²) of MTX administered. A clear trend of decreasing bioavailability with increasing oral dosage is evident. These clinical findings are consistent with animal studies demonstrating dose-dependent absorption of MTX.[24] This process is best described by Michaelis-Menten kinetics with typical K_m and V_{max} values of about 15 µmol/L and 0.48 µmol/min, respectively. Following oral dosages commonly used to treat acute lymphocytic leukemia (ALL) and other cancers (i.e., 25 mg/m^2), peak concentrations can occur from one to five hours after a dose, and peak concentrations can range from 0.25 to 1.25 μmol/L. Factors reported to affect the rate and/or extent of MTX absorption include food,[10] oral nonabsorbable antibiotics,[17] parenteral kanamycin,[25] and a shortened intestinal transit time.[26]

It is evident from published studies that the rate and extent of absorption are highly variable in patients. Studies published since the last edition of this text add further evidence of this variability. Teresi et al.[27] compared oral, intravenous (IV), and intramuscular (IM) administration in 12 children with ALL receiving MTX dosages of 13 to 120 mg/m^2. Oral bioavailability averaged 33% (range 13% to 76%) but averaged 76% (54% to 112%) for the same dose administered IM. There was a significant dose-dependent bioavailability for oral MTX with a mean of 42% versus 18% for dosages less than and greater than 40 mg/m^2, respectively. In a similar study, Balis et al.[28] compared oral and subcutaneous administration in Rhesus monkeys and 12 children with ALL receiving either 7.5 mg/m^2 biweekly or 40 mg/m^2 weekly. Four children also received IV MTX at the higher dosage.

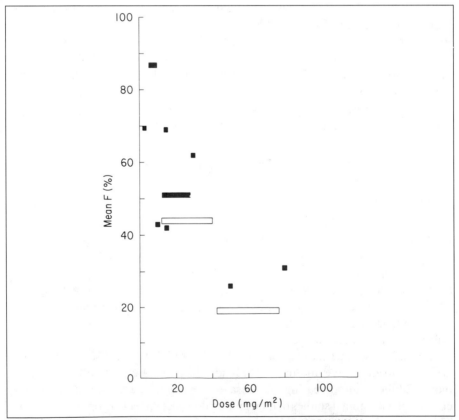

Figure 29-1. *Mean MTX bioavailability reported in literature*[3,6,7,11,12,20–23] *at various dosages or dosage ranges (solid symbols) compared with results from reference 27 (open symbols) for dosages ≤ 40 mg/m^2 and >40 mg/m^2 (reproduced with permission from reference 27).*

In the leukemia patients, the bioavailability of the subcutaneous and oral dosages was equivalent at the lower dosage level, but the area under the concentration-time curve (AUC) for the oral route was only about one-third that of the subcutaneous route at the higher dosage level. When compared to the IV route, the bioavailability of the oral dosage averaged only 42%. Subcutaneous administration of MTX appeared to represent a sustained release dosage form and was well tolerated in the children, with no evidence of local or systemic toxicity. Pearson et al.[26] compared oral absorption patterns in 28 children with ALL receiving 2.3 to 20.4 mg/m^2 to their small intestine transit time as measured by passage of lactulose to caecum. These investigators found that children with longer transit times had their peak MTX concentrations at later times and had more erratic absorption profiles with two peaks. There appeared to be an optimal transit time of 90 to 105 minutes with both faster and slower times producing lower peak concentrations relative to the dose.

The benefit of subdividing oral MTX doses to enhance bioavailability is not clear since contradictory results have been published.[2,4,5] Until these discrepancies are resolved, it seems prudent to assume that oral bioavailability of intermediate-dose ($\geq$100 mg/m^2) MTX will be relatively poor and not substantially improved by subdividing the dose as described above.

The clinical significance of intra- and intersubject variability in MTX absorption is not clearly defined. Craft et al.[13] have reported a lower rate of disease-free survival in children with ALL who absorb MTX "slowly" based on peak concentrations achieved. However, this observation must be evaluated more extensively in a prospective study that more completely characterizes MTX absorption and disposition before guidelines for dosage adjustments can be established. Routine measurement of MTX concentrations following oral doses is not currently recommended. In leukemia patients who require unusually large oral doses of MTX to maintain a white blood cell count between 2000 to 4000/μL (a biological measure of drug effect in acute leukemia patients receiving MTX maintenance therapy), a measurement of MTX concentrations may be useful to help distinguish incomplete absorption from noncompliance. In situations where complete bioavailability is essential, MTX may be given IM as an alternative to IV administration since essentially complete IM absorption occurs at doses up to at least 100 mg.[16,27] Similarly, subcutaneous administration[28] may provide another alternative to oral MTX since absorption from this route appears to be complete at least up to dosages of 40 mg/m^2.

Distribution

Following IV administration, MTX distributes within an initial volume approximating 18% (0.18 L/kg) of body weight[29] and exhibits a variable steady-state volume of approximately 40% to 80% of body weight.[20,30–32] MTX is approximately 50% bound to plasma protein,[20,21,33] primarily albumin, at serum concentrations ranging from 1 μmol/L to 100 μmol/L, (0.5 to 50 μg/mL). Other protein-bound organic acids such as sulfonamides and para-aminohippurate can displace MTX from protein binding sites,[33,34] but relatively high concentrations are necessary to substantially displace MTX. Relatively low concentrations of salicylate can also alter the protein binding of MTX, apparently by a noncompetitive mechanism that alters the binding affinity of albumin for MTX and other anionic drugs. The clinical significance of these drug-drug interactions is also difficult to assess, since many of these organic acids may also competitively inhibit renal tubular secretion of MTX.[33] The 7-hydroxy metabolite of MTX is more extensively bound to plasma proteins (i.e., >90%), but at concentrations seen clinically (<100 μmol), it does not appear to alter the protein binding of MTX.[35] This may be due to the relatively high capacity of MTX and 7-OH-MTX plasma protein binding sites and does not rule out a common binding site, since 7-OH-MTX concentrations of approximately 1000 μmol can displace MTX at equimolar concentrations.

In animals[36] and humans,[37] the highest tissue:plasma equilibrium distribution ratios are reported for the kidney and liver followed by the gastrointestinal tract and muscle. The gastrointestinal tract is apparently an important site of distribution and metabolism of both orally and intravenously administered MTX. Zaharko[36] and Bischoff,[37] in studies of MTX disposition in lower animals and humans, reported the persistence of higher MTX concentrations in gut lumen of the small intestine than in liver, kidney, muscle, or plasma. Their model predictions in mouse and human indicated that higher plasma levels in human are due to less rapid clearances by the kidney and bile and a longer residence time in the human small intestine. MTX in the gastrointestinal tract may be reabsorbed by a saturable process, excreted in the feces, or taken up and metabolized by bacteria in the large intestine. The differences between humans and smaller animals in the persistence of MTX in the gastrointestinal tract and the rate and extent of metabolism by gut bacteria are due in part to differences in transit time in the small and large intestine.[36] Decreased GI transit rate secondary to complete or partial gastrointestinal obstruction has been described as a potential mechanism for sustained concentrations of MTX in humans after high-dose infusions.[38,39]

Following the administration of high doses of MTX, distribution of MTX into pleural or ascitic fluid may have a substantial influence on MTX disposition.[40–42] The presence of a pleural effusion resulted in a significant increase in the terminal phase half-life in a patient extensively evaluated with and without a pleural effusion.[41] Beginning six hours after a high-dose MTX (HDMTX) infusion, MTX concentrations in pleural fluid were always greater than the simultaneous serum concentrations. These data support the observations that patients with ascites or pleural effusions are at increased risk for developing toxicity following HDMTX because of sustained MTX serum concentrations. The maximum concentration of MTX in pleural effusions and ascitic fluid is only about 10% of the maximum serum concentration but declines more slowly with an eventual pleural fluid:serum equilibrium ratio of approximately ten. This makes the influence of pleural effusions or ascites most important when high doses (>250 mg/m^2) of MTX are given, but of little importance at low doses (<50 mg/m^2). When such high doses are given to patients with "third spaces," MTX accumulated in these extravascular compartments acts as a "sustained-release" source, thereby maintaining higher serum concentrations of MTX. Such patients are at greater risk of having potentially cytotoxic MTX concentrations beyond the usual duration of leucovorin rescue. Although the effect of pleural effusion on the decline of serum concentrations may not be evident until 24 to 30 hours after the dose, serum concentrations at this time are still approximately 100-fold greater than the minimum concentration required for inhibition of DNA synthesis ($\approx$0.05 µmol/L).

An important consideration in the distribution of MTX is the process of membrane transport since the effects of MTX are dependent upon an intracellular concentration sufficient to inhibit DHFR activity. Intracellular transport can occur by two processes: simple transmembrane diffusion and a carrier-mediated active transport process. At low extracellular MTX concentrations (<5 µmol/L) a saturable (Michaelis-Menten) active transport process predominates, with a reported K_m value of about 5 µmol/L,[42] a value similar to that reported for naturally occurring reduced folates. However, a cell-surface receptor responsible for intracellular transport of reduced folates which also binds to methotrexate has more recently been described.[43,44] This receptor has a much lower K_m value for methotrexate (about 20 nmol/L) in cells grown in folate-depleted media, and the affinity for reduced folates is the same as for methotrexate. In addition, the receptor activity is regulated by intracellular folate content, and receptor expression is increased markedly in folate-depleted cells. It appears that this low affinity receptor is evident only in folate-depleted (physiological) media, and that previous reports of a 5 µmol/L K_m for MTX/folate membrane transport were due to the supraphysiologic folate content of the media.

Following the IV administration of high doses of MTX ($\geq$100 mg/kg), serum concentrations in the range of 100 to 1000 µmol/L are achieved. At these concentrations, the active transport process is clearly saturated, and passive diffusion becomes a major pathway by which higher intracellular concentrations can be achieved. This may be of particular importance in the treatment of malignant diseases which have an acquired or de novo resistance to MTX due to a reduced active transport process. Additionally, since MTX and reduced folates (i.e., leucovorin) share the same active transport process, high extracellular MTX concentrations can reduce or inhibit the intracellular transport of leucovorin.[45] Thus, leucovorin "rescue" following HDMTX can be a competitive process despite its apparent noncompetitive biochemical mechanism of circumventing the inhibition of DHFR with reduced folates. When MTX serum concentrations are approximately 0.1 µmol/L, MTX effects can be rescued with equimolar serum concentrations of leucovorin, whereas 1000 µmol/L concentrations of leucovorin may be required when MTX concentrations are 10 µmol/L.[45]

The anticancer agents teniposide (VM-26) and etoposide (VP-16) have been evaluated for their effects on MTX cellular transport and metabolism in Ehrlich ascites tumor cells *in vitro*.[46] It was found that these epipodophyllotoxins caused a net increase in cellular accumulation of MTX, mediated by an inhibition of MTX efflux. This also resulted in more extensive conversion of intracellular MTX to polyglutamate forms. VM-26 and VP-16 effects on MTX transport were qualitatively similar to those seen with vinca alkaloids (i.e., the effects were rapidly reversible when the epipodophyllotoxin was removed from the incubating media), and these effects were partially reversed by addition of the energy substrate, glucose. It remains unclear whether the high degree of protein binding of VM-26 and VP-16 will preclude this interaction from being clinically important. However, the teniposide-MTX combination has shown a therapeutic advantage when administered intraperitoneally to leukemia (L1210)-bearing mice.[47]

The blood-cerebrospinal fluid (CSF) barrier is relatively impermeable to MTX,[20,48,49] and CSF concentrations following IV administration of MTX are dose-related. Animal studies indicated that the brain:serum ratio for MTX after low dosages (10 mg/kg) is small (i.e., 0.11).[50,51] In humans, CSF MTX concentrations have been reported to range from 0.1 μmol/L after a 24-hour infusion of 500 mg/m^2 to greater than 10 μmol/L following 7500 mg/m^2 given as an IV bolus.[52-55] When MTX (1000 mg/m^2) was given IV over 24 hours, lumbar CSF concentrations averaged 2.3% (± 4.0%) of the steady-state serum concentrations at the end of the infusions.[56] A significant correlation was found between steady-state serum concentrations and CSF concentrations of MTX, with the correlation being better if the non-protein-bound MTX serum concentration was used.[56] Studies conducted in a small number of patients indicate that lumbar CSF and brain extracellular fluid concentrations are similar following HDMTX administration.[57] This is not the case when MTX is given by intrathecal (IT) injection into the lumbar CSF since MTX distribution into ventricular CSF is variable and unpredictable following IT administration and is influenced by body position.[58]

Ionizing radiation has been shown to alter permeability of the blood-brain barrier to MTX although these changes may vary from one region of the brain to another and from one species to another. It has been observed clinically that MTX-related leukoencephalopathy is most often a result of combined therapy with cranial irradiation and systemic MTX. It is postulated that radiation alters the integrity of the blood-brain barrier allowing MTX to diffuse more easily into the white matter.[20,59,60]

Metabolism

Although early studies with MTX indicated that this drug was not significantly metabolized,[20,61] it is now generally recognized that there are three routes for MTX metabolism and that the relative importance of each pathway is dependent on the dose and method of MTX administration. These pathways are summarized in Figure 29-2. First, MTX may be metabolized by intestinal bacteria, resulting in the removal of the glutamate residue and formation of 4-amino-4-deoxy-N^{10}-methylpteroic acid (DAMPA).[18,62] Although detection of this metabolite in plasma and urine has been reported,[62] it is usually undetectable and accounts for a very small percentage of the dose (i.e., <5%). DAMPA is an inactive metabolite with about 0.5% of the affinity of MTX for the target enzyme, DHFR.[18]

Secondly, MTX is metabolized by hydroxylation at C-7 of the pteridine moiety.[63] Although 7-hydroxymethotrexate (7-OH-MTX) is a less effective inhibitor of DHFR (about 1/100 of MTX)[64-67] and thus considered an inactive metabolite,[68] serum concentrations of 7-OH-MTX greater than MTX have been observed within hours after an IV dose.[69-77] Extensive conversion of MTX to 7-OH-MTX has been demonstrated in patients receiving high- or low-dose MTX therapy.[23,69,71,73,78]

Metabolic transformation of MTX to 7-OH-MTX is due mainly to a hepatic alde-hyde oxidase,[63] although this metabolite can be found in many other tissues.[79,80] Even if 7-OH-MTX is not formed in other tissues, the metabolite may enter by passive diffusion at the extremely high plasma concentrations (250 µmol/L) achieved in some patients.[81] Since 7-OH-MTX is much less soluble at neutral or acid pH than MTX,[63] the possibility exists that urine concentrations of the meta-bolite may exceed its solubility leading to tubular precipitation during renal elimination. Thus, 7-OH-MTX formation may contribute to the well-documented nephrotoxicity[82] that can occur with HDMTX therapy. In addition, it has been suggested that 7-OH-MTX competes with MTX for active renal tubular secretion and may therefore modulate MTX elimination.[83]

Several other mechanisms exist by which 7-OH-MTX may modulate both the pharmacokinetics and pharmacodynamics of MTX. First, the extensive protein binding of 7-OH-MTX (>90%) may alter the protein binding of MTX, but this appears to occur only at concentrations greater than 1000 µmol/L.[35] In addition, 7-OH-MTX inhibits MTX transport in Ehrlich ascites tumor cells[65,76] and in human KB cells.[76] Thus, when 7-OH-MTX is present in high concentrations relative to MTX (as occurs clinically), it may have an effect on MTX accumulation in cells and MTX's subsequent pharmacologic effects. Finally, 7-OH-MTX may compete with MTX for intracellular transformation to polyglutamate derivatives,[84] a con-version which represents the third major metabolic pathway for MTX.

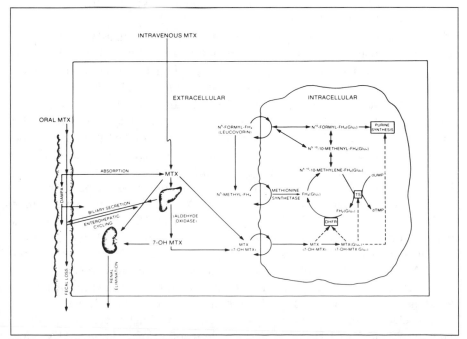

Figure 29-2. *Summary of MTX distribution, metabolism, excretion, and mechanisms of action, and leucovorin rescue. DHFR denotes dihydrofolate reductase, TS thymidylate synthetase, FH_4 tetrahydrofolate, FH_2 dihydrofolate, Glu glutamyl, dTMP thymidylate, and dUMP dioxyuridyl-ate. Broken lines indicate enzyme inhibition (adapted with permission from reference 158).*

Polyglutamate formation allows for selective retention of folates and antifolate (e.g., MTX) within cells[85–87] and has been shown to be an important determinant of antifolate toxicity and selectivity.[85] Since the initial reports in 1973 of the conversion of MTX to polyglutamate forms,[88,89] the intracellular formation of MTX polyglutamates has been well established in normal and malignant cells both *in vitro* and *in vivo*.[90–103] These metabolites are formed intracellularly by the enzyme, folyl polyglutamate synthetase (FPGS), which forms polyglutamates of naturally occurring folates.[104] Up to five additional glutamate residues may be added onto the MTX molecule[85,105] by FPGS. The substrate and cofactor specificities of this enzyme have been reported.[104,106] This enzyme will add glutamate residues to the terminal glutamate residue of folates or antifolates such as MTX. The amino acid polymer is formed by gamma carboxyl peptide linkage and is added sequentially. The importance of the MTX polyglutamate derivatives is thought to be due to their enhanced cellular retention. These polyanionic metabolites are not readily extruded from the cell by the carrier-mediated transport system known to operate for MTX and naturally occurring reduced folates. The transport system for MTX establishes an intracellular level of unmetabolized MTX substrate for FPGS to form polyglutamate derivatives. This results in a more prolonged level of antifolate above that of DHFR, which is critical for complete suppression of tetrahydrofolate production[107] and is thus of import for drug action.[108] There is some indication that the lower forms of MTX polyglutamates can be lost from the cell,[98] but it is unclear whether this represents direct loss of the polyglutamate forms or whether there is rapid breakdown by hydrolases with subsequent efflux of MTX monoglutamate.

The polyglutamyl derivatives of MTX are at least as potent as MTX as DHFR inhibitors,[99,109] which further underlines the importance of the selective retention of polyglutamate. The binding affinity of MTX polyglutamates (on-rate or association constant) is comparable to that of the parent drug. However, it has been demonstrated that the higher forms of MTX polyglutamates have a lower dissociation constant from DHFR.[105] In other words, MTX polyglutamates bind initially with the same affinity as MTX. Once the pteridine moiety of the antifolate is bound to the active site of DHFR, the long glutamate homopolymer tail may associate with sites outside the binding site which may result in a longer half-life for dissociation from the target enzyme. In a clinical situation in which malignant cells are exposed to MTX, antifolate accumulates and MTX polyglutamates are formed rapidly as soon as the DHFR binding capacity is exceeded and free MTX is available for FPGS to act on. Since binding affinities of the parent compound and polyglutamates for DHFR are similar, the proportions of free versus enzyme-bound MTX and MTX polyglutamates within the cell are comparable over time.[85,97] As MTX serum concentrations fall (following the termination of antifolate administration), intracellular MTX monoglutamate rapidly leaves the cell. There is selective retention of the polyglutamate forms which become the predominant form bound to DHFR.[85] Thus, the conversion of MTX to MTX-polyglutamates transforms a reversible inhibitor (MTX) into a selectively retained and much less rapidly reversible inhibitor of folate-dependent reactions.

If the retained MTX polyglutamates are produced differentially in malignant versus normal tissues, then the selectivity of this antifolate can be understood and perhaps improved. Several reports have, in fact, indicated that levels of MTX polyglutamates in malignant cells are greater relative to normal cells such as intestinal epithelial cells and bone marrow cells.[110–112] Evidence suggests that it is this differential accumulation of MTX polyglutamates in malignant cells versus the rapidly dividing normal cells which makes MTX an effective anticancer agent and partially accounts for the selectivity of leucovorin rescue. It has been shown that tissues such as intestinal epithelium, which do not accumulate MTX poly-glutamates, have a very active form of hydrolase enzyme which rapidly breaks down polyglutamates to the monoglutamate form.[113] One report[101] has demon-strated that the ability to accumulate polyglutamated methotrexate in lymphoblasts obtained at diagnosis has independent prognostic significance for children with acute lymphocytic leukemia. In a series of 43 children, those whose lymphoblasts accumulated higher levels of polyglutamates had a better five-year disease-free survival (65% versus 22%, P = 0.01). The ability to accumulate polyglutamates may be an inherent characteristic of some lymphoblasts, which results in increased sensitivity to treatment with this drug.

Another element of MTX metabolism relates to the recent finding that 7-OH-MTX can be polyglutamated.[65,80,84,106,114–116] 7-OH-MTX competes with MTX for entry into cells[65,76] and may also compete with the parent compound for the enzyme FPGS. In the chronic myelogenous leukemia cell line K562, selectively retained 7-OH-MTX polyglutamates have been shown to be cytotoxic.[114] Hence, during HDMTX regimens when 7-OH-MTX serum concentrations are in great excess of MTX concentrations, especially after termination of drug administration, the direct cytotoxic action of 7-OH-MTX (mediated through uptake and subsequent polyglutamation), may be an added determinant of MTX cytotoxicity.

Excretion

Renal excretion of unmetabolized drug is the major route of MTX elimina-tion.[28,61,117–120] Human and animal studies have demonstrated that MTX renal clearance involves glomerular filtration, tubular secretion, and tubular reabsorp-tion.[23,32,33,121,122] At low IV dosages, MTX total body clearance correlates with glomerular filtration estimated by creatinine or inulin clearance.[123] At the low steady-state serum concentrations achieved with such dosages (0.2 to 0.4 µmol/L), MTX total body clearance exceeds glomerular filtration rate (inulin clearance) by 6% to 49%[33] suggesting tubular secretion. At higher serum concentrations (2 to 1000 µmol/L), much lower net renal clearances of MTX (≤20 to 50 mL/min/m^2) have been reported.[23,123] These observations are consistent with saturation of renal tubular secretion of MTX at high serum concentrations and are in agreement with the lower net renal clearance of MTX previously observed in patients simulta-neously administered other organic acids such as para-aminohippurate (PAH), sulfonamides, or sodium salicylate.[33] The reduction of MTX renal clearance by PAH or sodium salicylate to values 30% to 35% lower than glomerular filtration (inulin clearance) also suggests extensive renal tubular reabsorption of MTX.[33]

Reabsorption may be saturated at lower concentrations than is tubular secretion resulting in overall nonlinear renal elimination and faster clearance with higher serum concentrations compared to the lower serum concentration range.[124] Based on these observations and the wide range in serum concentrations (0.1 to 1000 μmol/L) achieved with currently used dosages of 5 to 33,600 mg/m^2, renal clearance and total body elimination of MTX may vary extensively even in patients with normal renal function. Other variables which reportedly influence MTX renal clearances include concomitant hydration regimens,[125] urine flow, urine pH,[126] and severe vomiting and diarrhea.[127] However, the importance of these variables is not completely known and may depend on the MTX dosage administered.

Following six-hour IV infusions of high doses of MTX, greater than 40% of the administered dose can be recovered unchanged in urine within six hours and 90% within 24 hours.[20,69,118,128,129] In urinary recovery studies following MTX doses of 1000 mg/m^2 infused over 24 hours, only 62% ± 14% of the dose was recovered as unchanged drug in a 48-hour urine collection.[130] In these patients, renal clearance accounted for 61% ± 17% of the total systemic clearance during the infusion.[31,130] Cumulative 24-hour urinary recovery of lower IV doses of MTX (0.1 to 10 mg/kg) is reported to be 58% to 92% (median, 78%). As stated above, urinary recovery following oral administration is lower and dose dependent reflecting gut metabolism and incomplete absorption.

Serum concentrations of 7-OH-MTX are approximately equimolar to MTX by the end of a 24-hour infusion and decline more slowly postinfusion than MTX. Lankelma et al.[76] demonstrated a substantially longer plasma half-life (nine hours) for 7-OH-MTX compared to the usual half-life for MTX (<4 hours) in a volunteer to whom 7-OH-MTX was administered. This is consistent with lower 7-OH-MTX renal clearances measured in patients given HDMTX (140 to 350 mg/kg).[69]

The time course of MTX disappearance from plasma following high-dose IV infusions is essentially biexponential.[38,39,117,131,132] Mean half-lives for the initial phase have been reported to range from 1.5 to 3.5 hours,[32,117,128] whereas the terminal-phase half-life is about 8 to 15 hours in patients with normal total body clearance. Many of the early studies reporting half-lives were not designed as pharmacokinetic studies, and the reported initial-phase half-lives represent the rate of decline in serum concentrations (during the first 24 hours) and not $t\frac{1}{2}_\alpha$ (ln 2/α). However, Isacoff and co-workers[131] fit a biexponential equation to serum concentrations following 172 high-dose infusions and calculated parameters of a two-compartment model yielding a $t\frac{1}{2}_\alpha$ of 1.8 ± 0.5 hours. These values are similar to those reported by Stoller et al.[117] who also used a biexponential model. No significant differences in kinetic parameters were observed at dosages ranging from 50 to 200 mg/kg.[117] This half-life primarily reflects the renal elimination of MTX and correlates with creatinine clearance in patients with renal dysfunction.[123] Importantly, the terminal-phase half-life of MTX appears to correlate well with toxicity[30] as discussed below. When MTX is given as a rapid IV bolus, triphasic plasma disappearance can be observed with an initial distribution $t\frac{1}{2}_\alpha$ of about 0.75 ± 0.11 hours.[29,32] This early distribution half-life is generally not detected when MTX is given as a longer infusion since distribution essentially occurs during the infusion.

Because of the large amount of MTX excreted in urine (after high doses), urinary concentrations may exceed the 2 mmol/L solubility at pH 5.5. Therefore, hydration and urinary alkalinization have been recommended to prevent MTX precipitation and nephrotoxicity. The use of IV hydration of greater than 100 mL/ m^2/hr does not appear to alter the serum disposition curve of MTX when compared to maintenance IV hydration (40 mL/m^2/hr) given to the same patients.[133] However, we observed[125] a significant difference in the 21-hour and 44-hour MTX plasma concentrations in a group of patients who received two different hydration and alkalinization regimens with 2 gm/m^2 infused IV over two hours. Patients receiving the more vigorous hydration had lower plasma MTX concentrations and a lower incidence of severe toxicity, 6% versus 16%. The maintenance of a relatively alkaline urinary pH (>6.5) (using oral sodium bicarbonate) for 12 hours before and 48 hours after HDMTX reduces the risk of renal toxicity[53] and is currently recommended for all patients.[134,135]

Because of the extensive tissue binding and intracellular retention of MTX and its polyglutamate metabolites, hemodialysis has been of limited usefulness in lowering plasma MTX concentrations in patients with acute renal failure. However, the combination of hemodialysis with charcoal hemoperfusion has been successfully used to manage a patient with severe renal failure following HDMTX administration.[136] Despite a rebound in MTX plasma concentrations following hemodialysis, the persistent use of both combined hemodialysis and hemoperfusion, as well as hemoperfusion alone, significantly reduced plasma MTX concentrations and prevented any MTX-related toxicity in this patient.

Active biliary secretion of MTX probably occurs[23,137] but is a relatively minor excretory pathway. The total amount recovered in the gastrointestinal tract following IV administration is less than 10% of the administered dose.[24,32,138] After IV

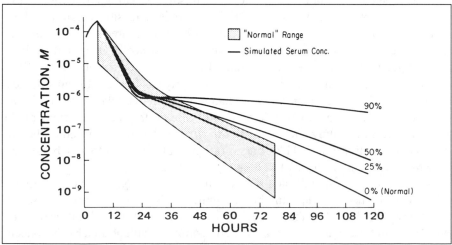

Figure 29-3. Simulation of MTX serum concentrations versus time (solid line) by a physiological pharmacokinetic model using normal gastrointestinal transit rate and transit rate reduced by 25%, 50%, and 90% from normal. Shaded area represents range of serum concentrations measured following 109 doses administered to 27 patients (6- to 24-hour measurements) and 38 doses administered to 21 patients (25- to 78-hour measurements) (reproduced with permission from reference 39).

doses of 30 to 80 mg/m^2, 0.4% to 20% of the MTX dose can be recovered in bile collected over 24 hours.[134,138,139] This relatively minor excretory pathway (<10% fecal excretion) may become clinically important (see Figure 29-3) when impaired (e.g., by GI obstruction)[38,39] due to biliary secretion and subsequent reabsorption of MTX, although studies to assess stereospecific biliary secretion are needed to fully quantitate the extent of enterohepatic cycling of MTX.

The enterohepatic recycling of MTX may be altered by oral administration of activated charcoal.[140,141] Studies in rats[140] have shown that MTX is readily bound to charcoal and subsequently secreted in bile, but the plasma pharmacokinetics of MTX did not appear to be altered. However, human studies[141] have demonstrated significantly lower serum concentrations, beginning 18 hours after a six-hour MTX IV infusion (1 gm/m^2) in patients treated with a single dose of 25 gm of charcoal. Oral administration of activated charcoal may increase elimination of MTX in patients with delayed MTX clearance.

PHARMACODYNAMICS

Clinical and Biochemical Effects

The cytotoxic effects of MTX are primarily the result of its competitive inhibition of intracellular DHFR. The K_i for this inhibition has not been precisely defined, although estimates of 0.0001 μmol/L have been made.[142] Extensive studies by Goldman[107,108] and others have demonstrated that a free intracellular MTX concentration in excess of that required to saturate the tight binding sites on DHFR is necessary for maximal suppression of DNA synthesis. It appears that only a small fraction of uninhibited DHFR is sufficient to maintain reduced folate pools adequate to sustain DNA synthesis,[107] thus necessitating intracellular concentrations of free MTX in excess of DHFR. There is no feasible means by which intracellular MTX concentrations can be routinely measured in target cells in clinical specimens. While the relationship between extracellular and intracellular MTX concentrations has been determined for several experimental tumors[143-146] and for intestinal mucosa,[145] it remains to be clearly established for most tissues. Since extracellular drug is in rapid exchange with intracellular free drug in the sensitive cells, it seems reasonable that extracellular drug concentrations might relate to intracellular drug effects. Studies *in vitro* have also established a relationship between extracellular MTX concentrations and the extent to which intracellular MTX exists in the form of MTX-polyglutamates.[93]

Animal studies have indicated that the inhibition of DNA synthesis in tumor cells, bone marrow, and intestinal epithelium requires the presence of a serum concentration of free MTX that is specific for each tissue.[145] The inhibition of DNA synthesis in mouse bone marrow is virtually complete with plasma MTX concentrations greater than 0.01 μmol/L, whereas intestinal epithelium shows similar inhibition of MTX levels above 0.005 μmol/L. Similar findings have been reported in humans in that resumption of DNA synthesis did not occur until serum concentrations were 0.02 μmol/L or below.[147] Pinedo and Chabner[148] have shown that at MTX concentrations greater than 0.01 μmol/L, the cytotoxic effects are a function of both drug concentration and duration of exposure. Their data demonstrated that exposure to an extracellular concentration of 0.05 μmol/L for 72 hours produces the same effect as exposure to 10 μmol/L for 12 hours. It therefore seems reasonable to assume that extracellular concentrations less than 0.01 μmol/L are not likely to produce pharmacologic or toxicologic effects. Although the absolute threshold appears to be organ dependent and a function of duration of exposure to suprathreshold concentrations, the relation between serum concentrations and pharmacologic effects remains to be precisely defined in human experiments.

In recent years, a relationship between plasma concentrations or total systemic clearance and clinical efficacy has been established for HDMTX in the treatment of ALL.[130,149-152] These studies have not established a concentration-effect profile *per se* but demonstrate that for some patient populations at an increased risk for relapse with ALL, higher plasma MTX concentrations increase the duration of continuous complete remission.

Adverse Effects

Intravenous Methotrexate. Oral or parenteral administration of low-dose MTX ($\leq$50 mg/m^2) generally produces peak serum concentrations of approximately 1 μmol/L. For cancer patients, the dosage of weekly low-dose MTX is often adjusted either up or down in accordance with individual tolerance to maintain total white blood counts in the range of 2000 to 4000/μL.[130] Serum MTX concentrations appear to be of little value for routine monitoring of low-dose MTX therapy other than to assess compliance or malabsorption.

Leucovorin is rarely administered when MTX dosages are less than 100 mg/m^2 although an occasional patient may experience toxicity which is severe enough to require leucovorin administration as a precautionary measure. Conversely, leucovorin administration or some other form of "rescue" is required for MTX dosages in excess of about 100 mg/m^2 to prevent severe toxicity (mucositis, pancytopenia, GI desquamation, renal and hepatic dysfunction), although one study demonstrated that children can often tolerate MTX dosages of 100 mg/m^2 without leucovorin rescue.[153] The relationship between serum MTX concentrations and toxicity is well established for MTX-leucovorin therapy,[38,40,154-160] and provides the basis for pharmacokinetic monitoring of MTX (see Clinical Application of Pharmacokinetic Data).

The classical view of the mechanism by which MTX toxicity is prevented by leucovorin is circumvention of the blocked tetrahydrofolate synthesis produced by MTX inhibition of DHFR. Rescue is accomplished by the transport of reduced folates into cells for utilization in tetrahydrofolate-dependent reactions. The nature of this rescue has been shown in *in vitro* studies to be competitive;[45] thus, extracellular reduced folate concentrations at least equal to extracellular MTX concentrations are required to prevent toxicity. Since the intracellular mechanism of rescue was believed to be noncompetitive (i.e., bypass of the blocked enzyme and repletion of the tetrahydrofolate pools), it was assumed that competition at the cell membrane level for the active transport sites which both MTX and leucovorin utilize was responsible for the competitive nature of rescue. Therefore, high extracellular MTX concentrations could block entry of reduced folates into the cell and prevent effective rescue. The competitive nature of leucovorin rescue is apparent at extracellular concentrations of 0.1 µmol/L for both MTX and leucovorin which is consistent with the K_m values reported by Kamen et al.[43] for both 5-methyltetrahydrofolate (5-CH$_3$-THF) and methotrexate.

It has also been suggested that exogenous leucovorin expands the total reduced folate pool as folylpolyglutamates.[161] Presence of high intracellular folylpolyglutamate concentrations reduces the inhibitory effect of MTX on thymidylate synthesis, resulting in normal thymidylate synthesis and conversion of tetrahydrofolates to dihydrofolates. Polyglutamate forms of dihydrofolates then accumulate to high concentrations and displace a small amount of MTX from sites on DHFR. A low level of free DHFR is sufficient to sustain normal tetrahydrofolate synthesis and prevent cell death. A critical step, therefore, in the protection of normal host tissues is the conversion of exogenously supplied leucovorin to polyglutamate forms and accumulation of total intracellular folates to higher than normal levels.[161]

Other work[162] has suggested that reduced folates which accumulate intracellularly following leucovorin rescue can compete directly with MTX at the level of DHFR and produce a net displacement of MTX from the enzyme. These studies lead us to conclude that while competition between MTX and reduced folates for intracellular transport may be important in some respects, some elements in the competitive nature of rescue may be subcellular. Certainly, at MTX concentrations near or above the K_m for transport, inhibition of leucovorin transport by MTX is important since all the proposed mechanisms for rescue require that leucovorin cross the cell membrane. However, at lower concentrations, where membrane transport is not saturated (thus noncompetitive), the competitive nature of leucovorin rescue may be due to displacement of MTX from DHFR by either dihydrofolate polyglutamates or reduced folates.

Toxicity may develop in patients with high serum MTX concentrations as a result of one or both of the following factors: 1) routine leucovorin rescue ends while cytotoxic MTX concentrations are present in serum, or 2) the usual leucovorin dosage produces reduced folate serum concentrations that are insufficient to prevent toxicity when MTX serum concentrations are high as a result of the competitive nature of leucovorin rescue.

Thus, rescue may be inadequate, allowing toxicity to develop, because leucovorin administration is discontinued too soon in patients who have cytotoxic MTX concentrations for a longer period than usual or because the usual leucovorin dosage produces serum concentrations of reduced folates that are too low to compete effectively with elevated MTX serum concentrations. These problems can be overcome and toxicity prevented by extending the duration of leucovorin administration or by increasing the dosage (and decreasing the dosage interval) of leucovorin, or both. Patients at high risk for MTX toxicity must be identified so that adequate leucovorin rescue can be initiated within 42 to 48 hours of continuous exposure,[163-165] after which the cytotoxic effects may not be reversible. However, excessive leucovorin administration should be avoided in patients with normal

MTX clearance, since both animal[166] and clinical[167] studies have demonstrated that both toxicity and antitumor effects may be prevented by progressive increases in leucovorin dosage.

Following reports[135,168,169] that documented a 6% mortality rate and an overall severe toxicity rate greater than 10% (morbidity plus mortality) in patients on HDMTX, a number of studies[40,154–157,159] were conducted to develop guidelines for monitoring serum MTX concentrations. The guidelines offered by these authors (see Figure 29-4) are remarkably similar considering that MTX dosages, length of infusion, IV hydration, urinary alkalinization, MTX assay methodology, and leucovorin dosage and schedule were not uniform. The optimum interval for measuring serum MTX concentrations and determining the risk of toxicity appears to be between 24 and 48 hours after initiation of MTX administration. Serum concentrations are very high over the first 24 hours, and low-dose leucovorin administration is essentially ineffective while serum MTX concentrations are high. In addition, serum MTX concentrations over the first 24 hours are primarily influenced by the MTX dosage and length of IV infusion. Even using the same MTX regimen, there is substantial interpatient variability in serum concentrations over this interval. It is important to note, however, that some pathologic factors, such as pleural effusion or gastrointestinal tract obstruction, may produce no alteration in serum concentrations or MTX half-life over the first 24 hours but may

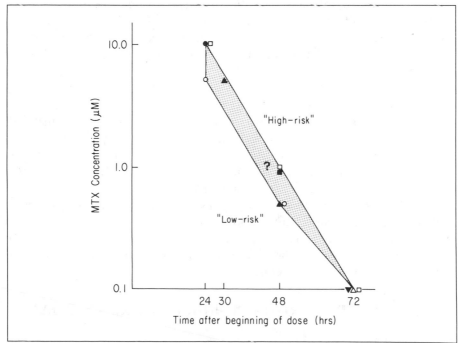

Figure 29-4. *Composite semi-logarithmic plot of serum MTX concentrations which have been proposed to identify patients at "high risk" to develop toxicity from HDMTX if conventional low-dose leucovorin is administered. Data obtained from reports of (▲) Evans,[38] (△) Tattersal,[40] (●) Isacoff,[154] (○) Isacoff,[155] (□) Nirenberg,[156] (■) Stoller,[157] and (▼) Rechnitzer.[159]*

nevertheless result in excessive toxicity due to cytotoxic serum concentrations which are sustained beyond the usual duration of leucovorin rescue (i.e., 72 to 96 hours).

By 24 to 48 hours, serum concentrations are generally comparable for patients receiving different dosages of MTX with different IV infusion rates. Serum concentrations are usually less than 10 µmol/L and 1 µmol/L at 24 hours and 48 hours, respectively. This is the interval in which intervention with high-dose leucovorin is most beneficial for high-risk patients, since serum concentrations of total reduced folates may be achieved which effectively compete with MTX to reduce toxicity. In addition, adequate leucovorin administration must be initiated within the first 42 to 48 hours of MTX exposure to prevent serious toxicity, as described above. Guidelines for adjusting leucovorin rescue are described below in the clinical applications section.

Intrathecal Methotrexate. Three general types of clinical manifestations of neurotoxicity have been reported following the use of IT MTX: meningeal irritation, transient or permanent paresis, and encephalopathy. The signs, symptoms, and proposed pathogenesis of each have been reviewed elsewhere in detail.[170] A number of potential mechanisms by which IT MTX may cause neurotoxicity have been proposed and include high concentrations of MTX in CSF, toxic preservatives in IT MTX solutions, and nonphysiological IT MTX solutions. Moreover, Bleyer and co-workers[171,172] have reported that CSF MTX concentrations are significantly higher in patients who develop neurotoxicity than in those who do not. In Bleyer's initial report,[171] mean CSF MTX concentrations were 13.8 times higher in five neurotoxic patients than in 20 asymptomatic patients at 48 hours after a dose. Patients developing neurotoxicity were significantly older than nontoxic patients, and four or five toxic patients had overt meningeal leukemia at the time of therapy. In a study[172] of 47 patients, CSF MTX concentrations measured from 48 to 192 hours post-dose were consistently higher in ten toxic patients than in nontoxic patients. This study also demonstrated that CSF MTX concentrations correlated directly with age (over the range of 3 to 26 years) when all patients were given the standard dosage of 12 mg/m^2 per dose. This is consistent with the fact that CSF volume increases very little after the age of three despite a continual increase in body surface area.[172] One study[173] suggests that elevated CSF MTX concentrations, following HDMTX infusions, may correlate with the presence or subsequent development of CNS leukemia in children with ALL. It has been proposed that this is due to delayed MTX outflow from the CSF due to meningeal leukemia. The clinical utility of monitoring CSF MTX concentrations remains to be clearly defined.

CLINICAL APPLICATION OF PHARMACOKINETIC DATA

Intrathecal Methotrexate

As shown in Figure 29-5, the data by Bleyer[172] indicate that MTX concentrations measured in lumbar CSF from two to eight days after an IT dose may correlate with both CNS response and toxicity. The inherent difficulties in obtaining CSF samples limit the usefulness of this approach to monitoring IT MTX therapy. We currently use CSF MTX concentrations only in patients who are at increased risk for neurotoxicity because of acute meningeal disease or in patients who exhibit signs or symptoms of MTX neurotoxicity in a temporal relationship to IT MTX therapy. In patients receiving several doses of IT MTX, CSF MTX concentrations obtained in the process of IT administration may be useful in adjusting the interval between subsequent IT doses.[174]

Following IT MTX administration, potentially cytotoxic serum concentrations of MTX (0.1 µmol/L) may result and persist for 24 to 48 hours.[48] This may result in systemic effects of MTX following IT administration and has led some clinicians to administer low doses of leucovorin to prevent any systemic effect. However, when leucovorin is given, the active metabolite (5-CH$_3$-THF) readily distributes into the CSF. Therefore, when leucovorin is given following IT MTX, its administration is usually delayed for 24 to 36 hours after the IT dose to minimize any potential compromise in IT therapy. Since one cannot be certain that leucovorin will not compromise the CNS effects of IT MTX, it is best to completely

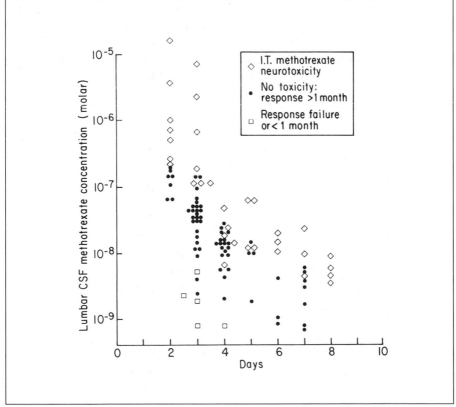

Figure 29-5. *CSF-antifolate concentration after intrathecal MTX (12 mg/m² of BSA). ◊ = patients with neurotoxic reactions to intrathecal MTX, □ = patients who failed to achieve CNS remission or who had a meningeal relapse within one month after therapy, and ● = patients who had neither neurotoxic reactions nor early CNS relapse (reprinted with permission from reference 172).*

avoid the administration of leucovorin after IT MTX. However, patients with renal dysfunction and others demonstrating systemic toxicity after IT MTX may require low-dose leucovorin rescue (i.e., 5 to 10 mg/m² every 6 to 12 hours over 24 hours).[231]

Intravenous Methotrexate

Prospective serum concentration monitoring of HDMTX has become a well-accepted method of identifying patients at high risk for MTX toxicity. At this time, it is the only routine application of pharmacokinetics in the clinical use of antineoplastic drugs, although the body of knowledge related to anticancer drug pharmacodynamics has expanded greatly in the last five years.[175] We have demonstrated that systemic MTX clearance has a statistically significant influence on the risk of early relapse following one treatment protocol for childhood ALL (see Figure 29-6).[130,149] In this study, children with median steady-state plasma MTX concentrations greater than 16 µmol/L following 1000 mg/m² administered IV over 24 hours had a significantly reduced risk of early relapse, compared to children with median concentrations less than 16 µmol/L. In addition, there was no significant difference between children with lower concentrations and historical control patients who had received almost identical therapy but did not receive HDMTX.[149] Other reports[176] have also reported a relationship between MTX serum concentrations and the clinical response to HDMTX therapy. A clear relationship between serum MTX concentration and therapeutic efficacy has been difficult to establish. This is not surprising in view of the multitude of other factors (e.g.,

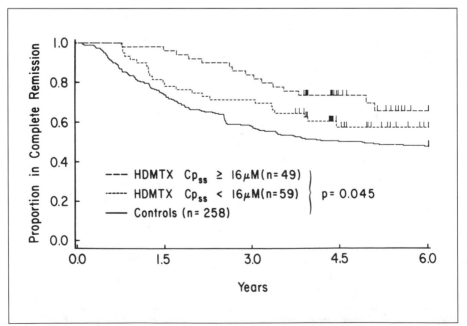

Figure 29-6. *Kaplan-Meier curves of complete remission for patients with median MTX steady-state plasma concentrations ≥16 µM (– – –), <16 µM (- - - -), and a control group that received no HDMTX (——) (adapted with permission from reference 150).*

membrane transport, DHFR levels, MTX binding affinity, folylpolyglutamate synthetase levels, tissue distribution of MTX, previous or concurrent anticancer therapy) which may also influence MTX's cytotoxicity and the overall efficacy of a treatment regimen.

There is a wealth of data demonstrating that serum concentration monitoring has had a significant impact on HDMTX-related toxicity and mortality.[38,157] At our institution, no HDMTX-induced deaths or serious toxicity have occurred since prospective pharmacokinetic monitoring was initiated in 1976, a period in which well over 3000 courses of HDMTX have been administered to over 300 patients.[38,131,149,177] This is in contrast to the overall 5% to 6% mortality rate reported nationally and at our institution prior to initiation of prospective serum concentration monitoring.[135,168] Greater attention to adequate hydration and urinary alkalinization may have also contributed to the decreased mortality during this period. Nevertheless, the contribution of pharmacokinetic monitoring has been important since delayed MTX clearance may occur in patients who have none of the clinical high-risk features, such as dehydration, aciduria, renal dysfunction, pleural effusion, ascites, or gastrointestinal tract obstruction.[135] It is this group of patients that benefits most from routine serum concentration monitoring.

The published criteria for identifying high-risk patients have been summarized above (see Pharmacodynamics: Adverse Effects). The exact criteria used may vary from one institution or investigator to another, but all monitoring strategies should have the following in common: 1) determination of MTX serum concentration at selected times (24, 48, or 72 hours) so that these concentrations can be related to the leucovorin dose being administered, and 2) an assessment of the rate of decline of MTX serum concentrations in order to determine how long leucovorin rescue should be continued. It is important that high-risk patients be identified within 48 hours after initiation of MTX administration since MTX toxicity may not be reversible if **adequate** leucovorin rescue is delayed for more than 42 to 48 hours after initiating MTX therapy. The criteria used at St. Jude Children's Research Hospital for three different dosages and administration schedules are summarized in Table 29-1. For dosages of 1 to 2 gm/m², we rely on a single serum concentration measured 42 to 48 hours after initiating therapy. For higher dosages (>5 gm/m²) we recommend measurement of MTX half-life over the first 24 hours postinfusion

Table 29-1. *High-Risk Concentrations for Three HDMTX Regimens Used at St. Jude Children's Research Hospital*

Regimen	Time from beginning of infusion (hr)	High-risk MTX concentration
1000 mg/m²–2000 mg/m² by IV bolus and 800 mg/m² as 24-hour IV infusion	42	>0.5 µmol/L
1500 mg/m²–2000 mg/m² by IV 1-hour and 1300 mg/m² as 23-hour IV infusion	42	>1.0 µmol/L
12,000 mg/m² as a 4-hour infusion	24	>10.0 µmol/L
	28	>5.0 µmol/L
	48	>1.0 µmol/L
	72	>0.2 µmol/L

as well as a serum concentration measurement at 48 hours. Patients with a half-life for decline in MTX serum concentrations that exceeds 3.5 hours during the first 24 hours postinfusion, or those individuals with a serum concentration exceeding 5 μmol/L at 28 hours after initiating therapy are considered at high risk for toxicity. With this approach, high-risk patients are identified early and intervention with escalated leucovorin dosages is initiated if required.

In addition to these pharmacokinetic risk criteria, an assessment of the patient for **clinical** risk features is critical. Some factors, such as pleural effusion, ascites, gastrointestinal tract obstruction, or other "third space" may not alter MTX disposition over the first 24 to 48 hours postinfusion (see Figures 29-3 and 29-7). These conditions tend to increase the terminal MTX half-life above the usual 8 to 15 hours, however, and may result in potentially cytotoxic serum concentrations (>0.05 μmol/L) for several days to weeks,[39,41] long after conventional leucovorin rescue is discontinued. We *a priori* consider such patients at high risk and monitor serum concentrations until MTX concentrations are less than 0.05 μmol/L; appropriate leucovorin dosage adjustments are made as necessary (see below).

Patients who have previously received cisplatin may also be at higher risk for toxicity,[177,178] particularly if they have received more than 300 mg/m^2 of cisplatin. This presumably is due to the cumulative renal toxicity of cisplatin. Delayed clearance may occur in patients with normal or only slightly elevated serum creatinine concentrations. However, these patients, as well as those with other causes of renal insufficiency, usually exhibit delayed MTX clearance within the first 24 hours postinfusion and therefore are identified by the pharmacokinetic risk criteria.

We have observed that children with Down's syndrome have altered pharmacokinetic disposition of MTX[179] as well as increased incidence of toxicity despite higher dosages and prolonged administration of leucovorin. A group of five patients with Down's syndrome and ALL had significantly higher plasma MTX concentrations and a higher incidence of high-risk courses than a matched control group of 15 ALL patients who did not have Down's syndrome. Down's syndrome patients must be treated cautiously with high-dose methotrexate and monitored carefully for hematologic and gastrointestinal toxicity.

The dosage of leucovorin usually needs to be increased, as well as continued for a longer duration, in patients with delayed MTX clearance and elevated serum MTX concentrations. As described in detail by Pinedo,[45] MTX and leucovorin share the same intracellular transport mechanisms. At high (>5 μmol/L) MTX serum concentrations, membrane transport of leucovorin may be inhibited because of competition with MTX, preventing effective rescue. At lower concentrations, transport inhibition is probably not important,[161] but other mechanisms result in competition between MTX and leucovorin, as described above. The net effect is that equimolar concentrations of total reduced folates and MTX are required to reverse MTX effects at concentrations less than 0.1 μmol/L. For MTX concentrations of 10 μmol/L, reduced folate concentrations of approximately 1000 μmol/L are required to prevent MTX toxicity. Therefore, the leucovorin dosage must be increased according to the serum MTX concentration. However, studies *in vitro* indicate that the toxic effects of 100 μmol/L MTX cannot be reversed by

1000 µmol/L reduced folate[45] suggesting the potential need for hemodialysis or hemoperfusion to lower persistent MTX serum concentrations greater than 100 µmol/L.[136]

In addition to the clinical pharmacokinetic studies of leucovorin published earlier,[180–188] a number of studies[189–194] focusing on the pharmacokinetics of the separate 6R- and 6S-diastereoisomers of leucovorin have been published since the last edition of this text. These studies have confirmed that orally administered leucovorin is rapidly and completely absorbed up to a dosage of about 50 mg in adults;[180,182–184,187,188] at higher doses it is more erratically and incompletely absorbed. The 6S-isomer of leucovorin (or l-leucovorin, the biologically active diastereoisomer) is rapidly converted to 5-CH$_3$-THF (which is also a biologically active reduced folate capable of reversing MTX toxicity) following oral leuco-

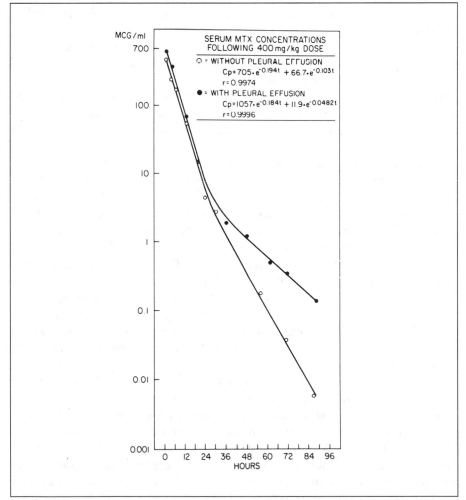

Figure 29-7. MTX serum concentrations in a 12-year-old boy with osteosarcoma, treated with 400 mg/kg both with and without a pleural effusion. MTX half-lives over the first 24 hours with and without the pleural effusion were 3.8 and 3.6 hours, respectively. Terminal serum half-lives were 14.4 and 6.7 hours, respectively (reproduced with permission from reference 41).

vorin administration and, to a lesser extent, after parenteral administration. The serum half-life of the 5-CH$_3$-THF is 2.2 to 3.8 hours.[182–184,188] The 6R-isomer (or d-leucovorin) is absorbed four to five times more slowly than the 6S-isomer, and the oral absorption process is saturable for both diastereoisomers.[188] The 6R-isomer is much more slowly eliminated with a plasma half-life of about six hours. This is probably due to much greater protein binding for 6R-leucovorin[189] with a mean free fraction of about 0.1 for this isomer compared to about 0.75 for 6S-leucovorin. The free fraction for the biologically active metabolite 5-CH$_3$-THF is about 0.5. Frequent doses of the racemic mixture could therefore result in accumulation of high concentrations of the 6R-isomer in plasma relative to those of the 6S-isomer. However, a recent study[190] suggests that concentrations of 6R-leucovorin up to 1 mmol/L do not interfere with the activity of 6S-leucovorin in lymphoblasts *in vitro*. These authors conclude that high plasma concentrations of 6R-leucovorin or 6R-5-CH$_3$-THF are unlikely to have significant clinical consequences.

At dosages of up to 50 mg, peak serum concentrations of active total reduced folates (6S-leucovorin plus 6S-5-CH$_3$-THF) are proportional to dose. Doses of 15 mg orally result in peak concentrations of about 0.5 µmol/L,[182,184] whereas the same dose given IM produces peak concentrations of about 2 µmol/L. Total reduced folate AUC is equivalent for IM or oral (liquid or tablet) doses of 20 mg, although the proportion converted to 5-CH$_3$-THF is much greater for the oral forms.[185]

Oral absorption appears to be saturated at doses of 50 mg[188] resulting in a decreased bioavailability of 6S-leucovorin from 75% at 50 mg to 37% at 100 mg. Therefore, doses greater than 50 mg ($\approx$30 mg/m^2) probably should be administered parenterally. However, since oral absorption is complete after about two hours,[188] frequent administration of small oral doses could be used to sustain serum concentrations of reduced folates.

Parenteral administration of larger doses ($\approx$100 mg/m^2) appears to produce proportional increases in serum reduced folate concentrations. A dose of 100 mg/m^2 given IV over 4.25 hours yielded steady-state reduced folate concentrations of about 4 µmol/L.[186] Therefore, assuming no change in the distribution of reduced folates at higher dosages, one would expect dosages of 1 gm/m^2 to yield peak reduced folate concentrations of about 100 µmol/L when administered as a short IV infusion.

Since the half-life of both active reduced folates is short (less than four hours), frequent administration (every two to three hours) or continuous IV infusion is necessary to maintain high serum concentrations in patients at high risk for MTX toxicity. Leucovorin administration should be continued, with progressive dosage decreases as the serum MTX concentration decreases, until the MTX concentration is less than 0.05 µmol/L. It is important to reserve high-dose leucovorin for only high-risk patients since progressive increases in leucovorin dosage may compromise the antitumor effect.[166,167] Table 29-2 summarizes our leucovorin dosage recommendations for patients at high risk for toxicity based on measured MTX serum concentrations and the length of time after initiation of MTX administration.

Currently, one pharmaceutical firm is conducting clinical tests of a single diastereoisomer product, 6S-leucovorin. The dosage administered is half of the racemic mixture, and clinical efficacy studies, as well as pharmacokinetic studies, are ongoing to determine the role and potential advantages of this product over currently marketed forms of racemic leucovorin. Administration of the single diastereoisomer would eliminate concerns about potential interaction and competition between the diastereoisomers.

The flow chart shown in Figure 29-8 summarizes our recommended comprehensive approach for monitoring high-dose MTX therapy.

ANALYTICAL METHODS

There are several methods by which MTX can be quantitated in biological fluids. These methods include radioimmune assay, fluorescence polarization immunoassay, competitive protein binding assay, radioenzymatic assay, enzyme immunoassay, enzyme inhibition assay, and high performance liquid chromatography with either UV or fluorescence detection. However, these assays differ with regard to specificity, sensitivity, length of procedure, sample preparation, cost, and ability to detect metabolites. No procedure is clearly superior in all respects (see Table 29-3), and the relative advantages and disadvantages of each are briefly reviewed.

Fluorescence Polarization Immunoassay (TDx)

Probably the most widely used clinical method for measuring MTX serum concentrations is fluorescence polarization immunoassay (FPIA), marketed as TDx by Abbott Laboratories, Diagnostics Division. The assay is based on the same

Table 29-2. *General Guidelines for Modification of Leucovorin Dosage Following HDMTX[d]*

MTX serum concentration ≥42 hr from beginning of infusion	Desired TRF Conc[a,b]	Approximate leucovorin dose required[c]
20–50 µmol/L	≈ 200–500 µmol/L	500 mg/m^2 IV Q 6 hr
10–20 µmol/L	≈ 100–200 µmol/L	200 mg/m^2 IV Q 6 hr
5–10 µmol/L	≈ 50–100 µmol/L	100 mg/m^2 IV Q 6 hr
1–5 µmol/L	≈ 5–10 µmol/L	30 mg/m^2 IV or PO Q 6 hr
0.6–1 µmol/L	≈ 0.6–1 µmol/L	15 mg/m^2 PO Q 6 hr
0.1–0.5 µmol/L	≈ 0.1–0.5 µmol/L	15 mg/m^2 PO Q 12 hr
0.05–0.1 µmol/L	≈ 0.05–0.1 µmol/L	5–10 mg/m^2 Q 12 hr

[a] Total reduced folates (active) = 1-formyl tetrahydrofolate and 5-methyl-tetrahydrofolate.
[b] Based on *in vitro* data from reference 45.
[c] Based on data from references 108–194.
   MTX concentrations should be monitored and leucovorin administration should be continued in "high-risk" patients until serum MTX concentrations are <0.05 µmol/L. Leucovorin dosages may be reduced, as indicated, as MTX serum concentrations decrease.
[d] To be applied only to "high-risk" patients as defined by critera in Table 29-1.

principles and procedure as other TDx assays for aminoglycosides, anticonvulsants, theophylline, vancomycin, antiarrhythmics, and digoxin.[195–197] Once patient samples, controls, cuvettes, and the reagent pack are placed in the instrument, it is totally automated. Required sample volume is 50 to 60 µL. The standard curve is determined from calibrators ranging in concentration from 0.05 to 1 µmol/L.

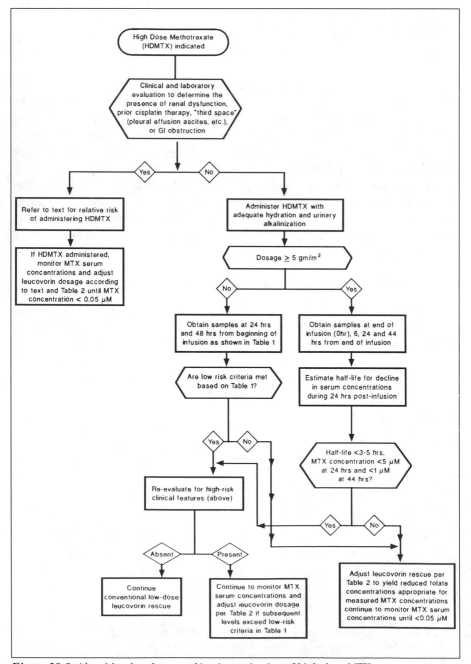

Figure 29-8. *Algorithm for pharmacokinetic monitoring of high-dose MTX.*

Table 29–3. Comparison of Relative Advantages and Disadvantages of the Various Methotrexate Assay Methods[e]

Analytical method[a]	Specificity for methotrexate	Limit of sensitivity	Metabolite analysis	Assayable samples				Minimum sample volume required[b]	Speed		Analysis costs[b]		Specialized operator training[c]	Preference & rank[d]			Comments
				Plasma/serum	Urine	Saliva	CSF		1–10 samples	10–100 samples	Estimated reagent and tech. cost per assay	Initial equipment costs		Small service	Large service	Research	
HPLC	1	0.1 µmol/L 0.05 µmol/L	Yes	Yes	Yes	Yes	Yes	1 mL for .01 µmol	30 min/sample	30 min/sample	3	3	5	4	3	1	UV Detection
EIA	3	0.05 µmol/L	No	Yes	Yes	?	Yes	50 µL	5 min	1–2 min/sample	4	3	2.5	2	3	4	Syva Co
RIA	3	0.01 µmol/L	No	Yes	Yes	Yes	Yes	100 µL	2 hr	2 hr	4	3	3	3	3	4	Diagnostic Biochemistry
REA	2	0.01 µmol/L	No	Yes	Yes	Yes	Yes	300 µL	2 hr	2 hr	4	3	3.5	3	3	3	New England Enzyme
ENZYME	2–3	0.02 µmol/L	No	Yes	?	?	Yes	20–50 µL	5 min	1–2 min/sample	4	3	4	4	3	3	
FPA	3	0.01 µmol/L	No	Yes	Yes	?	Yes	50 µL	10–20 min	1–2 min/sample	4	3	2	2	2	4	Abbott Diagnostics

[a] HPLC = High performance liquid chromatography; EIA = Enzyme immunoassay; RIA = Radioimmunoassay; REA = Radioenzymatic assay; ENZYME = Enzyme inhibition; FPA = Fluorescence polarization assay.

[b] 1 = Least expensive.

[c] 1 = Least training.

[d] 1 = Preferred method.

[e] Arbitrary Rating Scale of 1 (Excellent) to 5 (Poor).

We have established the lowest measurable concentration for our laboratory to be 0.05 μmol/L. Two automated dilution procedures are included in the microprocessor which controls the instrument. The first is used when the expected concentration of the sample is unknown to the operator. The instrument performs these serial tenfold dilutions and performs assays on all four specimens. This procedure can determine the concentration of the sample if it falls anywhere in the range of 0.05 to 1000 μmol/L. The second automated procedure is the interactive dilution protocol. This procedure allows the operator to specify into which concentration range the unknown is expected to fall, based on the drug dosage, clinical protocol, time of sample collection, and previous experience. This prevents wastage of reagents if the proper concentration range is selected.

Assay precision is good, with both within-run and between-run coefficients of variation less than 10% of all concentrations and less than 5% of concentrations other than the extremes (0.07 and 500 μmol/L). Accuracy, determined by assay of spiked serum samples, ranges from 93% to 100%. The only compounds producing significant cross-reactivity (>1%) in specificity studies were the MTX metabolites, 7-OH-MTX (1.5%) and 4-amino-4-deoxy-N^{10}-methylpteroic acid (DAMPA) (36%), and the MTX analog, aminopterin (4.6%).

Each 100-assay reagent kit will yield approximately 75 results with routine clinical use. Samples need not be run in duplicate, and calibration curve stability is very good (greater than two weeks). Control sera with MTX concentrations of 0.07, 0.40, 0.8, 5, 50, and 500 μmol/L are available from the manufacturer.

Enzyme Immunoassay (EMIT)

The homogeneous enzyme immunoassay for MTX[198] is based on the same principles and procedures as other EMIT assays for anticonvulsants, theophylline, lidocaine, and gentamicin. The reagents are available in kit form from Syva Corporation, Palo Alto, CA. Precise timing and pipetting are facilitated by an interfaced timer-printer and an automated pipetter diluter. The assay requires only 50 μL of sample and can detect concentrations as low as 0.1 μmol/L without modification of the standard procedures. The coefficient of variation for within-run and between-run precision is about 5%. The procedure is rapid, with a "turnaround" time of 5 to 30 minutes. The specificity of this method appears to be comparable to that of the radioimmune assay (Diagnostic Biochemistry, San Diego, CA) and the radioenzymatic assay (New England Enzyme Center, Boston, MA) with regard to interference by the 7-OH metabolite.[62] Unpublished observations suggest that the DAMPA metabolite may cross-react with the RIA (≈100%) and EMIT (≈100%) procedures significantly more than with the radioenzymatic assay (≈20%). However, a comparative study[199] evaluating results of clinical serum samples obtained within 24 hours after high-dose six-hour infusions of MTX demonstrated no significant difference using EMIT, REA, RIA, and HPLC. The advantages of this method are the rapid turnaround time, the low cost and versatility of necessary equipment, the stability of the standard curve and reagents, and the small volume of patient sample required. The major limitation at present is the inability to detect MTX concentrations less than 0.1 μmol/L. However, precise manipulation of the initial dilution techniques has permitted accurate and reproducible quantitation of concentrations as low as 0.03 µmol/L in our laboratory, and significant interference with DAMPA metabolites apparently does not occur within 24 hours following HDMTX administration. The accuracy of this assay and RIA for measuring low concentrations following IV or oral administration remains to be defined. Each 100-tube kit will yield 40 to 50 results (in duplicate) with routine clinical use.

Radioenzymatic Assay

This assay, previously described in detail by Meyers et al.,[200] employs competitive binding of unlabeled and[125] I-labeled MTX to the enzyme DHFR derived from *Lactobacillus casei*. The assay is commercially available in kit form from New England Enzyme Center (Boston, MA) and requires a gamma counter as the major equipment investment. The assay requires 300 µL of patient serum, two to four hours to complete, and precise manual timing and pipetting. The enzyme and reagents have a shelf-life of 30 to 60 days, and a new standard curve must be performed daily. The advantage of this method is that it can quantitate as little as 0.01 µmol/L of MTX. By using DHFR as the binding protein, any affinity of the MTX metabolites would be proportional to their relative activity against the target enzyme. The aminopteroic acid metabolite does not substantially interfere with the assay.[62] Trimethoprim does interfere with this assay, yielding spuriously high results for MTX. Each 100-tube kit will yield 20 to 40 results (in duplicate) with routine use.

Radioimmune Assay

A radioimmune assay utilizing[125] I-MTX as the radioactive hapten is commercially available from Diagnostic Biochemistry, Inc. (San Diego, CA). Like the radioenzymatic assay described above, this assay requires a gamma counter and precise timing and pipetting. The procedure requires 200 µL of patient serum to assay in duplicate and approximately two to three hours for completion. The commercially available kit has a shelf life of 30 to 60 days, and a new standard curve must be run daily. There is apparently more cross-reactivity with MTX metabolites (i.e., DAMPA, 7-OH-MTX) for this assay than for the radioenzymatic method.[62] The difference between results by this method and the other methods is probably not of any clinical significance when high concentrations are being measured following HDMTX.[199] However, significant interference may occur when low (0.01 to 0.1 µmol/L) concentrations are being measured at later times after high-dose therapy, or after oral administration, when metabolite concentrations may approach or exceed concentrations of the parent compound. Each 100-tube kit will yield 20 to 40 results (in duplicate) with routine clinical use.

High-Performance Liquid Chromatography (HPLC)

Several procedures for quantitating MTX and its metabolites in biological fluids by HPLC have been published.[201–204] The methods of Watson et al.[201] and

Wisnicki et al.[203] utilize an ultraviolet detector at 315 nm and 254 nm, respectively. The reported sensitivity for both MTX and 7-OH-MTX is 0.1 µmol/L. The method of Watson et al.[201] utilizes a strong anion exchange column for separation, while the Wisnicki method[203] uses a µBondapak C_{18} reverse-phase column for separation of urine samples, and a strong anion exchange column for aqueous solutions. The total retention time for all compounds was about 12 minutes for the method of Watson et al.[201] Plasma samples must also be extracted prior to analysis. The method of Watson appears to be useful for analysis of patient serum, while the method of Wisnicki was evaluated only for analysis of MTX solutions and urine. Nelson and co-workers[202] have reported on an HPLC procedure which utilizes a fluorescence detector to quantitate MTX in human plasma. This procedure requires oxidation of MTX to a fluorescent product by a five-minute incubation with potassium permanganate.

Cairnes and Evans[204] developed a HPLC-UV assay which separates and quantitates MTX, 7-OH-MTX, and DAMPA in serum, plasma urine, and cerebrospinal fluid. This assay is sensitive to a concentration of 0.1 µmol/L in serum or plasma, and the coefficient of variation for MTX is 9.7% at a concentration of 5 µmol/L.

Enzyme Inhibition Assay

The enzyme inhibition assay as described by Falk et al.[205] is based on inhibition by MTX of the enzyme DHFR derived from *Lactobacillus casei*. The change in absorbance of a mixture of NADPH, DHFR, and standards or unknowns is monitored over 120 seconds with a microsample spectrophotometer at 340 nm. The change in absorbance decreases linearly over the concentration range of 0.02 to 0.3 µmol/L. Within-run variability is reported to have a CV of 5%, and day-to-day variation is approximately 18%. Disadvantages of this assay are that it is not commercially available in kit form, the reaction mixture (NADPH, DHFR) must be freshly prepared each day, and other inhibitors of bacterial DHFR (trimethoprim) may interfere with the assay. Most of the reagents needed for this assay, including NADPH and DHFR, are commercially available.

Miscellaneous Assay Procedures

Several other methods for quantitating MTX in biological fluids have been published but are rarely used. These include fluorimetric,[206] microbiological,[207] and direct ligand-binding[208] methods.

PROSPECTUS

MTX has been in clinical use for over 30 years, but several aspects of its basic and clinical pharmacology are still under intense investigation and remain to be fully elucidated. Studies characterizing the formation of polyglutamates of MTX have altered our view of its cellular disposition and mechanisms of cytotoxicity. Recent work cloning and characterizing a low affinity receptor for membrane transport of MTX and folates has provided new insights to the cellular disposition of low-dose MTX. Although our understanding of the intracellular metabolism of folates and antifolates is incomplete, it is clear that these processes play an important and complex role in the pharmacodynamic action of MTX. This area remains exciting and fertile for future research.

Serum concentration monitoring has been well established for identifying patients at high risk for toxicity from HDMTX, but the relationship between serum concentrations and clinical response has not been conclusively established. Recent work by our laboratory and others has established a link between MTX pharmacokinetics and length of complete remission for children with ALL. A prospective, randomized trial is currently ongoing to assess the clinical importance of individualized dosages of HDMTX in treating ALL.

Leucovorin rescue has permitted the clinical use of a very wide range of MTX dosages and administration techniques. MTX dosages of more than 36 gm/m^2 have been used clinically in attempts to extend the spectrum of activity of MTX. It is unlikely that still higher dosages will be routinely used, simply because of the expenses and technical difficulties involved, and because dosages of 36 gm/m^2 do not appear to yield improvements in the MTX response rate observed with lower dosages (i.e., 5 to 8 gm/m^2). However, studies are underway to define more clearly the clinical activity and role of HDMTX and to identify patient populations and disease states that are most likely to benefit from HDMTX. Work with HDMTX to prevent and treat CNS relapses in ALL is likely to be extended to other CNS neoplasms, and HDMTX will most likely continue to be a fundamental component of adjuvant chemotherapy for osteosarcoma.

Studies are needed to more precisely define the optimal dosage, schedule, route, and duration of leucovorin administration following HDMTX. Current approaches are essentially empirical with an underlying philosophy of "use the least amount of leucovorin needed to prevent host toxicity." Development of more precise guidelines for determining the optimal approach to leucovorin rescue has been limited by the paucity of data on the clinical and cellular pharmacokinetics of leucovorin isomers and metabolites and by the incompletely defined mechanism(s) of leucovorin rescue. This clearly represents an area of research which could lead to substantial improvements in the clinical use of HDMTX with leucovorin rescue.

The recent development of chiral HPLC assays for quantitating the two isomers and the active 5-CH$_3$-THF metabolite[209,210] provide the tools needed to better characterize the pharmacokinetics and pharmacodynamics of leucovorin. The formulation of 6S-leucovorin product for clinical use is also providing a new tool for refining the process of leucovorin rescue.

Finally, it is noteworthy that the number and scope of clinical pharmacodynamic studies of anticancer drugs is rapidly expanding. As summarized in Table 29-4, there have now been over 25 published studies of the clinical pharmacodynamics of 13 different anticancer drugs establishing relationships between drug disposition and either toxicity or efficacy, or both. It is hoped that such studies will continue to expand in the coming years such that separate chapters on other anticancer drugs will be warranted in future editions of this text.

Table 29-4. Summary of Selected Clinical Pharmacodynamic Studies with Anticancer Drugs[b]

Drug	Type of study[a]	Pharmacokinetic parameter	Drug effect(s) measured	Pharmacodynamic relationship	References
Amsacrine (AMSA)	6 (of 19) adults with disseminated cancer given 30 or 40 mg/m²	CLs of ^{14}C-AMSA	Lowest measured granulocyte or platelet count	Lower CLs associated with lowest granulocyte count	211
Carboplatin	Adults with refractory tumors and renal dysfunction (n = 22)	Plasma AUC	Change in platelet count	Higher AUC associated with greater % drop in platelet count	212
	Adults with plasma AUC refractory tumors (n = 23)	Plasma AUC	Change in platelet count	Prospective validation of above relation between AUC and change in platelet count	213
Cisplatin	40 adults with various cancers given 80 mg/m²	Total plasma platinum concentration	>30% ↑ in serum creatinine or >30% ↓ in CL_{cr}	Higher C at 12 and 24 hr associated with nephrotoxicity	214
Cytosine arabinoside (ARA-C)	Adults with ANLL (n = 28)	4h Retention of ARA-CTP in leukemic blasts (after *in vitro* incubation)	Complete remission (CR)	Greater cellular retention of ARA-CTP associated with higher % achieving CR and a longer duration of CR	215, 216
Etoposide	Adults with refractory cancer (n = 18)	Steady-state plasma concentration (C_{SS})	Surviving fraction of WBCs	Lower surviving fraction of WBCs with higher Css	217
	Adults with solid tumors receiving etoposide and cisplatin	Plasma total AUC and unbound AUC	Change in WBC and platelet counts	Higher unbound AUC associated with greater ↓ in WBC count	232
5-Fluorouracil	Adults with liver metastases from colorectal cancer (n = 9)	Plasma AUC	Change in platelet and WBC count	Higher AUC associated with ↓ platelet and WBC count	218
	(n = 42)	Total cycle plasma AUC	Probability of toxicity (mucositis, diarrhea, leucopenia, or anemia)	AUC for cycle >30 mg/L/hr associated with toxicity	219
	(n = 6)	Plasma AUC corrected for dose	Hepatic tumor mass	↓ AUC associated with ↑ in hepatic metastases	220
	Colorectal cancer (n = 24)	CL and Css	Change in WBC count	Leucopenia more frequent with 120h C >1.5 μmol/L or with low clearance	221

Drug	Population	PK parameter	Effect	Correlation	Ref
Hexamethylene-bisacetamide	Adults with refractory solid tumors (n = 20)	Plasma AUC	Change in platelet count	Higher AUC associated with a greater % ↓ in platelet count	222
Menogaril	Patients with refractory malignancies (n = 24)	Plasma AUC	Change in WBC and neutrophil count	Higher AUC associated with greater % ↓ in WBC or absolute neutrophil counts	223
	Adults with liver dysfunction (n = 23)	Plasma AUC	Change in WBC and neutrophil count	Higher AUC associated with greater % ↓ in WBC and neutrophil count	224
Mercaptopurine (MP)	Children with ALL (n = 22, n = 19, and n = 120)	Red cell concentration of MP metabolite (6TG nucleotide)	Absolute neutrophil count 14 days post-dose	Higher 6TG nucleotide RBC concentration associated with neutropenia	225–227
Mercaptopurine (MP)	Children with ALL (n = 120)	Red cell concentration of MP metabolite (6 TG nucleotide)	Disease relapse	Lower 6TG nucleotide RBC concentration associated with higher risk at relapse	226
MTX (high-dose)	Children with ALL in first remission (n = 108)	Systemic clearance (CL_S)	Disease relapse	Higher CL_S associated with ↑ risk of early relapse	130
	Children with ALL in first remission (n = 108) longer follow-up of same patients as above	C_{SS}	Disease relapse	C_{SS} <16 µmol/L with 24 hr infusion of 1 gm/m^2 associated with ↑ risk of early relapse	149
	Children with ALL in first or second remission (n = 58)	CL_S	Disease relapse	Higher CL_S in those who relapsed	152
	Metastatic tumors and osteosarcoma (n >100)	Plasma concentration at 48 hours	Toxicity (mucositis), myelosuppression, renal dysfunction)	48 hr concentration >0.9 µmol/L associated with risk of toxicity	38, 40, 157
N-methylformamide	Adults with refractory solid tumors (n = 15)	Plasma AUC	Hepatotoxicity	Higher AUC associated with hepatotoxicity after IV doses	228

Table 29–4. *Summary of Selected Clinical Pharmacodynamic Studies with Anticancer Drugs[b] (cont.)*

Drug	Type of study[a]	Pharmacokinetic parameter	Drug effect(s) measured	Pharmacodynamic relationship	References
Teniposide	Children with refractory ALL or solid tumors (n = 23)	CL_S (C_{SS})	Oncolytic response (>75% ↓ in leukemic blasts or PR for solid tumors)	C_{SS} higher (CL_S lower) in responders versus non-responders	229
	Children with ALL in first remission or relapsed ALL	Plasma unbound AUC	% ↓ in WBC	Higher unbound AUC associated with greater ↓ in WBC count.	233
Vincristine	Adults (n = 24) and children (n = 3) with cancer of ITP	Plasma AUC	Neurological exam	Higher cumulative AUC associated with more severe neurotoxicity	230

[a] Patients and disease.
[b] ALL = Acute lymphocytic leukemia; ANLL = Acute nonlymphocytic leukemia; AUC = Area under the concentration-time curve; C = Plasma drug concentration; C_{SS} = Plasma drug concentration at steady state; CL_{cr} = Creatinine clearance; CL_S = Systemic clearance; ITP = Idiopathic thrombocytopenic purpura; PR = Partial response; RBC = Red blood cell; WBC = White blood cell; ARA-CTP= Cytosine arabinoside triphosphate; 6TG = 6 thioguanine.

REFERENCES

1. Bleyer WA. Methotrexate: clinical pharmacology, current status and therapeutic guidelines. Cancer Treat Rev. 1977;4:87.
2. Harvey VJ et al. The bioavailability of oral intermediate-dose methotrexate. Effect of dose subdivision, formulation, and timing in the chemotherapy cycle. Cancer Chemother Pharmacol. 1984;13:91.
3. Stuart JF et al. Bioavailability of methotrexate: implications for clinical use. Cancer Chemother Pharmacol. 1979;3:239.
4. Christophidis N et al. Comparison of intravenous and oral high-dose methotrexate in treatment of solid tumors. Br Med J. 1979;1:298.
5. Steele WH et al. Enhancement of methotrexate absorption by subdivision of dose. Cancer Chemother Pharmacol. 1979;3:235.
6. Pinkerton CR et al. Absorption of methotrexate under standardized conditions in children with acute lymphocytic leukemia. Br J Cancer. 1980;42:613.
7. Schornagel JH et al. Bioavailability of methotrexate tablets. Pharm Weekbl [Sci]. 1982;4:89.
8. Hendel J, Brodthagen H. Entero-hepatic cycling of methotrexate estimated by use of the D-isomer as a reference marker. Eur J Clin Pharmacol. 1984;26:103.
9. Kamen BA et al. Methotrexate and folate content of erythrocytes in patients receiving oral versus intramuscular therapy with methotrexate. J Pediatr. 1984;104:131.
10. Pinkerton CR et al. Can food influence the absorption of methotrexate in children with acute lymphocytic leukaemia? Lancet. 1980;2:944.
11. McVie JG et al. High-dose oral methotrexate. Cancer Treat Rep. 1981;65(Suppl):141.
12. Balis FM et al. Pharmacokinetics of oral methotrexate in children. Cancer Res. 1983;43:2342.
13. Craft AW et al. Methotrexate absorption in children with acute lymphoblastic leukemia. Cancer Treat Rep. 1981;65:77.
14. Forcast DJ et al. Clinical experience with oral high-dose methotrexate. Br J Cancer. 1981;43:719.
15. Smith DK et al. Clinical pharmacology of intermediate-dose oral methotrexate. Cancer Chemother Pharmacol. 1980;4:117.
16. Freeman-Narrod M et al. Comparison of serum concentrations of methotrexate after various routes of administration. Cancer 1975;36:1619.
17. Cohen MH et al. Effect of oral prophylactic broad spectrum nonabsorbable antibiotics on the gastrointestinal absorption of nutrients and methotrexate in small cell bronchogenic carcinoma patients. Cancer 1976;38:1556.
18. Valerino DM et al. Studies of the metabolism of methotrexate by intestinal flora. I: Identification and study of biological properties of the metabolite 4-amino-4-deoxy-N^{10}-methylpteroic acid. Biochem Pharmacol. 1972;21:821.
19. Evans WE, Rivera G. Pharmacokinetic studies of high-dose oral methotrexate in children with acute lymphocytic leukemia. Proc Am Assoc Cancer Res. 1979;20:266. Abstract.
20. Henderson ES et al. The metabolic fate of tritiated methotrexate. II: Absorption and excretion in man. Cancer Res. 1965;25:1018.
21. Wan K et al. Effect of route of administration and effusion on methotrexate pharmacokinetics. Cancer Res. 1974;34:3487.
22. Furst DE et al. Pharmacokinetics of low dose methotrexate (LD-MTX) in rheumatoid arthritis (RA). Clin Pharmacol Ther. 1986;29:193. Abstract.
23. Campbell MA et al. Methotrexate: bioavailability and pharmacokinetics. Cancer Treat Rep. 1985;69:833.
24. Chungi V et al. Drug absorption. VIII: Kinetics of GI absorption of methotrexate. J Pharm Sci. 1978;67:560.
25. Shen DD, Azarnoff DL. Clinical pharmacokinetics of methotrexate. Clin Pharmacokinet. 1978;3:1.
26. Pearson AD et al. Small intestinal transit time affects methotrexate absorption in children with acute lymphoblastic leukemia. Cancer Chemother Pharmacol. 1985;14:211.

27. Teresi ME et al. Methotrexate bioavailability after oral and intramuscular administration in children. J Pediatr. 1987;110:788.
28. Balis FM et al. Pharmacokinetics of subcutaneous methotrexate. J Clin Oncol. 1988;6:1882.
29. Lerne PR et al. Kinetic model for the disposition and metabolism of moderate and high-dose methotrexate (NSC-740) in man. Cancer Chemother Rep. 1975;59:811.
30. Pratt CB et al. High-dose methotrexate used alone and in combination for measurable primary or metastatic osteosarcoma. Cancer Treat Rep. 1980;64:11.
31. Evans WE et al. Disposition of intermediate dose methotrexate in children with ALL. Drug Intell Clin Pharm. 1982;16:839.
32. Huffman DH et al. Pharmacokinetics of methotrexate. Clin Pharmacol Ther. 1973;14:572.
33. Liegler DG et al. The effect of organic acids on renal clearance of methotrexate in man. Clin Pharmacol Ther. 1969;10:849.
34. Mandel MA. The synergistic effect of salicylates on methotrexate toxicity. Plast Reconstr Surg. 1976;57:733.
35. Abdelfattah E et al. Plasma protein binding of methotrexate and 7-hydroxymethotrexate. Drug Intell Clin Pharm. 1985;19:456.
36. Zaharko DS et al. Methotrexate tissue distribution: prediction by a mathematical model. J Natl Cancer Inst. 1971;46:775.
37. Bischoff KB et al. Methotrexate pharmacokinetics. J Pharm Sci. 1971;60:1128.
38. Evans WE et al. Pharmacokinetic monitoring of high-dose methotrexate: early recognition of high-risk patients. Cancer Chemother Pharmacol. 1979;3:161.
39. Evans WE et al. Pharmacokinetics of sustained serum methotrexate concentrations secondary to gastrointestinal obstruction. J Pharm Sci. 1981;70:1194.
40. Tattersall MHN et al. Clinical pharmacology of high-dose methotrexate (NSC-740). Cancer Chemother Rep. 1975;6(Pt. 3):25.
41. Evans WE, Pratt CB. Effect of pleural effusion on high-dose methotrexate kinetics. Clin Pharmacol Ther. 1978;23:68.
42. Goldman ID. Membrane transport of methotrexate (NSC-740) and other folate compounds: relevance to rescue protocols. Cancer Chemother Rep. 1975;6(Pt. 3):63.
43. Kamen BA, Capdevila A. Receptor-mediated folate accumulation is regulated by the cellular folate content. Proc Natl Acad Sci USA. 1986;83:5983.
44. Kane MA et al. The influence of extracellular folate concentration on methotrexate uptake by human KB cells. Partial characterization of a membrane-associated methotrexate binding protein. J Biol Chem. 1986;261:44.
45. Pinedo HM et al. The reversal of methotrexate cytotoxicity to mouse bone marrow cells by leucovorin and nucleosides. Cancer Res. 1976;36:4418.
46. Yalowich JC et al. Teniposide (VM-26)- and etoposide (VP-16-213)-induced augmentation of methotrexate transport and polyglutamylation in Ehrlich ascites tumor cells *in vitro*. Cancer Res. 1982;42:3648.
47. Wampler GL et al. Exploration of methods for demonstrating therapeutic synergism utilizing a time-interval between the interacting drugs methotrexate (MTX) and teniposide (VM-26). Proc Am Assoc Cancer Res. 1983;24:1060. Abstract.
48. Shapiro WR et al. Methotrexate: distribution in cerebrospinal fluid after intravenous, ventricular and lumbar injections. N Engl J Med. 1975;293:161.
49. Ushio Y et al. Uptake of tritiated methotrexate by mouse brain tumors after intravenous or intrathecal administration. J Neurosurg. 1974;40:706.
50. Griffin TW et al. The effect of photon irradiation on blood-brain barrier permeability to methotrexate in mice. Cancer 1977;40:1109.
51. Mellott LB. Physiochemical considerations and pharmacokinetic behavior in delivery of drugs to the central nervous system. Cancer Treat Rep. 1977;61:527.
52. Freeman AI et al. High-dose methotrexate in acute lymphocytic leukemia. Cancer Treat Rep. 1977;61:727.

53. Pitman SW, Frei E. Weekly methotrexate-calcium leucovorin rescue: effect of alkalinization on nephrotoxicity; pharmacokinetics in the CNS; and use in CNS non-Hodgkin's lymphoma. Cancer Treat Rep. 1977;61:695.

54. Bratlid D, Moe PJ. Pharmacokinetics of high-dose methotrexate treatment in children. Eur J Clin Pharmacol. 1978;14:143.

55. Tejada F et al. Methotrexate CSF levels during high dose methotrexate-leucovorin therapy. Proc Am Assoc Cancer Res. 1977;18:363. Abstract.

56. Evans WE et al. Methotrexate cerebrospinal fluid and serum concentrations after intermediate-dose methotrexate infusion. Clin Pharmacol Ther. 1983;33:301.

57. Rosen G et al. High-dose methotrexate with citrovorum factor rescue for the treatment of central nervous system tumors in children. Cancer Treat Rep. 1977;61:681.

58. Echelberger CK et al. Influence of body position on ventricular cerebrospinal fluid methotrexate concentrations following intralumbar administration. Proc Am Soc Clin Oncol. 1981;22:365. Abstract.

59. Fusner JE et al. Leukoencephalopathy following chemotherapy for rhabdomyosarcoma: reversibility of cerebral changes demonstrated by computed tomography. J Pediatr. 1977;91:77.

60. Price RA, Jamieson PA. The central nervous system in childhood leukemia. II: Subacute leukoencephalopathy. Cancer. 1975;35:306.

61. Freeman MV. The fluorometric measurement of the absorption, distribution and excretion of single doses of 4-amino-10-methyl-pteroylglutamic acid (amethopterin) in man. J Pharmacol Exp Ther. 1958;122:154.

62. Donehower RC et al. Presence of 2,4-diamino-N^{10}-methylpteroic acid after high-dose methotrexate. Clin Pharmacol Ther. 1979;26:63.

63. Jacobs SA et al. 7-Hydroxymethotrexate as a urinary metabolite in human subjects and rhesus monkeys receiving high dose methotrexate. J Clin Invest. 1976;57:534.

64. Johns DG, Loo TL. Metabolite of 4-amino-4-deoxy-N^{10}-methyl pteroylglutamic acid (methotrexate). J Pharm Sci. 1967;56:356.

65. Fabre G et al. Interactions between 7-hydroxymethotrexate and methotrexate at the cellular level in the Ehrlich ascites tumor *in vitro*. Cancer Res. 1984;44:970.

66. Chauvet M et al. Interaction of methotrexate metabolites with beef liver dihydrofolate reductase. I: Binary complex study. Biochem Pharmacol. 1983;32:1059.

67. Johns DG et al. Enzymatic oxidation of methotrexate and aminopterin. Life Sci. 1964;3:1383.

68. Redetzki HM et al. Resistance of the rabbit to methotrexate: isolation of a drug metabolite with decreased cytotoxicity. Biochem Pharmacol. 1966;15:425.

69. Breithaupt H, Kuenzlen E. Pharmacokinetics of methotrexate and 7- hydroxymethotrexate following infusions of high-dose methotrexate. Cancer Treat Rep. 1982;66:1733.

70. Wang YM et al. Effect of metabolism on pharmacokinetics and toxicity of high-dose methotrexate therapy in children. Proc Am Soc Clin Oncol. 1979;20:334. Abstract.

71. Chen ML et al. A specific HPLC assay to determine the pharmacokinetics of methotrexate in patients. Int J Clin Pharmacol Ther Toxicol. 1984;22:1.

72. Milano G et al. Plasma levels of 7-hydroxymethotrexate after high-dose methotrexate treatment. Cancer Chemother Pharmacol. 1983;11:29.

73. Chan KK et al. Metabolism of methotrexate in man after high and conventional doses. Res Commun Chem Pathol Pharmacol. 1980;28:551.

74. Breithaupt H, Kuenzlen E. High-dose methotrexate for osteosarcoma: toxicity and clinical results. Oncology 1983;40:85.

75. Collier CP et al. Analysis of methotrexate and 7-hydroxymethotrexate by high-performance liquid chromatography and preliminary clinical studies. Ther Drug Monit. 1982;4:371.

76. Lankelma J et al. The role of 7-hydroxymethotrexate during methotrexate anti-cancer therapy. Cancer Lett. 1980;9:133.

77. Canfell C, Sadee W. Methotrexate and 7-hydroxymethotrexate: serum level monitoring by high-performance liquid chromatography. Cancer Treat Rep. 1980;64:165.

78. Stewart AL et al. The pharmacokinetics of 7 hydroxymethotrexate following medium-dose methotrexate therapy. Cancer Chemother Pharmacol. 1985;14:165.

79. Chen ML, Chiou WL. Tissue metabolism and distribution of methotrexate in rabbits. Drug Metab Dispos. 1982;10:706.
80. Newton PA, Blakley RL. 7-Hydroxymethotrexate formation in a human lymphoblastic cell line. Biochem Biophys Res Commun. 1984;122:1212.
81. Howell SK et al. Plasma methotrexate as determined by liquid chromatography, enzyme-inhibition assay, and radio-immunoassay after high-dose infusion. Clin Chem. 1980;26:734.
82. Bertino JR. Methotrexate: clinical pharmacology and therapeutic application. In: Crooke ST, Prestayko AW, eds. Cancer and Chemotherapy. Vol 3. New York: Academic Press; 1981:359–75.
83. Christophidis N et al. Renal clearance of methotrexate in man during high-dose oral and intravenous infusion therapy. Cancer Chemother Pharmacol. 1981;6:59.
84. Fabre G et al. *In vitro* formation of polyglutamyl derivatives of methotrexate and 7-hydroxymethotrexate in human lymphoblastic leukemia cells. Cancer Res. 1983;43:4648.
85. Fry DW et al. Rapid formation of polyγglutamyl derivatives of methotrexate and their association with dihydrofolate reductase as assessed by high-pressure liquid chromatography in the Ehrlich ascites tumor cell *in vitro*. J Biol Chem. 1982;257:1890.
86. Schilsky RL et al. Methotrexate polyglutamate synthesis by cultured human breast cancer cells. Proc Natl Acad Sci USA. 1980;77:2919.
87. Balinska M et al. Efflux of methotrexate and its polyglutamate derivatives from hepatic cells *in vitro*. Cancer Res. 1981;41:2751.
88. Baugh CM et al. Polyγglutamyl metabolites of methotrexate. Biochem Biophys Res Commun. 1973;52:27.
89. Nair MG, Baugh CM. Synthesis and biological evaluation of polyγglutamyl derivatives of methotrexate. Biochemistry. 1973;12:3923.
90. Gewirtz DA et al. Transport, binding, and polyglutamation of methotrexate in freshly isolated rat hepatocytes. Cancer Res. 1980;40:573.
91. Zimmerman CL et al. Pharmacokinetics of the polyγglutamyl metabolites of methotrexate in skin and other tissues of rats and hairless mice. J Pharmacol Exp Ther. 1984;231:242.
92. Krakower GR, Kamen BA. *In situ* methotrexate polyglutamate formation in rat tissues. J Pharmacol Exp Ther. 1983;227:633.
93. Rosenblatt DS et al. Synthesis of methotrexate polyglutamates in cultured human cells. Mol Pharmacol. 1978;14:210.
94. Wilte A et al. Synthesis of methotrexate polyglutamates by bone marrow cells from patients with leukemia and lymphoma. Dev Pharmacol Ther. 1980;1:40.
95. Jacobs SA et al. Accumulation of methotrexate diglutamate in human liver during methotrexate therapy. Biochem Pharmacol. 1977;26:2310.
96. Kamen BA et al. Methotrexate accumulation and folate depletion in cells as a possible mechanism of chronic toxicity to the drug. Br J Haematol. 1981;49:355.
97. Galivan J. Evidence for the cytotoxic activity of polyglutamate derivatives of methotrexate. Mol Pharmacol. 1980;17:105.
98. Poser RG et al. Extracellular recovery of methotrexate polyglutamates following efflux from L1210 leukemia cells. Biochem Pharmacol. 1980;29:2701.
99. Whitehead VM. Synthesis of methotrexate polyglutamates in L1210 murine leukemia cells. Cancer Res. 1977;37:408.
100. Jolivet J, Schilsky RL. High-pressure liquid chromatography analysis of methotrexate polyglutamates in cultured human breast cancer cells. Biochem Pharmacol. 1981;30:1387.
101. Whitehead VM et al. Accumulation of methotrexate and methotrexate polyglutamates in lymphoblasts at diagnosis of childhood acute lymphoblastic leukemia: a pilot prognostic factor analysis. Blood. 1990;76:44.
102. Samuels LL et al. Detection by high-performance liquid chromatography of methotrexate and its metabolites in tumor tissue from osteosarcoma patients treated with high-dose methotrexate/leucovorin rescue. Biochem Pharmacol. 1984;33:2711.
103. Curt GA et al. Synthesis and retention of methotrexate polyglutamates by human small cell lung cancer. Biochem Pharmacol. 1984;33:1682.

104. McGuire JJ et al. Enzymatic synthesis of folylpolyglutamates. Characterization of the reaction and its products. J Biol Chem. 1980;255:5776.

105. Jolivet J, Chabner BA. Intracellular pharmacokinetics of methotrexate polyglutamates in human breast cancer cells. Selective retention and less dissociable binding of 4-NH_2-10-CH_3-pteroyl-glutamate$_4$ and 4-NH_2-10-CH_3-pteroylpteroylglutamate$_5$ to dihydrofolate reductase. J Clin Invest. 1983;72:773.

106. Moran RG et al. Structural features of 4-amino antifolates required for substrate activity with mammalian folylpolyglutamate synthetase. Mol Pharmacol. 1985;27:156.

107. Goldman ID. Analysis of the cytotoxic determinants for methotrexate: a role for free intracellular drug. Cancer Chemother Rep. 1975;6:51.

108. Goldman ID. Effects of methotrexate on cellular metabolism: some critical elements in the drug-cell interaction. Cancer Treat Rep. 1977;61:549.

109. Jacobs SA et al. Stoichiometric inhibition of mammalian dihydrofolate reductase by the γglutamyl metabolite of methotrexate, 4-amino-4-deoXy-N^{10}-methylpteroylglutamylγgluta-mate. Biochem Biophys Res Commun. 1975;63:692.

110. Fabre I et al. Polyglutamylation, an important element in methotrexate cytotoxicity and selectivity in tumor versus murine granulocytic progenitor cells *in vitro*. Cancer Res. 1984;44:3190.

111. Fry DW et al. Analysis of the role of membrane transport and polyglutamation of methotrexate in gut and the Ehrlich tumor *in vivo* as factors in drug sensitivity and selectivity. Cancer Res. 1983;43:1087.

112. Poser RG et al. Differential synthesis of methotrexate polyglutamates in normal profilerative and neoplastic mouse tissues *in vivo*. Cancer Res. 1981;41:4441.

113. Samuels LL et al. A comparison of hydrolase activity for 4-amino-folate polyglutamates in mouse small intestine and L1210 leukemia cells. Proc Am Assoc Cancer Res. 1984;25:1227. Abstract.

114. Fabre G, Goldman ID. Formation of 7-hydroxymethotrexate polyglutamyl derivatives and their cytotoxicity in human chronic myelogenous leukemia cells, *in vitro*. Cancer Res. 1985;45:80.

115. Fabre G et al. Synthesis and properties of 7-hydroxymethotrexate polyglutamyl derivatives in Ehrlich ascites tumor cells *in vitro*. J Biol Chem. 1984;259:5066.

116. McGuire JJ et al. Enzymatic synthesis of polyglutamate derivatives of 7-hydroxymethotrexate. Biochem Pharmacol. 1984;33:1355.

117. Stoller RG et al. Pharmacokinetics of high-dose methotrexate (NSC-740). Cancer Chemother Rep. 1975;6:19.

118. Pratt CB et al. Clinical trials and pharmacokinetics of intermittent high-dose methotrexate-"leucovorin rescue" for children with malignant tumors. Cancer Res. 1974;34:3326.

119. Zurek WK et al. Pharmacologic studies of methotrexate in man. Gynecol Obstet Invest. 1968;126:331.

120. Crom WR et al. Use of the automatic interaction detector method to identify patient characteristics related to methotrexate clearance. Clin Pharmacol Ther. 1986;39:592.

121. Williams WM, Huang KC. Renal tubular transport of folic acid and methotrexate in the monkey. Am J Physiol. 1982;242:F484.

122. Huang KC et al. Renal tubular transport of methotrexate in the Rhesus monkey and dog. Cancer Res. 1979;39:4843.

123. Kristensen LO et al. Renal function and the rate of disappearance of methotrexate from serum. Eur J Clin Pharmacol. 1975;8:439.

124. Hendel J, Nyfors A. Nonlinear renal elimination kinetics of methotrexate due to saturation of renal tubular reabsorption. Eur J Clin Pharmacol. 1984;26:121.

125. Christensen ML et al. Effect of hydration on methotrexate plasma concentrations in children with acute lymphocytic leukemia. J Clin Oncol. 1988;6:797.

126. Sand TE, Jacobsen S. Effect of urine pH and flow on renal clearance of methotrexate. Eur J Clin Pharmacol. 1981;19:453.

127. Van Den Berg HW et al. Rapid plasma clearance and reduced rate and extent of urinary elimination of parenterally administered methotrexate as a result of severe vomiting and diarrhea. Cancer Chemother Pharmacol. 1980;4:47.

128. Pratt CB et al. Response, toxicity and pharmacokinetics of high-dose methotrexate (NSC-740) with citrovorum factor (NSC-3500) rescue for children with osteosarcoma and other malignant tumors. Cancer Chemother Rep. 1975;6:13.

129. Wang Y et al. Methotrexate in blood, urine and cerebrospinal fluid of children receiving high doses by infusion. Clin Chem. 1976;22:1053.

130. Evans WE et al. Methotrexate systemic clearance influences the probability of relapse in children with standard-risk acute lymphocytic leukemia. Lancet 1984;1:359.

131. Isacoff WH et al. Pharmacokinetics of high-dose methotrexate with citrovorum factor rescue. Cancer Treat Rep. 1977;61:1665.

132. Reich SD et al. A pharmacokinetic model for high-dose methotrexate infusions in man. J Pharmacokinet Biopharm. 1977;5:421.

133. Romolo JL et al. Effect of hydration on plasma-methotrexate levels. Cancer Treat Rep. 1977;61:1393.

134. Bleyer WA. The clinical pharmacology of methotrexate: new applications of an old drug. Cancer 1978;41:36.

135. Chan H et al. Recovery from toxicity associated with high-dose methotrexate: prognostic factors. Cancer Treat Rep. 1977;61:797.

136. Relling MV et al. Removal of methotrexate, leucovorin, and their metabolites by combined hemodialysis and hemoperfusion. Cancer 1988;62:884.

137. Strum WB, Liem HH. Hepatic uptake, intracellular protein binding and biliary excretion of amethopterin. Biochem Pharmacol. 1977;26:1235.

138. Creaven PJ et al. Methotrexate in liver and bile after intravenous dosage in man. Br J Cancer. 1973;28:589.

139. Calvert AH et al. Some observations on the human pharmacology of methotrexate. Cancer Treat Rep. 1977;61:1647.

140. Scheufler E, Bos I. Influence of peroral charcoal on pharmacokinetics and intestinal toxicity of intravenously given methotrexate. Arch Int Pharmacodyn Ther. 1983;261:180.

141. Gadgil SD et al. Effect of activated charcoal on the pharmacokinetics of high-dose methotrexate. Cancer Treat Rep. 1982;66:1169.

142. Werkheiser WC. Specific binding of 4-amino folic acid analogues by folic acid reductase. J Biol Chem. 1961;2236:888.

143. Sirotnak FM, Donsback RC. Further evidence for a basis of selective activity and relative responsiveness during antifolate therapy of murine tumors. Cancer Res. 1975;35:1737.

144. Goldman ID et al. Exchangeable intracellular methotrexate levels in the presence and absence of vincristine at extracellular drug concentrations relevant to those achieved in high-dose methotrexate-folinic acid "rescue" protocols. Cancer Res. 1976;36:276.

145. Chabner BA, Young RC. Threshold methotrexate concentration for *in vivo* inhibition of DNA synthesis in normal and tumorous target tissues. J Clin Invest. 1973;52:1804.

146. Zaharko DS et al. Relative toxicity of methotrexate in several tissues of mice bearing Lewis lung carcinoma. J Pharm Exp Ther. 1974;189:585.

147. Young RC, Chabner BA. An *in vivo* method for monitoring differential effects of chemotherapy on target tissue in animals and man: correlation with plasma pharmacokinetics. Cancer Res. 1973;52:92a.

148. Pinedo HM, Chabner BA. Role of drug concentration, duration of exposure and endogenous metabolites in determining methotrexate cytotoxicity. Cancer Treat Rep. 1977;61:709.

149. Evans WE et al. Clinical pharmacodynamics of high-dose methotrexate in acute lymphocytic leukemia. Identification of a relation between concentration and effect. N Engl J Med. 1986;314:471.

150. Evans WE et al. Clinical pharmacodynamic studies of high-dose methotrexate in acute lympho-cytic leukemia. NCI Monogr. 1987;5:81.

151. Borsi JD et al. Prognostic importance of systemic clearance of methotrexate in childhood acute lymphoblastic leukemia. Cancer Chemother Pharmacol. 1987;19:261.

152. Borsi JD, Moe PJ. Systemic clearance of methotrexate in the prognosis of acute lymphoblastic leukemia in children. Cancer 1987;60:3020.

153. Pinkerton CR et al. Modified Capizzi maintenance regimen in children with relapsed acute lymphoblastic leukemia. Med Pediatr Oncol. 1986;14:69.

154. Isacoff WH et al. High-dose methotrexate therapy of solid tumors: observations relating to clinical toxicity. Med Pediatr Oncol. 1976;2:319.

155. Isacoff WH et al. Pharmacokinetics of high-dose methotrexate with citrovorum factor rescue. Cancer Treat Rep. 1977;61:1665.

156. Nirenberg A et al. High dose methotrexate with CF rescue: predictive value of serum methotrexate concentrations and corrective measures to avert toxicity. Cancer Treat Rep. 1977;61:779.

157. Stoller RC et al. Use of plasma pharmacokinetics to predict and prevent methotrexate toxicity. N Engl J Med. 1977;297:630.

158. Jolivet J et al. The pharmacology and clinical use of methotrexate. N Engl J Med. 1983;309:1094.

159. Rechnitzer C et al. Methotrexate in the plasma and cerebrospinal fluid of children treated with intermediate dose methotrexate. Acta Paediatr Scand. 1981;70:615.

160. Abelson HT et al. Methotrexate-induced renal impairment: clinical studies and rescue from systemic toxicity with high-dose leucovorin and thymidine. J Clin Oncol. 1983;1:208.

161. White JC. Predictions of a network thermodynamics computer model relating to the mechanism of methotrexate rescue by 5-formyltetrahydrofolate and to the importance of inhibition of thymidylate synthetase by methotrexate-polyglutamates. Adv Exp Med Biol. 1983;163:305.

162. Matherly LH et al. Role of methotrexate polyglutamylation and cellular energy metabolism in inhibition of methotrexate binding to dihydrofolate reductase by 5-formyltetrahydrofolate in Ehrlich ascites tumor cells *in vitro*. Cancer Res. 1983;43:2694.

163. Levitt M et al. Improved therapeutic index of methotrexate with "leucovorin rescue." Cancer Res. 1973;33:1729.

164. Bertino JR. "Rescue" techniques in cancer chemotherapy: use of leucovorin and other rescue agents after methotrexate treatment. Semin Oncol. 1977;4:203.

165. Goldie JH et al. Methotrexate toxicity: correlation with duration of administration, plasma levels, dose and excretion pattern. Eur J Cancer. 1972;8:409.

166. Sirotnak FM et al. Optimization of high-dose methotrexate with leucovorin rescue therapy in L1210 leukemia and sarcoma 180 murine tumor models. Cancer Res. 1978;38:345.

167. Browman GP et al. Modulation of the antitumor effect of methotrexate by low-dose leucovorin in squamous cell head and neck cancer: a randomized placebo-controlled clinical trial. J Clin Oncol. 1990;8:203.

168. Van Hoff DD et al. Incidence of drug-related deaths secondary to high-dose methotrexate and citrovorum factor administration. Cancer Treat Rep. 1977;61:745.

169. Jaffe N, Traggis D. Toxicity of high-dose methotrexate (NSC-740) and citrovorum factor (NSC-3590) in osteogenic sarcoma. Cancer Chemother Rep. 1975;6:31.

170. Pochedly C. Neurotoxicity due to CNS therapy for leukemia. Med Pediatr Oncol. 1977;3:101.

171. Bleyer WA et al. Pharmacokinetics and neurotoxicity of intrathecal methotrexate therapy. N Engl J Med. 1973;289:770.

172. Bleyer WA. Clinical pharmacology of intrathecal methotrexate. II: An improved dosage regimen derived from age-related pharmacokinetics. Cancer Treat Rep. 1977;61:1419.

173. Morse M et al. Altered central nervous system pharmacology of methotrexate in childhood leukemia: another sign of meningeal relapse. J Clin Oncol. 1985;3:19.

174. Strother DR et al. Variability in the disposition of intraventricular methotrexate: a proposal for rational dosing. J Clin Oncol. 1989;7:1741.

175. Evans WE, Relling MV. Clinical pharmacokinetics-pharmacodynamics of anticancer drugs. Clin Pharmacokinet. 1989;16:327.

176. Jurrgens H et al. Clinical and pharmacokinetic prognostic factors in the response of primary osteogenic sarcoma to pre-operative chemotherapy (high-dose methotrexate with citrovorum factor rescue). Proceedings of Symposium on Sarcoma of Soft Tissue and Bone in Childhood. Orlando, FL: 1979.

177. Crom WR et al. The effect of prior cisplatin therapy on the pharmacokinetics of high-dose methotrexate. J Clin Oncol. 1984;2:655.

178. Goren MP et al. Urinary N-acetylβD-glucosaminidase and serum creatinine concentrations predict impaired excretion of methotrexate. J Clin Oncol. 1987;5:804.

179. Garre ML et al. Pharmacokinetics and toxicity of methotrexate in children with Down's syndrome and acute lymphocytic leukemia. J Pediatr. 1987;111:606.

180. Nixon PF, Bertino JR. Effective absorption and utilization of oral formyltetrahydrofolate in man. N Engl J Med. 1972;286:175.

181. Mehta BM et al. Serum distribution of 5-methyltetrahydrofolate following high-dose methotrexate-leucovorin rescue regimen in osteogenic sarcoma. Proc Am Assoc Cancer Res. 1979;20:127. Abstract.

182. Mehta BM et al. Serum distribution of citrovorum factor and 5-methyltetrahydrofolate following oral and IM administration of calcium leucovorin in normal adults. Cancer Treat Rep. 1978;62:345.

183. Whitehead VM, Stein HA. Delay in metabolism of parenteral folinic acid to 5- methyltetrahydrofolate in man. Biochem Soc Trans. 1976;4:918.

184. Lankelma J et al. Determination of 5-methyltetrahydrofolic acid in plasma and spinal fluid by high-performance liquid chromatography using on-column concentration and electrochemical detection. J Chromatogr (Biomed Appl). 1980;183:35.

185. Hamel E et al. Pharmacokinetics of leucovorin rescue using a new methotrexate-independent biochemical assay for leucovorin and N^5-methyltetrahydrofolate. Cancer Treat Rep. 1981;65:545.

186. Mehta BM et al. Serum and cerebrospinal fluid distribution of 5-methyltetrahydrofolate after intravenous calcium leucovorin and intra-Ommaya methotrexate administration in patients with meningeal carcinomatosis. Cancer Res. 1983;43:435.

187. Lasseter KC et al. Bioavailability of oral and parenteral formulation of leucovorin. Clin Pharmacol Ther. 1983;33:222.

188. Straw JA et al. Pharmacokinetics of the diastereoisomers of leucovorin after intravenous and oral administration to normal subjects. Cancer Res. 1984;44:3114.

189. Newman EM et al. Pharmacokinetics of diastereoisomers of (6R,S)-folinic acid (leucovorin) in humans during constant high-dose intravenous infusion. Cancer Res. 1989;49:5755.

190. Bertrand R, Jolivet J. Lack of interference by the unnatural isomer of 5-formyltetrahydrofoate with the effects of the natural isomer in leucovorin preparation. J Natl Cancer Inst. 1989;81:1175.

191. Straw JA, Newman EM. Pharmacokinetic analysis of (6S)-5-formyltetrahydrofolate (l-CF), (6R)-5-formyltetrahydrofolate (d-CF) and 5-methyltetrahydrofolate (5-CH₃-THF) in patients receiving constant IV infusion of high-dose (6R,S)-5-formyltetrahydrofolate (leucovorin). Adv Exp Med Biol. 1988;244:53.

192. Greiner PO et al. Pharmacokinetics of (–)-folinic acid after oral and intravenous administration of the racemate. Br J Clin Pharmacol. 1989;28:289.

193. Straw JA et al. Pharmacokinetics of leucovorin (D,L-5- formyltetrahydrofolate) after intravenous injection and constant intravenous infusion. NCI Monogr. 1987;5:41.

194. Schilsky RL et al. Clinical pharmacology of the stereoisomers of leucovorin during repeated oral dosing. Cancer 1989;63:1018.

195. Weber G. Rotational Brownian movement and polarization of the fluorescence of solutions. Adv Protein Chem. 1953;8:415.

196. Dandliker WB, De Saussure VA. Review article: fluorescence polarization in immunochemistry. Immunochemistry 1970;7:799.

197. Dandliker WB et al. Fluorescence polarization immunoassay. Theory and experimental method. Immunochemistry 1973;10:219.

198. Gushaw JB, Miller JG. Homogenous enzyme immunoassay for methotrexate in serum. Clin Chem. 1978;24:1032.
199. Buice RG et al. Evaluation of the enzyme-mediated immunoassay (EMIT), radioenzyme assay (REA), and radioimmunoassay (RIA) of serum methotrexate, as compared with liquid chromatography. Clin Chem. 1980;26:1902.
200. Myers CE et al. Competitive protein binding assay for methotrexate. Proc Natl Acad Sci USA. 1975;72:3683.
201. Watson E et al. High-pressure liquid chromatographic determination of methotrexate and its major metabolite, 7-hdyroxymethotrexate, in human plasma. Cancer Treat Rep. 1978;62:381.
202. Nelson JA et al. Analysis of methotrexate in human plasma by high-pressure liquid chromatography with fluorescence detection. Cancer Res. 1977;37:3970.
203. Wisnicki JL et al. Analysis of methotrexate and 7-hydroxymethotrexate by high-pressure liquid chromatography. Cancer Treat Rep. 1978;62:529.
204. Cairnes DA, Evans WE. High-performance liquid chromatographic assay of methotrexate, 7-hydroxymethotrexate, 4-deoxy-4-amino-N^{10}-methylpteroic acid and sulfamethoxazole in serum, urine, and cerebrospinal fluid. J Chromatogr (Biomed Appl). 1982;231:103.
205. Falk LC et al. Enzymatic assay for methotrexate in serum and cerebrospinal fluid. Clin Chem. 1976;22:785.
206. Freeman MV. A fluorometric method for the measurement of a 4-amino-10- methylpteroyl-glutamatic acid (amethopterin) in plasma. J Pharmacol Exp Ther. 1957;120:1.
207. Noble WC et al. Assay of therapeutic doses of MTX in body fluids of patients with psoriasis. J Invest Dermatol. 1975;64:69.
208. Arons E et al. A direct ligand-binding radioassay for the measurement of methotrexate in tissues and biological fluids. Cancer Res. 1975;35:2033.
209. Wainer IW, Stiffin RM. Direct resolution of the stereoisomers of leucovorin and 5-methyl-tetrahydrofolate using a bovine serum albumin high-performance liquid chromatographic chiral stationary phase coupled to an achiral phenyl column. J Chromatogr. 1988;424:158.
210. Choi KE, Schilsky RL. Resolution of the stereoisomers of leucovorin and 5-methyltetrahydrofolate by chiral high-performance liquid chromatography. Anal Biochem. 1988;168:398.
211. Hall SW et al. Human pharmacokinetics of a new acridine derivative, 4'-(9-acrudubt-kanubi)methanesulfon-m-anisidide (NSC 249992). Cancer Res. 1983;43:3422.
212. Egorin MJ et al. Pharmacokinetics and dosage reduction of cisdiammine(1,1-cyclobutan-edicarboxylato)platinum in patients with impaired renal function. Cancer Res. 1984;44:5432.
213. Egorin MJ et al. Prospective validation of a pharmacologically based dosing scheme for the cisdiamminedichloroplatinum(II) analogue diamminecyclobutane dicarboxylatoplatinum. Cancer Res. 1985;45:6502.
214. Campbell AB et al. Plasma platinum levels: relationship to cisplatin dose and nephrotoxicity. Cancer Treat Rep. 1983;67:169.
215. Rustum YM, Preisler HD. Correlation between leukemic cell retention of 1-β-D-arabino-furanosylcytosine 5'-triphosphate and response to therapy. Cancer Res. 1979;39:42.
216. Rustum YM et al. Pharmacokinetic parameters of ara-C and their relationship to intracellular metabolism of ara-C, toxicity, and response of patients with acute nonlymphocytic leukemia treated with conventional and high-dose ara-C. Semin Oncol. 1987;14(Suppl. 1):141.
217. Bennett CL et al. Phase I clinical and pharmacological study of 72-hour continuous infusion of etoposide in patients with advanced cancer. Cancer Res. 1987;47:1952.
218. Goldberg JA et al. Pharmacokinetics and pharmacodynamics of locoregional 5- fluorouracil (5FU) in advanced colorectal liver metastases. Br J Cancer 1988;57:186.
219. Milano G et al. Dose versus pharmacokinetics for predicting tolerance to 5-day continuous infusion of 5-FU. Int J Cancer 1988;41:537.
220. Milano G et al. Relationship between systemic 5-FU passage and response in colorectal cancer patients treated with intrahepatic chemotherapy. Cancer Chemother Pharmacol. 1987;20:71.
221. Au JL et al. Clinical pharmacological studies of concurrent infusion of 5-fluorouracil and thymidine in treatment of colorectal carcinomas. Cancer Res. 1982;42:2930.

222. Egorin MJ et al. Phase I clinical and pharmacokinetic study of hexamethylene bisacetamide (NSC 95580) administered as a five-day continuous infusion. Cancer Res. 1987;47:617.

223. Egorin MJ et al. Human pharmacokinetics, excretion, and metabolism of the anthracycline antibiotic menogaril (7-DMEN, NSC 269148) and their correlation with clinical toxicities. Cancer Res. 1986;46:1513.

224. Egorin MJ et al. Phase I study and pharmacokinetics of menogaril (NSC 269148) in patients with hepatic dysfunction. Cancer Res. 1987;47:6104.

225. Lennard L et al. Childhood leukemia: a relationship between intracellular 6-mercaptopurine metabolites and neutropenia. Br J Clin Pharmacol 1983;16:359.

226. Lennard L et al. Oral 6-mercaptopurine in childhood leukemia: parent drug pharmacokinetics and active metabolite concentrations. Clin Pharmacol Ther. 1986;40:287.

227. Lennard L, Lilleyman JS. Variable mercaptopurine metabolism and treatment outcome in childhood lymphoblastic leukemia. J Clin Oncol. 1989;7:1816.

228. Rowinsky EK et al. Clinical pharmacology of oral and IV N-methylformamide: a pharmacologic basis for lack of clinical antineoplastic activity. J Natl Cancer Inst. 1988;80:671.

229. Rodman JH et al. Clinical pharmacodynamics of continuous infusion teniposide: systemic exposure as a determinant of response in a Phase I trial. J Clin Oncol. 1987;5:1007.

230. Desai ZR et al. Can severe vincristine neurotoxicity be prevented? Cancer Chemother Pharmacol. 1982;8:211.

231. Gregory RE et al. Raised plasma methotrexate concentrations following intrathecal administration in children with renal dysfunction. Leukemia. 1991;5:999.

232. Stewart CF et al. Relation of systemic exposure to unbound etoposide and hematologic toxicity. Clin Pharmacol Ther. 1991;50:385.

233. Evans WE et al. Differences in teniposide disposition and pharmacodynamics in patients with newly diagnosed and relapsed acute lymphocytic leukemia. J Pharmacol Exp Ther. 1992;260:71.

Chapter 30

Heparin

Robert J. Cipolle and Keith A. Rodvold

Heparin, named from its origin in the liver ("hepar"), is a mucopolysaccharide first discovered by McLean in 1916.[1-3] The development of commercial heparin for clinical use was not established until some 20 years after its discovery.[3-5] During the next 50 years, heparin established itself as a primary therapeutic agent for the prophylaxis and treatment of venous thromboembolism. Currently, low-molecular-weight heparin and other derivatives of heparin are being developed to improve the risk:benefit ratio of heparin therapy in an individual patient.

Despite its long history, several routine questions about heparin's clinical use remain:[6,7]

- By what route of administration (intravenous infusion, intermittent intravenous injection, subcutaneous injection) should heparin be administered?
- Should heparin be given in a standard dose or should the dose be adjusted by a coagulation test performed *in vitro*?
- How should heparin be monitored?
- How long should heparin be administered?
- Should the initial course of heparin be followed by longer-term anticoagulation therapy?

Because of these questions, the majority of patients continue to receive subtherapeutic doses of heparin and are monitored suboptimally.[8] This chapter will review how the application of clinical pharmacokinetic and pharmacodynamic data can be used to determine optimal dosage and monitoring of heparin therapy.

CLINICAL PHARMACOKINETICS

Absorption

Subcutaneous or intravenous administration is recommended when heparin is used for prophylaxis or treatment of patients with thromboembolic events. No data are available on the rate and extent of absorption of heparin following administration by the oral route. Studies have investigated the use of intrapulmonary instillation or inhalation of heparin in the treatment of thromboembolic disorders.

The total amount of heparin required to achieve the same degree of anticoagulant effect over the same time period does not appear to differ whether the agent is administered by intravenous, subcutaneous, or intrapulmonary routes.[9,10] The intramuscular administration is discouraged because of the high risk of serious localized bleeding complications.

No sophisticated pharmacokinetic studies have been conducted to determine the absorption rate constant following subcutaneous heparin administration. Data from normal subjects indicate that heparin is absorbed completely but slowly over the dosage interval. In patients who received individualized subcutaneous prophylactic heparin doses designed to maintain mid-interval activated partial thromboplastin times (APTTs) of 1.5 times control values, circulating heparin concentrations ranged from 0.1 to 0.3 units/mL throughout the dosing period. The mean dose required to achieve this effect was 10,000 units ($\pm$ 1000 units) administered subcutaneously every 12 hours. The peak heparin concentrations occurred at approximately two to four hours after injection.[11]

Although the subcutaneous route of administration is primarily used for prophylaxis of thromboembolism, it has been advocated for full therapeutic doses of heparin in patients in whom intravenous therapy is difficult. The application of pharmacokinetic data from patients receiving prophylactic heparin to patients treated with therapeutic subcutaneous doses may be confounded by variables such as body weight, site of injections, disease states, and concentrations of the heparin products used. Until the influence of these variables on the systemic availability of heparin is well-defined, caution must be applied in the decision to use the subcutaneous route for therapeutic treatment of patients with major thromboembolic disorders.

Clinical efficacy studies of subcutaneous heparin have used both the calcium and sodium salts. While some studies have demonstrated significantly lower peak plasma heparin concentrations or decreased anticoagulant effects from the calcium salts, other investigators have failed to find significant differences in plasma heparin concentrations or anticoagulant effects between the two salts.[12,13] The available data indicate that intravenously administered sodium and calcium salts exhibit similar anticoagulant potency *in vitro* and have essentially the same time-course of anticoagulant effect *in vivo*. Therefore, the observed differences in peak heparin concentrations between these two salts are probably related to differential absorption from the anterior abdominal wall.[12,13]

Distribution

Heparin is distributed primarily throughout the vascular system, and the apparent volume of distribution (V_d) quantitatively resembles that of plasma or blood volume. In blood, heparin binds to antithrombin III and several plasma constituents, including albumin, globulins, fibrinogen, lipoproteins, abnormal immunoglobulins, and platelet factor 4. Although no quantitative information has been reported, recent studies indicate that a substantial fraction of circulating heparin is bound to plasma constituents.[14]

Published data describing the apparent volume of distribution for heparin range from 40 to 100 mL/kg, with an average value of approximately 60 mL/kg. The apparent volume of distribution of heparin is directly related to body weight, and it has been suggested that heparin doses in obese patients should be based on ideal body weight (IBW).[15] However, several reports suggest that heparin dosage should be normalized to total body weight (TBW).[16-18] The volume of distribution of heparin varies widely between individual patients and does not seem to correlate with specific disease states (see Table 30-1).[16]

McDonald et al.[19,20] reported a larger volume of distribution of heparin in newborns. These results have been confirmed in piglets by measuring radioactivity of ^{125}I-heparin and antifactor X_a activity.[21,22] The heparin volume of distribution of human newborns varied inversely with gestational age. The largest mean volume of distribution of 81 mL/kg was reported in babies of 25 to 28 weeks gestation. These authors speculated that larger loading doses per kilogram of body weight would be required in newborns than adults to achieve desired degrees of antico-agulation.

The values obtained for individual pharmacokinetic parameters vary depending upon the heparin assay used. The apparent volume of distribution of heparin has been reported to be 1.5- to 2-fold larger when based on polybrene neutralizations of heparin than when based on bioassays using coagulation tests such as APTT or thrombin time (TT). Although animal studies have demonstrated a dose-dependent increase in apparent volume of distribution, this has not been verified in humans.[23]

Metabolism and Elimination

The metabolism and elimination of heparin are complex, but primarily involve metabolic processes of depolymerization and desulfation. Recent evidence demonstrates that the antithrombin III binding site of heparin resides in an oligosaccharide segment of the heparin molecule. Enzymes reported to be in-volved in heparin degradation include heparinase and desulfatase. Heparinase, which cleaves heparin into oligosaccharides, has been isolated from liver and spleen tissue. Dawes and Pepper[14] suggested that heparin is first desulfated by the reticuloendothelial system and subsequently broken down into oligosaccharides. Bjornsson et al. have suggested that depolymerization may be the rate-limiting step of heparin elimination since clearance of N-desulfated heparin is similar to that of standard heparin.[24] Their results also suggest that selective N-deacetylation and N-desulfation of the glucosamine residues of heparin significantly change the anticoagulant activities of heparin.

In humans, urinary excretion of unchanged heparin appears to be a minor route of elimination. Some urinary degradation products of heparin retain demonstrable anticoagulant activity. These degradation products appear to be partially de-sulfated species and provide some evidence of circulating heparin metabolites. Studies utilizing ^{35}S-heparin indicate that 80% of the radioactivity is recovered in the urine eight hours after intravenous injection. The majority of this radioactivity is in the form of inorganic sulfate; no radioactivity was detected in feces following intravenous heparin administration.[25,26]

Table 30–1. Summary of Heparin Pharmacokinetic Parameters[a]

Study population	No. of subjects	Coagulation test used	Heparin dose studied (unit/kg)	CL (mL/min/kg)	V_d (mL/kg)	$t\frac{1}{2}$ (hr)	References
Normal adults	17	X_a	75 ± 0	0.64 ± 0.11	70 ± 7	1.78 ± 0.28	29, 33
Normal adults	11	X_a	200 ± 0	0.38	50	1.51 ± 0.57	15
Normal adults	10	X_a	5000 units	0.68	45	0.76 ± 0.26	15
Normal adults	8	X_a	75 ± 0	0.43 ± 0.09	37 ± 7	1.06 ± 0.26	19, 20
Normal adults	6	APTT	70 ± 0	0.56 ± 0.10	45 ± 15	0.92 ± 0.22	16
Normal adults	4	TT	75 ± 0	0.69 ± 0.06	48 ± 13	0.82 ± 0.25	30
Normal adults	4	TT	50 ± 0	0.93 ± 0.16	55 ± 4	0.70 ± 0.08	30
Obese adults	10	X_a	200 ± 0	0.25	46	2.13 ± 0.56	15
Thrombophlebitis	15	APTT	70 ± 0	1.30 ± 0.57	123 ± 68	1.16 ± 0.27	27
Thrombophlebitis	14	X_a	76 ± 16	0.55 ± 0.19	62 ± 11	1.77 ± 0.47	29, 33
Thrombophlebitis	7	APTT	70 ± 0	0.69 ± 0.15	55 ± 16	0.93 ± 0.19	16
Pulmonary emboli	13	APTT	70 ± 0	0.70 ± 0.34	48 ± 24	0.86 ± 0.34	16
Pulmonary emboli	11	X_a	75 ± 0	0.80 ± 0.23	68 ± 15	1.33 ± 0.32	29, 33
Pulmonary emboli	4	APTT	70 ± 0	2.63 ± 0.98	141 ± 47	0.63 ± 0.03	27
Hepatic disease	7	X_a	70 ± 9	0.86 ± 0.28	78 ± 12	1.33 ± 0.35	29, 33
Renal disease	12	X_a	67 ± 7	0.60 ± 0.13	71 ± 12	1.83 ± 0.30	29, 33
Smoking adults	5	APTT	70 ± 0	0.87 ± 0.23	47 ± 17	0.62 ± 0.16	16
Newborns 33 to 36 wk G	8	X_a	100 ± 0	1.37 ± 0.46	58 ± 32	0.59 ± 0.15	19, 20
Newborns 29 to 32 wk G	7	X_a	100 ± 0	1.43 ± 0.39	73 ± 25	0.59 ± 0.11	19, 20
Newborns 25 to 28 wk G	10	X_a	100 ± 0	1.49 ± 0.87	81 ± 41	0.69 ± 0.24	19, 20

[a] Values are means; SD given when available.

The anticoagulant activity of heparin in plasma decreases exponèntially with time following intravenous administration; however, the half-life increases with increasing dose. The biological half-life of heparin in humans following a single intravenous injection has been reported to range from 0.4 to 2.5 hours. Heparin clearance ranges from 0.25 to 2 mL/min/kg. The reported values for both of these pharmacokinetic parameters vary widely between studies. Significant interpatient variation has been reported in individual half-life and clearance values for patients receiving therapeutic doses of heparin administered intravenously. Up to a tenfold range in heparin half-life has been reported within individual studies involving the administration of large doses. Other investigators have reported a six- and twelve-fold interpatient variability in heparin clearance values.[16,23,27–30] The disappearance of the anticoagulant activity follows nonlinear pharmacokinetics and has been described by a combination of a saturable and a linear process.[31,32]

The wide variation in heparin elimination data has prompted investigators to examine the effect of the following factors: body weight, age, gender, smoking, thromboembolic disorder, hepatic dysfunction, and renal dysfunction. In our investigation involving 20 patients with thromboembolic disorders, heparin clearances ranged from 14.7 to 65.9 mL/hr/kg.[16] When these values were standardized to IBW, clearance ranged from 21.2 to 84.8 mL/hr/kg IBW. Heparin clearance was related to both TBW and IBW ($r = 0.76$; $p > 0.001$). Clearance was found to be more rapid in males than females. Patients who smoked demonstrated a more rapid heparin clearance than did nonsmoking patients. A multiple-regression model was developed to predict heparin clearance from IBW, gender, and smoking ($r = 0.78$; $p > 0.005$), but the fraction of variance explained in heparin clearance by gender and smoking was substantially reduced after IBW was added to the multiple-regression model. Therefore, body weight was clearly the patient factor most highly associated with heparin clearance values.

The influence of age on heparin elimination and clearance has been investigated in pre-term newborns following a standardized 100 unit/kg intravenous bolus injection.[19,20] The newborn infants demonstrated a significantly shorter plasma half-life than did the normal adult comparison group. The heparin half-life and clearance values varied with gestational age in these pre-term newborns (see Table 30-1). In adult patients, changes in heparin clearance with respect to age have not been quantitated, but reports have demonstrated that patients over 60 years of age have a higher risk of bleeding than do younger adults and generally require lower doses per kilogram of TBW.[34,35] Whether this reduced dosage requirement is secondary to reduced heparin clearance or increased patient sensitivity to heparin is unclear.

The influence of the underlying thromboembolic process on heparin elimination half-life and clearance has been examined. Studies have indicated that patients with pulmonary embolism have shorter heparin elimination half-lives and more rapid total clearances than patients treated for venous thrombosis. Hirsh et al.[27] reported a 600% range in heparin clearances in 20 patients with thromboembolic disease. Four of these patients treated for pulmonary emboli had higher mean clearances than did the 16 patients with deep venous thrombosis. This observation was supported by investigators who have recommended larger heparin doses for patients with pulmonary emboli.[33] However, Elliott et al.[127] and Tenero et al.[35] reported no significant differences in dosage requirements between patients with pulmonary emboli and deep vein thrombosis. Similarly, White et al.[36] investigated the relationship between heparin dosage requirements and the presence or absence of thromboembolic disease. Although they also reported no significant difference in heparin requirements between patients with pulmonary emboli and deep vein thrombosis, patients with verified thromboembolic diseases required significantly larger mean heparin doses (25 units/kg/hr) than did patients without thromboembolic disease (15 units/kg/hr). In our series of 20 patients, there was a correlation between the time delay from onset of symptoms to initiation of treatment and the heparin dosage requirements.[16] These data indicate that patients with acute thromboembolic disorders have rapid clearance rates and require larger heparin doses to ensure adequate antithrombotic activity.

Studies examining the influence of renal and hepatic dysfunction on heparin elimination have yielded conflicting results. Most available data indicate that renal disease does not significantly affect the rate of disappearance of heparin or its anticoagulant effect.[33,37] Studies investigating the influence of hepatic dysfunction on heparin elimination have produced discordant results. Teien and Bjoornson[38] in 1976 reported a reduced heparin elimination in patients with advanced cirrhosis; however, in 1978 Simon et al.[33] reported a reduction in heparin half-life in seven patients with hepatic disease. Sette et al. reported a reduced mean elimination half-life in 15 patients with fulminant hepatic failure compared to 10 patients with chronic liver disease and 19 healthy volunteers measured by an anti-X_a assay (27.8 minutes versus 45.2 minutes and 50.2 minutes, respectively) or the whole blood activated clotting time (23.7 minutes versus 37.6 minutes and 37 minutes, respectively).[39] It is likely that the results of these investigations examining renal and hepatic effects on heparin elimination are confounded by the varying dosages and assay methodologies employed.

The most appropriate pharmacokinetic model to describe the disposition of heparin remains controversial. The vast majority of published reports have utilized a simple one-compartment model with first-order elimination. Bjornsson[40] reported that the biological half-life of heparin increases with increased doses in animals and humans. As heparin doses are increased, clearance decreases in a manner that does not seem to involve the classic Michaelis-Menten or capacity-limited pharmacokinetics. Bjornsson[41] reported that the biological half-life of heparin increased from a mean of 42 minutes to 153 minutes as doses were increased from 50 units/kg to 400 units/kg (see Figure 30-1). These investigations also indicated that increased doses did not cause an increase in the apparent volume of distribution. The mechanism underlying these observations is a matter of speculation, but it has been suggested that the decrease in heparin clearance resulting from increasing doses may be due to metabolite inhibition or to accumulation of a more active, slowly eliminated species of heparin.[23] Further experiments are needed to devise the appropriate model to describe these effects.

PHARMACODYNAMICS

As with many other agents, the interpatient variability in heparin dosage requirements is partly due to interpatient differences in its pharmacokinetics and partly due to interpatient variability in pharmacodynamics. Heparin pharmacodynamic indices of efficacy and safety are the prevention of thrombosis and the absence of hemorrhagic episodes due to excessive anticoagulation (see Tables 30-2a and 30-2b).

Clinical Response

The evidence that heparin is effective as an anticoagulant is well documented. The one randomized, controlled evaluation of anticoagulant versus placebo treatment of pulmonary embolism was abandoned after study of 35 patients, because 5 out of the 19 control patients died as a result of the embolism and another five had nonfatal recurrences. No recurrences arose among 16 patients given heparin.[42] In an appraisal of anticoagulation therapy for pulmonary embolism in 458 patients, 92% survived; this compares to a survival rate of only 42% in patients in whom anticoagulants were withheld due to medical contraindications.[43] Anticoagulation also lowered the incidence of recurrent pulmonary embolism from 47% to 8%.

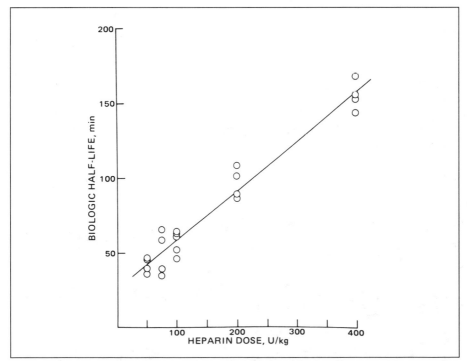

Figure 30-1. *Relationship between biological half-life and dose of heparin in humans when heparin activity in plasma is determined by a bioassay based on thrombin-induced clotting times. The line represents the best-fitted line for the relationship between these parameters (intercept, 26.2 minutes; slope, 0.323 min/kg/U^{-1}; $r^2 = 0.952$) (reprinted with permission from reference 41).*

Table 30–2a. Heparin Pharmacodynamics: Incidence of Bleeding Complications and Associated High Risk Groups[a]

No. of episodes treated	Mode of heparin therapy	Mean dosage (U/day)	Coagulation test used	Major bleeding (%)	Minor bleeding (%)	Patient groups with increased risk for bleeding	References
937	INT	45–90,000 (range)	—	0.5	1.0		44
82	INT	30–90,000 (range)	—	2.4	12.2	women	63
97	IV/SQ	—	CT	24.7		elderly, women	34
100	CONT	26,500	CT	1.0	3.0	CT >60 min	45
159	CONT	—	LWCT		6.3		64
147	INT	20–50,000	LWCT	10.9		elderly, women, CHF	65
42	CONT	—	CT	4.8	19.0		66
162	CONT	30,200	APTT	3.4	4.7	postoperative	46
72		28,300	APTT	11.1	15.3	elderly, women	
100	INT	—	WBCT	21.0	16.0	pre-existing anatomical or functional defects	56
72	INT	31,740	APTT	8.3	22.2	pre-existing anatomical or functional defects	56
68	INT	35,560	—	10.3	16.2	intermittent injections	
69	CONT	24,480	APTT	1.5	26.1		
36	INT	29,861	—	11.1	33.3	duration of therapy	55
40	CONT	33,074	APTT	15.0	22.5	elderly, women, trauma	
21	INT	32,808	APTT	33.3	47.6	elderly	47
20	CONT	25,488	APTT	0	30.0		
40	INT	37,015	WBCT, LWCT	10.0	27.5	soft tissue trauma	60
40	CONT	27,695	WBCT, LWCT	5.0	7.5	vascular damage, LWCTs >35 min for 2 consecutive days	
50	CONT	36,814	KCCT	8.0	8.0		67
19	CONT	<36,000	ACT, APTT	21.1			69
15	CONT	>36,000	ACT, APTT	0			
156	CONT	504[b]	ACT	6.4	21.1	surgery within 2 weeks, elderly, women	48

656	—	—		1.3	7.6	higher doses, elderly, women, severly ill, aspirin therapy, heavy alcohol use	62
13	INT	3,038[c]	APTT	30.8	—	elderly	61
15	CONT	3,270[c]	APTT	26.7	—	women	
29	INT	43,570	LWCT, APTT	17.3	13.8	high-risk patients receiving INT	49
36	CONT	28,440	LWCT, APTT	8.3	19.4	high-risk patients receiving INT	49
12	INT	360[b]	—	0	8.3		
16	CONT	360[b]	—	0	12.5		
7	INT	600[b]	—	14.3	14.3		
14	INT	600[b]	—	7.1	42.9		
67	CONT	510[b]	APTT	5.8	—		69
26	CONT	HIGH	—	7.7	15.4	major bleeding in 84.7% of patients with therapeutic ACT	53
95	CONT	CONV	ACT	11.6	12.6	major bleeding in 84.7% of patients with therapeutic ACT	53
131	CONT	19,700 MIN 25,600 MAX	APTT	9.9	7.6	serious concurrent disease	51
13	CONT	326[b]	—	7.7	30.8	elderly, women	
15	CONT	334[b]	APTT	6.7	53.3	higher doses	70
18	CONT	307[b]	TEG	0	33.3		
134	CONT	557[b]	ACT	1.5	11.9	ACT > 190 sec	54
280	CONT	370[b]	APTT	2.9	7.9	elderly, women	35
510	CONT	—	APTT	3.1	1.8	elderly	52

[a] Abbreviations: IV = Intravenous; SQ = Subcutaneous; INT = Intermittent injections; CONT = Continuous infusions; CT = Clotting time; APTT = Activated partial thromboplastin time; WBCT = Whole blood clotting time; LWCT = Lee White clotting time; KCCT = Kaolin cephalin clotting time; TEG = Thrombelastograph index; ACT = Activated clotting time; HIGH = 150 units/kg loading dose, 30–40 units/kg/hr maintenance dose; CONV = 25–50 units/kg loading dose, maintenance dose adjusted by ACT; MIN = Minimum mean daily dose; MAX = Maximum mean daily dose.

[b] Units/kg/day

[c] Units/kg in total therapy

Table 30–2b. Heparin Pharmacodynamics: Incidence of Thromboembolic Complications and Associated Mortality[a]

No. of episodes treated	Mode of heparin therapy	Mean dosage (U/day)	Coagulation test used	Recurrent thromboembolism (%)	Thromboembolic mortality (%)	References
54	INT	40,000	—	1.9	0	42
937	INT	45–90,000 (range)	—	2.6	0.5	44
82	INT	30–90,000 (range)	—	15.9	1.2	63
100	CONT	26,500	CT	3.0	1.0	45
159	CONT	—	LWCT	2.5	1.3	64
42	CONT	—	CT	2.4		66
162	CONT	30,200	APTT	3.1	0	46
100	INT	—	WBCT	2.0	2.0	56
72	INT	31,740	APTT	1.4	6.9	
68	INT	35,560	—	1.5	10.3	
69	CONT	24,480	APTT	1.5	8.7	
21	INT	32,808	APTT	0	2.5	47
20	CONT	25,488	APTT	2.5	10.0	
50	CONT	36,814	KCCT	20.0		67
19	CONT	<36,000	ACT, APTT	15.8	21.1	68
15	CONT	>36,000	ACT, APTT	0	20.0	
156	CONT	504[b]	ACT	0.6	0.6	48
29	INT	43,570	LWCT, APTT	3.4	10.3	49
36	CONT	28,440	LWCT, APTT	27.8	2.8	

12	INT	360[b]	—	16.7	8.3	
16	CONT	360[b]	—	25.0	12.5	
7	INT	600[b]	—	14.3	0	
14	INT	600[b]	—	0	0	
67	CONT	510[b]	APTT	1.5		69
26	CONT	HIGH	—	0	0	53
95	CONT	CONV	ACT	10.5	1.1	
13	CONT	326[b]	—	7.7		70
15	CONT	334[b]	APTT	0	0	
18	CONT	307[b]	TEG	0	0	
134	CONT	557[b]	ACT	0	0	54
280	CONT	370[b]	APTT	4.6	0.7	35

[a] Abbreviations: IV = Intravenous; SQ = Subcutaneous; INT = Intermittent injections; CONT = Continuous infusions; CT = Clotting time; APTT = Activated partial thromboplastin time; WBCT = Whole blood clotting time; LWCT = Lee White clotting time; KCCT = Kaolin cephalin clotting time; TEG = Thrombelastograph index; ACT = Activated clotting time; HIGH = 150 units/kg loading dose, 30–40 units/kg/hr maintenance dose; CONV = 25–50 units/kg loading dose, maintenance dose adjusted by ACT; MIN = Minimum mean daily dose; MAX = Maximum mean daily dose.

[b] Units/kg/day

[c] Units/kg in total therapy

The conclusions of these studies are supported by the results of many others which show a dramatically improved outcome in treated patients, and by studies relating outcome to the measured anticoagulant effect of treatment.[44-46]

High embolism and mortality rates are associated with venous thromboembolism that is not treated with anticoagulants. Zero percent to five percent of patients treated with adequate doses of intravenous heparin develop clinical evidence of recurrence, and the likelihood of fatal embolism during treatment is very low. There is good experimental evidence and persuasive clinical support that the risk of recurrence during treatment is greatest when the coagulation test results are consistently below the therapeutic range.[46-48] Basu et al.[46] found that recurrence of venous thromboembolism, based on clinical diagnosis, was related to an activated partial thromboplastin time (APTT) of less than 1.5 times the normal rate on two or more consecutive days during continuous intravenous heparin therapy. In a study by Wilson et al.[49] utilizing more objective diagnostic criteria, the same trend was found in patients being monitored with coagulation tests. Finally, Hull et al. demonstrated the need to maintain an adequate anticoagulation effect with heparin (APTT 1.5 to 2 times the control) for the initial treatment of patients with proximal vein thrombosis, no matter which route of heparin administration was used.[50]

Death from heparin-related hemorrhage is rare. Nelson et al.[51] reported three deaths in a collected series of 534 patients (0.56%), all due to intracerebral bleeding. Ramirez-Lassepas and Quinones[52] evaluated central nervous system hemorrhage in cerebral infarction patients treated with continuous intravenous heparin and found the risk to be low (0.8%). Because the reported rate of recurrent thromboembolism is as high as 18% with conventional heparin doses, several investigators have recommended aggressive, high-dose heparin therapy. Although higher doses of heparin have demonstrated lower recurrence rates and prompt resolution of symptoms, the incidence of hemorrhagic complications dramatically increases as doses are increased.[49,53] Wilson et al.[49] recommended that patients without risk factors for bleeding receive intermittent heparin therapy utilizing higher doses, because of fewer recurrences and no increase in hemorrhagic complications. Exceeding the normal values of "therapeutic" coagulation tests has been suggested to be predictive of these hemorrhagic complications.[45,48,49,54] However, Conti et al.[53] reported that 84.7% of patients experiencing major bleeding episodes had "therapeutic" activated clotting times (ACT). Mant et al.[55] found that neither heparin dose nor the APTT results could be related to bleeding complications (see Pharmacodynamics: Adverse Effects).

Several studies have described that a substantial part of the interpatient variation in heparin dosage requirements may be pharmacodynamic in nature.[45,46,56,57] This large interpatient variation in anticoagulant response to heparin can be demonstrated in vitro, when the anticoagulant effect is evaluated by APTT or activated clotting times (ACTs). Bjornsson demonstrated a twelvefold variation in the plasma heparin concentration required to yield a desired anticoagulant effect. The baseline APTT value accounted for more than 80% of the variability in the APTT-heparin slope values of sensitivity curves (r = 0.905; p <0.001).[40,58] The interpatient variability in heparin sensitivity is thought to be primarily due to varying concentrations or activities of the clotting factors involved. These studies suggest that the anticoagulant response to heparin can be predicted based on a pretherapy determination of APTT.[58,59]

Adverse Effects

The incidence of bleeding, particularly in patients with identified risk factors for bleeding, is significantly lower when heparin is administered by a continuous intravenous infusion than when it is given by intermittent injections.[47,49,56,60] In these studies, considerably larger total daily doses of heparin were given by the intermittent injections. By contrast, the heparin doses which Mant et al.[55] and Fagher et al.[61] used were larger in the continuous infusion group, and in these studies the frequency of major bleeding was higher in this group. What is apparent from these studies is that, in general, the risk of major bleeding increases sharply as doses increase. Regardless of differences in incidence of bleeding, continuous intravenous infusion is the recommended route of administration because it produces a more consistent degree of anticoagulation,[56] and it may be safer.

There is increasing evidence that the risk of bleeding is influenced not only by the dose and route of administration but also by several patient-related factors. When bleeding occurs during heparin therapy, it is often related to pre-existing hemostatic defects (uremia, drug-related defects of platelet aggregation, thrombocytopenia, liver disease) or to invasive procedures (cutdowns, arterial punctures, thoracenteses) and to patient factors such as gender and age.

It is essential that patients receiving heparin be monitored very closely to ensure an adequate degree of anticoagulation with minimal risk of heparin-associated bleeding. The most frequently encountered bleeding events include melena, hematomas, and hematuria, which occur in 2% to 3% of patients (see Table 30-3). In an extensive review of 2656 patients, Walker and Jick[62] identified numerous risk factors associated with both major and minor bleeding episodes in nonsurgical patients. These investigators determined the relative weight of each of these factors as a determinant of heparin bleeding risk.

Table 30-3. *Incidence and Type of Bleeding Episodes Associated with Heparin Therapy in Non-surgical Patients*[62]

Event	% of Patients
Melana	2.9
Hematoma	2.4
Hematuria	2.0
Ecchymosis	1.2
Epistaxis	0.8
Hematemesis	0.5
Intracranial hemorrhage	0.2
Pulmonary hemorrhage	0.2

The heparin dose (units/kg) was clearly the most important determinant of minor bleeding episodes.[62] When examined on a unit/kg/hr basis, there was over a threefold increase in the risk of bleeding in patients receiving 25 units/kg/hr as compared to patients who received less than 12.5 units/kg/hr. The linear regression analysis of six major heparin studies supports the relationship between total daily dose and the rate of major bleeding.[71] Heavy drinkers have nearly seven times the daily risk of moderate drinkers or nondrinkers in developing major bleeding complications associated with heparinization. Patients with substantial underlying morbidity have nearly a fourfold elevation in risk, and patients receiving concurrent aspirin therapy have a 1.5- to 2.5-fold increase in risk. Women have approximately a twofold greater risk of bleeding than their male counterparts. This gender difference is further exaggerated when age is examined as an additional risk factor. Jick[34] reported that elderly females have approximately a 50% risk of experiencing bleeding complications when receiving heparin. In general, the risk of bleeding not only varies with dose as well as numerous patient factors, but also increases with the length of heparin therapy. The seven-day cumulative risk of bleeding during heparin therapy is 9.1%. This cumulative risk increases with the length of therapy, and by three weeks of continuous heparin therapy, bleeding occurs in nearly 20% of patients (see Figure 30-2).[62] Wheeler et al. reported a cumulative

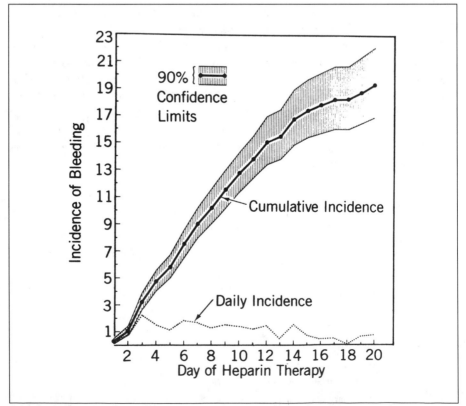

Figure 30-2. *Daily and cumulative risks of heparin sodium therapy (percent incidence of bleeding) as derived from a life table analysis (reprinted with permission from reference 62).*

bleeding incidence of 18.5%.[8] These authors found no correlation between the APTT or the rate of heparin infusion with major or minor bleeding, and no significant differences by gender among patients with and without bleeding.

Landefeld et al.[72] reported the following four predictors of major bleeding in hospitalized patients starting anticoagulant (warfarin or heparin) therapy:

• co-morbid conditions (heart, liver, or kidney dysfunction, cancer, and severe anemia)
• the use of heparin therapy in patients greater than 60 years of age
• the intensity of anticoagulation
• liver dysfunction that worsened during therapy

The risk of bleeding increased with the number of co-morbid conditions present and was more likely to occur in patients receiving intravenous heparin than warfarin. While the frequency of bleeding was similar among males and females, patients aged 60 to 79 years and those more than 80 years of age were 4.7 and 8.5 times more likely to develop major bleeding, respectively, than patients who received no heparin therapy or those less than 60 years of age.

Heparin-associated thrombocytopenia has been well documented as a serious complication necessitating careful monitoring of platelet counts.[73-76] This complication of heparin therapy can result in loss of limb and can be life threatening. The incidence has not been well established; however, it is reported to range from 1% to 30% in various patient populations receiving heparin.[73-77] It is unknown whether monitoring should focus on the absolute drop in platelet count or on the relative decrease in circulating platelets. Heparin-associated decreases in platelet count can result in cerebral infarction, acute myocardial infarction, arterial occlusions, hemorrhages, or death.[74,75,78,79] Careful monitoring of platelet counts can minimize the risk of heparin-associated thrombocytopenia. Before heparin administration, all patients should have a quantitative platelet count determined, and the platelet count should be monitored every two to three days for the duration of heparin therapy. The continuation of heparin and the need for alternative antithrombotic therapy must be evaluated in patients experiencing a substantial decline of platelet count (i.e., greater than 30%) and/or a drop in platelet count below 100,000/mm³.[79] Switching therapy to heparin manufactured from another source (e.g., beef lung or porcine mucosa) is not recommended because of the high incidence of cross-sensitivity between products.

CLINICAL APPLICATIONS OF PHARMACOKINETIC DATA

Interindividual differences in the *in vivo* anticoagulant response to heparin are largely a result of variations in heparin pharmacokinetic parameters and interindividual sensitivity. The lack of a reliable direct chemical assay for heparin has led several investigators to explore the relationship between *in vitro* coagulation test times (APTT or ACT) and heparin concentration in units/mL. Heparin sensitivity curves are graphic descriptions of the magnitude of an individual's anticoagulant response to heparin at various concentrations. The mathematical models used for heparin curves vary among investigators,[16,40,57,80] but in general, the slope and intercept of the separate sensitivity curves are used to quantitate interindividual variations in *in vitro* anticoagulant response and heparin concentrations (see Figures 30-3, 30-4, and 30-5).

In vitro sensitivity curves have been demonstrated to be highly correlated with an individual's *in vivo* response to varying heparin concentrations. There is wide variation in individual responses to heparin, which was first recognized by deTakats in 1943 as a major factor influencing heparin dosage requirements.[81] Until Estes[28] and Hirsh et al.[27] described methods to determine a patient's sensitivity to heparin, clinicians could only speculate about differences among patients. Hirsh[27] used a heparin sensitivity curve (change in APTT versus heparin concentration) to quantitate observed interindividual variations in response. In our investigation of patients, a pretreatment sensitivity curve was established for each patient to describe the relationship between a measured APTT and the corresponding heparin concentration.[16] These sensitivity curves allowed us to examine the relationships between patient variables, pharmacokinetic parameters, and heparin

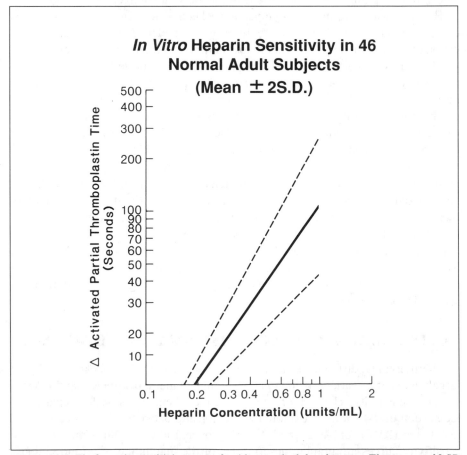

Figure 30-3. *The heparin sensitivity curves for 46 normal adult volunteers. The mean and 2 SD are represented. Intersubject variability is demonstrated by the wide ranges in APTT resulting from similar heparin concentrations. At 0.5 units/mL, the change in APTT ranged from approximately 22 seconds to 75 seconds.*

dosage requirements. Earlier work by Whitfield and Levy[59] employed a modification of a heparin sensitivity curve to determine whether individual differences in heparin sensitivity were predictable from certain physiological characteristics.

In normal volunteers, hematocrit and baseline APTT yielded the best correlation between predicted and actual slope values for the heparin sensitivity curves.[59] However, a test of the predictability of these two independent variables in hospitalized patients demonstrated an over-prediction of heparin sensitivity slope values. In this patient group, baseline APTT, total protein concentration, and factor XI were the best predictors of slope.[80] In a similar study of pregnant women, baseline APTT did not correlate with heparin sensitivity slopes.[82] The predictability of slope can vary with the patient population studied and may disappear as a function of altered physiological states.

Our investigations support the evidence that variability in patients' pretreatment heparin sensitivity is an important factor in determining dosage requirements.[16] Pretreatment heparin sensitivities varied widely among our 20 patients. Examination of the slopes and intercepts revealed a 500% range in heparin

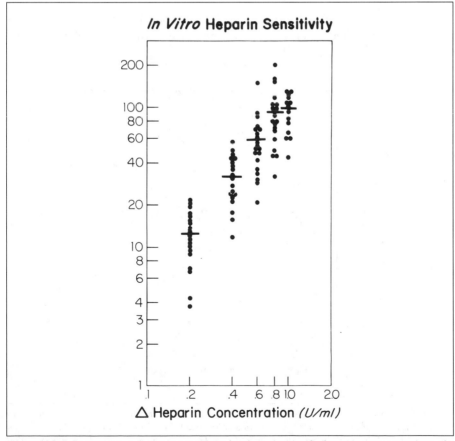

Figure 30-4. *Pretreatment heparin sensitivity* in vitro. *At specific heparin concentrations, the response as measured by APTT varied widely among 20 patients (reprinted with permission from reference 16).*

sensitivities. A heparin concentration of 0.4 units/mL resulted in a change in APTTs ranging from 11 to 57 seconds (see Figure 30-4). Heparin dosage regimens were calculated to produce an APTT of approximately twice baseline APTT and ranged from 500 to 2000 units/hr. The mean dose required, standardized to TBW, was 13.9 units/kg/hr (range, 8.6 to 19.8 units/kg/hr). A multiple-regression model was developed from TBW, gender, time delay from the onset of symptoms, and smoking. The multiple-regression model explained 78% of the variance in dosage requirements (see Equation 30-1). The use of pretreatment heparin sensitivity data to prospectively quantitate heparin dosage requirements is promising, but it needs much further examination.

$$\text{Dose in units/hr} = [(11.3)\,(\text{TBW in kg})] - [(255.7)\,(\text{gender})]$$

$$- [(2.5)\,(\text{onset in hours})] + [(211.9)\,(\text{smoking})] + 352.3 \qquad \text{(Eq. 30-1)}$$

where gender = 1 for males, 2 for females; smoking = 1 for nonsmokers, 2 for smokers; and onset = time between onset of signs (symptoms) and initiation of heparin therapy.

Hattersley et al.[54] demonstrated a log linear relationship between the ACT and heparin concentration. After a bolus injection of heparin, the ACT approaches

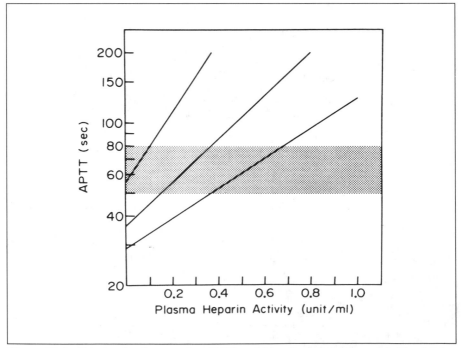

Figure 30-5. Relationship between log APTT and heparin activity (in units/mL) added to plasma. Shown are the best-fitted lines of this relationship for 3 of 20 subjects, the ones with the steepest and the shallowest slopes and a subject with an intermediate slope. The stippled area represents a range of commonly observed APTT values during heparin anticoagulation. Note that any given anticoagulant effect is caused by different plasma heparin activities in these three subjects (reprinted with permission from reference 58).

infinity and then falls by apparent first-order kinetics, with a half-life ranging from 30 to 200 minutes. Bull et al.[83] demonstrated that, even at very high doses, the ACT response to heparin remained linear to greater than 400 seconds. Thus, there is probably a linear relationship between the continuous infusion rate and the resultant plasma heparin concentration. This relationship has been used to derive an equation that relates the log of the anticoagulant effect of heparin (log ACT) to the amount of drug administered. The following equation has been proposed for calculating a required heparin infusion rate from a patient's initial infusion rate and coagulation times:

$$R_2 = R_1 \cdot \frac{(\log ACT_2 - \log ACT_0)}{(\log ACT_1 - \log ACT_0)} \qquad \text{(Eq. 30-2)}$$

where R_2 = required heparin administration rate; R_1 = initial heparin administration rate; ACT_2 = desired clotting time; ACT_1 = initial clotting time after the initial administration rate; and ACT_0 = baseline clotting time.

The application of this equation was applied retrospectively to 20 patients treated with continuous heparin infusion. The mean calculated dose (R_2) ranged from 15 to 36.3 units/kg/hr, with a corresponding mean ACT_2 of 173.5 seconds. These model-calculated doses compared closely with actual doses required to produce therapeutic ACTs (150 to 190 seconds). The mean calculated dose was 25.8 units/kg/hr, and the mean actual adjusted dose was 27.9 units/kg/hr. The correlation of calculated heparin dose to actual adjusted dose was significant ($r = 0.86$; $p > 0.05$). These investigators noted that their model is valid only if heparin clearance and sensitivity do not change with concentration or over the period of observation.

Groce et al. recently compared the conventional dosing of heparin based on APTT measurements with a method of individualizing heparin dosage requirements using whole blood heparin concentrations.[84] The individualized doses were calculated to maintain a steady-state heparin concentration of 0.45 units/mL using each patient's apparent heparin clearance. Clearance was determined from two non-steady-state heparin concentrations (C_1 and C_2, in units/mL) collected one hour (t_1) and four hours (t_2) after the beginning of a heparin infusion. Clearance (CL) was calculated by the method of Chiou et al.[85]

$$CL = \frac{2 R_o}{(C_1 + C_2)} + \frac{2 V_d (C_1 - C_2)}{(C_1 + C_2)(t_2 - t_1)} \qquad \text{(Eq. 30-3)}$$

where R_o is the heparin infusion rate (units/hr) and V_d is the apparent volume of distribution equal to the patient's estimated blood volume (mL). The mean heparin dose at 24 hours was 15.5 units/kg/hr for the 17 conventionally dosed patients and 20.5 units/kg/hr for the 15 individualized-dosed patients. Patients with individualized heparin doses had no APTT values less than 1.5 times control, faster symptomatic improvement (1.64 ± 0.5 versus 2.87 ± 0.95 days), and shorter hospital stays (6.43 ± 1.6 versus 8.76 ± 2.08 days) compared to the patients with conventionally derived dosage regimens. The authors concluded that the use of clinical pharmacokinetics to individualize heparin therapy offers substantial benefits over conventional dosing methods.[84]

Mungal and Floyd evaluated the use of a pharmacokinetic-pharmacodynamic Bayesian forecasting model to predict APTT response in 21 patients receiving continuous intravenous heparin, with and without concurrent warfarin administration.[86] A significant relationship was noted between observed and predicted APTT before warfarin therapy ($r = 0.82$; $p < 0.05$) and after starting warfarin therapy ($r = 0.69$; $p < 0.05$). Based on the predictive performance of the model, heparin dosages can be adjusted early in therapy with one or two APTTs to rapidly attain a therapeutic APTT. The model is useful in adjusting heparin doses in the presence of warfarin therapy by accounting for warfarin's effect to prolong APTT values.[87]

Several other dosing and monitoring protocols have been suggested.[87–89] The cost:benefit ratio of determining each patient's heparin requirements using a systematic and quantitative approach can be demonstrated by the following experience in our medical center. Over a four-year period, we followed the progress of 238 consecutive patients treated with intravenous heparin for thromboembolic events. The first 212 patients, 75 of whom were treated by our Medical/Surgical Services and 137 by Neurology Services, received traditional heparin therapy consisting of a loading dose of 5000 units followed by an initial infusion rate of 1000 units/hr. Dosages were then adjusted by monitoring APTT and/or TT tests. In 1982 we instituted an individualized approach to heparin therapy in Neurology Services. Each patient received a loading dose of 50 units/kg followed by an initial infusion of 15 units/kg/hr. Dosages were then adjusted by monitoring APTT and/or TT tests 6 to 12 hours after the continuous infusion was begun or changed. The efficiency of these dosages based on patient TBW was evaluated by determining the number of patients with therapeutic coagulation tests by the end of 24 and 48 hours of heparin therapy. We also evaluated the mean number of days required to therapeutically heparinize those patients. The results in Table 30-4 show that the mean number of days required to produce optimal heparin therapy based on coagulation times was reduced by 0.6 to 0.9 days by individualized dosing. The heparin doses based on patient TBW resulted in therapeutic coagulation tests in

Table 30-4. *Time Required for Therapeutic Heparinization*[a]

| | Traditionally dosed | | Individually dosed |
	Med-Surg	Neurology	Neurology
Number of patients	75	137	26
% Therapeutic			
by day 1	24%	39%	69%
by day 2	68%	82%	92%
Mean days to therapeutic	2.3 days	2.0 days	1.4 days

[a] There was a mean reduction of 0.6 days in the time required to therapeutically heparinize patients when initial doses were individually determined based on patient TBW. All individually dosed patients received loading doses of 50 units/kg and initial maintenance doses of 15 units/kg/hr TBW.

69% of patients in the first 24 hours compared to only 24% and 39% of patients receiving traditional doses. Wheeler et al.[8] reported that traditional fixed dose approaches to heparin therapy failed to produce therapeutic APTTs in 60% of patients during the critical first 24 hours of therapy. This simple, patient-specific approach exemplifies the value of applying the pharmacodynamic and pharmaco-kinetic heparin data that are presently available.

Cost considerations for the hospital management of heparin therapy have been reviewed at the Mayo Clinic.[91] Rooke and Osmundson concluded that measures such as shortening the duration of heparin therapy, minimizing the laboratory

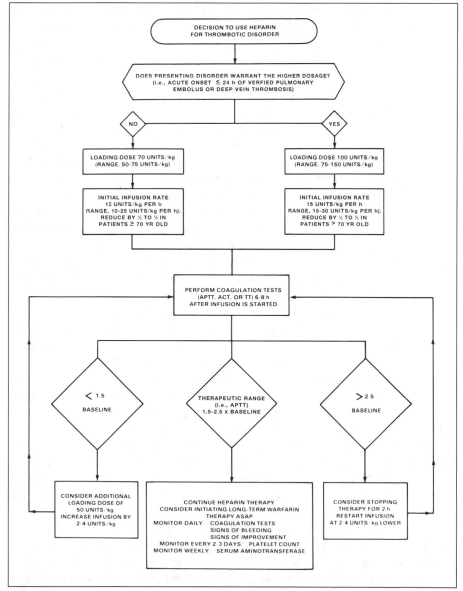

Figure 30-6. Algorithm.

monitoring of heparin in patients with low risk of bleeding, and administration of heparin by alternative routes (e.g., subcutaneous) can substantially reduce the cost of treating deep vein thrombosis. Two studies have now demonstrated the effectiveness and safety associated with a short course of continuous intravenous infusion heparin (four to five days, with warfarin started on the first day of therapy) compared to the traditional ten-day course of heparin (with warfarin started on the fifth day of therapy).[92,93] The effective use of a shorter course of heparin therapy can substantially reduce the cost of treating thromboembolic diseases.

To date, the most efficient method for providing patients with rapid and effective heparin anticoagulation is for the clinician to consider available heparin pharmacokinetic and pharmacodynamic data to determine individual initial dosages, systematically monitor coagulation studies, and then make quantitative dosage adjustments as indicated. Following a loading dose (50 to 150 units/kg) and an initial infusion rate (10 to 30 units/kg/hr), it is imperative that blood samples for coagulation tests (i.e., APTT) used to make heparin dosage adjustments be well planned and carefully timed (see Algorithm, Figure 30-6). Although heparin is most commonly administered by continuous infusion, it is essential that samples be collected as close to steady state as possible. This requires that after beginning the heparin infusion, or following any dosage change, the clinician wait at least six hours (and preferably eight hours) to draw coagulation tests to assess the effect of the heparin dose. Samples collected too early are often misleading, resulting in inappropriate dosage alteration; this can also start a costly cycle of "dosage change-coagulation test-another dosage change-another coagulation test" in a clinically stable patient. As described earlier, the risk of bleeding is minimal during the first 48 hours of heparin therapy (in patients without identified risk factors), and coagulation tests are primarily helpful to ensure adequate heparinization. Therefore, it is often most efficient to wait until steady-state conditions exist to monitor coagulation and make dosage alterations.

When a continuous infusion is not feasible, therapeutic heparin can be administered by intermittent intravenous injections. Heparin half-lives range from 0.4 to 2.5 hours; therefore, four-hour dosing intervals are appropriate for most patients. Coagulation tests are best performed 3.5 to 4 hours following the heparin injection. It is imperative to time and document carefully both the injection time and the time the coagulation test sample is drawn. The heparin dosage is considered adequate when the coagulation test collected 3.5 hours after an intravenous injection is in the therapeutic range for that test (i.e., APTT of 1.5 to 2.5 times baseline).

It is essential that blood for coagulation tests drawn just prior to one of the four-hour intermittent injections ("trough") is not assumed to represent a 3.5- to 4-hour sample. Because of the rapid clearance of heparin, any variation in the time after an injection that a sample is drawn can result in erroneous coagulation test results and substantial dosage errors.

Once a heparin dose has been determined which produces the desired degree of anticoagulation, daily monitoring of coagulation tests for minor dosage adjustments is indicated. Large variations in subsequent coagulation tests necessitate investigations to ensure that the patient's condition has not dramatically changed (i.e., extension or recurrence of the thromboembolic event) and that the patient is not developing thrombocytopenia. These two conditions can alter heparin dosage requirements. Additionally, before dosages are dramatically altered based on fluctuating coagulation test results, the clinician must ensure that the prescribed heparin dose is being administered accurately and that patient samples are being collected and assayed appropriately. If substantial heparin dosage changes are made, the new therapy needs to be monitored in a manner similar to initial heparin therapy (i.e., APTT six to eight hours after the new continuous infusion dose).

When monitoring a patient receiving intravenous heparin therapy, it is important to carefully collect information documenting adequate anticoagulation as well as data which can assist in minimizing the potential bleeding complications. Laboratory monitoring should be performed at the same time of the day (e.g., every morning) to minimize the influence of circadian variation on APTT values during heparin therapy.[94-98] Wheeler et al.[8] identified the following five common practices that led to delays or less intense anticoagulation (APTT less than 1.5 times control) in heparinized patients: 1) failure to start heparin therapy at the time of initial clinical impression; 2) suboptimal dosages; 3) delay in measuring the APTT; 4) inadequate response to an APTT less than 1.5 times the control; and 5) excessive and prolonged reductions in heparin dosing in response to an APTT greater than three times the control. These authors believe that the basis of these problems arises from the clinician's poor understanding of heparin's pharmacokinetics and the exaggerated fear of bleeding complications.

Coagulation tests should be performed before the initiation of heparin therapy for the following purposes: 1) to establish the patient's individual baseline value to determine the therapeutic endpoint of heparin therapy from a laboratory standpoint. For example, the usual therapeutic endpoint (range) using the APTT is 1.5 to 2.5 times the patient's baseline; 2) to establish a baseline prothrombin time (PT) as a guide for continued oral anticoagulation with warfarin.

Another baseline laboratory parameter is a platelet count which should be repeated every two or three days during therapy and following the discontinuation of therapy, to ascertain the risk of thrombosis and/or hemorrhage from heparin-associated thrombocytopenia. Hemoglobin and hematocrit measurements are indicated before heparinization and then every one to two days while the patient is receiving heparin to identify the presence of bleeding. These laboratory parameters are especially useful in determining the existence of retroperitoneal hemorrhage. Sputum, urine, and stool should be examined daily for the presence of blood.

Heparin-induced elevations in serum aminotransferases have been reported. Dukes et al.[99] reported that 95% of patients had elevations in their aminotransferase concentrations while exposed to heparin. These abnormalities return to normal after heparin is discontinued, and persistent hepatic damage has not been identified. Heparin-induced enzyme elevations do not appear to be related to the drug's interference with the laboratory test. This phenomenon has potential diagnostic implications in that serum aminotransferases are commonly used in the differential diagnosis of several thrombotic events, including pulmonary emboli and acute myocardial infarction.[99]

Patients should be examined twice daily for signs of bleeding which include hemorrhage at intravenous sites, hematomas, and ecchymosis. No intramuscular injections should be administered to patients receiving therapeutic heparinization. Additionally, invasive procedures which can be rescheduled should not be performed on heparinized patients.

The signs and symptoms of the thrombotic event requiring heparin therapy must be carefully monitored as well. The signs and symptoms of pulmonary embolism should be monitored frequently at first, followed by daily monitoring for changes in dyspnea, apprehension, cough, pleuritic chest pain, hemoptysis, and arterial blood gases. Additionally, repeat lung scans and/or perfusion-ventilation studies may be indicated to assess progress of antithrombotic therapy. Similarly, patients being treated for venous thrombosis should be initially monitored twice daily and then daily for changes in pain, tenderness, swelling, and redness. Patients being treated with heparin for cerebrovascular thrombotic disorders, including transient ischemic attacks (TIA), reversible ischemic neurologic deficits (RIND), and cerebral infarctions without hemorrhage, must be monitored every six to eight hours initially and then daily for changes in their neurologic status, including weakness, syncope, hemiparesis and hemiplegia.

In addition to the above-mentioned laboratory and clinical parameters, clinicians must be aware of other practical concerns in patients receiving heparin. Hattersley et al.[100] reported that the four most common errors associated with heparin therapy were: 1) lack of pump precision; 2) interruption in the continuous infusion; 3) errors in preparation of the solution containing the heparin dose; and 4) errors in charting the dose administered. For the intravenous administration of continuous-infusion heparin, reliable volumetric infusion pumps should be used. Every effort should be made not to interrupt the continuous infusions. During a one-hour interruption, the APTT can fall from 60 seconds (therapeutic) to less than 40 seconds; hence, interruptions in the infusion that exceed 30 to 60 minutes may require additional bolus injections. Any interruption needs to be well documented.

Unfortunately, errors in the preparation of heparin solutions for continuous intravenous administration still occur. The pharmacies preparing these solutions should initiate protocols to standardize the concentrations of all heparin solutions for adult patients. Heparin sodium can be administered in sodium chloride- or dextrose-containing solutions. Solutions containing either 50 units/mL or 100 units/mL are optimal in most situations. Standardized concentrations can reduce errors in calculating infusion rates while allowing maximum flexibility in adjusting individualized patient heparin doses. Utilizing the standard concentrations for heparin infusions, patient-specific doses should be rounded to the nearest 50 units/hr in adult patients. It is essential that when heparin is added to a flexible PVC container, thorough mixing occurs to assure even distribution of drug and to avoid potentially life-threatening overdoses. Bergman and Vellar[101] demonstrated that without thorough mixing (i.e., inverting and agitating the container six times before initiating the infusion) a patient might receive up to 70% of the total amount of heparin in the container during the first hour of infusion.

Finally, in order to interpret a coagulation test, it is essential to know the actual rate of infusion. Failure to adequately document and chart heparin infusion rates can lead to potentially serious errors. The importance of this problem is exemplified by the Boston Collaborative Drug Surveillance Program which involved 2656 heparinized patients. The actual heparin doses received could not be determined in 30% of the patients because of inadequate chart documentation.[62]

ADJUSTED-DOSE SUBCUTANEOUS HEPARIN

Several randomized trials now suggest that intermittent, adjusted-dose subcutaneous heparin is a safe and effective alternative route of therapy for the initial treatment of venous thrombosis (see Table 30-5).[50,67,102–104] Dosage and monitoring guidelines for subcutaneous heparin therapy are empiric. Most authors initiate heparin therapy with 15,000 units or 250 units/kg administered subcutaneously every 12 hours. Coagulation tests (APTT) are performed as follows: 1) before the initiation of heparin therapy; 2) four to six hours after the first subcutaneous dose; and 3) once daily at the middle of the dosing interval. The initial dose of subcutaneous heparin can be rapidly adjusted after the first 12 hours of therapy according to the APTT value drawn with the first dose. The mid-interval sampling period for subsequent monitoring has been chosen because this sampling period predicts the maximal response of APTT after subcutaneous injection and the sustained therapeutic response throughout the 12-hour dosing interval.

Major and minor hemorrhagic complications have been similar during intravenous and subcutaneous heparin administration (see Table 30-5). To minimize the excessive incidence of injection site bruising and hematoma, proper subcutaneous administration techniques must be employed. As with continuous intravenous heparin therapy, adjusted-dose subcutaneous heparin must be administered to maintain an APTT above 1.5 times the control value. Failure to rapidly achieve and maintain adequate anticoagulation significantly increases the risk of recurrent venous thromboembolic events.[50]

LOW-MOLECULAR-WEIGHT HEPARIN (LMWH)

Low-molecular-weight heparins (LMWHs) are undergoing extensive clinical trials.[105] LMWHs are prepared by fractionation or depolymerization, resulting in commercial products with a molecular weight between 4000 and 6000 Daltons. The LMWHs selectively enhance the inhibition of some proteases, including X_a, but have a weak effect on thrombin. Difficulty in comparing efficacy and toxicity of some of the early clinical LMWH trials[106] resulted in the establishment of the first international standard for LMWH.[107] The new LMWH standard was established by the World Health Organization (WHO) in 1986, with an assigned unitage of 1680 International Units (IU) per ampule by anti-X_a assay and 665 IU per ampule by anti-II_a assay.[108]

The pharmacokinetics of LMWH differ from those of conventional heparin (see Table 30-6).[109,110] The subcutaneous bioavailability of LMWH is greater than 90% compared to less than 20% of conventional heparin using a Factor X_a assay. The elimination half-lives of LMWH are two- to fourfold longer than conventional heparin, ranging from three to five hours. The elimination process of LMWH does not appear to be dose dependent. Although optimal dosage schedules for every

Table 30-5. Adjusted-Dose Subcutaneous Heparin Pharmacodynamics:: Incidence of Thromboembolic Complications and Bleeding Complications[a]

No. of episodes treated	Mode of heparin therapy	Mean dosage (units/day)	Recurrent thromboembolism (%)	Major bleeding (%)	Minor bleeding (%)	References
50	SQ	36,997	2	4	2	67
50	CONT	36,814	20	8	8	
72	SQ	500[b]	0	2.8	2.8	102
69	CONT	450[b]	0	2.9	0	
57	SQ	33,000	19.3	3.5	1.8	50
58	CONT	32,219	5	3.5	3.5	
51	SQ	29,180	10.6	7.8	2.0	103
52	CONT	29,260	10.2	3.9	5.8	
50	SQ	29,375	4.1	0	4	104
50	CONT	24,384	26.5	0	4	

[a] Abbreviations: SQ = Subcutaneous; CONT = Continuous infusions.
[b] Units/kg/day.

LMWH have not been established, initial investigations indicate that adequate anti-X_a activity can be maintained for 12 to 24 hours following a single subcutaneous injection; dosages should be based on an "unit/kg" basis.[111,112]

There is a significant relationship between the anti-X_a levels and bleeding.[113] In trials that measured anti-X_a levels and reported a low incidence of major bleeding (0% to 1%), the anti-X_a levels were between 0.1 units/mL and 0.2 units/mL. In trials reporting higher incidence of bleeding (2% to 10%), anti-X_a levels were 0.4 to 0.6 units/mL. While one of the initial intentions for the development of LMWHs was their very low risk of producing major bleeding, it must be emphasized that several trials have not demonstrated that LMWHs produce less bleeding than conventional heparin therapy.[114,115]

LMWHs can effectively be used for prophylaxis of thromboembolism.[116,117] LMWHs may serve as an alternative therapy for patients with heparin-induced thrombocytopenia, bleeding complications, and other side effects.[118,119] The data to support their use for the treatment of active thrombotic events are still lacking and need to be established.[117,120]

ANALYTICAL METHODS

The anticoagulant activity of heparin is the result of its interaction with the coagulation pathway at several steps. Heparin prolongs a number of tests which have been used to determine its pharmacokinetic parameters as well as to measure its anticoagulant activity. When reviewing data describing the pharmacokinetics of heparin, the clinician must recognize that heparin pharmacokinetic parameters

Table 30-6. *Difference of Low Molecular Weight Heparins (LMWHs) to Conventional Heparin and Differences Among LMWHs Deducted by Comparative Human Pharmacologic Studies*[a,109]

Pharmacologic property	Differences between LMWH and conventional	Differences among LMWHs
↑ factor X_a inhibition	+	+
Prolonged t½ on Factor X_a	+	+
>90% bioavailability Factor X_a	+	−
↑ anti-X_a / APTT ratio	+	+
↑ anti-X_a to anti-II_a ratio	+	+
100% protamine interaction	+	−
Protamine neutralization of APTT and thrombin	+	−
Release of glucosaminoglycans	+	+
↑ fibrinolytic potential	+	+/−
↑ lipolytic activities	+	+
↓ platelet factor 4 interaction	+	+
Less thrombocyte interaction	+	+/−
Less antigenic	+	+/−
Do not pass placenta	+	−

[a] + = Difference is present; − = Difference is not present.

are assay-dependent. It has been demonstrated that there are significant differences in pharmacokinetic parameters obtained from studies using similar patient populations and doses but different heparin assay methods. Heparin volumes of distribution and total clearances have been reported to be 1.5 to 2 times larger when heparin was assayed by polybrene neutralization than when APTT or TT tests were used.[23]

Tests most commonly used to monitor heparin therapy can be performed with whole blood, platelet-rich plasma, or platelet-poor plasma (see Table 30-7). Since platelets contain a cationic protein (platelet factor 4) which possesses antiheparin activity, an argument might be made for measuring the anticoagulant activity of heparin in whole blood or platelet-rich plasma. However, tests performed on platelet-poor plasma are convenient and appear to be quite satisfactory. Since clinical effectiveness depends in part on heparin activity, it is this measurement rather than a determination of heparin concentration that has been of most interest to clinicians. In general, coagulation assays either determine the effect of heparin on the clotting system in general or the effect of heparin on the rate of inactivation of specific clotting proteases. The whole blood clotting time and the APTT are examples of the most commonly used global tests for monitoring heparin therapy. Coagulation assays involving the inactivation of specific clotting proteases include the TT and the X_a inhibition test.

The APTT has become the most popular test for monitoring heparin therapy. This popularity is largely due to its suitability for use in routine clinical laboratories, the rapidity with which it can be performed, and its reproducibility. The APTT can also be used as a screening test for all coagulation factors except VII and XIII. It is most sensitive to intrinsic factors XII, XI, and VIII. The APTT can be disproportionately prolonged in the presence of fibrin degradation products and in patients with hypofibrinogenemia (i.e., less than 100 mg/dL). Patients with severe hepatic disease or vitamin K deficiencies as well as those undergoing warfarin therapy, those with lupus erythematosus, and those with deficiencies of factors VIII, IX, XI, or XII also will have prolonged APTTs. It is important to note that the APTT can be affected to a great extent by the various commercially available reagents, the instrument used, and the anticoagulant used in the sample collection system.[23,39,40,59] The two major disadvantages to using the APTT to monitor heparin therapy are its inability to distinguish between the anticoagulant activity of heparin and several clotting factor deficiencies and the fact that the instrumentation used requires that the APTT be performed in a laboratory. This latter fact significantly increases the turnaround time and delays adjustment in heparin dosages compared with the coagulation tests that can be performed at the bedside or within the operating room. Conversely, bedside coagulation tests do not lend themselves to standardized quality control procedures as do the laboratory-based APTT and TT. There is a high degree of interpatient variability in baseline APTT values and APTT-heparin slopes; therefore, it is more appropriate to use the individual patient's pretreatment baseline APTT as a reference point for treatment responses rather than a laboratory-determined normal range or control

Table 30-7. Comparison of Heparin Assay Methods

Global tests of coagulation system used to regulate heparin dosage	Performed at the bedside (B) or laboratory (L)	Sample material tested	Normal reference range[a]	Therapeutic range	Advantages	Disadvantages
Lee White–Whole Blood Clotting Time (WBCT)	B	Whole blood	6–14 min	1.5–3 × control	Standard with which newer tests are compared.	Time consuming; unreliable; insensitive.
Activated Coagulation Time (ACT)	B	Whole blood	80–130 sec	150–190 sec 400–600 sec[b]	Very rapid and readily available.	Lacks reproducibility with clotting times >600 seconds.
Activated Partial Thromboplastin Time (APTT)	L	Plasma	28–42 sec	1.5–3 × unheparinized baseline	Most commonly used test; nationally recognized standards available; rapid and readily automated.	Variable results with different reagents and instruments; each lab must establish its own therapeutic range.
Harem and BaSon Tests	B	Whole blood	120–150 sec	160–300 sec	Similar to APTT, but performed at bedside with good agreement with WBCT.	Wide normal range with no quality control; labor-intensive; insensitive; more complicated than ACT.

Tests used to estimate heparin concentrations

Thrombin time (TT)	L	Plasma	13–20 sec	50–100 sec at a 1:4 dilution	Sensitive to low concentrations of heparin, fibrinogen, fibrin split products; reliable.	Time consuming; labor-intensive.

Table 30–7. Comparison of Heparin Assay Methods (cont.)

Global tests of coagulation system used to regulate heparin dosage	Performed at the bedside (B) or laboratory (L)	Sample material tested	Normal reference range[a]	Therapeutic range	Advantages	Disadvantages
Protamine neutralization, polybren neutralization	L	Plasma	N/A	0.2–0.4 units/mL[c]	Sensitive to low concentrations of heparin.	Requires multiple steps and dilutions if high heparin concentrations present.
Fluorogenic substrate	L	Plasma	N/A	0.2–0.4 units/mL	More directly measures heparin concentration; automation possible.	Cannot indicate if patient is resistant to heparin; complicated; time consuming.
Chromogenic substrate	L	Plasma	N/A	0.2–0.4 units/mL	More directly measures heparin concentration; automation possible.	Cannot indicate if patient is resistant to heparin; complicated; time consuming.

[a] May vary with laboratory.

[b] This is for patients on extracorporeal circulation and represents the average effect of 2–5 units/mL of heparin.[78]

[c] Average range and may vary depending on variables such as antithrombin III, platelet factor 4 and circulating inhibitors.

values. This is especially important in patients with short APTTs due to elevated levels of clotting factors such as factor VIII. Normal adult reference values vary among laboratories and range from 28 to 42 seconds.

The TT also is frequently used to monitor heparin therapy. It is initiated by adding a known concentration of thrombin to an aliquot of plasma. The TT measures only Factor II_a conversion of fibrinogen to fibrin. The TT is affected by the amount and quality of fibrinogen in the plasma being tested and also by substances present in the plasma which inhibit the conversion of fibrinogen to fibrin, such as heparin, antithrombin III, and fibrinogen (fibrin) degradation products. Like the APTT, the TT utilizes platelet-poor plasma; however, it is extremely sensitive to low concentrations of heparin. Heparinized patient plasma can be diluted with standard normal plasma pool to improve the accuracy of the TT test. The specificity and sensitivity to heparin make the TT test very useful in the clinical setting.

Normal adult reference values vary with laboratories and range from 13 to 20 seconds. The thrombin time dilution is required when sufficient heparin is present to prolong the thrombin time to greater than 120 seconds. Most commonly used dilutions are 1:2, 1:4, and 1:8 using the standard normal plasma pool. Therapeutic heparinization is represented by a thrombin time of 50 to 100 seconds at a 1:4 dilution. A broader therapeutic range may be applied in certain clinical situations.

The ACT is a global test most frequently used to monitor heparin doses during hemodialysis, extracorporeal circulation for cardiac surgery, and extracorporeal membrane oxygenation therapy. Although less sensitive to low heparin concentrations than the APTT and TT tests, the ACT has the advantage of producing rapid results at the bedside or in the operating room. ACT systems vary, but they usually require small amounts of whole blood (0.2 to 2 mL) to which an activator is added. A controlled heating device is used to time the production of a clot which is detected photo-optically. Convenient and simple, the ACT does not have to be performed within the coagulation section of the laboratory. Thus, clinicians using the ACT to monitor heparin doses need to ensure that appropriate quality control procedures are followed in the setting in which the ACT is performed. The variability in ACT test results is significantly increased by variations in volume of blood tested, speed or direction of the agitation of the tubes, intermachine variability, and interpersonnel technique.[122] The relationship of change in ACT and heparin concentration, within the ranges useful in clinical practice, has recently been quantitated by the use of an automated system for monitoring heparin therapy. This linear relationship can be described by the equation:

$$\Delta ACT = 16.85 + 136.7 (C) \qquad \text{(Eq. 30-4)}$$

where C represents heparin concentration in units/mL.

With this type of technology and knowledge now available, rapid determination of pharmacokinetic and pharmacodynamic parameters and the relationships between these variables should help clinicians improve the efficacy and safety of heparin therapy.[123] Generally, normal adult values are 80 to 130 seconds. Heparin therapy is considered adequate when the ACT is 150 to 190 seconds. Heparin doses are commonly considered optimal when the ACT is 30 to 60 seconds above the pretreatment baseline value in hemodialysis patients.

The introduction of chromogenic substrates has also enhanced the possibility of using automated systems to determine heparin activity as well as concentrations. These assays are based on the inactivation of thrombin or Factor X_a by the heparin-antithrombin III complex. Anti-X_a assays are based on inhibition of a known amount of Factor X_a, which is measured using a synthetic peptide chromogenic or fluorogenic substrate. Since the inactivation rate of thrombin is dependent on the amount of antithrombin III present in the sample, two assay procedures are possible:

- **Heparin Activity.** Heparin exerts its inhibitory effect only through antithrombin III already present in the patient's sample. The thrombin activity measured after incubation with the patient's plasma sample reveals the biological activity of heparin.
- **Heparin Concentration.** Through addition of excess antithrombin III to the reaction mixture, the rate of inactivation of thrombin by heparin-antithrombin III becomes independent of the antithrombin III concentration in the plasma and dependent on the concentration of heparin in plasma; hence, heparin concentration can be determined.

When monitoring heparin therapy, one must determine that the plasma contains an adequate quantity of antithrombin III and that heparin has increased the reaction rate between antithrombin III and the clotting proteases. The APTT and anti-X_a assays can indirectly provide this information. What is not yet known, however, is the degree of heparin-induced increase in antithrombin III reactivity required to prevent the propagation of a thrombotic episode.

Determining the most appropriate coagulation assay to use is difficult. Clearly, clinicians must use the coagulation test which is the most reproducible within each institution. The choice of the APTT by many investigators and clinicians can be attributed to several reasons. Prolongation of the APTT is considered evidence that heparin therapy is producing an anticoagulant effect on the intrinsic coagulation pathway. Additionally, the APTT is convenient, is the most commonly available assay for heparin monitoring, and can be subjected to good laboratory quality control procedures. However, preliminary data indicate that quantitating the actual heparin concentration may be more helpful in predicting bleeding tendencies. Holm et al.[128] studied 237 patients with phlebographically documented deep vein thrombosis. Approximately 70% of the blood samples taken from patients with major blood loss had heparin concentrations (measured by chromogenic anti-X_a assay) that indicated excessive doses. Only 38 of these patients were identified by the APTT, and 22% of those with major blood loss were identified by excessive prolongation of the thrombin time.

PROSPECTUS

To achieve the maximal therapeutic response from a drug with complex pharmacological actions like those of heparin, rapid and effective patient monitoring tools are required. These types of technology and information are available to interpret pharmacokinetic data and support dosing decisions in clinical practice. However, most patients requiring heparin therapy still are given an empirically derived dose which is then adjusted based on an APTT, TT, or the ACT. These approaches to practice are semiquantitative and do not provide sufficient information to identify patients at risk of treatment failure or bleeding. Improved coagulation test methodology coupled with the incorporation of other patient factors such as weight, height, baseline coagulation status, pretreatment heparin sensitivity values and heparin concentrations can be used to improve the accuracy of heparin dose determination. Practitioners have been slow to adopt these improvements. Computer-based systems are now available to assist clinicians in quantitating dosage requirements, estimating bleeding risks, and storing patient dose-response relationships for future therapy modifications. Such computer programs allow the practitioner to predict the effect of various heparin doses on coagulation tests and, thereby, select an optimal patient-specific pharmacotherapeutic plan. The result should be a more systematic and quantitative approach to dosing heparin than changing the dose based solely on the last ACT or APTT value measured.

Several decades after worldwide use of heparin to treat and prevent serious and life-threatening thromboembolic disorders, common dosing and monitoring practices still result in subtherapeutic or potentially toxic heparin exposure in a substantial number of patients. In the report by Wheeler et al.,[124] 60% of patients did not have a single partial thromboplastin time greater than 1.5 times control within the critical first day of heparin therapy. Common practices which led to delays in achieving adequate heparinization included the inappropriate choice of an initial heparin bolus dose and continuous infusion dose insufficient to produce the desired outcome. Additionally, this report recognized the problem of ineffective heparin dosing changes in response to low or high APTT measurements.[124] Similarly, while heparin is the accepted anticoagulant during hemodialysis, there is considerable disagreement as to the optimum dosage regimen. A recent survey of the 33 dialysis units in the United Kingdom indicated no consensus regarding approaches to heparin dosage during dialysis and a fourfold difference in what was perceived to be the appropriate heparin dose. This lack of objective guidelines for anticoagulation makes comparison of various trials difficult and complicates any proposed evaluation of alternative approaches to anticoagulant therapy.[125] This ineffectiveness and inefficiency is still too common in practice and is a direct result of a poor understanding of heparin pharmacokinetics. Improvements are needed that will enhance patient outcomes, reduce laboratory expenditures, and minimize practitioner time required to monitor and adjust heparin therapy.

The standardization of heparin products on a unit basis has played an important role in the use of this naturally occurring substance. The purity of heparin has continually improved over the years, so that 10,000 international units of activity require approximately 50 to 60 mg of heparin based on the most current (i.e., 1984) standard, whereas formerly, comparable activity required about 100 mg.[126]

The most recent major development in the area of anticoagulation products is the introduction of low molecular weight heparins (LMWHs), which are now licensed for use in several countries. The development of these fractionated heparin products for clinical use will have a substantial impact on the treatment and prevention of thromboembolic disorders. The new LMWH Standard was established by the World Health Organization in 1986, with an assigned unitage of 1680 IU per ampule by anti-X_a assay and 665 IU per ampule by anti-II_a assay. A lack of early adherence to this proposed international standard has made it difficult to compare efficacy and toxicity results of some early clinical trials of LMWH products.[126] The pharmacokinetics of LMWH preparations are clearly different from those of the unfractionated heparin products. LMWH has a longer elimination half-life which has been exploited in early investigations to permit single daily dosing by subcutaneous injection. Research that compares the efficacy of LMWH preparations in the treatment of active thrombotic events to the established efficacy of unfractionated products is still lacking.[127]

Analytical methods are available to provide easy measurement of heparin concentrations and effect, allowing the determination of the relationship between heparin concentration and pharmacological response. Future improvements in automated coagulation technology will be extremely useful not only in the clinical environment, where rapid and accurate information is required, but also as a research tool to better define the therapeutic and toxic concentrations in various patient populations receiving heparin products for the treatment or prevention of thromboembolic disorders. There is a clinically significant relationship between LMWH levels determined by anti-X_a assay and bleeding. LMWH preparations have been demonstrated to provide effective prophylaxis and are associated with a low risk of major bleeding as long as their concentrations do not exceed 0.2 units/mL. LMWH doses which result in anti-X_a concentrations greater than 0.4 units/mL significantly increase the risk of post-operative bleeding.[113]

These LMWH products will improve our ability to control anticoagulation therapy because both drug concentrations as well as effect on the clotting system will be quantifiable in patients receiving these products. Additionally, if these products are demonstrated to produce more consistent, predictable anticoagulant responses, clinicians will have a new pharmacological tool which may readily lend itself to patient-controlled, home-based anticoagulant pharmacotherapy.

REFERENCES

1. McLean J. The thromboplastin action of cephalin. Am J Physiol. 1916;41:250–57.
2. Lam CR. The strange story of Jay McLean, the discoverer of heparin. Henry Ford Hosp Med J. 1985;33:18–23.
3. Bottiger LE. The heparin story: in search of the early history of heparin. Acta Med Scand. 1987;222:195–200.
4. Charles AF, Scott DA. Studies on heparin I. J Biol Chem. 1933;102:425–29.
5. Charles AF, Scott DA. Studies on heparin II. J Biol Chem. 1933;102:431–35.
6. Hyers TM et al. Antithrombotic therapy for venous thromboembolic disease. Chest. 1989;95(Suppl.):37S–51S.
7. Hirsh J. Heparin therapy in venous thromboembolism. Ann NY Acad Sci. 1989;556:378–85.
8. Wheeler AP et al. Physician practices in the treatment of pulmonary embolism and deep venous thrombosis. Arch Intern Med. 1988;148:1321–325.
9. Wright CJ, Jaques LB. Heparin via the lung. Can J Surg. 1979;22:317–19.
10. Mahadoo J et al. Vascular distribution of intratracheally administered heparin. Ann NY Acad Sci. 1981;370:650–55.

11. Hull R et al. Adjusted subcutaneous heparin versus warfarin sodium in the long-term treatment of venous thrombosis. N Engl J Med. 1982; 306:189–94.

12. Thomas DP et al. Plasma heparin levels after administration of calcium and sodium salts of heparin. Thromb Res. 1976;9:241–48.

13. Low J, Biggs JC. Comparative plasma heparin levels after subcutaneous sodium and calcium heparin. Thromb Haemost. 1978;40:397–406.

14. Dawes J, Papper DS. Catabolism of low-dose heparin in man. Thromb Res. 1979;14:845–60.

15. Beermann B, Lahnborg G. Pharmacokinetics of heparin in healthy and obese subjects and in combination with dihydroergotamine. Thromb Haemost. 1981;45:24–26.

16. Cipolle RJ et al. Heparin kinetics: variables related to disposition and dosage. Clin Pharmacol Ther. 1981;29:387–93.

17. Talstad I. Heparin therapy adjusted for body weight. Am J Clin Pathol. 1985;83:378–81.

18. Ellison MJ et al. Calculation of heparin dosage in a morbidly obese woman. Clin Pharm. 1989;8:65–68.

19. McDonald MM et al. Heparin clearance in the newborn. Pediatr Res. 1981;15:1015–18.

20. McDonald MM, Hathaway WE. Anticoagulant therapy by continuous heparinization in newborn and older infants. J Pediatr. 1982;101:451–57.

21. Andrew M et al. Heparin clearance and *ex vivo* recovery in newborn piglets and adult pigs. Thromb Res. 1988;52:517–27.

22. Andrew M et al. The comparison of the pharmacokinetics of a low molecular weight heparin in the newborn and adult pig. Thromb Res. 1989;56:529–39.

23. Bjornsson TD et al. Heparin kinetics determined by three assay methods. Clin Pharmacol Ther. 1982;31:104–13.

24. Bjornsson TD et al. Effects of N-deacetylation and N-desulfation of heparin on its anticoagulant activity and *in vivo* disposition. J Pharmacol Exp Ther. 1988;245:804–808.

25. Hoffmann JJ. The plasma concentration of heparin. In: Merkus FW, ed. The serum Concentration of drugs: Clinical Relevance, Theory and Practice. 1980:135–243.

26. Stau T et al. Exogenous ^{35}S-labeled heparin: organ distribution and metabolism. Naunyn Schmiedenbergs Arch Pharmacol. 1973;280:93.

27. Hirsh J et al. Heparin kinetics in venous thrombosis and pulmonary embolism. Circulation. 1976;53:691–95.

28. Estes JW. Clinical pharmacokinetics of heparin. Clin Pharmacokinet. 1980;5:204–20.

29. Simon TL. Heparin kinetic studies. In: Lundblad RL et al., eds. In: Chemistry and Biology of Heparin. New York: Elsevier North Holland; 1981:597–614.

30. Bjornsson TD. Clinical pharmacology of heparin. In: Turner P, Shand DG, eds. Recent Advances in Clinical Pharmacology. New York: Churchill Livingstone; 1983:129–55.

31. McAvoy TJ. Pharmacokinetics modeling of heparin and its clinical implications. J Pharmacokinet Biopharm. 1979;7:331–54.

32. de Swart CAM et al. Kinetics of intravenously administered heparin in normal humans. Blood. 1982;60:1251–258.

33. Simon TL et al. Heparin pharmacokinetics: Increased requirements in pulmonary embolism. Br J Haematol. 1978;39:111–20.

34. Jick H et al. Efficacy and toxicity of heparin in relation to age and sex. N Engl J Med. 1968;279:284–86.

35. Tenero DM et al. Comparative dosage and toxicity of heparin sodium in the treatment of patients with pulmonary embolism versus deep-vein thrombosis. Clin Pharm. 1989;8:40–53.

36. White TM et al. Continuous heparin infusion requirements: Diagnostic and therapeutic implications. JAMA. 1979;241:2717–720.

37. Perry PJ et al. Heparin half-life in normal and impaired renal function. Clin Pharmacol Ther. 1974;16:514–19.

38. Teien AN, Bjoornson J. Heparin elimination in uraemic patients on haemo-dialysis. Scand J Haematol. 1976;17:29–35.

39. Sette H et al. Heparin response and clearance in acute and chronic liver disease. Thromb Haemost. 1985;54:591–94.

40. Bjornsson TD, Wolfram KM. Intersubject variability in the anticoagulant response to heparin *in vitro*. Eur J Clin Pharmacol. 1982;21:491–97.

41. Bjornsson TD. Dose-dependent decreases in heparin elimination. J Pharm Sci. 1982;71:1186–188.

42. Barritt DW, Jordan SC. Anticoagulant drugs in the treatment of pulmonary embolism: a controlled trial. Lancet. 1960;1:1309–312.

43. Pollak EW et al. Pulmonary embolism: an appraisal of therapy in 516 cases. Arch Surg. 1973;107:66–68.

44. Bauer G. Clinical experience of a surgeon in the use of heparin. Am J Cardiol. 1964;14:29–35.

45. O'Sullivan EF et al. Heparin in the treatment of venous thromboembolic disease: administration, control, and results. Med J Aust. 1968;2:153–59.

46. Basu D et al. A prospective study of the value of monitoring heparin treatment with the activated partial thromboplastin time. N Engl J Med. 1972;287:324–27.

47. Glazier RL, Crowell EB. Randomized prospective trial of continuous vs intermittent heparin therapy. JAMA. 1976;236:1365–367.

48. Kashtan J et al. Heparin therapy for deep venous thrombosis. Am J Surg. 1980;140:836–40.

49. Wilson JE et al. Heparin therapy in venous thromboembolism. Am J Med. 1981;70:808–16.

50. Hull RD et al. Continuous intravenous heparin compared with intermittent subcutaneous heparin in the initial treatment of proximal-vein thrombosis. N Engl J Med. 1986;315:1109–114.

51. Nelson PH et al. Risk of complications during intravenous heparin therapy. West J Med. 1982;136:189–97.

52. Ramirez-Lassepas M, Quinones MR. Heparin therapy for stroke: hemorrhagic complications and risk factors for intracerebral hemorrhage. Neurology. 1984;34:114–17.

53. Conti S et al. A comparison of high-dose versus conventional-dose heparin therapy for deep vein thrombosis. Surgery. 1982;92:972–80.

54. Hattersley PG et al. Heparin therapy for thromboembolic disorders: a prospective evaluation of 134 cases monitored by the activated coagulation time. JAMA. 1983;250:1413–416.

55. Mant MJ et al. Haemorrhagic complications of heparin therapy. Lancet. 1977;1:1133–135.

56. Salzman EW et al. Management of heparin therapy: controlled prospective trial. N Engl J Med. 1975;292:1046–50.

57. Seifert R et al. Heparin kinetics during hemodialysis: variation in sensitivity, distribution volume, and dosage. Ther Drug Monit. 1986;8:32–36.

58. Bjornsson TD, Wolfram KM. Determinants of the anticoagulant effect of heparin in vitro. Ann NY Acad Sci. 1981;370:656–61.

59. Whitfield LR, Levy G. Relationship between concentration and anticoagulant effect of heparin in plasma of normal subjects: magnitude and predictability of interindividual differences. Clin Pharmacol Ther. 1980;28:509–16.

60. Wilson JR, Lampman J. Heparin therapy: a randomized prospective study. Am Heart J. 1979;97:155–58.

61. Fagher B, Lundh B. Heparin treatment of deep vein thrombosis: effects and complications after continuous or intermittent heparin administration. Act Med Scand. 1981;210:357–61.

62. Walker AM, Jick H. Predictors of bleeding during heparin therapy. JAMA. 1980;244:1209–212.

63. Kernohan PJ, Todd C. Heparin therapy in thromboembolic disease. Lancet. 1966;1:621–23.

64. Dale WA, Lewis MR. Heparin control of venous thromboembolism. Arch Surg. 1970;101:744–55.

65. Vieweg WVR et al. Complications of intravenous administration of heparin in elderly women. JAMA. 1970;213:1303–306.

66. Martyn DT, Janes JM. Continuous intravenous administration of heparin. Mayo Clin Proc. 1971;46:347–51.

67. Bentley PG et al. An objective study of alternative methods of heparin administration. Thromb Res. 1980;18:177–87.

68. Hunter G et al. Low- versus high-dose heparin in the treatment of pulmonary embolism. Vasc Surg. 1980;14:238–42.

69. Andersson G et al. Subcutaneous administration of heparin: a randomized comparison with intravenous administration of heparin to patients with deep-vein thrombosis. Thromb Res. 1982;27:631–39.

70. Caprini JA et al. Laboratory monitoring of continuous heparin therapy. Thromb Res. 1983;29:91–94.
71. Morabia A. Heparin doses and major bleedings. Lancet. 1986;1:1278–279. Letter.
72. Landefeld CS et al. Identification and preliminary validation of major bleeding in hospitalized patients starting anticoagulant therapy. Am J Med. 1987;82:703–13.
73. Ansell JE et al. Heparin-induced thrombocytopenia: what is its real frequency. Chest. 1985;88:878–82.
74. Warkentin TE, Kelton JG. Heparin-induced thrombocytopenia. Ann Rev Med. 1989;40:31–44.
75. Cola C, Ansell J. Heparin-induced thrombocytopenia and arteria thrombosis: alternative therapies. Am Heart J. 1990;119:368–74.
76. Powers PJ et al. Studies on the frequency of heparin-associated thrombocytopenia. Thromb Res. 1984;33:439–43.
77. Cipolle RJ et al. Heparin-associated thrombocytopenia: a prospective evaluation of 211 patients. Ther Drug Monit. 1983;5:205–11.
78. Silver D et al. Heparin-induced thrombocytopenia, thrombosis, and hemorrhage. Ann Surg. 1983;198:301–306.
79. Ramirez-Lassepas M et al. Heparin-induced thrombocytopenia in patients with cerebrovascular ischemic disease. Neurology. 1984;34:736–40.
80. Whitfield LR et al. Relationship between concentration and anticoagulant effect of heparin in plasma of hospitalized patients: magnitude and predictability of interindividual differences. Clin Pharmacol Ther. 1982;32:503–16.
81. deTakats G. Heparin tolerance. Surg Gynecol Obstet. 1943;77:31–39.
82. Whitfield LR et al. Effect of pregnancy on the relationship between concentration and anticoagulant effect of heparin. Clin Pharmacol Ther. 1983;34:23–28.
83. Bull BS et al. Heparin therapy during extracorporeal circulation. J Thorac Cardiovasc Surg. 1975;69:674–84.
84. Groce JB et al. Heparin dosage adjustment in patients with deep-vein thrombosis using heparin concentrations rather than activated partial thromboplastin time. Clin Pharm. 1987;6:216–22.
85. Chiou WL et al. Method for the rapid estimation of the total body drug clearance and adjustment of dosage regimens in patients during a constant-rate intravenous infusion. J Pharmacokinet Biopharm. 1978;6:135–51.
86. Mungall D, Floyd R. Bayesian forecasting of APTT response to continuously infused heparin with and without warfarin administration. J Clin Pharmacol. 1989;29:1043–47.
87. Hauser VM, Rozek SL. Effect of warfarin on the activated partial thromboplastin time. Drug Intell Clin Pharm. 1986;20:964–67.
88. Fennerty AG et al. Guidelines to control heparin treatment. Br Med J. 1986;292:579–78.
89. Felding P et al. Adjusted-dose intravenous heparin treatment evaluation of an automated and a nonautomated schedule. Thromb Res. 1988;51:447–52.
90. Saya FG et al. Pharmacist-directed heparin therapy using a standard dosing and monitoring protocol. Am J Hosp Pharm. 1985;42:1965–969.
91. Rooke TW, Osmundson PJ. Heparin and the in-hospital management of deep venous thrombosis: cost considerations. Mayo Clin Proc. 1986;61:198–204.
92. Gallus A et al. Safety and efficacy of warfarin started early after submassive venous thrombosis or pulmonary embolism. Lancet. 1986;2:1293–296.
93. Hull RD et al. Heparin for 5 days as compared with 10 days in the initial treatment of proximal venous thrombosis. N Engl J Med. 1990;322:1260–264.
94. Decousus HA et al. Circadian changes in anticoagulant effect on heparin infused at a constant rate. Br Med J. 1985;290:341–44.
95. Schved JF et al. Circadian changes in anticoagulant effect on heparin infused at a constant rate. Br Med J. 1985;290:1286. Letter.
96. Johnston KR et al. Circadian changes in anticoagulant effect on heparin infused at a constant rate. Br Med J. 1985;290:792. Letter.
97. Scully MF et al. Measurement of heparin in plasma: influence of intersubject and circadian variability in heparin sensitivity according to method. Thromb Res. 1987;46:447–55.

98. Fagrell B et al. Changes of activated partial thromboplastin time during constant intravenous and fixed intermittent subcutaneous administration of heparin. J Intern Med. 1989;225:257–60.

99. Dukes GE et al. Transaminase elevations in patients receiving bovine or porcine heparin. Ann Intern Med. 1984;100:646–50.

100. Hattersley PG et al. Sources of error in heparin therapy of thromboembolic disease. Arch Intern Med. 1980;140:1173–175.

101. Bergman N, Vellar ID. Potential life-threatening variations of drug concentrations in intravenous infusion systems. Med J Aust. 1982;2:270–72.

102. Andersson G et al. Subcutaneous administration of heparin: a randomized comparison with intravenous administration of heparin to patients with deep-vein thrombosis. Thromb Res. 1982;27:631–39.

103. Doyle DJ et al. Adjusted subcutaneous heparin or continuous intravenous heparin in patients with acute deep vein thrombosis: a randomized trial. Ann Intern Med. 1987;107:441–45.

104. Walker MG et al. Subcutaneous calcium heparin versus intravenous sodium heparin in treatment of established acute deep vein thrombosis of the legs: a multicentre prospective randomized trial. Br Med J. 1987;294:1189–192.

105. Johnson EA et al. Four heparin preparations: anti-X_a potentiating effect of heparin after subcutaneous injection. Thromb Haemost. 1976;35:586–91.

106. Thomas DP. Biologicals, standards and heparin. Thromb Haemostas. 1989;62:648–650.

107. Barrowcliffe TW et al. Standardization of low molecular weight heparins: a collaborative study. Thromb Haemost. 1985;54:675–79.

108. Barrowcliffe TW et al. An international standard for low molecular weight heparin. Thromb Haemost. 1988;60:1–7.

109. Harenberg J et al. Comparative human pharmacology of low molecular weight heparins. Semin Thromb Hemostas. 1989;15:414–23.

110. Bara L, Samana M. Pharmacokinetics of low molecular weight heparins. Acta Chir Scand. 1988;543(Suppl.):65–72.

111. Doutremepuich C et al. Is there an optimal therapeutic range for low molecular weight heparin? An experimental study. Thromb Res. 1988;50:575–81.

112. Vitoux JF et al. Should thromboprophylactic dosage of low molecular weight heparin be adapted to patient's weight. Thromb Haemost. 1988;59:120. Letter.

113. Levine MN, Hirsh J. An overview of clinical trials of low molecular weight heparin fractions. Acta Chir Scand. 1988;543:73–9.

114. Breddin HK. Low molecular weight heparins and bleeding. Semin Thromb Hemost. 1989;15:401–404.

115. Barrowcliffe TW, Thomas DP. Low molecular weight heparins: antithrombotic and haemorrhagic effects and standardization. Acta Chir Scand. 1988;543:57–64.

116. Salzman EW. Heparin for prophylaxis of venous thromboembolism. Ann NY Acad Sci. 1989;556:371–77.

117. Samana M et al. Clinical studies with low molecular weight heparins in the prevention and treatment of venous thromboembolism. Ann NY Acad Sci. 1989;556:386–405.

118. Messmore HL. Clinical potential of low molecular weight heparins. Semin Thromb Hemost. 1989;15:405–408.

119. ten Cate H et al. Clinical studies with low-molecular weigh heparin(oid)s: an interim analysis. Am J Hematol. 1988;27:146–53.

120. Levine MN, Hirsh J. Clinical use of low molecular weight heparins and heparinoids. Semin Thromb Hemost. 1988;14:116–25.

121. Gerson B. Essentials of Therapeutic Drug Monitoring. New York: Igaku-Shoin Medical Publishers;1983:273–83.

122. Uden DL et al. Procedural variables which affect activated clotting time test results during extracorporeal membrane oxygenation therapy. Critical Care Medicine. 1989;17:1048–51.

123. Cipolle RJ et al. Evaluation of a rapid monitoring system to study heparin pharmacokinetics and pharmacodynamics. Pharmacotherapy. 1990;10(6):367–72.

124. Wheeler AP et al. Physician practices in the treatment of pulmonary embolism and deep venous thrombosis. Arch Intern Med. 1988;148:1321–325.
125. Lane DA et al. Equivalent effective doses of heparin and low molecular weight heparin(oid)s in haemodialysis for chronic renal failure. Acta Chir Scand Suppl. 1988;543:101–104.
126. Duncan TP. Biologicals, standard and heparin. Thromb Haemost. 1989;62:648–50.
127. Elliott CG et al. Heparin requirements in pulmonary embolism and venous thrombosis: a prospective study. J Clin Pharmacol. 1982;22:102–109.
128. Holm HA et al. Heparin treatment of deep venous thrombosis in 280 patients: Symptoms related to dosage. Acta Med Scand. 1984;215:47–53.

Chapter 31

Warfarin

R. Stephen Porter and William T. Sawyer

Warfarin [1-(4'-hydroxy-3'coumarinyl)-1-phenyl-3 butanone] is one of a series of synthetic anticoagulant compounds (see Figure 31-1) developed at the University of Wisconsin in the 1940s.[1-3] Although the first report of its clinical use in 1941 described the compound as a therapeutic agent on the basis of very limited data, clinical and experimental evidence of warfarin's efficacy as an antithrombotic agent has since accumulated.[4-7] The pharmacodynamics and pharmacokinetics of warfarin also have been extensively studied, in part because of the relative ease with which the anticoagulant action of the drug can be quantified and the plasma warfarin concentration measured. The development of the prothrombin time assay provided a routinely available means of monitoring the drug-induced clotting defect in plasma.[8] It also has allowed for documentation and exploration of the interpatient variability in warfarin dose-response relationships and dosage requirements which have been observed in use.[5,9,10]

Notwithstanding almost 50 years of clinical experience, several important questions regarding warfarin use remain: 1) Which patients should receive warfarin therapy and for how long? 2) What procedures should be used to assess the risk-benefit ratio of warfarin therapy in an individual patient? 3) How should the individual therapeutic dosage of warfarin be determined? 4) How should drug effects be properly monitored? Certainly, in the current drug development environment these questions would have been answered before marketing. Furthermore, several issues not raised in 1941 are of particular concern today, including: 1) the need for a more complete understanding of the pathophysiology of the thrombotic process, as well as the way in which warfarin affects these processes; 2) the relevance of animal research data to drug effects in humans; 3) the questionable use of the prothrombin time as a measure of warfarin response when the test primarily predicts the risk of bleeding rather than demonstrating warfarin's antithrombotic effect; and 4) the scientific merit of the results of early investigations of the warfarin pharmacokinetics and pharmacodynamics when the limitations of the analytical techniques used are considered.[11]

When the logical extension of warfarin's pharmacological effect is hemorrhage, it is not surprising that the clinician is faced with a certain amount of "pharmaco-

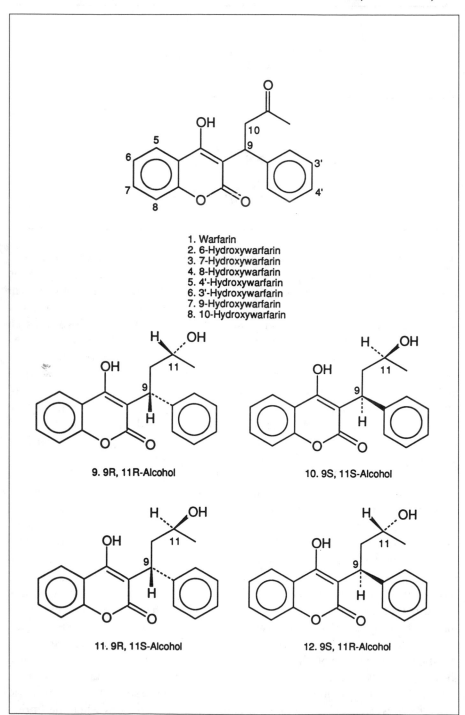

1. Warfarin
2. 6-Hydroxywarfarin
3. 7-Hydroxywarfarin
4. 8-Hydroxywarfarin
5. 4'-Hydroxywarfarin
6. 3'-Hydroxywarfarin
7. 9-Hydroxywarfarin
8. 10-Hydroxywarfarin

9. 9R, 11R-Alcohol

10. 9S, 11S-Alcohol

11. 9R, 11S-Alcohol

12. 9S, 11R-Alcohol

Figure 31-1. Warfarin metabolism in man is complex including: a) keto reduction to warfarin via NADH-catalyzed warfarin reductase to alcohols, each enantiomer yielding two diastereoisomers; b) hydroxylation reactions yielding regioisomeric products including 6, 7, 8, 3', 4' and 9' hydroxy (benzylic) warfarin; and c) dehydration of 9-hydroxywarfarin to yield 9,10 dehydrowarfarin.

logic catatonia." Therefore, it is important that three particular issues be explored: 1) Should the clinical use of warfarin anticoagulants be expanded, or should alternative agents be more aggressively investigated? 2) Can pharmacokinetic/ pharmacodynamic methods be routinely applied to the clinical management of warfarin therapy? 3) Should patients monitor their own therapy?

CLINICAL PHARMACOKINETICS

The pharmacokinetics of warfarin have been extensively studied, and several reviews of various pharmacokinetic characteristics of the drug have been published.[12-14] Commercially available warfarin is a racemic mixture of two optical stereoisomers of either the potassium or sodium salt. Warfarin potassium is a white crystalline powder; warfarin sodium is a white amorphous or crystalline powder. Both are very soluble in water and freely soluble in alcohol. Warfarin sodium powder was also previously available as a lyophilic compound which could be used for injection following reconstitution with sterile water.[15] However, commercial production of this preparation has been discontinued.

Absorption

Warfarin sodium is rapidly and extensively absorbed from the gastrointestinal tract.[16,17] Coumarin derivatives are also absorbed percutaneously, and cases of severe hemorrhagic toxicity and death in Vietnamese children exposed by repeated skin contact to contaminated talc have been reported.[18,19] However, the drug's oral absorption is of principal clinical interest. The absorption of oral warfarin is dissolution-rate-controlled, and the rate and extent of absorption of the drug may vary from one commercially available tablet to another.[15] Although early literature suggested a late-absorption pattern,[20] more recent data have demonstrated that peak absorption occurs between 60 to 90 minutes after oral tablet administration.[16] Breckenridge and Orme administered ^{14}C-warfarin to four subjects who ultimately were continued on warfarin therapy for deep vein thrombosis.[16] Eight normal volunteers were also given 20 mg vitamin K_1 by mouth prior to warfarin administration. In the four subjects given ^{14}C-warfarin, 61% to 92% of ^{14}C-warfarin radioactivity was measured in the urine. The wide variance in absorption most probably reflected the fact that the urine was collected for an inadequate period of time (four days) in two of the four subjects. Plasma warfarin concentrations peaked between 25 minutes and one hour in eight other subjects given warfarin tablets 0.5 mg/kg orally. These same eight subjects, after a two week period of time, were given a second warfarin dosage as an intravenous injection. Comparing the area under the curves of the oral and intravenous data, the mean bioavailability of the intravenous doses was between 77.6% and 100% of the oral dose. The completeness of warfarin absorption after oral administration has been further confirmed by pharmacodynamic studies showing similarity between hypoprothrombinemic response curves observed after oral and intravenous administration.[6] Warfarin does not exhibit dose dependency in the rate or extent of absorption, and enantiomer-specific differences in absorption patterns have not been reported.

In a study comparing bioavailability among four commercial products, the area under the warfarin plasma concentration-time curve (AUC) varied from 87% to 101% of the reference product and were considered "satisfactory."[21] However, variance of 5% to 10% of a warfarin sodium dosage may lead to an appreciable change in the degree of anticoagulation in the face of a small and seemingly acceptable difference in the bioavailability. An unwanted change in the patient's prothrombin times may also result if the brand of warfarin product is cross-prescribed, even though product bioavailability is considered to be comparable.[22] Comparative bioavailability trials between Panwarfarin and Coumadin and between Sofarin and Coumadin have shown no differences in clinical effectiveness, dissolution, or absorption.[23] However, changes in patient anticoagulant response have been noted after interchange of different brands of oral warfarin, and such practices may require additional monitoring immediately after such a change.[24]

Distribution

Extensive investigations of the *in vivo* and *in vitro* protein binding of warfarin analogs (see Table 31-1) have used plasma samples from patient populations and have noted protein binding to be 97.4% to 99.9% under normal physiologic conditions.[25-37] Many of these studies are methodologically flawed, however, because of nonspecific binding, use of impure radiolabelled warfarin,[38] and dilutional or Donnan effects associated with the equilibrium dialysis procedures employed.[39]

Albumin is the principal plasma protein fraction that binds warfarin. Warfarin binding sites on serum albumin include one primary and one secondary site.[40] Isomeric affinity for the primary binding sites appears to differ, with greater binding of the R-isomer than the S-isomer; therefore, warfarin protein binding has chirality.[31,37] Within the plasma concentration ranges associated with a therapeutic response, the degree of protein binding appears to be independent of the total

Table 31-1. Warfarin Binding to Plasma Proteins

Configuration	Concentration (µg/mL)	Bound %	Protein	Assay[a]	References
R/S warfarin	1.0	99.99	Undiluted serum	RED	31
	11.0	97.4	HSA	RED	32
	5.0	99.13	HSA	RED	33
	10.0	99.12	HSA	RED	33
	2–8	99.4	Plasma	RED	34
	4.6–9.2	98.91	Undiluted serum	SPF	35
	55.0	99	HSA	SPF	36
	2.0	99	HSA	SPF	36
R(+) warfarin	1.0	99.98	Undiluted serum	RED	31
	10.0	99.15	Plasma	SIST	37
S(−) warfarin	1.0	99.99	Undiluted plasma	SIST	37
	10.0	99.47			

[a] RED = Radioisotope equilibrium dialysis; SPF = Spectrofluorescent probes; SIST = Stable isotope technique.

plasma drug concentrations.[29] Yacobi et al. demonstrated significant intersubject variability in the extent of protein binding at therapeutic concentrations; however, the intrasubject variability was much less substantial.[30]

The ratio of the apparent volumes of distribution of the R- and S-enantiomers of 1.6 is almost identical to the "free" fraction ratios of 1.58.[37] Previous reports have suggested that the anticoagulant potency of the S-warfarin isomer is approximately four times that of its optical antipode.[41] However, this determination of anticoagulant potency did not consider the differential binding of the enantiomers and, thus, does not reveal the true intrinsic differences in potency between the enantiomers. When protein binding is taken into account, the S-enantiomer has an inherent potency approximately eight times greater than the R-enantiomer. For clinical purposes, it probably is sufficient to acknowledge the apparent differences in potency, rather than the magnitude of such differences. However, the intrinsic potency difference is important for understanding receptor-site interactions, drug interactions, and for consideration of structure-activity relationships.[32]

Concurrent administration of warfarin with other highly protein bound drugs may lead to changes in binding of either drug.[42,43] However, plasma is an open compartment, and drugs displaced from plasma proteins may readily redistribute to other tissue compartments, including organs of elimination. Consequently, a transient increase in the unbound fraction of warfarin produced by the displacing drug may or may not be of pharmacological significance. It is particularly important, however, to note that stereospecific changes in the free fraction of the two warfarin enantiomers may be associated with such concurrent drug administration. Failure to appreciate these isomer-specific changes in binding might foster the incorrect assumption that stereospecific changes in drug clearance (CL) originate at the enzymatic level (as measured by intrinsic clearance) as a result of changes in metabolic conduction or inhibition. Nonetheless, the stereoselective protein binding displacement of drugs that have poor hepatic extraction will manifest itself in an unequal change in the CL of the two enantiomers in the absence of any dynamic change in metabolism.[37] Clearly, the most significant drug interactions occur when the offending agent preferentially inhibits the metabolism of the more potent S-isomer. However, as previously described,[44] stereoselective changes in protein binding may be responsible for certain warfarin drug-drug interactions, particularly those associated with concurrent administration of sulfinpyrazone[37] and phenylbutazone.[45,46] Among the numerous drug interactions known to occur with warfarin, one of the more likely is that between warfarin and trimethoprim/sulfamethoxazole.[93]

Volume of distribution of racemic warfarin ranges from 0.09 to 0.17 L/kg, with mean values of 0.12 to 0.13 L/kg.[27,47–49] While early reports[26,48–50] show no enantiomeric differences in volume of distribution, more recent investigations have reported a larger volume of distribution for the R-isomer than the S-isomer,[32] which may well reflect altered protein binding.

Metabolism

The principal route of warfarin elimination in humans is hepatic metabolism within the smooth endoplasmic reticulum, producing two major metabolites: hydroxywarfarin and warfarin alcohols.[27,51,52] This hepatic metabolism represents the major determinant of intrasubject variability in the warfarin dose-concentration-response relationship. The development of precise liquid chromatographic assays[30,31,51,53] and chiral chromatographic analysis[54-56] have allowed the conduct of accurate pharmacokinetic evaluations of warfarin.

Warfarin metabolic disposition is stereospecific (see Figure 31-1). The R-isomer is oxidized to 6-hydroxywarfarin and further reduced to 9S,11R-warfarin alcohols. In contrast, the S-isomer is oxidized to 7-hydroxywarfarin and further reduced to 9S,11S warfarin alcohols.[51] Other possible mammalian stereoselection products have also been recently identified.[56] The stereoisomeric warfarin alcohol metabolites identified in humans have anticoagulant activity.[51,52] Single-dose administration of 3 mg/kg of all four warfarin stereoisomer alcohols produced measurable changes in vitamin K-dependent clotting factor concentrations. The S,S- and S,R-stereoisomer alcohols are the most pharmacologically active warfarin metabolites. In contrast to warfarin, which is eliminated only by metabolism, the warfarin alcohols appear to be eliminated only by renal excretion. Concurrent barbiturate administration producing hepatic enzyme induction did not affect the disposition of the warfarin alcohols.[51] However, this effect was only measured for one week, and perhaps, a longer period of time would be necessary to judge the effect of enzyme induction on warfarin stereoisomeric alcohols.

Demonstration of the anticoagulant activity of warfarin alcohols does not necessarily indicate what contribution these metabolites make to the drug's clinical anticoagulant effect. In a single patient receiving warfarin alcohol on a long-term basis, plasma warfarin alcohol concentrations between 4 and 7 μg/mL were associated with effective anticoagulation.[51] These concentrations are substantially greater than those observed in other studies involving racemic warfarin administration, suggesting that the metabolites are of little consequence in the total pharmacologic/pharmacodynamic action of warfarin. However, this conclusion is based on the (undocumented) assumption that exogenously administered alcohols have the same pharmacologic response as endogenously formed metabolites.

Warfarin's protein binding characteristics markedly affect the drug's total body clearance. The effect of protein binding on total body clearance was evaluated in 31 patients with cardiovascular disease receiving individualized fixed doses of warfarin. The bound fraction of racemic warfarin ranged from 99.1% to 99.6%.[29] The "free" fraction of racemic warfarin was essentially independent of the total warfarin concentration over a range of total warfarin concentrations from 0.6 to 8.7 μg/mL. In this study, a significant correlation was found between total body clearance and "free" fraction (r = 0.641).[29] Perhaps a stronger correlation of body clearance to "free" fraction would have been noted if the authors had obtained more than one steady state sample and if enantiomeric clearances had been determined. The Distribution section presents the effect of protein binding on clearance, and other sources of information provide a more exhaustive review of the subject.[39,44,58]

The rate of elimination of the two warfarin isomers differs substantially. The S-isomer half-life is approximately 33 hours while that of the R-isomer is 45.4 hours (see Figure 31-2).[41,50,54,59,60] Breckenridge et al. evaluated the pharmacokinetics and pharmacodynamics of enantiomeric warfarin in 11 male subjects, seven of whom were normal volunteers and four of whom were patients completing anticoagulant treatment for deep vein thrombosis.[41] No subjects were taking concurrent medication. The warfarin R-isomer plasma half-life after a single oral dose of 0.5 mg/kg ranged from 19.9 to 69.8 hours, while the S-warfarin plasma half-life ranged from 18.0 to 34.1 hours under the same conditions. The similarity in volume of distribution suggested the presence of a significant difference in the plasma clearance of the R-warfarin compared to that of the S-warfarin. Steady-state pharmacokinetic studies of the enantiomers in 8 of the 11 subjects demonstrated an R-warfarin half-life of 37.4 to 88.6 hours, with an S-warfarin half-life of 21.2 to 42.6 hours.[41]

In ten healthy men given single 1.5 mg/kg oral tablet doses of R-, S- and racemic warfarin at one-month intervals, a significant difference was noted in total body clearance between R- and S-warfarin and between R-warfarin and racemic warfarin.[60] Unfortunately, the volume of distribution was calculated based on extrapolation of the initial plasma concentration to time zero. Based on the results of the single-dose kinetic information, maintenance doses required to decrease pro-

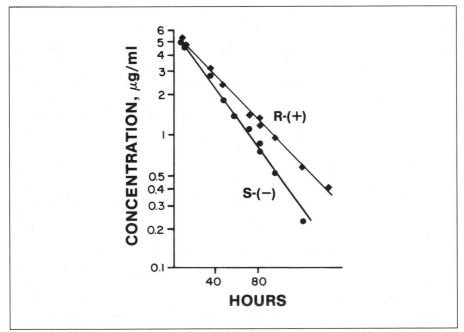

Figure 31-2. *Plasma concentration-time profile of R(+)-warfarin (R+)- and S(-)-warfarin (S-) following oral administration of R,S-warfarin (1.56 mg/kg) to a human subject (reproduced with permission from reference 54).*

thrombin complex activity to 30% of normal were calculated using previously described methods.[61] The mean calculated dose was 17.8 mg for R-warfarin, 6.6 for S-warfarin, and 9.4 mg for racemic warfarin. No correlation was observed between the clearances of R- and S-warfarin in individual subjects, as expected from rat studies.[31] Poor correlations were found between maintenance doses of racemic warfarin and doses of R-warfarin predicted to produce therapeutic anticoagulation.

With decreasing renal function, the non-renal clearance of warfarin is increased.[47] Although warfarin alcohols are renally eliminated and possess some intrinsic anticoagulant action,[52] the warfarin dose-response relationship is not altered significantly in chronic renal failure. This observation suggests the absence of accumulation of active warfarin metabolites. (See Table 31-2 for summary of warfarin kinetics.) Furthermore, in chronic renal failure, protein binding displacement appears to be associated with increased unbound drug concentrations which then become available for hepatic elimination; this decreases the anticoagulant effect.[29] Similarly, in patients with nephrotic syndrome and decreased serum albumin concentrations, increases in the free warfarin fraction in plasma and in plasma clearance have been observed after initial drug administration.[62] However, maintenance dose requirements are not substantially higher.

PHARMACODYNAMICS

Unlike the direct concentration-effect relationships identified for drugs such as digoxin, theophylline, and aminoglycoside antibiotics, the relationship between warfarin's anticoagulant effect and the drug's concentration in serum or plasma is complex and indirect. Warfarin produces two subtle but distinctly different pharmacologic effects: anticoagulation and *in vivo* antithrombotic activity. The anticoagulant action of warfarin is represented by its ability to prolong coagulation test results (e.g., the prothrombin time) while the drug's antithrombotic effect is reflected in decreases in the rate of occurrence/recurrence of thromboembolic disease. Based on the observation that concurrent administration of vitamin K analogs, particularly K_1, blocked the anticoagulant action of coumarin-type compounds (see Figure 31-3),[66] warfarin was originally considered to be a direct, competitive antagonist of vitamin K in the enzymatic processes leading to the synthesis of the four vitamin K-dependent clotting factors: II, VII, IX, and X. Subsequent investigations demonstrated that at least six vitamin K-dependent proteins are involved in the coagulation sequence. These include factors II, VII, IX, and X, and proteins C and S. Other vitamin K-dependent proteins (e.g., M, Z) have been isolated, although their clinical importance remains to be fully demonstrated. Inactive precursors of these proteins are modified through one or more vitamin K-dependent transcarboxylation reactions that alter glutamic acid residues,[67-70] which are subsequently bound to calcium ions and phospholipids. Warfarin inhibits this transcarboxylation, thereby preventing formation of gamma-carboxy glutamic acid residues[67,68] and maintaining the major procoagulant factors II, VII, IX and X in the inactive forms. Vitamin K_1-2,3-epoxide accumulates in the liver of rats receiving warfarin.[71] In the absence of warfarin, this vitamin K_1-2,3-

Table 31-2. Warfarin Pharmacokinetic Summary

Dose	N	t½ (hr)			Vd (L/kg)			Vd unbound (L/kg)			CL (mL/min/kg)			CL unbound (mL/min/kg)			References
		R[a]	S[b]	R/S[c]	R	S	R/S	R	S	R/S	R	S	R/S	R	S	R/S	
0.5 mg/kg[h]	9 NV[h]	35.0	23.9	—	0.15	0.16	—	—	—	—	0.058	0.81	—	—	—	—	41
Titrated[i]	9 p[e]	53.8	27.3	39.3	0.14	0.15	—	—	—	—	0.035	0.055	0.36	—	—	—	41
1.5 mg/kg[h]	2 NV[h]	37	25	—	0.14	0.14	—	25	33	—	0.04	0.07	—	8	16	—	46
0.75 mg/kg[h]	5 NV	—	—	44.8	0.17	—	—	—	—	—	—	—	0.04	—	—	—	47
	5 RF[g]	—	—	29.9	0.16	—	—	—	—	—	—	—	0.06	—	—	—	
100 mg[h]	4 NV[d]	45.4	32.5	—	10.4	10.9[j]	—	—	—	—	—	—	—	—	—	—	50
1.5 mg/kg[h]	10 NV	58	33	—	10	10	—	—	—	—	—	—	—	—	—	—	60
1.5 mg/kg[h]	8 NV	46	32	—	—	—	—	—	—	—	—	—	—	—	—	—	62
15 mg	5 NV	—	—	25	—	—	21	—	—	—	—	—	0.10	—	—	—	63
	5 H[f]	—	—	23	—	—	19	—	—	—	—	—	0.10	—	—	—	
1 mg[k]	5 NV	—	—	—	—	—	—	—	—	—	0.037	.054	—	—	—	—	64

[a] R(+) optical isomer of warfarin.
[b] S(−) optical isomer of warfarin.
[c] Racemate warfarin.
[d] Normal volunteers.
[e] Patients.
[f] Acute viral hepatitis; patient has own control.
[g] Chronic renal failure; mean creatinine clearance = 28 mL/min.
[h] Single-dose studies.
[i] Multiple-dose steady-state; racemate values calculation based on 4 patients only.
[j] Volume of distribution calculated on % body weight.
[k] Two weeks steady state.

epoxide is reduced to vitamin K_1 by two separate epoxide reductases. However, these enzymes are inhibited by warfarin, resulting in accumulation of vitamin K-epoxide which is not effective in the carboxylation reaction (see Figure 31-4).[71-74] This mechanism has provided an explanation for the observed time lag between warfarin administration and the onset of anticoagulant effect. An alternate pathway of warfarin action, involving vitamin K quinone, has also been identified. This pathway involves not only the reduction of vitamin K epoxides to the quinone, but also the reduction of the quinone to the hydroquinone.[76] The NADH-dependent quinone reductase is less sensitive to warfarin inhibition and may explain the ability of administered vitamin K to counteract the hemorrhagic effects of warfarin overdoses.

The effects of gamma-carboxy glutamic acid inhibition on the activities of the other, anticoagulant vitamin K-dependent compounds such as protein C have not been fully clarified.[70,77] However, it is apparent that familial protein C deficiency is a probable etiology of recurrent thromboembolism.[78] In addition, case reports of dermal and soft tissue necrosis (an uncommon but potentially disfiguring reaction associated with coumarin administration)[79-84] as well as recent studies evaluating protein C plasma concentrations in humans, have suggested that initial warfarin therapy leads to a depression of protein C and, possibly, protein S concentrations. Reduction of protein C plasma concentration occurs early in the

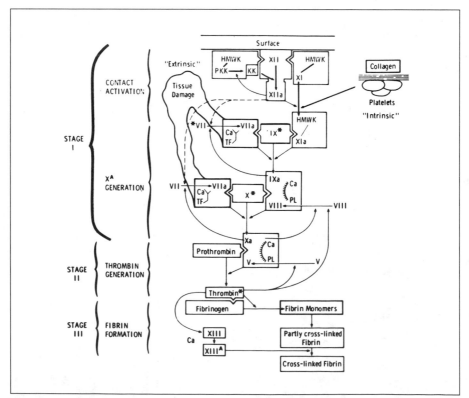

Figure 31-3. Activation of plasma coagulation mechanism via extrinsic and intrinsic systems with sites of warfarin activity indicated by * (adapted from reference 66).

course of warfarin administration (within the first 12 to 24 hours) when concentrations of factors X, IX, and XI are still near normal. This time course parallels the decline of factor VII concentration and is consistent with the similarity in half-lives of Factor VII and protein C (less than eight hours).[85] This time sequence retards development of warfarin's anticoagulant action leading to an initial and potentially dangerous thrombotic state.[86] (See also Clinical Application of Pharmacokinetic Data.) This effect appears to be dose-related, with more rapid and extensive depression of protein C concentrations associated with higher initial warfarin doses.[87] Suggested treatment of the dermatologic reaction includes concurrent administration of heparin[78] or vitamin K analogs.[88] The reaction may possibly be prevented by screening a patient's factor X to protein C ratios.[78] Normal factor X to protein C ratios are around 1, while ratios in patients with familial deficiencies of protein C are between 2.0 and 2.6.

The indirect relationship between warfarin plasma concentration and anticoagulant action can be mathematically described. Several pharmacodynamic models

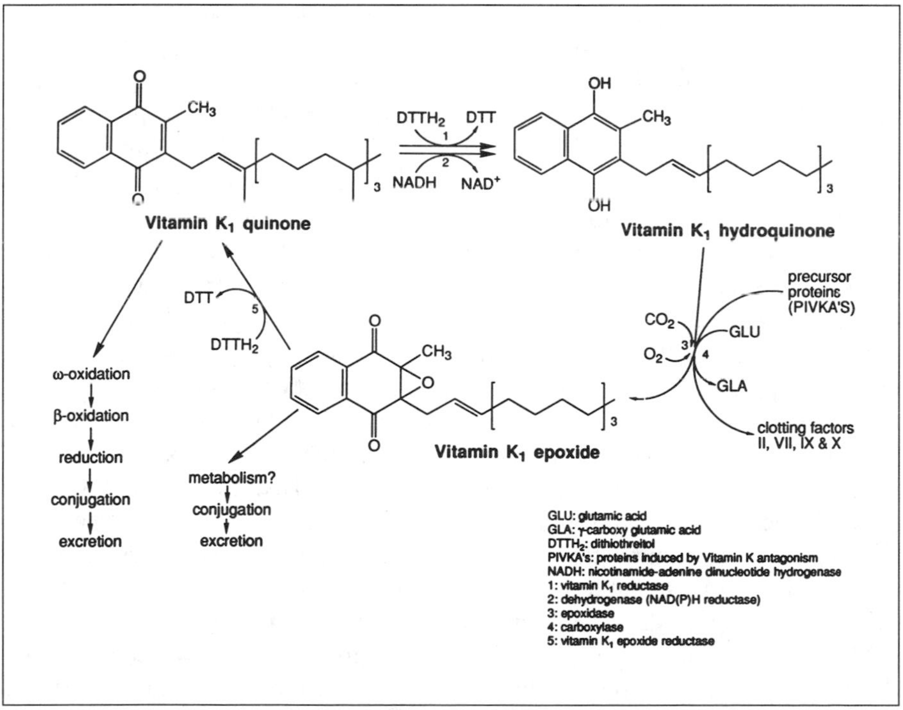

Figure 31-4. *The vitamin K cycle: metabolism of vitamin K and the carboxylation of GLU occurs on the rough endoplasmic reticulum of the liver. Epoxidation and carboxylation reactions of the vitamin K cycle are linked with both processes occurring via a common intermediate, a hydroperoxide of vitamin K. Vitamin K 2,3-epoxide may exist as two enantiomers. The physiologically predominant isomer is thought to be the 2R,3S vitamin K-2,3 epoxide. In the presence of anticoagulants or the absence of vitamin K, PIVKAs accumulate and are immunologically identical to clotting factors but lack activity because final carboxylation of GLU has not occurred. The generally accepted hypothesis is that warfarin exerts its effects on clotting factor synthesis by inhibiting enzyme vitamin K-epoxide reductase (reprinted with permission from reference 74).*

have been proposed to relate the rate of synthesis of vitamin K-dependent clotting factors, or laboratory indices of anticoagulant action such as prothrombin complex activity (PCA) or prothrombin time, to the warfarin plasma concentration (see Clinical Application of Pharmacokinetic Data).

Clinical Response

The limited number of studies describing warfarin dose-concentration-response relationships fall into one of three categories: 1) investigations in which patients receiving therapeutic, subtherapeutic and/or excessive doses of warfarin were prospectively identified, plasma concentrations measured, and the results tabulated in an attempt to identify a therapeutic range; 2) reports summarizing the results of episodic measurement of warfarin plasma concentration in selected patients because of apparent resistance to effect or unexpected toxicity; and 3) descriptions of warfarin plasma concentrations and anticoagulant effects measured in normal subjects during investigations of warfarin pharmacokinetics, isomer comparisons, or evaluations of drug interactions.

Studies in Therapeutically Anticoagulated Patients. Plasma warfarin concentrations and therapeutic effects have been compared in 133 outpatients being monitored on a routine basis during maintenance therapy.[89] Among these patients, the mean plasma warfarin concentration associated with therapeutic response (defined in that investigation as prothrombin time ratios (PR) between 1.5 and 2.5) was 2.64 µg/mL. The mean value among subtherapeutic observations (PR <1.5) was 2.07 µg/mL, while among excessively anticoagulated subjects the mean value (PR >2.5) was 3.68 µg/mL. Free warfarin concentrations were measured in 50 of the 133 subjects. The mean free warfarin concentration in patients with a therapeutic response was 9.4 ng/mL (mean total drug concentration 2.41 µg/mL). Mean values in patients with a subtherapeutic response were 5.9 µg/mL "free" warfarin and 1.64 mg/mL total warfarin, while those in patients who were overanticoagulated were 16.4 ng/mL "free" and 2.46 mg/mL total warfarin. Overall, these results are consistent with other observations in much smaller groups of patients.

In 15 patients receiving chronic maintenance therapy, a mean total warfarin plasma concentration of 0.67 µg/mL (range 0.19 to 1.03) was required to achieve a minimum prothrombin ratio of 1.8.[90] The mean "free" warfarin concentration in this group was 14.3 ng/mL (range 4.8 to 22.9). In another group of 39 patients, a mean total warfarin plasma concentration of 0.92 mg/mL was associated with a mean prothrombin ratio response of 2.0.[53] Among 31 cardiovascular disease patients receiving warfarin, in whom the mean measured prothrombin time was 20.7 seconds (range 15.6 to 29.8), the mean total warfarin concentration was 1.43 µg/mL (range 0.40 to 3.27), and the mean "free" warfarin concentration was 13.6 ng/mL (range 5.17 to 23.3).[26] In 23 patients described in a European report, a warfarin total plasma concentration range of 0.60 to 3.10 µg/mL was associated with a Thrombotest response of 5% to 8%.[41] Results obtained with this index of anticoagulation, used frequently in Europe, can be expressed as approximate prothrombin ratio equivalents.[91] The range of anticoagulation for the 23 patients expressed as prothrombin time was 2.0 to 2.3.

Only limited data describing the relationship between individual enantiomer concentrations and therapeutic effect in therapeutically anticoagulated patients are available. The ratio of the anticoagulant potency of S-warfarin to that of R-warfarin, determined by steady-state plasma concentration at the same level of anticoagulant control in four patients, has been reported to be approximately 3.8:1, with the ratio of doses of R- and S-warfarin associated with that degree of control of 1.59:1.[41] The mean total plasma concentration of racemic warfarin, R-warfarin, and S-warfarin associated with anticoagulant control in the four patients was 2.2, 4.7, and 1.3 µg/mL, respectively. Unfortunately, the sample size in this study was small and the specific level of anticoagulant control was not documented, although the reported statistical analysis showed no significant differences between Thrombotest percentages. Larger population studies are necessary to more fully characterize the relative differences between R- and S-warfarin anticoagulant and antithrombotic activity and therapeutic plasma concentrations.

The time-dependent relationship between individual enantiomer concentrations, total plasma warfarin concentration, and the anticoagulant effect associated with a given total plasma warfarin concentration merits specific consideration. A consequence of the marked differences in enantiomer half-life is a changing ratio of R-warfarin:S-warfarin concentrations during a dosing interval (usually 24 hours). While the ratio may approach one after dose administration at the beginning of an interval, it is higher at the interval's end, based on the relatively slower elimination of the R-isomer. At the same time, the substantial differences in enantiomer potency suggest that the anticoagulant effect associated with the sum of the concentrations of the two enantiomers will also vary. Therefore, a total warfarin concentration measured at a time when the R:S ratio is close to one will reflect greater intrinsic anticoagulant activity than an equivalent total concentration measured when the R:S ratio is substantially greater than one, because of the relatively lower potency of the R-isomer.

In addition, in routine clinical practice the warfarin product administered is a racemic mixture. The drug's pharmacologic action is therefore considered to reflect the effect of a homogeneous compound. Nonetheless, the relevance of isomer-specific pharmacokinetic characteristics and potency has become increasingly apparent in recent years. The stereoselective basis of a number of warfarin drug interactions has been documented.[92–97] Notably, several of these interactions are the result of selective alterations in the clearance of the less potent, but more slowly eliminated R-isomer.

Studies in Resistant/Toxic Patients. Several cases of hereditary warfarin resistance have been documented.[98,99] In one patient, remarkably large doses of warfarin (125 to 140 mg/day) were required to produce therapeutic anticoagulation, in association with a warfarin plasma concentration of 55 µg/mL. In a second patient, a daily warfarin dose of 75 to 80 mg (producing an average plasma concentration of 24 µg/mL) was required to maintain therapeutic effects. It is important to distinguish between such cases of altered concentration-response relationships (receptor affinity) and those of abnormal dose-concentration relationships where the concentration-response profile is unchanged. Several examples of the latter have been described in patients receiving concurrent barbiturate therapy.[26]

These patients may require extraordinary doses (50 to 200 mg/day) to achieve therapeutic anticoagulation, but their total warfarin plasma concentrations (2.0 to 2.5 µg/mL) are comparable to those normally observed. Ingestion of supplemental vitamin K contained in nutritional products, or disproportionate ingestion of leafy vegetables[100,101] may also contribute to abnormal dose-response relationships, although warfarin plasma concentration measurements have not been reported in these patients.

Studies in Normal Subjects. Steady-state total and free plasma warfarin concentrations and prothrombin time response were measured in five normal adult subjects during stable daily warfarin administration.[102] A mean total warfarin plasma concentration of 2.6 µg/mL (range 1.8 to 3.0) was associated with a mean prothrombin time response of 20.9 seconds (range 18.1 to 21.9). The mean free warfarin concentration was 2.35 ng/mL (range 2.06 to 2.61).

In a report (see Figures 31-5 and 31-6) describing the use of a log linear mathematical model for characterization of warfarin effect (see Clinical Application of Pharmacokinetic Data: Computer-Assisted Characterization of Anticoagulant Response and Dose Estimation), it was noted that warfarin plasma concentrations above 1 µg/mL were necessary for depression of the synthesis rate of prothrombin complex activity below 80%.[61] Concentrations above 11.3 µg/mL were associated with complete inhibition of PCA synthesis (C_{max}). Although individual response varied among the six subjects studied, these results suggested that the lower end of the therapeutic range for total plasma warfarin concentration was approximately 1 µg/L, while the upper range was below 11 µg/L (since ther-

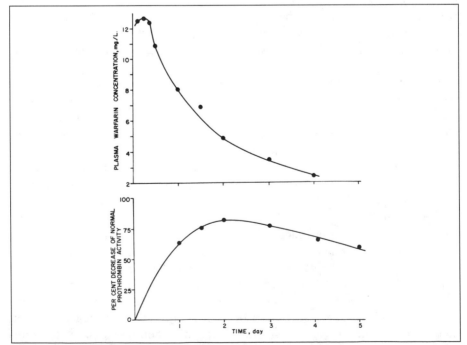

Figure 31-5. *Relationship between plasma warfarin concentration and depression of prothrombin complex activity (reprinted with permission from reference 61).*

apeutic anticoagulation does not require complete inhibition of clotting factor synthesis). In a subsequent study in a larger patient population, the identified range was somewhat lower, with reported mean values of C_{max} of 5.7 μg/mL in 26 inpatients and 6.5 μg/mL in 30 outpatients. The mean minimum warfarin concentration necessary for any inhibition of active clotting factor synthesis (C_{min}) was 0.39 and 0.36 μg/mL in the two groups, respectively.[103]

The effects of single doses of individual warfarin enantiomers on clotting factor synthesis in a single normal subject have been described.[59] The clotting factor synthesis rate was reduced to 80% by S-isomer concentrations of 0.3 to 0.4 μg/mL, whereas R-isomer concentrations of almost 5 μg/mL were required to produce an equivalent degree of inhibition. The extrapolated C_{max} values were 4 to 5 μg/mL for the S-isomer and 17 to 19 μg/mL for the R-isomer.

Concentration-Dependent Adverse Effects

Attempts have not been made to identify minimum toxic plasma warfarin concentrations or to correlate onset or degree of excessive anticoagulation with a particular warfarin plasma concentration range. The absence of readily available warfarin concentration assays has limited such efforts as has the routine practice of managing excessive anticoagulation by drug discontinuation, dosage reduction

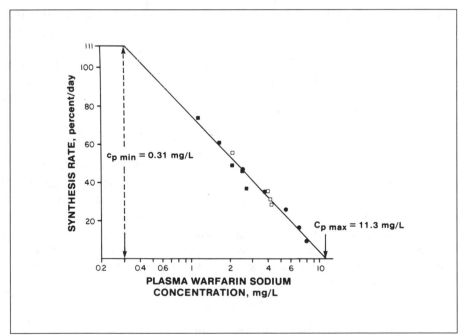

Figure 31-6. *Synthesis rate of prothrombin complex activity as a function of plasma-warfarin concentration, based on the average data from six normal subjects ("N-average"). Warfarin sodium dosing schedules:* ● = *a single oral dose of 1.5 mg/kg;* ■ = *daily oral doses of 10 mg for five days;* ❑ = *daily oral doses of 15 mg for four days.* Cp_{min} *is the apparent minimum effective plasma warfarin-sodium concentration.* Cp_{max} *is the concentration of warfarin sodium in the plasma which apparently suppresses totally the synthesis of prothrombin complex activity (reprinted with permission from reference 61).*

and/or vitamin K administration. In the majority of studies of warfarin pharmaco-kinetics in normal subjects, prophylactic administration of 10 to 50 mg of vitamin K has been employed. Alternatively, drug administration was discontinued when excessive anticoagulation occurred because of the serious potential consequences of severe hypoprothrombinemia.

Summary

Definition of a therapeutic plasma concentration range for warfarin on the basis of published data is difficult. The results of limited assessments in patients suggest that a total warfarin plasma concentration range of 0.5 to 3.0 µg/mL is most likely to be associated with therapeutic anticoagulation. The values reported for free warfarin plasma concentrations suggest a therapeutic range of 5 to 15 ng/mL.[30,90]

It is also possible theoretically to define a therapeutic total plasma warfarin concentration range using a log linear concentration-effect model and mean model parameter values.[103,104] A therapeutic effect range defined as a prothrombin ratio value of 1.5 to 2.5 can be described by an equivalent range of PCA (35.5% to 15.5%). Warfarin concentrations necessary to achieve the upper and lower limits of this range of anticoagulation can be computed (0.7 to 2.7 µg/mL). This range notably is consistent with that described in actual patient studies, suggesting that there is both clinical and theoretical validity for this range.

It is important to reiterate that warfarin plasma concentration measurements are only infrequently applied in clinical practice. They have potential value in the assessment of unusual responses (e.g., possible surreptitious ingestion or apparent resistance) or management of warfarin-associated drug interactions. However, even in these instances, the therapeutic concentration range serves only as a guide to optimizing therapy, not a mandate.

CLINICAL APPLICATION OF PHARMACOKINETIC DATA

Traditional pharmacokinetic methods have limited applicability to the optimi-zation of warfarin therapy because there is no direct relationship between drug concentration and therapeutic effect and the total and free warfarin plasma con-centration ranges associated with therapeutic response and toxicity are poorly defined. Warfarin dose determination in patients is most appropriately based on assessment of an individual's initial or sustained response to the drug. Dose selection using only pharmacokinetic parameters (individual or population) or reported mean doses may predispose the patient to a subtherapeutic outcome or toxicity.

Dose Estimation Based on Initial Anticoagulant Response

Evaluation of a patient's initial response to warfarin may provide an approxi-mate predictive guide to maintenance therapy dose requirements as well as steady-state response. A variety of simple methods have been developed to assess initial response in the clinical setting.[105-110] Methods for dose determination based on initial response generally represent maintenance dose as a linear function, usually determined by simple regression analysis of three independent variables: 1) initial dose administered; 2) the quantitative pharmacologic endpoint used to assess response; and 3) the timing of endpoint measurement in relation to initiation of therapy. Four general categories of dose prediction methods have been described, and these are characterized by the flexibility present in each of the three parameters: fixed dose/time, variable endpoint; fixed dose/endpoint, variable time; fixed time, variable dose/endpoint; and fixed endpoint, variable dose/time.

Fixed Dose/Time, Variable Endpoint. A number of published prediction methods employ the initial use of three 10 mg doses, administered at 24-hour intervals, with an endpoint prothrombin ratio measured 16 to 20 hours after administration of the third dose.[105–109] Dose projections vary according to the prothrombin ratio endpoint (PR) value. Five representative equations relating maintenance dose requirements to initial response are shown below:

$$\text{DOSE} = (7.6)\left[(\log_{10})\left[\frac{68.9}{(3.636)\,(PR) - 2.636}\right] - 7.13\right] - 3.33 \qquad \text{(Eq. 31-1)}$$

$$\text{DOSE} = 11.17 - \left[(21.08)\,(\log_{10} PR)\right] \qquad \text{(Eq. 31-2)}$$

$$\text{DOSE} = (-10)\,(PR - 2.4) \qquad \text{(Eq. 31-3)}$$

$$\text{DOSE} = (0.322)\left[\frac{100}{(3.636)\,(PR - 2.636)} - 11.6\right] \qquad \text{(Eq. 31-4)}$$

$$\text{DOSE} = 14.87 - \left[(34.08)\,(\log_{10} PR)\right] \qquad \text{(Eq. 31-5)}$$

Doses predicted by these methods for a given range of prothrombin ratio response are quite similar (see Figures 31-7 and 31-8) and have been compared in an 86-patient, multicenter investigation.[111] In this study, doses predicted using Equation 31-5 were closer to actual maintenance dose requirements than doses estimated with the other four techniques (see Figure 31-9). Although the observed correlation between actual and predicted doses with this method ($r = 0.5$) was somewhat lower than that reported in individual studies, a therapeutic response was nonetheless achieved in 80% of patients placed on a maintenance dose that was within 2.5 mg of the predicted dose. It is equally important to note that the calculated doses are those predicted to produce a steady-state prothrombin ratio of 1.5:1 to 2.5:1. Thus, these doses may be higher than those required to achieve the more modest increase in PR (1.2:1 to 2:1) currently considered to represent therapeutic anticoagulation.

Fixed Dose/Endpoint, Variable Time. A fixed dose/endpoint, variable time method for dose estimation was developed in a study of 18 patients in whom the time required to achieve therapeutic anticoagulation (PCA $\leq$ 40%) during daily 15 mg dose administration was compared to daily maintenance dose requirements during chronic therapy.[112] Patients in whom therapeutic response was achieved with the initial dosing regimen in less than three days required lower daily maintenance doses (≤ 2.5 mg) than those in whom either three days (7.5 mg) or four or more days (≥10 mg) were required. This approach has been theoretically substantiated by computer simulation of a hypothetical patient's response to daily administration of 10 mg doses;[108] however, variability in maintenance dose requirements was also projected for each level of response time (see Identification of a Therapeutic Endpoint: Intensity of Anticoagulation). Therefore, while these methods may have some conceptual merit, the equations derived from these earlier studies are invalid for current practice and should no longer be directly applied to patient care.

Fixed Time, Variable Dose/Endpoint. A modification of the original fixed dose/time, variable endpoint has been developed to reduce the risk of excessive anticoagulation by administration of three 10 mg doses.[113,114] This procedure employs an initial 10 mg dose, but the second dose is determined according to response to the first 10 mg, and the third dose is determined by response to the first two doses. The maintenance dose is calculated from the measured PT ratio on day four. Although the results of this study were expressed in terms of an International Normalized Ratio (INR), the published table can be easily adapted for use in any institution by using the potency index [International Sensitivity Index (ISI)] of the thromboplastin employed in that facility to convert the INR criteria to facility-specific prothrombin ratio criteria (see Identification of a Therapeutic Endpoint: Intensity of Anticoagulation). In contrast to the previously noted limitations of the "fixed dose/time, variable endpoint" methods, this approach is based upon a currently valid therapeutic range of anticoagulation (INR 2.0 to 3.0).

Fixed Endpoint, Variable Dose/Time. Warfarin maintenance dose estimation has also been based on measurement of the area under the prothrombin time-cumulative warfarin dose curve during initial therapy, up to a prothrombin time of

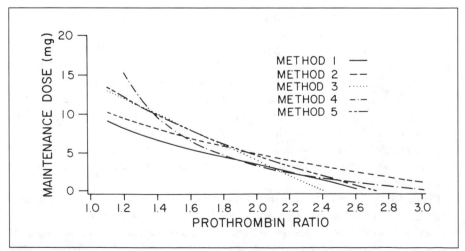

Figure 31-7. Comparison of maintenance dose projections estimated from Methods 1 through 5.

20 seconds.[110] This method predicted precise maintenance dose requirements among patients described in the original report, although subsequent evaluations of the method have produced less encouraging results.[111]

Computer-Assisted Characterization of Anticoagulant Response and Dose Estimation

More sophisticated computer-assisted methods are now available to characterize individual patient responses to warfarin administration during initial or maintenance therapy.[104,115–118] With microcomputer implementation, these techniques may assist the clinician in routine dose determination as well as with the assessment of unusual warfarin responses, including apparent sensitivity or resistance. Several approaches have been described for the clinical application of mathematical models in the optimization of warfarin therapy. The methods differ primarily in the pharmacodynamic (concentration-response) model relationship employed in each; a similar pharmacokinetic (dose-concentration) model, one-compartment, zero-order input and first-order output, is used in each. Warfarin absorption after oral administration is considered to be both rapid and essentially complete,[16] and a zero-order input function can be used without clinically significant loss of precision.

$$C(t) = [C(0)]\left[e^{(-K_{el})(t)}\right] \qquad \text{(Eq. 31-6)}$$

where $C(t)$ is the warfarin plasma concentration at any time, t, after dose administration, $C(0)$ is the warfarin plasma concentration immediately after dose administration, and K_{el} is the warfarin elimination rate constant.

The derivation of a number of models describing warfarin pharmacodynamics has been summarized in a comprehensive review.[13] Three representative models are discussed here.

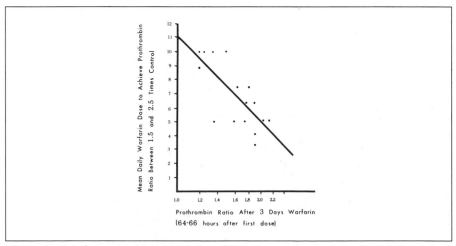

Figure 31-8. *Relationship between prothrombin ratio on third day and mean daily warfarin dose. Regression equation: Maintenance dose (in mg) = 11.17 – 21.08 (log 10 prothrombin ratio). (r = –0.74) (Reprinted with permission from reference 106.)*

Model A. A non-physiological model to characterize patient anticoagulant response has been reported.[119] Prothrombin ratio (PR) changes were described by a differential equation that incorporates warfarin plasma concentration and a function that represents return of ratio values to normal in the absence of drug:

$$\frac{dPR}{dt} = (K_2 \times C) - (K_3 \times PR)$$

(Eq. 31-7)

where K_2 is a constant representing the relationship between warfarin concentration and change (increase) in PR, and K_3 is a constant representing return of prothrombin ration to normal in the absence of drug. Integration of this expression after substitution of drug concentration (C) described by Equation 31-6, provides an expression that describes prothrombin ratio as a function of time following warfarin administration:

$$PR(t) = (K_2) \left[\frac{C(0)}{K_{el} - K_3} \right] \left[e^{(-K_3)(t)} - e^{(-K_{el})(t)} \right]$$

(Eq. 31-8)

Although this model was initially implemented on an analog computer, it is also applicable to digital systems.[116] However, there has been only limited evaluation of its clinical utility, and a quantitative assessment of its precision when used during chronic/maintenance therapy has not been made. One report compared its performance, on the basis of the time required to achieve anticoagulant dose stabilization after initiation of therapy, to that of a linear regression method (see Equation 31-5) and empiric physician dosing.[120] While superior to the linear regression method, the analog computer method was not observed to be better than

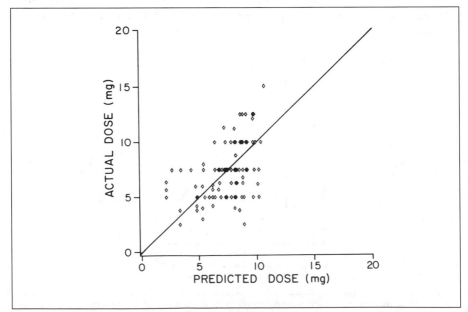

Figure 31-9. *Comparison of actual and predicted warfarin maintenance doses in 86 anti-coagulated patients (reprinted with permission from reference 111).*

empiric physician performance. It should be noted, however, that the definition of "stabilization" utilized in that report was limited to the perceived need for dosage adjustment before inpatient discharge, and no assessment of post-discharge response was made. In a subsequent evaluation of the analog model,[188] it was shown that the prothrombin ratio response to a given dose predicted by the model was "very close" to the actual measured ratio value. Unfortunately, the ability of the model to support the prospective control of therapy was neither demonstrated nor assessed.

Model B. A differential equation based on an enzyme-substrate model has also been used to describe warfarin action:[115]

$$\frac{dPCA}{dt} = [K_d]\,[PCA\,(0)]\left[1 - \frac{(0.01)(C)}{(0.01)(C) + K_m}\right] - [(K_d)\,(PCA)] \qquad \text{(Eq. 31-9)}$$

Where PCA, PCA (0), and C are constants as previously described, K_d is the degradation rate constant for prothrombin complex activity and K_m represents the plasma warfarin concentration (free) of half maximal prothrombin complex activity. Frequently referred to an E_{max} model, this equation has been evaluated in a retrospective study of 58 patients and a subsequent prospective assessment of 99 additional patients, using a digital microcomputer implementation (see Figure 31-10). However, the accuracy of dose estimation during long-term therapy has not been assessed.

Model C. A log-linear pharmacodynamic model describing the relationship between drug effect and plasma drug concentration has been described:

$$R_{SYN} = [K_d]\,[PCA\,(0)] + [M_p]\,[(\log C_{min})\,(\log C)] \qquad \text{(Eq. 31-10)}$$

where R_{SYN} is the aggregate synthesis rate of vitamin K-dependent clotting factors, K_d is the degradation rate constant for the activity of these factors, expressed as percentage prothrombin complex activity (PCA), M_p is the constant relating warfarin plasma concentration to the rate of clotting factor synthesis; PCA(0) is the level of prothrombin complex activity before warfarin administration (i.e., 100%); C_{min} is the minimum warfarin plasma concentration necessary for inhibition of clotting factor synthesis; and C is the warfarin plasma concentration at any particular time after administration.

Integration of Equation 31-10, with substitution of Equation 31-6 for C, produces an expression which describes the time course of warfarin effect on prothrombin complex activity after administration of a single dose (see Figure 31-5):

$$PCA(t) = PCA(0) \times e^{-K_d \times t} - \left(\frac{M_p \times K_{el}}{K_d^2}\right) \times 1 - K_d \times t - e^{-K_d \times t}$$

$$- \left(\frac{MP}{K_d}\right) \times \left(1 - e^{-K_d \times t}\right) \times \log\left(\frac{C(0)}{C_{max}}\right) \qquad \text{(Eq. 31-11)}$$

Several applications of the basic log-linear model have been reported, although different nomenclature has been used by various investigators.[104,116,117,121]

As with the previously described equation, coagulation activity is represented as a percentage of prothrombin complex activity. In environments where the prothrombin time and ratio are employed, a simple, arbitrary expression can be used to relate the prothrombin ratio to percentage prothrombin complex activity:[116,117]

$$\text{PCA (\%)} = \frac{100}{3.636 \times \text{PR} - 2.636} \qquad \text{(Eq. 31-12)}$$

This model has been implemented on both digital mainframe and microcomputers for clinical application (see Figure 31-11).[104,116,121,122] Prospective evaluations of the model have demonstrated its ability to describe patient response to warfarin administration during initial or chronic therapy. In one trial, inclusion of patient-specific pharmacokinetic variables (volume of distribution and clearance) did not improve the model's predictive performance over that observed when literature-derived estimates were used.[122] Evaluation of this model, using mean population values for the model parameters, in a Bayesian forecasting approach has been reported.[121,122,123,189] This approach was capable of providing reasonable prospective estimates of future (i.e., next day) prothrombin time responses based on previous dose-response information. At least two commercial applications of this model have also been developed by private firms. (Anticoagulation Dosing Service, Data-Med, Inc., Minneapolis, Minnesota; DRUGCALC, MediFore, Inc. Lansing, Michigan.)

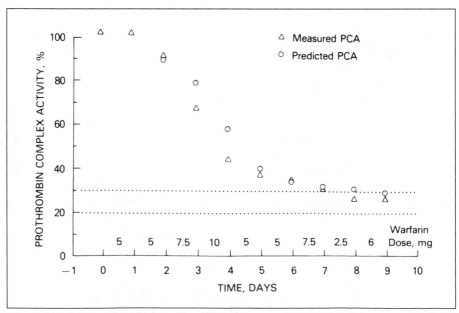

Figure 31-10. *Model B computer-projected and measured anticoagulant response to warfarin administration (reprinted with permission from reference 115).*

Unfortunately, while initial evaluations of the clinical application of this model have been encouraging, limitations to the precision of either dosage estimation or prothrombin ratio response prediction are apparent in virtually every report. Not inconsequentially, the evaluation methodologies employed could not establish the clinical value of these methods. Frequently, retrospective investigations have been used where precision of response prediction was indirectly or only qualitatively assessed. Bayesian-based log linear models bias estimates of next-day prothrombin time values unless at least three (and preferably four or five) dose-prothrombin time response data pairs are used as the basis for prediction. While estimates of anticoagulant response using three or more data pairs are reasonably precise, meaningful interpatient and intrapatient variability exists; this is reflected in substantial errors in individual ratio predictions. Clearly, these predictive pharmacodynamic models are subject to error due to the simplistic assumptions inherent in the model. Therefore, they cannot be expected to perform less flawlessly than any predictive pharmacokinetic technique. However, the imprecision or bias inherent in these models should not obscure their relative accuracy when compared to more traditional empiric dosage adjustment methods used clinically.

Comparative evaluation of the three models is made difficult by the limited availability of data from direct comparative clinical studies. Model A, run on a digital mainframe computer, has been compared to Model B in a 12-patient study; the two methods were comparable in performance.[116] In a comparison of Model B

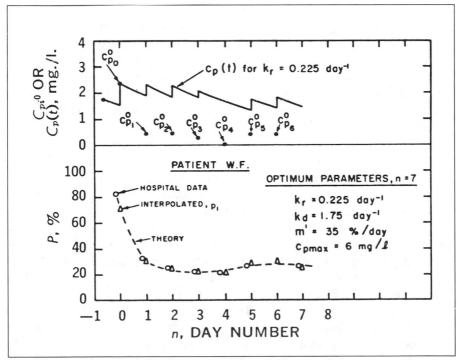

Figure 31-11. *Model C computer-projected and measured anticoagulant response to warfarin administration (reprinted with permission from reference 104).*

and Model C, the latter method provided somewhat more precise fits of actual patient data, with substantially less computer time required for the iterative fitting process.[124]

The clinical precision of these models is subject to certain assumptions and limitations which should be recognized. First, several models consider warfarin plasma concentration to be adequately characterized by a one-compartment, open, linear pharmacokinetic model. The pharmacokinetics of warfarin may be more precisely described by a two-compartment model, but a one-compartment model is acceptable for routine purposes of representation of effect. Second, the total plasma concentration of warfarin is frequently used as a model variable. However, because the free fraction is normally so small, an absolute change of 0.5% in the free fraction could result in a 33% to 100% increase in the total free drug concentration. Therefore, warfarin action may be substantially altered in certain cases (e.g., drug interactions) with little if any appreciable change in total plasma concentrations. Third, the models generally represent warfarin pharmacodynamics as the action of a homogeneous drug entity. The two warfarin optical enantiomers present in commercial racemic products differ in both pharmacokinetic characteristics and pharmacodynamic properties, as noted. These issues should be considered in any evaluation of data describing the relationship between warfarin anticoagulant action and plasma concentration, particularly when the measured plasma concentration values represent the sum of varying ratios of the individual isomer concentrations. For routine clinical purposes, however, warfarin's anticoagulant action may be considered to represent the homogeneous effect of a single drug entity. Fourth, the optimal index of anticoagulant action remains to be determined. Several models represent coagulation test results as prothrombin complex activity (PCA), a composite of clotting factor effects, rather than as individual factor concentrations or activity. Similarly, the anticoagulant action of warfarin is normally assessed by measurement of the prothrombin time which also reflects the composite activity of clotting factors rather than individual factor activity. The time course and magnitude of warfarin's effect on the synthesis of the active forms of the vitamin K-dependent clotting factors may vary among factors and among individuals. Although measurement of the prothrombin time and prothrombin ratio are the ways warfarin's effects are assessed clinically, this does not preclude the use of a model that characterizes the time course of warfarin's effects based on the activity of individual clotting factors. The response of factor II and factor X activity to warfarin administration in normal subjects, using one model, are described in a subsequent section (see Identifying a Therapeutic Endpoint: Clotting Factor Assays). Fifth, the complexity of warfarin's mechanism of action and its influence on the dose-effect relationship must not be overlooked. Warfarin most directly inhibits the activity of one or more enzymes responsible for vitamin K regeneration. This indirectly decreases the availability of vitamin K, which results in decreased synthesis of not one, but several coagulation factors. The models currently used to measure drug effect only capture a part of the complexity which characterizes warfarin's action. Finally, the difference between warfarin's anticoagulant and antithrombotic effect must be considered. Most studies have assessed the relationship between the drug's plasma concentration and its more readily quantifiable anticoagulant effect, not its antithrombotic effect. To a certain extent this is a reflection of the variability among factors in the time course of warfarin action.

OPTIMIZING WARFARIN THERAPY

Identifying a Therapeutic Endpoint: Index of Anticoagulation

Prothrombin Time/Ratio. Various indices of coagulation have been used to assess warfarin's anticoagulant action. For all of these, a known quantity of procoagulant (thromboplastin) is added to patient plasma which is then agitated to produce a clot. Results are reported as the time required to produce a clot or as percent activity. The latter is derived from a percentage activity curve constructed from the serial dilution of normal plasma. The thromboplastin used to measure the prothrombin time initiates the coagulation process by activating factor VII and the extrinsic coagulation system. Therefore, this index reflects the activity of vitamin K-dependent clotting factors that participate in the common pathway (factors II and X) as well as factor VII. The procedure may not accurately reflect the status of the intrinsic coagulation system, including factor IX. Nonetheless, the pro-thrombin time is the test routinely used to monitor warfarin therapy. Other tests may be of greater value in the future, however.

In North America, prothrombin time values are ordinarily reported as the prothrombin ratio which is calculated by dividing the patient's prothrombin time by a control prothrombin time. Traditionally, the control value represents the prothrombin time of a pooled plasma sample. The control test is performed on the same day and under the same conditions as the patient sample. The source of pooled plasma may vary from day to day. Unfortunately, this control value is an inappropriate denominator to use because it has no relation to values measured in any particular patient and the daily variability that exists is unrelated to laboratory or patient conditions. More recently, a "normal" PT value that represents the midpoint of the normal PT range for the particular reagent used (e.g., a value of 12 seconds if the reported normal range is 11 to 13 seconds) has been substituted for the measured control. Although the "normal" PT is not necessarily related to values in an individual patient, it is not subject to the variability associated with control values obtained from pooled plasma. Perhaps, the best approach would be to use each individual patient's pre-therapy baseline prothrombin time as the denominator value. However, this approach has not been adequately evaluated and its potential value is theoretical.

A portable whole blood capillary prothrombin time monitor (CoumaTrak) is now available.[125-127] The monitor uses a disposable cartridge with rabbit brain thromboplastin in a reagent well to activate the clotting sequence. The progress of clot formation is tracked by laser; using technology similar to that employed in compact disk players, the results are displayed in seconds. Precision and accuracy are sufficient to monitor anticoagulation under routine clinical conditions. Using fingerstick samples, such devices allow rapid determination of the prothrombin time at the bedside in hospitalized patients and eliminate the need for venipuncture.

More importantly, because the devices are easy to use and quite small, patients can monitor PTs in their homes. Although use of these devices is not yet widespread, they may increase the efficiency of monitoring patients in organized anticoagulation clinics and in hospitals.

Clotting Factor Assays. Assays of clotting factors (II, VII, IX, and X) may be a more precise way to directly assess the pharmacodynamic and pharmacokinetic endpoints of warfarin administration than prothrombin time.[128–135] In one study, concentrations of clotting factors II, VII, IX, and X were spectrophotometrically determined (chromogenic assay) in samples from 33 healthy subjects and 98 patients receiving long-term anticoagulant therapy. There were strong correlations between Thrombotest activity and the factor concentrations. Factor X concentration has also been used to predict acenocoumarol maintenance dose requirements in 19 patients during initial heparin treatment (see Figure 31-12).[131] In another investigation, ten normal volunteers received three 10 mg doses of oral warfarin, followed by 5 to 12 mg/day to maintain the prothrombin time within 1 to 1.5 times control.[136] A strong correlation among prothrombin time ratios, the plasma concentration of factors II and X, and total warfarin plasma concentrations was noted. The data were fit to a mathematical model using a microcomputer-based iterative statistical fitting procedure. A slight, but not statistically significant, improvement

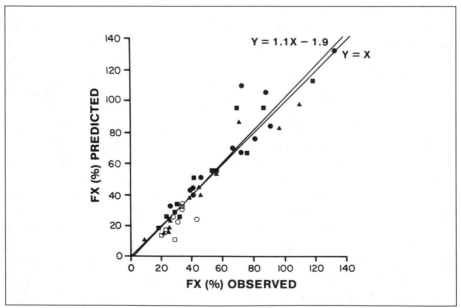

Figure 31-12. *Overall correlation between observed (horizontal axis) and predicted (vertical axis) values of Factor X (FX) activity (in % of normal) in two groups of patients. Predicted values were extrapolated from those actually measured at Day 0, Day 1, and Day 2 using the equation: log e (FX) = b − a (Day). There is a linear correlation between the observed and predicted values at Day 4 ●, Day 6 ■, and Day 8 ▲. Y = X: identity line; Y = 1.1 X − 1.9: regression line (r = 0.948). Three patients (n 2 to n 4 dosage modification on Day 4) are represented only at Day 4 ○, and 3 patients (n 5 to n 7, dosage modification on Day 6), only at Day 4 ○ and Day 6 ❑ (reprinted with permission from reference 131).*

in the correlation between measured and predicted coagulation parameter values was observed when clotting factor concentrations were used instead of prothrombin time ratios (r = 0.970, r = 0.919).[136]

Currently, therapeutic factor concentration ranges have not been documented in substantial numbers of patients nor have therapeutic endpoints for maintenance therapy been determined. In the few investigations reported to date, therapeutic concentration ranges for factor X (reported as a percentage of normal values) are similar to those for prothrombin activity (10% to 30%).[130–131] The values correlated with the intensity of oral anticoagulant activity in patients in over 70% of the cases evaluated.[130] Potential advantages to the use of factor concentration assays to monitor oral anticoagulant therapy are their ease of automation and the smaller assay variations relative to the prothrombin test. The suitability of the four different chromogenic assays to monitor oral anticoagulant therapy can be compared on the basis of general criteria: 1) the assay should be technically simple; 2) biological variation in the normal plasma activity should be small; 3) the biological half-life of the clotting factors should be short, because plasma activity of the clotting factors that have short half-lives better reflect the momentary state of anticoagulation of the patient; and 4) it should be possible to define a concentration zone that reflects optimal anticoagulation. Table 31-3 summarizes the findings of this report.[128] Factor VII has a short half-life; however, its concentrations in the plasma vary widely making it unsuitable for monitoring patients receiving oral anticoagulants. Factors II and X are, therefore, the preferred chromogenic assays for monitoring oral anticoagulation.

Native Prothrombin Assays. The native prothrombin antigen has been compared to prothrombin time as a means of monitoring oral anticoagulant therapy.[137] Native prothrombin is secreted into the plasma and contains 10 gamma-carboxy glutamic acid residues. In the absence of vitamin K or in the presence of vitamin K antagonists like warfarin, an undercarboxylated prothrombin known as abnormal prothrombin circulates in the blood.[137] In contrast to the native prothrombins, abnormal prothrombin lacks clotting activity and does not bind to calcium or to membrane surfaces.[138] Abnormal prothrombin is not a component of normal blood,

Table 31-3. *Criteria to Evaluate the Suitability of Different Chromogenic Assays to Monitor Oral Anticoagulant Therapy*[a]

Assay	Assay Variation (%)	Simplicity of the assay[b]	Biological t½ (hr)	Biological variation (%)	Relation to TT, PTR
Factor II chromogenic assay	3.6	2	48–96	11.7	0.88
Factor X chromogenic assay	3.0	3	40–60	14.8	0.78
Factor IX chromogenic assay	5.1	5	18–30	9.7	0.72
Factor VII chromogenic assay	3.5	4	4–6	21.23	0.72
Thrombotest	3.8	1			

[a] Ideal assay: one-step; small assay variation; short biological t½; small biological variation.
[b] Simplicity of the assays is graded on a scale from 1–5, where 1 can be carried out fast in a few steps, while 5 is a more complicated and time-consuming assay.

but appears in patients with vitamin K deficiency, acute hepatitis, cirrhosis, or primary hepatocellular carcinoma.[137] Abnormal prothrombin and native prothrombin can be quantified in the blood of patients treated with warfarin.[139,140] Although no correlation was observed between abnormal prothrombin antigen and the risk for bleeding or thromboembolic complications, a very strong correlation was found between the concentrations of native prothrombin and the incidence of bleeding and thrombosis.[137] Unfortunately, a direct comparison between native prothrombin antigen and prothrombin time as a means of monitoring oral anticoagulant therapy was not made. Instead, the native prothrombin antigen was measured in blood samples obtained from patients who had been controlled and monitored using the prothrombin time.[137] Based on a retrospective analysis, the use of prothrombin times to predict the risk of bleeding or thromboembolic disorders was successful in only 30% to 60% of the samples. However, use of native prothrombin resulted in successful prediction of these risks in 95% of samples.[137] While such results are encouraging, the application of native prothrombin assays to routine clinical use has not been adequately evaluated and such techniques remain, for the present, investigational.

Intensity of Anticoagulation

The optimal intensity of anticoagulation to manage thromboembolic disease has been difficult to determine. The results of an international survey of oral anticoagulant prescribing practices in 23 countries illustrated the problem. When the Quick prothrombin time test was compared to the British Comparative Thromboplastin (BCT), a wide variation in the intensity of anticoagulation was demonstrated.[141] The overall mean dose of warfarin was 5.34 mg for all 23 countries based on a therapeutic prothrombin time, and 5.54 mg based on the Thrombotest. However, the mean reported doses varied markedly according to country. In particular, a markedly dissimilar warfarin dosage pattern observed in Hong Kong patients compared to that used in other countries suggested that local variables may influence the response to warfarin. These variables could include the use of different laboratory reagents as well as patient variables such as diet, pharmacogenetics, or differences in body weight.

Variability in observed therapeutic prothrombin time or ratio ranges, and the associated difficulty establishing a therapeutic prothrombin time ratio or range reflects two potential problems. One is the differing potencies of thromboplastins used to determine the prothrombin time. Much of the published literature describing the relationship between degree of anticoagulation and therapeutic and toxic effects has come from experience in European centers where less potent thromboplastins have been used. Consequently, therapeutic prothrombin time values reported in these studies are substantially higher (three to four times control) than those observed in the United States. In the United States, clinical guidelines for warfarin therapy inappropriately suggested that prolongation of the prothrombin ratio to values 2.0 to 2.5 times control was necessary for therapeutic anticoagulation.[142] However, a number of studies have demonstrated that this intensity of anticoagulation is associated with a higher incidence of untoward bleeding without providing additional antithrombotic protection. At present in the United States, more potent rabbit tissue reagents (e.g. Simplastin) are routinely used, and lesser degrees of prothrombin time prolongation are considered therapeutic (1.3 to 1.5 times control for the majority of indications).

The well-documented[141] variability in reported therapeutic anticoagulation ranges has been a source of considerable confusion and debate for a number of years. This problem has been successfully addressed by the European Community Bureau of Reference and the World Health Organization through adoption of the International Normalized Ratio (INR) as the reference index for prothrombin time reporting and interpretation.[143] The INR represents the prothrombin ratio measured using a standardized reference thromboplastin (WHO/IRP 67/40) of known potency. All other reported prothrombin ratio values, measured using thromboplastins of different potencies, can be converted to INR equivalents, using a quantitative index of the thromboplastin potency, the International Sensitivity Index (ISI). The ISI of the reference thromboplastin is considered to be 1. For any measured prothrombin ratio (PR), the INR can be determined by raising the value of that PR to the power of the sensitivity index of the thromboplastin used in its determination:

$$INR = PR^{ISI}$$ (Eq. 31-13)

For example, if the ISI of a particular thromboplastin is 2.1, and the measured prothrombin ratio is 1.5, the INR would be 2.3. Thromboplastin manufacturers have been encouraged to label all reagent products with an appropriate ISI value calibrated to that of the reference thromboplastin. Practitioners should become familiar with the ISI values for the reagent(s) used in their respective institutions in order to appropriately interpret prothrombin time and ratio results. The current ACCP/NHLBI recommendations are specific for a particular ISI and are therefore not uniformly applicable to all measured PT values. As a consequence, PT results are best evaluated through consideration of the calculated INR.

The other difficulty associated with identifying an optimal range of anticoagulation intensity is the variability in results that cannot be attributed to a variation in thromboplastin potency. Currently, for therapy of deep venous thrombosis in the lower extremity, a rabbit tissue-thromboplastin prothrombin ratio of 1.3 to 1.5 times control (INR 2 to 3) is recommended when a thromboplastin with an ISI of 2.4 is used.[144-146] The therapy required for other patients — including those with prosthetic devices (e.g., cardiac valves) — may be more intense, with a goal of achieving a prothrombin ratio of 1.5 to 2.0 (INR 3.0 to 4.5). Nonetheless, some investigators have suggested more intensive oral anticoagulation in combination with shorter heparin therapy in the treatment of deep vein thrombosis.[147] In a randomized study, 129 patients were stratified into low-dose and high-dose groups. The low-dose group received 15 mg of warfarin on the first day of therapy and 7.5 mg/day or less subsequently. The high-dose group received 15 mg of warfarin until the prothrombin complex activity (PCA) fell below 30%. Concurrent heparin therapy was also administered; the low-dose group received 5.4 days of heparin versus 4.4 days in the high-dose group. No hemorrhagic side effects of any clinical significance were found in either group.

The results also documented the appropriateness of continuing heparin administration for a short period of time. At least four and as many as seven days are required to achieve a clinically significant degree of antithrombosis after initiation of oral anticoagulant therapy.[132,148–150] During this period concomitant heparin administration is indicated. Coon suggested that "every patient with thromboembolism receive heparin therapy concurrently with anticoagulant therapy, administered orally, for at least seven to ten days."[148] One study gave strong statistical support for the effectiveness of adjusting warfarin dosages to prevent recurrent venous thromboembolism; all of their patients, however, were treated with continuous intravenous heparin for 14 days, and warfarin therapy was begun on day ten.[151] On the other hand, with the more intensive warfarin therapy regimen described above, heparin infusions averaged five days; despite this shortened therapy, there were no significant thromboembolic complications.[147] Additional compelling evidence which supports the use of concurrent heparin and oral anticoagulant administration for the initial five days in the management of deep venous thrombosis has been presented.[152]

The relationship between risk of hemorrhage and intensity of anticoagulation was retrospectively evaluated in 541 patients receiving warfarin, using a prothrombin time ratio of 1.8 to 2.6:1 as a target therapeutic range.[154] The actuarial analysis of the probability of hemorrhage for each completed year of therapy appears to show no increased evidence of risk for hemorrhage for the first three years but a marked increase in risk between years four and eight. The relative risk of hemorrhage between years five and eight was over three times greater than that in the first three years. Aspirin ingestion was a factor that contributed to the risk of hemorrhage. The risk of hemorrhage during maintenance warfarin therapy has been evaluated in relation to the prothrombin time in two United States studies.[155,156] In a retrospective analysis of patient data from the years 1970 to 1980, hemorrhage was observed with substantially greater frequency in patients in whom the prothrombin ratio was above 2.[156] In another study, the incidence of bleeding was found to be very low when the prothrombin time was maintained below 1.5. This observation is consistent with the revised understanding of the appropriate range of anticoagulation intensity.[155] Similarly, in another evaluation of 272 patients, major hemorrhage was observed more frequently in patients with INR values greater than 4.0, while thromboembolic events were recorded in patients without malignancy only when the INR was less than 2.0.[157]

Appropriate Methods for Initiating Therapy and Determining the Maintenance Dose

In 1968, O'Reilly and Aggeler[112] showed that when patients received 10 mg of warfarin daily, they reached a putative therapeutic prothrombin time (PT) in five days; at 15 mg/day three days were required, and with a 1.5 mg/kg loading dose one day was required. The shortened time required for therapeutic prolongation of the PT after loading dose administration was principally the result of a precipitous decrease in factor VII concentration, since the concentrations of factors II, IX, and X decreased at equivalent rates with all three regimens. This rapidly induced prolongation in the prothrombin time predominantly reflected an anticoagulant effect rather than an antithrombotic action. The major disadvantage of a large loading dose is that an increased incidence of hemorrhage has been associated with this method of administration.[158] The rate of decrease of the four measurable vitamin K clotting factors is a function of their intrinsic half-life (factor II 100 hours; factor VII 3 to 6 hours; factor IX 15 to 24 hours; factor X 40 hours).[116] Generally, after 10 to 14 days of therapy, the concentrations of all four factors (as a percentage of normal) have reached equivalent values, as has the ratio of protein C concentration to that of the other vitamin K-dependent factors.[159] As noted above, during initial phases of warfarin administration, the prothrombin time does not necessarily reflect the drug's antithrombotic action. As emphasized by Gurewich[158] and experimentally confirmed by Deykin[132] and Jewell,[160] the antithrombotic effect of warfarin may not be fully apparent until the concentrations of each of the vitamin K-dependent clotting factors have decreased to 20% to 30%.

Justification no longer exists for initial administration of a 50 to 75 mg loading dose followed by daily dose adjustment based on prothrombin time response. Administration of a large loading dose places the patient at risk of hemorrhage from precipitous declines in Factor VII concentration and may precipitate the uncommon, but potentially serious, dermatologic reaction (necrosis) believed to be associated with acute protein C depletion.[78,80,81,86] Initial use of three 10 mg doses administered at 24-hour intervals is a safer and more efficient approach. However, even though such an initiation regimen is appropriate for many patients, it may represent an unnecessarily excessive dosage in selected patient populations, specifically those who have undergone cardiac valve replacement.[162] This observation provides additional support for the practice of initial daily prothrombin time measurements. In addition, it should be noted that concurrent initiation of warfarin and heparin therapy is not only feasible but preferred. Although it has previously been common practice to delay initiation of warfarin therapy for several days after beginning heparin administration, current evidence supports the efficacy, safety, and efficiency of concurrent initial administration.[163,164]

The prothrombin time should be determined before initiation of therapy, to document pre-existing coagulation disorders as well as the possibly excessive effect of heparin therapy on the prothrombin time.[153] Daily prothrombin time measurements should then be made for the first four days of therapy. Although a therapeutic antithrombotic effect cannot be expected to develop during this initial period, patients may nonetheless, manifest excessive anticoagulant response (necessitating adjustment of the initiation regimen) or blunted responsiveness. In addition, although approximations of maintenance dose requirements can be computed from a prothrombin time measured on day four of therapy, use of a single prothrombin time value provides only a very limited cross-sectional view of the patient's response. In contrast, daily measurements allow one to characterize the slope of the dose-response curve in individual patients. Recognizing an inaccurate laboratory measurement on day four is also more feasible when a series of earlier measurements is available for comparison. In addition, input of at least four dose-prothrombin time-response measurements is necessary for computer modeling of an individual patient's response using MODEL C[31,115] (although the model can certainly be used from the start of therapy to provide gross approximations of next-day response, as patient-specific dose-response experience accumulates). A gross initial estimate of maintenance dose requirements can be calculated using the "Fixed Time, Variable Dose/Endpoint" approach, on the basis of prothrombin time response on day four. Administration of daily 10 mg doses can then be continued until a therapeutic degree of anticoagulation is achieved, or administration of the projected maintenance dose can be begun immediately. It must be noted, however, that the regression-based dose projection method estimates a maintenance dose, but does not guarantee that a therapeutic prothrombin time response will be achieved after the first three (e.g., 10 mg) doses or at a particular point in therapy (e.g., day four to five). Instead, this method provides an index of the anticoagulant dose required to provide a therapeutic response during stable maintenance therapy. The mean response to the administration of three 10 mg doses in one trial (86 patients) was a prothrombin ratio of 1.5, with a range of 1.1 to 2.4 and a median value of 1.4.[111] This also suggests there is a limited potential for excessive anticoagulation with this initial regimen. This has been noted in several other reports, although it differs from the experience in certain European centers where a more pronounced anticoagulant response to the regimen has been observed.[113] The discrepancy may reflect the variability in the thromboplastin previously noted or differences in patient groups. These observations underscore the importance of daily PT measurements during initial therapy to allow for early detection of exaggerated response in warfarin-sensitive patients.

The role of computer modeling in the design of individual drug dosage regimens is increasingly important. The increased availability of microcomputers and commercial software products utilizing MODEL C encourages their routine application. At a minimum, patients exhibiting a blunted (PR 1.0 to 1.2) or exaggerated (PR >2.2) response to the fixed initial regimen are certainly candidates for computer modeling. In reality, all patients are candidates for computer-assisted dosing, subject to its availability of hardware and software resources. This is justified on the basis of warfarin's narrow therapeutic index, the serious consequences of dose-related toxicities or subtherapeutic response, and the documented interpatient variability in response. Although the previously noted caveats relative to the accuracy and potential bias of predictive pharmacodynamic models require that appropriate clinical judgment be exercised in their application and results interpretation, the value of the experience gained from their expanded use may contribute to adaptive improvement in their performance.

Of particular interest is a report which describes the application of a warfarin dosing nomogram developed from population parameter values previously identified for MODEL C.[190] Although the nomogram is appropriate only for steady-state dosage adjustment, it represents a potentially useful tool for management of anticoagulant therapy.

Appropriate Techniques for Monitoring Therapy

Frequency of Coagulation Measurement. After initial administration of warfarin and estimation of maintenance dose requirements, the majority of patients can be discharged on a projected maintenance dose for outpatient follow up. During chronic ambulatory therapy, specific attention to individual patient dose-response relationships is necessary, although the specific frequency of monitoring is a somewhat arbitrary decision. Maintenance doses that have been based on the patient's initial response are approximations and should be thought of, therefore, as absolute requirements.

During the first week of post-discharge maintenance therapy, two prothrombin time measurements should be taken to monitor for the possibility that plasma warfarin concentrations and effects may still be increasing. It is also possible to assess the potential impact of diet changes on anticoagulant response and any problems with poor compliance to the prescribed regimen which may indicate a need for patient education. Weekly PT determinations for the next three weeks are recommended, after which time measurements can be made less frequently (every two to four weeks) if the patient's response is stable, dietary habits are regular, and compliance is consistent (see Figure 31-13). Unfortunately, validated guidelines for patient-specific sampling frequency are not available. Studies that have attempted to predict the required frequency of measurement, or the risks associated with varying frequencies of monitoring have not demonstrated the superiority of any particular schedule.[165] An approach to the determination of an optimal PT sampling strategy for initial estimation of pharmacokinetic and pharmacodynamic parameters has been reported.[166] While the presented results are encouraging, details of the method have not been fully described and its clinical value remains to be determined.

Assessing an Unusual Response

Several specific factors should be considered when assessing an unusual response to warfarin:
1) Inaccurate or spurious laboratory results.
2) Alterations in the dose-plasma concentration relationship.
   • Drug-disease interactions.
   • Drug-drug interactions.
3) Alterations in the plasma concentration-anticoagulant response relationship.
   • Altered receptor site sensitivity to warfarin (e.g., hereditary resistance, pharmacogenetics).
   • Change in nutritional status.
4) Alterations in drug administration or patient compliance.
5) Abnormal product performance or interchange of products from various manufacturers.

Among these, variability in the precision of laboratory test results is probably the most common source of an apparently abnormal or unusual response to war-

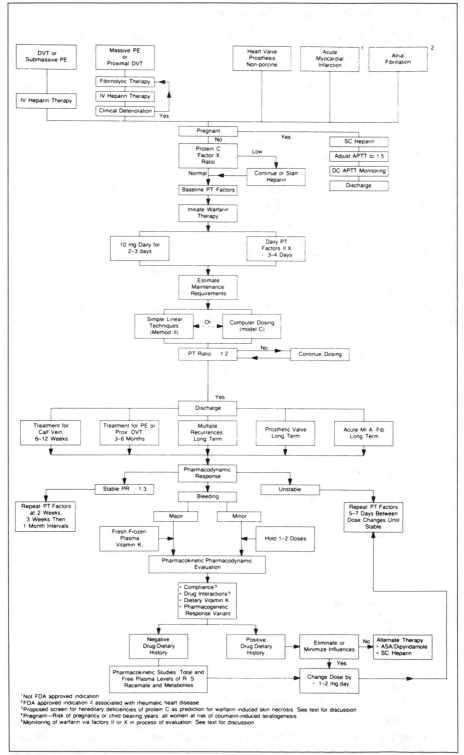

Figure 31-13. *Algorithm for management of warfarin therapy.*

farin administration. It is also the easiest to document (by repeated prothrombin time measurement), although it is not always the first possibility evaluated. Because so many drugs interact with warfarin, one should routinely consider drug interaction as a possible source of an unusual anticoagulant response (see Figure 31-14).[42,43,167-169] An analysis of the relationship of smoking history to warfarin maintenance dose requirements has failed to identify a substantive association.[170] Much of the newer information regarding warfarin drug interactions has emphasized their stereoselective basis.[37,45,46,92-97,171,172] The most clinically important warfarin drug interactions occur when there is stereoselective inhibition of the clearance of the more potent S-isomer, leading to an exaggerated hypoprothrombinemic response.[46]

The influence of changes in dietary vitamin K content on warfarin effect has been repeatedly demonstrated. Patients who are receiving nutritional supplements high in vitamin K content may demonstrate a markedly reduced anticoagulant response.[100,101,173-176] Altered response is less likely to occur with limited ingestion, and sustained changes in diet are usually required before a substantial change in response is detectable.[178]

Documented hereditary resistance to warfarin's effect is rare, although the actual incidence may be higher than reported[99] since warfarin plasma concentration measurements (necessary to document resistance) are not readily available. Unfortunately, problems associated with drug administration, including patient compliance, are not adequately explored in the assessment of unusual response. It is routinely assumed that patient noncompliance is principally a matter of failure to take the prescribed dose in an ambulatory environment, resulting in subtherapeutic response. However, the possibility of noncompliance while in the hospital or noncompliance manifested by excessive ingestion of prescribed warfarin should be considered as well.[178] Currently, problems with variable drug product performance do not appear to be clinically significant. However, as previously noted, product brand interchange may result in substantial intrapatient variance in the dose-response profile. Bentley et al. have provided an excellent, humorous review of practical clinical approaches to the assessment of abnormal response to warfarin therapy using simple algorithms (see Figures 31-15 and 31-16).[180]

Timing of Sample Collection. The timing of prothrombin time measurement, relative to changes in the daily dose as well as to administration of the most recent dose, is important. After administration of a single dose of warfarin, the peak depression of coagulation occurs in approximately 36 hours (see Figure 31-5). Unfortunately, this observation has been used to support the notion that it is necessary to wait 36 hours after a dose to assess the magnitude of that particular dose's effect. It is not possible to selectively differentiate between the effects of several previous doses on prothrombin time during a given dosing interval. It is more appropriate to select a particular time during a dosing interval (e.g., three hours before the next scheduled dose administration) and perform coagulation studies consistently at that time. Additionally, after the first four to five doses, the fluctuation in prothrombin time response observed over a 24 hour time interval is limited. Simulation studies have demonstrated a variation in the prothrombin ratio of only 0.1 to 0.3 over a 24 hour dosing interval at steady state.[181]

The time course of stabilization of warfarin plasma concentrations and coagulation response during continued administration of a stable maintenance dose is less clearly resolved. When both the extended plasma half-life of warfarin (36 hours) and observed patterns of response are considered, a minimum time of approximately ten days would appear to be necessary before the dose-response curve shows interval-to-interval stability. In some patients, a longer period may be necessary to fully assess the steady-state anticoagulant response to a given maintenance dose.

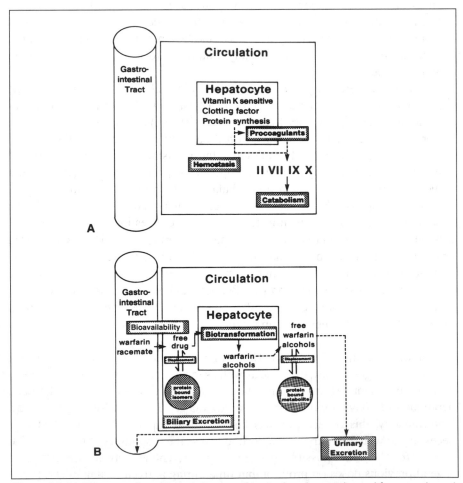

Figure 31-14. Pharmacodynamic and pharmacokinetic drug interactions with coumarin anticoagulants. 14A indicates schematically the mechanisms of pharmacodynamic interactions (i.e., pharmacological actions of coumarins which may be altered by other drugs affecting clotting factor synthesis or the hemostatic process). 14B indicates schematically the mechanisms of pharmacokinetic interactions (i.e., interactions in which the absorption, biotransformation or disposition of coumarin anticoagulants may be altered). Adapted from reference 169.

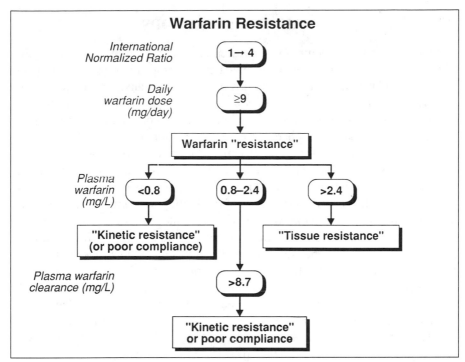

Figure 31-15. *Algorithm for evaluation of warfarin resistance (reprinted with permission from reference 180).*

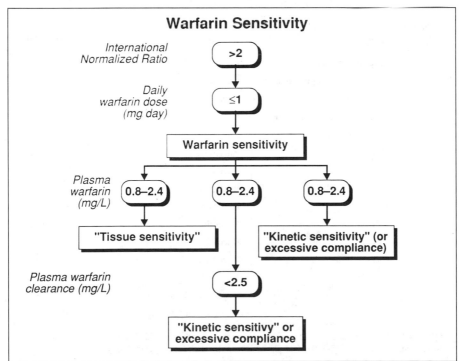

Figure 31-16. *Algorithm for evaluation of warfarin sensitivity (reprinted with permission from reference 180).*

ANALYTICAL METHODS

Plasma warfarin concentration measurement is not a routine clinical practice. The availability of a pharmacologic indicator of therapeutic effect (prothrombin time) has obviated the need, in the minds of many clinicians, for routine warfarin plasma concentration measurement. Nonetheless, plasma concentration determinations may be of particular value in patients who exhibit an unusual response to warfarin. In these patients, concentration determination may help rule out factors such as hereditary resistance or identify mechanisms of a drug-drug interaction.

Table 31-4 summarizes the assay methodologies that have been used by investigators to measure plasma warfarin concentration. The majority of the assays involved difficult extraction procedures; further, they were imprecise, the reproducibility among investigators was inconsistent, and the assay procedures were subject to interference from concurrently administered drugs. High-performance liquid chromatographic procedures currently represent the methods of choice for racemic warfarin determination.[40,55,181–186] Major deficiencies of all these assays have been the inability to measure low concentrations of "free" warfarin. For the racemic assays, a direct comparison of methodologies[40,186] lends substantial documentation to their superiority as an assay methodology. Recently, Banfield and Rowland[54] have described a relatively simple high-performance liquid chromatographic analysis of the stereoisomers of warfarin in plasma.

Table 31-4. Warfarin Analytical Assay Methods

Number of subjects	Assay[a]	Resolution	References
14	Spectrophotometric	Racemic	20
8 (4)	TLC with spectrophotometric	Racemic, R S	45
10	Spectrophotometric	Racemic, R S	60
12	Spectrophotometric and HPLC	Racemic	40
5	Spectrophotometric	Racemic	47
1	HPLC	Racemic	181
1	GLC	Racemic	53
6	HPLC with SIST	Racemic, R S	149
3	HPLC	Racemic	184
	HPLC	Racemic, metabolites	183
	HPLC	Racemic	185
	HPLC, chiral	Racemic, R S	54
	GC-MS	Racemic, R S	37
	HPLC	Racemic, R S metabolites	186
	HPLC, chiral	Phenprocoumon R S, Warfarin R S	55

[a] HPLC = High-performance liquid chromatography; GLC = Gas liquid chromotography; SIST = Stable isotope; GC-MS = Gas chromotography with mass spectroscopy.

PROSPECTUS

The future for research in antithrombotic therapy offers promise for a better understanding of 1) basic mechanisms of coagulation and thrombosis; 2) stereo-specific warfarin pharmacokinetics and pharmacodynamics; 3) risk-benefit criteria based on indications for therapy; 4) optimal therapeutic endpoints for evaluation of warfarin response; 5) the routine applicability of microcomputer-based techniques for warfarin dosage regimen design and modification; and 6) better trial designs for comparing alternative or adjunctive antithrombotic therapies.

The availability of reliable assays for R- and S-warfarin may allow a more careful evaluation of previously described warfarin drug interactions, especially those involving the possible metabolic inhibition or displacement of the more potent S-isomer. As new drugs are introduced into the market, it will be critical to apply this analytical technology to the prediction of potential drug interactions. The previous assumption that warfarin resistance is a rare occurrence must be re-evaluated in light of new information and the ready availability of new assays to assess not only racemic but also R- and S-warfarin isomers. Trends toward dietary narcissism have led to life-threatening instances of hypercoagulability from excessive ingestion of vitamin K. Warfarin assays will continue to help sort out this puzzling problem.

The use of newer, more sophisticated and technically precise techniques to assess warfarin response, including the more widespread use of the INR in the assessment of warfarin response, protein C:factor X ratios, clotting factor II and X concentration assays, and native prothrombin immunoassays should provide an added dimension to the safety and accuracy of predicting warfarin response. Microcomputer-based dosing programs utilizing existing or new monitoring assays should greatly improve the empiricism which continues to be associated with warfarin dosing. However, their expanded clinical use must be critically evaluated, with documentation of both rates of failure and of success in achieving optimal anticoagulation.

REFERENCES

1. Schoefield FW. A brief account of a disease of cattle simulating hemorrhagic septicaemia due to feeding sweet clover. Can Vet Rec. 1922;3:74.
2. Link K. The discovery of dicumarol and its sequels. Circulation. 1959;19:97–107.
3. Meyer O. Historical data regarding the experiences with coumarin anticoagulants at the University of Wisconsin Medical School. Circulation. 1959;19:114–17.
4. Butt H et al. A preparation from spoiled sweet clover, 3,3'-methylenebis-(4-hydroxycoumarin) which prolongs coagulation and prothrombin time of the blood: preliminary report of experimental and clinical studies. Mayo Clin Proc. 1941;16:388–95.
5. Fremont R, Jagendorf B. Clinical observations on use of warfarin (coumadin) sodium, a new anticoagulant. JAMA. 1957;165:1381–388.
6. Pollock B. Clinical experience with warfarin (coumadin) sodium, a new anticoagulant. JAMA. 1955;159:1094–97.
7. Shapiro S, Ciferri F. Intramuscular administration of the anticoagulant warfarin (coumadin) sodium. JAMA. 1957;165:1377–380.

8. Quick A et al. A study of the coagulation defect in hemophilia and in jaundice. Am J Med Sci. 1935;190:501–11.
9. O'Reilly RA, Aggeler PM. Determinants of the response to oral anticoagulant drugs in man. Pharmacol Rev. 1970;22:35–95.
10. Coon W, Willis P. Some aspects of the pharmacology of oral anticoagulants. Clin Pharmacol Ther. 1973;11:312–35.
11. Wessler S, Gitel SN. Warfarin. From bedside to bench. N Engl J Med. 1984;311(10):645–52.
12. Kelly J, O'Malley K. Clinical pharmacokinetics of oral anticoagulants. Clin Pharmacokinet. 1979;4:1–15.
13. Holford NHG. Clinical pharmacokinetics and pharmacodynamics of warfarin: understanding the dose-effect relationship. Clin Pharmacokinet. 1986;11:483–504.
14. Shetty HGM et al. Clinical pharmacokinetic considerations in the control of anticoagulant therapy. Clin Pharmacokinet 1989; 16:238–53.
15. Anticoagulants: coumarin and indandione derivatives. In: McEvoy GK, McQuarrie GM, eds. Bethesda, MD: American Hospital Formulary Service – Drug Information 85. American Society of Hospital Pharmacists, Inc. 1985;559–65.
16. Breckenridge AM, Orme M. Kinetics of warfarin absorption in man. Clin Pharmacol Ther. 1984;14:955–61.
17. Wagner J et al. *In vivo* and *in vitro* availability of commercial warfarin tablets. J Pharm Sci. 1971;60:656–76.
18. Martin-Bouyer G et al. Epidemic of haemorrhagic disease in Vietnamese infants caused by warfarin-contaminated talcs. Lancet. 1983;1(8318):230–32.
19. Fristedt B, Sterner N. Warfarin intoxication from percutaneous absorption. Arch Environ Health. 1965;11:205–8.
20. O'Reilly RA et al. Studies on the coumarin anticoagulant drugs: the pharmacodynamics of warfarin in man. J Clin Invest. 1963;42:1542–551.
21. Ruedy J et al. Drug bioavailability. Can Med Assoc J 1976;115:105.
22. Loeliger EA, Broekmans AW. Drugs affecting blood clotting, fibrinolysis, and hemostasis. In: Westerholhm B, section ed. Meylers's Side Effects of Drugs. Amsterdam: Elsevier. 1984;648–93.
23. Personal communication: Abbott Laboratories, Inc. 1985 May.
24. Richton-Hewwett S et al. Medical and economic consequences of a blinded oral anticoagulant brand change at a municipal hospital. J Am Med Assoc. 1988;148:806–8.
25. Breckenridge AM. Oral anticoagulant drugs: pharmacokinetic aspects. Semin Hematol. 1978;15:19–26
26. O'Reilly RA. The pharmacodynamics of oral anticoagulant drugs. In: Spaet TH, ed. Progress in Hemostasis and Thrombosis. New York: Grune & Stratton. 1974;2:175–213.
27. O'Reilly RA et al. Studies on the coumarin anticoagulant drugs: a comparison of the pharmacodynamics of dicumarol and warfarin in man. Thromb Haemostas. 1964;11:1–22.
28. Shepherd A et al. Age as a determinant of sensitivity to warfarin. Br J Clin Pharmacol. 1977;14:315–20.
29. Yacobi A et al. Serum protein binding as a determinant of warfarin body clearance and anticoagulant effect. Clin Pharmacol Ther. 1976;19:552–58.
30. Yacobi A et al. Intrasubject variation of warfarin binding to protein in serum of patients with cardiovascular disease. Clin Pharmacol Ther. 1976;20:300–3.
31. Yacobi A, Levy G. Protein binding of warfarin enantiomers in serum of humans and rats. J Pharmacokin Biopharm. 1977;5(2):123–31.
32. Solomon H, Schrogie J. The effect of various drugs on the binding of warfarin-14C to human albumin. Biochem Pharmacol. 1967;16:1219–226.
33. Wosilait W, Garten S. Computation of unbound anticoagulant values in plasma. Res Comm Chem Path Pharmacol. 1972;3:285–91.
34. Bachman K. Rapid determination of the concentration of unbound warfarin in human plasma. Res Comm Chem Path Pharmacol. 1974;9:379–82.

35. Sudlow G et al. Spectroscopic techniques in the study of protein binding: a fluorescence technique for the evaluation of the albumin binding and displacement of warfarin and warfarin-alcohol. Clin Exper Pharmacol Physio. 1975;2:129–40.

36. Oester Y et al. Effect of temperature on binding of warfarin by human serum albumin. J Pharm Sci. 1976;65:1173–677.

37. Toon S, Trager WF. Pharmacokinetic implications of stereo-selective changes in plasma-protein binding: warfarin/sulfinpyrazone. J Pharm Sci. 1984;73(11):1671–673.

38. Mungall D et al. Plasma protein binding of warfarin: methodological considerations. J Pharm Sci. 1984;73(7):1000–1.

39. Wandell M, Wilcox-Thole WL. Protein binding and free drug concentrations. In: Mungall D, ed. Applied Clinical Pharmacokinetics. New York: Raven Press. 1983;17–48.

40. Vessell E, Shively C. Liquid chromatographic assay of warfarin: similarity of warfarin half-lives in human subjects. Science. 1974;184:466–68.

41. Breckenridge AM et al. Pharmacokinetics and pharmacodynamics of the enantiomers of warfarin in man. Clin Pharmacol Ther. 1974;15:424–30.

42. Koch-Wesser J, and Sellers E. Drug interactions with coumarin anticoagulants. N Engl J Med. 1971;285:547–58.

43. Serlin MJ, Breckenridge AM. Drug interactions with warfarin. Drugs. 1983;25:610–20.

44. Rowland M et al. Clearance concepts in pharmacokinetics. J Pharmacokinet Biopharm. 1973;1:123–35.

45. Lewis RJ et al. Warfarin: stereochemical aspects of its metabolism and the interaction with phenylbutazone. J Clin Invest. 1974;53:1607–617.

46. Banfield C et al. Phenylbutazone-warfarin interaction in man: further stereochemical and metabolic considerations. Br J Clin Pharmacol. 1983;16:669–75.

47. Bachmann K et al. Warfarin elimination and responsiveness in patients with renal dysfunction. J Clin Pharmacol. 1977;30:292–99.

48. O'Reilly RA et al. Stereoselective interaction of phenylbutazone with (12C/13C) warfarin pseudoracemates in man. J Clin Invest. 1980;65:746–53.

49. O'Reilly RA et al. Pharmacokinetics of warfarin following intravenous administration to man. Thromb Haemostas. 1971;25:178–86.

50. Hewick D, McEwen J. Plasma half-lives, plasma metabolites and anticoagulant efficacies of the enantiomers of warfarin in man. J Pharm Pharmacol. 1983;25:458–65.

51. Lewis RJ, Trager WF. Warfarin metabolism in man: identification of metabolites in urine. J Clin Invest. 1970;49:907–13.

52. Lewis RJ et al. Warfarin metabolites: the anticoagulant activity and pharmacology of warfarin alcohols. J Lab Clin Med. 1973;81:925–31.

53. Hotraphinyo K et al. Warfarin sodium: steady-state plasma levels and patient age. Clin Exp Pharmacol Physiol. 1978;5:143–49.

54. Banfield C, Rowland M. Stereospecfic high-performance liquid chromatographic analysis of warfarin in plasma. J Pharm Sci. 1983;72(8):921–24.

55. DeVries JX, Volker U. Separation of the enantiomers of phenprocoumon and warfarin by high-performance liquid chromatography using a chiral stationary phase determination of the enantiomeric ratio of phenprocoumon in human plasma and urine. J Chromatog. 1989;493:149–56.

56. Wong YWJ, Davis PJ. Analysis of warfarin and its metabolites by reversed-phase ion-pair liquid chromatography with fluorescence detection. J Chromatog. 1989;469:281–91.

57. Wong YWJ, Davis PJ. Microbial models of mammalian metabolism: stereoselective metabolism of warfarin in the fungus cunninghamella elegans. Pharm Res. 1989;6(11):982–87.

58. Rowland M. Protein binding and drug clearance. Clin Pharmacokin. 1984;9(Suppl. 1):10–7.

59. Levy G, Wingard L. Relationship between the kinetics of the anticoagulant effects of racemic warfarin and its individual enantiomers in man. Res Commun Chem Pathol Pharmacol. 1974;7:359–65.

60. O'Reilly RA. Studies on the optical enantiomorphs of warfarin in man. Clin Pharmacol Ther. 1974;16:348–54.

61. Nagashima R, O'Reilly RA. Kinetics of pharmacologic effects in man: the anticoagulant action of warfarin. Clin Pharmacol Ther. 1969;10:22–34.

62. Ganeval D et al. Pharmacokinetics of warfarin in the nephrotic syndrome and the effects on vitamin K-dependent clotting factors. Clin Nephrol. 1986;25:75–80.

63. O'Reilly RA. The stereoselective interaction of warfarin and metronidazole in man. N engl J Med. 1976;295:354–57.

64. Williams RL et al. Influence of acute viral hepatitis on disposition and pharmacologic effect of warfarin. Clin Pharmacol Ther. 1976;20(1):90–7.

65. Choonara IA et al. Enantiomers of warfarin and vitamin K metabolism. Br J Clin Pharmacol. 1986;22:729–32.

66. Hall R, Mailia RG, eds. Medical Laboratory Haematology. Boston: Butterworth's. 1983;53–4.

67. Suttie JW, Jackson CM. Prothrombin structure, activation, and biosynthesis. Physiol Rev. 1977;57:1–70.

68. Stenflo J, Suttie JW. Vitamin K-dependent formation of gamma-carboxyglutamic acid. Ann Rev Biochem. 1977;46:157–72.

69. Hemker HC, Muller AD. Kinetic aspects of the interaction of blood-clotting enzymes. VI. Localization of the site of blood coagulation inhibition by the protein induced by vitamin K absence (PIVKA). Thromb Diath Haemorrh. 1968;20:78–87.

70. Burnier JP et al. Gamma-carboxy-glutamic acid. Mol Cell Biochem. 1981;39:191–99.

71. Fasco MJ et al. Warfarin inhibition of vitamin K_2, 3-epoxide reductase in rat liver microsomes. Biochemistry. 1983;22(24):5655–660.

72. Bell RG, Ren P. Inhibition by warfarin enantiomers of prothrombin synthesis, protein carboxylation, and the regeneration of vitamin K from vitamin K epoxide. Biochem Pharmacol. 1981;30:1953–958.

73. Ren P et al. Mechanism of action of anticoagulants: correlation between the inhibition of prothrombin synthesis and the regeneration of vitamin K from vitamin K_1-epoxide. J Pharmacol Exp Ther. 1977;201:541–46.

74. Bovill EG, Mann KG. Warfarin and the biochemistry of the vitamin K-dependent proteins. In: Wessler S, Becker DG, Memerson Y, eds. The New Dimensions of Warfarin Prophylaxis. New York and London: Plenum Press. 1987;17–46.

75. Sutcliffe FA et al. Aspects of anticoagulant action: a review of the pharmacology, metabolism and toxicology of warfarin and congeners. Drug Metab Drug Interact. 1987;5:225–73.

76. Suttie JW. The biochemical basis of warfarin therapy. In: Wessler S, Becker CG, Memerson Y, eds. The New Dimensions of Warfarin Prophylaxis. New York and London: Plenum Press. 1987;17–46.

77. Esmon CT et al. Anticoagulation Proteins C and S. In: Wessler S, Becker CG, Memerson Y, eds. The New Dimensions of Warfarin Prophylaxis. New York and London: Plenum Press. 1987;17–46.

78. McGehee WG et al. Coumarin necrosis associated with hereditary protein C deficiency. Ann Intern Med. 1984;101(1):59–60.

79. Chua F et al. Dermal gangrene: an unpredictable complication of coumarin therapy. J Thor Cardiovasc Surg. 1973;65:238–40.

80. Horn J et al. Warfarin-induced skin necrosis: Report of four cases. Am J Hosp Pharm. 1981;38:1763–768.

81. Jones R, Cunningham J. Warfarin skin necrosis. Br J Dermatol. 1979;100:561–65.

82. Engler AM, Weiss PR. Coumadin-induced necrosis of the breast. Plastic Resconstr Surg. 1987;9:469–70.

83. Zauber NP, Stark MW. Successful warfarin anticoagulation despite protein C deficiency and a history of warfarin necrosis. Ann Intern Med. 1986;104:659–60.

84. Hyman BT et al. Warfarin-related purple toes syndrome and cholesterol microembolization. Am J Med. 1987;82:1233–237.

85. Epstein DJ et al. Radioimmmunoassays for protein C and Factor X. Am J Clin Pathol. 1984;82:573–81.

86. Broekmans AW et al. Protein C and development of skin necrosis during anti-coagulant therapy. Thromb Haemost. 1983;49:251.

87. Weiss P et al. Decline of protein C and S and factors II, VII, IX, and X during the initiation of warfarin therapy. Thromb Res. 1987;45:783–90.

88. Van Amstel WJ et al. Successful prevention of coumarin-induced hemorrhagic skin necrosis by timely administration of vitamin K_1. Blut. 1978;36:89–93.

89. Mungall D et al. Relationships between steady-state warfarin concentrations and anticoagulant effect. Clin Pharmacokin. 1984;9(1):99–100.

90. Routledge P et al. Pharmacokinetics and pharmacodynamics of warfarin at steady state. Br J Clin Pharmacol. 1979;8:245–47.

91. Canaday BR, Sawyer WT. A pocket calculator program for prediction of warfarin maintenance dose. Comp Biol Med. 1982;12:179–87.

92. Toon S et al. The warfarin-sulfinpyrazone interaction: Stereochemical considerations. Clin Pharmacol Ther. 1986;39:15–24.

93. Okino K, Weibert RT. Warfarin-griseofulvin interaction. Drug Intell Clin Pharm. 1986;20:291–93.

94. Heimark LD et al. The mechanism of the warfarin-rifampin drug interaction in humans. Clin Pharmacol Ther. 1987;42:388–94.

95. Kates RE et al. Interaction between warfarin and propafenone in healthy volunteer subjects. Clin Pharmacol Ther. 1987;42:305–11.

96. O'Reilly RA et al. Interaction of amiodarone with racemic warfarin and its separated enantiomorphs in humans. Clin Pharmacol Ther. 1987;42:290–94.

97. Toon S et al. Enoxacin-warfarin interaction: pharmacokinetic and stereochemical aspects. Clin Pharmacol Ther. 1987;42:33–41.

98. O'Reilly RA. Vitamin K in hereditary resistance to oral anticoagulant drugs. Am J Physiol. 1971;221:1327–330.

99. Berenberg JC, Peck CC. Hereditary warfarin resistance. Arch Intern Med. 1985;145:499–501.

100. Walker FB IV. Myocardial infarction after diet-induced warfarin resistance. Arch Intern Med. 1984;144:2089–90.

101. Qureshi G et al. Acquired warfarin resistance and weight-reducing diet. Arch Intern Med. 1981;141:507–9.

102. Jain A et al. Effect of naproxen on the steady-state serum concentration and anticoagulant activity of warfarin. Clin Pharmacol Ther. 1979;25:61–6.

103. Murray B et al. Pharmacodynamics of warfarin. Clin Pharmacol Ther. 1985;37:215.

104. Theofanous T, Barile R. Multiple-dose kinetics of oral anticoagulants: methods of analysis and optimized dosing. J Pharm Sci. 1973;62:261–66.

105. Routledge P et al. Predicting patient's warfarin requirements. Lancet. 1977;2:854–55.

106. Miller D, Brown M. Predicting warfarin maintenance dosage based on initial response. Am J Hosp Pharm. 1979;36:1351–355.

107. McGhee J et al. Predictability of warfarin maintenance dosage based upon initial response. JAOA. 1981;80:335–38.

108. Sawyer WT. Predictability of warfarin dose requirements: theoretical considerations. J Pharm Sci. 1979;68:432–34.

109. Carter B, Reinders T. Prediction of maintenance warfarin dosage from initial patient response. Drug Intell Clin Pharm. 1983;17:23–6.

110. Williams D, Karl R. A simple technique for predicting daily maintenance dose of warfarin. Am J Surg. 1979;137:572–76.

111. Sawyer WT et al. Predictability of warfarin maintenance dose, comparison of six methods. Clin Pharm. 1985;4:440–46.

112. O'Reilly RA, Aggeler PM. Studies on coumarin anticoagulant drugs: initiation of warfarin therapy without a loading dose. Circulation. 1968;38:169–77.

113. Fennerty A et al. Flexible induction dose regimen for warfarin and prediction of maintenance dose. Brit Med J. 1984;288:1208–210.

114. Cosh DG et al. Prospective evaluation of a flexible protocol for starting treatment with warfarin and predicting its maintenance dose. Aust NZ J Med. 1989;19:191–97.

115. Albrecht PH et al. Evaluation of a computer-assisted method for individualized anticoagulant therapy: retrospective and prospective studies using a pharmacodynamic model. Clin Pharmacol Ther. 1982;32:129–36.

116. Sawyer WT, Finn AL. Digital computer-assisted warfarin therapy: comparison of two models. Comput Biomed Res. 1979;12:221–31.

117. Sheiner L. Computer-aided long-term anticoagulation therapy. Comp Biomed Res. 1969;2:507–18.

118. Wiegman H, Vossepoel A. A computer program for long-term anticoagulation control. Comput Programs Biomed. 1977;7:71–84.

119. Rock WL et al. Evaluation of computer-assisted pharmacist consultation during initiation and stabilization of warfarin therapy. Presented at the 14th Annual ASHP Midyear Clinical Meeting. Las Vegas, NV; 1979.

120. Carter BL et al. Evaluation of three dosage-prediction methods for initial in-hospital stabilization of warfarin therapy. Clin Pharm. 1987;6:37–45.

121. Boyle DA et al. Evaluation of a Bayesian regression program for predicting warfarin response. Ther Drug Monit. 1989;11:276–84.

122. Lee C et al. Effect of using warfarin plasma concentrations in Bayesian forecasting of prothrombin-time response. Clin Pharm. 1987;6:406–12.

123. Svec JM et al. Bayesian pharmacokinetic/pharmacodynamic forecasting of prothrombin time response to warfarin therapy: preliminary evaluation. Ther Drug Monitor. 1985;7:174–80.

124. O'Quinn S, Sawyer WT. Comparison of two computer-assisted pharmacodynamic models for characterization of warfarin effect. Honors Essay: School of Pharmacy, University of North Carolina at Chapel Hill, 1990.

125. Lucas FV et al. A novel whole blood capillary technic for measuring the prothrombin time. Am J Clin Path. 1987;88:442–46.

126. White RH et al. Home prothrombin time monitoring after initiation of warfarin therapy. Ann Intern Med. 1989;111:730–37.

127. Weibert RT, Adler DS. Evaluation of a capillary whole-blood prothrombin time measurement system. Clin Pharm. 1989;8:864–67.

128. van Dieijen-Visser MP et al. Use of chromogenic peptide substrates in the determination of clotting factors II, VII, IX and X in normal plasma and in plasma of patients treated with oral anticoagulants. Haemostasis. 1982;12:241–55.

129. van Wijk EM et al. Mechanized amidolytic technique for determination of factor X and factor-X antigen, and its application to patients being treated with oral anticoagulants. Clin Chem. 1980;26(7):885–90.

130. Lammle B et al. Monitoring of oral anticoagulation by an amidolytic factor X assay. Thromb Haemostas. 1980;44:150–53.

131. Aiach M et al. Kinetic study of factor X during oral anticoagulation with acenocoumarol: potential value for the initiation of treatment. Thromb Haemostas. 1982;47(1):69–71.

132. Deykin D et al. Evidence for an antithrombotic effect of dicumarol. Am J Physiol. 1984;199:1161–164.

133. Kazmier FJ et al. Effect of oral anticoagulants on Factors VII, IX, X and II. Arch Intern Med. 1965;115:667–73.

134. Owren PA. Critical study of tests for control of anticoagulant therapy. Thromb Diath Haemorrh. 1962;7(Suppl. 1):294–305.

135. Loeliger EA et al. Behavior of Factors II, VII, IX and X during long-term treatment with coumarin. Thromb Diath Haemorrh. 1963;9:74–89.

136. Porter RS et al. Pharmacokinetic and pharmacodynamic analysis of warfarin in human subjects. Clin Pharmacol Ther. 1985;37:221. Abstract.

137. Furie B et al. Comparison of the native prothrombin antigen and the prothrombin time for monitoring oral anticoagulant therapy. Blood. 1984;64:445–51.

138. Esmon CT et el. The functional significance of vitamin K action. Difference in phospholipid binding between normal and abnormal prothrombin. J Biol Chem. 1975;250:4095–99.

139. Blanchard RA et al. Acquired vitamin K-dependent carboxylation deficiency in liver disease. N Engl J Med. 1981;305:242–48.

140. Blanchard RA et al. Immunoassay of human prothrombin species which correlate with fractional coagulant activities. J Lab Clin Med. 1983;101:242–55.
141. Poller L, Taberner DA. Dosage and control of oral anticoagulants: An international collaborative survey. Br J Haematol. 1982;51:479–85.
142. Aledort LM. Effective use of anticoagulants. Drug Therapy. 1982;22:107–17.
143. Loeliger EA et al. Reliability and clinical impact of the normalization of the prothrombin times in oral anticoagulant control. Thromb Haemostas. 1985;53:148–54.
144. Loeliger EA. ICSH/ICTH Recommendation for reporting prothrombin time in oral anticoagulant control. Thromb Haemost. 1985;53:155–56.
145. Hirsh J et al. Optimal therapeutic range for oral anticoagulants. Chest. 1989;95(Suppl. 2):5S–10S.
146. Hull R et al. Different intensities of oral anticoagulation therapy in the treatment of proximal-vein thrombosis. N Engl J Med. 1982;307:1676–681.
147. Schulman S et al. Intensive initial oral anticoagulation and shorter heparin treatment in deep vein thrombosis. Thromb Haemostas. 1984;52:276–80.
148. Coon W, Willis P. Thromboembolic complications during anticoagulant therapy. Arch Surg. 1972;105:209–12.
149. Hoak J et al. The anti-thrombotic properties of coumarin drugs. Ann Intern Med. 1961;54:73–81.
150. Wessler S et al. An assay of the antithrombotic action of warfarin: its correlation with the inhibition of stasis thrombosis in rabbits. Thromb Haemost. 1979;40:486–98.
151. Hull R et al. Warfarin sodium versus low-dose heparin in the long-term treatment of venous thrombosis. N Engl J Med. 1979;301:855–58.
152. Hull R et al. Heparin for 5 days compared to 10 days in the initial treatment of proximal vein thrombosis. N Engl J Med. 1990;322:1260–264.
153. Sawyer WT, Raasch RH. Effect of heparin on prothrombin time. Clin Pharm. 1984;3:192–94.
154. Forfor JC. Prediction of hemorrhage during long-term oral coumarin anticoagulation by excessive prothrombin ratio. Am Heart J. 1982;103(3):445–46.
155. Landefeld CS et al. Bleeding in outpatients treated with warfarin: relation to the prothrombin time and important remediable lesions. Am J Med. 1989;87:153–59.
156. Petitti DB et al. Prothrombin time and other factors associated with bleeding in patients treated with warfarin. J Clin Epidemiol. 1989;42:759–64.
157. Schulman S et al. Haemorrhagic and thromboembolic complications versus intensity of treatment of venous thromboembolism with oral anticoagulants. Acta Med Scand. 1988;224:425–30.
158. Gurewich V. Guidelines for the management of anticoagulant therapy. Sem Thromb Hemostasis. 1976;II:176–92.
159. Takahashi H et al. Plasma levels of protein C and vitamin K-dependent coagulation factors in patients on long-term oral anticoagulant therapy. Tohoku J Exp Med. 1986;149:351–57.
160. Jewell P et al. Heparin and ethyl-biscoumacetate in prevention of experimental venous thrombosis. Br Med J. 1954;1:1013–19.
161. Bays RP. Unusual sensitivity to warfarin sodium. J La State Med Soc. 1965;117:55–9.
162. Killilea TA et al. Increased response to warfarin in valve-replacement patients compared to PE/DVT patients. Clin Pharmacol Therap. 1988;43:161.
163. Westbloom TU, Marienfield RD. Prolonged hospitalization because of inappropriate delay of warfarin therapy in deep venous thrombosis. Southern Med J. 1985;78:1164–167.
164. Gallus A et al. Safety and efficacy of warfarin started early after submassive venous thrombosis or pulmonary embolism. Lancet. 1986;II:1293–296.
165. Rospond RM et al. Evaluation of factors associated with stability of anticoagulant therapy. Pharmacother. 1989;9(4):207–13.
166. Boyle DA, Ludden TM. Optimal sampling strategy for warfarin therapy. Clin Pharmacol Ther. 1988;43:131.
167. O'Reilly RA. The stereoselective interaction of warfarin and metronidazole in man. N Engl J Med. 1976;295:354–57.
168. Williams J et al. Effect of concomitantly administered drugs on the control of long-term anticoagulant therapy. Quart J Med. 1976;45:63–73.

169. MacLeod SM, Sellers EM. Pharmacodynamic and pharmacokinetic drug interactions with coumarin anticoagulants. Drugs. 1976;11:461–70.

170. Weiner B et al. Warfarin dosage following prosthetic valve replacement: effect of smoking history. Drug Intell Clin Pharm. 1984;18:904–6.

171. Yacobi A et al. Pharmacokinetic and pharmacodynamic studies of acute interaction between warfarin enantiomers and metronidazole in rats. J Pharmacol Exp Ther. 1984;231(1):72–9.

172. Yacobi A et al. Pharmacokinetic and pharmacodynamic studies of acute interaction between warfarin enantiomers and chloramphenicol in rats. J Pharmacol Exp Ther. 1984;231(1):80–4.

173. Fletcher D. Do clotting factors in vitamin K-rich vegetables hinder anticoagulant therapy? J Am Med Assoc. 1977;237:1871.

174. Lader E et al. Warfarin dosage and vitamin K in Osmolite. Ann Intern Med. 1980;93:373–74.

175. Udall J. Human sources and absorption of vitamin K in relation to anticoagulation stability. J Am Med Assoc. 1965;194:127–29.

176. Walker FB IV. Myocardial infarction after diet-induced warfarin resistance. Arch Intern Med. 1984;144(10):2089–90.

177. Richmond R et al. Extreme warfarin intoxication secondary to covert drug ingestion. Drug Intell Clin Pharm. 1988;22:696–99.

178. Karlson B et al. On the influence of vitamin K-rich vegetables and wine on the effectiveness of warfarin treatment. Acta Med Scand. 1986;220:347–50.

179. Bentley DP et al. Investigation of patients with abnormal response to warfarin. Br J Clin Pharmacol. 1986;22:37–41.

180. Wingard L, Levy G. Comparative pharmacokinetics of coumarin anticoagulants XXXVI: predicted steady-state patterns of prothrombin complex activity produced by equieffective doses of (R) - (+) and (S) - (-) warfarin in humans. J Pharm Sci. 1977;66:1790–791.

181. Bjornsson T et al. High-pressure liquid chromatographic analysis of drugs in biological fluids, I: Warfarin. J Pharm Sci. 1977;66:142–44.

182. Forman W, Shlaes J. Comparison of high performance liquid chromatography and a spectrophotometric technique for determining plasma warfarin. J Chromatogr. 1978;146:522–26.

183. Lee S et al. High performance liquid chromatographic separation and fluorescence detection of warfarin and its metabolites by postcolumn acid/base manipulation. Anal Chem. 1981;53:467–71.

184. Robinson CA et al. Quantitation of plasma warfarin concentrations by high performance liquid chromatography. Ther Drug Mon. 1981;3(3):287–90.

185. Tasker RAR, Nakatsu K. Rapid, reliable and sensitive assay for warfarin using normal-phase high-performance liquid chromatography. J Chromat. 1982;28:346–49.

186. Banfield C, Rowland M. Stereospecific fluorescence high-performance liquid chromatographic analysis of warfarin and its metabolites in plasma and urine. J Pharm Sci. 1984;73(10):1000–1.

187. Carter BL, et al. Warfarin dosage predictions assisted by the analog computer. Ther Drug Monit. 1988;10:69–73.

188. Farrow L et al. Predicting the daily prothrombin time response to warfarin. Ther Drug Monit. 1990;12:246–49.

189. Fredriks DA. Coleman RW. Nomogram for dosing warfarin at steady state. Clin Pharm. 1991;10:923–27.

Chapter 32

Salicylates

Sydney H. Dromgoole and Daniel E. Furst

There are many different derivatives of salicylic acid commercially available which can be classified into two groups: acetylated and nonacetylated salicylates. Acetylsalicylic acid (aspirin) and benorylate are the two representatives of the acetylated class of salicylates, whereas the other derivatives belong to the nonacetylated class of salicylates. There are important differences between the acetylated and nonacetylated salicylate preparations with respect to their effects on platelet function, prostaglandin synthesis inhibition, and gastrointestinal bleeding.[1]

The structures of the salicylate derivatives are shown in Figure 32-1. The most important ester derivative of salicylic acid is acetylsalicylic acid or aspirin. Choline salicylate is the salt of the strongly basic choline ion and salicylic acid. Because of its hygroscopic nature, it is marketed in a liquid form (Arthropan). Choline magnesium trisalicylate (Trilisate) is a combination of choline salicylate and magnesium salicylate. Salicylic acid (Disalcid) is a salicylate derivative which on hydrolysis produces two molecules of salicylate. Benorylate (4-[acetamido] phenyl-2-acetoxy-benzoate) is the acetaminophen ester of aspirin which is absorbed and broken down to its active constituents in the gastrointestinal tract. Diflunisal (2,4-difluoro-4-hydroxy-3-biphenylcarboxylic acid) is a derivative of salicylic acid which differs from aspirin in having a difluorophenyl group and lacks the acetyl groups. It is not, however, metabolized to salicylic acid and will not be discussed further. All the other salicylate derivatives are rapidly hydrolyzed to salicylic acid. They circulate in the blood in the ionized form, salicylate. Conversion factors for estimating aspirin equivalent doses (AED) for various salicylates have been published.[2]

In this chapter, the words salicylic acid and salicylate will be used interchangeably while the term salicylates will refer to the group of drugs that produce salicylate *in vivo* (e.g., aspirin, sodium salicylate, Trilisate).

Despite the widespread use of salicylates as antipyretic, analgesic, and anti-inflammatory agents for over 100 years, it was only after the elucidation of the complicated pharmacokinetics of salicylates that a more rational approach to therapy could be attained. The therapeutic concentration range of plasma salicylates is narrow, and small changes in dosage can have a nonproportional effect on steady-state concentrations; regular dosing rate adjustments must be made based on plasma salicylate concentration monitoring and the patient's clinical status. The disproportionate effects of changes in dosage upon plasma salicylate concentrations are related to the complicated and unusual pharmacokinetics of salicylates.

CLINICAL PHARMACOKINETICS

Absorption

Salicylic acid and its derivatives are absorbed rapidly from the stomach and intestine by passive diffusion of undissociated molecules. Absorption from conventional tablets and capsules is usually complete within two to four hours, and the rate of absorption is determined more by the physical characteristics of the particular formulation than by any other feature.[3-6] Gastrointestinal intolerance to salicylates in some individuals is well documented.[8-21] This problem has been reduced by employing salicylate formulations with enteric coatings,[22,23] or buffers,[24] or in suppository form,[25,26] or by chemically modifying the salicylate molecule.[27-29] Some of these formulations (e.g., salicylic acid) preferentially dissolve in the small intestine where the pH is neutral rather than in the stomach where the pH is acidic. Optimum absorption of salicylates in the human stomach occurs in the pH range of 2.5 to 4.0.[30] The low pH of the stomach, as compared with the higher pH in the intestinal tract, favors gastric absorption of salicylates. Aspirin,

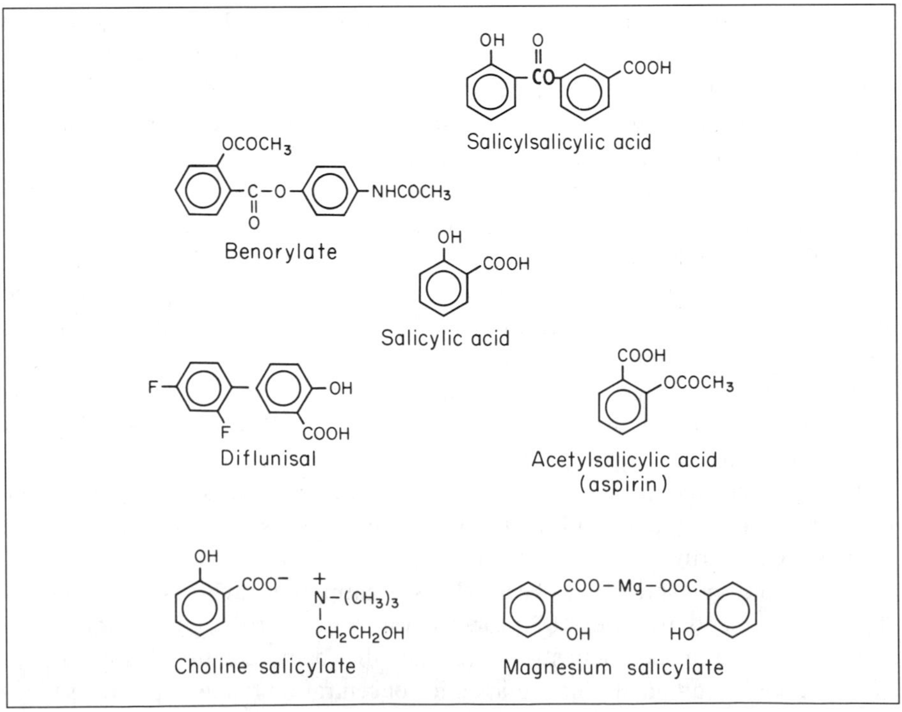

Figure 32-1. *Chemical structures of salicylic acid and derivatives.*

salicylic acid, and choline salicylate are absorbed to some extent in the stomach; however, the small intestine is the optimum site for rapid absorption because of its much larger surface area. Stomach emptying time is also a critical determinant of the absorption rate of drugs, and large doses of salicylate may decrease the emptying time and lead to a decreased rate of drug absorption.[31] Evidence to support this is found in patients with salicylate overdoses where there may be a significant amount of salicylates in the stomach nine to ten hours after an overdose.[32]

Food and antacids can affect the absorption of aspirin from the gastrointestinal tract.[33,34] Antacids decreased the maximum concentrations of both aspirin and salicylic acid, and the effect was maximal when antacids were administered two hours before aspirin. Food significantly prolonged the mean gastric residence time of aspirin as well as the time to reach peak salicylate concentrations. Women exhibited greater prolongation in the gastric residence time and a greater delay in the lag time than men.[34]

The rate of absorption determines the time to peak blood levels, but it is the extent of absorption which determines the effective bioavailability of a drug. Strictly, bioavailability is defined as the availability of a drug at the actual site of action; however, this would require measurement of drug at a cellular level, and direct measurement of bioavailability is not possible in human subjects. Instead, serum, blood, or plasma concentrations are used. The chemical form of salicylate can influence its bioavailability.[35-38] Although the enteric-coated formulations are more slowly absorbed than uncoated aspirin tablets, the bioavailability of the coated preparations is, in general, equivalent to uncoated (buffered or unbuffered) aspirin.[22,23,39-41] However, erratic, delayed and incomplete absorption has been observed with some enteric coated formulations.[42] Rectal suppositories have been used to circumvent the gastrointestinal irritation caused by oral administration of aspirin. The absorption half-life from suppositories is much longer (three hours) than the oral absorption half-life (15 to 30 minutes), and such slow absorption may result in prolonged low subtherapeutic salicylate blood levels over the dosage interval.[25] Gibaldi and Grundhofer[43] have shown that the bioavailability of aspirin from five commercially available suppositories was much less than orally administered aspirin. Bioavailability from suppositories increases markedly with retention time.[25]

Absorption of salicylates can also be influenced by disease. Patients with celiac disease absorb salicylates faster than do normal subjects.[44] It has been suggested that the difference is caused by changes in gastric emptying or by altered small intestinal permeability. Salicylate bioavailability is impaired in patients with Kawasaki disease.[45,46] Bioavailability was only 47.7% during the febrile phase of the disease but increased to 75.1% in the afebrile phase. The reason for the impaired absorption is unknown.

Miaskiewicz et al.[47] have reported gender differences in the absorption kinetics of sodium salicylate. In a group of young, healthy nonsmoking women and an age- and weight-matched group of men, the time to reach maximum plasma levels of salicylate (T_{max}) following a 9 mg/kg oral dose of sodium salicylate was significantly shorter (p <0.01) in men (31.5 ± 3.1 minutes) than women (54.0 ± 6.5 minutes), although the Cp_{max}, AUC, plasma t½, and plasma protein binding values were similar in the two groups.

Distribution

The distribution of salicylates in the body is a reflection of the manner in which the drug is bound to albumin and equilibrates with the tissues.

It is interesting to note that the distribution of the acetyl group of aspirin has been reported to be different from that of the salicyl moiety.[69] It has been demonstrated that the labile acetyl group is bound to a variety of proteins, glycoproteins, and lipids of the glandular and nonglandular regions of the stomach, kidney, liver, and bone marrow (organs in which side-effects are frequently encountered). The significance of this widespread acetylation has been discussed elsewhere.[69]

With salicylates, the fraction bound to albumin decreases with increasing total salicylate concentration.[48–61] At low therapeutic salicylate concentrations in plasma (100 µg/mL), about 90% is bound, while at higher concentrations of salicylate (400 µg/mL), only 76% of the salicylate is bound on the average.[48]

The protein binding of salicylates is also influenced by age[56,58,62,64] and disease.[63–67] For example, low albumin concentrations in nephrotic syndrome, liver disease, or protein-losing enteropathy can change distribution, since less albumin is present to bind salicylate.[63,66] Uremia may alter protein binding by affecting the affinity and/or number of binding sites.[65] The clinical significance of the concentration-dependent protein binding of salicylates has been discussed elsewhere.[68]

Salicylates and other nonsteroidal anti-inflammatory agents can cross the placental barrier[70–74] and, if they are ingested just before delivery, plasma salicylate concentrations in the newborn remain elevated longer than the corresponding values in the maternal plasma, indicating slower elimination of salicylate in newborns than in adults.[75] This may in turn be related to the fact that the ductus venosus allows drugs to escape exposure to the metabolic enzymes in the liver.[76] During chronic oral administration of salicylates to pregnant women, salicylates may be distributed throughout fetal tissues in concentrations that are higher than those in the mother.[77,78]

Salicylates are also distributed into breast milk, but the extent of distribution is not clearly established. One study has shown that the peak concentrations of salicylate in milk were 2% to 5% of the peak maternal plasma salicylate concentrations.[79] An important point to remember is that since salicylates can transfer across the placental barrier, can distribute into breast milk, and can inhibit the synthesis of prostaglandins which are important to fetal cardiovascular hemostasis and other fetal functions, salicylates and other nonsteroidal anti-inflammatory drugs (NSAIDs) should be administered with caution to pregnant or nursing mothers.

Salicylates rapidly distribute into semen following the administration of a single dose of aspirin.[80] Both aspirin and salicylurate were also present in semen in concentration ratios (semen:plasma) of 0.12 and 0.15, respectively.

One report indicated that there was no correlation between plasma and cerebro-spinal fluid salicylate levels.[81] The authors suggest that this finding, typical of hydrophilic NSAIDs, may be due to bulk absorption of the salicylate at the arachnoidal villi and/or the presence of a weak organic acid transport system, putatively located in the choroidal plexus epithelium.

Metabolism

Irrespective of the parent source of salicylic acid, once the drug is absorbed and rapidly hydrolyzed (in the bowel wall and liver) to salicylic acid, the metabolism and elimination is essentially that of salicylic acid. Consequently, blood and urinary concentrations of salicylic acid or salicylate are usually more meaningful than blood and urine concentrations of the parent source of salicylate.

The major metabolic and elimination pathways of salicylic acid are now well characterized[82–116] and are diagrammed in Figure 32-2. Salicylic acid (SA) is eliminated from the body: 1) by renal excretion of salicylic acid; 2) by conjugation with glycine to form salicyluric acid (SU); 3) by conjugation with glucuronic acid to form salicyl phenolic glucuronide (SPG), salicyl acyl glucuronide (SAG), and salicyluric acid phenolic glucuronide (SUPG); 4) by oxidation to gentisic acid (GA); and 5) by the formation of gentisuric acid (GU) from either SU (via microsomal oxidation) or GA (via glycine conjugation). 2,3-dihydroxybenzoic acid (DBA) has been identified in urine and plasma following the ingestion of aspirin.

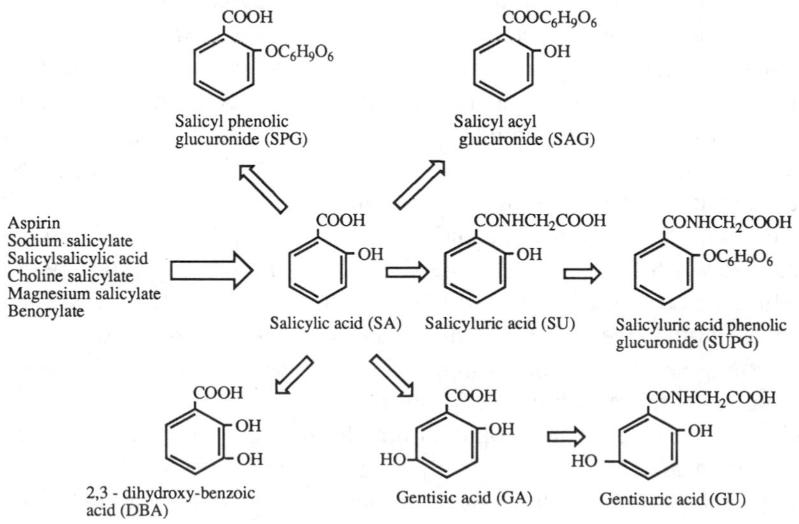

Figure 32-2. Metabolism of salicylic acid.

The elimination pathways of salicylic acid involve two processes that are saturable and follow Michaelis-Menten type kinetics (SU and SPG) and three linear or first-order pathways, all acting in parallel.[87,91,92] The kinetics of the minor elimination pathways of GU and 2,3-dihydroxybenzoic acid have not yet been characterized. The predominant pathway for salicylic acid elimination is the conjugation with glycine and excretion as salicyluric acid. After a small dose of aspirin (i.e., 300 mg or less) about 90% is excreted as salicyluric acid and SPG.[98] However, after moderate doses, when the amount of salicylate in the body is more than about 600 mg, the maximum rates of formation of salicyluric acid, SUPG, and SPG are reached.[97,98,120] As the capacities of these major pathways are approached, the linear pathways become more important in the elimination of salicylates. This means that the amount of salicylic acid in the body increases nonlinearly with increasing dosage. Consequently, the half-life of salicylate in serum becomes longer with increasing dosage, and the blood level of salicylate increases disproportionately as the salicylate dosage is increased. Thus, when the amount of salicylate increases from 250 mg (equivalent to one aspirin tablet) to 10 gm, the time required for the first 50% of the dose to be removed from the body increases from 3 to 20 hours (see Table 32-1).

Patel et al.[120,227] observed that patients with aspirin overdose (plasma salicylates of 240 to 870 µg/mL on admission) had lower percentages of total salicylate recovered as SU and SUPG than those in volunteers who had ingested 600 mg aspirin. In patients with plasma salicylate concentrations of 240 to 600 µg/mL, SU and SPG accounted for 46.7% and 22.9% respectively, while those with plasma salicylates between 715 and 870 µg/mL excreted 21.6% and 15.9% as SU and SPG, respectively.

Several studies have shown that there is much intersubject variation with respect to the relative contribution of the different salicylate pathways.[104,105] These data suggest that salicylate metabolism is extremely variable among subjects, and this variability, in turn, may affect the intensity and duration of pharmacological effect of the drug. The metabolism of SA and ASA is gender-dependent, and the metabolism as well as the excretion of salicylates can be influenced by concomitant use of oral contraceptive steroids.[61] Ho et al.[123] have reported age- and gender-related differences in the disposition of ASA and its metabolites. They observed significantly higher plasma levels of ASA and SA in females, while the plasma levels of SU were found to be significantly higher in the elderly groups. These findings confirmed the results of other studies.[124-126] Ho et al. suggested that the higher plasma levels observed in females were related to the lower intrinsic aspirin esterase activity in this group, while the lower clearance of SU led to the accumulation of this metabolite in the elderly.

Evidence indicates that autoinduction of salicylate metabolism occurs on chronic administration.[101,110,111] This phenomenon could account for the decrease in steady-state serum salicylate concentrations observed on chronic administration of high doses of aspirin.[106-109] Day et al.[110] observed that the SU formation rates in patients with rheumatoid arthritis receiving aspirin significantly increased during the first two weeks of high-dose therapy. They further characterized the autoinduction phenomenon in normal subjects.[111] Significant increases in the maximal

Table 32-1. Summary of Pharmacokinetic Variables

Variable	Mean ± SD[a]	n	Comments[a]	Reference
T_{maxSA} (min) absorption	31.5 ± 3.1 (M)	20	D = 9 mg/kg NaSa	42
	54.0 ± 6.5 (F)	20		
T_{maxSA} (min)	2.15 ± 0.56	5	D = 160 mg ASA	33
	2.33 ± 0.59	5	D = 160 mg ASA + antacid	33
	2.5 ± 0.3	5	D = 975 mg ASA tabs	80
	3.9 ± 0.6	6	D = 50 mg ASA (modified release)	118
	0.56 ± 0.02	6	D = 50 mg ASA soln	118
	0.62 ± 0.25	6	D = 50 mg ASA intravenously	118
	3.02 ± 1.91	6	D = 50 mg ASA (modified release)	118
	8.3 ± 2.9	8	D = 648 mg ASA (enteric coated)	34
	13.8 ± 4.5	8	D = 648 mg ASA (enteric coated) + food	34
	0.94 ± 0.33	6YM	D = 600 mg ASA	123
	0.93 ± 0.12	7YF	D = 500 mg ASA	123
	0.71 ± 0.19	6OM	D = 500 mg ASA	123
	0.72 ± 0.17	6OF	D = 600 mg ASA	123
T_{maxASA} (min)	50 ± 15	5	D = 160 mg ASA	33
	60 ± 14	5	D = 160 mg ASA + antacid	33
	24.0 ± 7.2	6	D = 500 mg ASA (single dose)	41
	244.2 ± 42.6	6	D = 500 mg ASA (enteric coated)	41
	26 ± 8	5	D = 975 mg ASA tabs	80
	22.8 ± 12.6	6YM	D = 600 mg ASA	123
	18.6 ± 6.0	7YF	D = 600 mg ASA	123
	21.0 ± 6.0	6OM	D = 600 mg ASA	123
	17.4 ± 7.2	6OF	D = 600 mg ASA	123
V_d (L/kg)	0.18 ± 0.03	20	D = 9 mg/kg NaSA	42
	0.17 ± 0.03	16	D = 1.2 gm ASA	37
	0.15 ± 0.02	36	D = 1.3 gm ASA; 1 gm SSA	36
	0.16 ± 0.35	11	V ↑ with ↑ dose	16

Table 32-1. *Summary of Pharmacokinetic Variables (cont.)*

Variable	Mean ± SD[a]	n	Comments[a]	Reference
V_d (L/kg)	0.19 ± 0.05	6	D = 50 mg ASA IV	118
	0.16 ± 0.02	8M	D = 900 mg ASA	61
	0.15 ± 0.02	8F	D = 900 mg ASA	61
	0.16 ± 0.02	8F (BCP)	D = 900 mg ASA	61
	0.22 ± 0.07	6YM	D = 600 mg ASA	123
	0.18 ± 0.03	7YF	D = 600 mg ASA	123
	0.24 ± 0.07	6OM	D = 600 mg ASA	123
	0.24 ± 0.11	6OF	D = 600 mg ASA	123
V_{maxSU} (mg/hr)	57.3 ± 11.7	8	D = 1.8 gm ASA	103
	71.4 ± 9.4	8	D > 2.7 gm ASA	103
	43.4 ± 10.1	5	D = 1.2 gm to 1.5 gm ASA, NaSA	104
	66.3 ± 4.1	12	D = 40 mg/kg ASA	91
	60.3 ± 5.3	4	D = 3 gm NaSA	84
K_{mSU} (mg)	338 ± 47	4	D = 3 gm NaSA	84
	143 ± 34	5	D = 1.2 gm to 1.5 gm ASA, NaSA	104
V_{maxSPG} (mg/hr)	32.3 ± 12.4	4	D = 3 gm NaSA	84
K_{mSPG} (mg)	629 ± 376	4	D = 3 gm NaSA	84
K_{SA} (hr^{-1})	0.010 ± 0.005	4	D = 3 gm NaSA	84
K_{SAG} (hr^{-1})	0.0075 ± 0.0016	4	D = 3 gm NaSA	84
K_{GA} (hr^{-1})	0.0025 ± 0.0007	4	D = 3 gm NaSA	84
F	0.98 ± 0.28	4	D = 3 gm NaSA	84
	0.90 ± 0.12	6	D = 1.3 gm ASA	36
	0.86 ± 0.32	6	D = 1.0 gm SSA	36
F	0.46–0.51	5	D = 20–1300 mg ASA	193

Parameter	Value	Dose	n	Ref
$t\frac{1}{2}_{ASA}$ (min)	26.5 ± 5.7	D = 160 mg ASA	5	33
	41.0 ± 24.0	D = 160 mg ASA + antacid	5	33
	19.8 ± 4.41	D = 500 mg ASA (single dose)	6	41
	23.4 ± 4.41	D = 500 mg ASA (enteric coated)	6	41
	10.6 ± 1.9	D = 900 mg ASA	8M	61
	15.5 ± 3.2	D = 900 mg ASA	8F	61
	16.0 ± 3.7	D = 900 mg ASA	8F (BCP)	61
$t\frac{1}{2}_{SA}$ (hr)	2.9 ± 0.17	D = 0.25 gm ASA	4	78
	2.4 ± 0.1 (Y)	D = 1.0 gm ASA	7	189
	3.7 ± 0.4 (O)		15	
	4.1 ± 0.3 (F)	D = 9 mg/kg NaSA	20	42
	4.5 ± 0.3 (M)		20	
	5.1 ± 0.5 (M)	D = 1.2 gm ASA	7	157
	5.8 ± 0.3 (F)		5	
	19.0	D = 10–20 gm NaSA		78
$t\frac{1}{2}_{SA}$ (hr)	3.4 ± 0.5	D = 500 mg ASA (single dose)	6	41
	4.4 ± 1.5	D = 500 mg ASA (enteric coated)	6	41
	5.39 ± 1.84	D = 1300 mg ASA soln	6	122
	3.03 ± 0.74	D = 900 mg ASA	8M	61
	4.53 ± 1.19	D = 900 mg ASA	8F	61
	3.36 ± 0.85	D = 900 mg ASA	8F (BCP)	61
T_{LSA} (hr)	2.7 ± 0.8	D = 648 mg ASA (enteric coated)	8	34
	8.9 ± 3.7	D = 648 mg ASA (enteric coated) + food	8	34
MRT (hr)	0.8 ± 0.5	D = 648 mg ASA (enteric coated)	8	34
	5.9 ± 3.3	D = 648 mg ASA (enteric coated) + food	8	34

Table 32-1. *Summary of Pharmacokinetic Variables (cont.)*

Variable	Mean ± SD[a]	n	Comments[a]	Reference
% excreted in urine as				
unchanged SA	8.3 ± 5.9	129	D = 0.9 gm ASA	119
	3.4 ± 1.2	4	D = 0.25 gm ASA	78
	6.8 ± 3.5	10	D = 0.6 gm ASA	
	5.3 ± 1.7	4	D = 1.0 gm NaSA	
	8.8 ± 0.6	45	D = 0.6 gm ASA	227
	14.0 ± 7.1	4	D = 3.0 gm NaSA	84
	34.0 ± 21.9	9	Acute ASA overdose	120
SU	83.2 ± 5.2	4	D = 0.25 gm ASA	78
	63.1 ± 8.4	10	D = 0.6 gm ASA	120
	70.3 ± 7.1	4	D = 1.0 gm NaSA	
	75.0 ± 1.2	45	D = 0.6 gm ASA	227
	45.0 ± 10.6	129	D = 0.9 gm ASA	119
	50.2 ± 4.4	4	D = 3.0 gm NaSA	84
	30.0 ± 8.2	9	Acute ASA overdose	120
Salicyl glucuronides	13.5 ± 5.2	4	D = 0.25 gm ASA	78
	24.3 ± 5.7	4	D = 1.0 gm NaSA	
	30.5 ± 4.4	4	D = 3.0 gm NaSA	84
SPG	7.2 ± 7.6	129	D = 0.9 gm ASA	119
	9.7 ± 3.1	10	D = 0.6 gm ASA	120
	13.7 ± 6.0	9	Acute ASA overdose	120
	11.5 ± 0.6	45	D = 0.6 gm ASA	227
SAG	8.3 ± 2.3	10	D = 0.6 gm ASA	120
	5.6 ± 2.4	115	D = 0.9 gm ASA	119
	14.4 ± 6.0	9	Acute ASA overdose	120
SUPG	9.3 ± 3.9	10	D = 0.6 gm ASA	120
	2.0 ± 2.2	9	Acute ASA overdose	120
	3.2 ± 1.3	114	D = 0.9 gm ASA	119

GA	3.5 ± 3.4	10	D = 0.6 gm ASA	120
	0.9 ± 0.5	5	D = 1.2 gm to 1.5 gm ASA, NaSA	104
	5.1 ± 0.4	45	D = 0.6 gm ASA	227
	3.1 ± 0.6	4	D = 3.0 gm NaSA	84
	1.0 ± 0.4	117	D = 0.9 gm ASA	119
GU	5.3 ± 2.7	9	Acute overdose ASA	120
CL_{PASA} (mL/hr/kg)	560 ± 75	6	D = 50 mg ASA IV	118
CL_{RSU} (mL/min)	382 ± 192	8	D = 1.8 gm ASA	103
	340 ± 51	5	D = 1.2 gm to 1.5 gm ASA, NaSA	104
CL_{RGA} (mL/min)	64 ± 10	8	D = 1.8 gm ASA	103
	65 ± 10	5	D = 1.2 gm to 1.5 gm ASA, NaSA	104
CL_{PSA} (mL/kg/hr)	9.7 ± 2.2	6	D = 1.3 gm ASA	36
	12.9 ± 5.1	6	D = 1.0 gm SSA	36
CL_{PSA} (mL/hr/kg)	73 ± 24	6	D = 50 mg ASA IV	118
	33.8 ± 6.6	8M	D = 900 mg ASA	61
	21.0 ± 3.8	8F	D = 900 mg ASA	61
	29.6 ± 6.6	8F (BCP)	D = 900 mg ASA	61
CL_{MSU} (mL/min/kg)	0.390 ± 0.056	8M	D = 900 mg ASA	61
	0.241 ± 0.044	8F	D = 900 mg ASA	61
	0.334 ± 0.073	8F (BCP)	D = 900 mg ASA	61
CL_{MSG} (mL/min/kg)	0.101 ± 0.038	8M	D = 900 mg ASA	61
	0.064 ± 0.022	8F	D = 900 mg ASA	61
	0.110 ± 0.040	8F (BCP)	D = 900 mg ASA	61
CL_{SA} (mL/hr)	89 ± 57	6YM	D = 600 mg ASA	123
	88 ± 60	7YF	D = 600 mg ASA	123
	18 ± 18	6OM	D = 600 mg ASA	123
	20 ± 24	6OF	D = 600 mg ASA	123

[a] (M) = Male; (F) = Female; (Y) = Young subjects (ave age 21); (O) = Elderly subjects (ave age 77); D = Dose of salicylate; NaSA = Sodium salicylate; ASA = Acetylsalicylic acid (aspirin); SSA = Salicylsalicylic acid (salsalate); BCP = Birth control pill; YM = Young males (mean age: 20.8 years); OM = Elderly males (mean age: 75.2 years); YF = Young females (mean age: 26.7 years); OF = Elderly females (mean age: 78.7 years).

formation rates (V_{max}) for both SU and SPG occurred during multiple dosing, while the first-order rate constants for the formation of SAG, GA, and excretion of unchanged SA remained constant. Rate constants for the SUPG, DBA, and GU pathways have yet to be determined. A study of salicylate pharmacokinetics in patients with rheumatoid arthritis confirmed earlier reports of declining plasma salicylate levels during chronic dosing and significant increases in the V_{max} for the formation of salicyluric acid, while K_m and clearance of this metabolite remained constant.[127]

Decreased formation of salicyluric acid has been noted in children with Down's syndrome,[102] but the disposition of salicylates in patients with rheumatoid arthritis appears to be similar to that in healthy subjects.[112,113] Patients with acute, active Kawasaki disease manifested decreased bioavailability (48% versus 75%) and increased renal clearance of salicylate (15.8 mL/kg/min versus 7.1 mL/kg/min) compared to their values after recovery.[46]

Excretion

Renal excretion of salicylate is the summation of glomerular filtration, active proximal tubular secretion, passive tubular secretion, and passive tubular absorption.[114] The excretion of salicylic acid is markedly pH-dependent, and as the urinary pH changes from 5 to 8, the amount of free ionized salicylate excreted increases from 2% to 3% of the total salicylate dose to more than 80%.[103,114] Possible mechanisms to account for the pH-dependent enhancement of salicylate excretion have been discussed elsewhere.[68]

There are several reports of circadian rhythms in the urinary excretion of salicylate, with excretion being faster after the drug is ingested between 7:00 and 11:00 p.m.[116,128] This increase may in part be related to the circadian changes in urinary pH or the increased clearance of salicylate during bed rest or prolonged supination.[129] Although preliminary evidence[130,131] suggested that females excrete salicylate faster than males, additional studies have demonstrated that renal clearance of SA in males is higher than in females.[61,123] It is also interesting to note that females taking oral contraceptives had increased rates of salicylate excretion (similar to males) compared to those not using oral contraceptives. This suggests the influence of hormonal factors in salicylate disposition.

The effect of alkalinizing the urine (with the administration of sodium bicarbonate or antacids) on salicylate excretion and plasma salicylate concentrations has been well documented,[33,132–138] but its effect is probably underestimated or overlooked during plasma salicylate monitoring. Studies have shown that the administration of 120 to 150 mL of antacids such as magnesium-aluminum hydroxide (Maalox) significantly reduces the steady-state plasma salicylate concentrations by antacid-induced alkalinization of urine which, in turn, increases renal salicylate clearance. In addition, clinicians should be aware that salicylate intoxication may occur when antacids are discontinued.

Salicylate renal clearance in patients with Kawasaki disease was significantly higher during the febrile stage of the disease.[46] The increased clearance was postulated to be due to decreased protein binding of the drug during the febrile stage.

The various pharmacokinetic parameters describing the absorption, distribution, metabolism and excretion of salicylates are listed in Table 32-1.

PHARMACODYNAMICS

Therapeutic and Toxic Concentrations

Salicylate concentrations in the blood generally correlate with the pharmacological actions and adverse effects observed. Figure 32-3 shows the approximate relationship of plasma salicylate levels to pharmacodynamic effects. The therapeutic plasma salicylate concentrations are only approximations, because the analgesic and anti-inflammatory effects of salicylates in patients are subjective and cannot be measured objectively in a graded manner.[139] Salicylate serum concentrations up to 100 µg/mL are required for effective analgesia,[140] whereas steady-state serum concentrations of 150 to 300 µg/mL are generally accepted as correlating with the anti-inflammatory effects needed for the management of rheumatoid arthritis.[141] The Ritchie articular index in patients with rheumatoid arthritis significantly improved at steady-state plasma salicylate levels (Cp_{ss}) greater than 70 µg/mL indicating that the anti-inflammatory effects of salicylates may occur at low plasma concentrations.[112] In adults, symptoms of intoxication can appear at serum salicylate concentrations of 300 µg/mL and are associated with more severe salicylate intoxication. Nevertheless, levels of 300 to 400 µg/mL

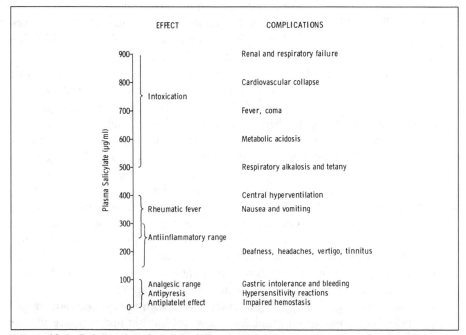

Figure 32-3. *Relationships between plasma salicylate levels, effects, and complications.*

are frequently used to manage acute rheumatic fever.[142,143] From the above data, one can easily see that therapeutic concentrations of salicylates are frequently very close to those at which toxic manifestations may appear.

Because salicylates have unusual pharmacokinetics, there are numerous exceptions and limitations to these therapeutic and toxic plasma concentrations. First, the volume of distribution (V_d) increases with increasing dose. Levy and Yaffe[144] studied children who had ingested large doses of salicylate and found that the volume of distribution increased from 162 mL/kg to 345 mL/kg as the dose increased from 50 mg/kg to greater than 300 mg/kg. This change in V_d should be remembered when treating salicylate intoxication because it means that a given plasma concentration in an individual may reflect a much larger amount of drug in the body than the same plasma concentration in another who had taken a smaller dose of salicylate. This explains why some patients are clinically ill when overdosed despite relatively low salicylate levels. Factors which contribute to the increased distribution are: 1) decreases in plasma pH, resulting in increased amounts of nonionized salicylate available to cross membranes;[145] 2) decreased plasma albumin and protein concentrations,[48,146,147] which result in an increased amount of the free, pharmacologically active drug; and 3) increased amounts of unbound salicylate secondary to drug- or disease-induced conformational changes in the albumin molecule.[85,148-151]

Drug Interactions. Interactions of salicylates with other NSAIDs is a subject of continued dispute.[152-171] In general, the area under the plasma concentration-time cure (AUC) of NSAIDs is decreased in humans when the NSAIDs and aspirin are taken together.[156-158,163,171-173] Brooks and others were unable to demonstrate significant increases in efficacy when indomethacin, tolmetin, ibuprofen, or flurbiprofen were added to high dose aspirin regimens.[154,164-167,173] One careful study compared salicylate (adjusted to serum salicylate concentrations greater than 150 μg/mL), naproxen 1500 mg daily, salicylate (at the therapeutic doses above) plus naproxen 1500 mg daily, and half doses of both, in RA patients. The full dose combination was only 4% better than full dose naproxen and 10% better than full dose salicylate or half dose of both drugs together (these were not statistically different). While toxicity was uncommon, it was twice as frequent in the full dose combination as other regimens (7.5% versus 1.8% to 3.7%) and nearly twice as expensive.[152]

Verbeeck has recently published an extensive review of pharmacokinetic drug interactions with NSAIDs.[202] Table 32-2 lists the numerous documented drug interactions with the salicylate group of drugs and their relative clinical significance.

The *influence of corticosteroids on salicylate elimination* is also important, since these drugs are often administered concomitantly in patients with severe rheumatoid arthritis. Corticosteroids appear to decrease steady-state concentrations of salicylates during long-term aspirin administration. Klinenberg and Miller[174] suggested this was due to increased renal salicylate acid clearance, whereas Graham et al.[175] suggested it was secondary to induction of salicylic acid metabolism. Therefore, etiology of this interaction is still unresolved.

Salicylates and sulfonamides can interact *in vivo* with endogenous substances such as bilirubin. These drugs can compete with bilirubin and displace it from

Table 32-2. *Drug Interactions with Salicylates*

Drug	Possible Effects and Clinical Significance
Acetaminophen	Concurrent administration may provide a cytoprotective effect to GI tissues. It may also ↑ plasma levels of unhydrolyzed aspirin.
Acetazolamide[202]	Aspirin significantly ↓ the plasma protein binding and renal tubular secretion of acetazolamide.
Activated charcoal[203]	Coadministration can ↓ absorption of salicylates.
Alcohol[202]	May enhance the gastric damage induced by salicylates. Avoid in subjects with history of GI bleeding.
Ammonium chloride Ascorbic acid[68]	May ↑ plasma concentrations because of ↓ urinary clearance. Use caution when giving drugs to acidify the urine of subjects on high doses of salicylates.
Antacids[132–138,202]	May ↓ plasma concentrations by ↓ the systemic absorption of salicylates or ↑ urinary clearance of salicylates. May cause subtherapeutic salicylate levels which may require salicylate dosage adjustment.
Anticoagulants (warfarin, acenocoumarol, anisindione, heparin)[202,203,204]	Aspirin may potentiate the hypothrombinemic effects of anticoagulants. The inhibition of platelet function by aspirin can impair one of the hemostatic mechanisms which prevents bleeding in heparin-treated subjects. In addition, aspirin can produce gastric mucosal damage, which may ↑ the risk of GI bleeding in anticoagulated subjects. Aspirin should be used with caution in these subjects.
Antidepressants (nortriptyline, imipramine)	Plasma levels and side effects of antidepressants may be ↑ if aspirin is given concurrently.
Antidiabetic drugs (chlorpropamide, tolbutamide)[202,203]	Aspirin may enhance the hypoglycemic effect of these drugs by competitive interference in tubular secretion or displacement from protein binding sites. Large doses of salicylate may have intrinsic hypoglycemic activity.
Antihypertensive agents[203]	Antihypertensive action of angiotensin-converting enzyme inhibitors and β-adrenergic blockers may be ↓ by concomitant use of salicylates.
Caffeine[206]	Caffeine may significantly ↑ the rate of appearance, the maximum plasma concentration, and the bioavailability of aspirin.
Carbonic anhydrase inhibitors[203]	Salicylate intoxication may occur and/or action of carbonic anhydrase inhibitor may be ↓.
Corticosteroids[174,175,202]	May cause ↑ renal clearance of salicylates.
Dipyridamole	Concurrent administration can inhibit thromboxane B_2 production without change in prostacyclin production.
Indomethacin[200]	Can block the irreversible acetylation of platelets by aspirin, probably by competitive protein binding.

Table 32-2. Drug Interactions with Salicylates (cont.)

Drug	Possible Effects and Clinical Significance
Methotrexate (MTX)[202,203]	Salicylates may cause elevated and/or prolonged serum concentrations of free methotrexate, ↑ the potential for methotrexate toxicity.
Metoprolol (Lopressor)[207]	Plasma salicylate concentrations may ↑ with concomitant administration of metoprolol.
Nicotinic acid[208]	Coadministration of aspirin ↓ total nicotinic acid clearance and saturates the nicotinuric acid conjugation pathway. Nicotinic acid concentrations are prolonged. Clinical significance unknown—may diminish nicotinic acid induced-flushing.
Nitroglycerin (NTG)[203]	May result in unexpected hypotension.
Nizatidine[203]	↑ drug levels have occurred in patients receiving high doses of salicylates.
Nonsteroidal anti-inflammatory drugs (NSAIDs) (fenoprofen, indomethacin, ibuprofen, ketoprofen, pirprofen, diclofenac, diflunisal, naproxen, isoxicam, tenoxican)[152,156,157,158, 168,169,202]	May alter salicylate and/or NSAID pharmacokinetics and consequently affect efficacy and/or toxicity. Salicylates ↓ the AUC of numerous NSAIDs by 8% to 48%. Salicylates also ↓ serum naproxen concentrations 26% and ↑ serum naproxen clearance by 56%. Naproxen had little effect on serum salicylate concentrations.
Oral Contraceptives[61,202]	Metabolism and excretion of salicylates is changed in women taking birth control pills. Clinical significance is unknown.
Phenytoin[209]	Concomitant administration can ↑ the serum concentration of phenytoin and can influence thyroid function tests. Changes are consistent with ASA-induced displacement of T_4 from its binding proteins and phenytoin-induced clearance of FT_4. Thyroid function tests should be interpreted with caution in subjects taking this combination.
Spironolactone[203]	Possible inhibition of natriuresis.
Thyroid function tests[209,210]	Concomitant administration of salicylates may influence thyroid function tests. Use caution in interpretation of thyroid function tests of patients taking salicylates.
Uricosuric agents (phenylbutazone, probenicid, sulfinpyrazone)[202.203,211]	Large doses of salicylates can inhibit the uricosuric effect of these drugs. In addition, probenecid and sulfinpyrazone can also inhibit the uricosuric effect which usually follows large doses of aspirin.
Valproate (VPA)[212]	Concomitant administration of aspirin can displace VPA from protein binding sites and cause ↑ free VPA and potential VPA-induced toxicity.

plasma protein binding sites. In neonates, the displaced, unbound, and unconjugated bilirubin readily passes the poorly developed blood-brain barrier and may lead to kernicterus.[201]

Antiplatelet Effects. The interaction of NSAIDs (particularly aspirin) with platelets has been widely studied.[176–198,275] NSAIDs inhibit the second wave of platelet aggregation by blocking the formation of the powerful platelet aggregator, thromboxane A_2 (T_xA_2), in platelets. They also affect prostacyclin (PGI_2) synthesis in the blood vessel wall. Prostacyclin both inhibits substances which promote platelet aggregation and stimulates vasodilation. Thus, the NSAIDs alter the balance between the synthesis of PGI_2 and T_xA_2.[177,179,180] The inhibitory effect on platelets of NSAIDs, including nonacetylated salicylates, is reversible; if platelets are washed to remove the drug, aggregation returns to normal.[181,182,185,190,191] Aspirin, however, causes irreversible inhibition of platelet aggregation by acetylation of the platelets.[177,180,187,190,192,194] This inhibition lasts seven to ten days, the lifetime of the platelet.[195] Evidence[192,193] suggests that as little as 20 mg of aspirin can reduce serum thromboxane B_2 levels (a measure of T_xA_2) dramatically and that these remain inhibited with long-term maintenance therapy using low aspirin doses. However, since women have lower T_xB_2 in serum, aspirin affects them less than it affects men.[188] Some evidence[192] suggests that at these low aspirin doses PGI_2 synthesis is not affected, indicating that the most beneficial aspect of aspirin with respect to antithrombotic therapy may be achieved with very low dose aspirin regimens. Salicylic acid, aspirin's major metabolite, may protect prostacyclin from inhibition by aspirin *per se*.[196–198] These effects, plus increased clot lysis due to N-acetylation of fibrinogen, can lead to increased postoperative bleeding.[178,199] Both sodium salicylate and indomethacin, when given before aspirin *in vivo* prevent or decrease the inhibition of platelet aggregation by aspirin.[200]

Reye's Syndrome. Reye's syndrome, a pediatric illness characterized by progressive encephalopathy and liver abnormalities, was first described in 1963.[213] Epidemiologic studies in the 1980s implicated aspirin therapy as a significant predisposing factor in this disease.[213,214] Thus, prior aspirin use was associated with a relative risk ratio of Reye's syndrome of 26 (lower 95% confidence interval = 6.4) in a U.S. Public Health Service study.[214] Aspirin use in young children decreased after publication of this report. Strangely, however, the incidence of this illness was unchanged in countries (e.g., Australia) where aspirin use had decreased previously, thus calling the above relationship into question.[215] The actual cause of Reye's syndrome and the relationship of aspirin to Reye's syndrome require further clarification.

Gastrointestinal Effects. While rare, major gastrointestinal (GI) bleeding and ulcers have been associated with chronic aspirin use.[216,217,218] Although no prospective study is likely to be performed, because GI bleeding from aspirin is so rare, case control studies indicate a relative risk ratio of 15 for regular aspirin use in hospitalized GI bleeders.[217] The elderly, particularly, are prone to this complication. The cause of the damage is probably direct damage of the gastric mucosa by salicylate and secondary effects of aspirin via inhibition of cyclo-oxygenase.[219]

Aspirin Intolerance. Aspirin intolerance occurs in 4% to 19% of asthma patients.[220] It is associated with a "classical triad" of nasal polyps, asthma, and aspirin sensitivity. This syndrome, called Samter's syndrome, is related to cyclo-oxygenase inhibition, with more potent cyclo-oxygenase inhibition being associated with more sensitivity.[221] Treatment includes avoidance of aspirin, desensitization with increasing aspirin doses (given under close, in-hospital observation), and the use of prednisone.[220,222]

Comparative Toxicity of Aspirin and Salicylate. Since salicylate is a good anti-inflammatory compound, as shown in a large multicenter trial of 233 RA patients,[223] it is possible that salicylate could be substituted for aspirin. In this context, salicylate's side-effect profile, as separate from aspirin, is of interest. Salicylate inhibits platelet functions much less potently than aspirin (about 2% as effective).[224] It causes less gastroduodenal damage than enteric-coated aspirin. For example, only one of ten volunteers taking 3 gm/day of salicylate developed endoscopic gastric mucosal damage, compared to six of ten using 2.6 gm/day of enteric-coated aspirin.[225] In addition, salicylate does not affect prostaglandins, renal blood flow, or glomerular filtration rate in sodium-restricted dogs, while aspirin profoundly suppresses these measures.[226] Thus, salicylate may be a useful alternative to aspirin in circumstances where the use of aspirin is associated with a high risk of toxicity.

CLINICAL APPLICATION OF PHARMACOKINETIC DATA

Individual variability in response to drugs is a crucial and often neglected fact in pharmacotherapeutics. Many drugs are still habitually prescribed in "usual" or "average" doses, and an inadequate dose may be interpreted as ineffectiveness of the drug, while excessive dosages may be judged as intolerance. Such variability has been reported with salicylate therapy[228–232] and is in part due to the unusual and variable metabolism and elimination kinetics of salicylate. In addition, there is considerable uncertainty among physicians concerning the optimal salicylate dosage for achieving analgesic or anti-inflammatory effects.

For anti-inflammatory effects, a reasonable and relatively conservative approach is to initiate therapy with a daily aspirin dose of 45 mg/kg, taken every four to six hours during the day.[148,233,234] While there is considerable latitude with respect to the timing and size of the salicylate dose fractions, the total daily salicylate dose is critical.[233] Steady-state concentrations will only be achieved after five to seven days, and it may be misleading to measure plasma salicylate levels before this time. Serum salicylate concentrations of 150 to 300 µg/mL are generally accepted as correlating with anti-inflammatory effect.[141,148,233,234]

Another important factor for patients using salicylates chronically is that serum salicylate concentrations may decrease during long-term therapy.[106–111] The decrease may be due to autoinduction of salicylate metabolism[110,111] rather than poor compliance.[235] One report states that presence of autoinduction reinforces the need to perform periodic serum salicylate measurements on patients using salicylates long term.[148]

Low salicylate levels may also be observed in some patients who are receiving concomitant antacids. Alkalinization of urine secondary to antacid use may result in marked increases in salicylic acid excretion and consequent apparent loss of anti-inflammatory effect.[132-138] Conversely, patients whose salicylate dosing regimens have been adjusted to produce therapeutic salicylate concentrations while taking antacid may become intoxicated upon withdrawal of the antacid.

The effect of age on the pharmacokinetics of salicylates has been reported. Buchanec et al.[238] found higher C_{ss} and delayed excretion in three- to five-week-old neonates compared to 10- to 15-year-old children. Berman et al.[75] reported that newborns eliminated salicylates more slowly than adults. Two groups, Montgomery and Sitar[236] and Cuny et al.[237] reported increased serum half-lives (both absorption and elimination), increased salicylate metabolites (GA and SU), and increased volume of distribution among the elderly.[236,238] Grigor noted that the elderly developed as many side effects as the young, despite ingesting lower salicylate doses (39 mg/kg/dL versus 50 mg/kg/dL, p = 0.02).[239]

Gender also seems to affect salicylate kinetics as salicylate acid clearance was 61% higher among eight men than eight women (not on oral contraceptives).[61] Further, AUC for aspirin and aspirin elimination half-life were significantly greater (33% to 46%) and aspirin hydrolysis was slower (31%) among women than men. The use of oral contraceptives partially obliterated these differences.[61]

In light of these comments, it is important to individualize salicylate dosing regimens to the needs and tolerance of each patient; individual differences in metabolism and elimination kinetics are not taken into account with standard dosing regimens. The ideal method is to titrate the dose against the direct clinical effect. The onset of tinnitus has been used as an indicator of toxicity but has proved an unreliable guide in patients with pre-existing hearing loss. Mongan et al. noted that the serum salicylate level was always greater than 196 µg/mL (average, 304 µg/mL in 59 subjects experiencing tinnitus; however, 15 of 22 patients with pre-existing hearing loss did not experience tinnitus, despite an average serum salicylate concentration of 431 µg/mL.[240] One report states that some patients on placebo reported tinnitus.[241] Another study demonstrated a better relationship between subjective hearing loss and salicylate concentration than between tinnitus and salicylate concentration. Further, 25% of the patients had ototoxic symptoms (e.g., decreased hearing, tinnitus, etc.) but serum salicylate concentrations less than 250 µg/mL.[242] Individualization of dosage can be achieved by monitoring serum salicylate concentrations. However, these levels *per se* should be used only in conjunction with clinical assessment of the patient. The possibility of drug interactions must always be kept in mind, as must concomitant disease, patient age, and gender. Further, the dose-related and relatively complicated pharmacokinetics of the salicylates must be understood to obtain meaningful information from serum salicylate concentrations.

Nomograms have been described for both therapeutic and toxic salicylate dosage estimation.[243-246] With the therapeutic nomogram described by Ross et al., therapeutic salicylate concentrations were safely attained within two weeks by 80% of patients.[243,246] Furst et al.[148] achieved similar salicylate concentrations in 72% of their patients by simply starting them on a weight-adjusted salicylate dose of 45 mg/kg/day. However, 11% of the patients had salicylate concentrations greater than 350 µg/mL.[148] These approaches depend on several important factors, including good absorption of the salicylate from the GI tract, urinary acidification to reduce salicylic acid excretion and, most importantly, good patient compliance. Nomograms have also been used to monitor and predict salicylate concentrations during acute salicylate intoxication, but such nomograms are reliable only if complete absorption of salicylate from GI tract has occurred.[244,245] It should be pointed out that Done's nomogram applies only to cases of acute intoxication and does not pertain to therapeutic overdosage where chronic ingestion has taken place.[244] Done's nomogram also does not take into account the following: the increase in volume of distribution with increased dosing as a result of decreased protein binding at the higher concentrations;[144] changes in salicylate clearance with disease;[248,249] the age of the subject, which can influence the excretion and protein binding of salicylates;[145] changes in blood pH;[145] or the gender of the patient.[61,239]

Renal salicylate excretion can be enhanced by alkaline diuresis but should be performed with caution, particularly in infants, older children and adults with respiratory alkalosis, since fluid and electrolyte imbalances may result.[248]

ALGORITHM FOR THE MONITORING OF SALICYLATE THERAPY

The major variation in the dose-effect relationship of salicylates is due to interindividual differences in the absorption, distribution, metabolism, and excretion processes. These processes are under the influence of genetic and environmental factors as well as disease, age, gender, urine and blood pH, and concomitant drug therapy.

The pharmacological response to salicylates is not directly quantifiable in the usual clinical situation, but in general, anti-inflammatory therapy can be optimized by adjusting the therapy to achieve steady-state serum salicylate concentrations of 150 to 300 μg/mL. If for any reason subtherapeutic salicylate levels (less than 150 μg/mL) are measured in patients undergoing anti-inflammatory salicylate therapy, the scheme outlined in Figure 32-4 should be followed to identify the source of the low serum salicylate levels. The major limitation of this approach is that the pharmacological effect of salicylates (as well as many other drugs) may correlate better with the unbound molecules than with the protein-bound fraction.[249] Thus, monitoring should ideally measure unbound or free salicylate rather than total salicylate. Some patients may have apparently low serum total salicylate concentrations even when free drug concentration is within the therapeutic range. Unfortunately, the therapeutic range of unbound salicylate concentrations has not been established. Nevertheless, as Levy has pointed out, it is better to monitor the total salicylate concentration than not to monitor at all.[248]

The results from several studies have suggested the possibility that monitoring of salicylate therapy may be achieved by measuring drug levels in saliva.[250–254] While potentially useful, in children with juvenile arthritis, salivary salicylate concentrations were extremely variable when compared to concomitant serum unbound salicylate concentrations.[254]

The ingestion of aspirin can interfere with drug and commonly performed biochemical assays;[255–260] significant changes in chloride, total protein, calcium, cholesterol, uric acid, bilirubin, and thyroxine have been observed in normal subjects on aspirin therapy. These abnormalities reverted toward normal when the drug was discontinued.[255] Hoeldtke[257] reported that aspirin, salicylic acid, and an unidentified metabolite of salicylic acid interfere with the assay of homovanillic acid, which is used to diagnose dopamine-secreting tumors. Salicylates can interfere with the measurement of acetaminophen[258,260] and 5-HIAA (fluorescent determination)[203] and can mimic an abnormal creatine kinase isoenzyme.[254] Results of thyroid tests

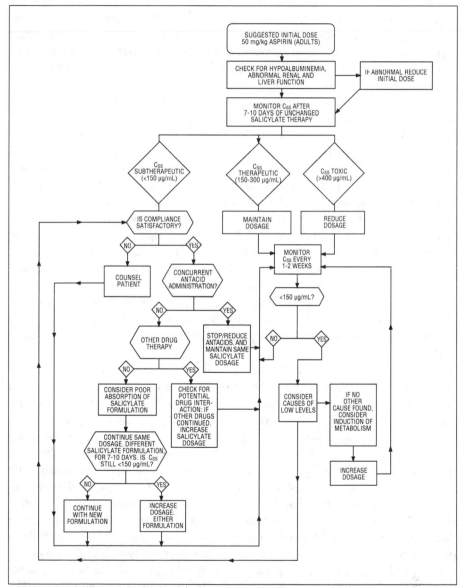

Figure 32-4. *Diagrammatic approach to salicylate therapy by monitoring serum salicylate levels. M = Measurement of salicylate levels in plasma after five to seven days of unchanged salicylate therapy. The subtherapeutic serum salicylate levels assume that the protein binding of salicylate is normal.*

should be interpreted with caution in patients taking salicylates.[209,210] Anti-inflammatory doses of salicylates can cause both false-positive and false-negative glucose tests, depending on the assay methodology.[203]

ANALYTICAL METHODS

Numerous methods are available for the qualitative and quantitative estimation of salicylate derivatives, salicylic acid, and its metabolites in biological fluids and pharmaceutical preparations. These include various colorimetric, ultraviolet, fluorescent, gas-liquid chromatographic, thin-layer and paper chromatographic, and high-performance liquid chromatographic fluorescent polarization immunoassays and enzymatic techniques.[68,261,262,263] Table 32-3 compares the relative advantages and disadvantages of these various assay methods.

The choice of method for measuring salicylates depends on the nature of the biological fluid to be examined (since the relative concentrations of salicylic acid, its metabolites, and parent source of salicylate vary with the biological matrix) and the type of instrumentation available to the analyst. In general, the colorimetric methods, although not as sensitive and specific as the ultraviolet and fluorometric techniques, are sufficiently accurate to measure steady-state salicylate concentrations in plasma and total salicylates in urine. However, it is important to remember that if patients are taking other drugs that interfere with the colorimetric assay, a falsely high reading may be observed. The sensitive fluorometric techniques are ideal for measuring low concentrations of salicylate in saliva and unbound salicylate in plasma. The various chromatographic assays can also be used to measure steady-state salicylate levels, but these assays require more sophisticated, expensive equipment. Chromatographic assays are usually employed to determine the concentrations of the metabolites of salicylic acid as well as salicylic acid, or to characterize the rate of hydrolysis of the parent source of salicylate to salicylic acid.[261,262]

Methods for the estimation of salicylates in various biological fluids have been reviewed.[68,261,262] Following the publication of these reviews, several additional noteworthy publications have appeared. Siebert and Bochner[264] have reported a sensitive HPLC assay to determine aspirin and salicylic acid in plasma using post-column hydrolysis and fluorescence detection. The sensitivity of the assay was reported to be 2 ng/mL. Ion-pair and partition-liquid chromatography have been used to simultaneously measure acetaminophen, theophylline, and salicylate levels in toxicological samples.[265] A nonextraction HPLC method for the determination of serum paracetamol and salicylate has also been reported by Dawson et al.[266] Salicylate levels obtained with this method correlated well with those determined by enzymatic and colorimetric methods. Retention of chemicals in patients with renal dysfunction can sometimes interfere with HPLC assays, but Gaspari and Locatelli[267] have reported a simple method involving hexane extraction for the determination of aspirin and salicylic acid in uremic plasma. The performance of chromatographic techniques in analytical laboratories can vary tremendously between laboratories and problems associated with such technology transfer have been reviewed.[268] A sensitive, selective HPLC method for the determi-

Table 32-3. Comparison of the Relative Advantages and Disadvantages of the Various Salicylate Assay Methods

Analysis method[d]	Specificity for salicylate	Limit of sensitivity (µg/mL)	Metabolite analysis	Serum and urine	Tissue and other	Minimum sample Volume (µL)	Speed[a] 1–10	Speed[a] 10–100	Estimated reagents and tech.	Equipment	Small	Large	Research	References
Colorimetric														
Ferric salts		11	no	yes		200–1000	1	1	5	3	3	3	5	261,262
Folin Ciocalteu reagent		75	no	yes		200–1000	1	1	5	3	3	3	5	261,262
Ultraviolet	yes	2.5	yes	yes	yes	300–2000	2	2	4	3	3	4	4	202,254, 261,262
Fluorometric		0.5–20	yes	yes	yes	10–2000	2	3	3	2	2	4	2	261,262
TLC	yes	0.001	yes	yes	yes	10–50	3	2	3	3	4	5	3	261,262
GLC	yes	0.2–2	yes	yes	yes	500–1000	3	4	2	1	2	2	2	261,262
HPLC	yes	0.2–1	yes	yes	yes	3–1000	2	2	1	1	1	1	1	261–268
Enzyme Assays[e]	yes	36–70	no	yes	yes	40–50	1	1	3	3	1	1	3	262

(Headers: **Assayable samples**, **Speed[a]**, **Analysis cost[b]**, **Preference and rank[c]** with subcolumns Small / Large / Research)

[a] Most rapid = 1.
[b] Highest cost = 1.
[c] Arbitrary ranking scale of 1 (excellent) to 5 (poor) with a score of 3 being average or nominal.
[d] TLC = Thin layer chromatography; GLC = Gas liquid chromatography; HPLC = High performance liquid chromatography.
[e] Based on reduction of SA to catechol by bacterial enzymes.

nation of salicylate glucuronide conjugates in human urine recently has been reported by Shen et al.[263] This assay allows for the simultaneous determination of three salicylate glucuronides (SUPG, SPG, SAG) as well as GA, SU, and SA. This methodology should facilitate accurate pharmacokinetic studies of the phenolic glucuronides, SUPG and SPG.

PROSPECTUS

Quantification of appropriate concentration-response relationships in the measurement of pain and inflammation would help to establish the therapeutic range for salicylate therapy. In the field of joint inflammation, for example, changes in inflammation can be quantitated by measuring changes in the concentrations of inflammatory indicators in synovial fluid. This approach has been used to measure changes in prostaglandin levels in the synovial fluid and tissues during salicylate therapy.[269,270] However, the prostaglandins represent only one of the many inflammatory indicators present in the fluid. In fact, the poor inhibition of prostaglandin synthesis by salicylate *in vitro*[271,272] has caused many to speculate that salicylates (nonacetylated) inhibit inflammation via other mechanisms, as yet unidentified.[273,274] Clearly, the mechanism(s) by which salicylates modulate the inflammatory cascade must be elucidated before quantitation of a concentration-response relationship for salicylate anti-inflammatory therapy can occur.

REFERENCES

1. Dromgoole SH et al. Rational approaches to the use of salicylates in the treatment of rheumatoid arthritis. Seminars in Arthritis and Rheumatism 1981;11:257–83.
2. Vandenberg SA et al. Non-aspirin salicylates: conversion factors for estimating aspirin equivalency. Vet Hum Toxicol. 1989;31:49.
3. Levy G. Comparison of dissolution and absorption rates of different commercial aspirin tablets. J Pharm Sci. 1961;50:388–92.
4. Leonards JR. The influence of solubility on the rate of gastrointestinal absorption of aspirin. Clin Pharmacol Ther. 1963;4:476–79.
5. Cooke AR, Hunt JN. Absorption of acetylsalicylic acid from unbuffered and buffered gastric contents. Am J Dig Dis. 1970;15:95–102.
6. Lieberman SV, Wood JH. Aspirin formulation and absorption rate II. Influence on serum levels of tablets, antacids and solutions. J Pharm Sci. 1964;53:1492–496.
7. Levy G et al. The effect of dosage form upon the gastrointestinal absorption rate of salicylate. Canad Med Assoc J. 1961;85:414–19.
8. Alvarez AS, Summerskill WHJ. Gastrointestinal hemorrhage and salicylates. Lancet 1958;2:920–25.
9. Keith JD, Ross A. Observations on salicylate therapy in rheumatic fever. Can Med Assoc J. 1945;52:554–59.
10. Barager FD, Duthie JJR. Importance of aspirin as a cause of anemia and peptic ulcer in rheumatoid arthritis. Br Med J. 1960;1:1105–106.
11. Gyory AZ, Steil JN. Effect of particle size on aspirin induced gastrointestinal bleeding. Lancet. 1968;2:300–301.
12. Mielants H et al. Salicylate-induced gastrointestinal bleeding. Comparison between soluble buffered, enteric coated and intravenous administration. J Rheumatol. 1979;6:210–18.
13. Leonards JR, Levy G. Effect of pharmaceutical formulation on gastrointestinal bleeding from aspirin tablets. Arch Intern Med. 1972;129:457–60.

14. Arvidson B et al. Acetylsalicylic acid and gastrointestinal bleeding. Measurement of blood loss using a modified radioactive chromium method. Scand J Gastroenterol. 1975;10:155–60.
15. Leonards JR, Levy G. Gastrointestinal blood loss from aspirin and sodium salicylate tablets in man. Clin Pharmacol Ther. 1973;14:62–6.
16. Davenport AW. Salicylate damage to the gastric mucosal barrier. N Engl J Med. 1967;276:1307–312.
17. Frenkel EP et al. Fecal blood loss following aspirin and coated aspirin microspherule administration. J Clin Pharmacol. 1968;8:347–51.
18. Kuiper DH et al. Gastroscopic findings and fecal blood loss following aspirin administration. Am J Dig Dis. 1969;14:161–69.
19. Ivey DJ et al. Effect of intravenous salicylates on the gastric mucosal barrier in man. Am J Dig Dis. 1972;17:1055–64.
20. Leonards JR et al. Gastrointestinal blood loss during prolonged aspirin administration. N Engl J Med. 1973;289:1020–22.
21. Leonards JR, Levy G. The role of dosage form in aspirin-induced gastrointestinal bleeding. Clin Pharmacol Ther. 1967;8:400–408.
22. Leonards JR, Levy G. Absorption and metabolism of aspirin administered in enteric-coated tablets. JAMA. 1965;193:99–104.
23. Canada AT et al. The bioavailability of enteric-coated acetylsalicylic acid: a comparison with buffered ASA in rheumatoid arthritis II. Curr Ther Res. 1976,19:544–56.
24. Leonards JR, Levy G. Reduction or prevention of aspirin-induced occult gastrointestinal blood loss in man. Clin Pharmacol Ther. 1965;10:571–75.
25. Nowak M et al. Rectal absorption from aspirin suppositories in children and adults. Pediatrics 1974;54:23–6.
26. Parrott EJ. Salicylate absorption from rectal suppositories. J Pharm Sci. 1971;60:867–72.
27. Cohen A, Garber HE. Comparison of choline magnesium trisalicylate and acetylsalicylic acid in relation to fecal blood loss. Curr Ther Res. 1978;23:187–93.
28. Leonards JR. Absence of gastrointestinal bleeding following administration of salicylsalicylic acid. J Lab Clin Med. 1969;74:911–14.
29. Cohen A. Fecal blood loss and plasma salicylate study of salicylsalicylic acid and aspirin. J Clin Pharmacol. 1979;19:242–47.
30. Cohen LS. Clinical pharmacology of acetylsalicylic acid. Semin Thromb Hemost. 1976;2:146–75.
31. Rushton DG. Discussion of the toxicity of salicylates. In: Dixon ASJ et al., eds. Salicylates. London: Churchill; 1963;253–54.
32. Matthew H et al. Gastric aspiration and lavage in acute poisoning. Br Med J. 1966;1:1333–337.
33. Gaspari F et al. Influence of antacid administrations on aspirin absorption in patients with chronic renal failure on maintenance hemodialysis. Am J Kidney Dis. 1988;11:338.
34. Mojaverian P et al. Effect of food on the absorption of enteric-coated aspirin: correlation with gastric residence time. Clin Pharmacol Ther. 1987;41:11.
35. Levy G, Gagliardi B. Gastrointestinal absorption of aspirin anhydride. J Pharm Sci. 1963;52:730–32.
36. Levy G, Sahli B. Comparison of the gastrointestinal absorption of aluminum acetylsalicylate and acetylsalicylic acid in man. J Pharm Sci. 1962;51:58–62.
37. Cohen A. A comparative blood salicylate study in two salicylate tablet formulations utilizing normal volunteers. Curr Ther Res. 1978;23:772–78.
38. Dromgoole SH et al. Availability of salicylate from salsalate and aspirin. Clin Pharmacol Ther. 1983;34:539–45.
39. Paull P et al. Single-dose evaluation of a new enteric-coated aspirin preparation. Med J Aust. 1976;1:617–19.
40. Baum J. Blood salicylate levels and clinical trials with a new form of enteric-coated aspirin: studies in rheumatoid arthritis and degenerative joint diseases. J Clin Pharmacol. 1970;10:132–37.
41. Anttila M et al. The absorption of acetylsalicylic acid from an enteric-coated formulation and the inhibition of thromboxane formation. J Clin Pharmacol, Ther Toxicol. 1988;26:88.

42. Bogentoft C et al. Influence of food on the absorption of acetylsalicylic acid from enteric-coated dosage forms. Eur J Clin Pharmacol. 1978;14:351–55.

43. Gibaldi M, Grundhofer B. Bioavailability of aspirin from commercial suppositories. J Pharm Sci. 1975;64:1064–66.

44. Parsons RL et al. Pharmacokinetics of salicylate and indomethacin in celiac disease. Eur J Clin Pharmacol. 1973;11:473–77.

45. Koren G et al. Salicylates in Kawasaki disease—a review of clinical pharmacokinetics and efficacy. Prog Clin Biol Res. 1987;250:415–24.

46. Koren G et al. Determinants of low serum concentrations of salicylates in patients with Kawasaki disease. J Pediatr. 1988;112:663–67.

47. Miaskiewicz SL et al. Sex differences in absorption kinetics of sodium salicylate. Clin Pharmacol Ther. 1982;31:30–7.

48. Wosilait WD. Theoretical analysis of the binding of salicylate by human serum albumin. Eur J Clin Pharmacol. 1976;9:285–90.

49. Yacobi A, Levy G. Intraindividual relationships between serum protein binding of drugs in normal human subjects, patients with impaired renal function and rats. J Pharm Sci. 1977;66:1285–288.

50. Kucera JL, Bullock FJ. The binding of salicylate to plasma protein from several animal species. J Pharm Pharmacol. 1969;21:293–96.

51. McArthur JN et al. The binding of indomethacin, salicylate and phenobarbitone to human whole blood *in vitro*. J Pharm Pharmacol. 1971;23:32–6.

52. Sturman JA, Smith MJH. The binding of salicylates to plasma proteins from several animal species. J Pharm Pharmacol. 1967;19:621–22.

53. McArthur JN, Smith MJ. The determination of the binding of salicylate to serum proteins. J Pharm Pharmacol. 1969;21:589–94.

54. Kramer E, Routh JI. The binding of salicylic acid and acetylsalicylic acid to human serum albumin. Clin Biochem. 1973;6:98–105.

55. Zaroslinski JF et al. Effect of temperature on the binding of salicylate by human serum albumin. Biochem Pharmacol. 1974;23:1767–776.

56. Windorfer A et al. The influence of age on the activity of acetylsalicylic acid-esterase and protein salicylate binding. Eur J Clin Pharmacol. 1974;7:227–31.

57. Otagiri M, Perrin H. Circular dichroic investigations of the binding of salicylate and related compounds to human serum albumin. Biochem Pharmacol. 1977;26:283–88.

58. Windorfer A et al. Investigations on salicylate protein binding in newborns and infants. Eur J Pediatr. 1978;127:163–72.

59. Furst DE et al. Salicylate clearance, the resultant of protein binding and metabolism. Clin Pharmacol Ther. 1979;26:380–89.

60. Ekstrand R et al. Concentration-dependent plasma protein binding of salicylate in rheumatoid patients. Clin Pharmacokinet. 1979;4:137–43.

61. Miners JO et al. Influence of gender and oral contraceptive steroids on the metabolism of salicylic acid acetylsalicylic acid. Br J Clin Pharmacol. 1986;22:135–42.

62. Alvan G et al. High unbound fraction of salicylate in plasma during intoxication. Br J Clin Pharmacol. 1981;11:625–26.

63. Wallace S, Brodie MJ. Decreased drug binding in serum from patients with chronic hepatic disease. Eur J Clin Pharmacol. 1976;9:429–32.

64. Wallace S, Whiting B. Factors affecting drug binding in plasma of elderly patients. Br J Clin Pharmacol. 1976;3:327–30.

65. Borga O et al. Protein binding of salicylate in uremic and normal plasma. Clin Pharmacol Ther. 1976;20:464–75.

66. Perez-Mateo M, Erill S. Protein binding of salicylate and quinidine in plasma from patients with renal failure, chronic liver disease and chronic respiratory insufficiency. Eur J Clin Pharmacol. 1977;11:225–31.

67. Steele WH et al. Protein binding of salicylate in cutaneous hepatic porphyria. Eur J Clin Pharmacol. 1978;13:309–18.

68. Dromgoole SH, Furst DE. Salicylates. In: Evans WE et al, eds. Applied Pharmacokinetics: Principles of Therapeutic Drug Monitoring. Vancouver, WA: Applied Therapeutics, Inc. 1986.

69. Rainsford KD et al. Distribution of the acetyl compared with the salicyl moiety of acetylsalicylic acid. Biochem Pharmacol. 1983;32:1301–308.

70. Altshuler G et al. Premature onset of labor, neonatal patent ductus arteriosus, and prostaglandin synthetase antagonists—a rat model of the human problem. Am J Obstet Gynecol. 1979;135:261–65.

71. Anderson DF et al. The placental transfer of acetylsalicylic acid in near-term ewes. Am J Obstet Gynecol. 1980;136:814–18.

72. Garrettson LK et al. Fetal acquisition and neonatal elimination of a large amount of salicylate. Clin Pharmacol Ther. 1975;17:98–103.

73. Harris WH. The effects of repeated doses of indomethacin on fetal rabbit mortality and on the potency of the ductus arteriosus. Can J Physiol Pharmacol. 1980;58:212–16.

74. Parks BR et al. Indomethacin: studies of absorption and placental transfer. Am J Obstet Gynecol. 1977;129:464–65.

75. Berman W et al. Pharmacokinetics of inhibitors of prostaglandin synthesis in the perinatal period. Semin Perinatol. 1980;4:67–72.

76. Green TP et al. Determinants of drug disposition and effect in the fetus. Ann Rev Pharmacol Toxicol. 1979;19:285–322.

77. Corby DG. Aspirin in pregnancy: maternal and fetal effects. Pediatrics 1978;130:930–37.

78. Levy G et al. Distribution of salicylate between neonatal and maternal serum at diffusion equilibrium. Clin Pharmacol Ther. 1975;18:210–14.

79. Nonsteroidal anti-inflammatory agents: salicylates. In: American Hospital Formulary Service. Bethesda, MD: American Society of Hospital Pharmacists; 1991;1055–145.

80. Kershaw et al. Disposition of aspirin and its metabolites in the semen of man. J Clin Pharmacol. 1987;27:304–309.

81. Bannwarth B et al. Clinical pharmacokinetics of nonsteroidal anti-inflammatory drugs in the cerebrospinal fluid. Pharmacother. 1989;43:121–26.

82. Kapp EM, Coburn AF. Urinary metabolites of sodium salicylate. J Biol Chem. 1942;145:549–65.

83. Lester D et al. The fate of acetylsalicylic acid. J Pharmacol Exp Ther. 1946;87:329–42.

84. Roseman S, Dorfman A. The determination of metabolism of gentisic acid. J Biol Chem. 1951;192:105–14.

85. Cummings AJ, Martin BK. Factors influencing the plasma salicylate concentration and urinary salicylate excretion after oral dosage with aspirin. Biochem Pharmacol. 1964;13:767–76.

86. Hollister L, Levy G. Some aspects of salicylate distribution and metabolism in man. J Pharm Sci. 1965;54:1126–129.

87. Levy G. Pharmacokinetics of salicylate elimination in man. J Pharm Sci. 1965;54:959–67.

88. Cummings AJ et al. The elimination of salicylic acid in man: serum concentrations and urinary excretion rates. Br J Pharmacol. 1966;26:461–67.

89. Rowland M, Riegelman S. Pharmacokinetics of acetylsalicylic acid and salicylic acid after intravenous administration in man. J Pharm Sci. 1968;57:1313–319.

90. Boreham DR, Martin BK. The kinetics of elimination of salicylic acid and the formation of gentisic acid. Br J Pharmacol. 1969;37:294–300.

91. Levy G et al. Capacity limited salicylurate formation during prolonged administration of aspirin to healthy human subjects. J Pharm Sci. 1969;58:503–504.

92. Levy G, Tsuchiya T. Salicylate accumulation kinetics in man. N Engl J Med. 1972;287:430–32.

93. Levy G et al. Limited capacity for salicyl phenolic glucuronide formation and its effect on the kinetics of salicylate elimination in man. Clin Pharmacol Ther. 1972;13:258–68.

94. Schachter D, Manis JG. Salicylate and salicyl conjugates: fluorometric estimation, biosynthesis and renal excretion in man. J Clin Invest. 1958;37:800–807.

95. Levy G, Garrettson LK. Kinetics of salicylate elimination by newborn infants of mothers who ingested aspirin before delivery. Pediatrics. 1974;53:201–10.

96. Levy G, Procknal JA. Drug biotransformation interactions in man. I: Mutual inhibition in glucuronide formation of salicylic acid and salicylamide in man. J Pharm Sci. 1968;57:1330–335.

97. Levy G et al. Kinetics of salicyluric acid elimination in man. J Pharm Sci. 1969;58:827–29.

98. Tsuchiya T, Levy G. Biotransformation of salicylic acid to its acyl and phenolic glucuronides in man. J Pharm Sci. 1972;61:800–801.

99. Gupta N et al. Correlation of plateau serum salicylate level with rate of salicylate metabolism. Clin Pharmacol Ther. 1975;18:350–55.

100. Furst DE et al. Salicylate metabolism in twins. Evidence suggesting a genetic influence and induction of salicylurate formation. J Clin Invest. 1977;60:32–42.

101. Wilson JT et al. Gentisuric acid: metabolic formation in animals and identification as a metabolite of aspirin in man. Clin Pharmacol Ther. 1978;23:635–43.

102. Ebadi MS, Kugel RB. Alteration in metabolism of acetylsalicylic acid in children with Down's syndrome: decreased plasma binding and formation of salicyluric acid. Pediatr Res. 1970;4:187–93.

103. Smith PK et al. Studies on the pharmacology of salicylates. J Pharmacol Exp Ther. 1946,87:237–55.

104. Alpen EL et al. The metabolism of C^{14}-carboxyl salicylic acid in the dog and in man. J Pharm Exp Ther. 1951;102:150–56.

105. Caldwell J et al. Interindividual differences in the glycine conjugation of salicylic acid. Br J Clin Pharmacol. 1980;9:114.

106. Muller FO et al. Decreased steady-state salicylic acid plasma levels associated with chronic aspirin ingestion. Curr Med Res Opin. 1975;3:417.

107. Muller FO et al. Pharmacokinetic and pharmacodynamic implications of long-term administration of nonsteroidal anti-inflammatory agents. Int J Clin Pharmacol Biopharm. 1976;14:234.

108. Rumble RH et al. Metabolism of salicylate during chronic aspirin therapy. Br J Clin Pharmacol. 1980;9:41.

109. Aarons LJ et al. A chronic dose ranging kinetic study of salicylate in man. Br J Clin Pharmacol. 1977;7:456–57.

110. Day RO et al. Induction of salicyluric acid formation in rheumatoid arthritis patients treated with salicylates. Clin Pharmacokinet. 1983;8:263–71.

111. Day RO et al. Changes in salicylate serum concentration and metabolism during chronic dosing in normal volunteers. Biopharm Drug Dispos. 1988;9:273–83.

112. Gunsberg M et al. Disposition of and clinical response to salicylates in patients with rheumatoid disease. Clin Pharmacol Ther. 1984;35:585–93.

113. Bochner F et al. Salicylate metabolite kinetics after several salicylates. Clin Pharmacol Ther. 1981;30:266–75.

114. MacPherson CR et al. The excretion of salicylate. Br J Pharmacol. 1955;10:484–89.

115. Roch-Ramel F, Peters G. Micropuncture techniques as a tool in renal pharmacology. Ann Rev Pharmacol Toxicol. 1979;19:323–45.

116. Reinberg A et al. Circadian rhythms in the urinary excretion of salicylate (chronopharmacokinetics) in healthy adults. C R Seances Acad Sci [III]. 1975;280:1697–699.

117. Grootveld M, Halliwell B. 2,3-dihydroxybenzoic acid is a product of human aspirin metabolism. Biochem Pharmacol. 1988;37:271–80.

118. Bochner F et al. Pharmacokinetics of low-dose oral modified release, soluble and intravenous aspirin in man, and effects on platelet function. Eur J Clin Pharmacol. 1988;35:287.

119. Hutt AJ et al. The metabolism of aspirin in man: a population study. Xenobiotica. 1986;16:239–49.

120. Patel DK et al. Comparative metabolism of high doses of aspirin in man and rat. Xenobiotica. 1990;20:847–54.

121. Notarianni LJ et al. Glycane conjugation of salicylic acid after aspirin overdose. Br J Clin Pharmacol. 1983;15:587P.

122. Ho JL et al. An evaluation of the effect of repeated doses of oral activated charcoal on salicylate elimination. J Clin Pharmacol. 1989;29:366.

123. Ho FC et al. The effects of age and sex on the disposition of acetylsalicylic acid and its metabolites in man. Br J Clin Pharmacol. 1985;19:675.

124. Kelton JG et al. Sex-related differences in the efficacy of acetylsalicylic acid (ASA): the absorption of ASA and its effect on collagen-induced thrombaxane B_2 generation. Thromb Res. 1981;24:163.

125. Buchanan MR et al. The sex-related differences in aspirin pharmacokinetics in rabbits and men and its relationship to antiplatelet effects. Thromb Res. 1983;29:125.

126. Montgomery PR, Sitar DS. Increased serum salicylate metabolites with age in patients receiving chronic acetylsalicylic acid therapy. Gerontol. 1981;27:329.

127. Owen SG et al. Salicylate pharmacokinetics in patients with rheumatoid arthritis. Br J Clin Pharmacol. 1989;28:449.

128. Ayres JW et al. Circadian rhythm of urinary pH in man with and without chronic antacid administration. Eur J Clin Pharmacol. 1977;12:415–20.

129. Levy G. Effect of bed rest on the distribution and elimination of drugs. J Pharm Sci. 1967;56:928–29.

130. Menguy R et al. Evidence for a sex-linked difference in aspirin metabolism. Nature. 1972;239:102–103.

131. Seahserova M et al. Sexual differences in the metabolism of salicylates. Arzneimittelforschung. 1975;25:1581–582.

132. Smull K et al. The effect of sodium bicarbonate on the serum salicylate level. JAMA. 1944;125:1173–175.

133. Levy G, Leonards JR. Urine pH and salicylate therapy. JAMA. 1971;217:81.

134. Strickland-Hodge B et al. The effects of antacids on enteric-coated salicylate preparations. Rheumatol Rehab. 1976;15:148–52.

135. Hansten PD, Hayton WL. Effect of antacid and ascorbic acid on serum salicylate concentration. J Clin Pharmacol. 1980;20:326–31.

136. Gibaldi M et al. Effects of antacid on pH of urine. Clin Pharmacol Ther. 1974;16:520–25.

137. Gibaldi M et al. Time course and dose dependence of antacid effect on urine pH. J Pharm Sci. 1975;64:2003–2004.

138. Levy G et al. Decreased serum salicylate concentrations in children with rheumatic fever treated with antacid. N Engl J Med. 1975;293:323–25.

139. Levy G. Pharmacokinetics of salicylates. Drug Metab Rev. 1979;9:3–19.

140. Ventafridda V, Martino G. Observations on the relationships between plasma concentration and analgesic activity of a soluble acetylsalicylic acid derivative after intravenous administration in man. Adv PA Res Ther. 1976;1:529–36.

141. Koch-Weser J. Serum drug concentrations as therapeutic guides. N Engl J Med. 1972;287:227–31.

142. Bywaters EGL. Rheumatic fever (including chorea). In: Scott JT, ed. Copeman's Textbook of the Rheumatic Diseases. New York: Churchill; 1978:764–807.

143. Bencher KJ. Salicylate intoxication. Drug Intell Clin Pharm. 1975;9:350–60.

144. Levy G, Yaffe J. Relationship between dose and apparent volume of distribution of salicylate in children. Pediatrics. 1974;54:713–17.

145. Hill JB. Experimental salicylate poisoning: observation of the effects of altering blood pH on tissue and plasma salicylate concentrations. Pediatrics. 1971;47:658–65.

146. Cockel R et al. Serum biochemical values in rheumatoid disease. Ann Rheum Dis. 1971;30:166–70.

147. Jusko WJ. Pharmacokinetics in disease states changing protein binding. In: Benet LZ, ed. The Effect of Disease States on Drug Pharmacokinetics. Washington, DC: Am Pharm Assoc; 1976:99–123.

148. Furst DE et al. A strategy for reaching therapeutic salicylate levels in patients with rheumatoid arthritis using standardized dosing regimens. J Rheumatol. 1987;342–47.

149. Reid RT, Farr RS. Further evidence for albumin alterations in some patients with rheumatic disease. Arthritis Rheum. 1964;7:747–48.

150. Hawkins D et al. Acetylation of human serum albumin by acetylsalicylic acid. Science. 1966;160:780–81.

151. Denko CW et al. Albumin amino acids in patients with rheumatoid arthritis. Arthritis Rheum. 1970;13:311–12.

152. Furst DE et al. A controlled study of concurrent therapy with a non-acetylated salicylate and naproxen in rheumatoid arthritis. Arthritis Rheum. 1987;30:146–54.

153. Wilkens RF, Segre EJ. Combination therapy with naproxen and aspirin in rheumatoid arthritis. Arthritis Rheum. 1976;19:677–82.

154. Brooks PM et al. Indomethacin-aspirin interaction: a clinical appraisal. Br Med J. 1975;3:69–71.
155. Rubin A et al. Interaction of aspirin and nonsteroidal anti-inflammatory drugs in man. Arthritis Rheum. 1973;16:635–45.
156. Selley ML et al. Protein binding of tolmetin. Clin Pharmacol Ther. 1978;24:694–705.
157. Segre EJ et al. Naproxen aspirin interactions in man. Clin Pharmacol Ther. 1974;15:374–79.
158. Rubin A et al. Physiological disposition of fenoprofen in man III. J Pharmacol Exp Ther. 1972;183:449–57.
159. Moller PW. Anti-inflammatory drugs and their interaction. NZ Med J. 1973;78:79.
160. Chignell CF, Starkweather DK. Optical studies of drug protein complexes. Mol Pharmacol. 1971;7:229–37.
161. Champion GD et al. The effect of aspirin on serum indomethacin. Clin Pharmacol Ther. 1972;13:239–44.
162. Lindquist B et al. Effect of concurrent administration of aspirin and indomethacin on serum concentrations. Clin Pharmacol Ther. 1974;15:247–52.
163. Kwan KC et al. Effects of concomitant aspirin administration on the pharmacokinetics of indomethacin in man. J Pharmacokinet Biopharm. 1978;6:451–76.
164. Robinson DS. Pharmacokinetic mechanism of drug interactions. Postgrad Med. 1975;57:55–62.
165. Grennan DM et al. The aspirin-ibuprofen interaction in rheumatoid arthritis. Br J Clin Pharmacol. 1979;8:497–503.
166. Brooks PM, Khong TK. Flurbiprofen-aspirin interaction. A double-blind crossover study. Curr Med Res Opin. 1977;5:53–7.
167. Chalmers A, Robinson HS. A double-blind controlled study comparing the use of aspirin and tolmetin with aspirin and placebo in the treatment of rheumatoid arthritis. Curr Ther Res. 1978;24:517–23.
168. Hansten PD. Interactions involving nonsteroidal anti-inflammatory drugs. Pharmacy International. 1984;5:300–303.
169. Day RO et al. The effect of concurrent aspirin upon plasma concentrations of tenoxicam. Br J Clin Pharmacol. 1988;26:455–62.
170. Furst DE et al. Serum concentrations of salicylates and naproxen during concurrent therapy in patients with rheumatoid arthritis. Arthritis Rheum. 1987;30:1157–161.
171. Brogden RN et al. Diclofenac sodium: a review. Drugs. 1980;20:20–48.
172. Davies RO. Review of the animal and clinical pharmacology of diflunisal. Pharmacotherapy. 1983;3:9S–22S.
173. Lewis AJ, Furst DE. Nonsteroidal anti-inflammatory drugs: mechanisms and clinical use. New York: Marcel-Dekker; 1987.
174. Klinenberg JR, Miller F. Effect of corticosteroids on blood salicylate concentration. JAMA. 1965;194:601–604.
175. Graham GG et al. Patterns of plasma concentrations and urinary excretion of salicylate in rheumatoid arthritis. Clin Pharmacol Ther. 1978;22:410–20.
176. Weiss HJ, Aledort LM. Impaired platelet-connective tissue reaction in man after aspirin ingestion. Lancet. 1967;2:495–97.
177. Hircsh J et al. Aspirin and other platelet active drugs. Chest 1989;95(Suppl. R):125–85.
178. Bjornsson T et al. Aspirin acetylates fibrinogen and enhances fibrinolysis. Fibrinolytic effect is independent of changes in plasminogen activator levels. J Pharmacol Exp Ther. 1989;250:154–61.
179. Weiss HJ et al. The effect of salicylates on hemostatic properties of platelets in man. J Clin Invest. 1968;47:2169–180.
180. O'Brien JR. Effect of salicylates on human platelets. Lancet. 1968;1:779–83.
181. O'Brien JR. Effect of anti-inflammatory agents on platelets. Lancet. 1968;1:894–95.
182. O'Brien JR et al. A comparison of an effect of different anti-inflammatory drugs on human platelets. J Clin Pathol. 1970;23:522–25.
183. Al-Mondhiry H et al. On the mechanism of platelet function and inhibition by ASA. Proc Soc Exp Biol Med. 1970;133:632–36.
184. Zucker MB, Peterson J. Effect of acetylsalicylic acid, other nonsteroidal anti-inflammatory agents and dipyridamole on human blood platelets. J Lab Clin Med. 1970;76:66–75.

185. Zucker MB, Rothwell KG. Differential influences of salicylate compounds on platelet aggregation and serotonin release. Curr Ther Res. 1978;23:194–99.

186. Patrono C et al. Low-dose aspirin and inhibition of thromboxane B_2 production in healthy subjects. Thromb Res. 1980;17:317–27.

187. Paccioretti MJ, Block LH. Effects of aspirin on platelet aggregation as a function of dosage and time. Clin Pharmacol Ther. 1980;27:803–809.

188. Escolar G et al. Sex-related differences in the effects of aspirin on the interaction of platelets with subendothelium. Thrombosis Research. 1986;44:837–47.

189. Thiessen JJ et al. Human platelet response to three salicylate dosage forms. Biopharm Drug Dispos. 1983;4:43–51.

190. Burch JW et al. Inhibition of platelet prostaglandin synthetase by oral aspirin. J Clin Invest. 1978;61:314–19.

191. Estes D, Kaplan K. Lack of platelet effect with the aspirin analog, salsalate. Arthritis Rheum. 1980;23:1303.

192. Sinzinger H et al. Evidence for 20 mg aspirin (ASA) being optimal. New York: Raven Press; 1989.

193. Pedersen AK, Fitzgerald GA. Dose-related kinetics of aspirin. Presystemic acetylation of platelet cyclooxygenase. New Eng J Med. 1984;311:1206–211.

194. Siebert DJ et al. Aspirin kinetics and platelet aggregation in man. Clin Pharmacol Ther. 1983;33:367–74.

195. Ali M et al. Plasma acetylsalicylate and salicylate and platelet cyclooxygenase activity following plain and enteric-coated aspirin. Stroke 1980;11:9–13.

196. Dejena E et al. "Aspirinated" platelets are hemostatic in thrombocytopenic rats with "non-aspirinated" vessel walls—evidence from an exchange transfusion model. Blood 1980;56:959–62.

197. Dejena E et al. Salicylate-aspirin interaction in the rat. Evidence that salicylate accumulating during aspirin administration may protect vascular prostacyclin from aspirin-induced inhibition. J Clin Invest. 1981;68:1108–112.

198. Dejena E et al. Interaction of salicylate and other nonsteroidal anti-inflammatory drugs with aspirin on platelet and vascular cyclo-oxygenase activity. Thromb Res. 1983;4:153–59.

199. Ferraris V et al. Preoperative aspirin ingestion increases operative blood loss after coronary artery bypass grafting. Ann Thorac Surg. 1988;45:71–4.

200. Livio M et al. Indomethacin prevents the long-lasting inhibitory effect of aspirin on human platelet cyclooxygenase activity. Prostaglandins 1982;23:787–96.

201. Odell GB. The dissociation of bilirubin from albumin and its clinical implications. J Pediatr. 1959;55:268–79.

202. Verbeeck RK. Pharmacokinetic drug interactions with nonsteroidal anti-inflammatory drugs. Clin Pharmacokinet. 1990;19:44–66

203. Facts and Comparisons. St. Louis, MO: JB Lippincott; 1990; 248b.

204. Hansten, PD, Horn JR. Clinical significance of drug-drug interactions and drug effects on clinical laboratory tests. In: Drug Interactions and Updates. 3rd Ed. Philadelphia: Lea and Febiger; 1976.

205. American Pharmaceutical Association. Evaluation of Drug Interactions. 2nd ed. Washington; 1976.

206. Yoovathaworn K et al. Influence of caffeine on aspirin pharmacokinetics. Eur J Drug Met Pharmacokinetics. 1986;11:71–6.

207. Spahn H et al. Pharmacokinetics of salicylates administered with metoprolol. Arzneimittel-forschung. 1986;36:1697–699.

208. Ding RW et al. Pharmacokinetics of nicotinic acid-salicylic acid interaction. Clin Pharm Ther. 1989;46:642–47.

209. Baranetsky NG et al. Combined phenytoin and salicylate effects on thyroid function. Tests Arch Int Pharmacodyn Ther. 1986;284:166–76.

210. McConnell RJ. Salsalate alters thyroid function test results. Arthritis Rheum. 1989;32:1344.

211. Salicylates (systemic). In: 1984 Drug Information for the Health Care Professional. United States Pharmacopeial Convention Inc. Volume 1B. Oradell, New Jersey: Medical Economics Books. 1991;2279–300.

212. Goulden KJ et al. Clinical valproate toxicity induced by acetylsalicylic acid. Neurology. 1987;37:1392–394.

213. Glen-Bott AM. Aspirin and Reye's syndrome, a reappraisal. Medical Toxicology. 1987;2:161–65.

214. Hurwitz ES et al. Public health service study of Reye's syndrome and medications. JAMA. 1987;257:1905–911.

215. Baral J, Orlowski JP. Aspirin and Reye's syndrome. Pediatrics 1988;82:135–36. Letter.

216. Prichard PJ, Hawkey CJ. Aspirin and gastroduodenal injury. Dig Dis. 1989;7:28–38.

217. Faulkner G et al. Aspirin and bleeding peptic ulcers in the elderly. Brit Med J. 1988;297:1311–313.

218. Levy M et al. Major upper gastrointestinal tract bleeding. Arch Intern Med. 1988:148.

219. Kauffman G. Aspirin-induced gastric mucosal injury: lessons learned from animal models. Gastroenterology 1989;606–14.

220. Morassut P et al. Aspirin intolerance. Seminars Arthritis Rheum. 1989;19(1):22–30.

221. Zeitz HJ. Bronchial asthma, nasal polyps, and aspirin sensitivity: Samter's syndrome. Clin Chest Med. 1988;9(4).

222. Nizankowska E, Szczeklik A. Glucocorticosteroids attenuate aspirin-precipitated adverse reactions in aspirin-intolerant patients with asthma. Ann Allergy 1989;63:159–62.

223. April PA et al. Does the acetyl group of aspirin contribute to the anti-inflammatory efficacy of salicylic acid in the treatment of rheumatoid arthritis? J Rheumatol. 1989;16:321–27.

224. Higgs GA et al. Pharmacokinetics of aspirin and salicylate in relation to inhibition of arachinonate cyclo-oxygenase and anti-inflammatory activity. Medical Sciences 1987;84:1417–420.

225. Scheiman JM et al. Salicylsalicylic acid causes less gastroduodenal mucosal damage than enteric-coated aspirin—an endoscopic comparison. Dig Dis Sci. 1989;34(2):229–32.

226. Zambraski EJ et al. Effects of salicylate versus aspirin on renal prostaglandins and function in normal and sodium-depleted dogs. J Pharmacol Exp Ther. 1988.

227. Patel DK et al. Metabolism of aspirin after therapeutic and toxic doses. Hum Exp Toxicol. 1990;9:131–136.

228. Paulus HE et al. Variations of serum concentrations and half-life of salicylate in patients with rheumatoid arthritis. Arthritis Rheum. 1971;14:527–31.

229. Champion GD et al. Salicylate in rheumatoid arthritis. Clin Rheum Dis. 1975;1:245–65.

230. Barraclough DRE et al. Salicylate therapy and drug interaction in rheumatoid arthritis. Aust NZ J Med. 1975;5:518–23.

231. Perez-Mateo M et al. Blood and saliva salicylate measurement in the monitoring of salicylate therapy. Int J Clin Pharmacol. 1977;15:113–15.

232. Bardare M et al. Value of monitoring plasma salicylate levels in treating juvenile rheumatoid arthritis: observations in 42 cases. Arch Dis Child. 1978;53:381–85.

233. Levy G, Giacomini KM. Rational aspirin dosage regimens. Clin Pharmacol Ther. 1978;23:247–52.

234. Cassel S et al. Steady-state serum salicylate levels in hospitalized patients with rheumatoid arthritis receiving two dosage schedules of choline-magnesium trisalicylate. Arth Rheum. 1979;22:384–89.

235. Gerstein HR et al. Patient compliance within the context of seeking medical care for arthritis. J Chronic Dis. 1973;26:689–98.

236. Montgomery PR, Sitar DS. Increased serum salicylate metabolites with age in patients receiving chronic acetylsalicylic acid therapy. Gerontology 1981. 27:329–33.

237. Cuny G et al. Pharmacokinetics of salicylates in the elderly. Gerontology 1979;25:49–55.

238. Buchanec J et al. Effect of age on pharmacokinetics of salicylate. J Pediatr. 1981;99:833–34.

239. Grigor RR et al. Salicylate toxicity in elderly patients with rheumatoid arthritis. J Rheumatol. 1987;14:60–6.

240. Mongan E et al. Tinnitus as an indication of therapeutic serum salicylate levels. JAMA. 1973;226:142–45.

241. Champion GD et al. Clinical pharmacology and efficacy of benorylate in patients with RA. Aust NZ J Med. 1978;8:22–8.

242. Halla JT, Hardin JG. Salicylate ototoxicity in patients with rheumatoid arthritis: a controlled study. Ann Rheum Dis. 1988;47:134–37.

243. Ross M et al. Salicylate nomogram. XIV International Congress of Rheumatology. 1977;118:470. Abstract.

244. Done AK. Salicylate intoxication: significance of measurements of salicylate in blood in cases of acute ingestion. Pediatrics 1960;26:800–807.

245. Spector S. Management of acute aspirin poisoning in children. Q Rev Pediatr. 1958;13:179–87.

246. Dromgoole SH, Furst DE. Salicylates. In: Evans WE et al., eds. Applied Pharmacokinetics. Vancouver, WA: Applied Therapeutics, Inc. 1980;486–517.

247. Lesko LJ et al. Salicylate protein binding in young and elderly as measured by ultrafiltration. Clin Res. 1982;33:257.

248. Levy G. Clinical pharmacokinetics of aspirin. Pediatrics 1978;62:867–72.

249. Reynolds RC, Cluff LE. Interaction of serum and sodium salicylate: changes during acute infection and its influence on pharmacological activity. Bull Johns Hopkins Hosp. 1960;105:278–90.

250. Graham G, Rowland M. Application of salivary salicylate data to biopharmaceutical studies of salicylates. J Pharm Sci. 1972;61:1219–222.

251. Borzelleca JF, Doyle CH. Excretion of drugs in the saliva. Salicylate, barbiturate, sulphonamide. J Oral Ther Pharmacol. 1966;3:104–11.

252. Borzelleca JF, Putney JW. A model for the movement of salicylate across the parotid epithelium. J Pharmacol Exp Ther. 1970;174:527–34.

253. Poe TE et al. Total and free salicylate concentrations in juvenile rheumatoid arthritis. J Rheumatol. 1980;7:717–23.

254. Levy G et al. Relationship between saliva salicylate concentration and free or total salicylate concentration in serum of children with juvenile rheumatoid arthritis. Clin Pharmacol Ther. 1980;27:619–27.

255. Routh JI, Paul WD. Assessment of interference by aspirin with some assays commonly done in the clinical laboratory. Clin Chem. 1976;22:837–42.

256. Singh HP et al. Effect of some drugs on clinical laboratory values as determined by the Technicon SMA 12/60. Clin Chem. 1972;18:137–44.

257. Hoeldtke R. Effect of aspirin on the assay of homovanillic acid. Am J Clin Pathol. 1972;57:324–25.

258. Rosenbaum JM et al. Misleading results in cases of coexisting acetaminophen and salicylate overdose. Clin Chem. 1980;26:673–74.

259. McCoy MT et al. Salicylate mimicking an abnormal CK-isoenzyme. Clin Chem. 191;27:1622–623.

260. Reed RG et al. Salicylate interference with measurement of acetaminophen. Clin Chem. 1982;28:2178–179.

261. Dromgoole SH, Furst DE. Salicylates. In: Evans WE et al., eds. Applied Pharmacokinetics: Principles of Therapeutic Drug Monitoring. 2nd ed. Vancouver, WA: Applied Therapeutics, Inc. 1988;944–977.

262. Stewart MJ, Watson ID. Analytical reviews in clinical chemistry; methods for the estimation of salicylate and paracetamol in serum, plasma and urine. Ann Clin Biochem. 1987;24:552.

263. Shen J et al. Novel direct high-performance liquid chromatographic method for the determination of salicyl glucuronide conjugates in human urine. J Chromotog. 1991;565:309–20.

264. Siebert DM, Bochner F. Determination of plasma aspirin and salicylic acid concentrations after low aspirin doses by high-performance liquid chromatography with post-column hydrolysis and fluorescence detection. J Chromatog. 1987;420:425.

265. Osterloh J, Yu S. Simultaneous ion-pair and partition liquid chromatography of acetaminophen, theophylline and salicylate with application to 500 toxicologic specimens. Clin Chem Acta. 1988;175:239.

266. Dawson CM et al. A non-extraction HPLC method for the simultaneous determination of serum paracetamol and salicylate. Ann Clin Biochem. 1988;25:661.

267. Gaspari G, Locatelli M. Determination of aspirin and salicylic acid in uremic patients plasma using reversed phase high-performance liquid chromatography. Drug Monitoring 1987;9:243.

268. Kirschenbaum JJ. Inter-laboratory transfer of HPLC methods; problems and solutions. J Pharm Biomedical Analysis 1989;7:813.

269. Robinson DR, Levine L. Prostaglandin concentrations in synovial fluid in rheumatic diseases: action of indomethacin and aspirin in prostaglandin synthetase inhibitors. In: Prostaglandin Synthetase Inhibitors: Their Effects on Physiological Functions and Pathological States. Robinson HJ and Vane JR, eds. New York: Raven Press; 1974:223.

270. Patrono C et al. Comparative evaluation of the inhibitory effects of aspirin-like drugs on prostaglandin production by human platelets and synovial tissue in advances in prostaglandin and thromboxane research. In: Samuelsson B, Paoletti R, eds. New York: Raven Press; 1976.

271. Vane JR. Inhibition of prostaglandin synthesis as a mechanism of action of aspirin-like drugs. Nature 1971;231:232–35.

272. Crook D et al. Prostaglandin synthetase activity from human rheumatoid synovial microsomes. Effect of "aspirin-like" drug therapy. Ann Rheum Dis. 1976;35:327–32.

273. Packham MA. Mode of action of acetylsalicylic acid in acetylsalicylic acid: new uses for an old drug. In: Barnett HJM et al., eds. New York: Raven Press; 1982.

274. Atkinson DC, Collier HOJ. Salicylates: molecular mechanism of therapeutic action. Adv Pharmacol Chemother. 1980;17:233–88.

275. Coppe P et al. Sex differences in the platelet response to aspirin. Thromb Res. 1981;23:1.

Chapter 33

Cyclic Antidepressants

C. Lindsay DeVane and C. Rick Jarecke

The tricyclic antidepressants were introduced into clinical practice in the 1950s. Controlled clinical trials documented that they provided an effective means to ameliorate various symptoms of depression. However, the percentage of patients who completely recovered during a therapeutic trial varied, generally between 50% and 80%, with an average efficacy of about 70%. In the 1960s analytical methodology became available to quantitate plasma concentrations of these drugs. A large variability, at times exceeding a 30-fold difference, was noted in the steady-state concentration among patients taking similar doses.[3] In addition, there was no apparent relationship between the concentration of parent drug in plasma and that of known active metabolites. This pharmacokinetic variability can be appreciated by observing the lack of relationship between steady-state imipramine concentration and its active metabolite, desipramine, an antidepressant in its own right (see Figure 33-1). These observations made difficult the application of tricyclic pharmacokinetics to the treatment of depressed patients.

Subsequently, numerous studies tested the hypothesis that a clinically useful relationship existed between steady-state tricyclic plasma concentrations and clinical response.[5] This issue has been widely debated and reviewed.[8] There is evidence for existence of a therapeutic range for some tricyclics. However, it can be concluded that plasma concentration monitoring on a routine basis is only justified for a few patients. This chapter identifies the types of patients most likely to benefit from antidepressant concentration monitoring.

Much has been learned about the clinical pharmacokinetics of the tricyclic antidepressants since the appearance of the first edition of this text.[9] Unfortunately, the therapeutic range for some tricyclics remains equivocal, and it is unlikely that further concentration-versus-effect studies for these drugs will be performed. Instead, attention is now being focused on a new generation of antidepressants. In clinical trials, these drugs frequently show efficacy comparable to that of the tricyclics. Moreover, the side-effect profile of the second generation drugs is improved.[11]

Cyclic Antidepressants

No longer can the group of drugs used to treat depression be labeled the tricyclics. Newer drugs, representative of more diverse chemical entities, are appearing on the market. Fluoxetine and bupropion are the most recent additions to this class of drugs. Clomipramine, structurally related to imipramine, has recently been marketed as the only FDA-approved pharmacologic treatment for obsessive-compulsive disorder. These drugs can be distinguished by the classification proposed in Table 33-1. Excluding the traditional tricyclics, the remaining compounds are classified according to the number of benzene rings in their structure, except when drugs have one or more rings containing a non-hydrocarbon atom. These drugs are classified as the heterocyclics.

Bupropion is a chloropropiophenone whose antidepressant efficacy has been established in open and double-blind, placebo-controlled studies.[12] Investigations of its autonomic and cardiovascular pharmacology show bupropion to be free of significant sympathomimetic, sympatholytic, anticholinergic, or cardiovascular effects, thereby conferring important clinical advantages over the tricyclics.[13] Paroxetine, sertraline, and fluvoxamine are selective serotonin reuptake inhibitors which are undergoing clinical trials.[14,15,16] These compounds are neither sedating nor stimulating and may possess an earlier onset of action than the tricyclics. Fluoxetine is an effective antidepressant which also has a low incidence of side effects.[11] Maprotiline is a dibenzobicyclo-octadiene which has an efficacy comparable to that of the tricyclics but has a similar spectrum of side effects.[17]

The heterocyclics consist of drugs from distinctly different chemical classes. Trazodone is a triazolopyridine derivative with some antidepressant effectiveness in outpatients and a high degree of sedative effect.[18] Alprazolam was the first

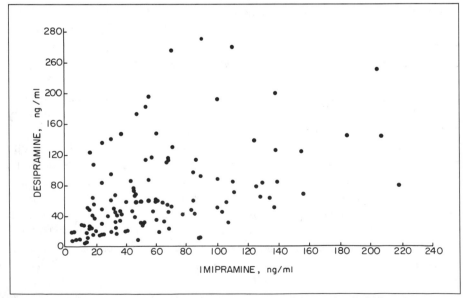

Figure 33-1. *Plasma concentrations of imipramine and desipramine in 119 patients treated with imipramine. Data from reference 216.*

benzodiazepine to demonstrate possible antidepressant properties in clinical trials at doses two to four times those approved for anti-anxiety effects.[19] Amoxapine, a dibenzoxazepine compound, is an effective antidepressant that possesses no striking advantages over the tricyclics and has been associated with extra-pyramidal side effects.[20]

Since the first edition of *Applied Pharmacokinetics: Principles of Therapeutic Drug Monitoring* in 1980, the pharmacokinetic properties of the tricyclics have been better elucidated, the role of active metabolites has been further defined, and concentration-versus-effect studies have included children. Overall, our ability to apply pharmacokinetic theory has improved, with better predictive methods for achieving a desired steady-state dose early in therapy. Because the second-generation antidepressants have only recently become available, much work remains to be done on their pharmacokinetics and concentration-response relationships. Commercial laboratories are offering plasma concentration measurements for the newer cyclic antidepressants in conjunction with purported therapeutic ranges. However, we lack enough information to quote reliable concentration-effect relationships for most of these agents. This chapter updates our knowledge of tricyclic pharmacokinetics and surveys the present state of our knowledge of the remaining cyclic antidepressants.

CLINICAL PHARMACOKINETICS

The pharmacokinetic characteristics of some cyclic antidepressants are displayed in Table 33-2. Many similarities exist between the newer drugs and the traditional tricyclics. Overall, the cyclic antidepressants are characterized by nearly complete oral absorption, substantial presystemic elimination, extensive distribu-

Table 33-1. Classification of Cyclic Antidepressants

Classification	Drug
Unicyclics	bupropion
	fluvoxamine
Bicyclics	fluoxetine
Tricyclics	amitriptyline
	clomipramine
	desipramine
	doxepin
	imipramine
	nortriptyline
	protriptyline
	trimipramine
Tetracyclics	maprotiline
Heterocyclics	alprazolam
	amoxapine
	mianserin
	paroxetine
	sertraline
	trazodone

Table 33-2. *Pharmacokinetic Properties of Cyclic Antidepressants in Healthy Adults*

Drugs	Percent bioavailable	Percent unbound	Half-life (hr)[a]	V_d (L/kg)[b]	CL_M (L/hr)[c]	References
Alprazolam	>95	26–32	7–18	0.9–1.9	6.6–40	45,218
Amitriptyline	30–60	3–15	9–46	6.4–36	19–72	219–221
Amoxapine	46–82	—	8.8–14	—	41.7–73.5	1
Bupropion	>90	20	9.6–20.9	27–63	126–140	222
Clomipramine	36–62	2–10	15–62	9–25	23–122	223,224
Desipramine	33–51	8–27	12–28	24–60	78–168	215,219,226
Doxepin	13–45	15–32	8–25	9–33	41–61	227
Fluoxetine	≈72	5	26–220	12–42	5.6–42	228
Fluvoxamine	>90	33	13–19	>5	—	43
Imipramine	22–77	4–37	6–28	9.3–23	32–102	24,229
Maprotiline	79–87	12	27–50	16–32	17–34	16,46,63
Nortriptyline	46–70	7–13	18–56	15–23	17–79	25,225
Paroxetine	>90	5	7–37	3–28	15–92	43
Protriptyline	75–90	6–10	54–198	15–31	8.4–23.4	230,231
Sertraline	—	5	≈25	—	—	43
Trazodone	70–90	5–11	6.3–13	0.8–1.5	1.8 ± 1.0	18,232,249
Trimipramine	18–63	3–7	16–40	17–48	40–105	233,234

[a] Biologic half-life in slowest phase of elimination.
[b] Volume of distribution, either in the steady-state or the slowest phase of elimination.
[c] CL_M = Plasma clearance.

tion with avid plasma protein and tissue binding, and hepatic clearance which approaches values for liver blood flow. Metabolism produces biologically active metabolites for nearly all of these drugs.

Absorption

Tricyclic Antidepressants. After oral administration, the tricyclics are ionized in the stomach, and no absorption is assumed to take place until the drug reaches the more alkaline environment of the intestines. The rate of appearance of drug in the blood is rapid. Peak concentrations have often been observed from two to eight hours following a single oral dose.[24] The lag time before absorption begins is usually less than 20 minutes. Pharmacokinetic theory predicts that peak concentrations will occur sooner in the multiple-dosing situation than following single doses.[26] However, Gram et al.[27] found imipramine peak concentrations to occur two to six hours after drug dosing at steady state; this finding was no different from single dose observations. Therefore, the clinical significance of earlier peak concentrations at steady state is doubtful.

The absorption characteristics of tricyclics have most often been observed in single-dose studies in which food was restricted for several hours before and after dosing. Abernethy et al.[28] studied the influence of food on the bioavailability of imipramine. Concurrent ingestion of a standardized meal had no effect on imipramine's absolute bioavailability, the peak concentration attained after an oral dose, or the time to peak concentration.

The systemic bioavailability of tricyclics is low (see Table 33-2). Comparison of the area under the concentration-versus-time curve (AUC) for oral and intravenous doses of imipramine in the same subjects indicates an availability of 30% to 70%.[28] Nevertheless, studies which have determined the urinary excretion of tricyclic metabolites indicate that oral absorption is nearly complete.[24,30] When imipramine was administered intramuscularly and orally in a crossover fashion to healthy volunteers, similar total fractions of the doses were recovered in urine, indicating complete absorption of the oral doses.[24] A high degree of presystemic elimination is well documented for the tricyclics. While this is mostly hepatic in origin,[31] imipramine metabolism by microsomes of small intestine obtained from guinea pigs suggests that the first-pass effect may also occur in other organs.[32] These factors contribute to the intersubject variation in bioavailability after oral doses (see Table 33-2).

Parenteral dosage forms of amitriptyline, clomipramine, and imipramine are available in some countries. Oral and parenteral routes of tricyclic administration produce differences in parent drug and metabolite concentration-time profiles. This finding is of potential clinical importance because active metabolites often have effects on neurotransmitters that are different from those of their precursors. For example, desipramine inhibits the reuptake of norepinephrine to a greater extent and inhibits the reuptake of serotonin to a lesser extent than does imipramine.[33] It has been suggested that the onset of antidepressant effects for amitriptyline and clomipramine is faster when they are given intravenously than when given orally.[34] Some pharmacokinetic considerations are pertinent to this suggestion. Compared to parenteral drug administration, oral administration will produce earlier and higher metabolite concentrations, because of the first-pass elimination of tricyclics. Mellstrom et al.[35] found that the peak concentration of nortriptyline, the demethylated metabolite of amitriptyline, occurred 8 to 24 hours after oral dosing of the parent drug; intramuscular administration of amitriptyline produced lower nortriptyline peak plasma concentrations, occurring 24 to 48 hours after administration. However, no difference in the fraction of drug doses converted to metabolites from different routes of administration would be expected if the following assumptions are valid: complete oral absorption, elimination only by hepatic biotransformation, and linear pharmacokinetics.[26] This theory has been supported by experimental data.[24,36] Sutfin et al.[24] found the average fraction of single imipramine doses recovered as imipramine and metabolites in urine to be similar following single oral and intramuscular doses. Mellstrom et al.[35] found that the AUC of nortriptyline from intramuscular amitriptyline was similar to the AUC from oral amitriptyline. Thus, if clinical outcomes differ when tricyclics are administered by different routes of administration, these should not relate to differences in the fraction of drug converted to metabolites.

Do different oral formulations result in differences in total absorption? This is an important clinical concern. In a multiple-dose study of four different amitriptyline formulations with variable dissolution rates, amitriptyline trough concentrations at steady state did not significantly differ.[37] Differences in absorption rate were apparent between imipramine syrup and tablets[38] and between an amitriptyline sustained-release preparation and conventional tablets,[39] although the total absorption appeared similar. Very little information is available on tricyclic absorption by rectal administration. However, extemporaneously compounded amitriptyline suppositories have produced apparently good clinical effects in one patient.[40] Overall, bioequivalence among tricyclic products has been demonstrated in several studies.

Non-tricyclic Antidepressants. The newer cyclic antidepressants show a greater diversity in their absorption characteristics than do the tricyclics. The absorption of amoxapine is rapid and virtually complete, and maximum serum concentrations have been observed one to four hours following an oral dose.[41] A similar profile applies to bupropion[22] and alprazolam.[45] Trazodone also exhibits rapid absorption, reaching peak concentrations within two hours.[249] Unlike that of the tricyclic, imipramine,[28] trazodone absorption appears to be influenced by food. The peak concentration is reported to be lower and delayed when drug is taken in the nonfasting state;[18] however, the total AUC is reported to be increased when trazodone is administered in the nonfasting state.[4] The absorption of maprotiline appears to be relatively slow.[46] The lag time for absorption of oral tablets is at about 1.4 hours with an absorption half-life of approximately two hours. This slow absorption pattern explains why peak concentrations are observed between 8 and 24 hours after a drug dose.[46] Fluoxetine is rapidly absorbed with peak plasma concentrations occurring within four to eight hours after oral administration.[6] A relatively low first-pass effect occurs based on limited data from dogs.[2] The extent of fluoxetine absorbed is not influenced by food, but the rate of absorption may be decreased.[6] Paroxetine and fluvoxamine are both well absorbed when taken orally. Sertraline may undergo a significant interaction with food.[43]

Distribution

Tricyclic Antidepressants. The tricyclics are highly lipophilic compounds which distribute widely in the body. Octanol:water partition coefficients are on the order of log 3–5.[48] This characteristic partly explains their extensive distribution beyond the vascular system. Figure 33-2 shows the concentration-time course of imipramine in plasma and various tissues after a single administration to pregnant rats. Maternal brain concentrations are an order of magnitude greater than concentrations in plasma or whole blood. Even though the partition coefficients for the tricyclics are high, lipophilicity alone does not account for their extensive tissue distribution. Using rats as a model, Bickel et al.[49] found that following single and

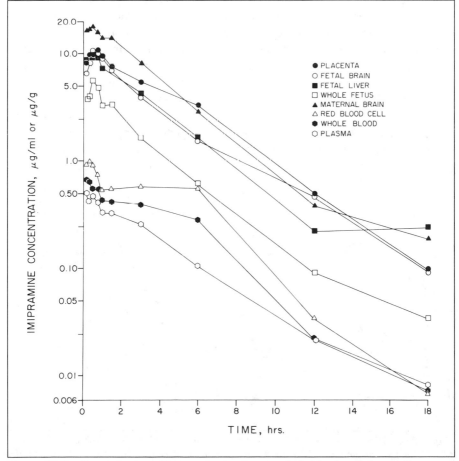

Figure 33-2. *Concentration of imipramine in plasma, whole blood, and tissues of pregnant rats treated with an acute imipramine dose. Points represent the mean value obtained from three to five animals.*

chronic imipramine doses, the lowest concentrations in 12 tissues occurred in plasma and adipose tissue. The highest concentrations were found in lung, followed by kidney, brain, small intestine, liver, skeletal muscle, and skin. While obesity has been incompletely studied as a specific factor affecting tricyclic pharmacokinetics, these animal data suggest that adipose tissue is not a sink for tricyclic accumulation as would be intuitively presumed for highly lipophilic compounds. Thus, until specific investigations prove otherwise, one may not generalize that obese subjects will have longer tricyclic half-lives due to a larger volume of distribution.

Steady-state volumes of distribution may be as large as 60 L/kg (see Table 33-2) and may show considerable intersubject variation. This extensive distribution beyond the vascular system partly explains why extracorporeal methods of treating tricyclic intoxication, such as hemodialysis and hemoperfusion, have been largely unsuccessful in removing significant amounts of the body's total drug burden following overdosage.[51] Figure 33-3 shows that six hours of hemoperfusion had a minimal effect on decreasing the plasma concentration of imipramine and its three major metabolites following an imipramine overdose. Calculations using data represented by the lower curves in Figure 33-3, which represent venous drug concentrations returning to the body, indicate that drug extraction efficiency is between 75% and 95%; yet, less than 1% of the estimated ingested dose is removed.

Protein Binding. Several groups have examined the protein binding of tricyclics. Kristensen and Gram[52] and Bertilsson et al.[250] have reviewed the potential artifacts in the methodology used in these determinations. Important factors which influence the precision in measuring protein binding include equilibrium dialysis time and temperature. The studies of imipramine binding, the prototype tricyclic,

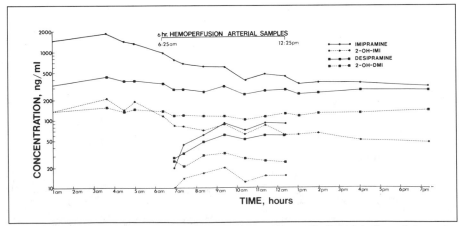

Figure 33-3. *Plasma concentrations of imipramine and its metabolites, 2-hydroxy-imipramine (2-OH-IMI), desipramine, and 2-hydroxy-desipramine (2-OH-DMI) over an 18-hour period in a patient who ingested an overdose one hour previously. The lower drug concentration curves between 7:00 a.m. and 1:00 p.m. represent venous samples returning to the body from the hemoperfusion apparatus. Data redrawn from reference 51.*

are summarized in Table 33-3 and reflect the variability in reported results. Most studies have not compared binding *in vitro* with cerebrospinal fluid:plasma ratios which may serve as a better reflection of binding *in vivo*.

Several factors affect tricyclic protein binding. Pike et al.[54] examined the effect of plasma albumin, α_1-acid glycoprotein (AAG), and lipoprotein concentrations. They found that the degree of binding for amitriptyline and nortriptyline was strongly dependent on the serum concentrations of cholesterol and triglycerides. Other studies have shown that tricyclics bind to AAG with high affinity and low capacity, whereas they bind to albumin with low affinity.[56] Imipramine binding is increased in cardiac patients with elevated concentrations of AAG after myocardial infarction.[57] Alcoholics, who were found to have a greater concentration of AAG than normals, were also found to have a greater degree of imipramine protein binding.[58] Thus, alcoholics may have binding characteristics that differ from depressed patients who have no significant history of alcohol abuse. Baumann et al.[59] found that a three-week treatment of amitriptyline significantly increased the AAG concentration in depressed patients . This finding suggests that the degree of tricyclic binding might change over the course of therapy, thus altering the fraction of free drug in plasma. Inflammatory processes have also been reported to increase AAG levels. Total plasma drug concentration would therefore be elevated, however, doses may not need to be altered as the free drug concentration should not change. Overall, real evidence of altered protein binding as a source of altered response to cyclic antidepressants is practically nonexistent.

The question arises whether estimates of free drug concentrations would be useful for improving the quality of therapeutic drug monitoring. Although the results across studies have been more variable, a two- to fourfold interindividual variability in free fractions of tricyclics have been found within studies (see Table 33-3). Some investigators have found relatively strong relationships between unbound drug concentration and total concentration in plasma.[54,60] However, occasional outlyers—usually high binders—have been noted in some studies.[61]

Table 33-3. Summary of Imipramine Protein Binding Studies in Human Plasma

Mean percent free	Range (SD)	Number of subjects	Method	Reference
4.2	(0.8)	5	Ultrafiltration	219
41.0	—	—	ED,[a] 2–3 hr	240
14.3	5.4–23	26	ED, 36–48 hr	241
7.9	6–11	23	ED, 6 hr	56
5.2	(1.3)	8	Gel filtration	242
11.5	8–14	43	ED, 6 hr	220
	(1.4)			
30.1	24–37	19	ED, 36 hr	60
10.4	8.5–12	5	ED, 5–6 hr	52
	(1.4)			
8.3	5–18	36	ED, 4 hr	57
16.5	(1.79)	6	ED, 5 hr	28

[a] Equilibrium dialysis.

For most patients, drug protein binding differences are relatively small compared to the much larger intersubject variability in total plasma concentrations. Protein binding is of lesser importance than the much larger variability found in total body clearance. Breyer-Pfaff et al.[62] evaluated both free and total amitriptyline concentrations and found that protein binding measurements were not helpful in clarifying the relationship between antidepressant response and plasma concentration. Perry et al. found no statistically significant relationship between free nortriptyline concentrations and clinical response but noted that free nortriptyline levels greater than 10 ng/mL suggested a tendency toward a negative clinical response.[10] Given the low concentrations expected for free drug (10 to 20 ng/mL), measurement of free concentrations does not appear to be a practical way to improve the value of therapeutic drug monitoring with tricyclics.

Non-tricyclic Antidepressants. Most of the newer cyclic antidepressants behave as lipophilic bases. With the exception of alprazolam, all have high volumes of distribution far exceeding body weight (see Table 33-2). In tissue distribution studies of animals, maprotiline,[63] amoxapine,[64] trazodone,[65] and bupropion[66] all produce higher tissue than plasma concentrations. In tissue taken from a suicide case due to an overdose of maprotiline, drug concentrations were highest in liver, lung, and kidney, followed by the brain, heart, muscle, and plasma.[63] Since these drugs are widely distributed and readily pass into the central nervous system, it can be presumed that they also cross the placenta. Amoxapine and its 8-hydroxy metabolite have been found in human breast milk, although in lower concentrations than in plasma.[67] Fluoxetine is also reported to be highly protein bound (95%) in healthy human subjects and in subjects with renal insufficiency.[228]

Metabolism and Elimination

Tricyclic Antidepressants. The tricyclics are extensively metabolized. Overall, renal clearance accounts for elimination of less than 5% of administered doses as unchanged drug.[24,68] The major metabolic pathways include oxidation and conjugation; N-oxidation and dealkylation are minor pathways. The most important reactions in man are N-demethylation and hydroxylation, followed by glucuronide coupling.

Imipramine is the most thoroughly studied tricyclic. Figure 33-4 shows the major pathways of imipramine metabolism in man. Following oral administration of imipramine, demethylation produces desmethylimipramine (desipramine). Aromatic hydroxylation occurs at the 2-carbon positions, resulting in 2-hydroxy-imipramine and 2-hydroxy-desipramine. It is likely that formation of 2-hydroxy-imipramine may also be an intermediate pathway to formation of 2-hydroxy-desipramine. These reactions probably occur in a sequential fashion during imipramine's first pass through the liver. Minor pathways of imipramine metabolism include dealkylation of the entire side chain to form imidodibenzyl; further demethylation of desipramine to the primary amine, didesmethylimipramine, and hydroxylation at the 10-carbon position. N-oxidation, by which imipramine-N-oxide is formed, occurs as a reversible reaction. Additional metabolic pathways in the rat have been elucidated.[70]

The other tricyclics are biotransformed in a manner analogous to that of imipramine, with some minor differences. For example, the major pathways of amitriptyline metabolism are demethylation and hydroxylation, but the latter reaction occurs preferentially at the 10-carbon position.[72] The tricyclics appear to be metabolized by several hepatic enzyme systems, including the microsomal P-450 system.[72,73] Some evidence exists for biliary excretion and reabsorption of imipramine (i.e., enterohepatic circulation).[74] The review by Gram[72] presents an extensive discussion of tricyclic metabolism.

Non-tricyclic Antidepressants. The metabolism of maprotiline is similar to that of the tricyclics. The principal metabolite is the desmethyl derivative, but both this metabolite and the parent drug may be further biotransformed into multiple minor metabolites by aromatic hydroxylation and oxidative modification of the side chain. [63,75] The desmethyl metabolite accumulates to substantial proportions of its precursor upon chronic maprotiline dosing.[63] Unchanged maprotiline in the urine accounts for less than 2% of the administered dose.

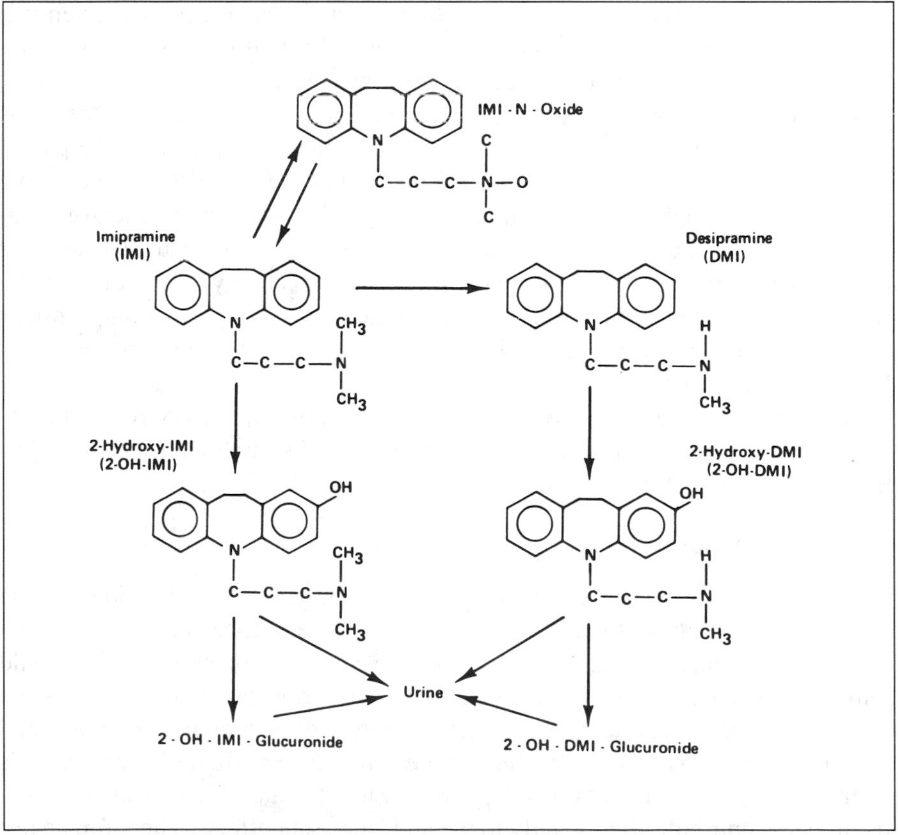

Figure 33-4. *Major pathways of imipramine metabolism in man.*

The major route of amoxapine metabolism is by aromatic hydroxylation to 7-hydroxy-amoxapine and 8-hydroxy-amoxapine.[64] About 3% of an amoxapine dose is excreted in an unchanged form. The metabolites may be further conjugated and eliminated in the urine. The terminal elimination half-life of 8-hydroxy-amoxapine exceeds that of amoxapine. This metabolite accumulates at steady state to plasma concentrations exceeding those of amoxapine.[77]

Trazodone is extensively metabolized, with less than 1% of a dose excreted unchanged in the urine.[78] Major metabolic transformations occur by hydroxylation and N-oxidation. An active metabolite is m-chlorophenylpiperazine. Little is known of its plasma concentration profile. Excretion of the inactive propionic acid derivative in the urine accounts for approximately 20% of an ingested dose.

Bupropion undergoes extensive hepatic metabolism, with less than 1% of a dose excreted unchanged.[66] The major basic metabolites are the erythro-amino alcohol, the threo-amino alcohol and the hydroxy metabolite. In man, two metabolites have accumulated to several times the bupropion concentration in plasma.[80] Investigation of the hydroxylated metabolite from a single bupropion dose in normal volunteers indicates that the apparent half-life for elimination of the metabolite is approximately twice that of bupropion.[22] All three major metabolites appeared in greater concentration than did bupropion in the cerebrospinal fluid of patients receiving antidepressant therapy with bupropion.[22] In non-depressed subjects with alcoholic liver disease, the half-life of bupropion's metabolites was extended, although the disposition of the parent compound did not differ substantially when compared with data from healthy, age- and weight-matched volunteers.

Fluoxetine, a specific serotonin reuptake inhibitor, undergoes N-desmethylation to produce a pharmacologically active metabolite, norfluoxetine. The parent drug exhibits an elimination half-life of one to three days, whereas the active metabolite has a half-life of seven to nine days.[6] Schenker et al. found that in patients with alcoholic cirrhosis, the mean half-life was 6.6 versus 2.2 days for patients with cirrhosis versus normal volunteers, respectively.[25] In addition, norfluoxetine formation and clearance was decreased. In patients with compromised hepatic function, it would be advisable to lower the dosage to avoid drug accumulation and concentration-dependent side effects.

Neither paroxetine nor fluvoxamine produce pharmacologically active metabolites.[43] Desmethylsertraline is an active metabolite of sertraline, but its contribution to the clinical effects of sertraline is unknown.

Active Metabolites

Pharmacologically active metabolites are important when considering the cyclic antidepressants. Table 33-4 summarizes the evidence for antidepressant activity of the major metabolites for some cyclic antidepressants. One should remember that activity *in vitro* does not necessarily translate into antidepressant effects *in vivo*. However, many of these metabolites accumulate to substantial degree in the plasma and are present in the cerebrospinal fluid of humans. This distribution pattern suggests that they may reach the site of action in sufficient quantity to contribute significantly to the antidepressant effects. The ultimate test of antidepressant activity would be separate administration of the metabolites to depressed patients; however, such studies are unlikely to be performed for many of these compounds. Nevertheless, because these metabolites have presumptive antidepressant and/or toxicological activity, they should be included in pharmacokinetic studies.

The 2-hydroxy metabolite of imipramine (2-OH-IMI) and desipramine (2-OH-DMI) and the 10-hydroxy metabolite of amitriptyline (2-OH-AMI) and nortriptyline (2-OH-NOR) have been of particular interest, and their pharmacologic role has been extensively examined. Since these metabolites are presumed to possess antidepressant activity,[87-89] accounting for their presence during antidepressant therapy should enhance correlations between plasma concentration and response. Before well-controlled antidepressant studies were performed which included measurements of these hydroxy metabolites, their plasma concentrations were first assessed in relationship to steady-state concentrations of the parent drugs. As can be seen in Table 33-5, the concentration of 2-OH-DMI might be important in producing clinical effects, since it usually accumulates to about 50% of the DMI concentration from both IMI or DMI administration. Also, the steady-state concentration of 10-OH-NOR usually predominates over that of NOR. For this reason, 10-OH-NOR may be of more practical importance than the other hydroxy metab-

Table 33-4. *Basis for Suspected Antidepressant Activity of Some Cyclic Antidepressant Metabolites*

Parent drug	Metabolite	Evidence of activity
Alprazolam	Alpha-hydroxy alprazolam	High-affinity binding to benzodiazepine receptors; seizure protection in mice.[244]
Amitriptyline	Nortriptyline 10-hydroxy-nortriptyline	Nortriptyline active as preformed compound; hydroxy metabolite inhibits reuptake of noradrenaline; accumulation in plasma; present in cerebrospinal fluid of man.[89]
Amoxapine	7-hydroxy-amoxapine 8-hydroxy-amoxapine	Both metabolites accumulate in plasma; 7-hydroxy exhibits dopamine blocking activity similar to haloperidol.[245]
Bupropion	Hydroxy-bupropion	Accumulation in plasma often greater than bupropion; present in CSF of man; LD_{50} in mice is less than that of bupropion; approximately 50% activity compared to parent compound in *in vitro* antidepressant screening test.[246]
Fluoxetine	Norfluoxetine	As an inhibitor of 5-HT reuptake, norfluoxetine is less potent than the parent compound.[29]
Imipramine	2-hydroxy-imipramine Desipramine 2-hydroxy-desipramine	Desipramine active as pre-formed compound; both hydroxy metabolites present in CSF of man; inhibit reuptake of catecholamines *in vitro*; cardiotoxic in dogs; some accumulation in plasma and brain.[88]
Maprotiline	Desmethylmaprotiline	Some accumulation in plasma; distributes to animal brain tissue.[63]
Trazodone	m-chlorophenylpiperazine	Metabolite is a direct serotonin receptor agonist; present in brain of animals after trazodone dosing; the preformed compound has pharmacologic activity when directly administered to humans.[247, 248]

olites and merits additional study. The 10-hydroxy metabolite of amitriptyline and the 2-OH-IMI metabolite are presumably of lesser importance, based on their steady-state accumulation ratios.

Some exceptions to the usual accumulation patterns shown in Table 33-5 have been noted. Garvey et al.[90] and DeVane et al.[91] observed that some patients accumulated unusually high concentrations of parent drugs and very low concentrations of the hydroxy metabolites. Studies of genetic polymorphism attempt to explain the basis behind altered clearance of specific drugs undergoing oxidative metabolism. Sparteine and debrisoquine oxidative polymorphism allows us to define those patients who exhibit compromised oxidative metabolic processes and are therefore at increased risk for concentration-dependent side effects and/or toxicity. Steiner et al.[42] have estimated that approximately 7% of the Caucasian population can be classified as poor oxidative metabolizers (PM) of sparteine and debrisoquine. Brosen and Gram,[44] in a review of the current literature, describe the pharmacokinetic consequences of genetic polymorphism for tricyclic antidepressants eliminated by the sparteine/debrisoquine oxygenase (P-450-db1 isozyme) system (see Table 33-6).

Brosen and Gram[44] have also shown how extensive metabolizers (EMs) and PMs, vary in their first-pass metabolism of imipramine and its demethylated metabolite, desipramine. They demonstrated that the first-pass metabolism of imipramine and desipramine was greater in EMs than in PMs and that different isozymes of CP-450 are responsible for 2-hydroxylation and demethylation.[44] Phenotyping patients into those that rapidly metabolize and those that slowly

Table 33-5. *Steady-State Ratios of Tricyclic Hydroxy Metabolite to Parent Drug Concentrations*

Drug treatment	Subject group	Number of subjects	Mean metabolite: parent ratio[a] (with range)
Desipramine[243]	depressed elderly	4	2-OH-DMI:DMI 0.86 ± 0.05 (0.75–1.00)
Desipramine[243]	depressed	9	2-OH-DMI:DMI 0.38 ± 0.06 (0.05–0.62)
Desipramine[243]	depressed	61	2-OH-DMI:DMI 0.48 ± 0.26
Desipramine[243]	normals	6	2-OH-DMI:DMI 0.55 ± 0.09 (0.15–0.62)
Imipramine[81]	enuretic boys	32	2-OH-IMI:IMI 0.23 2-OH-DMI:DMI 0.38
Imipramine[216]	depressed	126	2-OH-IMI:IMI 0.27 ± 0.19 2-OH-DMI:DMI 0.56 ± 0.30
Amitriptyline[114]	depressed	27	10-OH-AMI:AMI 0.17 ± 0.09 10-OH-NOR:NOR 1.65 ± 1.12
Amitriptyline or Nortriptyline[89]	depressed	87	10-OH-NOR:NOR 1.40 ± 0.86 (0.32–5.03)

[a] Abbreviations: AMI = amitriptyline; NOR = nortriptyline. DMI = desipramine; IMI = imipramine; 10-OH-AMI = 10-hydroxy-amitriptyline; 10-OH-NOR = 10-hydroxy-nortriptyline; 2-OH-IMI = 2-hydroxy-imipramine; 2-OH-DMI = 2-hydroxy-desipramine.

metabolize drugs oxidized via the CP-450 system may be prudent to identify slow metabolizers who may develop toxic serum concentrations following "normal" doses. Also, differences in first-pass metabolism could alter metabolite:parent drug ratios which, in turn, may contribute to therapeutic drug efficacy. The urinary ratio of debrisoquine to 4-hydroxy-debrisoquine correlated well with the total plasma clearance of nortriptyline. Such data support other observations[95] that the elimination of tricyclics is strongly genetically influenced.

In a series of investigations on depressed inpatients, Nelson et al.[96] considered the role of 2-OH-DMI in correlating desipramine plasma concentrations to both antidepressant and adverse effects. Drug responders had desipramine plasma concentrations that were substantially different from those of nonresponders, but the mean 2-OH-DMI concentration did not differ between the groups. While desipramine concentrations correlated positively with response, as found previously,[99] the 2-OH-DMI concentration alone provided no useful correlation. Furthermore, adding the parent drug and metabolite (desipramine + 2-OH-DMI) concentrations did not improve the correlation over that achieved with desipramine alone. The 2-OH-DMI concentration was not helpful in differentiating patients with or without major adverse reactions or subjective side effects. These investigators could find no practical value in measuring plasma concentrations of 2-OH-DMI. Nevertheless, these data do not disprove the activity of 2-OH-DMI, which is active *in vitro* and *in vivo* (see Table 33-4).

An explanation for the lack of relationship between 2-OH-DMI concentration and effects may be the low proportion in plasma of 2-OH-DMI compared to DMI (see Table 33-5). The relationship with nortriptyline as the test drug might be different since plasma concentrations of 10-OH-NOR are generally higher than those of nortriptyline (see Table 33-5). Breyer-Pfaff et al.[67] indirectly addressed

Table 33-6. *Pharmacokinetic Consequences of Polymorphism for Drugs Eliminated via the Sparteine/Debrisoquine Oxygenase, P450-dbl[a,b]*

Biotransformation	Consequence for poor metabolizers	Drug	Reference
D ➤ *M$_a$ ↓ M$_b$	Accumulation of drug, D	Tricyclic antidepressants Nortriptyline Desipramine Clomipramine	110 122 123**
D ➤ M$_a$ * ↓ ▼* M$_b$ M$_c$	Accumulation of active metabolite, M$_a$	Imipramine (active metabolite: desipramine)	124,127
D ➤ *M$_a$ * ↓ ▼* M$_b$ M$_c$	Accumulation of drug, D, and active metabolite, M$_a$	Amitriptyline (active metabolite: nortriptyline)	130, 131

[a] ➤ = important pathway; ↓ = less important pathway; * = pathway catalyzed by the P-450 which oxidized sparteine and debrosoquine; ** = only urine data available.
[b] Adapted from reference 44 with permission.

this point in a study of the antidepressive effect of amitriptyline. In 27 depressed inpatients, the inclusion of 10-OH-NOR measurements only slightly improved the distinction of a concentration range associated with improvement when amitriptyline and nortriptyline concentrations were combined. There have been no controlled clinical trials of nortriptyline administration which have specifically examined the utility of including plasma concentration measurements of 10-OH-NOR. However, 10-OH-NOR has been administered as a preformed compound and found to have antidepressant effects. At this time there is little evidence to suggest that monitoring the hydroxy tricyclic plasma concentrations has any practical value in improving therapy.

Table 33-7. *Factors Reported to Affect Cyclic Antidepressant Plasma Concentration*

Factor	Effect on plasma concentration	Mechanism
Acute ethanol ingestion	↓	Hepatic enzyme induction
Barbiturates	↓	Hepatic enzyme induction
Smoking	↓	Hepatic enzyme induction
Carbamazepine	↓	Hepatic enzyme induction
Chloral hydrate	↓	Enzyme induction
Trihexyphenidyl	↓	Interference with absorption
Acidic urine pH	↓	Reduces renal tubular reabsorption
Phenytoin	↓	Hepatic enzyme induction
Benzodiazepines	No effect	
L-triiodothyronine	No effect	
Aging	No effect or ↑	Decreased metabolic clearance
Methylphenidate	↑	Competitive enzyme inhibition of hydroxylation pathways
Chloramphenicol	↑	Enzyme inhibition
Haloperidol	↑	Enzyme inhibition
Phenothiazines	↑	Mutual hepatic enzyme competition
Disulfiram	↑	Hepatic enzyme inhibition
Basic urine pH	↑	Increased urinary reabsorption
Cimetidine	↑	Decreased hepatic blood flow and (or) hepatic enzyme inhibition
Fluoxetine	↑	Hepatic enzyme inhibition
Alcoholic liver disease	↑	Decreased metabolic capacity in advanced disease state
Renal failure	↑	Decreased excretion of conjugated metabolites
Oral contraceptives	↑	Enzyme inhibition

Factors Affecting Plasma Concentration

The metabolism of cyclic antidepressants is remarkably variable among individuals and is subject to perturbation by social and environmental influences. Unfortunately, it is impossible to quantitatively predict the extent of their influence on metabolic clearance. Table 33-7 is provided to alert the reader to factors that may influence antidepressant plasma concentrations. In practice, these factors may negate each other (e.g., in an elderly patient who smokes).

As highly metabolized drugs, the tricyclics could be expected to interact with cimetidine because it inhibits hepatic microsomal enzymes and decreases hepatic blood flow.[100] When coadministered with cimetidine, the bioavailability of imipramine increased from 40.2% to 75.3%,[102] and its systemic clearance dropped from 15.1 to 9.0 mL/min/kg. This effect of cimetidine was reflected by an increased AUC and a prolonged elimination half-life. That desipramine AUC was increased during cimetidine therapy after oral imipramine doses suggests that desipramine clearance was inhibited as well. Cimetidine had no effect on plasma protein binding. Similar results were reported in another cimetidine-tricyclic interaction study,[103] but a lack of effect was noted when nortriptyline was the test drug. However, plasma concentrations of the major active metabolite, 10-hydroxy-nortriptyline, were increased. In our laboratory, cimetidine has also been found to increase the systemic availability of amitriptyline. Volunteers who took this drug combination as opposed to amitriptyline alone demonstrated impaired mental functioning as measured by a battery of psychological rating scales. A case report of imipramine toxicity associated with the combined use of cimetidine has appeared.[104] Taken together, these findings suggest that the pharmacologic and toxic effects of tricyclic drugs may be enhanced when cimetidine is co-prescribed. In this situation, the initial tricyclic doses should be appreciably reduced, unless plasma concentration monitoring is available. It should be noted that when amitriptyline was coadministered with ranitidine, another commonly used H_2 blocker, no pharmacokinetic changes were noted.[47]

Omeprazole, a proton pump inhibitor, may interact with drugs metabolized by the mixed function oxidase systems (e.g., warfarin, disulfiram). Phenytoin and diazepam AUCs increase following coadministration of omeprazole, presumable through the latter's inhibition of the microsomal CP-450 enzyme system.[50] At this time, it is unknown to what extent this new class of drugs will alter the pharmacokinetics of other highly metabolized drugs. Until the interaction between omeprazole and the tricyclics has been specifically studied, however, their coadministration warrants caution and monitoring of tricyclic plasma concentration.

Care should be taken if fluoxetine is combined with other antidepressants. Fluoxetine is a metabolic inhibitor and has raised the plasma concentration of several coadministered drugs, including desipramine, nortriptyline, haloperidol, and diazepam.[43] The interaction of fluoxetine with monamine oxidase inhibitors has produced a fatal outcome.

Alcohol consumption is important to consider in patients taking cyclic antidepressants. The incidence of depression is greater in patients with alcoholic liver disease than in the normal population.[105] Thus, the generally recognized detrimental effects of alcohol on the liver might alter the pharmacokinetics of cyclic antidepressants. Ciraulo et al.[106] compared imipramine pharmacokinetic and therapeutic response variables in depressed alcoholics and depressed nonalcoholic male inpatients. Drug clearance appeared to be faster in the alcoholics and was accompanied by lower plasma concentrations. Hamilton Rating Scale measurements also indicated that the alcoholics were less improved after equal periods of therapy. While these data suggest that alcoholics might require higher-than-normal doses of tricyclics because hepatic enzymes are induced by alcohol, cautious interpretation is warranted because of the multiple effects of alcohol. In another study which used amitriptyline as the test drug, Sandoz et al.[107] found that alcoholic depressed patients had lower amitriptyline plus nortriptyline steady-state plasma concentrations than did nonalcoholics. In the alcoholics, the mean level of hydroxylated compounds was significantly higher. DeVane et al.[252] found that the mean elimination half-life of bupropion's active metabolite was significantly prolonged in subjects with alcoholic liver disease. The meaning of these data is unclear.

More subtle effects of alcohol have been reported by Dorian et al.[108] In the presence of ethanol, plasma concentrations of unbound amitriptyline were dramatically increased during the drug absorption phase. This resulted in a free AUC increase of $48\% \pm 13\%$ over an eight-hour period. This pharmacokinetic interaction was accompanied by an increase in postural sway over baseline and a decrease in short-term memory recall. This effect could be a result of a pharmacokinetic or pharmacodynamic interactions. Overall, these data suggest that the combination of a tricyclic and alcohol may markedly impair mental function. No studies have examined the effects of either alcoholic hepatitis or cirrhotic liver disease on tricyclic pharmacokinetics. The effect of acute or chronic alcohol ingestion concurrent with cyclic antidepressant administration must be regarded as unpredictable.

Concurrent administration of phenothiazines may also alter tricyclic metabolism.[112] It is likely that a mutual metabolic inhibition occurs with this drug combination. Nelson and Jatlow[113] found that among 30 patients taking similar mg/kg doses of desipramine, 15 who also took an antipsychotic drug had mean steady-state DMI concentrations twice as high as those of patients who were not taking these agents. In another group of 82 depressed patients, 35 who were taking an antipsychotic drug along with desipramine had higher DMI concentrations and a lower proportion of 2-OH-DMI compared to the remaining patients taking only DMI.[98] These investigators have also determined that antipsychotic usage affects the extent of amitriptyline hydroxylation.[114] Loga et al.[115] found that the use of nortriptyline in schizophrenic patients taking chlorpromazine resulted in increased plasma chlorpromazine concentrations and a prolonged half-life. Overall, the studies demonstrating an interaction between antipsychotics and tricyclic antidepressants strongly suggest that tricyclic doses should be appreciably reduced if they are added to a regimen that already includes an antipsychotic and that addition of an antipsychotic to a cyclic antidepressant regimen could potentially result in loss of drug efficacy and/or production of toxicity through a pharmacokinetic interaction.

The renal clearance of the tricyclics is low, with less than 2% of a dose excreted in the urine. This percentage does not apply to metabolites. Sutfin et al.[24] found that following a single imipramine dose, approximately 8% was excreted as free 2-hydroxy-desipramine and 33% as imipramine or desipramine glucuronide conjugates. While the latter metabolites are inactive, the appreciable renal clearance of unconjugated 2-OH-DMI implies that accumulation might occur in chronic renal failure. This could alter the concentration-response relationship of the parent drug. There is an added concern that conjugates may break down, releasing pharmacologically active drug. In a study comparing two groups of depressed patients on long-term amitriptyline therapy, Sandoz et al.[109] found that plasma concentrations of conjugated metabolites were extremely high in uremic patients, while concentrations of amitriptyline, nortriptyline, and their unconjugated 10-hydroxy-metabolites were decreased compared to those in patients with normal kidney function. Dawling et al.[111] have previously determined that nortriptyline kinetics were unaltered in chronic renal failure but that the elimination of the metabolites was reduced. While these findings suggest that no specific alteration of tricyclic dosing is required in patients who have renal failure, plasma concentration monitoring is recommended.

Nonlinearity in tricyclic disposition has been suggested. The terminal half-life of imipramine in the study of Sutfin et al.[24] was 1.5 to 2 times longer after an intramuscular dose than after an oral dose. However, it is possible that this effect resulted from slow release of drug from strong tissue binding sites. The hydroxylated metabolite of trimipramine has also been shown to increase in a nonlinear fashion compared to the parent compound after dosing increases, suggesting saturation of the enzyme responsible for hydroxylation.[55] Bjerre et al.[116] found that in a group of elderly depressed patients treated with usual daily doses of imipramine, a dose increase resulted in a greater-than-proportional rise in the steady-state plasma concentrations of desipramine. In a separate report on these same patients,[117] it was noted that the 2-OH-IMI concentrations remained almost unchanged following a substantial increase in imipramine dose. This finding suggests that the desipramine hydroxylation pathway might become saturated in some patients. Nelson and Jatlow[253] found that one-third of patients receiving a stable dose of desipramine who had a dose increase displayed some evidence of nonlinearity. Preliminary reports suggest some linearity in the disposition of the selective serotonin reuptake inhibitors;[43] however, the clinical significance is unclear. The generally accepted idea of limited metabolic capacity of the elderly implies that plasma concentration monitoring would be helpful to decrease the risk of disproportionate increases in plasma concentration that may result from nonlinear metabolism in this group of patients. However, it should be noted that considerable evidence exists for the linear metabolism of the tricyclics.

Several studies have addressed the hypothesis that cyclic antidepressant disposition is reduced in the elderly. Table 33-8 lists some pharmacokinetic parameters for several tricyclics and the tetracyclic compound maprotiline in elderly and younger subjects. The results vary substantially, but overall there are strong trends suggesting reduced clearance of the tricyclics in the elderly. When small numbers of patients are studied, as in the study of desipramine concentrations in elderly

Table 33-8. *Pharmacokinetic Parameters of Antidepressants in the Elderly and Healthy Young Volunteers*

Subject characteristics and pharmacokinetic parameters	Amitriptyline		Nortriptyline		Imipramine		Maprotiline	
	Young	Elderly	Young	Elderly	Young	Elderly	Young	Elderly
Age range studied (years)	21–35	72–83	20–35	68–100	21–36	75–83	38–58	75–83
Number of subjects	15	11	17	20	7	5	12	5
CL (L/hr)[a]	19.4–71.8	12.5–65.2	16–115	8–38.5	50–88	16.5–28.2	16.9–34.4	16.7–31.4
V_d (L/kg)[b]	6.4–36.5	9–28.1	—	—	9.3–23	9.6–21	16.1–32.6	14.8–28.5
Half-life (hr)[c]	10.1–46.6	16.7–44.6	14–51	23.5–79	6–28	21–35	27.4–50	20.6–51.8
References	235, 236, 222, 237		238		239, 229, 24, 116		239, 46, 63	

[a] Plasma clearance.
[b] Volume of distribution—either in steady state or during the slowest phase of elimination.
[c] Biologic half-life determined from the terminal portion of the plasma concentration-time curve.

women by Cutler et al.,[118] the data suggest that aging does not seem to alter tricyclic pharmacokinetics. On closer examination,[119] the ratio of 2-OH-DMI to DMI at steady state was higher than expected in younger patients. Previous studies[120,121] and those listed in Table 33-8 suggest that elderly patients will require lower doses of cyclic antidepressants to obtain targeted steady-state plasma concentrations than younger adults. The documented nonlinearity in the elderly, as discussed above,[116] further implies that pharmacokinetic monitoring may be of particular benefit in this population. Finally, it should be recognized that the decrease in renal function that accompanies aging can adversely influence cyclic antidepressant clearance.

PHARMACODYNAMICS

Tricyclic Concentration versus Antidepressant Response

The practical utility of using tricyclic plasma concentrations to guide therapy is controversial and has been widely debated and reviewed.[71] If critical therapeutic ranges existed and regular plasma concentration measurements improved the outcome of therapy, then routine monitoring would be justified. However, relatively few studies have addressed this issue. Furthermore, the problems of uniform diagnostic criteria, assay quality control, reliability of rating scales, and criteria of response make inter-study comparisons difficult.[125] Even for the most widely studied drugs (imipramine, amitriptyline, and nortriptyline), therapeutic ranges remain equivocal. Ironically, although fewer than 50 patients have been investigated for some of the newer cyclic antidepressants, therapeutic ranges have been proposed for all, including those not yet available on the market. This situation results partly from the rapid proliferation of assay methodology and the entry of commercial laboratories into the field of biological psychiatry. In general, cyclic antidepressant plasma concentration monitoring is beneficial only for a few patients.

The concept of a therapeutic range is discussed in Chapter 1: General Principles of Applied Pharmacokinetics. As a probability range within which the best clinical effect is observed, two types of relationships have emerged with the tricyclics. Imipramine appears to demonstrate the usual sigmoidal dose-response curve, with no particular upper limit associated with loss of response.[129] The upper limit is defined by intervening toxicity. For nortriptyline, a curvilinear response between concentration and effect has been repeatedly demonstrated.[134] The curvilinear nature of the relationship is called a "therapeutic window" where concentrations above the upper limit are associated with a declining, but not necessarily a toxic, response. These two are the only cyclic antidepressants for which a clear relationship exists between plasma concentration and improvement in depressive symptoms. Amitriptyline has also been extensively studied, but no clear relationship between concentrations and therapeutic response has emerged. Several studies have found a sigmoidal response[135,136] and a curvilinear response,[137] whereas others have found no apparent relationship between concentration and effect.[138,139] Table 33-9 lists the therapeutic ranges for those antidepressants for which a relationship between plasma concentration and therapeutic response has been suggested.

Imipramine. The results of several well-controlled studies have demonstrated a positive, significant correlation between the steady-state plasma concentration of imipramine (combined with its metabolite desipramine) and an antidepressant response.[128,129] The lower threshold concentration appears to be about 120 ng/mL with at least 45 ng/mL of imipramine and 75 ng/mL of desipramine. Studies have demonstrated good clinical response when combined concentrations were higher than 85 ng/mL,[140] 120 ng/mL,[69] 180 ng/mL,[129] and 240 ng/mL.[128] Simpson et al.[141] reported a clinical trial of imipramine involving 27 patients. Dividing the patients into good or poor responders according to four different rating scales and using the minimum plasma concentration ranges cited above, the authors were unable to demonstrate the value of monitoring steady-state plasma concentration. The only significant differentiation between responders and nonresponders was a combined imipramine plus desipramine threshold of 240 ng/mL. It is interesting that 12 of the 27 patients on an imipramine dose of 200 mg/day had concentrations below a total of 120 ng/mL; about half of these patients were poor responders. These data can be compared to that of Matuzas et al.[142] in a trial of depressed outpatients taking 150 mg/day of imipramine, in which the mean total plasma concentration was 122 ng/mL. Note that 150 mg/day of imipramine is regarded as an adequate dose for testing drug responsiveness.[143] Since there is considerable evidence that combined plasma concentrations of greater than 180 ng/mL are associated with an increased probability of clinical response, one can speculate that some nonresponders in the Simpson study might have benefited from an increase in dose.

Table 33-9. *Antidepressant Plasma Concentrations and Clinical Response*[256]

Drug	Total patients studied	Usual dosage range	Type of correlation	Therapeutic range (ng/mL)
Imipramine	259	75–300	Linear	≥ 225–240[a]
Nortriptyline	414	50–150	Curvilinear	50–150
Amitriptyline	321	75–300	Uncertain	120–250[a]
Desipramine	63	75–300	Probably Linear	≥ 115–180
Doxepin	42	75–300	Uncertain	110–250[a]
Protriptyline	49	15–60	Probably Curvilinear	70–250
Imipramine[b]	30	Average: 4.3 mg/kg/day	Linear	155–284
Nortriptyline[b]	40	0.5–1.6 mg/kg/day	Curvilinear	45–130
Nortriptyline[c]	26	45 mg/day	Curvilinear	80–120

[a] Parent drug plus N-desmethyl metabolite.
[b] Prepubertal major depressive disorder.
[c] Geriatric major depressive disorder.

There is uncertainty about the existence of an upper threshold for response. Anecdotal case reports[90,91] and close examination of controlled trials show that some patients may respond at much higher concentrations: up to 500 ng/mL. The risk of cardiac conduction disturbances, however, is increased at this concentration.[144] A practical upper limit would be 350 ng/mL, but this should not be regarded as absolute.

Nortriptyline. For nortriptyline, additional studies[134] have confirmed the initial observation that endogenously depressed patients showed a curvilinear response, with the best antidepressant effect in the concentration range of 50 to 150 ng/mL.[130] The upper limit of 150 ng/mL represents a concentration above which the therapeutic effect is less assured. In the study of Kragh-Sorensen,[134] plasma concentrations were specifically manipulated to be either within the range of 50 to 150 ng/mL or above this presumed window. Patients with plasma concentrations greater than 180 ng/mL improved when plasma concentrations were lowered to 655 than 150 ng/mL.

Recently, Lipsey et al.[146] demonstrated for the first time in a placebo-controlled, double-blind trial that a tricyclic antidepressant, nortriptyline, was effective in treating post-stroke depression. By the end of the study, all successfully treated patients had nortriptyline plasma concentrations between 50 and 140 ng/mL. While the trial was not specifically designed to assess the therapeutic range of nortriptyline, the separation between nortriptyline and placebo response became evident when serum concentrations of nortriptyline were consistently in the presumed therapeutic range. These results lend further support to the recommendation that this tricyclic be dosed to achieve a target concentration range.

Amitriptyline. Many studies illustrate a positive relationship between amitriptyline plasma concentration and response. Whether this relationship is linear or curvilinear is unclear. When the results of the studies supporting a linear response are taken together,[135,136] the combined amitriptyline and nortriptyline concentration corresponding to patient response is between 80 and 220 ng/mL. The lower threshold concentration is approximately 80 to 120 ng/mL, and there is no decrease in response when serum concentrations exceed 220 ng/mL. The studies supporting a curvilinear response[137] limit the upper level to 220 to 250 ng/mL. Investigators in the two largest amitriptyline studies[138] found no useful relationship between concentration and effect. However, since only one-third of the patients in the multicenter trial responded, a high proportion of tricyclic nonresponders may have been included; the study has been criticized on that basis.[147] Recently, it has been suggested that the nortriptyline:amitriptyline concentration ratio may help define clinical response,[148] but the data are inconclusive at this time.

Desipramine. The earliest concentration-versus-response studies with desipramine were small and included mostly outpatients.[150] The results suggested a probable therapeutic range between 75 and 160 ng/mL, with a "therapeutic window" effect similar to that of nortriptyline. Results of a well-controlled study of 30 depressed inpatients[99] strongly support the concept of a therapeutic range for desipramine. Eighty-nine percent of patients with plasma concentrations above 115 ng/mL responded, while only 14% responded when plasma concentrations were below this level. The data show that ten initial nonresponders were converted to responders when dosage increases raised the desipramine plasma concentration to 125 ng/mL or greater. Other well-conducted studies have produced equivocal results. In the study of Stewart et al.[151] desipramine responders spanned a broad concentration range between 48 and 712 ng/mL. Neither Brunswick et al.,[152] nor Simpson et al.[153] could find a useful relationship between desipramine concentration and antidepressant effect. Optimistically, the overall data suggest that if a therapeutic window exists with desipramine, it is not as narrow as that for nortriptyline, since patients have responded across a broad concentration range. However, a threshold concentration appears to exist, whereby the probability of responding is increased when concentrations are greater than 115 ng/mL.[99]

Other Tricyclic Antidepressants. Despite its widespread use, very few investigators have studied doxepin plasma concentration relationships.[154,155] Friedel and Raskind reported that improvement was related to a plasma concentration greater than 110 ng/mL.[154] Linnoila et al.[156] found that serum doxepin concentrations were higher among responders than among non-responding, neurotically depressed patients. In contrast, Brunswick et al.[152] found no relationship between plasma concentration and clinical response. While most studies have included measurements of the active desmethyl metabolite of doxepin, another complexity exists with this drug: its cis and trans isomers possess different pharmacologic effects and accumulate to different degrees at steady-state.[157]

Clomipramine has been examined for a relationship between plasma concentration and response in the treatment of depression[158,159] as well as in the treatment of obsessive-compulsive behavior.[160] These studies, however, lack agreement because a therapeutic plasma concentration range cannot be defined. The data relating concentration to response for other tricyclics are unclear. In general, one can only state that therapeutic responses occur between 50 and 350 ng/mL.

Newer Cyclic Antidepressants and Clinical Response. No significant relationship between plasma maprotiline concentration and clinical response has been found.[163] Unfortunately, investigators have not included measurements of desmethylmaprotiline concentrations, either separately or combined with maprotiline. There is inadequate information available on the relationship between plasma concentration and antidepressant response for the remaining cyclic antidepressants. Two limited investigations with trazodone,[164,165] and one with amoxapine,[77] failed to find a relationship between concentration and response. It is clear from experience with the tricyclics that future investigations should use an assay methodology which quantitates the metabolites as well as the parent compound (see Table 33-4). Preliminary evidence from Preskorn indicates that a curvilinear relationship exists between antidepressant response and bupropion plasma levels between 5 and 100 ng/mL.[79] However, this was not a fixed-dose study, and more research is needed before a curvilinear range *is defined* for bupropion, if one truly exists. Based upon our present understanding of cyclic antidepressant pharmacokinetics, the "therapeutic" plasma ranges proposed for the newer antidepressants by commercial laboratories are questionable. Some concentration ranges represent uncontrolled data obtained from patients responsive to therapy.

Only preliminary data are available for the new serotonin reuptake inhibitors. Several groups have reported fluoxetine plasma concentrations in relation to antidepressant effects.[43] Most reports have found no usable relationship between steady-state concentration and antidepressant effect. Fluoxetine doses between 20 and 60 mg/day produce plasma concentrations of fluoxetine between 50 and 450 ng/mL while norfluoxetine concentrations usually vary between 50 and 350 ng/mL. Montgomery et al.[76] found a negative relationship between high metabolite concentrations and antidepressant response. Larger studies are needed to draw conclusions about a therapeutic range for fluoxetine.

Clinical Response in Pediatrics

Major depressive disorders in children have been the studied systematically. Imipramine has been primarily used in the treatment of childhood depression, but few attempts have been made to correlate plasma concentration with clinical response. Preskorn et al.[166] studied 20 hospitalized children 7 to 12 years of age. When steady-state concentrations of imipramine plus desipramine were correlated to clinical response, there was an 80% remission rate for children in the 125 to 225 ng/mL range versus no remissions for those outside this range. The data suggest a lower concentration threshold of 125 ng/mL, similar to that for adults.[69] Four patients whose steady-state concentrations were above 225 ng/mL responded only when doses were reduced. This observation, unlike the adult data, argues for a curvilinear relationship, but the number of patients is too small for us to draw this conclusion. Overall, this well-controlled study supports previous data[168] and the practice of monitoring plasma imipramine concentrations in children whose therapeutic response to a usual therapeutic regimen is unsatisfactory. One can exclude low plasma concentrations as a basis for nonresponsiveness by this method.

For indications other than depression, little information exists in the relationship between plasma concentration and response for cyclic antidepressants in children. Imipramine's anti-enuretic effects have only recently been investigated in relation to plasma drug concentration. Jorgensen et al.[169] studied 22 hospitalized children with nocturnal enuresis and found a significant correlation between the steady-state plasma concentration of imipramine plus desipramine or desipramine concentration alone and the reduction in enuresis frequency. The effect was optimal when the plasma imipramine plus desipramine concentration was above 60 ng/mL. However, in this study, only 30% of the patients achieved this concentration. Rapoport et al.[170] studied a larger sample of 40 patients and also found a significant relationship between desipramine plasma concentrations and its anti-enuretic effect. Their data suggest that the optimal effect occurs when the steady-state plasma drug concentration is greater than 150 ng/mL. This relationship, however, did not hold for a few patients evaluated at follow-up. Some responders developed an apparent tolerance to imipramine's anti-enuretic effect, despite sustained drug plasma concentrations. This observation suggests that the pharmacokinetics and/or pharmacodynamic variables change with continued dosing. We were unable to find a positive correlation between concentrations of imipramine and its three major metabolites with anti-enuretic response in 14 patients.[171] Most patients, however, demonstrated a good drug therapeutic response at a relatively low plasma concentration. Therefore, the role of monitoring imipramine plasma concentrations in enuretic children remains unclear. Because of the large variability in imipramine pharmacokinetics, plasma concentration monitoring may be warranted whenever avoidance of toxicity is of major concern.

Concentration versus Toxicity

The tricyclics produce troublesome anticholinergic and cardiovascular adverse effects and can be fatal in overdosage situations. Correlations have been reported between objectively measured or subjectively reported side effects and plasma concentrations. Asberg et al.[172] found a weak positive correlation between common side effects scored on a rating scale and plasma nortriptyline concentrations. Ziegler et al.[173] correlated increased perspiration and dry mouth to nortriptyline plasma concentrations; however, these findings are of little practical value since many subjective effects of tricyclics are also symptoms of depression. Objective measures such as change in visual accommodation[174] or reduction in salivary flow[175] reportedly correlate to plasma concentration but are impractical to measure. Of greater practical value would be strong positive correlations between plasma concentration and major adverse effects such as orthostatic hypotension or anticholinergic delirium. Crome and Braithwaite[176] found that tricyclic concentrations greater than 500 ng/mL were associated with anticholinergic effects and that concentrations greater than 1000 ng/mL were associated with convulsions, coma, and cardiac arrhythmias. Preskorn and Simpson[177] examined 14 patients receiving amitriptyline who had concentrations above 300 ng/mL. A drug-induced delirium was present in six of seven patients whose concentration was greater than 450 ng/mL, while none of the seven with a concentration between 300 and 450 ng/mL developed delirium. While these data suggest that adverse effects could be avoided by monitoring tricyclic concentrations and reducing doses when appropriate, the range at which side effects appear is variable. For example, Nelson et al.[178] examined the relationship between desipramine plasma concentrations and major adverse effects that occurred in 16 of 84 patients undergoing a clinical trial with desipramine. Desipramine plasma concentrations in patients having side effects did not differ significantly from those in patients without side effects. In addition, the concentrations at which side effects developed were variable. Four patients who experienced orthostatic hypotension had a desipramine concentration of less than 100 ng/mL, while the concentrations encountered in patients with no side effects ranged up to 683 ng/mL.

There is convincing evidence that tricyclic plasma concentrations greater than 1000 ng/mL are associated with severe toxicity.[145] A QRS complex on the electrocardiogram of greater than 100 milliseconds is pathognomonic of a potentially lethal overdose and is correlated with concentrations greater than 1000 ng/mL.[179] This concentration is also associated with greater frequency of need for respiratory support, development of coma, seizures, and cardiac arrhythmias. While severe symptoms of overdosage can occur at lower concentrations, patients with persistently elevated concentrations are at greater risk for sudden death.

Glassman et al.[180] found no relationship between the development of orthostatic hypotension, which may occur with therapeutic doses, and particular tricyclic plasma concentrations. The overall data suggest that routine monitoring of plasma concentrations to avoid side effects is of little clinical value; however, a plasma concentration measurement might be useful to confirm a tricyclic-induced anticholinergic delirium.

CLINICAL APPLICATION OF PHARMACOKINETIC DATA

The response of recalcitrant depressed patients to pharmacotherapy can be so unsatisfactory that any monitoring tool which improves therapy would be a welcome advance. It was anticipated that the ability to monitor tricyclic plasma concentrations would improve efficacy and decrease side effects. Unfortunately, these benefits have not yet been realized. It can be assumed that, for those patients who respond to antidepressants, there is some relationship between drug concentration and effect. The studies which have found a lack of relationship between concentration and effect serve to moderate the application of clinical pharmacokinetics in psychiatry. They illustrate that the concentration-effect relationships in small group studies are so variable that no uniform relationship will emerge. However, these negative or equivocal findings do not prove that plasma concentrations will be less useful than empirical dosing to titrate tricyclic therapy to response. Similarly, those studies in which a good correlation between concentration and effect was observed may only have succeeded because the subjects studied were more homogeneous than those in other studies. The greater the number of patients studied (e.g., with imipramine and nortriptyline), the clearer the therapeutic range becomes. This information can be used to guide therapy when empiric

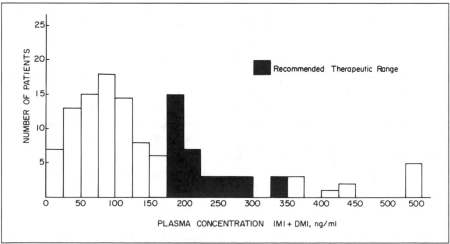

Figure 33-5. *Plasma imipramine plus desipramine concentrations in 126 patients receiving routine treatment with different daily doses of imipramine. The shaded area represents the usually recommended target range for antidepressant effect. Data from reference 216.*

dosage adjustment is unsuccessful. In contrast, therapeutic concentrations for some less-studied tricyclics, such as doxepin, trimipramine, and protriptyline, are not well documented and should not be used to establish therapeutic response.

Indications for Cyclic Antidepressants Monitoring

Clinicians who do not routinely monitor tricyclic concentrations will often exceed or fall below the purported therapeutic ranges. In Figure 33-5 it can be observed that a number of patients on empirical imipramine therapy have combined imipramine plus desipramine concentrations which fall outside the recommended target range. The pronounced intersubject pharmacokinetic variability, problems with drug interactions, noncompliance, the probable nonlinearity in tricyclic metabolism, and the delayed onset of clinical response in relation to initiation of therapy are all reasons why therapeutic drug monitoring should be useful for patients on antidepressant pharmacotherapy. This may be due to a number of mitigating factors which may include noncompliance, inappropriate drug, wrong diagnosis, insufficient duration of therapy and subtherapeutic plasma drug concentrations.

Noncompliance. The most obvious indication for a cyclic antidepressant measurement is suspected noncompliance. Only by recourse to previous measurements can noncompliance be accurately assessed. The broad variability (see Figure 33-5) in concentrations occurring with usual daily doses means that some patients who are fully compliant may have cyclic antidepressant concentrations which are relatively low. For the tricyclics, a concentration below 30 ng/mL when adequate doses have been prescribed (150 mg/day or more) should suggest noncompliance and/or rapid clearance. With a previous measurement, such an aberrant value will further suggest noncompliance or irregular drug intake.

Nonresponders. The second indication for therapeutic drug monitoring is in patients who fail to respond to therapy. The suggested therapeutic ranges listed in Table 33-9 can be used to adjust doses in those individuals who do not respond satisfactorily to prolonged therapy with usual clinical doses. For imipramine and nortriptyline, a plasma concentration measurement may indicate a need to increase or decrease the dose. For the remaining antidepressants, one can determine whether the patient's plasma concentration is equivalent to those purported to be approximately therapeutic.

Toxicity. A case of suspected toxicity is another indication for obtaining a plasma concentration. Valuable diagnostic information can be gained if the plasma concentration is excessively high (e.g., greater than 500 ng/mL for the tricyclics). However, one should remember that the relationship between side effects and drug concentrations is equivocal. In overdose cases, concentrations above 1000 ng/mL with or without prolonged QRS intervals indicate the need for continued clinical monitoring.

Cardiovascular Disease. In depressed patients with pre-existing heart disease, plasma concentration monitoring may be beneficial. ECG changes occasionally occur at therapeutic plasma concentrations. Excellent reviews on this subject are available.[181,182] While Burrows et al.[183] suggested on the basis of ECG studies that doxepin was a better choice than nortriptyline for patients with cardiac disease, this recommendation can be questioned because nortriptyline concentrations were higher during the comparison than were those of doxepin. The drug of choice in patients with cardiac disease is one of the newer cyclic antidepressants such as fluoxetine or bupropion, both of which appear to be safer than amitriptyline.

Clinicians should be aware that tricyclics are occasionally used therapeutically in patients with concurrent heart disease. Imipramine has antiarrhythmic effects similar to those of quinidine and has been used for prophylactic treatment of ventricular premature depolarizations.[186] Giardina et al.[187] determined in 15 cardiac patients that maximal suppression occurred when the combined imipramine and desipramine concentration ranged from 74 to 385 ng/mL. Fenster et al. examined the antiarrhythmic efficacy of desipramine in seven patients with chronic ventricular ectopy. They found that desipramine was effective in reducing the number of ventricular ectopic depolarizations by 75% in three patients treated with 150 mg and one patient treated with 75 mg. However, the clinical utility of using desipramine for this purpose was limited by adverse reactions, most notably anticholinergic side effects.[92] This use of tricyclics should be accompanied by plasma concentration monitoring.

Drug Interactions. The addition of another drug to an established antidepressant dosage regimen may result in alterations in clearance (see Table 33-7). If side effects occur, or if therapeutic response decreases, a plasma concentration measurement will be useful to assess whether the individual's therapeutic and/or toxic concentration range has been exceeded.

Elderly Patients. Conventional wisdom suggests that in patient populations where clearance differs from that in the majority of patients who receive the drug, benefits may accrue from closely monitoring therapy. The elderly have decreased clearance compared to younger depressed patients (see Table 33-8) and a higher incidence of side effects. In addition, because the metabolism of tricyclics is nonlinear in the elderly, they are more likely to experience a disproportionate increase in plasma concentration when doses are increased. Plasma concentration monitoring is also justified by the increased susceptibility of the elderly to antidepressant side effects.[96]

Children. Similarly to the elderly population, pharmacokinetics of drugs in children differ from those in the normal healthy adult population. Children tend to have increased metabolic capacity and a trend toward shorter elimination half-lives of drugs. Because children may require higher daily doses relative to body weight as compared to the general population, pharmacokinetic monitoring is justified. Pharmacokinetic data derived from single dose studies of nortriptyline have been obtained in the child and adolescent population. Weller et al.[167] found in a population of 5- to 12-year-olds a shorter mean half-life (range 11.2 to 42.5 hours) compared to a group of 13- to 16-year olds with a half-life ranging from 14.2 to 89.4 hours. Altered clearance may also lead to variable steady-state concentrations and concentration dependent side effects. Preskorn et al.[166] found that in a group of depressed children aged 6 to 12 years, toxicity developed in 3.75% (3 out of 80 children) while taking standard doses. Two of these subjects were on a fixed dose of 75 mg/day. Side effects at supratherapeutic levels, while

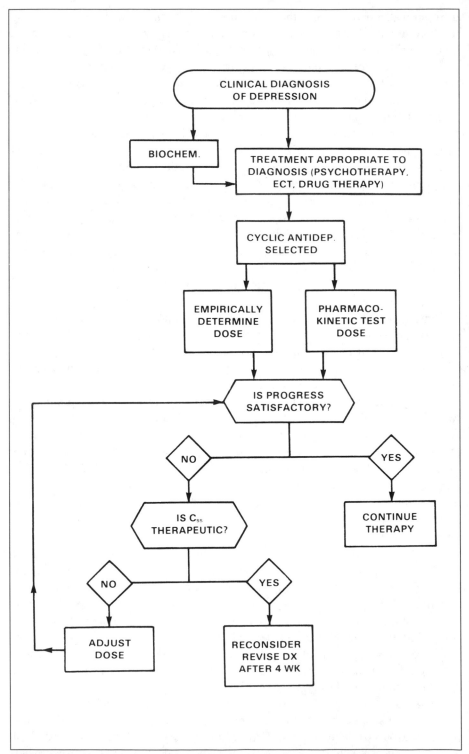

Figure 33-6. Algorithm for use of pharmacokinetics in the treatment of depression.

on standard doses, may not only impair cognitive performance in this population but may also be confused with worsening depression.[101] Because of large differences in oral clearance leading to highly variable elimination half-lives in the pediatric population, plasma level monitoring is warranted.

Treatment of Depression

The schematic diagram in Figure 33-6 outlines the use of pharmacokinetic data in the treatment of depression. Remember that most of the concentration-response relationships for the tricyclics were determined in patients closely fitting the criteria for major depressive disorder described in the third edition of the Diagnostic and Statistics Manual of the American Psychiatric Association (DSM-III-R). Because depression is a heterogeneous disorder, it is difficult to apply the purported therapeutic ranges (which were determined most often in endogenously depressed patients) to the variety of patients who receive cyclic antidepressants. For example, depression often occurs in schizophrenic patients as their psychosis improves upon treatment with antipsychotics. No studies have examined the plasma concentration range associated with therapeutic effects in this type of patient. While milder forms of depression, such as those formerly classified as reactive depression, are likely to respond to cyclic antidepressant therapy, the proposed therapeutic ranges (see Table 33-9) are less applicable.

The selection of a particular drug may be made on the basis of a history of previous response, the response of an immediate family member or other close relative, or on the basis of side-effects profiles. As yet, there are few indications that specific symptoms of depression are predictors of response to pharmacotherapy. The dexamethasone suppression test helps to identify depressed patients,[188] but, like catecholamine studies of urine, has no proven practical value for identifying responders to specific drugs.[189] Nevertheless, the possibility of identifying depressive predisposition with genetic markers sustains the hope of identifying specific drug responders through biochemical tests.

Treatment appropriate to diagnosis is mandatory. Supportive care should be given to all patients. In addition, many will benefit from treatment with a cyclic antidepressant. Once a drug is chosen, small initial doses may be beneficial to test drug acceptability and to accustom the patient to the occurrence of side effects (which often dissipate). A pharmacokinetic test dose may be given and serial plasma samples collected to predict the maintenance dose for a targeted steady-state concentration. This procedure is generally limited to research settings and is more thoroughly discussed below. Approximate steady-state concentrations will occur within four to five half-lives, or between four and seven days, for most of the drugs listed in Tables 33-1 and 33-2. It is likely that some elderly patients will require a longer time to attain steady-state concentrations, because of greater variability in their half-lives (see Table 33-8). There is little reason to check steady-state concentrations for most patients, especially if they are responding adequately. However, for patients who do not respond, a plasma concentration measurement may indicate irregular drug intake or rapid clearance. Once a steady-state concentration is determined, the dose can be adjusted proportionately to achieve a new steady state.

If the patient is responsive to cyclic antidepressants and is not experiencing unacceptable side effects, no adjustment in dose is necessary unless excessive plasma concentrations happen to be noted. When therapeutic concentrations are observed in unresponsive patients, one should maintain the dose for at least four weeks to allow for the usual lag in full efficacy before reconsidering the diagnosis or changing therapy. It should be remembered that the correlations between response and concentration reflected in Table 33-9 were observed after two to four weeks of therapy and one to three weeks after steady-state concentrations were likely to have been achieved. One should also consider the factors in Table 33-7 when continuing patients on maintenance therapy and recheck plasma concentrations when symptoms recur or when unexpected side effects occur.

Predictive Test Doses

Following the initial work of Alexanderson with nortriptyline,[95] Cooper et al.[190] demonstrated that the serum concentration of lithium determined shortly after a test dose could be empirically correlated with a steady-state measurement. Several groups of investigators have subsequently explored the application of this technique to the tricyclic antidepressants.[191-202] As a result, nomograms using initial plasma concentrations to determine maintenance doses which will achieve a desired steady-state concentration have been proposed. Many of these studies present impressive data supporting the accuracy of these nomograms.[254]

All the methods were developed in research centers where tricyclic assays were either being developed or performed routinely with rigorous quality control. Based on the nomograms, the lower the concentration at the initial measurement point, the higher the maintenance dose; this is because the clearance is likely to be greater in patients with lower initial concentrations. An analytical problem arises because the lower the measured plasma concentration, the greater the difficulty in achieving precision and reproducibility of tricyclic assays. All of the studies routinely encountered tricyclic concentrations less than 10 ng/mL. Only when quality control is rigorously maintained can plasma concentration measurements at this low level be assured to be accurate. Most studies have shown that the longer the time interval between the first dose and the first concentration measurement, the better the predictive accuracy of these nomograms.

The concentration-response studies from which the prediction studies have taken their targeted steady-state concentrations all included patients who improved at steady-state concentrations below the ultimately defined mean therapeutic range. Thus, the routine use of a nomogram or predictive test dose to achieve a target concentration will automatically result in the overtreatment of some patients who responded to lower concentrations. The use of higher-than-necessary doses in these individuals could lead to a higher incidence of side effects. The therapeutic concentration range should be approached from the low end in most patients. Use of routine dosing schedules undermines identification of individual therapeutic and/or toxic thresholds. Although the nortriptyline therapeutic range of 50 to 150 ng/mL represents a probability of improvement, each patient will have his or her own "therapeutic range." It is possible to overshoot this range in patients by following steady-state protocols.

All of the methods assume that the patient will be drug free at the time of the test dose. Thus, these methods are not applicable to anyone who has a measurable plasma concentration at the time the test drug is administered. This situation would artifactually increase the test dose concentration, leading to an inaccurate dose prediction. To avoid this error, a blood sample should be taken immediately before as well as after the test dose.

Few studies have documented the success of these methods in centers other than those in which they were developed. Therefore, it is recommended that clinicians thoroughly test these methods in their own settings to confirm their practical utility for the intended patient population. The recommended dosing procedure for the majority of patients is to adjust doses on the basis of random plasma concentration measurements by assuming linear pharmacokinetics. An increase or decrease in dose based on a steady-state plasma concentration should result in a proportional change in concentration.

In summary, the advantages of a predictive dosing method must be balanced against the risk of instituting an inappropriate maintenance dose, with the attendant possibility of losing definition of the patient's lowest dose requirement. Reliance upon these predictive methods compromises our ability to define subgroups of depressed patients who may respond at therapeutic ranges different from those assumed in the development of the nomograms. More widespread application of predictive approaches to dosage regimen design of antidepressants may lead to reduced hospitalization and cost savings. Studies are needed to document these benefits.[254]

ANALYTICAL METHODS

The various methods used to measure have been thoroughly reviewed,[203,204] and the most common ones are summarized in Table 33-10. No single assay is best for all purposes. The selection of a particular method will depend on such factors as cost, ease of operation, availability of equipment, and applicability to research as well as clinical monitoring. The overall quality of analytical results is also influenced by timing of the blood sample collection, the type of container, separation procedures, and storage conditions.

Collection and Storage of Samples

Both serum and plasma are used to determine cyclic antidepressant concentrations. While one report has shown no difference in antidepressant concentrations between serum and plasma determinations,[205] there is a large difference between erythrocyte and plasma drug concentrations, with red blood cell concentrations exceeding those in plasma[206] (see Figure 33-2). While use of vacuum-stoppered glass tubes has greatly simplified collection of blood in clinical chemistry, several

Table 33-10. Analytical Methodologies for Cyclic Antidepressant Plasma Concentrations

Method[a]	Sample[b] requirement	Speed	Sensitivity	Specificity	Difficulty of operation	Cost
GC-MS	1-4 mL	15 samples/hr	1.0 ng/mL	Excellent	High	High
GC-AFID	1-2 mL	6-8 samples/hr	5 ng/mL	Good	Moderate	Moderate
GC-EC	1-3 mL	6-8 samples/hr	1.0 ng/mL	Good	Moderate	Moderate
HPLC	1-3 mL	4-6 samples/hr	2-5 ng/mL	Good	Low	Moderate
RIA	<1.0 mL	>10 samples/hr	<1 ng/mL	Low[c]	Low	Low

[a] For abbreviations see text.
[b] Serum or plasma.
[c] Assays may not distinguish between parent compound and metabolites.

reports have documented that the use of some manufacturers' tubes introduces a laboratory error in the measurements.[207,208] Spurious reductions in measured plasma concentrations result from interference by tris(2-butoxyethyl) phosphate, a plasticizer contained within the rubber stoppers. This agent displaces basic drugs from their plasma protein binding sites,[209] resulting in a re-equilibration with red cells and a lower measurable concentration when plasma is separated. This problem has been presumably corrected for the Vacutainer brand of tubes and does not exist with the Venoject brand.[208] Thus, it behooves the investigator to compare drug concentrations obtained using an all-glass system to those obtained using blood collection aids when the effects of a specific collection method are in question.

For routine monitoring at steady-state, blood samples should be collected during the terminal elimination phase of drug disposition which usually occurs eight to twelve hours after a dose. The best time to obtain a sample is in the morning before the first dose of the day.

The effect that cooling of the blood sample has on the analysis of cyclic antidepressant concentrations has not been thoroughly investigated. However, because erythrocyte drug concentrations exceed those of plasma, temperature changes may alter re-equilibration of the antidepressants with plasma. Thus, without specific data on this effect, it is preferable to centrifuge blood samples without delay after collection. The tricyclics appear to be stable in plasma at room temperature for at least one week.[210] This suggests that samples can be shipped unfrozen to other laboratories; however, this degree of stability does not hold for some of the newer drugs. Bupropion was found to have a 54-hour half-life in plasma at room temperature; thus, it should be frozen soon after sample collection to prevent drug degradation.[251] The effect of prolonged frozen storage is another unknown area in the clinical pharmacokinetics of the newer cyclic antidepressants. Imipramine and desipramine samples re-analyzed after one year of frozen storage in our laboratory gave results which were essentially identical to those of the initial analysis. Analysis of any samples stored for longer than one month should ideally be supported with a stability study.

Indwelling heparin locks are commonly used to collect multiple cyclic antidepressant samples for pharmacokinetic studies. Since the tricyclics bind strongly to lipoproteins,[211] heparin-induced release of lipoprotein lipase may lead to artifacts in protein-binding studies.[212] When multiple samples must be collected, a saline drip, rather than heparin, is recommended to keep the catheter patent.

Extraction of Samples

Most chromatographic methods for measuring antidepressant concentrations require sample preparation, including organic solvent extraction. The tricyclics are lipophilic compounds which are extractable as free bases at high pH with various organic solvents, including heptane, hexane, and ether. Silanization of glassware, the addition of 2% to 5% isoamyl alcohol to the solvent, or the use of polypropylene instead of glass will minimize drug loss during the extraction procedure. Depending on the specificity of the detection method, sample clean-up may be improved by back-extracting the base at low pH into an aqueous phase. If an evaporation step is required, meticulous attention to laboratory technique is helpful to prevent losses during this step. Most extraction procedures report reproducible recovery values in the range of 85% to 95%. The polar hydroxylated metabolites of tricyclics have different extraction properties than do their secondary and tertiary amine precursors. Assaying these metabolites may require a precise adjustment of pH during the extraction process. The partitioning of imipramine and its metabolites into various organic solvents has been reported by Weder and Bickel and can serve as a guide for developing extraction procedures.[213]

Standard Curves

A standard curve which incorporates an internal standard should be run with each set of unknown samples. Use of at least four points encompassing the expected range is recommended, with the lowest standard being 5% to 10% of the concentration of the highest standard. A blank sample should be included in each run, and the standards should be prepared in tissues of the same type as those to be analyzed. For example, analysis of unknown whole-blood concentrations should be referenced to a standard curve prepared in whole blood. In our laboratory, we found that recovery of imipramine's hydroxylated metabolites varied greatly between different tissue types.[214]

Analytical Instruments

For identification of compounds in research, the combination of a mass spectrometer with gas chromatography (GC-MS) is the recognized standard. This method is highly reliable but requires expensive equipment and a knowledgeable operator. Gas chromatography (GC) has been extensively used in clinical chemistry, and several different detection systems can be used together for quantitation of cyclic antidepressants. An alkali flame ionization detector (AFID), sometimes called a nitrogen detector, has the selectivity and sensitivity for research use and is not as difficult to operate as GC-MS. Electron-capture (GC-EC) is another detection system for GC and is more sensitive than AFID; however, its operation requires more technical skill, and poor specificity is a drawback.

High-performance liquid chromatography (HPLC) is the most popular and versatile analytical technique and can be applied to the measurement of all the cyclic antidepressants. When coupled with a fluorescence detector, it is a highly sensitive and specific assay. While moderately expensive, HPLC is a good tool for research and clinical monitoring due to its ease of operation. When an HPLC can be dedicated to cyclic antidepressant analysis, this is probably the best choice of the available methods.

Non-chromatographic methods such as radioimmunoassay (RIA) and enzyme immunoassay (EMIT) require only a small quantity of blood but do not have the requisite specificity for research use because of interferences from metabolites. Ultimately, these methods may become widely used, due to ease of sample preparation and low cost of analysis.

Quality Control

The results of studies comparing the analyses of cyclic antidepressants by various methods indicate that there is a need for external quality control.[215,217] Serum standards for some tricyclics are available from national sources, but quality control programs for the remaining cyclic antidepressants are essentially nonexistent. All laboratories measuring cyclic antidepressant concentrations should have an internal quality control program in place. When a method is first developed, it should be compared to another analytical technique. For HPLC, this should ideally be another HPLC technique of reversed polarity. An alternative is another chromatographic method such as GC. Once good precision and accuracy data have been generated, quality control samples should be included in each assay run. Large pools of drug-free plasma should be spiked at a high and low concentration with the drugs of interest and stored at $-20°$ to $-70°$ C. With each assay run, one or preferably two aliquots of these samples should be included as unknown samples and the results recorded. After 10 to 15 such runs, a mean and standard deviation can be calculated. Thereafter, the quality control sample should be within ± 2 standard deviations of the mean.

Laboratories running a large number of unknowns should save the residual plasma from these assays to form a pool for each drug. These pools can be collected until an adequate volume is obtained (e.g., 100 mL). These pools should then be aliquoted and run as quality control samples. These samples serve as better controls than spiked samples because of the presence of metabolites. Generation of the pools should be a continuous process.

PROSPECTUS

The number and type of antidepressant compounds available to the clinician is increasing. Some of the "second-generation" drugs may allow the clinician to avoid certain side effects, such as weight gain or drowsiness, attendant with the use of the older drugs. However, it should be emphasized that the newer compounds have no proven superiority in efficacy to the standard tricyclics, amitriptyline and imipramine. Additional clinical experience is needed, and within-class drug comparisons need to be performed before "drug-of-choice" preferences can be confidently stated. In addition, our knowledge of the basic and applied pharmacokinetics for many of the newer drugs is rudimentary. An especially important lesson gained from experience with tricyclics is that one should not overlook the identification and study of active metabolites.

We now have a good perspective on tricyclic antidepressant disposition. Because of basic pharmacokinetic investigations, drug metabolism studies in twins and genetically slow hydroxylators, investigations of drug interactions, and limited forays into plasma concentration monitoring at the two extremes of age, many variables have been identified which affect antidepressant clearance. Unfortunately, within patients, these variables are sometimes opposed to one another as, for example, in an elderly patient who smokes. Even though many variables are identified, our ability to predict individual clearances is largely retrospective and occurs only after a patient with aberrant drug absorption or elimination is identified. The creation of large computerized databases which could correlate patient factors with pharmacokinetic information might help alleviate this situation, but this is unlikely to occur soon.

In the absence of reliable concentration-effect relationships, pharmacokinetic surveillance has limited use. An American Psychiatric Association Task Force on the Use of Laboratory Tests in Psychiatry concluded that plasma concentration measurements of imipramine, desipramine, and nortriptyline are unequivocally clinically useful in certain situations.[71] This consensus report could have the effect of elevating the standard of care for patients receiving these drugs. The report also emphasizes the equivocal nature of plasma concentration measurements for the remaining cyclic antidepressants. Additional research may improve this situation.

REFERENCES

1. Calvo B et al. Pharmacokinetics of amoxipine and its active metabolites. Int J Clin Pharmacol Ther Toxicol. 1985;23:180–85.
2. Bergstrom RF et al. Absolute bioavailability of fluoxetine in beagle dogs. Abstracts of the APhA 133rd annual meeting and exposition. Amer Pharm Assoc, Washington D.C. 1986;16:126.
3. Hammer W, Sjoqvist F. Plasma levels of monomethylated tricyclic antidepressants during treatment with imipramine-like compounds. Life Sci. 1967;6:1895–903.
4. Mead Johnson. Data on file, Evansville, IN.
5. Risch SC et al. Plasma levels of tricyclic antidepressants and clinical efficacy: review of the literature—Parts I and II. J Clin Psychiatry. 1979;40:4–16,58–69.
6. Lemberger L et al. Fluoxetine: clinical pharmacology and physiologic disposition. J Clin Psychiatry. 1985;46:14–9.
7. Kragh-Sorenson P, Larsen NE. Factors influencing notriptyline steady-state kinetics: plasma and saliva levels. Clin Pharmacol Ther 1980;28:796–803.
8. Gram LF et al. Drug level monitoring in psychopharmacology: usefulness and clinical problems, with special reference to tricyclic antidepressants. Ther Drug Monit. 1982;4:17–25.
9. DeVane CL. Tricyclic antidepressants. In: Evans WE et al., eds. Applied Pharmacokinetics: Principles of Therapeutic Drug Monitoring. Spokane: Applied Therapeutics;1980:549–85.
10. Perry PJ et al. Relationship of free notriptyline level to therapeutic response. Acta Psychiatr Scand. 1985;72:120–25.
11. Feighner JP. Clinical efficacy of the newer antidepressants. J Clin Psychopharmacol. 1981;1(Suppl.):235–65.
12. Zung WWK. Review of placebo-controlled trials with bupropion. J Clin Psychiatry. 1983;44:104–14.
13. Van Wyck et al. Overview of clinically significant adverse reactions to bupropion. J Clin Psychiatry. 1983;44:191–96.
14. Bascara L. A double-blind study to compare the effectiveness and tolerability of paroxetine and amitriptyline in depressed patients. Act Psychiatr Scan Suppl. 1989; 350:141–42.
15. Feldmann HS, Denber HCB. Long-term study of fluvoxamine: a new rapid-acting antidepressant. Int Pharmacopsychiatry. 1982;17:114–22.
16. Amin M et al. A double-blind, placebo-controlled dose finding study with sertraline. Psychopharmacol Bull. 1989;25:164–67.
17. Wells BG, Gelenberg AJ. Chemistry, pharmacology, pharmacokinetics, adverse effects, and efficacy of the antidepressant maprotiline hydrocholoride. Pharmacotherapy. 1981;1:121–39.
18. Bryant SG, Ereshefsky L. Antidepressant properties of trazodone. Clin Pharm. 1982;1:406–17.
19. Evans RL. Alprazolam. Drug Intell Clin Pharm. 1981;15:633–38.

20. Lydiard RB, Gelenberg AJ. Amoxapine—an antidepressant with some neuroleptic properties: a review of its chemistry, animal pharmacology and toxicology, human pharmacology, and clinical efficacy. Pharmacotherapy. 1981;1:163–75.

21. Ross DR et al. Akathisia induced by amoxapine. Am J Psychiatry. 1983;140:115–16.

22. Laizure SC et al. Pharmacokinetics of bupropion and its major metabolites in normal subjects after a single dose. Clin Pharmacol Ther. 1985;38:586–89.

23. Golden RN et al. Bupropion in depression: the role of metabolites in clinical outcome. Arch Gen Psychiatry. 1988;45:145–49.

24. Sutfin TA et al. The analysis and disposition of imipramine and its active metabolites in man. Psychopharmacology. 1984;82:310–17.

25. Schenker S et al. Fluoxetine disposition and elimination in cirrhosis. Clin Pharmacol Ther. 1988;44:353–59.

26. Gibaldi M, Perrier D. Pharmacokinetics, 2nd ed. Revised and expanded. New York: Marcel Dekker;1982.

27. Gram LF et al. Steady-state kinetics of imipramine in patients. Psychopharmacology. 1977;154:255–61.

28. Abernethy DR et al. Absolute bioavailability of imipramine: influence of food. Psychopharmacology. 1984;83:104–6.

29. Horng JS, Wong DT. Effects of serotin uptake inhibitor, Lilly 110140, on transport of serotonin in rat and human blood platelets. Biochemical Pharmacology. 1976;25:865–67.

30. Alexanderson B et al. The availability of orally administered nortriptyline. Eur J Clin Pharmacol. 1973;5:181–85.

31. Minder R et al. Hepatic and extrahepatic metabolism of the psychoactive drugs, chlorpromazine, imipramine and imipramine-N-oxide. Naunyn-Schmiedeberg's Arch Pharmacol. 1971;268:334–47.

32. Christ W et al. Phase I metabolism of imipramine by microsomes of small intestine in comparison with metabolism by liver microsomes. Naunyn-Schmiedebergs Arch Pharmacol. 1983;323:176–82.

33. Randrup A, Braestrup C. Uptake inhibition of biogenic amines by newer antidepressant drugs: relevance to the dopamine hypothesis of depression. Psychopharmacology. 1977;53:309–14.

34. Escobar JI et al. Chlorimipramine: a double-blind comparison of intravenous versus oral administration in depressed patients. Psychopharmacologia. 1973;33:111–16.

35. Mellstrom B et al. Nortriptyline formation after single oral and intramuscular doses of amitriptyline. Clin Pharmacol Ther. 1982;32:664–67.

36. Burch JE, Herries DG. The demethylation of amitriptyline administered by oral and intramuscular routes. Psychopharmacology. 1983;80:249–53.

37. Giller EL et al. Steady-state bioequivalence and therapeutic equivalence of different amitriptyline compounds with variable dissolution rates. J Clin Psychopharmacol. 1984;4:299–300.

38. Gagnon MA et al. Comparative biopharmaceutical performance of imipramine formulations in man. J Clin Pharmacol. 1980;20:151–58.

39. Jorgensen A. Comparative bioavailability of a sustained release preparation of amitriptyline and conventional tablets. Eur J Clin Pharmacol. 1977;12:187–90.

40. Adams S. Amitriptyline suppositories. N Engl J Med. 1982;306:996.

41. Cooper TB, Kelly RG. GLC analysis of loxapine, amoxapine, and their metabolites in serum and urine. J Pharm Sci. 1979;68:216–19.

42. Steiner E et al. Polymorphic desbrisoquine hydroxylation in 757 Swedish subjects. Clin Pharmacol Ther. 1988;44:431–35.

43. DeVane CL. Pharmacokinetics of the selective serotonin reuptake inhibitors. J Clin Psychiatry (in press).

44. Brosen K, Gram LF. First pass metabolism of imipramine and desipramine: impact of the sparteine oxidation phenotype. Clin Pharmacol Ther. 1988;43:400–6.

45. Cohon MS et al. Pharmacokinetic profile for alprazolam tablets. UpJohn Company. October, 1982. Unpublished study.

46. Alkalay D et al. Bioavailability and kinetics of maprotiline. Clin Pharmacol Ther. 1980;27:697–703.

47. Curry SH et al. Lack of interaction of ranitidine with amitriptyline. Eur J Clin Pharmacol. 1987;32:317–20.
48. Embil K, Torosian G. Solubility and ionization characteristics of doxepin and desmethyl-doxepin. J Pharm Sci. 1982;71:191–93.
49. Bickel MH et al. Distribution of chlorpromazine and imipramine in adipose and other tissues of rats. Life Sci. 1983;33:2025–31.
50. Prichard PJ et al. Oral phenytoin pharmacokinetics during omeprazole therapy. Br J Clin Pharmacol. 1987;24:543–45
51. Pentel PR et al. Hemoperfusion for imipramine overdose: elimination of active metabolites. J Toxicol Clin Toxicol. 1982;19:239–48.
52. Kristensen CB, Gram LF. Equilibrium dialysis for determination of protein binding of imipramine—evaluation of a method. Acta Pharmacol Toxicol. 1982;50:130–36.
53. Gugler R, Jensen JC. Omeprazole inhibits oxidative drug metabolism studeis with diazepam and phenytoin in vivo and 7-ethoxycoumarin in vitro. Gastroenterology. 1985;89:1235–241.
54. Pike E, Skuterud B. Plasma binding variations of amitriptyline and nortriptyline. Clin Pharmacol Ther. 1982;32:228–34.
55. Musa MN. Nonlinear kinetics of trimipramine in depressed patients. J Clin Pharmacol. 1989;29:746–47.
56. Piafsky KM, Borga O. Plasma binding of basic drugs II. Importance of alpha-l-acid glycoprotein for interindividual variation. Clin Pharmacol Ther. 1977;22:545–49.
57. Freilich DI, Giardina E-GV. Imipramine binding to alpha-l-acid glycoprotein in normal subjects and cardiac patients. Clin Pharmacol Ther. 1984;35:670–74.
58. Javaid JI et al. Binding of imipramine to plasma in alcoholic patients. Fed Proc. 1982;41:1556.
59. Baumann P et al. Increase of alpha-l-acid glycoprotein after treatment with amitriptyline. Br J Clin Pharmacol. 1982;14:102–3.
60. Potter WZ et al. Binding of imipramine to plasma protein and to brain tissue: relationship to CSF tricyclic levels in man. Psychopharmacology. 1979;63:187–92.
61. Virtanen R et al. Protein binding of doxepin and desmethyldoxepin. Acta Pharmacol Toxicol. 1982;51:159–64.
62. Breyer-Pfaff U et al. Antidepressive effect and pharmacokinetics of amitriptyline with consideration of unbound drug and 10-hydroxynortriptyline plasma levels. Psychopharmacology. 1982;76:240–44.
63. Riess W et al. The pharmacokinetic properties of maprotiline in man. J Int Med Res. 1975;3:16–41.
64. Jue SG et al. Amoxapine: a review of its pharmacology and efficacy in depressed states. Drugs. 1982;24:1–23.
65. Brogden RN et al. Trazodone: a review of its pharmacological properties and therapeutic use in depression and anxiety. Drugs. 1981;21:401–29.
66. Schroeder DH. Metabolism and kinetics of bupropion. J Clin Psychiatry. 1983;44:5:79–81.
67. Gelenberg AJ. Amoxapine, a new antidepressant, appears in human milk. J Nerv Ment Dis. 1979;167:635–36.
68. Gram LF et al. Imipramine metabolism: pH-dependent distribution and urinary excretion. Clin Pharmacol Ther. 1970;12:239–44.
69. Gram LF et al. Plasma levels and antidepressive effect of imipramine. Clin Pharmacol Ther. 1976;19:318–24.
70. Bickel MH, Weder HJ. The total fate of a drug: kinetics of distribution, excretion and formation of 14 metabolites in rats treated with imipramine. Arch Int Pharmacodyn Ther. 1968;173:433–63.
71. Task Force on the Use of Laboratory Tests in Psychiatry. Tricyclic antidepressants—blood level measurements and clinical outcome: an APA task force report. Am J Psychiatry. 1985;142:155-162.
72. Gram LF. Metabolism of tricyclic antidepressants: a review. Dan Med Bull. 1974;21:218–28.
73. Von Bahr C, Orrenius S. Spectral studies on the interaction of imipramine and some of its oxidized metabolites with rat liver microsomes. Xenobiotica. 1971;1:69–78.
74. Dencker H et al. Intestinal absorption, demethylation, and enterohepatic circulation of imipramine. Clin Pharmacol Ther. 1976;19:584–86.

75. Pinder RM et al. Maprotiline: a review of its pharmacological properties and therapeutic efficacy in mental depressive states. Drugs. 1977;13:321–52.

76. Montgomery SA et al. Plasma level response relationships with fluoxetine and zimelidine. Clin Neuropharmacol. 1990;13(Suppl. 1):71–5.

77. Boutelle WE. Clinical response and blood levels in the treatment of depression with a new antidepressant drug, amoxapine. Neuropharmacology. 1980;19:1229–231.

78. Koss FW, Busch U. Trazodone as an example—drug levels in the blood and brain. In: Gersho, eds. Trazodone–A New Broad-spectrum Antidepressant. Proceedings of the 11th Congress of the Collegium Internationale Neuro-Psychopharmacologicum. Amsterdam: Excerpta Medica; 1980:27–33.

79. Preskorn SH. Antidepressant response and plasma concentrations of bupropion. J Clin Psychiatry. 1983;44(Sec. 2):137–39.

80. Cooper TB et al. Determination of bupropion and its major basic metabolites in plasma by liquid chromatography with dual-wavelength ultraviolet detection. J Pharm Sci. 1984;73:1104–107.

81. Potter WZ et al. Active metabolite of imipramine and desipramine in man. Clin Pharmacol Ther. 1982;31:393–401.

82. Brogden RN et al. Nomifensine: a review of its pharmacological properties and therapeutic efficacy in depressive illness. Drugs. 1979;18:1–24.

83. Dawling S, Braithwaite R. The stability of the antidepressant nomifensine in human plasma. J Pharm Pharmacol. 1980;32:304–5.

84. Ringoir S et al. Pharmacokinetics of nomifensine in impaired renal function. Br J Clin Pharmacol. 1977;4(Suppl. 2):129S–34S.

85. Lundstrom J et al. Metabolism of zimelidine in rat, dog, and man. Arzneimittelforschung. 1981;31:486–94.

86. Potter WZ et al. Zimelidine, a pro-drug? Short and long term pharmacokinetic studies in man. Clin Pharmacol Ther. 1980;27:278–79.

87. Javaid JI et al. Inhibition of biogenic amines uptake by imipramine, desipramine, 2-OH-imipramine and 2-OH-desipramine in rat brain. Life Sci. 1979;24:21–8.

88. Potter WZ et al. Hydroxylated metabolites of tricyclic antidepressants: pre-clinical assessment of activity. Biol Psychiatry. 1979;14:601–13.

89. Bertilsson L et al. Pronounced inhibition of noradrenaline uptake by 10-hydroxymetabolites of nortriptyline. Life Sci. 1979;25:1285–292.

90. Garvey MJ et al. Elevated plasma tricyclic levels with therapeutic doses of imipramine. Am J Psychiatry. 1984;141:853–56.

91. DeVane CL et al. Excessive plasma concentrations of tricyclic antidepressants resulting from usual doses: a report of six cases. J Clin Psychiatry. 1981;42:143–47.

92. Fenster PE et al. Antiarrhythmic efficacy of desipramine. J Clin Pharmacol. 1989;29:114–17.

93. Bertilsson L et al. Nortriptyline and antipyrine clearance in relation to debrisoquine hydroxylation in man. Life Sci. 1980;27:1673–677.

94. Mellstrom B et al. E- and Z-10-hydroxylation of nortriptyline: relationship to polymorphic debrisoquine hydroxylation. Clin Pharmacol Ther. 1981;30:189–93.

95. Alexanderson B. Prediction of steady-state plasma levels of nortriptyline from single oral dose kinetics: A study in twins. Eur J Clin Pharmacol. 1973;6:44–53.

96. Nelson JC et al. Major adverse reactions during desipramine treatment. Arch Gen Psychiatry. 1982;39:1055–61.

97. Nelson JC et al. Clinical implications of 2-hydroxydesipramine plasma concentrations. Clin Pharmacol Ther. 1983;33:183–89.

98. Bock JL et al. Desipramine hydroxylation: variability and effect of antipsychotic drugs. Clin Pharmacol Ther. 1983;33:322–28.

99. Nelson JC et al. Desipramine plasma concentration and antidepressant response. Arch Gen Psychiatry. 1982;39:1419–422.

100. Feely J et al. Reduction of liver blood flow and propranolol metabolism by cimetidine. N Engl J Med. 1981;304:692–95.

101. Preskorn SH et al. Depression in children: concentration-dependent CNS toxicity of tricyclic antidepressants. Psychopharmacol Bull. 1988;24:140–42.
102. Abernethy DR et al. Imipramine-cimetidine interaction: impairment of clearance and enhanced absolute bioavailability. J Pharmacol Exp Ther. 1984;229:702–5.
103. Henauer SA, Hollister LE. Cimetidine interaction with imipramine and nortriptyline. Clin Pharmacol Ther. 1984;35:183–87.
104. Miller DD, Macklin M. Cimetidine-imipramine interaction: a case report. Am J Psychiatry. 1983;140:351–52.
105. Ciraulo DA, Jaffe JH. Tricyclic antidepressants in the treatment of depression associated with alcoholism. J Clin Psychopharmacol. 1981;1:146–50.
106. Ciraulo DA et al. Imipramine disposition in alcoholics. J Clin Psychopharmacol. 1982;2:2–7.
107. Sandoz M et al. Biotransformation of amitriptyline in alcoholic depressive patients. Eur J Clin Pharmacol. 1983;24:615–21.
108. Dorian P et al. Amitriptyline and ethanol: pharmacokinetic and pharmacodynamic interaction. Eur J Clin Pharmacol. 1983;25:325–31.
109. Sandoz M et al. Metabolism of amitriptyline in patients with chronic renal failure. Eur J Clin Pharmacol. 1984;26:227–32.
110. Bertilsson L et al. Nortriptylin and antipyrine clearance in relation to debrisoquine hydroxylation in man. Life Sci. 1980;27:1673–677.
111. Dawling S et al. Nortriptyline metabolism in chronic renal failure: metabolite elimination. Clin Pharmacol Ther. 1982;32:322–29.
112. Gram LF, Overo KF. Drug interaction: inhibitory effect of neuroleptics on metabolism of tricyclic antidepressants in man. Br Med J. 1972;1:463–65.
113. Nelson JC, Jatlow PI. Neuroleptic effect on desipramine steady-state plasma concentrations. Am J Psychiatry. 1980;137:1232–234.
114. Bock JL et al. Steady-state plasma concentrations of cis-and trans-10-OH amitriptyline metabolites. Clin Pharmacol Ther. 1982;31:609–16.
115. Loga S et al. Interaction of chlorpromazine and nortriptyline in patients with schizophrenia. Clin Pharmacokinet. 1981;6:454–62.
116. Bjerre M et al. Dose-dependent kinetics of imipramine in elderly patients. Psychopharmacology. 1981;75:354–57.
117. Gram LF et al. Imipramine metabolites in blood of patients during therapy and after overdose. Clin Pharmacol Ther. 1983;33:335–42.
118. Cutler NR et al. Concentrations of desipramine in elderly women. Am J Psychiatry. 1981;138:1235–237.
119. Kitanaka I et al. Altered hydroxydesipramine concentrations in elderly patients. Clin Pharmacol Ther. 1982;31:51–5.
120. Nies A et al. Relationship between age and tricyclic antidepressant plasma levels. Am J Psychiatry. 1977;134:790–93.
121. Musa MN. Imipramine: relationship of age to steady-state plasma level in endogenous depression. Res Commun Psychol Psychiatr Behavior. 1979;4:205–8.
122. Bertilsson L et al. The debrisoqine hydroxylation test predicts steady-state plasma levels of desiprmaine. Br J Clin Pharmacol. 1983;15:388–90.
123. Balant-Gorgia AE et al. Importance of oxidative polymorphism and levomepromazine treatment on the steady-state blood concentrations of clomipramine and its major metabolites. Eur J Clin Pharmacol. 1986;31:449–55.
124. Brosen K et al. Imipramine demethylation and hydroxalation: impact of the sparteine oxidation phenotype. Clin Pharmacol Ther. 1986;40:543–49.
125. Kupfer DJ, Rush AJ. Recommendations for scientific reports on depression. Am J Psychiatry. 1983;140:1327–328.
126. Evans WE. General principles of applied pharmacokinetics. In: Evans WE et al., eds. Applied Pharmacokinetics: Principles of Therapeutic Drug Monitoring, 3rd edition. Vancouver: Applied Therapeutics; 1991.

127. Brosen K et al. Steady state concentrations of imipramine and its metabolites in relation to the sparteine/debrisoquine polymorphism. Eur J Clin Pharmacol. 1986;30:678–84.

128. Reisby N et al. Imipramine: clinical effects and pharmacokinetic variability. Psychopharmacology. 1977;54:263–72.

129. Glassman AH et al. Clinical implications of imipramine plasma levels for depressive illness. Arch Gen Psychiatry. 1977;34:197–204.

130. Mellstrom B et al. Amitriptyline metabolism: relationship to polymorphic debrisoquine hydroxalation. Clin Pharmacol Ther. 1983;34:516–20.

131. Bowman P et al. Amitriptyline pharmacokinetics and clinical response: II metabolic polymorphism assessed by hydroxylation of debrisoquine and mephenytoin. Int Clin Psychopharmacol. 1986;1:102–12.

132. Montgomery S et al. High plasma nortriptyline levels in the treatment of depression. Clin Pharmacol Ther. 1978;23:309–14.

133. Ziegler VE et al. Nortriptyline levels and therapeutic response. Clin Pharmacol Ther. 1976;20:458–63.

134. Kragh-Sorensen P et al. Self-inhibiting action of nortriptyline's antidepressant effect at high plasma levels. Psychopharmacologia. 1976;45:305–12.

135. Ziegler VE et al. Amitriptyline plasma levels and therapeutic response. Clin Pharmacol Ther. 1976;19:795–801.

136. Kupfer DJ et al. Amitriptyline plasma levels and clinical response in primary depression. Clin Pharmacol Ther. 1977;22:904–11.

137. Montgomery SA et al. Amitriptyline plasma concentration and clinical response. Br Med J. 1979;1:230–31.

138. Robinson DS et al. Plasma tricyclic drug levels in amitriptyline-treated depressed patients. Psychopharmacology. 1979;63:223–31.

139. Mendelwicz J et al. A double-blind comparison of dothiepin and amitriptyline in patients with primary affective disorder: serum levels and clinical response. Br J Psychiatry. 1980;136:154–60.

140. Costa D et al. Endogenous depression and imipramine levels in the blood. Psychopharmacology. 1980;70:291–94.

141. Simpson GM et al. Relationship between plasma antidepressant levels and clinical outcome for inpatients receiving imipramine. Am J Psychiatry. 1982;139:358–60.

142. Matuzas W et al. Plasma concentrations of imipramine and clinical response among depressed outpatients. J Clin Psychopharmacol. 1982;2:140–42.

143. Avery D, Winokur G. The efficacy of electroconvulsive therapy and antidepressants in depression. Biol Psychiatry. 1977;12:507–23.

144. Langou RA et al. Cardiovascular manifestations of tricyclic antidepressant overdose. Am Heart J. 1980;100:458–64.

145. Pedersen OL et al. Overdosage of antidepressants: clinical and pharmacokinetic aspects. Eur J Clin Pharmacol. 1982;23:513–21.

146. Lipsey JR et al. Nortriptyline treatment of poststroke depression: a double-blind study. Lancet. 1984;1:297–300.

147. Potter WZ, Goodwin FK. Antidepressant drug levels and clinical response. Lancet. 1978;1:1049–50.

148. Jungkunz G, Kuss HJ. On the relationship of nortriptyline: amitriptyline ratio to clinical improvement of amitriptyline treated depressive patients. Pharmakopsychiatr Neuropsychopharmakol. 1980;13:111–16.

149. Khalid R et al. Desipramine plasma levels and therapeutic response. Psychopharmacol Bull. 1978;14:43–44.

150. Friedel RO et al. Desipramine plasma levels and clinical response in depressed outpatients. Commun Psychopharmacol. 1979;3:81–7.

151. Stewart JW et al. Efficacy of desipramine in endogenomorphically depressed patients. J Affective Disord. 1980;2:165–76.

152. Brunswick DJ et al. Relationship between tricyclic antidepressant plasma levels and clinical response in patients treated with desipramine or doxepin. Acta Psychiatr Scand. 1983;67:371–77.

153. Simpson GM et al. Relationship between plasma desipramine levels and clinical outcome for RDC major depressive inpatients. Psychopharmacology. 1983;80:240–42.

154. Friedel RO, Raskind MA. Relationship of blood levels of Sinequan to clinical effects in the treatment of depression in aged patients. In: Mendels J, ed. Sinequan (Doxepin HC1): a monograph of recent clinical studies. Excerpta Medica; 1975:51–3.

155. Kline NS et al. Doxepin and desmethyldoxepin serum levels and clinical response. In: Gottschalk LA, Merlis SD, eds. Pharmacokinetics of Psychoactive Drugs—Blood Levels and Clinical Response. New York: Spectrum; 1976:221–28.

156. Linnoila M et al. Clomipramine and doxepin in depressive neurosis: plasma levels and therapeutic response. Arch Gen Psychiatry. 1980;37:1295–299.

157. Bogaert MG et al. Plasma levels of the cis- and transisomers of doxepin and desmethyldoxepin after administration of doxepin to patients. Arzneimittelforschung. 1981;31:113–15.

158. Reisby N et al. Clomipramine: plasma levels and clinical effects. Commun Psychopharmacol. 1979;5:341–51.

159. Traskman L et al. Plasma levels of chlorimipramine and its demethyl metabolite during treatment of depression. Differential biochemical and clinical effects of the two compounds. Clin Pharmacol Ther. 1979;26:600–10.

160. Stern RS et al. Clomipramine and exposure for compulsive rituals II: plasma levels, side effects and outcome. Br J Psychiatry. 1980;136:161–66.

161. Mulgirigama LD et al. Clinical responses in depressed patients in relation to plasma levels of tricyclic antidepressants and tyramine pressor response. Postgrad Med J. 1977;53(Suppl. 4):155–59.

162. Montgomery SA et al. Pharmacokinetics and efficacy of maprotiline and amitriptyline in endogenous depression: a double-blind controlled trial. Clin Ther. 1980;3:292–310.

163. Gwirtsman HE et al. Therapeutic superiority of maprotiline versus doxepin in geriatric depression. J Clin Psychiatry. 1983;44:449–53.

164. Putzolu S et al. Trazodone: clinical and biochemical studies II. Blood levels and therapeutic responsiveness. Psychopharmacol Bull. 1976;12:40–1.

165. Mann JJ et al. A controlled study of trazodone, imipramine, and placebo in outpatients with endogenous depression. J Clin Psychopharmacol. 1981;1:75–80.

166. Preskorn SH et al. Depression in children: relationship between plasma imipramine levels and response. J Clin Psychiatry. 1982;43:450–53.

167. Weller EB et al. Childhood depression: imipramine levels and response. Psychopharmacol Bull. 1983;19:59–61.

168. Puig-Antich J et al. Plasma levels of imipramine (IMI) and desmethylimipramine (DMI) and clinical response in prepubertal major depressive disorder. J Am Acad Child Psychiatry. 1979;18:616–27.

169. Jorgensen OS et al. Plasma concentrations and clinical effect in imipramine treatment of childhood enuresis. Clin Pharmacokinet. 1980;5:386–93.

170. Rapoport JL et al. Childhood enuresis III. Psychopathology, tricyclic concentration in plasma, and anti-enuretic effect. Arch Gen Psychiatry. 1980;37:1146–152.

171. DeVane CL et al. Concentrations of imipramine and its metabolites during enuresis therapy. Pediatr Pharmacol. 1984;4:245–51.

172. Asberg M et al. Correlation of subjective side effects with plasma concentrations of nortriptyline. Br Med J. 1970;4:18–21.

173. Ziegler VE et al. Nortriptyline plasma levels and subjective side effects. Br J Psychiatry. 1978;132:55–60.

174. Asberg M, Germanis M. Ophthalomological effects of nortriptyline—relationship to plasma level. Pharmacology. 1972;7:349–56.

175. Bertram U et al. Saliva secretion following long-term antidepressant treatment with nortriptyline controlled by plasma levels. Scand J Dent Res. 1979;87:58–64.

176. Crome P, Braithwaite RA. Relationship between clinical features of tricyclic antidepressant poisoning and plasma concentrations in children. Arch Dis Child. 1978;53:902–5.

177. Preskorn SH, Simpson S. Tricyclic-antidepressant-induced delirium and plasma drug concentration. Am J Psychiatry. 1982;139:822–23.
178. Nelson JC et al. Major adverse reactions during desipramine treatment, relationship to plasma drug concentrations, concomitant antipsychotic treatment, and patient characteristics. Arch Gen Psychiatry. 1982;39:1055–61.
179. Bailey DN et al. Tricyclic antidepressants: plasma levels and clinical findings in overdose. Am J Psychiatry. 1978;135:1325–328.
180. Glassman AH et al. Clinical characteristics of imipramine-induced orthostatic hypotension. Lancet. 1979;1:468–72.
181. Glassman AH, Bigger JT. Cardiovascular effects of therapeutic doses of tricyclic antidepressants. Arch Gen Psychiatry. 1981;38:815–20.
182. Smith RC et al. Cardiovascular effects of therapeutic doses of tricyclic antidepressants: importance of blood level monitoring. J Clin Psychiatry. 1980;41:57–63.
183. Burrows GD et al. Cardiac effects of different tricyclic antidepressant drugs. Br J Psychiatry. 1976;129:335–41.
184. Burgess CD et al. Cardiovascular effects of amitriptyline, mianserin, zimelidine, and nomifensine in depressed patients. Postgrad Med J. 1979;55:704–708.
185. Wenger TL, Stern WC. The cardiovascular profile of bupropion. J Clin Psychiatry. 1983;44:176–82.
186. Giardina EG, Bigger JT Jr. The antiarrhythmic effect of imipramine hydrochloride in cardiac patients with ventricular premature complexes without psychological depression. Am J Cardiol. 1982;50:172–79.
187. Giardina EG et al. Antiarrhythmic plasma concentration range of imipramine against ventricular premature depolarizations. Clin Pharmacol Ther. 1983;34:284–89.
188. Carroll BJ. Dexamethasone suppression test for depression. In: Usdin E et al, eds. Frontiers in biochemical and pharmacological research in depression. New York: Raven Press; 1984.
189. Maas JW. Relationships between central nervous system noradrenergic function and plasma and urinary concentrations of norepinephrine metabolites. In: Usdin E et al, eds. Frontiers in biochemical and pharmacological research in depression. New York: Raven Press; 1984.
190. Cooper TB et al. The 24-hour serum lithium level as a prognosticator of dosage requirements. Am J Psychiatry. 1973;130:601–3.
191. Dawling S et al. Nortriptyline therapy in elderly patients: Dosage prediction after single dose pharmacokinetic study. Eur J Clin Pharmacol. 1980;18:147–50.
192. Redmond FC et al. Single dose prediction of amitriptyline and nortriptyline requirement in unipolar depression. Curr Ther Res. 1980;27:635–42.
193. Brunswick DJ et al. Prediction of steady-state plasma levels of amitriptyline and nortriptyline from a single dose 24 hour level in depressed patients. J Clin Psychiatry. 1980;41:337–40.
194. Brunswick DJ et al. Prediction of steady-state imipramine and desmethylimipramine plasma concentrations from single-dose data. Clin Pharmacol Ther. 1979;25:605–10.
195. Potter WZ et al. Single-dose kinetics predict steady-state concentrations of imipramine and desipramine. Arch Gen Psychiatry. 1980;37:314–20.
196. Cooper TB et al. Prediction of steady-state plasma and saliva levels of desmethylimipramine using a single dose, single time point procedure. Psychopharmacology. 1981;74:115–21.
197. Cooper TB, Simpson GM. Prediction of individual dosage of nortriptyline. Am J Psychiatry. 1978;135:333–35.
198. Montgomery SA et al. Dosage adjustment from simple nortriptyline spot level predictor tests in depressed patients. Clin Pharmacokinet. 1979;4:129–36.
199. Madakasira S et al. Single dose prediction of steady-state plasma levels of amitriptyline. J Clin Psychopharmacol. 1982;2:136–39.
200. Clothier J, Reed K. Targeting therapeutic plasma levels of nortriptyline from test dose plasma concentrations. J Clin Psychopharmacol. 1984;4:216–17.
201. Dawling S et al. Nortriptyline therapy in elderly patients: dosage prediction from plasma concentration at 24 hours after a single 50 mg dose. Br J Psychiatry. 1981;139:413–16.

202. Browne JL et al. Pharmacokinetic protocol for predicting plasma nortriptyline levels. J Clin Psychopharmacol. 1983;3:351–56.
203. Gupta R, Molnar G. Measurement of therapeutic concentrations of tricyclic antidepressants in serum. Drug Metab Rev. 1979;9:79–97.
204. Scoggins BA et al. Measurement of tricyclic antidepressants. Part I. A review of methodology. Clin Chem. 1980;26:5–17.
205. Saady JJ et al. A comparison of plasma and serum levels of two tricyclic antidepressants: imipramine and desipramine. Psychopharmacology. 1981;75:173–74.
206. Linnoila M et al. Plasma and erythrocyte levels of tricyclic antidepressants in depressed patients. Am J Psychiatry. 1978;135:557–61.
207. Brunswick DJ, Medels J. Reduced levels of tricyclic antidepressants in plasma from vacutainers. Commun Psychopharmacol. 1977;1:131–34.
208. Veith RC et al. The clinical impact of blood collection methods on tricyclic antidepressants as measured by GC/MS-SIM. Commun Psychopharmacol. 1978;2:491–94.
209. Borga O et al. Plasma protein binding of basic drugs I. Selective displacement from alpha-1-acid glycoprotein by tris(2-butoxyethyl) phosphate. Clin Pharmacol Ther. 1977;22:539–44.
210. Zetin M et al. Tricyclic antidepressant sample stability and the vacutainer effect. Am J Psychiatry. 1981;138:1247–248.
211. Bickel MH. Binding chlorpromazine and imipramine to red cells, albumin, lipoproteins, and other blood components. J Pharm Pharmacol. 1975;27:733–38.
212. Brown JE et al. The artifactual nature of heparin-induced drug protein-binding alterations. Clin Pharmacol Ther. 1981;30:636–43.
213. Weder HJ, Bickel MH. Separation and determination of imipramine and its metabolites from biological samples by gas-liquid chromatography. J Chromatogr. 1968;37:181–89.
214. Stout SA, DeVane CL. Quantification of imipramine and its major metabolites in whole blood, brain, and other tissues of the rat by liquid chromatography. Psychopharmacology. 1984;84:39–41.
215. Orsulak PJ, Gerson B. Clinical laboratory quality control, application to analysis of tricyclic antidepressants. Clinical Pharmacology in Psychiatry. New York: Elsevier; 1981:43–57.
216. DeVane CL, Jusko WJ. Plasma concentration monitoring of hydroxylated metabolites of imipramine and desipramine. Drug Intell Clin Pharm. 1981;15:263–66.
217. Baumann P et al. Quality control of amitriptyline and nortriptyline plasma level assessments: a multicenter study. Pharmacopsychiatria. 1982;15:156–60.
218. Abernethy DR et al. Interaction of cimetidine with the triazolobenzodiazepines, alprazolam, and triazolam. Psychopharmacology. 1983;80:275–78.
219. Borga O et al. Plasma protein binding of tricyclic antidepressants in man. Biochem Pharmacol. 1969;18:2135–143.
220. Brinkschulte M, Breyer-Pfaff U. Binding of tricyclic antidepressants and perazine to human plasma. Naunyn-Schmiedeberg's Arch Pharmacol. 1979;308:1–7.
221. Jorgensen A, Hanson V. Pharmacokinetics of amitriptyline infused intravenously in man. Eur J Clin Pharmacol. 1976;10:337–41.
222. Lai AA, Schroeder DH. Clinical pharmacokinetics of bupropion: a review. J Clin Psychiatry. 1983;44:5:82–4.
223. Evans LEJ et al. The bioavailability of oral and parenteral chlorimipramine (Anafranil). Prog Neuropsychopharmacol. 1980;4:293–302.
224. Dawling S et al. Single oral dose pharmacokinetics of clomipramine in depressed patients. Postgrad Med J. 1980;56(Suppl. 1):115–16.
225. Alexanderson B. Pharmacokinetics of desmethylimipramine and nortriptyline in man after single and multiple oral doses—a cross-over study. Eur J Clin Pharmacol. 1972;5:1–10.
226. DeVane CL et al. Desipramine and 2-hydroxy-desipramine pharmacokinetics in normal volunteers. Eur J Clin Pharmacol. 1981;19:61–4.
227. Ziegler VE et al. Doxepin kinetics. Clin Pharmacol Ther. 1978;23:573–79.
228. Aronoff GR et al. Fluoxetine kinetics and protein binding in normal and impaired renal function. Clin Pharmacol Ther. 1984;36:138–44.

229. Gram LF et al. Comparison of single dose kinetics of imipramine, nortriptyline, and antipyrine in man. Psychopharmacology. 1976;50:21–7.
230. Ziegler VE et al. Protriptyline kinetics. Clin Pharmacol Ther. 1978;23:580–84.
231. Moody JP et al. Pharmacokinetic aspects of protriptyline plasma levels. Eur J Clin Pharmacol. 1977;11:51–6.
232. Abernethy DR et al. Plasma levels of trazodone: methodology and applications. Pharmacology. 1984;28:42–6.
233. Abernethy DR et al. Trimipramine kinetics and absolute bioavailability: use of gas-liquid chromatography with nitrogen-phosphorus detection. Clin Pharmacol Ther. 1984;35:348–53.
234. Caille G et al. Pharmacokinetic characteristics of two different formulations of trimipramine determined with a new GLC method. Biopharm Drug Dispos. 1980;1:187–94.
235. Henry JF et al. Pharmacokinetics of amitriptyline in the elderly. Int J Clin Pharmacol Ther Toxicol. 1981;19:1–5.
236. Ziegler VE et al. Contribution to the pharmacokinetics of amitriptyline. J Clin Pharmacol. 1978;18:462–67.
237. Schulz P et al. Amitriptyline disposition in young and elderly normal men. Clin Pharmacol Ther. 1983;33:360–66.
238. Dawling S et al. Pharmacokinetics of single oral doses of nortriptyline in depressed elderly hospital patients and young healthy volunteers. Clin Pharmacokinet. 1980;5:394–401.
239. Hrdina PD et al. Comparison of single-dose pharmacokinetics of imipramine and maprotiline in the elderly. Psychopharmacology. 1980;70:29–34.
240. Weder HJ, Bickel MH. Interactions of drugs with proteins. I. Binding of tricyclic thymoleptics to human and bovine plasma proteins. J Pharm Sci. 1970;59:1505–507.
241. Glassman AJ et al. Plasma binding of imipramine and clinical outcome. Am J Psychiatry. 1973;130:1367–369.
242. Danon A, Chen Z. Binding of imipramine to plasma proteins: effect of hyperlipoproteinemia. Clin Pharmacol Ther. 1979-,25:316–21.
243. Kitanaka I et al. Altered hydroxydesipramine concentrations in elderly depressed patients. Clin Pharmacol Ther. 1982;31:51–5.
244. Sethy VH, Harris DW. Determination of biological activity of alprazolam, triazolam, and their metabolites. J Pharm Pharmacol. 1982;34:115–16.
245. Cohen BM et al. Amoxapine—neuroleptic as well as antidepressant? Am J Psychiatry. 1982;139:1165–167.
246. Schroeder DH. Metabolism and kinetics of bupropion. J Clin Psychiatry. 1983;44:5:79–81.
247. Fong MH et al. 1-m-chlorophenylpiperazine is an active metabolite common to the psychotropic drugs trazodone, etoperidone, and mepiprazole. J Pharm Pharmacol. 1982;34:674–75.
248. Sansone M et al. Reversal of depressant action of trazodone on avoidance behavior by its metabolite m-chlorophenylpiperazine. J Pharm Pharmacol. 1983;35:189–90.
249. Bayer AJ et al. Pharmacokinetic and pharmacodynamic characteristics of trazodone in the elderly. Br J Clin Pharmacol. 1983;16:371–76.
250. Bertilsson L et al. Techniques for plasma protein binding of demethylchlorimipramine. Clin Pharmacol Ther. 26:265–71.
251. Laizure SC, DeVane CL. The stability of bupropion and its major metabolites in human plasma under varying storage conditions. Ther Drug Monit. 1985;7:447–50.
252. DeVane CL et al. Disposition of bupropion in healthy volunteers and subjects with alcoholic liver disease. J Clin Psychopharmacol. 1990;10:328–32.
253. Nelson JC, Jatlow PI. Nonlinear desipramine kinetics: prevalence and importance. Clin Pharmacol Ther. 1987;41:666-70.
254. DeVane CL et al. Dosage regimen design for cyclic antidepressants: a reveiw of pharmacokinetic methods. Psychopharm Bull. (in press).
255. Brosen K, Gram LF. Clinical significance of sparteinel debrisoquine oxidation polymorphism. Eur J Clin Pharmacol. 1989;36:537–47.
256. Pollock BG, Perel JM. Tricyclic antidepressants: contemporary issues for therapeutic practice. Can J Psychiatry. 1989;34:609–71.

Chapter 34

Lithium

Stanley W. Carson

L ithium is well established as the drug of choice for the treatment and prophylaxis of bipolar (manic-depressive) disorders. It can also be used prophylactically against schizo-affective disorders and unipolar (recurrent) depressive disorders.[1,2] Many hypotheses have been proposed to explain the mechanisms for lithium's pharmacological effects. These range from relatively simple theories of partial substitution for various anions (Na^+, K^+, Mg^{++}, Ca^{++}) to more complex hypotheses involving inhibition of intracellular messengers. Although there are conflicting data on lithium's effect on serotonergic and noradrenergic neurotransmitter function, preclinical and clinical studies do suggest that lithium causes a subsensitivity of α_2-adrenergic receptors.[130] There is also evidence that lithium's primary site of action may be on intracellular signal transduction mechanisms.[130] Direct inhibition of hormone-activated adenyl cyclase and cyclic AMP-mediated processes as well as intracellular ion transport mechanisms have received considerable attention.[2] However, these hypotheses cannot satisfactorily explain why lithium seems to selectively affect or even "search out" those neurotransmitter systems which may be overactive (e.g., in patients with bipolar disorder) but has little or no effect on these systems in normal subjects.

The "inositol depletion hypothesis" has been proposed to explain the neuronal and developmental effects of lithium and is based on its ability to inhibit signal transduction indirectly by reducing concentrations of inositol. Lithium blocks the formation of inositol and thus indirectly decreases the formation of the second messengers, diacylglycerol and inositol 1,4,5-triphosphate which regulate intracellular calcium mobilization.[3,4,5] Risby et al. have reported that lithium may interfere with guanine nucleotide binding (G) protein function. These proteins transduce signals from receptors to second messenger systems, including adenyl cyclase and inositol.[130] Although lithium may be selective in its therapeutic effects by dampening only those receptors that are overactive, side effects and toxicities are dose and concentration dependent in both normal subjects and patients resulting in a narrow therapeutic index. This situation is reflected in the warning statement that appears in the product labeling:

WARNING: *Lithium toxicity is closely related to serum lithium levels and can occur at doses close to therapeutic levels. Facilities for prompt and accurate serum lithium determination should be available before initiating therapy.*

The use of serum lithium concentrations (S_{Li}) is therefore necessary for all patients treated with lithium. This chapter focuses on the pharmacokinetic basis for the rational use of S_{Li} concentrations to optimize lithium therapy.

CLINICAL PHARMACOKINETICS

One year following Cade's 1949 report on the therapeutic use of lithium in mania, Talbott used plasma lithium concentrations as a monitoring tool in lithium treatment. In 1951, Noack and Trautner reported no correlation between clinical effects (including toxicity) and plasma and urine concentrations determined *at random*. They, therefore, saw no utility in monitoring plasma lithium concentrations during its use to treat psychiatric disorders. In 1954, Schou et al. also reported no correlation between lithium concentration and effect in their patients; however, since most lithium concentrations in their patients were between 0.5 and 2 mEq/L, they recommended 2 mEq/L as the upper safety limit. Ever since these early reports, it has been assumed that to achieve therapeutic effects without toxicity, near-toxic doses must be used.[6,7,8] It should be noted that in the 1950s, clinical pharmacokinetic principles were not generally appreciated. Consequently, blood samples were often obtained at random times following a dose, ensuring that any concentration-effect or concentration-adverse effect relationship would remain obscured.

Gradually, it was recognized that safe lithium treatment required continuous observation for side effects (by the patient and/or close relative), careful patient education, and monitoring of S_{Li} concentrations in the blood serum or plasma.[8] These procedures should help the clinician identify impending toxicity and therapeutic failure due to noncompliance.

A prerequisite for individualization of dosage regimens is that S_{Li} concentrations are interpreted in the context of lithium absorption, distribution, and elimination. These pharmacokinetic properties are significantly different between species and significant variations are observed between individuals of the same species.[9] In humans, both the interindividual and the intraindividual variations in S_{Li} concentrations are wide compared to the narrow therapeutic index.[10] Consequently, the therapeutic doses needed by one patient may be toxic to another. The best known and probably most important causes of these variations are the wide ranges in renal clearance (10 to 40 mL/min) and the apparent distribution volume (50% to 120% of the body weight). Within an individual, both may also change with age[11,12] and possibly with duration of treatment.[13] However, the varying dissolution, rate of absorption from the gastrointestinal tract, and bioavailability of the drug formulation may also play decisive roles.[14]

Absorption

In practice, lithium is only given orally. Lithium carbonate is the most commonly used salt form because it has a longer shelf-life and contains more lithium on a weight for weight basis than other salts (e.g., citrate, sulfate, glutamate, gluconate, and aspartate). The effects of the different salts are similar since the therapeutic and adverse effects fundamentally depend on the lithium ion itself. Although lithium has been administered intravenously under research conditions, an intravenous formulation is not available for clinical use in the United States Moreover, rectal lithium preparations invoke painful diarrhea and are not available.[15]

The absorption of lithium from a dilute solution (e.g., lithium citrate in the United States or lithium chloride in Europe) is rapid with considerably less variability between individuals and within the same subject than from solid dosage forms. In fasting normal volunteers, the absorption half-life ranges from 6 to 17 minutes.[16,17] After about 15 to 40 minutes a peak concentration is usually reached and the serum concentration declines biexponentially (see Figure 34-1). Significant absorption of lithium occurs in the jejunum and ileum with negligible absorption in the colon.[18,19] This partially explains the difficulties encountered in manufacturing a sustained-release tablet that maintains a consistent release rate over a specific period of time as well as high bioavailability. These influencing factors are exemplified by the fundamental differences between the concentration-time curves following liquid, ordinary tablets or capsules, and sustained release dosage forms.

If S_{Li} is used as a monitoring tool, one must consider variations in the bioavailability and dissolution of the various products since these may alter the time course of S_{Li} significantly. In current practice, the average bioavailability for tablets and capsules ranges from 80% to 104% (see Table 34-1). The variability in S_{Li} is greatest shortly after the ingestion of a lithium dose and is minimal in the post-absorption and post-distributive phases.[9,10] Thus, a sampling time standard-

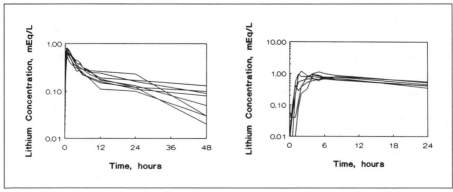

Figure 34-1. *Lithium concentration-time profiles following a 16 mEq dose of lithium citrate syrup (equivalent to 600 mg lithium carbonate) in eight healthy young male volunteers (data from reference 17) following an overnight fast (left panel). The right panel illustrates the slower absorption from a 1200 mg (32 mEq) dose of lithium carbonate from a regular tablet dosage form in seven elderly male volunteers.*

ized to 12 hours post-dose (also called the 12-hour standardized serum lithium concentration, 12 h–stS$_{Li}$) is strongly recommended to minimize this variability and thereby maximize the precision with which S$_{Li}$ can be assessed.[9,10]

Distribution

Lithium disposition is classically described using the open, two-compartment model. The central compartment volume has been found to be 25% to 40% of the body weight[16,20] and the combined central and peripheral compartments are equivalent to a mean of 123% of the body weight.[21] The apparent volume of distribution (V$_{d_\beta}$ or V$_{d_{area}}$) is approximately 0.8 L/kg with micro-rate constants of 0.24 h^{-1} (k$_{12}$) and 0.19 h^{-1} (k$_{21}$) in normal volunteers.[16] Often, this distribution phase is obscured by absorption of lithium from solid dosage forms and elimination appears to be monoexponential. Population pharmacokinetic parameters of lithium were deter-

Table 34–1. *Bioavailability of Lithium Preparations*

Product	Manu-facturer	Peak Time (hr)	Peak Conc.[a] (mEq/L)	Bioavail-ability (%)
Capsules				
150 mg lithium carbonate, 4.06 mEq Li				
Lithium carbonate	Roxane	e	e	e
300 mg lithium carbonate, 8.12 mEq Li				
Lithium carbonate	Roxane	1–2	0.45–0.85	100[b]
Eskalith	SKF	1–2	0.42–0.80	95–100[c]
Lithonate	Rowell	1–3	0.44–0.75	100[d]
600 mg lithium carbonate, 16.24 mEq Li				
Lithium carbonate	Roxane	e	e	e
Syrup				
8 mEq lithium as citrate/5mL				
Lithium citrate	Roxane	e	e	e
	My-K	e	e	e
Cibalith-S	Ciba	e	e	e
Tablets				
Regular				
300 mg lithium carbonate, 8.12 mEq Li				
Lithium carbonate	Roxane	1–2	0.6–0.9	104[d]
	Goldline	e	e	e
Eskalith	SKF	0.5–2	0.5–0.98	98[b]
Lithane	Miles	e	e	e
Controlled-release				
450 mg lithium carbonate, 12.18 mEq Li				
Eskalith CR	SKF	2–5	e	97[b]
Film-coated				
300 mg lithium carbonate 8.12 mEq Li				
Lithotabs	Reid-Rowell	1.5–3	0.5–0.88	99[b]–103[c]
Slow-release				
300 mg lithium carbonate, 8.12 mEq Li				
Lithobid	Ciba	3.5–5.5	0.24–0.43	80[d]

[a] Normalized to a 600 mg dose of lithium carbonate.
[b] Fast-release capsule as reference product.
[c] Solution as reference product.
[d] Fast-release tablet as reference product.
[e] Data unavailable from company.

mined with the nonlinear mixed-effects model (NONMEM) in 79 psychiatric inpatients who received lithium two or three times a day. The volume of distribution averaged 39.5 L with a 15.6% standard error, and the patient weights averaged 70.5 kg (range 44.5 to 111 kg).[131]

A 20% to 30% age-dependent reduction of the apparent distribution volume in those patients aged 67 to 88 years compared to normal volunteers aged 18 to 48 years (perhaps secondary to a decrease in total body water and lean body mass) has been reported by several groups.[11,12] This, along with concomitant reductions in renal clearance with age results in prolonged elimination half-lives in the elderly patients.[12,13] After absorption, lithium is unevenly distributed among several tissue compartments[22] in a pattern which differs among species.[23] It is not bound to plasma proteins. Uneven distribution of lithium into the brain[24] might explain the rare cases of cerebral intoxication which may have been observed in patients with a S_{Li} below the range usually associated with toxicity. Antidepressants and neuroleptics may significantly influence lithium distribution between plasma and tissue compartments by altering lithium transport mechanisms for cellular influx and efflux.[25,26]

Lithium is distributed slowly and proportionally to both the brain and erythrocytes. For this reason, a high or low erythrocyte (RBC) lithium concentration has been suggested as a measure of toxicity or noncompliance, even if plasma lithium levels are within the usual therapeutic range. However, the clinical usefulness of this test may be limited because of the pronounced interindividual variability of erythrocyte lithium concentrations.[27,28] The measurement of lithium concentrations in erythrocytes has yet to emerge from the research lab into routine clinical practice.

Elimination

Lithium is eliminated renally as the free ion and is not bound by plasma proteins nor metabolized. Consequently, it is considered to be freely diffusible across the glomerular membrane like sodium and potassium and is 80% reabsorbed. Radomski et al.[29] and Foulks et al.[30] regarded renal lithium reabsorption as a passive process in consideration of the large concentration gradient. It has been hypothesized that lithium is reabsorbed solely in the proximal renal tubules to the same extent as both sodium and water. In contrast to sodium and water, lithium is not reabsorbed in the distal nephron except, possibly, in connection with an extremely low sodium intake.[31] Lithium is completely eliminated through renal clearance with negligible elimination via saliva, sweat, and feces under normal circumstances.[29,30,32]

Renal lithium clearance in humans varies from about 10 to 40 mL/min and is closely correlated with creatinine clearance, averaging about 20% of glomerular filtration rate (GFR).[10,33] Jermain et al.,[131] using the computer program NONMEM, found population clearance to be a function of creatine clearance (CL_{cr}) and lean body weight (LBW). Their model was $CL_{Li} = (0.0093\ [L/hr/kg] \times LBW) + (0.0885 \times CL_{cr})$. Like GFR, renal lithium clearance is subject to circadian variations. In humans, it has been demonstrated that the mean renal clearance at night is 78% of the daytime value (20.7 mL/min versus 26.4 mL/min)[34] and the night:day ratio of lithium half-life varies from 1 hour to as high as 2.5 hours.[10] This is further complicated by a pronounced decrease in lithium clearance as posture is changed from a recumbent to an upright position.[35,36] These facts, together with considerations of convenience, are the reasons to obtain blood samples for monitoring S_{Li} in the morning 12 hours following the previous evening's dose.

Recent reports on long-term lithium therapy do not support earlier concerns that chronic lithium therapy could result in renal insufficiency.[37,38,39] However, the most frequent side-effects of chronic lithium treatment are a reduced urine concentrating ability in about one-half of patients and chronic polyuria in about 20% of patients chronically treated with lithium. These side effects are probably caused by a reversible inhibition of antidiuretic hormone (ADH)-mediated water transport in the collecting tubule of the nephron.[37] Amelioride may specifically inhibit the epithelial uptake of lithium and prevent lithium's inhibition of ADH-mediated water transport.[37] Amelioride is also less likely to elevate S_{Li} concentrations. Protocols for monitoring renal function during long-term lithium therapy are available.[40] To prevent an elevated S_{Li} and any resultant toxicity, lithium patients should be thoroughly informed about the risk of dehydration, the danger of a negative sodium balance, and the need for caution if natriuretic diuretics or nonsteroidal anti-inflammatory drugs (NSAIDs) are used concomitantly.[41,42]

A reduction of renal lithium clearance parallels a reduction of creatinine clearance with increasing age, averaging about 0.5% per year in adults. It also diminishes with the duration of lithium treatment by about 1% per year after age 30.[43] Thus, elderly people usually need lower lithium dosages to achieve a target S_{Li} concentration. In particular, it should be noted that the consequence of the simultaneous reduction of renal clearance and distribution volume may result in a more rapid development of intoxication in elderly patients. It may be assumed that any renal impairment which reduces GFR will also reduce the lithium excretion. Many renal disorders develop insidiously and may produce a gradual increase in the lithium concentration which may eventually lead to chronic toxicity.

The elimination rate or half-life of S_{Li} depends upon the apparent distribution volume and the total body (renal) clearance. As is the case for many other psychotropic drugs, there is tremendous interindividual variation in lithium disposition. The half-life typically varies from 18 to 27 hours in subjects with normal renal function but has ranged between 5 and 79 hours.[10,13,16]

Treatment with natriuretic drugs, many NSAIDs, and sodium-poor diets may rapidly induce a pronounced reduction of the renal lithium clearance. Either aminophylline[44] or sodium in large doses[33] may enhance renal lithium elimination, reduce the S_{Li}, and produce a loss in the therapeutic effect. Neither of these agents has been found useful in the treatment of lithium-intoxicated patients who are normally hydrated. Sodium loading[45,46] may even be dangerous because of sodium-induced hyperosmolality.[41,46] Protracted diarrhea and profuse sweating are potentially hazardous not only because extra lithium is lost, but also because elimination is decreased due to dehydration and temporarily impaired renal clearance. The question of the effect of protracted diarrhea has not yet been investigated, but acute, profuse sweating has led to a reduced S_{Li}[32,47] in spite of simultaneous dehydration. However, extrapolation of results from these studies of acute medical conditions to chronic cases where adaptation in the composition of sweat may have taken place is not warranted.[47] When lithium treatment is carried out concurrently with any of the above conditions, cautious monitoring is essential.

Factors Affecting Serum Concentration

The disposition of lithium varies considerably between subjects, but is relatively stable within any given individual with consistent renal function. This necessitates individualization of dosage regimens and monitoring adverse effects. The within-subject stability of lithium disposition allows estimation of chronic dosage requirements using population and pharmacokinetic prediction techniques. However, alterations in fluid or electrolyte balance, renal function, and/or sodium intake may complicate dosage regimen design. Table 34-2 summarizes a number of factors that have been reported to affect lithium disposition and S_{Li} concentrations.

Compliance. As with any chronic drug regimen, patient noncompliance is a major factor affecting serum concentration monitoring. The variability in S_{Li} concentrations (12-hour post-dose) in a 42-year-old male with bipolar disorder is illustrated in Figure 34-2. During the first 40 months of treatment, he received a standard-release preparation and no counseling on dosage compliance, had a coefficient of variation (CV) of 23.4%. This variability was reduced to 11.3% and eventually to 8.3% by using a controlled release lithium preparation and by taking into account patient-specific information regarding compliance and timing of blood sampling (see reference 45 for more details).

Menstrual Cycle. Another possible source of variability is the menstrual cycle. Most of the available reports are conflicting and limited to examination of trough S_{Li} concentrations.[48,49,50] Chamberlain et al.[132] reported no change in lithium concentrations over 24 hours following single 300 mg doses of lithium carbonate during three phases of the menstrual cycle in six healthy female volunteers and in seven healthy female volunteers on oral contraceptives. Another study found no significant effect of the menstrual cycle on lithium disposition in six women

Table 34-2. *Factors Reported to Affect Serum Lithium Concentration*

Lower	Variable or no effect	Raise
Acetazolamide	Amelioride	ACE inhibitors
Aminophylline	Aspirin	Ibuprofen
Caffeine	Furosemide	Indomethacin
Osmotic diuretics	Sulindac	Chronic lithium
Pregnancy[a]		Phenylbutazone
Sodium supplement		Thiazide diuretics
		Dehydration
		Renal impairment
		Sodium loss
		Increasing age

[a] Lithium clearance and serum concentrations return to pre-pregnancy values after delivery.

treated for bipolar disorder.[51] The average between-subject variability for oral clearance was 45%; however, the average within-subject variability was 13.4%, a figure quite similar to the variability in trough S_{Li} concentrations seen in the clinic setting (see Figure 34-2).

Diuretics. It is well established that thiazide diuretics will reduce the renal clearance of lithium with a resultant increase in S_{Li} concentration and increased likelihood of toxicity if the lithium dose is not reduced. This interaction is reported for hydrochlorothiazide,[133] but is best documented for chlorothiazide which reduces lithium renal clearance by 40% to 70% depending on the diuretic dose.[52-55] With careful monitoring of S_{Li} concentrations, however, this combination can be used successfully.[56] Conflicting reports on the concomitant use of furosemide or potassium-sparing diuretics suggest cautious monitoring of S_{Li} concentrations is also warranted.[57,58,59,133]

Methylxanthines. Variability between and within subjects is also related to sodium excretion rates.[60] Theoretically, any drug capable of influencing the proximal tubular reabsorption of sodium such as thiazide diuretics,[64] phenylbutazone,[65] and angiotensin converting enzyme (ACE) inhibitors[66] may affect lithium renal clearance. Methylxanthines such as theophylline and caffeine may increase the elimination of lithium by altering sodium disposition in the kidney.[33] Theophylline has been reported to increase lithium renal clearance and decrease

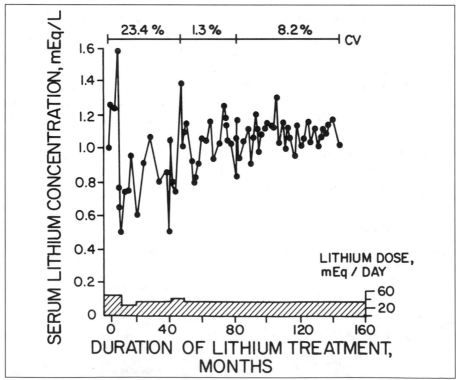

Figure 34-2. *The long-term variability in steady-state 12-hour post-dose S_{Li} concentrations, expressed as percent coefficient of variation, %(CV), in a 42-year-old male clinic patient with bipolar disorder (see text for further details).*

trough S_{Li} concentrations by 20% to 30%.[59,62,63] Caffeine has been reported to increase urinary sodium excretion[67] and case reports further suggest an effect on lithium disposition.[68] The effects of caffeine on lithium pharmacokinetics were evaluated in a double-blinded crossover study in eight normal male volunteers.[17] Caffeine in doses of 300 mg significantly (p <0.01) increased the renal excretion rate of sodium (24.7 ± 5.7 versus 13.4 ± 6.2 mEq/hr) and increased lithium renal clearance by 26% (28.9 ± 8.1 to 36.5 ± 8.2 mL/min) as compared to placebo during the first four hours following concomitant administration of single doses (see Figure 34-3).

Nonsteroidal Anti-inflammatory Drugs (NSAIDs). Another important mediator of renal excretion of sodium is prostaglandin E_2 (PGE_2). Frolich et al.[69] reported that 150 mg/day of indomethacin increased the mean 12-hour S_{Li} concentration by 30% to 59%, reduced mean renal clearance by 30%, and decreased the urinary excretion of the main metabolite of PGE_2 by 55%. Increases in the S_{Li} concentrations of 20% to 50% along with decreases in renal clearance and/or decreases in urinary PGE_2 excretion have been reported for diclofenac,[70] piroxicam,[71] naproxen,[72] and to a lesser extent with ibuprofen.[73,74] Conflicting data suggest sulindac may not significantly reduce lithium renal clearance.[72,75] Sulindac has been used as the NSAID of choice for patients who need alleviation of arthritic symptoms, but clinicians should be aware of an initial decrease in S_{Li} concentrations during the first two weeks, followed by a return to baseline concentrations with continued sulindac therapy.[75]

PHARMACODYNAMICS

The primary aim of pharmacodynamic studies has been to identify the concentration versus response and concentration versus toxicity relationships for lithium therapy and to identify therapeutic ranges for the acute and prophylactic treatment of bipolar disorders. The concept of a therapeutic range is based on statistical

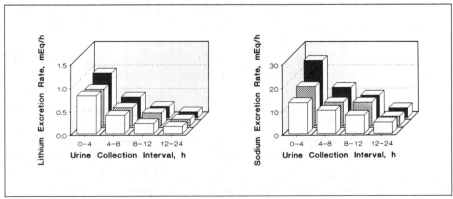

Figure 34-3. *The excretion rate of lithium (left panel) and sodium (right panel) in four urine collections over 24 hours following a 16 mEq dose of lithium citrate (equivalent to 600 mg lithium carbonate) concurrently with a placebo (white bars), 100 mg dose of caffeine (hatched bars), or a 300 mg dose of caffeine (dark bars) in a double-blind crossover fashion to eight healthy male volunteers (data from reference 17).*

theory. It also assumes a relatively homogeneous group of patients and a response variable that can be easily measured, preferably with a direct and reversible continuous effect. This is rarely the case in psychopharmacology.

Concentration Versus Clinical Response

Lithium concentrations often vary by a factor of two to three during a dosage interval, depending on the time interval and the magnitude of the dose (see Figure 34-4). For this reason, a representative single time point for S_{Li} concentration monitoring was established at 12 hours post-dose (12 hr–stS_{Li}),[9] usually in the morning following the evening dose. This time point was essentially arbitrary, but it did avoid the absorption and distribution phases where most of the between-subject variability exists. However, even the within-subject variability can be significant as illustrated in Figure 34-4. Therefore, all references to a therapeutic range assume divided daily doses. No therapeutic range data exist for once daily dosage regimens. When monitoring drug therapy for a "chronic disease," an indicator of the total or average daily exposure to the drug (i.e., the pharmacokinetic parameters of area-under-the-curve (AUC) or average concentration at steady state ($C_{ss\,ave}$)) rather than a trough serum concentration might best define a therapeutic range for lithium treatment of bipolar disorders. The pharmacokinetic basis for the individualization of lithium dosage regimens to a target therapeutic concentration is illustrated by Equation 34-1

$$C_{ss\,ave} = \frac{F \cdot Dose}{\tau \cdot CL_R}$$

(Eq. 34-1)

where the average steady-state target concentration ($C_{ss\,ave}$) is determined by two factors that are clinician determined—the available dose (F · Dose) and the dosing interval (τ)—and one patient-specific factor: renal lithium clearance (CL_R). However, the 12-hour trough S_{Li} concentration is the usual parameter used in clinical practice. The use of several nomograms has been proposed to convert the S_{Li} to the $C_{ss\,ave}$, taking into account the dosage schedule and sampling time.[76] Nomograms for general monoexponential decline can also be used to convert $C_{ss\,ave}$ to trough S_{Li} concentrations and vice versa.[77]

Some disagreement exists regarding the therapeutic range for lithium and this issue is complicated by a lack of standardized time for determining S_{Li} concentrations in past studies. Target S_{Li} concentrations of 0.8 to 1.2 mEq/L for acute therapy and 0.6 to 0.8 mEq/L for maintenance therapy are widely accepted. Prien and Caffey found that periodically depressed patients responded less satisfactorily between 0.5 and 0.8 mEq/L and that manic patients needed 0.9 to 1.4 mEq/L.[78] They used S_{Li} concentrations sampled between 8 and 12 hours after the dose, and their ranges would probably have been 15% lower if a standardized 12-hour time point had been used. Jerram and McDonald[79] found equally good suppression of relapses at S_{Li} concentrations between 0.50 and 0.69 mEq/L, but the sampling times were 12 to 16 hours after the dose. Their range probably would have been

15% higher with a standardized 12-hour sampling time. Stokes et al.[80] found an increasing response in manic patients as the S_{Li} concentration increased from 0.2 to 2 mEq/L; samples were drawn in the morning before the next dose.

Currently, lower therapeutic ranges are recommended. The National Institute of Mental Health Consensus Development Conference[81] has recommended a therapeutic range of 0.6 to 0.8 mEq/L to maintain bipolar disorders. In an effort to help clarify response at the lower end of the therapeutic range for lithium prophylaxis, Gelenberg et al.[82] evaluated 94 patients with bipolar disorder in a randomized, double-blind prospective trial. S_{Li} concentrations (12 hours post-dose)[83] were maintained between 0.4 and 0.6 mEq/L in the low-dose group and between 0.8 and 1 mEq/L in the standard-dose group. In actuality, the S_{Li} concentrations for each group tended to merge during the study. The median value was 0.53 mEq/L for the low-dose group and 0.83 mEq/L for the standard-dose group with 25th and 75th percentile ranges of 0.51 to 0.62 mEq/L and 0.75 to 0.90 mEq/L, respectively. Even so, the risk of relapse was 2.6 times higher (95% confidence interval, 1.3 to 5.2) in the low-dose group. Doses resulting in S_{Li} concentrations between 0.8 and 1 mEq/L were more effective but also resulted in more frequent side effects. This study suggests that small changes in S_{Li} concentrations can significantly affect relapse rates and that lithium maintenance doses need to be targeted to produce S_{Li} concentrations more precisely than the typical 0.6 to 1.2 mEq/L range. This is where the application of pharmacokinetic principles can effectively impact lithium therapy.

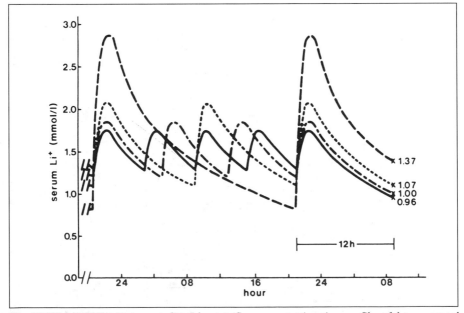

Figure 34-4. *Computer-generated steady-state S_{Li} concentration-time profiles of the same total daily dosage of lithium divided into one, two, three, or four doses illustrating the variability of 12-hour S_{Li} concentration due solely to differences in dosage interval.*

Concentration Versus Toxicity

S_{Li} concentrations (at least 12 hours post-dose) greater than 1.5 mEq/L are potentially toxic, and dialysis should be considered for concentration values greater than 3.5 to 4 mEq/L.[41,46] Lithium intoxication primarily presents as neurotoxicity and acute intoxication involves both the central nervous system and the kidneys. The clinical management of lithium intoxication has been previously reviewed.[41,46,84] Hemodialysis and peritoneal dialysis are the only effective means to remove lithium (i.e., an extrarenal clearance of an additional 50 and 15 mL/min, respectively);[84,85] charcoal is ineffective. Since distributional rebound will occur, the goal of dialysis is to keep the six- to eight-hour post-dialysis S_{Li} concentration below 1 mEq/L.[41]

CLINICAL APPLICATION OF PHARMACOKINETIC DATA

Traditionally, patients are initiated on low, divided doses of lithium which are then adjusted on the basis of multiple S_{Li} concentration determinations until the desired concentration is achieved.[16] In contrast, one group used a 30 mg/kg loading dose of a sustained-release lithium carbonate formulation given in three divided doses over six hours. All 38 patients achieved S_{Li} concentrations between 0.45 and

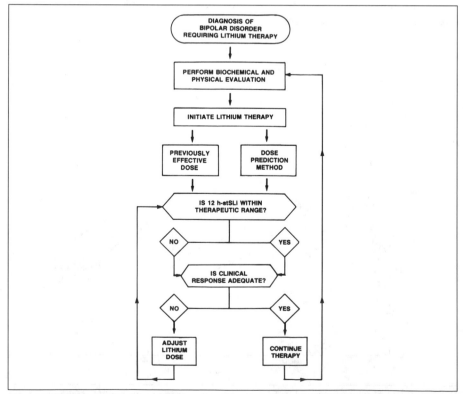

Figure 34-5. *General scheme for pharmacokinetic monitoring of lithium therapy in bipolar disorders.*

1.4 mEq/L by 12 hours.[86] The package insert recommends a daily dose of 1800 mg of lithium carbonate to treat acute mania and 900 mg to 1200 mg for long-term control, divided into two or three doses. These doses are said to produce trough S_{Li} concentrations in the range of 1 to 1.5 mEq/L and 0.6 to 1.2 mEq/L, respectively, although periodic S_{Li} concentration monitoring is required. This empirical approach may cause undue delay in determining the optimum dosage for some patients as well as toxicity in other patients; however, the application of pharmacokinetic principles may allow a more accurate and quicker prediction of lithium dosages requirements. A general algorithm for pharmacokinetic monitoring of lithium is shown in Figure 34-5 and a more comprehensive algorithm is reported by Johnston et al.[87]

Pharmacokinetic Dosing Methods

Numerous dosing methods have been reported for lithium and many are based on pharmacokinetic principles. One exception is the use of a statistical model using multiple linear regression that incorporates the S_{Li} concentration; the subject's age, weight, gender, and inpatient/outpatient status; and the concurrent use of tricyclic antidepressants.[88] Regardless of the dosing method used, clinicians must be cognizant of their implicit assumptions and limitations and use sound clinical judgment.

There is a direct proportionality between lithium renal clearance and the dosage required to achieve a certain S_{Li} concentration. This principle was exploited by Cooper et al.[89] who developed the classic dosing guidelines following the use of a single-dose pretest. While investigating the pharmacokinetics of lithium, they observed that the 24-hour S_{Li} concentration following the first 600 mEq dose correlated highly (r = 0.97) with the steady-state trough S_{Li} concentration when patients were placed on a fixed-dose regimen (see Figure 34-6).[90]

Each dosage range (labels A through G in Figure 34-6 and Table 34-3) was calculated by extrapolating from the regression line developed from data from the

Table 34–3. Recommended Dosages Required to Achieve a Serum Level of 0.6 to 1.2 mEq/L[89,a]

Range	24-hour serum level after single loading dose	Patients (n)	Dosage required
A	< 0.05	0	1200 mg TID
B	0.05–0.09	4	900 mg TID
C	0.10–0.14	4	600 mg TID
D	0.15–0.19	2	300 mg QID
E	0.20–0.23	3	300 mg TID
F	0.24–0.30	3	300 mg BID
G	> 0.30	1	300 mg QD[b]

[a] The regimen selected minimizes fluctuation in the plasma level while maintaining a schedule the patient can adhere to. Variation in the regimen can be made at the choice of the clinician, but the total daily dose must remain the same. All "steady-state" values are collected just before the next medication is to be taken.

[b] Use extreme caution.

first 17 patients studied. The dosage recommendations are intended to produce trough S_{Li} concentrations of 0.6 to 1.2 mEq/L. The reliability of this method has been tested by several groups,[91,92,93,94] in patients taking doses other than the fixed-dose regimen of 600 mg three times daily from which the relationship was generated. Under controlled research conditions, results generally have been acceptable. However, it should be noted that critically important assumptions for the use of pretests include the following: linearity and stationarity (stable renal clearance and volume of distribution) of lithium disposition; blood sampling in the terminal post-absorptive/post-distributive phase; consistency of lithium content, dissolution and bioavailability of the dosage form; precise assay methodology to minimize the variability that exists as the 24-hour concentrations following a single dose approach the limit of assay sensitivity; and the cautious use of initial lithium doses which are estimated through the pretest method.[94-96] It is important to recheck the S_{Li} concentration 48 to 72 hours after starting the maintenance dose to identify patients with unusual pharmacokinetic characteristics, especially if the patient is switched to another lithium preparation shortly after treatment has been initiated.

The prediction of steady-state serum concentrations following a single test dose is based on the principle of superposition[97] and on the accumulation ratio (R), which is a nonlinear function of the terminal elimination rate (λ_z) and the dosage interval (τ) as depicted in Equation 34-2.

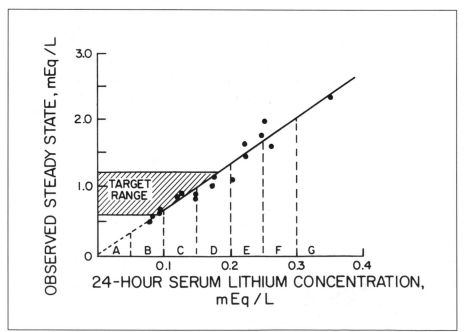

Figure 34-6. *Relationship between 24-hour concentrations following a 600 mg test-dose of lithium carbonate and steady-state S_{Li} concentrations following maintenance doses of 600 mg three times a day. The 24-hour concentrations are divided into six ranges (A through G) to be used with the accompanying dosing table to result in steady-state S_{Li} concentrations within the target range of 0.6 to 1.2 mEq/L (modified with permission from reference 89).*

$$R = \frac{C_{ss} \, min}{C_1^p \, min} = \frac{1}{1 - e^{\lambda \cdot \tau}}$$

(Eq. 34-2)

This relationship was determined for the antidepressant imipramine at two different doses and illustrates that nonlinearity can be expected at each extreme of the therapeutic range (see Figure 34-7).[95] Detailed theoretical considerations are discussed by DeVane and Jusko[95] and by Slattery and Gibaldi.[96]

The nonlinearity of R occurs at the extremes of the serum concentration range where data are often scarce; however, within the therapeutic range R is often linear, as illustrated by the data of Cooper et al.[89] Thus, test-dose concentrations at the extremes may account for the under- or overpredictions reported by several investigators.[91,98] This pharmacokinetic-based dosing technique further assumes that the next dose is given after absorption and distribution from the previous dose is complete. If this assumption does not hold, the recommended dose could result in toxic drug accumulation as in the case reported by Gengo et al.[99] This situation occurred when the 24-hour post-dose S_{Li} concentration occurred during the more rapidly declining distribution phase, instead of the expected slower terminal phase (see Figure 34-8).

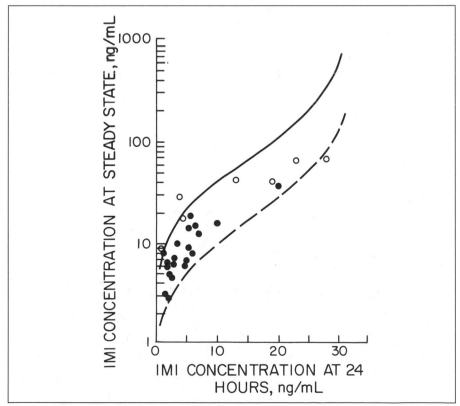

Figure 34-7. *Theoretical relationships between 24-hour serum concentration following a 50 mg test-dose and steady-state serum concentrations from a daily maintenance dose of 2.5 mg (- - - -) and 100 mg (————). (Reproduced with permission from reference 95.)*

These conditions limit our ability to estimate a maintenance dose by the one-dose pretest methods.[89,94,100] Since the lithium content of products may be variable, any single-dose pretest should be used cautiously.[94] Techniques which utilize multiple test doses are less likely to be limited by this factor.[101,102]

Patients with unusual pharmacokinetic characteristics may be better managed with a pretest method in which the patient's own terminal elimination rate constant (λ_z) is determined from two or three serum concentration measurements following the test dose. One can then directly calculate the maintenance dose using standard pharmacokinetic equations or dosing nomograms and can be more accurate and precise.[97,100,103]

An implicit assumption of these techniques is rapid absorption of the test drug. However sustained-released products may exhibit "flip-flop" kinetics and invalidate the assumption that the 24-hour sample is collected in the post-distributive, post-absorptive phase. Karki et al.[104] compared a two-point method and the Cooper dosing chart for predicting lithium maintenance dosages in 20 patients using a slow-release tablet. The two-point method predicted the actual maintenance dosage within clinically acceptable limits, but dosages from the dosing chart would have yielded higher steady-state S_{Li} concentrations. Moreover, the time of sample collection affected the strength of the correlation between predicted and observed S_{Li} concentrations. The time combinations that allowed a 24-hour interval between samples (e.g., 12 and 36 hours following the test dose) resulted in correlation coefficients (r) of -0.919 and -0.894 versus -0.775 and -0.603 for the 24, 36 hour and 12, 24 hour time combinations, respectively. This may in part reflect the circadian changes[10,34] in lithium disposition and, therefore, violation of the assump-

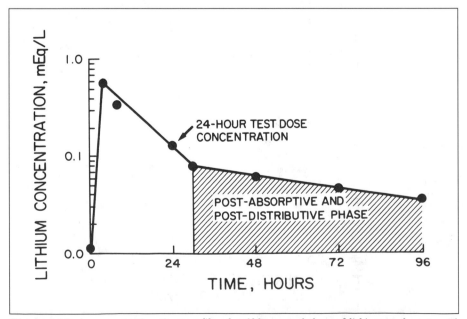

Figure 34-8. *A concentration-time profile of a 600 mg oral dose of lithium carbonate with 0.13 mEq/L 24-hour test dose concentration erroneously obtained before post-absorptive and post-distributive phase. (Adapted from reference 99 with permission.)*

tion of stationarity. It must be noted that better correlations have been reported with rapid-release formulations using the single (r = −0.97) or two-point methods (r = −0.96).

Pretest methods can be used to estimate maintenance doses with sufficient accuracy if their limitations are appreciated and if there is adequate analytical support. These techniques may minimize the number of lithium determinations and time required to achieve a therapeutic maintenance dose. Pretests are especially useful for patients who are being placed on lithium therapy for the first time and for whom a history of a therapeutic lithium dosage is unavailable.[107] Table 34-4 summarizes some requirements of the various pharmacokinetic test-dose methods used to predict lithium maintenance dosages. Interested readers can find additional evaluations and comparisons of these dosing methods in several reports[105–108] as well as in the excellent review of Lobeck.[109]

A limited number of studies have suggested that computer-aided dosing methods can improve the clinical response and decrease the toxicity of drugs such as gentamicin, digoxin, phenytoin, theophylline, and lidocaine.[110] Similar computer-aided techniques that forecast individualized dosing regimens for lithium are also available. One approach uses sophisticated iterative nonlinear least-squares procedures.[103,111,112] This approach which is based on classic monoexponential or biexponential decline equations generates the distribution volume, clearance and/or half-life. Usually, parameters such as absorption rate and bioavailability are obtained from population data and are fixed as constants. These methods usually do not use patient-specific demographic data, test doses, or serum creatinine concentrations, but often require at least two S_{Li} concentration values obtained at flexible time points. A major advantage of these techniques is their capacity to accommodate irregular dosing intervals and non-steady-state S_{Li} concentrations.

A second forecasting approach is the use of *a priori* population data and patient specific information along with Bayesian decision making applications to generate

Table 34–4. *Requirements of Lithium Dosage-Prediction Methods*[109]

Method	Demographics[a]	Test dose	S_{Cr}[b]	# of serum samples	Sample timing	Computer needed
Single-Point Methods						
Cooper et al[89]	No	Yes	No	1	24 hr	No
Slattery et al[96]	No	Yes	No	1	24 hr	Helpful
Modified Slattery[138]	Yes	Yes	Yes	1	24 hr	Helpful
Simplified[98,100,106]	No	Yes	No	1	24 hr	No
Multipoint Methods						
Perry 2-point[109]	No	Yes	No	2	12 and 36 hr	Helpful
Repeated 1-point[102]	No	Yes	No	2	12 and 34 hr	Helpful
Computer Based Methods						
Iteration[103]	No	No	No	>1	Flexible[c]	Required
Bayesian[114,115]	Yes/No	No	Yes	≥1	Flexible[c]	Required

[a] Variables such as age, weight, concomitant medication, etc.

[b] Requires the results of serum creatinine determination.

[c] Sample collections must be made such that different parts of time concentration curve are represented.

pharmacokinetic parameter estimates that are unique to an individual patient (See Chapter 3: Strategies for Using Clinical Pharmacokinetic Data to Individualize Drug Dosage Regimens for additional details).[113-115] Williams et al.[114] retrospectively evaluated a single-point method, a multiple-point method, a nonlinear regression method, and a Bayesian method and found equivalent bias and precision among all in the estimation of measured steady-state S_{Li} concentrations for 21 patients with bipolar disorder.

Computer Software for Pharmacokinetic Consultations

Several commercial pharmacokinetic software programs for IBM-compatible personal computers are designed to generate patient-specific pharmacokinetic consults based upon S_{Li} concentrations. The theoretical basis for these programs is generally a linear or nonlinear iterative procedure that uses standard pharmacokinetic equations or a Bayesian feedback technique to estimate individualized pharmacokinetic parameters by minimizing an objective function which compares actual patient S_{Li} concentrations with predicted concentrations. The intent is to generate dosing recommendations that maintain the S_{Li} concentration within a specific target range.

The programs generally use patient-specific data such as age, gender, weight, height, concomitant drugs, other disease states, dietary factors, and serum creatinine concentrations to estimate lithium clearance, volume of distribution, and/or half-life values. Individualized parameters are then determined as serum lithium concentrations become available. The *Computer Assisted Dosing Program* (Therapeutic Software, Inc., Charlotte, NC) uses the Bayesian technique to fit lithium clearance and volume of distribution values and calculates the elimination half-life. A unique aspect of this program is the fitting of an outpatient compliance factor. The initial value for each of the fitted parameters can be modified by the user. A consultation listing patient demographic data, modifying factors such as classes of drug interactions, dosing history, measured serum concentrations, pharmacokinetic parameters, curve-fitting analysis, and dosing recommendations can be printed.

The *Pharmacokinetic Consultation System*, Version 6.0. (Cedar Systems Limited, Charlottesville, VA) also uses the Bayesian technique with the Marquardt-Livenberg algorithm for least-squares estimation to estimate the lithium distribution volume and the elimination rate constant. The system is designed to print both a clinical consultation and a graphical output.

The *Simkin Pharmacokinetics Simulation System*, Version 4.2 (Simkin Inc., Gainesville, FL) also produces a written and graphic consultation. This program is based on simulation of lithium's pharmacokinetic disposition. The system uses one- and two-point linear and nonlinear iterative regression techniques (e.g., a simplex and a Bayesian method). The system fits the distribution volume and half-life by minimizing the sum of the squared error for the linear and nonlinear Simplex methods and by minimizing the weighted sum of the squared error for the Bayesian method. Patient demographic data, specific interacting drugs, disease interactions, dietary factors, and specific lithium products are used to generate suggested dosing regimens. A simulated graphic output of S_{Li} that is likely to be produced by a specific dosing recommendation can also be generated as part of the individualized consult. Patient data may be stored, revised, and statistically evaluated.

The contribution of these programs to the design of lithium regimens awaits evaluation. Many of these programs provide individualized consultations for an array of other drugs that have narrow therapeutic ranges and are used in the acutely ill patient. One limitation of all the programs and especially the graphically based programs is their inability to incorporate the extensive dosing histories often available for chronically treated patients. The strength and challenge of these programs may lie in their ability to accurately fit serum drug concentrations and to generate appropriate dosing recommendations in the context of concurrent drug, disease, dietary, and compliance conditions.

Lithium Concentrations in Other Biological Fluids

Application of pharmacokinetic principles to lithium treatment is primarily based on serum or plasma concentrations. There may be an exceptional case in which the determination of saliva lithium concentrations may be used as a noninvasive method, but only for intra-individual control. Simple routine determinations of lithium concentrations in red cells, spinal fluid, and urine have been suggested, but none of these has gained sufficient experimental support for practical, safe, and routine use in therapeutic monitoring.[116]

In spite of a large number of published studies, considerable uncertainty exists regarding the validity of the saliva to plasma concentration ratio (S:P) and its use in therapeutic drug monitoring. The major concern relates to the between- and within-subject stability of the S:P ratio.[117] The average ratio is usually between two and three; yet, it can be as high as three to four in some patients. Although regression correlations are often significant between the concentration of lithium in paired saliva and plasma samples, the variability is often too great to accurately predict plasma concentrations from a single population S:P ratio. Many patients exhibit considerably less variability in their own S:P ratios.[118] Several studies have attempted to relate the large between-subject variability to the type of saliva sampled (mixed versus parotid), the use of secretagogues (paraffin, pebbles, sour chewing gum, or citric acid solution), the saliva flow rate, the time of sampling following the last dose, and the concomitant drug therapy. Moreover, the stability of lithium in saliva, the viscosity of saliva, and the type of assay methodology (correction for K^+ concentration with flame photometry) may contribute to the uncertainty. Although problems still exists for the routine use of saliva concentration monitoring, it may prove helpful in a subgroup of patients who have stable S:P ratios over time. Sampling near peak concentrations and at trough concentrations which may fall below the lower limits of assay sensitivity should be avoided.

Saliva lithium concentrations have been shown to parallel the fluctuations in plasma concentrations and can be used in pharmacokinetic disposition studies.[119] Shimizu and Smith[120] found that saliva concentrations do not reflect the changes in urinary clearance following abrupt changes in posture in two volunteers. Since plasma concentrations did not change either, the implications of this observation for therapeutic drug monitoring are unknown.

Urine lithium concentrations depend on both the amount of water and lithium excreted during the urine collection period and therefore have no role in therapeutic monitoring. However, the urinary excretion rate can be used to determine the terminal disposition slope and half-life;[119] also, the amount of lithium excreted in the urine can be used to determine maintenance doses directly or by means of renal clearance (CL_R) according to Equation 34-1.

Periodic determination of renal lithium clearance to monitor renal function during long-term treatment has been suggested. However, since lithium clearance closely correlates with creatinine clearance, measuring the serum creatinine concentration is probably sufficient.[40] Interestingly, the renal clearance of lithium has recently been considered as a potential tool for simultaneous but separate testing of renal proximal tubular reabsorption of water and sodium.[31,121]

ANALYTICAL METHODS

An analytical method with an accuracy and precision corresponding to a coefficient of variation (CV) of 1% to 3% or less is necessary to monitor lithium intoxication and patient noncompliance and to predict the maintenance dosage after a one-dose pretest.[90,122] A CV of 1.5% is reasonable when the S_{Li} is above 0.25 mEq/L, and it is a prerequisite for measuring 12-hour S_{Li} concentrations with a between-day CV of 7% to 8% (see Figure 34-2).

The method of choice for determining serum lithium concentrations is photometry. Three methods are available (see Table 34-5): atomic emission flame photometry (FP),[122] which is by far the most widespread method; flame atomic absorption spectrophotometry (Flame-AA), which is more demanding and in less widespread use, although it is equally accurate;[123,124] and flameless furnace atomic absorption spectrophotometry (Furnace AA), which is a seldom-used, sophisticated method. The absorption methods are generally more expensive than the emission methods. The basic principle of these methods is that the lithium content

Table 34–5. Comparison of Lithium Assay Methodologies[a]

Method[b]	Specificity	Sensitivity	Sample volume	Speed	Cost	Difficulty of operation
FP	1	2	25 µL–2 mL	2	1	1
Flame AA	2	1	25 µL–1 mL	1	2	2
Furnace AA	2	3	1 µL–0.1 mL	1	2	3–2
ISE	1	1	<0.1 mL	3	1	1

[a] 1 = Least.
[b] Abbreviations as in text.

of a test sample is measured against a series of lithium reference samples in an appropriately matched matrix (with regard to background substances and viscosity) to form a standard calibration curve.

The ion-selective electrode (ISE) technique measures the Li^+ ion concentration similar to the way a pH electrode measures H^+ ions. Generally, the available electrodes for lithium are not as specific as those available for sodium or potassium. Therefore, some ISE assays simultaneously measure sodium and utilize specific correction algorithms to correct for background ion concentrations. The advantages of this assay include rapid speed, low cost, small sample size, ability to measure concentrations in various biological fluids, and portability. One study has compared the ISE assay with FP and found similar S_{Li} values at concentrations above 0.15 mEq/L. However, at lower concentrations the assay differences were significant and this may affect estimations of pharmacokinetic parameters or perhaps test-dose methods following small, single oral doses (see Figure 34-9).[125]

Several other techniques which are unavailable for clinical application include the neutron-activation method and the mass spectrophotometry method, both of which are very accurate but also very expensive. Nuclear magnetic resonance spectrophotometry has been used to measure brain and muscle concentrations of lithium in normal volunteers and bipolar patients.[127,128] Lithium concentrations can be determined from small volumes (1 to 100 μL) of blood, saliva, and urine with appropriate dilutions and sample preparations.[116,123,129]

PROSPECTUS

The relationship between S_{Li} concentrations and prophylactic effectiveness in the treatment of bipolar disorders (mania) has been more clearly defined at the lower range. Although considerable progress has been made regarding the use of serum concentration to monitor therapy, refinements are still needed. The significance of lithium concentration in various biological tissues such as brain and muscle can now be addressed. Moreover, the significance of erythrocyte to plasma concentrations and the influence of posture, affective disorder phase, and circadian rhythms on lithium pharmacokinetics is still uncertain. Research needs to shift from acute treatment to long-term pharmacologic treatment. Prospective longitu-

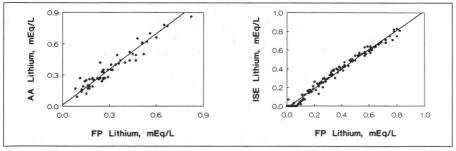

Figure 34-9. *Relationship between S_{Li} concentrations determined by flame photometry and atomic absorption spectrophotometry (left panel) and ion-selective electrode assay (right panel). (data from reference 125 and 126).*

dinal studies should address the cost-effectiveness of pharmacokinetic monitoring of lithium when used to prevent the relapse and recurrence of bipolar disorders. Concentration monitoring of lithium is an integral part of lithium therapy, but must be tempered by appropriate clinical judgment. Both written and repeated verbal instructions addressing the importance of compliance and symptoms of toxicity are essential throughout treatment.

ACKNOWLEDGMENTS

This work was supported in part by Grant #MH33127-11 from the National Institute of Mental Health and Grant #RR 00046 from the National Institutes of Health.

REFERENCES

1. Tyrer S, Shaw DM. Lithium carbonate. In: Tyrer PJ, ed. Drugs in Psychiatric Practice. London: Butterworth;1983.
2. Lydiard RB, Pearsall R. Lithium: predicting response/maximizing efficacy. In: Gold MS, Lydiard RB, Carman JS, eds. Advances in Psychopharmacology: Predicting and Improving Treatment Response. Boca Raton: CRC Press;1984.
3. Berridge MJ. Inositol triphosphate and diacylglycerol: two interacting second messengers. Ann Rev Biochem. 1987;56:159.
4. Berridge MJ, Irvine RF. Inositol phosphates and cell signaling. Nature. 1989;21:197.
5. Avissar S et al. Lithium inhibits adrenergic and cholinergic increase in GTP binding in rat cortex. Nature. 1988;331:440.
6. Johnson FN. The history of lithium therapy. London: MacMillan;1984.
7. Schou M. Lithium: Personal reminiscences. Psychiatr J Univ Ottawa. 1989;14(1):260.
8. Johnson FN. The Psychopharmacology of Lithium. London: MacMillan;1984.
9. Amdisen A, Carson SW. Lithium. In: Evans WE, Schentag JJ, Jusko WJ, eds. Applied Pharmacokinetics: Principles of Therapeutic Drug Monitoring. 2nd ed. Spokane, WA: Applied Therapeutics;1984.
10. Amdisen A. Monitoring of lithium treatment through determination of lithium concentration. Dan Med Bull. 1975;22(7):277.
11. Chapron DJ et al. Observations on lithium disposition in the elderly. J Am Geriatr Soc. 1982;30:651.
12. Hardy BG et al. Pharmacokinetics of lithium in the elderly. J Clin Psychopharmacol. 1987;7:153.
13. Goodnick PJ et al. Lithium pharmacokinetics, duration of therapy, and the adenylate cyclase system. Int Pharmacopsychiatry. 1982;17:65.
14. Reed JV et al. An investigation of the bioavailability of lithium preparations in relation to their release characteristics. CINP. 1984;361. Abstract.
15. Amdisen A. Sustained release preparations of lithium. In: Johnson FN, ed. Lithium Research and Therapy. London, New York, San Francisco: Academic Press;1975.
16. Nielsen-Kudsk F, Amdisen A. Analysis of the pharmacokinetics of lithium in man. Eur J Clin Pharmacol. 1979;16:271.
17. Carson SW et al. Pharmacokinetic and pharmacodynamic effects of caffeine on lithium disposition. Pharmacotherapy. 1989;9:196. Abstract.
18. Diamond JM et al. Lithium absorption in tight and leaky segments of intestine. J Membr Biol. 1983;72:153.
19. Amdisen A, Sjorgren J. Lithium absorption from sustained-release tablets (Duretter). Acta Pharm Suec. 1968;5:465.
20. Lehmann K. Die Kinetik des Lithiums im menschlichen Organismus. Int J. Clin Pharmacol. 1974;10:283.

21. Thornhill DP. Comparison of ordinary and sustained release lithium carbonate in manic patients. Br J Clin Pharmacol. 1978;5:352.
22. Amdisen A et al. Grave lithium intoxication with fatal outcome. Acta Psychiatr Scand. (Suppl.) 1974;255:25.
23. Balfour D et al. Comparison of plasma, erythrocyte, and brain lithium concentrations in the guinea-pig and rat. Proceedings of the BPS; July 1979:474.
24. Smith DF, Amdisen A. Lithium distribution in rat brain after long-term central administration by minipump. J Pharm Pharmacol. 1981;33:805.
25. Ostrow DG et al. Lithium-drug interactions altering the intracellular lithium level; an *in vitro* study. Biol Psychiatry. 1980;15:723.
26. Samoilov NN et al. Effect of psychotropic drugs on the pharmacokinetics of lithium. (English translation) Bull Exp Biol Med. 1980;89:784.
27. Mendels J, Frazer A. Intracellular lithium concentrations and clinical response: towards a membrane theory of depression. J Psychiatr Res. 1973;10:9.
28. Gengo FM et al. The lithium ratio as a guide to patient compliance. Compr Psychiatry. 1980;21(4):276.
29. Radomski JL et al. The toxic effects, excretion and distribution of lithium chloride. J Pharmacol Exp Ther. 1950;100:429.
30. Foulks J et al. Renal excretion of cation in the dog during infusion of isotonic solutions of lithium chloride. Am J Physiol. 1952;168:642.
31. Thomsen K. Lithium clearance: a new method for determining proximal and distal tubular reabsorption of sodium and water. Nephron. 1984;37:217.
32. Jefferson JW et al. Effect of strenuous exercise on serum lithium levels in man. Am J Psychiatry. 1982;139:1593.
33. Thomsen K, Schou M. Renal lithium excretion in man. Am J Physiol. 1968;215:823.
34. Lauritsen BJ et al. Serum lithium concentrations around the clock with different treatment regimens and the diurnal variation of the renal lithium clearance. Acta Psychiatr Scan. 1981;64:314.
35. Solomon LR et al. Effect of posture on plasma immunoreactive atrial natriuretic peptide concentrations in man. Clin Sci. 1986;71:299.
36. Kamper AL et al. The influence of body posture on lithium clearance. Scand J Clin Lab Invest. 1988;48:509.
37. Boton R et al. Prevalence, pathogenesis, and treatment of renal dysfunction associated with chronic lithium therapy. Am J Kidney Dis. 1987;10:329.
38. Schou M. Effects of long-term lithium treatment on kidney function: an overview. J Psychiatr Res. 1988;22:287.
39. Jorkasky DK. Lithium-induced renal disease; a prospective study. Clin Nephrol. 1988;30:293.
40. Waller DG, Edwards JG. Lithium and the kidney: an update. Psychol Med. 1989;19:825.
41. Hansen HE, Amdisen A. Lithium intoxication. Q J Med. 1978;47:123.
42. Hansen HE. Renal toxicity of lithium. Drugs. 1981;22:461.
43. Wallin L et al. Impairment of renal function in patients on long-term lithium treatment. Clin Nephrol. 1982;18:23.
44. Danion JM et al. Theophylline et elimination urinaire du lithium chez le chien anesthesie. J Pharmacol. 1983;14:295.
45. Thomsen K, Olesen OV. Determination of lithium-induced impairment of distal water reabsorption. J Psychiatr Res. 1981;16:79.
46. Thomsen K, Schou M. Treatment of lithium poisoning. In: Johnson FN, ed. Lithium Research and Therapy. London, New York, San Francisco: Academic Press;1975.
47. Aref A et al. Lithium loss in sweat. Psychomosomatics. 1982;23;407.
48. Kukopulos A et al. The influence of mania and depression on the pharmacokinetics of lithium: a longitudinal case study. J Affective Disord. 1985;8:159.
49. Conrad CD, Hamilton JA. Recurrent premenstrual decline in serum lithium concentration; clinical correlates and treatment implications. J Am Acad Child Psychiatry. 1986;26(6):852.

50. Libusova E, et al. Lithium therapy and the hormonal cycle in women. Actica Nerv Super (Praha). 1975;17(4):267.
51. Carson SW et al. Influence of hormonal fluctuations associated with the menstrual cycle on lithium pharmacokinetics in bipolar disorder. Presented to the 26th Annual ACNP Meeting, San Juan, PR; 1987 December 7.
52. Himmelhoch JM et al. Adjustment of lithium dose during lithium-chlorothiazide therapy. Clin Pharm Ther. 1977;22(2):225.
53. Solomon K. Combined use of lithium and diuretics. South Med J. 1978;71(9):1098.
54. Dorevitch A, Baruch E. Lithium toxicity induced by combined amiloride HCl-hydrochlorothiazide administration. Am J Psychiatry. 1986;143(2):257.
55. Chambers G et al. Lithium used with a diuretic. Br Med J. 1977;24:805.
56. Lippmann S et al. A practical approach to management of lithium concurrent with hyponatremia, diuretic therapy and/or chronic renal failure. J Clin Psychiatr. 1981;42:304.
57. Shalmi M et al. Effect of chronic oral furosemide administration on the 24-hour cycle of lithium clearance and electrolyte excretion in humans. Eur J Clin Pharmacol. 1990;38:275.
58. Colussi G et al. Effects of acute administration of acetazolamide and frusemide on lithium clearance in humans. Nephrol Dial Transplant. 1989;4:707.
59. Bruun NE et al. Unchanged lithium clearance during acute amiloride treatment on sodium-depleted man. Scand J Clin Lab Invest. 1989;49:259.
60. Boer WH et al. Small intra- and large inter-individual variability in lithium clearance in humans. Kidney Int. 1989;35:1183.
61. Perry PJ et al. Theophylline precipitated alterations of lithium clearance. Acta Psychiatr Scand. 1984;69:528.
62. Cook BL. Theophylline-lithium interaction. J Clin Psychiatry. 1985;46:278.
63. Holstad SG et al. The effects of intravenous theophylline infusion versus intravenous sodium bicarbonate infusion on lithium clearance in normal subjects. Psychiatry Res. 1988;25:203.
64. Peterson V et al. Effect of prolonged thiazide treatment on renal lithium clearance. Br Med J. 1974;2:143.
65. Ibms JL et al. Urinary elimination of lithium: drug interactions. Kidney Int. 1979;16:96.
66. Mahieu M et al. Lithium-inhibiteurs de l'enzyme de conversion: une association a eviter? La Presse Med. 1988;17:281.
67. Passmore AP et al. Renal and cardiovascular effects of caffeine: a dose-response study. Clin Sci. 1987;72:749.
68. Jefferson J. Lithium tremor and caffeine intake: two cases of drinking less and shaking more. J Clin Psychiatry. 1988;42:72.
69. Frolich JC et al. Indomethacin increases plasma lithium. Br Med J. 1979;l:1115.
70. Reiman IW, Frolich JC. Effects of diclofenac on lithium kinetics. Clin Pharmacol Ther. 1981;20:348.
71. Ketty RJ et al. Possible toxic interaction between lithium and piroxicam. Lancet. 1983;1:418. Letter.
72. Ragheb M, Powell AL. Lithium interaction with sulindac and naproxen. J Clin Psychopharmacol. 1986;6(3):150.
73. Kristoff CA et al. Effect of ibuprofen on lithium plasma and red blood cell concentrations. Clin Pharm. 1986;5:51.
74. Furnell MM, Davis J. The effect of sulindac on lithium therapy. Drug Intell Clin Pharm. 1985;19:374.
75. Ragheb MA, Powell AL. Failure of sulindac to increase serum lithium levels. J Clin Psychiatry. 1986;47(1):33.
76. Swartz CM. Correction of lithium levels for dose and blood sampling times. J Clin Psychiatry. 1987;48(2):60.
77. Carson SW, DeVane CL. Estimation of half-life and exponential decay using a nomogram. Am J Hosp Pharm. 1983;40:1696.
78. Prien RF et al. Relationship between serum lithium level and clinical response in acute mania treated with lithium. Br J Psychiatry. 1972;120:409.

79. Jerram TC, McDonald R. Plasma lithium control with particular reference to minimum effective levels. In: Johnson FN, Johnson S, eds. Lithium in Medical Practice. Lancaster: MTP Press;1978.

80. Stokes PE et al. Relationship of lithium chloride dose to treatment response in acute mania. Arch Gen Psychiatry. 1976;33:1080.

81. Consensus Development Panel. Mood disorders: pharmacologic prevention of recurrences. Am J Psychiatry. 1985;142:469.

82. Gelenberg AJ et al. Comparison of standard and low serum levels of lithium for maintenance treatment of bipolar disorder. N Engl J Med. 1989;321:1489.

83. Gelenberg AJ et al. Serum lithium during treatment of bipolar disorder. N Engl J Med. 1990;322:1160. Letter.

84. Simard M et al. Lithium carbonate intoxication. Arch Intern Med. 1989;149:36.

85. Jacobsen D et al. Lithium intoxication: pharmacokinetics during and after terminated hemodialysis in acute intoxications. Clin Toxicol. 1987;25:81.

86. Kook KA et al. Accuracy and safety of *a priori* lithium loading. J Clin Psychiatry. 1984;6:49.

87. Johnston JA et al. Protocols for the use of psychoactive drugs: Part III. Protocol for the treatment of bipolar affective disorder with lithium. J Clin Psychiatry. 1984;45:210.

88. Zetin M et al. Prediction of lithium dose: A mathematical alternative to the test-dose method. J Clin Psychiatry. 1986;47(4):175.

89. Cooper TB et al. The 24-hour serum lithium level as a prognosticator of dosage requirements. Am J Psychiatry. 1973;130:601.

90. Cooper TB. Pharmacokinetics of lithium. In: Meltzer HY, ed. Psychopharmacology. Raven Press;1987.

91. Naiman IF et al. Practicality of a lithium dosing guide. Am J Psychiatry. 1981;138(10):1369.

92. Cooper TB, Simpson GM. The 24-hour lithium level as a prognosticator of dosage requirements: a 2-year follow-up study. Am J Psychiatry. 1976;133(4):440.

93. Fava GA et al. The lithium loading dose method in a clinical setting. Am J Psychiatry. 1984;141:812.

94. Tyrer SP et al. Estimation of lithium dose requirement by lithium clearance, serum lithium, and saliva lithium following a loading dose of lithium carbonate. Neuropsychobiology. 1981;7:152.

95. DeVane CL et al. Pharmacokinetic basis for predicting steady-state serum drug concentrations of imipramine from single dose data. Commun Psychopharmacol. 1980;3:353.

96. Slattery JT et al. Prediction of maintenance dose required to attain a desired drug concentration at steady-state from a single determination of concentration after an initial dose. 1980;5:377.

97. Gibaldi M, Perrier D. Prediction of drug concentrations on multiple dosing using the principle of superposition. Pharmacokinetics, 2nd ed. New York: Marcel Dekker;1982.

98. Palladino A Jr et al. Lithium test-dose methodology using flame photometry: problem and alternatives. J Clin Psychiatry. 1983;44:7.

99. Gengo F et al. Prediction of dosage of lithium carbonate: Use of a standard predictive method. J Clin Psychiatry. 1980;41:319.

100. Perry PJ et al. Prediction of lithium maintenance doses using a single point prediction protocol. J Clin Psychopharmacol. 1983;3:13.

101. Amdisen A. Serum level monitoring and clinical pharmacokinetics of lithium. Clin Pharmacokinet. 1977;2:73.

102. Marr MA et al. Prediction of lithium carbonate dosage in psychiatric inpatients using the repeated one-point method. Clin Pharm. 1983;2:243.

103. Swartz CM, Wilcox CO. Characterization and prediction of lithium blood levels and clearances. Arch Gen Psychiatry. 1984;41:1154.

104. Karki SD et al. Evaluation of a two-point method for prediction of lithium maintenance dosage. Inter Clin Psychopharmacol. 1987;2:343.

105. Lobeck F et al. Evaluation of four methods of predicting lithium dosage. Clin Pharm. 1987;6:230.

106. Perry PJ et al. The utility of a single-point dosing protocol for predicting steady-state lithium levels. Br J Psychiatry. 1986;148:401.

107. Nelson MV. Comparison of three lithium dosing methods in 950 "subjects" by computer simulation. Ther Drug Monit. 1988;10:269.

108. Browne JL et al. A comparison of pharmacokinetic versus empirical lithium dosing techniques. Ther Drug Monit. 1989;11:149.

109. Lobeck F. A review of lithium dosing methods. Pharmacotherapy. 1988;8(4):248.

110. Burton ME et al. Comparison of drug dosing methods. Clin Pharmacokinet. 1985;10:1.

111. Alda M. Method for prediction of serum lithium levels. Biol Psychiatry. 188;24:218.

112. Gaillot J et al. *A priori* lithium dosage regimen using population characteristics of pharmacokinetic parameters. J Pharmacokinet Biopharm. 1979;7(6):579.

113. Schumacher GE, Barr JT. Bayesian approaches in pharmacokinetic decision making. Clin Pharm. 1984;3:525.

114. Williams PJ et al. Bayesian forecasting of serum lithium concentrations. Clin Pharm. 1989;17(1):45.

115. Higuchi S et al. PEDA: A microcomputer program for parameter estimation and dosage adjustment in clinical practice. J Pharmacobiodyn. 1987;10:703.

116. Cooper TB, Carroll BJ. Monitoring lithium dose levels: estimation of lithium in blood and other body fluids. J Clin Psychopharmacol. 1981;1:53.

117. McKeage MJ, Maling TJB. Saliva lithium: a poor predictor of plasma and erythrocyte levels. N Z Med J. 1989;102:559.

118. Khare CB et al. Saliva lithium levels for monitoring lithium prophylaxis of manic depressive psychosis. Int J Clin Pharmacol Ther Toxicol. 1983;21:541.

119. Groth U et al. Estimation of pharmacokinetic parameters of lithium from saliva and urine. Clin Pharmacol Ther. 1974;16:490.

120. Shimizu M, Smith DF. Salivary and urinary lithium clearance while recumbent and upright. Clin Pharmacol Ther. 1977;21:212.

121. Kamper AL et al. Lithium clearance in chronic nephropathy. Clin Sci. 1989;77:311.

122. Amdisen A. Serum lithium determinations for clinical use. Scand J Clin Lab Invest. 1967;60:104.

123. Amdisen A. The estimation of lithium in urine. In: Johnson FN, ed. Lithium Research and Therapy. London, New York, San Francisco: Academic Press;1975.

124. Fry S. Lithium – analytical techniques. In: Richen A, Marks V, eds. Therapeutic Drug Monitoring. Edinburgh, London, Melbourne, New York: Churchill Livingstone;1981.

125. Carson SW et al. Utility of an ion selective electrode assay for lithium pharmacokinetic studies. Pharmacotherapy. 1990;10:256.

126. Karki SD et al. Effect of assay methodology on the prediction of lithium maintenance dosages. DICP Ann Pharmacother. 1988;23:372.

127. Gyulai L et al. Measurement of tissue lithium concentration by lithium magnetic resonance spectroscopy in patients with bipolar disorder. Biol Psychiatry. 1990;27:41A. Abstract.

128. Renshaw PF, Wicklund S. *In vivo* measurement of lithium in humans by nuclear magnetic resonance spectroscopy. Biol Psychiatry. 1988;23:465.

129. Cooper TB. Monitoring lithium dose levels: Estimation of lithium in blood. In: Johnson FN, ed. Handbook of Lithium Therapy. Lancaster: MTP Press;1980.

130. Risby ED et al. The mechanism of action in lithium. II: Effects on adenyl cyclase activity and beta adrenergic receptor binding in normal subjects. Arch Gen Psychiatry. 1991;48:513.

131. Jermain DM et al. Population pharmacokinetics of lithium. Clin Pharm. 1991;10:376.

132. Chamberlain S et al. Effect of menstrual cycle phase and oral contraceptive use on serum lithium levels after a loading dose of lithium in normal women. Am J Psychiatry. 1990;147:907.

133. Crabtree BL et al. Comparison of the effects of hydrochlorothiazide and furosemide on lithium disposition. Am J Psychiatry. 1991;148;1060.

Index

A